D1426385

Fourth Edition

Plastic Surgery

Craniofacial, Head and Neck Surgery

Pediatric Plastic Surgery

Volume Three

Content Strategist: Belinda Kuhn
Content Development Specialists: Louise Cook, Sam Crowe, Alexandra Mortimer
e-products, Content Development Specialist: Kim Benson
Project Managers: Anne Collett, Andrew Riley, Julie Taylor
Designer: Miles Hitchen
Illustration Managers: Karen Giacomucci, Amy Faith Heyden
Marketing Manager: Melissa Fogarty
Video Liaison: Will Schmitt

Fourth Edition

Plastic Surgery

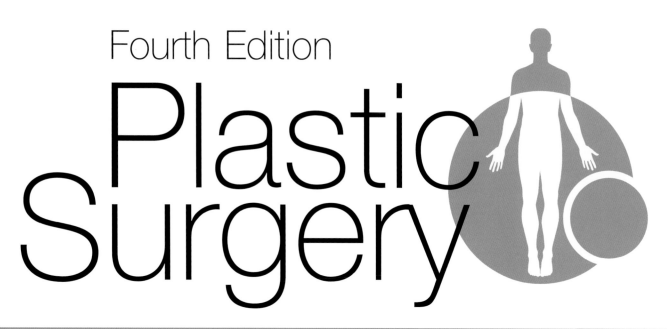

Craniofacial, Head and Neck Surgery

Pediatric Plastic Surgery

Volume Three

Part 1 Volume Editor

Eduardo D. Rodriguez

MD, DDS
Helen L. Kimmel Professor of Reconstructive
Plastic Surgery
Chair, Hansjörg Wyss Department of Plastic
Surgery
NYU School of Medicine
NYU Langone Medical Center
New York, NY, USA

Editor-in-Chief

Peter C. Neligan

MB, FRCS(I), FRCSC, FACS
Professor of Surgery
Department of Surgery, Division of Plastic Surgery
University of Washington
Seattle, WA, USA

Part 2 Volume Editor

Joseph E. Losee

MD
Ross H. Musgrave Professor of Pediatric
Plastic Surgery
Department of Plastic Surgery
University of Pittsburgh Medical Center;
Chief Division of Pediatric Plastic Surgery
Children's Hospital of Pittsburgh
Pittsburgh, PA, USA

Multimedia Editor

Daniel Z. Liu

MD
Plastic and Reconstructive Surgeon
Cancer Treatment Centers of America at
Midwestern Regional Medical Center
Zion, IL, USA

For additional online figures, videos and video lectures visit Expertconsult.com

ELSEVIER   London, New York, Oxford, Philadelphia, St Louis, Sydney 2018

ELSEVIER

First edition 1990
Second edition 2006
Third edition 2013
Fourth edition 2018

Notices

Knowledge and best practice in this field are constantly changing. As new research and experience broaden our understanding, changes in research methods, professional practices, or medical treatment may become necessary.

Practitioners and researchers must always rely on their own experience and knowledge in evaluating and using any information, methods, compounds, or experiments described herein. In using such information or methods they should be mindful of their own safety and the safety of others, including parties for whom they have a professional responsibility.

With respect to any drug or pharmaceutical products identified, readers are advised to check the most current information provided (i) on procedures featured or (ii) by the manufacturer of each product to be administered, to verify the recommended dose or formula, the method and duration of administration, and contraindications. It is the responsibility of practitioners, relying on their own experience and knowledge of their patients, to make diagnoses, to determine dosages and the best treatment for each individual patient, and to take all appropriate safety precautions.

To the fullest extent of the law, neither the Publisher nor the authors, contributors, or editors, assume any liability for any injury and/or damage to persons or property as a matter of products liability, negligence or otherwise, or from any use or operation of any methods, products, instructions, or ideas contained in the material herein.

Volume 3 ISBN: 978-0-323-35698-5
Volume 3 Ebook ISBN: 978-0-323-35699-2
6 volume set ISBN: 978-0-323-35630-5

ELSEVIER your source for books, journals and multimedia in the health sciences
www.elsevierhealth.com

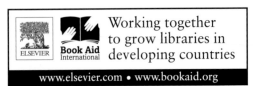

Working together to grow libraries in developing countries

www.elsevier.com • www.bookaid.org

The publisher's policy is to use **paper manufactured from sustainable forests**

Printed in Canada
Last digit is the print number: 9 8 7 6 5 4 3 2 1

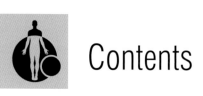

Contents

Volume Three: Craniofacial, Head and Neck Surgery, and Pediatric Plastic Surgery

Part 1: Head, neck, and craniofacial surgery: edited by Eduardo D. Rodriguez

Part 2: Pediatrics: edited by Joseph E. Losee

Section I: Clefts

Volume Four: Lower Extremity, Trunk, and Burns

edited by David H. Song

Volume Five: Breast
edited by Maurice Y. Nahabedian

Section I: Aesthetic Breast Surgery

Section II: Reconstructive Breast Surgery

Volume Six: Hand and Upper Extremity

edited by James Chang

Video Contents

Lecture Video Contents

Preface to the Fourth Edition

When I wrote the preface to the 3rd edition of this book, I remarked how honored and unexpectedly surprised I was to be the Editor of this great series. This time 'round, I'm equally grateful to carry this series forward. When Elsevier called me and suggested it was time to prepare the 4th edition, my initial reaction was that this was way too soon. What could possibly have changed in Plastic Surgery since the 3rd edition was launched in 2012? As it transpires, there have been many developments and I hope we have captured them in this edition.

We have an extraordinary specialty. A recent article by Chadra, Agarwal and Agarwal entitled "Redefining Plastic Surgery" appeared in *Plastic and Reconstructive Surgery—Global Open*. In it they gave the following definition: "Plastic surgery is a specialized branch of surgery, which deals with deformities, defects and abnormalities of the organs of perception, organs of action and the organs guarding the external passages, besides innovation, implantation, replantation and transplantation of tissues, and aims at restoring and improving their form, function and the esthetic appearances." This is an all-encompassing but very apt definition and captures the enormous scope of the specialty.[1]

In the 3rd edition, I introduced volume editors for each of the areas of the specialty because the truth is that one person can no longer be an expert in all areas of this diverse specialty, and I'm certainly not. I think this worked well because the volume editors not only had the expertise to present their area of subspecialty in the best light, but they were tuned in to what was new and who was doing it. We have continued this model in this new edition. Four of the seven volume editors from the previous edition have again helped to bring the latest and the best to this edition: Drs Gurtner, Song, Rodriguez, Losee, and Chang have revised and updated their respective volumes with some chapters remaining, some extensively revised, some added, and some deleted. Dr. Peter Rubin has replaced Dr. Rick Warren to compile the Aesthetic volume (Vol. 2). Dr. Warren did a wonderful job in corralling this somewhat disparate, yet vitally important, part of our specialty into the Aesthetic volume in the 3rd edition but felt that the task of doing it again, though a labor of love, was more than he wanted to take on. Similarly, Dr. Jim Grotting who did a masterful job in the last edition on the Breast volume, decided that doing a major revision should be undertaken by someone with a fresh perspective and Dr. Maurice Nahabedian stepped into that breach. I hope you will like the changes you see in both of these volumes.

Dr. Allen Van Beek was the video editor for the last edition and he compiled an impressive array of movies to complement the text. This time around, we wanted to go a step further and though we've considerably expanded the list of videos accompanying the text (there are over 170), we also added the idea of lectures accompanying selected chapters. What we've done here is to take selected key chapters and include the images from that chapter, photos and artwork, and create a narrated presentation that is available online; there are annotations in the text to alert the reader that this is available. Dr. Daniel Liu, who has taken over from Dr. Van Beek as multimedia editor (rather than video editor) has done an amazing job in making all of this happen. There are over 70 presentations of various key chapters online, making it as easy as possible for you, the reader, to get as much knowledge as you can, in the easiest way possible from this edition. Many of these presentations have been done by the authors of the chapters; the rest have been compiled by Dr. Liu and myself from the content of the individual chapters. I hope you find them useful.

The reader may wonder how this all works. To plan this edition, the Elsevier team, headed by Belinda Kuhn, and I, convened a face-to-face meeting in San Francisco. The volume editors, as well as the London based editorial team, were present. We went through the 3rd edition, volume by volume, chapter by chapter, over an entire weekend. We decided what needed to stay, what needed to be added, what needed to be revised, and what needed to be changed. We also decided who should write the various chapters, keeping many existing authors, replacing others, and adding some new ones; we did this so as to really reflect the changes occurring within the specialty. We also decided on practical changes that needed to be made. As an example, you will notice that we have omitted the complete index for the 6 Volume set from Volumes 2-6 and highlighted only the table of contents for that particular volume. The complete index is of course available in Volume 1 and fully searchable online. This allowed us to save several hundred pages per volume, reducing production costs and diverting those dollars to the production of the enhanced online content.

In my travels around the world since the 3rd edition was published, I've been struck by what an impact this publication has had on the specialty and, more particularly, on training. Everywhere I go, I'm told how the text is an important part of didactic teaching and a font of knowledge. It is gratifying to see that the 3rd edition has been translated into Portuguese, Spanish, and Chinese. This is enormously encouraging. I hope this 4th edition continues to contribute to the specialty, remains a resource for practicing surgeons, and continues to prepare our trainees for their future careers in Plastic Surgery.

Peter C. Neligan
Seattle, WA
September, 2017

---

[1] Chandra R, Agarwal R, Agarwal D. Redefining Plastic Surgery. *Plast Reconstr Surg Glob Open*. 2016;4(5):e706.

List of Editors

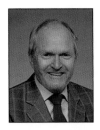

Editor-in-Chief
Peter C. Neligan, MB, FRCS(I), FRCSC, FACS
Professor of Surgery
Department of Surgery, Division of Plastic Surgery
University of Washington
Seattle, WA, USA

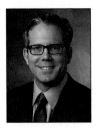

Volume 1: Principles
Geoffrey C. Gurtner, MD, FACS
Johnson and Johnson Distinguished Professor of
Surgery and Vice Chairman,
Department of Surgery (Plastic Surgery)
Stanford University
Stanford, CA, USA

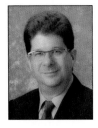

Volume 2: Aesthetic
J. Peter Rubin, MD, FACS
UPMC Professor of Plastic Surgery
Chair, Department of Plastic Surgery
Professor of Bioengineering
University of Pittsburgh
Pittsburgh, PA, USA

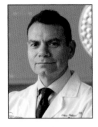

Volume 3: Craniofacial, Head and Neck Surgery
Eduardo D. Rodriguez, MD, DDS
Helen L. Kimmel Professor of Reconstructive
Plastic Surgery
Chair, Hansjörg Wyss Department of Plastic
Surgery
NYU School of Medicine
NYU Langone Medical Center
New York, NY, USA

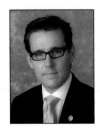

Volume 3: Pediatric Plastic Surgery
Joseph E. Losee, MD
Ross H. Musgrave Professor of Pediatric Plastic
Surgery
Department of Plastic Surgery
University of Pittsburgh Medical Center;
Chief Division of Pediatric Plastic Surgery
Children's Hospital of Pittsburgh
Pittsburgh, PA, USA

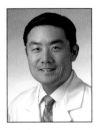

Volume 4: Lower Extremity, Trunk, and Burns
David H. Song, MD, MBA, FACS
Regional Chief, MedStar Health
Plastic and Reconstructive Surgery
Professor and Chairman
Department of Plastic Surgery
Georgetown University School of Medicine
Washington, DC, USA

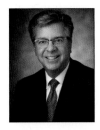

Volume 5: Breast
Maurice Y. Nahabedian, MD, FACS
Professor and Chief
Section of Plastic Surgery
MedStar Washington Hospital Center
Washington, DC, USA;
Vice Chairman
Department of Plastic Surgery
MedStar Georgetown University Hospital
Washington, DC, USA

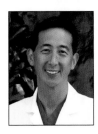

Volume 6: Hand and Upper Extremity
James Chang, MD
Johnson & Johnson Distinguished
Professor and Chief
Division of Plastic and Reconstructive Surgery
Stanford University Medical Center
Stanford, CA, USA

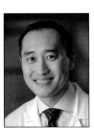

Multimedia editor
Daniel Z. Liu, MD
Plastic and Reconstructive Surgeon
Cancer Treatment Centers of America at Midwestern Regional Medical Center
Zion, IL, USA

List of Contributors

The editors would like to acknowledge and offer grateful thanks for the input of all previous editions' contributors, without whom this new edition would not have been possible.

VOLUME ONE

Hatem Abou-Sayed, MD, MBA
Vice President
Physician Engagement
Interpreta, Inc.
San Diego, CA, USA

Paul N. Afrooz, MD
Resident
Plastic and Reconstructive Surgery
University of Pittsburgh Medical Center
Pittsburgh, PA, USA

Claudia R. Albornoz, MD, MSc
Research Fellow
Plastic and Reconstructive Surgery
Memorial Sloan Kettering Cancer Center
New York, NY, USA

Nidal F. Al Deek, MD
Doctor of Plastic and Reconstructive Surgery
Chang Gung Memorial Hospital
Taipei, Taiwan

Amy K. Alderman, MD, MPH
Private Practice
Atlanta, GA, USA

Louis C. Argenta, MD
Professor of Plastic and Reconstructive Surgery
Department of Plastic Surgery
Wake Forest Medical Center
Winston Salem, NC, USA

Stephan Ariyan, MD, MBA
Emeritus Frank F. Kanthak Professor of Surgery,
Plastic Surgery, Surgical Oncology,
Otolaryngology
Yale University School of Medicine;
Associate Chief
Department of Surgery;
Founding Director, Melanoma Program
Smilow Cancer Hospital, Yale Cancer Center
New Haven, CT, USA

Tomer Avraham, MD
Attending Plastic Surgeon
Mount Sinai Health System
Tufts University School of Medicine
New York, NY, USA

Aaron Berger, MD, PhD
Clinical Assistant Professor
Division of Plastic Surgery
Florida International University School of
Medicine
Miami, FL, USA

Kirsty Usher Boyd, MD, FRCSC
Assistant Professor Surgery (Plastics)
Division of Plastic and Reconstructive Surgery
University of Ottawa
Ottawa, Ontario, Canada

Charles E. Butler, MD, FACS
Professor and Chairman
Department of Plastic Surgery
Charles B. Barker Endowed Chair in Surgery
The University of Texas MD Anderson Cancer
Center
Houston, TX, USA

**Peter E. M. Butler, MD, FRCSI, FRCS,
FRCS(Plast)**
Professor
Plastic and Reconstructive Surgery
University College and Royal Free London
London, UK

Yilin Cao, MD, PhD
Professor
Shanghai Ninth People's Hospital
Shanghai Jiao Tong University School of
Medicine
Shanghai, China

Franklyn P. Cladis, MD, FAAP
Associate Professor of Anesthesiology
Department of Anesthesiology
The Children's Hospital of Pittsburgh of UPMC
Pittsburgh, PA, USA

Mark B. Constantian, MD
Private Practice
Surgery (Plastic Surgery)
St. Joseph Hospital
Nashua, NH, USA

Daniel A. Cuzzone, MD
Plastic Surgery Fellow
Hanjörg Wyss Department of Plastic Surgery
New York University Medical Center
New York, NY, USA

Gurleen Dhami, MD
Chief Resident
Department of Radiation Oncology
University of Washington
Seattle, WA, USA

Gayle Gordillo, MD
Associate Professor
Plastic Surgery
The Ohio State University
Columbus, OH, USA

Geoffrey C. Gurtner, MD, FACS
Johnson and Johnson Distinguished Professor
of Surgery and Vice Chairman,
Department of Surgery (Plastic Surgery)
Stanford University
Stanford, CA, USA

Phillip C. Haeck, MD
Surgeon
Plastic Surgery
The Polyclinic
Seattle, WA, USA

The late Bruce Halperin†, MD
Formerly Adjunct Associate Professor of
Anesthesia
Department of Anesthesia
Stanford University
Stanford, CA, USA

Daniel E. Heath
Lecturer
School of Chemical and Biomedical Engineering
University of Melbourne
Parkville, Victoria, Australia

Joon Pio Hong, MD, PhD, MMM
Professor
Plastic Surgery
Asan Medical Center, University of Ulsan
Seoul, South Korea

Michael S. Hu, MD, MPH, MS
Postdoctoral Fellow
Division of Plastic Surgery
Department of Surgery
Stanford University School of Medicine
Stanford, CA, USA

C. Scott Hultman, MD, MBA
Professor and Chief
Division of Plastic and Reconstructive Surgery
University of North Carolina
Chapel Hill, NC, USA

Amir E. Ibrahim
Division of Plastic Surgery
Department of Surgery
American University of Beirut Medical Center
Beirut, Lebanon

Leila Jazayeri, MD
Microsurgery Fellow
Plastic and Reconstructive Surgery
Memorial Sloan Kettering Cancer Center
New York, NY, USA

Brian Jeffers
Student
Bioengineering
University of California Berkeley
Berkeley, CA USA

Lynn Jeffers, MD, FACS
Private Practice
Oxnard, CA, USA

Mohammed M. Al Kahtani, MD, FRCSC
Clinical Fellow
Division of Plastic Surgery
Department of Surgery
University of Alberta
Edmonton, Alberta, Canada

Gabrielle M. Kane, MB, BCh, EdD, FRCPC
Associate Professor
Radiation Oncology
University of Washington
Seattle, WA, USA

Raghu P. Kataru, PhD
Senior Research Scientist
Memorial Sloan-Kettering Cancer Center
New York, NY, USA

Carolyn L. Kerrigan, MD, MSc, MHCDS
Professor of Surgery
Surgery
Dartmouth–Hitchcock Medical Center
Lebanon, NH, USA

Timothy W. King, MD, PhD, FAAP, FACS
Associate Professor with Tenure
Departments of Surgery and Biomedical
Engineering;
Director of Research, Division of Plastic Surgery
University of Alabama at Birmingham (UAB)
Craniofacial and Pediatric Plastic Surgery
Children's of Alabama – Plastic Surgery;
Chief, Plastic Surgery Section
Birmingham VA Hospital
Birmingham, AL, USA

Brian M. Kinney, MD, FACS, MSME
Clinical Assistant Professor of Plastic Surgery
University of Southern California
School of Medicine
Los Angeles, CA, USA

W. P. Andrew Lee, MD
The Milton T. Edgerton MD, Professor and
Chairman
Department of Plastic and Reconstructive
Surgery
Johns Hopkins University School of Medicine
Baltimore, MD, USA

**Sherilyn Keng Lin Tay, MBChB, MSc,
FRCS(Plast)**
Consultant Plastic Surgeon
Canniesburn Plastic Surgery Unit
Glasgow Royal Infirmary
Glasgow, UK

Daniel Z. Liu, MD
Plastic and Reconstructive Surgeon
Cancer Treatment Centers of America at
Midwestern Regional Medical Center
Zion, IL, USA

Wei Liu, MD, PhD
Professor
Plastic and Reconstructive Surgery
Shanghai Ninth People's Hospital
Shanghai Jiao Tong University School of
Medicine
Shanghai, China

Michael T. Longaker, MD, MBA, FACS
Deane P. and Louise Mitchell Professor and Vice
Chair
Department of Surgery
Stanford University
Stanford, CA, USA

H. Peter Lorenz, MD
Service Chief and Professor, Plastic Surgery
Lucile Packard Children's Hospital
Stanford University School of Medicine
Stanford, CA, USA

Susan E. Mackinnon, MD
Sydney M. Shoenberg Jr. and Robert H.
Shoenberg Professor
Department of Surgery, Division of Plastic and
Reconstructive Surgery
Washington University School of Medicine
St. Louis, MO, USA

Malcolm W. Marks, MD
Professor and Chairman
Department of Plastic Surgery
Wake Forest University School of Medicine
Winston-Salem, NC, USA

Diego Marre, MD
Fellow
O'Brien Institute
Department of Plastic and Reconstructive
Surgery
St. Vincent's Hospital
Melbourne, Australia

David W. Mathes, MD
Professor and Chief of the Division of Plastic
and Reconstructive Surgery
University of Colorado
Aurora, CO, USA

Evan Matros MD, MMSc
Plastic Surgeon
Memorial Sloan-Kettering Cancer Center
New York, NY, USA

Isabella C. Mazzola, MD
Attending Plastic Surgeon
Klinik für Plastische und Ästhetische Chirurgie
Klinikum Landkreis Erding
Erding, Germany

Riccardo F. Mazzola, MD
Plastic Surgeon
Department of Specialistic Surgical Sciences
Fondazione Ospedale Maggiore Policlinico, Ca'
Granda IRCCS
Milano, Italy

Lindsay D. McHutchion, MS, BSc
Anaplastologist
Institute for Reconstructive Sciences in Medicine
Edmonton, Alberta, Canada

Babak J. Mehrara, MD, FACS
Associate Member, Associate Professor of
Surgery (Plastic)
Memorial Sloan Kettering Cancer Center
Weil Cornell University Medical Center
New York, NY, USA

Steven F. Morris, MD, MSc, FRCSC
Professor of Surgery
Department of Surgery
Dalhousie University
Halifax, Nova Scotia, Canada

Wayne A. Morrison, MBBS, MD, FRACS
Professorial Fellow
O'Brien Institute
Department of Surgery, University of Melbourne
Department of Plastic and Reconstructive
Surgery, St. Vincent's Hospital
Melbourne, Australia

**Peter C. Neligan, MB, FRCS(I), FRCSC,
FACS**
Professor of Surgery
Department of Surgery, Division of Plastic
Surgery
University of Washington
Seattle, WA, USA

Andrea J. O'Connor, BE(Hons), PhD
Associate Professor
Department of Chemical and Biomolecular
Engineering
University of Melbourne
Parkville, Victoria, Australia

Rei Ogawa, MD, PhD, FACS
Professor and Chief
Department of Plastic
Reconstructive and Aesthetic Surgery
Nippon Medical School
Tokyo, Japan

Dennis P. Orgill, MD, PhD
Professor of Surgery
Harvard Medical School
Medical Director, Wound Care Center;
Vice Chairman for Quality Improvement
Department of Surgery
Brigham and Women's Hospital
Boston, MA, USA

Cho Y. Pang, PhD
Senior Scientist
Research Institute
The Hospital for Sick Children;
Professor
Departments of Surgery/Physiology
University of Toronto
Toronto, Ontario, Canada

Ivo Alexander Pestana, MD, FACS
Associate Professor
Plastic and Reconstructive Surgery
Wake Forest University
Winston Salem, NC, USA

Giorgio Pietramaggior, MD, PhD
Swiss Nerve Institute
Clinique de La Source
Lausanne, Switzerland

Andrea L. Pusic, MD, MHS, FACS
Associate Professor
Plastic and Reconstructive Surgery
Memorial Sloan Kettering Cancer Center
New York, NY, USA

Russell R. Reid, MD, PhD
Associate Professor
Surgery/Section of Plastic and Reconstructive
Surgery
University of Chicago Medicine
Chicago, IL, USA

Neal R. Reisman, MD, JD
Chief
Plastic Surgery
Baylor St. Luke's Medical Center
Houston, TX, USA

Joseph M. Rosen, MD
Professor of Surgery
Plastic Surgery
Dartmouth–Hitchcock Medical Center
Lebanon, NH, USA

Sashwati Roy, MS, PhD
Associate Professor
Surgery, Center for Regenerative Medicine and
Cell based Therapies
The Ohio State University
Columbus, OH, USA

J. Peter Rubin, MD, FACS
UPMC Professor of Plastic Surgery
Chair, Department of Plastic Surgery
Professor of Bioengineering
University of Pittsburgh
Pittsburgh, PA, USA

Karim A. Sarhane, MD
Department of Surgery
University of Toledo Medical Center
Toledo, OH, USA

David B. Sarwer, PhD
Associate Professor of Psychology
Departments of Psychiatry and Surgery
University of Pennsylvania School of Medicine
Philadelphia, PA, USA

Saja S. Scherer-Pietramaggiori, MD
Plastic and Reconstructive Surgeon
Plastic Surgery
University Hospital Lausanne
Lausanne, Vaud, Switzerland

Iris A. Seitz, MD, PhD
Director of Research and International
Collaboration
University Plastic Surgery
Rosalind Franklin University;
Clinical Instructor of Surgery
Chicago Medical School
Chicago, IL, USA

Jesse C. Selber, MD, MPH, FACS
Associate Professor, Director of Clinical
Research
Department of Plastic Surgery
MD Anderson Cancer Center
Houston, TX, USA

Chandan K. Sen, PhD
Professor and Director
Center for Regenerative Medicine and Cell-
Based Therapies
The Ohio State University Wexner Medical
Center
Columbus, OH, USA

Wesley N. Sivak, MD, PhD
Resident in Plastic Surgery
Department of Plastic Surgery
University of Pittsburgh
Pittsburgh, PA, USA

M. Lucy Sudekum
Research Assistant
Thayer School of Engineering at Dartmouth
College
Hanover, NH, USA

**G. Ian Taylor, AO, MBBS, MD, MD(Hon
Bordeaux), FRACS, FRCS(Eng), FRCS(Hon
Edinburgh), FRCSI(Hon), FRSC(Hon
Canada), FACS(Hon)**
Professor
Department of Plastic Surgery
Royal Melbourne Hospital;
Professor
Department of Anatomy
University of Melbourne
Melbourne, Victoria, Australia

Chad M. Teven, MD
Resident
Section of Plastic and Reconstructive Surgery
University of Chicago
Chicago, IL, USA

Ruth Tevlin, MB BAO BCh, MRCSI, MD
Resident in Surgery
Department of Plastic and Reconstructive
Surgery
Stanford University School of Medicine
Stanford, CA, USA

E. Dale Collins Vidal, MD, MS
Chief
Section of Plastic Surgery
Dartmouth–Hitchcock Medical Center
Lebanon, NH, USA

Derrick C. Wan, MD
Associate Professor
Division of Plastic Surgery
Department of Surgery
Director of Maxillofacial Surgery
Lucile Packard Children's Hospital
Stanford University School of Medicine
Stanford, CA, USA

Renata V. Weber, MD
Assistant Professor Surgery (Plastics)
Division of Plastic and Reconstructive Surgery
Albert Einstein College of Medicine
Bronx, NY, USA

Fu-Chan Wei, MD
Professor
Department of Plastic Surgery
Chang Gung Memorial Hospital
Taoyuan, Taiwan

Gordon H. Wilkes, BScMed, MD
Clinical Professor of Surgery
Department of Surgery University of Alberta
Institute for Reconstructive Sciences in Medicine
Misericordia Hospital
Edmonton, Alberta, Canada

**Johan F. Wolfaardt, BDS,
MDent(Prosthodontics), PhD**
Professor
Division of Otolaryngology – Head and Neck
Surgery
Department of Surgery
Faculty of Medicine and Dentistry;
Director of Clinics and International Relations
Institute for Reconstructive Sciences in Medicine
University of Alberta
Covenant Health Group
Alberta Health Services
Alberta, Canada

Kiryu K. Yap, MBBS, BMedSc
Junior Surgical Trainee & PhD Candidate
O'Brien Institute
Department of Surgery, University of Melbourne
Department of Plastic and Reconstructive
Surgery, St. Vincent's Hospital
Melbourne, Australia

Andrew Yee
Research Assistant
Division of Plastic and Reconstructive Surgery
Washington University School of Medicine
St. Louis, MO, USA

Elizabeth R. Zielins, MD
Postdoctoral Research Fellow
Surgery
Stanford University School of Medicine
Stanford, CA, USA

VOLUME TWO

Paul N. Afrooz, MD
Resident
Plastic and Reconstructive Surgery
University of Pittsburgh Medical Center
Pittsburgh, PA, USA

Jamil Ahmad, MD, FRCSC
Director of Research and Education
The Plastic Surgery Clinic
Mississauga;
Assistant Professor
Surgery
University of Toronto
Toronto, Ontario, Canada

Lisa E. Airan, MD
Aesthetic Dermatologist NYC
Private Practice;
Associate Clinical Professor Department of
Dermatology
Mount Sinai School of Medicine
New York, NY, USA

Gary J. Alter, MD
Assistant Clinical Professor
Division of Plastic Surgery
University of California
Los Angeles, CA, USA

Al S. Aly, MD
Professor of Plastic Surgery
Aesthetic and Plastic Surgery Institute University
of California Irvine
Orange, CA, USA

Khalid Al-Zahrani, MD, SSC-PLAST
Assistant Professor
Consultant Plastic Surgeon
King Khalid University Hospital
King Saud University
Riyadh, Saudi Arabia

Bryan Armijo, MD
Plastic Surgery Chief Resident
Department of Plastic and Reconstructive
Surgery
Case Western Reserve/University Hospitals
Cleveland, OH, USA

Daniel C. Baker, MD
Professor of Surgery
Institute of Reconstructive Plastic Surgery
New York University Medical Center
Department of Plastic Surgery
New York, NY, USA

Fritz E. Barton Jr., MD
Clinical Professor
Department of Plastic Surgery
UT Southwestern Medical Center
Dallas, TX, USA

Leslie Baumann, MD
CEO
Baumann Cosmetic and Research Institute
Miami, FL, USA

Miles G. Berry, MS, FRCS(Plast)
Consultant Plastic and Aesthetic Surgeon
Institute of Cosmetic and Reconstructive
Surgery
London, UK

Trevor M. Born, MD
Division of Plastic Surgery
Lenox Hill/Manhattan Eye Ear and Throat
Hospital North Shore-LIJ Hospital
New York, NY, USA;
Clinical Lecturer
Division of Plastic Surgery
University of Toronto Western Division
Toronto, Ontario, Canada

Terrence W. Bruner, MD, MBA
Private Practice
Greenville, SC, USA

Andrés F. Cánchica, MD
Chief Resident of Plastic Surgery
Plastic Surgery Service Dr. Osvaldo Saldanha
São Paulo, Brazil

Joseph F. Capella, MD
Chief Post-bariatric Body Contouring
Division of Plastic Surgery
Hackensack University Medical Center
Hackensack, NJ, USA

Robert F. Centeno, MD, MBA
Medical Director
St. Croix Plastic Surgery and MediSpa;
Chief Medical Quality Officer
Governor Juan F. Luis Hospital and Medical
Center
Christiansted, Saint Croix, United States Virgin
Islands

Ernest S. Chiu, MD, FACS
Associate Professor of Plastic Surgery
Department of Plastic Surgery
New York University
New York, NY, USA

Jong Woo Choi, MD, PhD, MMM
Associate Professor
Department of Plastic and Reconstructive
Surgery
Seoul Asan Medical Center
Seoul, South Korea

Steven R. Cohen, MD
Senior Clinical Research Fellow, Clinical
Professor
Plastic Surgery
University of California
San Diego, CA;
Director
Craniofacial Surgery
Rady Children's Hospital, Private Practice,
FACES+ Plastic Surgery, Skin and Laser Center
La Jolla, CA, USA

Sydney R. Coleman, MD
Assistant Clinical Professor
Plastic Surgery
New York University Medical Center
New York;
Assistant Clinical Professor
Plastic Surgery
University of Pittsburgh Medical Center
Pittsburgh, PA, USA

Mark B. Constantian, MD
Private Practice
Surgery (Plastic Surgery)
St. Joseph Hospital
Nashua, NH, USA;
Adjunct Clinical Professor
Surgery (Plastic Surgery)
University of Wisconsin School of Medicine
Madison, WI, USA;
Visiting Professor
Plastic Surgery
University of Virginia Health System
Charlottesville, VA, USA

Rafael A. Couto, MD
Plastic Surgery Resident
Department of Plastic Surgery
Cleveland Clinic
Cleveland, OH, USA

Albert Cram, MD
Professor Emeritus
University of Iowa
Iowa City Plastic Surgery
Coralville, IO, USA

Phillip Dauwe, MD
Department of Plastic Surgery
University of Texas Southwestern Medical
School
Dallas, TX, USA

Dai M. Davies, FRCS
Consultant and Institute Director
Institute of Cosmetic and Reconstructive
Surgery
London, UK

Jose Abel De la Peña Salcedo, MD, FACS
Plastic Surgeon
Director
Instituto de Cirugia Plastica S.C.
Huixquilucan
Estado de Mexico, Mexico

Barry DiBernardo, MD, FACS
Clinical Associate Professor, Plastic Surgery
Rutgers, New Jersey Medical School
Director New Jersey Plastic Surgery
Montclair, NJ, USA

Felmont F. Eaves III, MD, FACS
Professor of Surgery, Emory University
Medical Director, Emory Aesthetic Center
Medical Director, EAC Ambulatory Surgery
Center
Atlanta, GA, USA

Marco Ellis, MD
Director of Craniofacial Surgery
Northwestern Specialists in Plastic Surgery;
Adjunct Assistant Professor
University of Illinois Chicago Medical Center
Chicago, IL, USA

Dino Elyassnia, MD
Associate Plastic Surgeon
Marten Clinic of Plastic Surgery
San Francisco, CA, USA

Julius Few Jr., MD
Director
The Few Institute for Aesthetic Plastic Surgery;
Clinical Professor
Plastic Surgery
University of Chicago Pritzker School of
Medicine
Chicago, IL, USA

Osvaldo Ribeiro Saldanha Filho, MD
Professor of Plastic Surgery
Plastic Surgery Service Dr. Osvaldo Saldanha
São Paulo, Brazil

Jack Fisher, MD
Associate Clinical Professor
Plastic Surgery
Vanderbilt University
Nashville, TN, USA

Nicholas A. Flugstad, MD
Flugstad Plastic Surgery
Bellevue, WA, USA

James D. Frame, MBBS, FRCS, FRCSEd, FRCS(Plast)
Professor of Aesthetic Plastic Surgery
Anglia Ruskin University
Chelmsford, UK

Jazmina M. Gonzalez, MD
Bitar Cosmetic Surgery Institute
Fairfax, VA, USA

Richard J. Greco, MD
CEO
The Georgia Institute For Plastic Surgery
Savannah, GA, USA

Ronald P. Gruber, MD
Adjunct Associate Clinical Professor
Division of Plastic and Reconstructive Surgery
Stanford University
Stanford, CA
Clinical Association Professor
Division of Plastic and Reconstructive Surgery
University of California San Francisco
San Francisco, CA, USA

Bahman Guyuron, MD, FCVS
Editor in Chief, Aesthetic Plastic Surgery Journal
Emeritus Professor of Plastic Surgery
Case School of Medicine
Cleveland, OH, USA

Joseph P. Hunstad, MD, FACS
Associate Consulting Professor
Division of Plastic Surgery
The University of North Carolina at Chapel Hill;
Private Practice
Huntersville/Charlotte, NC, USA

Clyde H. Ishii, MD, FACS
Assistant Clinical Professor of Surgery
John A. Burns School of Medicine;
Chief, Department of Plastic Surgery
Shriners Hospital
Honolulu Unit
Honolulu, HI, USA

Nicole J. Jarrett, MD
Department of Plastic Surgery
University of Pittsburgh
Pittsburgh, PA, USA

Elizabeth B. Jelks, MD
Private Practice
Jelks Medical
New York, NY, USA

Glenn W. Jelks, MD
Associate Professor
Department of Ophthalmology
Department of Plastic Surgery
New York University School of Medicine
New York, NY, USA

Mark Laurence Jewell, MD
Assistant Clinical Professor Plastic Surgery
Oregon Health Science University
Portland, OR, USA

David M. Kahn, MD
Clinical Associate Professor of Plastic Surgery
Department of Surgery
Stanford University School of Medicine
Stanford, CA, USA

Michael A. C. Kane, BS, MD
Attending Surgeon
Plastic Surgery
Manhattan Eye, Ear, and Throat Hospital
New York, NY, USA

David L. Kaufman, MD, FACS
Private Practice Plastic Surgery
Aesthetic Artistry Surgical and Medical Center
Folsom, CA, USA

Jeffrey Kenkel, MD
Professor and Chairman
Department of Plastic Surgery
UT Southwestern Medical Center
Dallas, TX, USA

Kyung S. Koh, MD, PhD
Professor of Plastic Surgery
Asan Medical Center, University of Ulsan School
of Medicine
Seoul, South Korea

Tracy Leong, MD
Dermatology
Rady Children's Hospital - San Diego;
Sharp Memorial Hospital;
University California San Diego Medical Center
San Diego;
Private Practice, FACES+ Plastic Surgery, Skin
and Laser Center
La Jolla, CA, USA

Steven M. Levine, MD
Assistant Professor of Surgery (Plastic)
Hofstra Medical School, Northwell Health,
New York, NY, USA

Michelle B. Locke, MBChB, MD
Senior Lecturer in Surgery
Department of Surgery
University of Auckland Faculty of Medicine and
Health Sciences;
South Auckland Clinical Campus
Middlemore Hospital
Auckland, New Zealand

Alyssa Lolofie
University of Utah
Salt Lake City, UT, USA

Timothy J. Marten, MD, FACS
Founder and Director
Marten Clinic of Plastic Surgery
San Francisco, CA, USA

Bryan Mendelson, FRCSE, FRACS, FACS
The Centre for Facial Plastic Surgery
Toorak, Victoria, Australia

Constantino G. Mendieta, MD, FACS
Private Practice
Miami, FL, USA

Drew B. Metcalfe, MD
Division of Plastic and Reconstructive Surgery
Emory University
Atlanta, GA, USA

Gabriele C. Miotto, MD
Emory School of Medicine
Atlanta, GA, USA

Foad Nahai, MD
Professor of Surgery
Division of Plastic and Reconstructive Surgery
Department of Surgery
Emory University School of Medicine
Emory Aesthetic Center at Paces
Atlanta, Georgia, USA

Suzan Obagi, MD
Associate Professor of Dermatology
Dermatology
University of Pittsburgh;
Associate Professor of Plastic Surgery
Plastic Surgery
University of Pittsburgh
Pittsburgh, PA, USA

Sabina Aparecida Alvarez de Paiva, MD
Resident of Plastic Surgery
Plastic Surgery Service Dr. Ewaldo Bolivar de
Souza Pinto
São Paulo, Brazil

Galen Perdikis, MD
Assistant Professor of Surgery
Division of Plastic Surgery
Emory University School of Medicine
Atlanta, GA, USA

Jason Posner, MD, FACS
Private Practice
Boca Raton, FL, USA

Dirk F. Richter, MD, PhD
Clinical Professor of Plastic Surgery
University of Bonn
Director and Chief
Dreifaltigkeits-Hospital
Wesseling, Germany

Thomas L. Roberts III, FACS
Plastic Surgery Center of the Carolinas
Spartanburg, SC, USA

Jocelyn Celeste Ledezma Rodriguez, MD
Private Practice
Guadalajara, Jalisco, Mexico

Rod J. Rohrich, MD
Clinical Professor and Founding Chair
Department of Plastic Surgery
Distinguished Teaching Professor
University of Texas Southwestern Medical Center
Founding Partner
Dallas Plastic Surgery Institute
Dallas, TX, USA

E. Victor Ross, MD
Director of Laser and Cosmetic Dermatology
Scripps Clinic
San Diego, CA, USA

J. Peter Rubin, MD, FACS
Chief
Plastic and Reconstructive Surgery
University of Pittsburgh Medical Center;
Associate Professor
Department of Surgery
University of Pittsburgh
Pittsburgh, PA, USA

Ahmad N. Saad, MD
Private Practice
FACES+ Plastic Surgery
Skin and Laser Center
La Jolla, CA, USA

Alesia P. Saboeiro, MD
Attending Physician
Private Practice
New York, NY, USA

Cristianna Bonnetto Saldanha, MD
Plastic Surgery Service Dr. Osvaldo Saldanha
São Paulo, Brazil

Osvaldo Saldanha, MD, PhD
Director of Plastic Surgery Service Dr. Osvaldo
Saldanha;
Professor of Plastic Surgery Department
Universidade Metropolitana de Santos
- UNIMES
São Paulo, Brazil

Renato Saltz, MD, FACS
Saltz Plastic Surgery
President
International Society of Aesthetic Plastic Surgery
Adjunct Professor of Surgery
University of Utah
Past-President, American Society for Aesthetic
Plastic Surgery
Salt Lake City and Park City, UT, USA

Paulo Rodamilans Sanjuan MD
Chief Resident of Plastic Surgery
Plastic Surgery Service Dr. Ewaldo Boliar de
Souza Pinto
São Paulo, Brazil

Nina Schwaiger, MD
Senior Specialist in Plastic and Aesthetic
Surgery
Department of Plastic Surgery
Dreifaltigkeits-Hospital Wesseling
Wesseling, Germany

Douglas S. Steinbrech, MD, FACS
Gotham Plastic Surgery
New York, NY, USA

Phillip J. Stephan, MD
Clinical Faculty
Plastic Surgery
UT Southwestern Medical School;
Plastic Surgeon
Texoma Plastic Surgery
Wichita Falls, TX, USA

David Gonzalez Sosa, MD
Plastic and Reconstructive Surgery
Hospital Quirónsalud Torrevieja
Alicante, Spain

James M. Stuzin, MD
Associate Professor of Surgery
(Plastic) Voluntary
University of Miami Leonard M. Miller School of
Medicine
Miami, FL, USA

Daniel Suissa, MD, MSc
Clinical Instructor
Section of Plastic and Reconstructive Surgery
Yale University
New Haven, CT, USA

Charles H. Thorne, MD
Associate Professor of Plastic Surgery
Department of Plastic Surgery
NYU School of Medicine
New York, NY, USA

Ali Totonchi, MD
Assistant Professor
Plastic Surgery
Case Western Reserve University;
Medical Director Craniofacial Deformity Clinic
Plastic Surgery
MetroHealth Medical center
Cleveland, OH, USA

Jonathan W. Toy, MD, FRCSC
Program Director, Plastic Surgery Residency
Program Assistant Clinical Professor
University of Alberta
Edmonton, Alberta, Canada

Matthew J. Trovato, MD
Dallas Plastic Surgery Institute
Dallas, TX, USA

Simeon H. Wall Jr., MD, FACS
Director
The Wall Center for Plastic Surgery;
Assistant Clinical Professor
Plastic Surgery
LSU Health Sciences Center at Shreveport
Shreveport, LA, USA

Joshua T. Waltzman, MD, MBA
Private Practice
Waltzman Plastic and Reconstructive Surgery
Long Beach, CA, USA

Richard J. Warren, MD, FRCSC
Clinical Professor
Division of Plastic Surgery
University of British Columbia
Vancouver, British Columbia, Canada

Edmund Weisberg, MS, MBE
University of Pennsylvania
Philadelphia, PA, USA

Scott Woehrle, MS BS
Physician Assistant
Department of Plastic Surgery
Jospeh Capella Plastic Surgery
Ramsey, NJ, USA

**Chin-Ho Wong, MBBS, MRCS, MMed(Surg),
FAMS(Plast Surg)**
W Aesthetic Plastic Surgery
Mt Elizabeth Novena Specialist Center
Singapore

Alan Yan, MD
Former Fellow
Adult Reconstructive and Aesthetic
Craniomaxillofacial Surgery
Division of Plastic and Reconstructive Surgery
Massachusetts General Hospital
Boston, MA, USA

Michael J. Yaremchuk, MD
Chief of Craniofacial Surgery
Massachusetts General Hospital;
Clinical Professor of Surgery
Harvard Medical School;
Program Director
Harvard Plastic Surgery Residency Program
Boston, MA, USA

James E. Zins, MD
Chairman
Department of Plastic Surgery
Dermatology and Plastic Surgery Institute
Cleveland Clinic
Cleveland, OH, USA

VOLUME THREE

Neta Adler, MD
Senior Surgeon
Department of Plastic and Reconstructive
Surgery
Hadassah University Hospital
Jerusalem, Israel

Ahmed M. Afifi, MD
Assistant Professor of Plastic Surgery
Department of Surgery
University of Wisconsin
Madison, WI, USA;
Associate Professor
Department of Plastic Surgery
Cairo University
Cairo, Egypt

Marta Alvarado, DDS, MS
Department of Orthodontics
Facultad de Odontología
Universidad de San Carlos de Guatemala
Guatemala

Eric Arnaud, MD
Pediatric Neurosurgeon and Co-Director
Unité de Chirurgie Craniofaciale
Hôpital Necker Enfants Malades
Paris, France

Stephen B. Baker, MD, DDS
Associate Professor and Program Director
Co-Director Inova Hospital for Children
Craniofacial Clinic
Department of Plastic Surgery
Georgetown University Hospital
Georgetown, WA, USA

Scott P. Bartlett, MD
Professor of Surgery
Surgery
University of Pennsylvania;
Chief Division of Plastic Surgery
Surgery
Children's Hospital of Philadelphia
Philadelphia, PA, USA

Bruce S. Bauer, MD
Chief
Division of Plastic Surgery
NorthShore University HealthSystem
Highland Park;
Clinical Professor of Surgery
Department of Surgery
University of Chicago Pritzker School of
Medicine
Chicago, IL, USA

Adriane L. Baylis, PhD
Speech Scientist
Section of Plastic and Reconstructive Surgery
Nationwide Children's Hospital
Columbus, OH, USA

Mike Bentz, MD, FAAP, FACS
Interim Chairman
Department of Surgery
University of Wisconsin;
Chairman Division of Plastic Surgery
Department of Surgery
University of Wisconsin
Madison, WI, USA

Craig Birgfeld, MD, FACS
Associate Professor, Pediatric Plastic and
Craniofacial Surgery
Seattle Children's Hospital
Seattle, WA, USA

William R. Boysen, MD
Resident Physician, Urology
University of Chicago Medicine
Chicago, IL, USA

James P. Bradley, MD
Professor and Chief
Section of Plastic and Reconstructive Surgery
Temple University
Philadelphia, PA, USA

Edward P. Buchanan, MD
Division of Plastic Surgery
Baylor College of Medicine
Houston, TX, USA

Michael R. Bykowski, MD, MS
Plastic Surgery Resident
Plastic Surgery
University of Pittsburgh Medical Center
Pittsburgh, PA, USA

Edward J. Caterson, MD, PhD
Director of Craniofacial Surgery
Division of Plastic Surgery
Brigham and Women's Hospital
Boston, MA, USA

Rodney K. Chan, MD
Chief Plastic and Reconstructive Surgery
Clinical Division and Burn Center
United States Army Institute of Surgical
Research
Joint Base San Antonio, TX, USA

Edward I. Chang, MD
Assistant Professor
Department of Plastic Surgery
The University of Texas M. D. Anderson Cancer
Center
Houston, TX, USA

Constance M. Chen, MD, MPH
Director of Microsurgery
Plastic and Reconstructive Surgery
New York Eye and Ear Infirmary of Mt Sinai;
Clinical Assistant Professor
Plastic and Reconstructive Surgery
Weil Medical College of Cornell University;
Clinical Assistant Professor
Plastic and Reconstructive Surgery
Tulane University School of Medicine
New York, NY, USA

Yu-Ray Chen, MD
Professor of Surgery
Plastic and Reconstructive Surgery
Chang Gung Memorial Hospital
Taoyuan City, Taiwan

Philip Kuo-Ting Chen, MD
Professor
Craniofacial Center
Chang Gung Memorial Hospital
Taoyuan City, Taiwan

Ming-Huei Cheng, MD, MBA
Professor
Division of Reconstructive Microsurgery
Department of Plastic and Reconstructive
Surgery
Chang Gung Memorial Hospital
Taoyuan City, Taiwan

Gerson R. Chinchilla, DDS MS
Director
Department of Orthodontics
Facultad de Odontología
Universidad de San Carlos de Guatemala
Guatemala

Peter G. Cordeiro, MD
Chief
Plastic and Reconstructive Surgery
Memorial Sloan Kettering Cancer Center;
Professor of Surgery
Surgery
Weil Medical College of Cornell University
New York, NY, USA

Alberto Córdova-Aguilar, MD, MPH
Attending Plastic Surgeon
Surgery
Faculty of Medicine Ricardo Palma University
Lima, Peru

Edward H. Davidson, MA(Cantab), MBBS
Resident Plastic Surgeon
Department of Plastic Surgery
University of Pittsburgh
Pittsburgh, PA, USA

Sara R. Dickie, MD
Clinician Educator
Surgery
University of Chicago Hospital Pritzker School of Medicine;
Attending Surgeon
Section of Plastic and Reconstructive Surgery
NorthShore University HealthSystem
Northbrook, IL, USA

Risal S. Djohan, MD
Microsurgery Fellowship Program Director
Plastic Surgery
Cleveland Clinic;
Surgery ASC Quality Improvement Officer
Plastic Surgery
Cleveland Clinic
Cleveland, OH, USA

Amir H. Dorafshar, MBChB, FACS, FAAP
Associate Professor
Plastic and Reconstructive Surgery
Johns Hopkins Medical Institute;
Assistant Professor
Plastic Surgery
R Adams Cowley Shock Trauma Center
Baltimore, MD, USA

Jeffrey A. Fearon, MD
Director
The Craniofacial Center
Dallas, TX, USA

Alexander L. Figueroa, DMD
Craniofacial Orthodontist
Rush Craniofacial Center
Rush University Medical Center
Chicago, IL, USA

Alvaro A. Figueroa, DDS, MS
Co-Director
Rush Craniofacial Center
Rush University Medical Center
Chicago, IL, USA

David M. Fisher, MB, BCh, FRCSC, FACS
Medical Director Cleft Lip and Palate Program
Plastic Surgery
Hospital for Sick Children;
Associate Professor
Surgery
University of Toronto
Toronto, Ontario, Canada

Roberto L. Flores, MD
Associate Professor of Plastic Surgery
Director of Cleft Lip and Palate
Hansjörg Wyss Department of Plastic Surgery
NYU Langone Medical Center
New York, NY, USA

Andrew Foreman, B. Physio, BMBS(Hons), PhD, FRACS
Consultant Surgeon, Department of Otolaryngology - Head and Neck Surgery
University of Adelaide,
Royal Adelaide Hospital,
Adelaide, SA, Australia

Patrick A. Gerety, MD
Assistant Professor of Surgery
Division of Plastic and Reconstructive Surgery
Indiana University and Riley Hospital for Children
Philadelphia, PA, USA

Jesse A. Goldstein, MD
Chief Resident
Department of Plastic Surgery
Georgetown University Hospital
Washington, DC, USA

Arun K. Gosain, MD
Chief
Division of Plastic Surgery
Ann and Robert H. Lurie Children's Hospital of Chicago
Chicago, IL, USA

Lawrence J. Gottlieb, MD
Professor of Surgery
Department of Surgery
Section of Plastic and Reconstructive Surgery
University of Chicago
Chicago, IL, USA

Arin K. Greene, MD, MMSc
Department of Plastic and Oral Surgery
Boston Children's Hospital;
Associate Professor of Surgery
Harvard Medical School
Boston, MA, USA

Patrick J. Gullane, MD, FRCS
Wharton Chair in Head and Neck Surgery
Professor of Surgery, Department of Otolaryngology - Head and Neck Surgery
University of Toronto
Toronto, Ontario, Canada

Mohan S. Gundeti, MB, MCh, FEBU, FRCS(Urol), FEAPU
Associate Professor of Urology in Surgery and Pediatrics, Director Pediatric Urology, Director Centre for Pediatric Robotics and Minimal Invasive Surgery
University of Chicago and Pritzker Medical School Comer Children's Hospital
Chicago, IL, USA

Eyal Gur, MD
Professor of Surgery, Chief
Department of Plastic and Reconstructive Surgery
The Tel Aviv Sourasky Medical Center
Tel Aviv, Israel

Bahman Guyuron, MD, FCVS
Editor in Chief, Aesthetic Plastic Surgery Journal;
Emeritus Professor of Plastic Surgery
Case School of Medicine
Cleveland, OH, USA

Matthew M. Hanasono, MD
Associate Professor
Department of Plastic Surgery
The University of Texas MD Anderson Cancer Center
Houston, TX, USA

Toshinobu Harada, PhD
Professor in Engineering
Department of Systems Engineering
Faculty of Systems Engineering
Wakayama University
Wakayama, Japan

Jill A. Helms, DDS, PhD
Professor
Surgery
Stanford University
Stanford, CA, USA

David L. Hirsch, MD, DDS
Director of Oral Oncology and Reconstruction
Lenox Hill Hospital/Northwell Health
New York, NY, USA

Jung-Ju Huang, MD
Associate Professor
Division of Microsurgery
Plastic and Reconstructive Surgery
Chang Gung Memorial Hospital
Taoyuan, Taiwan

William Y. Hoffman, MD
Professor and Chief
Division of Plastic and Reconstructive Surgery
UCSF
San Francisco, CA, USA

Larry H. Hollier Jr., MD
Division of Plastic Surgery
Baylor College of Medicine
Houston, TX, USA

Richard A. Hopper, MD, MS
Chief
Division of Craniofacial Plastic Surgery
Seattle Children's Hospital;
Surgical Director
Craniofacial Center
Seattle Children's Hospital;
Associate Professor
Department of Surgery
University of Washington
Seattle, WA, USA

Gazi Hussain, MBBS, FRACS
Clinical Senior Lecturer
Macquarie University
Sydney, Australia

Oksana Jackson, MD
Assistant Professor
Plastic Surgery
Perelman School of Medicine at the University of Pennsylvania;
Assistant Professor
Plastic Surgery
The Children's Hospital of Philadelphia
Philadelphia, PA, USA

Syril James, MD
Clinic Marcel Sembat
Boulogne-Billancourt
Paris, France

Leila Jazayeri, MD
Microsurgery Fellow
Plastic and Reconstructive Surgery
Memorial Sloan Kettering Cancer Center
New York, NY, USA

Sahil Kapur, MD
Assistant Professor
Department of Plastic Surgery
University of Texas - MD Anderson Cancer
Center
Houston, TX, USA

Henry K. Kawamoto Jr., MD, DDS
Clinical Professor
Surgery Division of Plastic Surgery
UCLA
Los Angeles, CA, USA

David Y. Khechoyan, MD
Division of Plastic Surgery
Baylor College of Medicine
Houston, TX, USA

Richard E. Kirschner, MD
Section Chief
Plastic and Reconstructive Surgery
Nationwide Children's Hospital;
Senior Vice Chair
Plastic Surgery
The Ohio State University Medical College
Columbus, OH, USA

John C. Koshy, MD
Division of Plastic Surgery
Baylor College of Medicine
Houston, TX, USA

Michael C. Large, MD
Urologic Oncologist
Urology of Indiana
Greenwood, IN, USA

Edward I. Lee, MD
Division of Plastic Surgery
Baylor College of Medicine
Houston, TX, USA

Jamie P. Levine, MD
Chief of Microsurgery
Associate Professor
Plastic Surgery
NYU Langone Medical Center
New York, NY, USA

Jingtao Li, DDS, PhD
Consultant Surgeon
Oral and Maxillofacial Surgery
West China Hospital of Stomatology
Chengdu, Sichuan, People's Republic of China

Lawrence Lin, MD
Division of Plastic Surgery
Baylor College of Medicine
Houston, TX, USA

Joseph E. Losee, MD
Ross H. Musgrave Professor of Pediatric Plastic
Surgery
Department of Plastic Surgery
University of Pittsburgh Medical Center;
Chief, Division of Pediatric Plastic Surgery
Children's Hospital of Pittsburgh
Pittsburgh, PA, USA

David W. Low, MD
Professor of Surgery
Division of Plastic Surgery
Perelman School of Medicine at the University
of Pennsylvania;
Clinical Associate
Department of Surgery
Children's Hospital of Philadelphia
Philadelphia, PA, USA

Ralph T. Manktelow, MD, FRCSC
Professor of Surgery,
The University of Toronto,
Toronto, Ontario, Canada

Paul N. Manson, MD
Distinguished Service Professor
Plastic Surgery
Johns Hopkins University
Baltimore, MD, USA

David W. Mathes, MD
Professor and Chief of the Division of Plastic
and Reconstructive Surgery
Surgery Division of Plastic and Reconstructive
Surgery
University of Colorado
Aurora, CO, USA

Frederick J. Menick, MD
Private Practitioner
Tucson, AZ, USA

Fernando Molina, MD
Director
Craniofacial Anomalies Foundation A.C.
Mexico City;
Professor of Plastic Reconstructive and
Aesthetic Surgery
Medical School
Universidad La Salle
Mexico City, Distrito Federal, Mexico

Laura A. Monson, MD
Division of Plastic Surgery
Baylor College of Medicine
Houston, TX, USA

Reid V. Mueller, MD
Associate Professor
Plastic Surgery
Oregon Health and Science University
Portland, OR, USA

John B. Mulliken, MD
Professor
Department of Plastic and Oral Surgery
Boston Children's Hospital
Harvard Medical School
Boston, MA, USA

Gerhard S. Mundinger, MD
Assistant Professor
Craniofacial, Plastic, and Reconstructive Surgery
Louisiana State University Health Sciences
Center
Children's Hospital of New Orleans
New Orleans, LA, USA

Blake D. Murphy, BSc, PhD, MD
Craniofacial Fellow
Plastic Surgery
Nicklaus Children's Hospital
Miami, FL, USA

**Peter C. Neligan, MB, FRCS(I), FRCSC,
FACS**
Professor of Surgery
Department of Surgery, Division of Plastic
Surgery
University of Washington
Seattle, WA, USA

M. Samuel Noordhoff, MD, FACS
Emeritus Professor in Surgery
Chang Gung University
Taoyuan City, Taiwan

Giovanna Paternoster, MD
Unité de chirurgie crânio-faciale du departement
de neurochirurgie
Hôpital Necker Enfants Malades
Paris, France

Jason Pomerantz, MD
Assistant Professor
Surgery
University of California San Francisco;
Surgical Director
Craniofacial Center
University of California San Francisco
San Francisco, CA, USA

Julian J. Pribaz, MD
Professor of Surgery
University of South Florida, Morsani College of
Medicine
Tampa General Hospital
Tampa, FL, USA

Chad A. Purnell, MD
Division of Plastic Surgery
Lurie Children's Hospital of Northwestern
Feinberg School of Medicine
Chicago, IL, USA

Russell R. Reid, MD, PhD
Associate Professor
Surgery/Section of Plastic and Reconstructive
Surgery
University of Chicago Medicine
Chicago, IL, USA

Eduardo D. Rodriguez, MD, DDS
Helen L. Kimmel Professor of Reconstructive
Plastic Surgery
Chair, Hansjörg Wyss Department of Plastic
Surgery
NYU School of Medicine
NYU Langone Medical Center
New York, NY, USA

Craig Rowin, MD
Craniofacial Fellow
Plastic Surgery
Nicklaus Children's Hospital
Miami, FL, USA

Ruston J. Sanchez, MD
Plastic and Reconstructive Surgery Resident
University of Wisconsin
Madison, WI, USA

Lindsay A. Schuster, DMD, MS
Director Cleft-Craniofacial Orthodontics
Pediatric Plastic Surgery
Children's Hospital of Pittsburgh of UMPC;
Clinical Assistant Professor of Plastic Surgery
Department of Plastic Surgery
University of Pittsburgh School of Medicine
Pittsburgh, PA, USA

Jeremiah Un Chang See, MD
Plastic Surgeon
Department of Plastic and Reconstructive
Surgery
Penang General Hospital
Georgetown, Penang, Malaysia

Pradip R. Shetye, DDS, BDS, MDS
Assistant Professor (Orthodontics)
Hansjörg Wyss Department of Plastic Surgery
NYU Langone Medical Center
New York, NY, USA

Roman Skoracki, MD
Plastic Surgery
The Ohio State University
Columbus, OH, USA

Mark B. Slidell, MD, MPH
Assistant Professor of Surgery
Department of Surgery
Section of Pediatric Surgery
University of Chicago Medicine Biological
Sciences
Chicago, IL, USA

Michael Sosin, MD
Research Fellow
Department of Plastic Surgery Institute of
Reconstructive Plastic Surgery
NYU Langone Medical Center
New York, NY, USA;
Research Fellow
Division of Plastic Reconstructive and
Maxillofacial Surgery
R Adams Cowley Shock Trauma Center
University of Maryland Medical Center
Baltimore, MD, USA;
Resident
Department of Surgery
Medstar Georgetown University Hospital
Washington, DC, USA

**Youssef Tahiri, MD, MSc, FRCSC, FAAP,
FACS**
Associate Professor
Pediatric Plastic & Craniofacial Surgery
Cedars Sinai Medical Center
Los Angeles, CA, USA

Peter J. Taub, MD
Professor
Surgery Pediatrics Dentistry and Medical
Education
Surgery Division of Plastic and Reconstructive
Surgery
Icahn School of Medicine at Mount Sinai
New York, NY, USA

Jesse A. Taylor, MD
Mary Downs Endowed Chair of Pediatric
Craniofacial Treatment and Research;
Director, Penn Craniofacial Fellowship;
Co-Director, CHOP Cleft Team
Plastic, Reconstructive, and Craniofacial Surgery
The University of Pennsylvania and
Children's Hospital of Philadelphia
Philadelphia, PA, USA

Kathryn S. Torok, MD
Assistant Professor
Pediatric Rheumatology
University of Pittsburgh
Pittsburgh, PA, USA

Ali Totonchi, MD
Assistant Professor
Plastic Surgery
Case Western Reserve University;
Medical Director Craniofacial Deformity Clinic
Plastic Surgery
MetroHealth Medical Center
Cleveland, OH, USA

Kris Wilson, MD
Division of Plastic Surgery
Baylor College of Medicine
Houston, TX, USA

S. Anthony Wolfe, MD
Plastic Surgery
Miami Children's Hospital
Miami, FL, USA

Akira Yamada, MD, PhD
Professor of Plastic Surgery
World Craniofacial Foundation
Dallas, TX, USA;
Clinical Assistant Professor
Plastic Surgery
Case Western Reserve University
Cleveland, OH, USA

Peirong Yu, MD
Professor
Plastic Surgery
M. D. Anderson Cancer Center;
Adjunct Professor
Plastic Surgery
Baylor College of Medicine
Houston, TX, USA

**Ronald M. Zuker, MD, FRCSC, FACS,
FRCSEd(Hon)**
Professor of Surgery
Department of Surgery
University of Toronto;
Staff Plastic and Reconstructive Surgeon
Department of Surgery
SickKids Hospital
Toronto, Ontario, Canada

VOLUME FOUR

Christopher E. Attinger, MD
Professor, Interim Chairman
Department of Plastic Surgery
Center for Wound Healing
Medstar Georgetown University Hospital
Washington, DC, USA

Lorenzo Borghese, MD
Plastic Surgeon
Chief of International Missions
Ospedale Pediatrico Bambino Gesù
Rome, Italy

Charles E. Butler, MD, FACS
Professor and Chairman
Department of Plastic Surgery
Charles B. Barker Endowed Chair in Surgery
The University of Texas M. D. Anderson Cancer
Center
Houston, TX, USA

David W. Chang, MD
Professor of Surgery
University of Chicago
Chicago, IL, USA

Karel Claes, MD
Department of Plastic and Reconstructive
Surgery
Ghent University Hospital
Ghent, Belgium

Mark W. Clemens II, MD, FACS
Associate Professor
Plastic Surgery
MD Anderson Cancer Center,
Houston, TX, USA

Shannon M. Colohan, MD, MSc
Assistant Professor of Surgery
University of Washington
Seattle, WA, USA

Peter G. Cordeiro, MD
Chief
Plastic and Reconstructive Surgery
Memorial Sloan Kettering Cancer Center
New York, NY, USA

Salvatore D'Arpa, MD, PhD
Department of Plastic and Reconstructive
Surgery
Ghent University Hospital
Ghent, Belgium

Michael V. DeFazio, MD
Department Plastic Surgery
MedStar Georgetown University Hospital
Washington, DC, USA

A. Lee Dellon, MD, PhD
Professor of Plastic Surgery
Professor of Neurosurgery
Johns Hopkins University
Baltimore, MD, USA

Sara R. Dickie, MD
Clinical Associate of Surgery
University of Chicago Hospitals
Pritzker School of Medicine
Chicago, IL, USA

Ivica Ducic, MD, PhD
Clinical Professor of Surgery
GWU Washington Nerve Institute
McLean, VA, USA

Gregory A. Dumanian, MD
Stuteville Professor of Surgery
Division of Plastic Surgery
Northwestern Feinberg School of Medicine
Chicago, IL, USA

John M. Felder III, MD
Fellow in Hand Surgery
Plastic Surgery
Washington University in Saint Louis
St. Louis, MO, USA

Goetz A. Giessler, MD, PhD
Professor Director
Plastic-Reconstructive, Aesthetic and Hand
Surgery
Gesundheit Nordhessen
Kassel, Germany

Kevin D. Han, MD
Department of Plastic Surgery
MedStar Georgetown University Hospital
Washington, DC, USA

Piet Hoebeke
Department of Urology
Ghent University Hospital
Ghent, Belgium

Joon Pio Hong, MD, PhD, MMM
Professor of Plastic Surgery
Asan Medical Center, University of Ulsan
Seoul, South Korea

Michael A. Howard, MD
Clinical Assistant Professor of Surgery
Plastic Surgery
NorthShore University HealthSystem/University
of Chicago
Chicago, IL, USA

Jeffrey E. Janis, MD, FACS
Professor of Plastic Surgery, Neurosurgery,
Neurology, and Surgery;
Executive Vice Chairman, Department of Plastic
Surgery;
Chief of Plastic Surgery, University Hospitals
Ohio State University Wexner Medical Center
Columbus, OH, USA

Leila Jazayeri, MD
Microsurgery Fellow
Plastic and Reconstructive Surgery
Memorial Sloan Kettering Cancer Center
New York, NY, USA

Grant M. Kleiber, MD
Assistant Professor of Surgery
Division of Plastic and Reconstructive Surgery
Washington University School of Medicine
St. Louis, MO, USA

Stephen J. Kovach III, MD
Assistant Professor
Division of Plastic Surgery
University of Pennsylvania
Philadelphia, PA, USA

Robert Kwon, MD
Southwest Hand and Microsurgery
3108 Midway Road, Suite 103
Plano, TX, USA

**Raphael C. Lee, MS, MD, ScD, FACS,
FAIMBE**
Paul and Allene Russell Professor
Plastic Surgery, Dermatology, Anatomy and
Organismal Biology, Molecular Medicine
University of Chicago
Chicago, IL, USA

L. Scott Levin, MD, FACS
Chairman of Orthopedic Surgery
Department of Orthopaedic Surgery
University of Pennsylvania School of Medicine
Philadelphia, PA, USA

Otway Louie, MD
Associate Professor
Surgery
University of Washington Medical Center
Seattle, WA, USA

Nicolas Lumen, MD, PhD
Head of Clinic
Urology
Ghent University Hospital
Ghent, Belgium

Alessandro Masellis, MD
Plastic Surgeon
Euro-Mediterranean Council for Burns and Fire
Disasters
Palermo, Italy

Michele Masellis, MD
Former Chief of Department of Plastic and
Reconstructive Surgery and Burn Therapy
Department of Plastic and Reconstructive
Surgery and Burn Therapy - ARNAS Ospedale
Civico e Benfratelli
Palermo, Italy

Stephen M. Milner, MB BS, BDS
Professor of Plastic Surgery
Surgery
Johns Hopkins School of Medicine
Baltimore, MD, USA

Arash Momeni, MD
Fellow, Reconstructive Microsurgery
Division of Plastic Surgery
University of Pennsylvania Health System
Philadelphia, PA, USA

Stan Monstrey, MD, PhD
Department of Plastic and Reconstructive
Surgery
Ghent University Hospital
Ghent, Belgium

**Venkateshwaran N, MBBS, MS, DNB, MCh,
MRCS(Intercollegiate)**
Consultant Plastic Surgeon
Jupiter Hospital
Thane, India

Rajiv P. Parikh, MD, MPHS
Resident Physician
Department of Surgery, Division of Plastic and
Reconstructive Surgery
Washington University School of Medicine
St. Louis, MO, USA

Mônica Sarto Piccolo, MD, MSc, PhD
Director
Pronto Socorro para Queimaduras
Goiânia, Goiás, Brazil

Nelson Sarto Piccolo, MD
Chief
Division of Plastic Surgery
Pronto Socorro para Queimaduras
Goiânia, Goiás, Brazil

Maria Thereza Sarto Piccolo, MD, PhD
Scientific Director
Pronto Socorro para Queimaduras
Goiânia, Goiás, Brazil

Vinita Puri, MS, MCh
Professor and Head
Department of Plastic, Reconstructive Surgery
and Burns
Seth G S Medical College and KEM Hospital
Mumbai, Maharashtra, India

Andrea L. Pusic, MD, MHS, FACS
Associate Professor
Plastic and Reconstructive Surgery
Memorial Sloan Kettering Cancer Center
New York, NY, USA

Vinay Rawlani, MD
Division of Plastic Surgery
Northwestern Feinberg School of Medicine
Chicago, IL, USA

Juan L. Rendon, MD, PhD
Clinical Instructor Housestaff
Department of Plastic Surgery
The Ohio State University Wexner Medical
Center
Columbus, OH, USA

Michelle C. Roughton, MD
Assistant Professor
Division of Plastic and Reconstructive Surgery
University of North Carolina at Chapel Hill
Chapel Hill, NC, USA

Hakim K. Said, MD, FACS
Associate Professor
Division of Plastic surgery
University of Washington
Seattle, WA, USA

Michel Saint-Cyr, MD, FRSC(C)
Professor
Plastic Surgery
Mayo Clinic
Rochester, MN, USA

Michael Sauerbier, MD, PhD
Professor, Chair
Department for Plastic, Hand, and
Reconstructive Surgery
Academic Hospital Goethe University Frankfurt
am Main
Frankfurt am Main, Germany

Loren S. Schechter, MD
Associate Professor and Chief
Division of Plastic Surgery
Chicago Medical School
Morton Grove, IL, USA

David H. Song, MD, MBA, FACS
Regional Chief, MedStar Health
Plastic and Reconstructive Surgery
Professor and Chairman
Department of Plastic Surgery
Georgetown University School of Medicine
Washington, DC, USA

Yoo Joon Sur, MD, PhD
Associate Professor
Department of Orthopedic Surgery
The Catholic University of Korea, College of
Medicine
Seoul, Korea

Chad M. Teven, MD
Resident
Section of Plastic and Reconstructive Surgery
University of Chicago
Chicago, IL, USA

VOLUME FIVE

Jamil Ahmad, MD, FRCSC
Director of Research and Education
The Plastic Surgery Clinic
Mississauga, Ontario, Canada;
Assistant Professor of Surgery
University of Toronto
Toronto, Ontario, Canada

Robert J. Allen Sr., MD
Clinical Professor of Plastic Surgery
Department of Plastic Surgery
New York University Medical Center
Charleston, NC, USA

Ryan E. Austin, MD, FRCSC
Plastic Surgeon
The Plastic Surgery Clinic
Mississauga, ON, Canada

Brett Beber, BA, MD, FRCSC
Plastic and Reconstructive Surgeon
Lecturer, Department of Surgery
University of Toronto
Toronto, Ontario, Canada

Philip N. Blondeel, MD
Professor of Plastic Surgery
Department of Plastic Surgery
University Hospital Ghent
Ghent, Belgium

Benjamin J. Brown, MD
Gulf Coast Plastic Surgery
Pensacola, FL, USA

Mitchell H. Brown, MD, MEd, FRCSC
Plastic and Reconstructive Surgeon
Associate Professor, Department of Surgery
University of Toronto
Toronto, Ontario, Canada

M. Bradley Calobrace, MD, FACS
Plastic Surgeon
Calobrace and Mizuguchi Plastic Surgery Center
Departments of Surgery, Divisions of Plastic
Surgery
Clinical Faculty, University of Louisville and
University of Kentucky
Louisville, KY, USA

Grant W. Carlson, MD
Wadley R. Glenn Professor of Surgery
Emory University
Atlanta, GA, USA

Bernard W. Chang, MD
Chief of Plastic and Reconstructive Surgery
Mercy Medical Center
Baltimore, MD, USA

Mark W. Clemens II, MD, FACS
Assistant Professor Plastic Surgery
M. D. Anderson Cancer Center
Houston, TX, USA

Robert Cohen MD, FACS
Medical Director
Plastic Surgery
Scottsdale Center for Plastic Surgery
Paradise Valley, AZ and;
Santa Monica, CA, USA

Amy S. Colwell, MD
Associate Professor
Harvard Medical School
Massachusetts General Hospital
Boston, MA, USA

Edward H. Davidson, MA(Cantab), MB, BS
Resident Plastic Surgeon
Department of Plastic Surgery
University of Pittsburgh Medical Center
Pittsburgh, PA, USA

Emmanuel Delay, MD, PhD
Unité de Chirurgie Plastique et Reconstructrice
Centre Léon Bérard
Lyon, France

Francesco M. Egro, MB ChB, MSc, MRCS
Department of Plastic Surgery
University of Pittsburgh Medical Center
Pittsburgh, PA, USA

Neil A. Fine, MD
President
Northwestern Specialists in Plastic Surgery;
Associate Professor (Clinical) Surgery/Plastics
Northwestern University Fienberg School of
Medicine
Chicago, IL, USA

Jaime Flores, MD
Plastic and Reconstructive Microvascular
Surgeon
Miami, FL, USA

Joshua Fosnot, MD
Assistant Professor of Surgery
Division of Plastic Surgery
The Perelman School of Medicine
University of Pennsylvania Health System
Philadelphia, PA, USA

Allen Gabriel, MD
Clinical Associate Professor
Department of Plastic Surgery
Loma Linda University Medical Center
Loma Linda, CA, USA

Michael S. Gart, MD
Resident Physician
Division of Plastic Surgery
Northwestern University Feinberg School of
Medicine
Chicago, IL, USA

Matthew D. Goodwin, MD
Plastic Surgeon
Plastic Reconstructive and Cosmetic Surgery
Boca Raton Regional Hospital
Boca Raton, FL, USA

Samia Guerid, MD
Cabinet
50 rue de la République
Lyon, France

Moustapha Hamdi, MD, PhD
Professor of Plastic and Reconstructive Surgery
Brussels University Hospital
Vrij Universitaire Brussels
Brussels, Belgium

Alexandra M. Hart, MD
Emory Division of Plastic and Reconstructive
Surgery
Emory University School of Medicine
Atlanta, GA, USA

Emily C. Hartmann, MD, MS
Aesthetic Surgery Fellow
Plastic and Reconstructive Surgery
University of Southern California
Los Angeles, CA, USA

Nima Khavanin, MD
Resident Physician
Department of Plastic and Reconstructive
Surgery
Johns Hopkins Hospital
Baltimore, MD, USA

John Y. S. Kim, MD
Professor and Clinical Director
Department of Surgery
Division of Plastic Surgery
Northwestern University Feinberg School of
Medicine
Chicago, IL, USA

Steven Kronowitz, MD
Owner, Kronowitz Plastics
PLLC;
University of Texas, M. D. Anderson Medical
Center
Houston, TX, USA

John V. Larson, MD
Resident Physician
Division of Plastic and Reconstructive Surgery
Keck School of Medicine of USC
University of Southern California
Los Angeles, CA, USA

Z-Hye Lee, MD
Resident
Department of Plastic Surgery
New York University Medical Center
New York, NY, USA

Frank Lista, MD, FRCSC
Medical Director
The Plastic Surgery Clinic
Mississauga, Ontario, Canada;
Assistant Professor Surgery
University of Toronto
Toronto, Ontario, Canada

Albert Losken, MD, FACS
Professor of plastic surgery and Program
Director
Emory Division of Plastic and Reconstructive
Surgery
Emory University School of Medicine
Atlanta, GA, USA

**Charles M. Malata, BSc(HB), MB ChB,
LRCP, MRCS, FRCS(Glasg), FRCS(Plast)**
Professor of Academic Plastic Surgery
Postgraduate Medical Institute
Faculty of Health Sciences
Anglia Ruskin University
Cambridge and Chelmsford, UK;
Consultant Plastic and Reconstructive Surgeon
Department of Plastic and Reconstructive
Surgery
Cambridge Breast Unit at Addenbrooke's
Hospital
Cambridge University Hospitals NHS
Foundation Trust
Cambridge, UK

Jaume Masià, MD, PhD
Chief and Professor of Plastic Surgery
Sant Pau University Hospital
Barcelona, Spain

G. Patrick Maxwell, MD, FACS
Clinical Professor of Surgery
Department of Plastic Surgery
Loma Linda University Medical Center
Loma Linda, CA, USA

James L. Mayo, MD
Microsurgery Fellow
Plastic Surgery
New York University
New York, NY, USA

Roberto N. Miranda, MD
Professor
Department of Hematopathology
Division of Pathology and Laboratory Medicine
MD Anderson Cancer Center
Houston, TX, USA

**Colin M. Morrison, MSc (Hons) FRCSI
(Plast)**
Consultant Plastic Surgeon
St. Vincent's University Hospital
Dublin, Ireland

Maurice Y. Nahabedian, MD, FACS
Professor and Chief
Section of Plastic Surgery
MedStar Washington Hospital Center
Washington DC, USA;
Vice Chairman
Department of Plastic Surgery
MedStar Georgetown University Hospital
Washington DC, USA

James D. Namnoum, MD
Clinical Professor of Plastic Surgery
Atlanta Plastic Surgery
Emory University School of Medicine
Atlanta, GA, USA

Maria E. Nelson, MD
Assistant Professor of Clinical Surgery
Department of Surgery, Division of Upper GI/
General Surgery, Section of Surgical Oncology
Keck School of Medicine
University of Southern California
Los Angeles, CA, USA

Julie Park, MD
Associate Professor of Surgery
Section of Plastic Surgery
University of Chicago
Chicago, IL, USA

Ketan M. Patel, MD
Assistant Professor of Surgery
Division of Plastic and Reconstructive Surgery
Keck Medical Center of USC
University of Southern California
Los Angeles, CA, USA

**Nakul Gamanlal Patel, BSc(Hons),
MBBS(Lond), FRCS(Plast)**
Senior Microsurgery Fellow
St. Andrew's Centre for Plastic Surgery
Broomfield Hospital
Chelmsford, UK

Gemma Pons, MD, PhD
Head
Microsurgery Unit
Plastic Surgery
Hospital de Sant Pau
Barcelona, Spain

Julian J. Pribaz, MD
Professor of Surgery
Brigham and Women's Hospital
Harvard Medical School
Boston, MA, USA

**Venkat V. Ramakrishnan, MS, FRCS,
FRACS(Plast Surg)**
Consultant Plastic Surgeon
St. Andrew's Centre for Plastic Surgery
Broomfield Hospital
Chelmsford, UK

Elena Rodríguez-Bauzà, MD
Plastic Surgery Department
Hospital Santa Creu i Sant Pau
Barcelona, Spain

Michael R. Schwartz, MD
Board Certified Plastic Surgeon
Private Practice
Westlake Village, CA, USA

Stephen F. Sener, MD
Professor of Surgery, Clinical Scholar
Chief of Breast, Endocrine, and Soft Tissue
Surgery
Department of Surgery, Keck School of
Medicine of USC
Chief of Surgery and Associate Medical Director
Perioperative Services
LAC+USC (LA County) Hospital
Los Angeles, CA, USA

Joseph M. Serletti, MD, FACS
The Henry Royster–William Maul Measey
Professor of Surgery and Chief
Division of Plastic Surgery
University of Pennsylvania Health System
Philadelphia, PA, USA

Deana S. Shenaq, MD
Chief Resident
Department of Surgery - Plastic Surgery
The University of Chicago Hospitals
Chicago, IL, USA

Kenneth C. Shestak, MD
Professor, Department of Plastic Surgery
University of Pittsburgh Medical Center
Pittsburgh, PA, USA

Ron B. Somogyi, MD MSc FRCSC
Plastic and Reconstructive Surgeon
Assistant Professor, Department of Surgery
University of Toronto
Toronto, ON, Canada

David H. Song, MD, MBA, FACS
Regional Chief, MedStar Health
Plastic and Reconstructive Surgery
Professor and Chairman
Department of Plastic Surgery
Georgetown University School of Medicine
Washington, DC, USA

The late Scott L. Spear†, MD
Formerly Professor of Plastic Surgery
Division of Plastic Surgery
Georgetown University
Washington, MD, USA

Michelle A. Spring, MD, FACS
Program Director
Glacier View Plastic Surgery
Kalispell Regional Medical Center
Kalispell, MT, USA

W. Grant Stevens, MD, FACS
Clinical Professor of Surgery
Marina Plastic Surgery Associates;
Keck School of Medicine of USC
Los Angeles, CA, USA

Elizabeth Stirling Craig, MD
Plastic Surgeon and Assistant Professor
Department of Plastic Surgery
University of Texas
MD Anderson Cancer Center
Houston, TX, USA

Simon G. Talbot, MD
Assistant Professor of Surgery
Brigham and Women's Hospital
Harvard Medical School
Boston, MA, USA

Jana Van Thielen, MD
Plastic Surgery Department
Brussels University Hospital
Vrij Universitaire Brussel (VUB)
Brussels, Belgium

Henry Wilson, MD, FACS
Attending Plastic Surgeon
Private Practice
Plastic Surgery Associates
Lynchburg, VA, USA

Kai Yuen Wong, MA, MB BChir, MRCS, FHEA, FRSPH
Specialist Registrar in Plastic Surgery
Department of Plastic and Reconstructive
Surgery
Cambridge University Hospitals NHS
Foundation Trust
Cambridge, UK

VOLUME SIX

Hee Chang Ahn, MD, PhD
Professor
Department of Plastic and Reconstructive
Surgery
Hanyang University Hospital School of Medicine
Seoul, South Korea

Nidal F. Al Deek, MD
Surgeon
Plastic and Reconstructive Surgery
Chang Gung Memorial Hospital
Taipei, Taiwan

Kodi K. Azari, MD, FACS
Reconstructive Transplantation Section Chief
Professor
Department of Orthopedic Surgery
UCLA Medical Center
Santa Monica, CA, USA

Carla Baldrighi, MD
Staff Surgeon
Pediatric Surgery Meyer Children's Hospital
Pediatric Hand and Reconstructive Microsurgery
Unit
Azienda Ospedaliera Universitaria Careggi
Florence, Italy

Gregory H. Borschel, MD, FAAP, FACS
Assistant Professor
University of Toronto Division of Plastic and
Reconstructive Surgery;
Assistant Professor
Institute of Biomaterials and Biomedical
Engineering;
Associate Scientist
The SickKids Research Institute
The Hospital for Sick Children
Toronto, Ontario, Canada

Kirsty Usher Boyd, MD, FRCSC
Assistant Professor
Division of Plastic Surgery, University of Ottawa
Ottawa, Ontario, Canada

Gerald Brandacher, MD
Scientific Director
Department of Plastic and Reconstructive
Surgery
Johns Hopkins University School of Medicine
Baltimore, MD, USA

Lesley Butler, MPH
Clinical Research Coordinator
Charles E. Seay, Jr. Hand Center
Texas Scottish Rite Hospital for Children
Dallas, TX, USA

Ryan P. Calfee, MD
Associate Professor
Department of Orthopedic Surgery
Washington University School of Medicine
St. Louis, MO, USA

Brian T. Carlsen, MD
Associate Professor
Departments of Plastic Surgery and Orthopedic
Surgery
Mayo Clinic
Rochester, MN, USA

David W. Chang, MD
Professor
Division of Plastic and Reconstructive Surgery
The University of Chicago Medicine
Chicago, IL, USA

James Chang, MD
Johnson & Johnson Distinguished Professor
and Chief
Division of Plastic and Reconstructive Surgery
Stanford University Medical Center
Stanford, CA, USA

Robert A. Chase, MD
Holman Professor of Surgery – Emeritus
Stanford University Medical Center
Stanford, CA, USA

**Alphonsus K. S. Chong, MBBS, MRCS,
MMed(Orth), FAMS (Hand Surg)**
Senior Consultant
Department of Hand and Reconstructive
Microsurgery
National University Health System
Singapore;
Assistant Professor
Department of Orthopedic Surgery
Yong Loo Lin School of Medicine
National University of Singapore
Singapore

David Chwei-Chin Chuang, MD
Senior Consultant, Ex-President, Professor
Department of Plastic Surgery
Chang Gung University Hospital
Tao-Yuan, Taiwan

Kevin C. Chung, MD, MS
Chief of Hand Surgery
Michigan Medicine
Charles B G De Nancrede Professor, Assistant
Dean for Faculty Affairs
University of Michigan Medical School
Ann Arbor, Michigan, USA

Christopher Cox, MD
Attending Surgeon
Kaiser Permanente
Walnut Creek, CA, USA

Catherine Curtin, MD
Associate Professor
Department of Surgery Division of Plastic
Surgery
Stanford University
Stanford, CA, USA

Lars B. Dahlin, MD, PhD
Professor and Consultant
Department of Clinical Sciences, Malmö – Hand
Surgery
University of Lund
Malmö, Sweden

Kenneth W. Donohue, MD
Hand Surgery Fellow
Division of Plastic Surgery
Department of Orthopedic Surgery
Baylor College of Medicine
Houston, TX, USA

Gregory A. Dumanian, MD, FACS
Stuteville Professor of Surgery
Division of Plastic Surgery
Northwestern Feinberg School of Medicine
Chicago, IL, USA

William W. Dzwierzynski, MD
Professor and Program Director
Department of Plastic Surgery
Medical College of Wisconsin
Milwaukee, WI, USA

Simon Farnebo, MD, PhD
Associate Professor and Consultant Hand
Surgeon
Department of Plastic Surgery, Hand Surgery
and Burns
Institution of Clinical and Experimental
Medicine, University of Linköping
Linköping, Sweden

Ida K. Fox, MD
Assistant Professor of Plastic Surgery
Department of Surgery
Division of Plastic and Reconstructive Surgery
Washington University School of Medicine
St. Louis, MO, USA

Paige M. Fox, MD, PhD
Assistant Professor
Department of Surgery, Division of Plastic and
Reconstructive Surgery
Stanford University Medical Center
Stanford, CA, USA

Jeffrey B. Friedrich, MD
Professor of Surgery and Orthopedics
Department of Surgery, Division of Plastic
Surgery
University of Washington
Seattle, WA, USA

Steven C. Haase, MD, FACS
Associate Professor
Department of Surgery, Section of Plastic
Surgery
University of Michigan Health
Ann Arbor, MI, USA

Elisabet Hagert, MD, PhD
Associate Professor
Department of Clinical Science and Education
Karolinska Institute;
Chief Hand Surgeon
Hand Foot Surgery Center
Stockholm, Sweden

Warren C. Hammert, MD
Professor of Orthopedic and Plastic Surgery
Chief, Division of Hand Surgery
Department of Orthopedics and Rehabilitation
University of Rochester
Rochester, NY, USA

Isaac Harvey, MD
Clinical Fellow
Department of Pediatric Plastic and
Reconstructive Surgery
Hospital for SickKids
Toronto, Ontario, Canada

Vincent R. Hentz, MD
Emeritus Professor of Surgery and Orthopedic
Surgery (by courtesy)
Stanford University
Stanford, CA, USA

Jonay Hill, MD
Clinical Assistant Professor
Anesthesiology, Perioperative and Pain Medicine
Stanford University School of Medicine
Stanford, CA, USA

Steven E. R. Hovius, MD, PhD
Former Head, Department of Plastic,
Reconstructive and Hand Surgery
Erasmus MC
University Medical Center
Rotterdam, the Netherlands;
Xpert Clinic, Hand and Wrist Center
The Netherlands

Jerry I. Huang, MD
Associate Professor
Department of Orthopedics and Sports
Medicine
University of Washington;
Program Director
University of Washington Hand Fellowship
University of Washington
Seattle, WA, USA

Marco Innocenti, MD
Associate Professor of Plastic Surgery,
University of Florence;
Director, Reconstructive Microsurgery
Department of Oncology
Careggi University Hospital
Florence, Italy

Neil F. Jones, MD, FRCS
Professor and Chief of Hand Surgery
University of California Medical Center;
Professor of Orthopedic Surgery;
Professor of Plastic and Reconstructive Surgery
University of California Irvine
Irvine, CA, USA

Ryosuke Kakinoki, MD, PhD
Professor of Hand Surgery and Microsurgery,
Reconstructive, and Orthopedic Surgery
Department of Orthopedic Surgery
Faculty of Medicine
Kindai University
Osakasayama, Osaka, Japan

Jason R. Kang, MD
Chief Resident
Department of Orthopedic Surgery
Stanford Hospital & Clinics
Redwood City, CA, USA

Joseph S. Khouri, MD
Resident
Division of Plastic Surgery, Department of
Surgery
University of Rochester
Rochester, NY, USA

Todd Kuiken, MD, PhD
Professor
Departments of PM&R, BME, and Surgery
Northwestern University;
Director, Neural Engineering Center for Artificial
Limbs
Rehabilitation Institute of Chicago
Chicago, IL, USA

Donald Lalonde, BSC, MD, MSc, FRCSC
Professor of Surgery
Division of Plastic and Reconstructive Surgery
Saint John Campus of Dalhousie University
Saint John, New Brunswick, Canada

W. P. Andrew Lee, MD
The Milton T. Edgerton MD, Professor and
Chairman
Department of Plastic and Reconstructive
Surgery
Johns Hopkins University School of Medicine
Baltimore, MD, USA

Anais Legrand, MD
Postdoctoral Research Fellow
Plastic and Reconstructive Surgery
Stanford University Medical Center
Stanford, CA, USA

Terry Light, MD
Professor
Department of Orthopedic Surgery
Loyola University Medical Center
Maywood, IL, USA

Jin Xi Lim, MBBS, MRCS
Senior Resident
Department of Hand and Reconstructive
Microsurgery
National University Health System
Singapore

Joseph Lopez, MD, MBA
Resident, Plastic and Reconstructive Surgery
Department of Plastic and Reconstructive
Surgery
Johns Hopkins University School of Medicine
Baltimore, MD, USA

Susan E. Mackinnon, MD
Sydney M. Shoenberg, Jr. and Robert H.
Shoenberg Professor
Department of Surgery, Division of Plastic and
Reconstructive Surgery
Washington University School of Medicine
St. Louis, MO, USA

Brian Mailey, MD
Assistant Professor of Surgery
Institute for Plastic Surgery
Southern Illinois University
Springfield, IL, USA

Steven J. McCabe, MD, MSc, FRCS(C)
Director of Hand and Upper Extremity Program
University of Toronto
Toronto Western Hospital
Toronto, Ontario, Canada

Kai Megerle, MD, PhD
Assistant Professor
Clinic for Plastic Surgery and Hand Surgery
Technical University of Munich
Munich, Germany

Amy M. Moore, MD
Assistant Professor of Surgery
Division of Plastic and Reconstructive Surgery
Department of Surgery
Washington University School of Medicine
St. Louis, MO, USA

Steven L. Moran, MD
Professor and Chair of Plastic Surgery
Division of Plastic Surgery, Division of Hand and
Microsurgery;
Professor of Orthopedics
Rochester, MN, USA

Rebecca L. Neiduski, PhD, OTR/L, CHT
Dean of the School of Health Sciences
Professor of Health Sciences
Elon University
Elon, NC, USA

David T. Netscher, MD
Program Director, Hand Surgery Fellowship;
Clinical Professor, Division of Plastic Surgery
and Department of Orthopedic Surgery
Baylor College of Medicine;
Adjunct Professor of Clinical Surgery (Plastic
Surgery)
Weill Medical College
Cornell University
Houston, TX, USA

Michael W. Neumeister, MD
Professor and Chairman
Division of Plastic Surgery
Springfield Illinois University School of Medicine
Springfield, IL, USA

Shelley Noland, MD
Assistant Professor
Division of Plastic Surgery
Mayo Clinic Arizona
Phoenix, AZ, USA

Christine B. Novak, PT, PhD
Associate Professor
Department of Surgery, Division of Plastic and
Reconstructive Surgery
University of Toronto
Toronto, Ontario, Canada

Scott Oates, MD
Deputy Department Chair;
Professor
Department of Plastic Surgery, Division of
Surgery
The University of Texas MD Anderson Cancer
Center
Houston, TX, USA

Kerby Oberg, MD, PhD
Associate Professor
Department of Pathology and Human Anatomy
Loma Linda University School of Medicine
Loma Linda, CA, USA

Scott Oishi, MD
Director, Charles E. Seay, Jr. Hand Center
Texas Scottish Rite Hospital for Children;
Professor, Department of Plastic Surgery and
Department of Orthopedic Surgery
University of Texas Southwestern Medical Center
Dallas, TX, USA

William C. Pederson, MD, FACS
President and Fellowship Director
The Hand Center of San Antonio;
Adjunct Professor of Surgery
The University of Texas Health Science Center at
San Antonio
San Antonio, TX, USA

Dang T. Pham, MD
General Surgery Resident
Department of Surgery
Houston Methodist Hospital
Houston, TX, USA

Karl-Josef Prommersberger, MD, PhD
Chair, Professor of Orthopedic Surgery
Clinic for Hand Surgery
Bad Neustadt/Saale, Germany

Carina Reinholdt, MD, PhD
Senior Consultant in Hand Surgery
Center for Advanced Reconstruction of
Extremities
Sahlgrenska University Hospital/ Mölndal
Mölndal, Sweden;
Assistant Professor
Department of Orthopedics
Institute for Clinical Sciences
Sahlgrenska Academy
Goteborg, Sweden

Justin M. Sacks, MD, MBA, FACS
Director, Oncological Reconstruction;
Assistant Professor
Department of Plastic and Reconstructive
Surgery
Johns Hopkins School of Medicine
Baltimore, MD, USA

Douglas M. Sammer, MD
Associate Professor of Plastic and Orthopedic
Surgery
Chief of Plastic Surgery at Parkland Memorial
Hospital
Program Director Hand Surgery Fellowship
University of Texas Southwestern Medical Center
Dallas, TX, USA

Subhro K. Sen, MD
Clinical Associate Professor
Plastic and Reconstructive Surgery
Robert A. Chase Hand and Upper Limb Center
Stanford University School of Medicine
Stanford, CA, USA

**Pundrique R. Sharma, MBBS, PhD and
FRCS (Plast)**
Consultant Plastic Surgeon
Department for Plastic and Reconstructive
Surgery
Alder Hey Children's Hospital
Liverpool, UK

Randolph Sherman, MD, FACS
Vice Chair
Department of Surgery
Cedars-Sinai Medical Center
Los Angeles, CA, USA

Jaimie T. Shores, MD
Clinical Director, Hand/Arm Transplant Program
Department of Plastic and Reconstructive
Surgery
Johns Hopkins University School of Medicine
Baltimore, MD, USA

Vanila M. Singh, MD, MACM
Clinical Associate Professor
Anesthesiology, Perioperative and Pain Medicine
Stanford University School of Medicine
Stanford, CA, USA

Jason M. Souza, MD, LCDR, MC, USN
Staff Plastic Surgeon, United States Navy
Walter Reed National Military Medical Center
Bethesda, MD, USA

Amir Taghinia, MD, MPH
Attending Surgeon
Department of Plastic and Oral Surgery
Boston Children's Hospital;
Assistant Professor of Surgery
Harvard Medical School
Boston, MA, USA

David M. K. Tan, MBBS
Senior Consultant
Department of Hand and Reconstructive
Microsurgery
National University Health System
Singapore;
Assistant Professor
Department of Orthopedic Surgery
Yong Loo Lin School of Medicine
National University Singapore
Singapore

Jin Bo Tang, MD
Professor and Chair
Department of Hand Surgery;
Chair, The Hand Surgery Research Center
Affiliated Hospital of Nantong University
Nantong, The People's Republic of China

Johan Thorfinn, MD, PhD
Senior Consultant of Plastic Surgery, Burn Unit;
Co-Director
Department of Plastic Surgery, Hand Surgery
and Burns
Linköping University Hospital
Linköping, Sweden

**Michael Tonkin, MBBS, MD, FRACS(Orth),
FRCS(Ed Orth)**
Professor of Hand Surgery
Department of Hand Surgery and Peripheral
Nerve Surgery
Royal North Shore Hospital
The Children's Hospital at Westmead
University of Sydney Medical School
Sydney, New South Wales, Australia

Joseph Upton III, MD
Staff Surgeon
Department of Plastic and Oral Surgery
Boston Children's Hospital;
Professor of Surgery
Harvard Medical School
Boston, MA, USA

Francisco Valero-Cuevas, PhD
Director
Brain-Body Dynamics Laboratory;
Professor of Biomedical Engineering;
Professor of Biokinesiology and Physical
Therapy;
(By courtesy) Professor of Computer Science
and Aerospace and Mechanical Engineering
The University of Southern California
Los Angeles, CA, USA

Christianne A. van Nieuwenhoven, MD, PhD
Plastic Surgeon/Hand Surgeon
Plastic and Reconstructive Surgery
Erasmus Medical Centre
Rotterdam, the Netherlands

Nicholas B. Vedder, MD
Professor of Surgery and Orthopedics
Chief of Plastic Surgery Vice Chair
Department of Surgery
University of Washington
Seattle, WA, USA

Andrew J. Watt, MD
Attending Hand and Microvascular Surgeon;
Associate Program Director, Buncke Clinic Hand
and Microsurgery Fellowship;
Adjunct Clinical Faculty, Stanford University
Division of Plastic and Reconstructive Surgery
The Buncke Clinic
San Francisco, CA, USA

Fu-Chan Wei, MD
Professor
Department of Plastic Surgery
Chang Gung Memorial Hospital
Taoyuan, Taiwan

Julie Colantoni Woodside, MD
Orthopedic Surgeon
OrthoCarolina
Gastonia, NC, USA

Jeffrey Yao, MD
Associate Professor
Department of Orthopedic Surgery
Stanford Hospital & Clinics
Redwood City, CA, USA

Acknowledgments

My wife, Gabrielle Kane, has always been my rock. She not only encourages me in my work but gives constructive criticism bolstered by her medical expertise as well as by her knowledge and training in education. I can never repay her. The editorial team at Elsevier have made this series possible. Belinda Kuhn leads the group of Alexandra Mortimer, Louise Cook, and the newest addition to the team, Sam Crowe. The Elsevier production team has also been vital in moving this project along. The volume editors, Geoff Gurtner, Peter Rubin, Ed Rodriguez, Joe Losee, David Song, Mo Nahabedian, Jim Chang, and Dan Liu have shaped and refined this edition, making vital changes to keep the series relevant and up-to-date. My colleagues in the University of Washington, headed by Nick Vedder, have provided continued encouragement and support. Finally, and most importantly, the residents and fellows who pass through our program keep us on our toes and ensure that we give them the best possible solutions to their questions.

Peter C. Neligan, MB, FRCS(I), FRCSC, FACS

Driven by constant innovation, the field of head, neck, and craniofacial surgery has truly evolved and made noteworthy advances over the last several decades. The diverse expertise of the renowned contributors has provided the latest clinical evidence and surgical techniques to facilitate the decision-making process, which ultimately impacts the outcomes of patients with conditions involving congenital, oncologic, traumatic, and acquired deformities. This volume is a comprehensive resource for specialists of all levels. It has been a true privilege to work with such a distinguished faculty willing to share their vast experience and insights in their respective fields. It is with great admiration that I sincerely thank the contributors for their generous donation of time, commitment to excellence, dedication to education, and advancement of the field.

Eduardo D. Rodriguez, MD, DDS

This volume represents the expertise of the current leaders within pediatric plastic surgery; and I am grateful for their dedication and efforts in making this "labor of love" a reality and the standard within the field. This work is dedicated to my families – at work and at home – and serves as a living example of work–life integration for me. "Thank you" to my work family – my colleagues, staff, patients and their families; and, to my home family – Franklyn P. Cladis, MD and our son Hudson. You all have and continue to provide significant meaning to my life.

Joseph E. Losee, MD, FACS, FAAP

Dedicated to future plastic surgeons. Take up the torch and lead us forward!

PART 1

Head, neck, and craniofacial surgery

1

Anatomy of the head and neck

Ahmed M. Afifi, Ruston J. Sanchez and Risal S. Djohan

SYNOPSIS

■ The superficial fascial layer of the face and neck is formed by the superficial cervical fascia (enclosing the platysma), the superficial facial fascia (synonymous with the superficial musculo-aponeurotic system (SMAS)), the superficial temporal fascia (often called the temporoparietal fascia), and the galea.

■ The deep fascial layer of the face and neck is formed by the deep cervical fascia (or the general investing fascia of the neck), the deep facial fascia (also known as the parotideomasseteric fascia), and the deep temporal fascia. The deep temporal fascia is continuous with the periosteum of the skull.

■ The deep temporal fascia splits into two layers at the level of the superior orbital rim. The two layers insert into the superficial and deep surfaces of the zygomatic arch.

■ The facial nerve is initially deep to the deep fascia, eventually penetrating it towards the superficial fascia. The fat and connective tissue filling the space between the superficial temporal fascia and the superficial layer of the deep temporal fascia is a subject of significant debate. Its importance stems from the temporal branch of the facial nerve crossing from deep to superficial in this layer.

■ Most surgeons believe that it is the superficial temporal fat pad that fills this space. Others believe there is a distinct fascial layer in this region, named the parotideomasseteric fascia.

■ The facial nerve is at significant risk of injury in the area right above the zygomatic arch.

■ Pitanguy's line describes the course of the largest branch of the temporal division of the facial nerve.

■ The marginal mandibular nerve can be located above or below the level of the mandible. It is usually located between the platysma and the deep cervical fascia and is always superficial to the facial vessels.

■ There are multiple fat pads in the face. They can be superficial to the SMAS, between the SMAS and the deep fascia, or deep to the deep fascia.

■ Knowledge of the sensory nerves is important, especially within the context of evaluating and treating migraine headaches.

Aesthetic and reconstructive surgery of the head and neck depends on appreciating the three-dimensional anatomy and the functional and cosmetic methods of rearranging the different structures. This chapter is not intended to be a detailed description of the head and neck anatomy, which is beyond such a limited space. It rather offers a different perspective on the anatomy that is more relevant to the plastic surgeon and highlights certain anatomical regions that have fundamental importance or are more controversial.

The fascial planes of the head and neck and the facial nerve

A peculiar feature of the anatomy of the head and neck is the concentric arrangement of the facial soft tissues in layers. These layers have different names and characteristics from one area of the head and neck to the other, but they maintain their continuity across boundaries (Fig. 1.1). Unfortunately, inconsistent nomenclature has been used to describe these layers leading to significant confusion among readers. The facial nerve usually passes in defined planes in between these layers, crossing from one layer to the other only in specific well-described zones. Knowledge of these planes and their relation to the facial nerve is vital if plastic surgeons are to safely access the soft tissues and bony structures of the head and neck.[1,2] In the following discussion, we will not only describe the anatomy and nomenclature of these layers as mostly agreed upon, but also try to elucidate the sources of deliberation and confusion in describing this crucial anatomy.[3]

The bordering regions of neck, cheek (lower face), temple, and the scalp are arbitrarily divided by the lower border of the mandible, the zygomatic arch, and the temporal line, respectively. Topographically, there are two layers of fascia covering the face, a superficial and deep, which cover these regions and extend over other structures, such as the eyelid and the nose (see Fig. 1.1).

The superficial layer of fascia is formed by the superficial cervical fascia (platysma), the superficial facial fascia (SMAS), the superficial temporal fascia (temporoparietal fascia), and

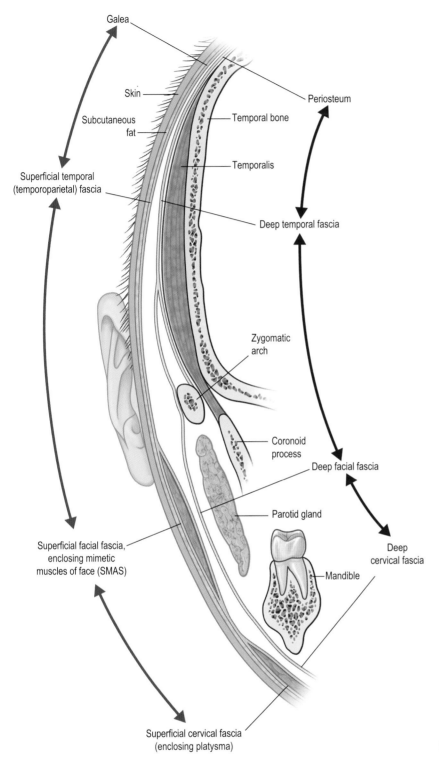

Fig. 1.1 The facial layers of the scalp, face, and neck.

the galea aponeurotica (Figs. 1.1 & 1.2). To be more precise, this superficial fascia splits to enclose many of the facial muscles. This is a consistent pattern seen all over the head and neck region; e.g., the superficial cervical fascia splits into a deep and superficial layer to enclose the platysma, the superficial facial fascia splits to enclose the midfacial muscles, and the galea splits to enclose the frontalis. The two layers of the superficial fascia then rejoin at the other end of the muscle, before splitting again to enclose the next muscle and so on.

The deep layer of fascia is formed by the deep cervical fascia, the deep facial fascia (parotideomasseteric fascia), the deep temporal fascia, and the periosteum. This layer is superficial to the muscles of mastication, the salivary glands and the main neurovascular structures (see Figs. 1.1 & 1.2). Over bony areas, such as the skull and the zygomatic arch, this deep fascia is inseparable from the periosteum.

The facial fat pads are localized collections of fat present deep to the superficial layer of fascia. These are anatomically

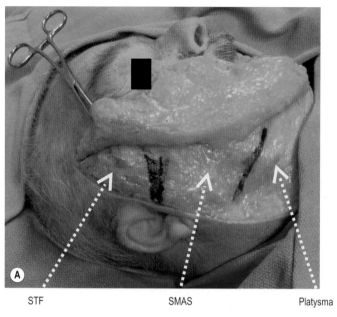

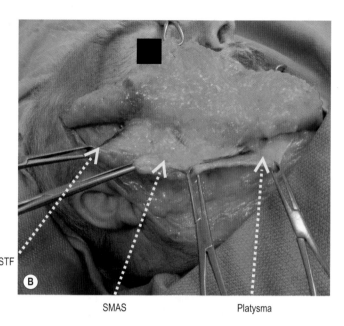

STF

SMAS

Platysma

STF

SMAS

Platysma

Superficial layer reflected

Zygomatic
ligament
and nerve

Mandibular
ligament
and
buccal
nerve

The nerves penetrate the deep fascia towards their
innervation of the SMAS and platysma

Fig. 1.2 The different fascial layers of the face and neck.
(A) Dissection in the superficial plane, between the skin and the
superficial fascia. **(B)** Elevation of the superficial fascial layer,
formed of the superficial cervical fascia (platysma), the superficial
facial fascia (SMAS), and the superficial temporal fascia
(temporoparietal fascia). **(C)** Note the proximity of the nerve (on
the blue background) to the zygomatic and mandibular ligaments
(at the tips of the left and right surgical instruments, respectively).

and histologically distinct structures from the subcutaneous
fat present between the skin and the superficial fascia (which
will be discussed later). These fat pads include the superficial
temporal fat pad, the galeal fat pad, suborbicularis oculi fat
pad (SOOF), the retro-orbicularis oculi fat pad (ROOF), and
the preseptal fat of the eyelids. Deep to the deep fascia are
several other fat pads: the deep temporal fat pads, the buccal
fat pads, and the postseptal fat pads of the eyelids.[4]

The fascia in the face

The first layer the surgeon encounters in the face deep to
the skin and its associated subcutaneous fat is the SMAS
(superficial musculo-aponeurotic system) (see Figs. 1.1 &
1.2).[5] The SMAS varies in thickness and composition between
individuals and from one area to another, and it can be fatty,
fibrous, or muscular.[6] The muscles of facial expression, e.g.,

orbicularis oculi, oris, zygomaticus major and minor, frontalis,
and platysma, are enclosed by (or form part of) the SMAS.
The SMAS is often referred to as the superficial facial fascia.
In reality, the superficial facial fascia covers the superficial
and deep surfaces of the muscles. However, these layers are
hard to separate intraoperatively (except in certain areas such
as the neck). Dissection superficial to the superficial facial
fascia (just under the skin) will generally avoid injury to
the underlying facial nerve. However, such dissection can
compromise the blood supply of the overlying skin flaps.
Often, the surgeon can safely maintain this superficial fascia
in the lower face and neck (whether it is the platysma or
the SMAS) with the skin, allowing a secure double layer
closure and maintaining skin vascularity (e.g. during a neck
dissection). In the anterior (medial) face, the facial nerve
branches become more superficial just under or within the
SMAS layer.

The next layer in the face is the deep facial fascia, which is also known as the parotideomasseteric fascia (see Figs. 1.1 & 1.2). Over the parotid gland, this layer is adherent to the capsule of the gland. The facial nerve is initially (i.e., right after it exits the parotid gland) deep to the deep facial fascia. Most of the muscles of facial expression are superficial to the planes of the nerve. The nerve branches pierce the deep fascia to innervate the muscles from their deep surface, with the exception of the mentalis, levator anguli oris, and the buccinators (see Fig. 1.2). These three muscles are deep to the facial nerve and are thus innervated on their superficial surface.

The fascia in the temporal region

The cheek and lower face are separated from the temporal region by the zygomatic arch. There are two layers of fascia in the temporal region (below the skull temporal lines): the superficial temporal fascia (also known as the temporoparietal fascia (TPF)) and the deep temporal fascia (Figs. 1.3 & 1.4A).[7–9] The deep temporal fascia lies on the superficial surface of the temporalis muscle. Between the superficial and deep temporal fascia is a loose areolar plane that is relatively avascular and easily dissected. However, the frontal branch of the facial nerve is within or directly beneath the superficial temporal

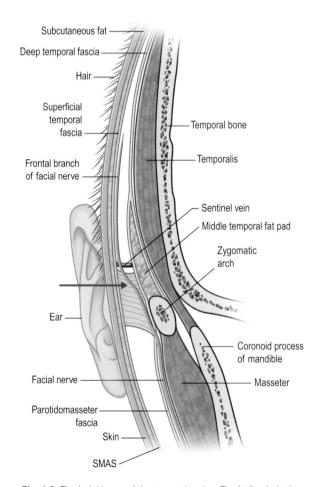

Fig. 1.3 The facial layers of the temporal region. The fat/fascia in the subaponeurotic plane (arrow; between the temporal fascia and deep temporal fascia) is intimately related to the facial nerve. Some authors believe that there is a separate fascial layer in this space, referred to as the parotideomasseteric fascia.

Labels in figure:
Subcutaneous fat
Deep temporal fascia
Hair
Superficial temporal fascia
Frontal branch of facial nerve
Ear
Facial nerve
Parotidomasseter fascia
Skin
SMAS
Temporal bone
Temporalis
Sentinel vein
Middle temporal fat pad
Zygomatic arch
Coronoid process of mandible
Masseter

fascia (see Fig. 1.4A).[5] Therefore, dissection in this plane should be strictly on the deep temporal fascia, which can be identified by its bright white color and sturdy texture. To ensure that the surgeon is in the right plane, he or she can attempt to grasp the areolar tissues over the deep temporal fascia using an Adson forceps; if in the right plane, one will not catch any tissue. Once deep enough and right on the deep temporal fascia, dissection can proceed quickly using a periosteal elevator hugging the tough deep temporal fascia (Fig. 1.5).

In the region right above the zygomatic arch the space between the superficial TPF and the deep temporal fascia (sometimes referred to as the subaponeurotic space) and the fat/fascia it contains is both a debatable and an important subject (see Fig. 1.4). Its importance stems from the facial nerve crossing this space from deep to superficial right above the zygomatic arch. A third layer of fascia has been described in this space (between the superficial and deep temporal fascia) and is referred to as the parotidotemporal fascia, the subgaleal fascia, or the innominate fascia.[10,11] The term "fascial layer" is used loosely, as there is no general consensus as to how thick connective tissue must be before it can be considered a "fascial layer". What some authors refer to as "loose connective tissue" may be called a "fascial layer" or a "fat pad" by others. Our own cadaver dissection showed that this third fascial layer could often be identified. It extends for a short distance above and below the arch. Directly superficial to the arch, the facial nerve is deep to this layer, piercing it to become more superficial 1–2 cm cephalad to the arch (see below).

Above the zygomatic arch and at the same horizontal level as the superior orbital rim, the deep temporal fascia splits into two layers: the superficial layer of the deep temporal fascia (sometimes referred to as the middle temporal fascia, intermediate fascia, or the innominate fascia) and the deep layer of the deep temporal fascia (see Fig. 1.3).[7] The deep and superficial layers of the deep temporal fascia attach to the superficial and deep surfaces of the zygomatic arch. There are three fat pads in this region.[7,12] The superficial fat pad is located between the superficial temporal fascia and superficial layer of the deep temporal fascia and, as described above, is analogous with the parotidotemporal fascia, subgaleal fascia, and/or the loose connective tissue between the superficial and deep temporal fascia. The middle fat pad is located directly above the zygomatic arch between the superficial and deep layers of the deep temporal fascia. Finally, the deep fat pad (also known as the buccal fat pad) is deep to the deep layer of the deep temporal fascia, superficial to the temporalis muscles and extends deep to the zygomatic arch. It is considered an extension of the buccal fat pad.

Most of the controversy in describing the fascial layers in the temporal region arises from confusing the *superficial temporal fascia* with the *superficial layer of the deep temporal fascia*. This is very significant since the facial nerve is deep to or within the former and superficial to the latter. The second point is the location of the *deep temporal fascia superficial* to the temporalis muscle. There is another fascial layer on the deep surface of the muscle; this is not the deep temporal fascia and is of little significance from a surgical standpoint. The final controversy is what exactly is the *innominate* fascia? This term is often used to describe the superficial layer of the deep temporal fascia above the arch. Other surgeons reserve the

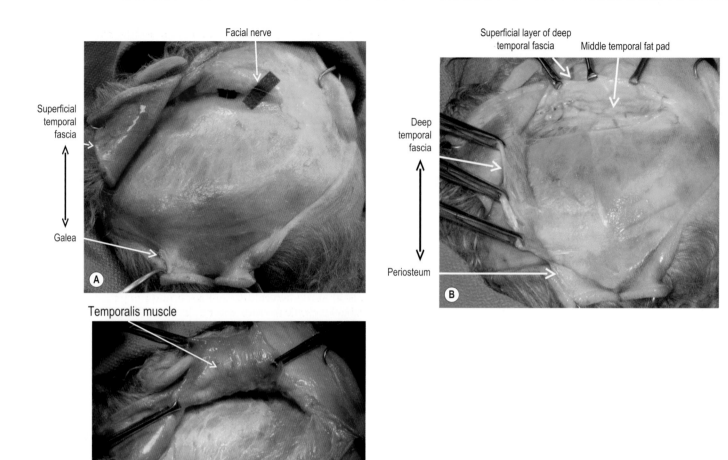

Fig. 1.4 The different planes of dissection in the temporal region. **(A)** Dissection between the superficial temporal fascia (temporoparietal fascia) and the deep temporal fascia. In this plane, the surgeon should try to stay right on the deep temporal fascia. **(B)** Dissection deep to the deep temporal fascia. This is a safe plan that will lead to the zygomatic arch. The facial nerve will be protected by the superficial layer of the deep temporal fascia. **(C)** Dissection deep to the temporalis muscle. The muscle can be left as part of the skin flap. This is a safe and easy plan if no exposure of the arch is needed.

term to the areolar tissue between the superficial layer of the deep temporal fascia and the superficial temporal fascia (i.e., the innominate fascia can be synonymous with the parotidotemporal fascia or subgaleal fascia or the superficial temporal fat pad).[13]

The plane of dissection in the temporal region depends on the goal of the surgery (see Fig. 1.4). In general, the surgeon should avoid the superficial temporal fascia as it harbors the frontal branch of the facial nerve. During surgery to expose the orbital rims and the forehead musculature, the dissection plane is between the superficial temporal fascia and deep temporal fascia (see Fig. 1.4A). To expose the arch, the superficial layer of the deep temporal fascia is divided and dissection proceeds between it and the middle fat pad (the superficial layer of the deep temporal fascia will act as an extra layer protecting the nerve) (see Fig. 1.4B). Finally, when a coronal approach is used, but the arch does not need to be exposed, dissection can proceed deep to the temporalis muscles, elevating them with the coronal flap (see Fig. 1.4B). Using this avascular plane avoids potential traction or injury to the frontal nerve and ensures good aesthetic results as it prevents possible fat atrophy or retraction of the temporalis muscle.

While the fascial layers in the temporal region are well described, there is more debate and variability of the anatomy of the fascial layers and the facial nerve directly superficial to the arch.[12,14,15] The superficial facial fascia (SMAS) is continuous with the TPF, but it is not clear if the deep facial and deep temporal fasciae are continuous to each other or attach and arise from the periosteum of the arch separately. In addition, the thickness of the soft tissues from the periosteum to skin is minimal and the tissues are tightly adherent, making identification of the fascial planes and the facial nerve hazardous in this region.[16] The frontal branch of the facial nerve pierces the deep temporal fascia to become more superficial near the vicinity of the upper border of the arch, and this area constitutes one of the danger zones of the face (see below).

The fascia in the neck

The nomenclature used to describe the different fascial layers in the neck also creates significant confusion. There are two different fascias in the neck: the superficial and the deep (Figs. 1.3 & 1.6). The latter is composed of three different layers: (1) the superficial layer of the deep cervical fascia, also known as

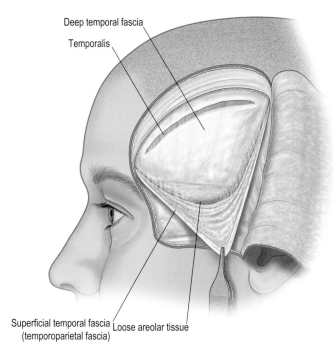

Deep temporal fascia

Temporalis

Superficial temporal fascia (temporoparietal fascia)   Loose areolar tissue

Fig. 1.5 Dissection in the temporal layer.

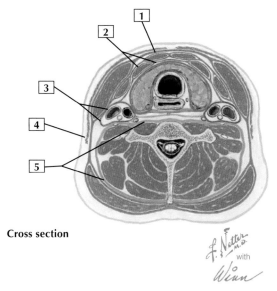

Cross section

Fig. 1.6 Fascial layers of the neck. 1, Investing layer of deep cervical fascia; 2, pretracheal fascia; 3, carotid sheath; 4, superficial fascia; 5, prevertebral fascia. *(Reprinted with permission from www.netterimages.com © Elsevier Inc. All rights reserved.)*

the general investing layer of deep cervical fascia; (2) the middle layer, commonly named the pretracheal fascia; and (3) the deep layer, or the prevertebral fascia (see Figs. 1.3 & 1.6). The pretracheal fascia encircles the trachea, thyroid, and the esophagus, while the prevertebral fascia encloses the prevertebral muscles and forms the floor of the posterior triangle of the neck. For practical purposes, it is the superficial cervical fascia and the superficial layer of the deep cervical fascia that the plastic surgeon encounters.[17,18]

The superficial cervical fascia encloses the platysma muscle and is closely associated with the subcutaneous adipose tissue. The platysma muscle and its surrounding superficial

cervical fascia represent the continuation of the SMAS into the neck. In general, when skin flaps are raised in the neck, the platysma muscle is maintained with the skin to enhance its blood supply (e.g. during neck dissections). However, in necklifts the skin is raised off the platysma to allow platysmal shaping and skin redraping. Tissue expanders placed in the neck could be placed either deep or superficial to the platysma. Placing them superficially will create thinner flaps that are more suitable for facial resurfacing, while placing them deeper allows a more secure coverage of the expander.[19,20]

The superficial layer of deep cervical fascia, or the general investing layer of deep cervical fascia, is what plastic surgeons commonly refer to simply as the "deep cervical fascia". It encircles the whole neck and has attachments to the spinous processes of the vertebrae and the ligamentum nuchae posteriorly. It splits to enclose the sternocleidomastoid and the trapezius muscles. It also splits to enclose the parotid and the submandibular glands. The deep facial fascia, or parotideomasseteric fascia, is therefore considered the continuation of the deep cervical fascia into the face.

Retaining ligaments and adhesions of the face

The ligaments of the face maintain the skin and soft tissues of the face in their normal positions, resisting gravitational changes. Knowledge of their anatomy is important for both the craniofacial and the aesthetic surgeon for several reasons. For the aesthetic surgeon, these ligaments play an important role in maintaining facial fat in its proper positions. For ideal aesthetic repositioning of the skin and soft tissues of the face, numerous surgeons recommend releasing the ligaments. For the craniofacial surgeon, the zones of adherence represent coalescence between different fascial layers, possibly luring the surgeon into an erroneous plane of dissection. In facial reconstruction or face transplants, reconstructing or maintaining these ligaments is important to prevent sagging of the soft tissues with its functional and aesthetic consequences.

Various terms have been used to describe these ligamentous attachments. Moss *et al.* classified them into ligaments (connecting deep fascia/periosteum to the dermis), adhesions (fibrous attachments between the deep and the superficial fascia), and septi (fibrous wall between layers).[21]

In the periorbital and temporal region, various ligaments and adhesions have been described with numerous names given to each (Fig. 1.7). Along the skull temporal line lies the temporal line of fusion, also known as the superior temporal septum, which represents the coalition of the temporal fascia with the skull periosteum. These adhesions end as the temporal ligamentous adhesions (TLA) at the lateral third of the eyebrow.[21] The TLA measure approximately 20 mm in height and 15 mm in width and begin 10 mm cephalad to the superior orbital rim. Both the temporal line of fusion and the TLA are sometimes referred to collectively as temporal adhesions. The inferior temporal septum extends posteriorly and inferiorly from the TLA on the surface of the deep temporal fascia towards the upper border of the zygoma. It separates the upper temporal region superiorly from the lower temporal region inferiorly and represents the upper boundary of the parotideomasseteric fascia (the fascial layer between the superficial and the deep temporal fascia in the region just

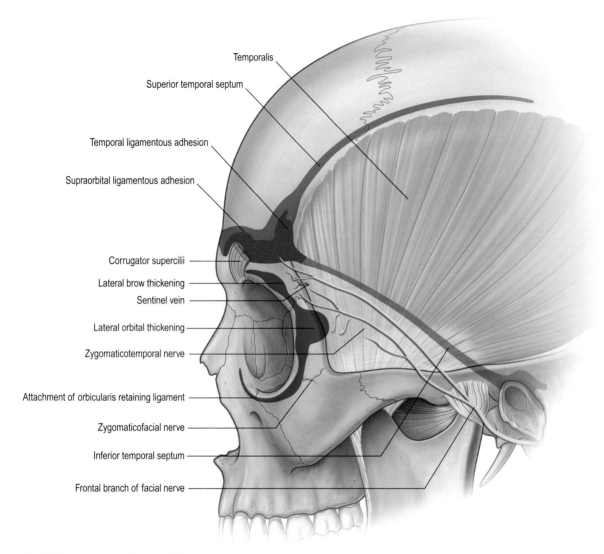

Temporalis

Superior temporal septum

Temporal ligamentous adhesion

Supraorbital ligamentous adhesion

Corrugator supercilii

Lateral brow thickening

Sentinel vein

Lateral orbital thickening

Zygomaticotemporal nerve

Attachment of orbicularis retaining ligament

Zygomaticofacial nerve

Inferior temporal septum

Frontal branch of facial nerve

Fig. 1.7 The ligaments of the periorbital region.

above the zygomatic arch).[22] The supraorbital ligamentous adhesions extend from the TLA medially along the eyebrow.

The orbicularis retaining ligament (ORL) lies along the superior, lateral, and inferior rims of the orbit, extending from the periosteum just outside the orbital rim to the deep surface of the orbicularis oculi muscle (Fig. 1.8).[23,24] This ligament serves to anchor the orbicularis oculi muscle to the orbital rims. The orbicularis oculi muscle attaches directly to the bone from the anterior lacrimal crest to the level of the medial limbus. At this level the ORL replaces the bony origin of the muscle, continuing laterally around the orbit. Initially short, it reaches its maximum length centrally near the lateral limbus.[25] It then begins to diminish in length laterally, until it finally blends with the lateral orbital thickening (LOT). The LOT is a condensation of the superficial and deep fascia on the frontal process of the zygoma and the adjacent deep temporal fascia. The ORL and the orbital septum both attach to the arcus marginalis, a thickening of the periosteum of the orbital rims.[24] The ORL is also referred to as the periorbital septum and, in its inferior portion, as the orbitomalar ligament. The ORL attaches to the undersurface of the orbicularis oculi muscle at the junction of its pretarsal and orbital components.

In the midface, the retaining ligaments have been divided into direct, or osteocutaneous, ligaments and indirect ligaments. Direct ligaments run directly from the periosteum to the dermis, and include the zygomatic and mandibular ligaments. Indirect ligaments represent a coalescence between the superficial and deep fascia and include the parotid and the masseteric cutaneous ligaments (Fig. 1.9; see Fig. 1.2C). The retaining ligaments indirectly fix the mobile skin and its intimately related superficial fascia (SMAS) to the relatively immobile deep fascia and underlying structures (masseter and parotid).

The zygomatic and the masseteric ligaments together form an inverted L, with the angle of the L formed by the major zygomatic ligaments (Fig. 1.9; see Fig. 1.2C). These ligaments are typically around 5–15 mm wide and are located 4.5 cm in front of the tragus and 5–9 mm behind the zygomaticus minor muscle.[26–30] Anterior to this main ligament are multiple other bundles that form the horizontal limb of the inverted L. There have been different descriptions of the anatomy of these

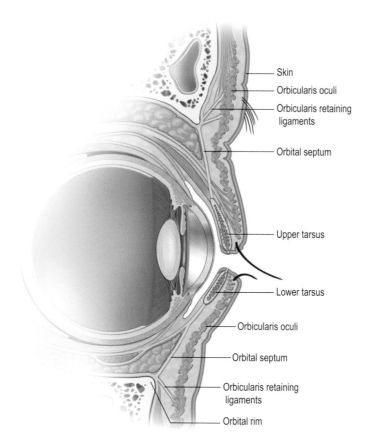

Skin
Orbicularis oculi
Orbicularis retaining ligaments
Orbital septum
Upper tarsus
Lower tarsus
Orbicularis oculi
Orbital septum
Orbicularis retaining ligaments
Orbital rim

Fig. 1.8 The orbicularis retaining ligaments.

zygomatic ligaments, likely related to the variability in their thickness and location, as well as the different criteria used by different authors to define what is truly a "ligament". Often the surgeon will encounter these ligaments along the whole length of the zygomatic arch.[30] The vertical limb of the L is formed by the masseteric ligaments, which are stronger near their upper end (at the zygomatic ligaments), and extend along the entire anterior border of the masseter as far as the mandibular border.[5,31] The parotid ligaments, also referred to as preauricular ligaments, represent another area of firm adherence between the superficial and deep fascia.[26,28,29] The mandibular ligaments originate from the parasymphyseal region of the mandible around 1 cm above the lower mandibular border.[28,29] There are several descriptions of other retaining ligaments in the face, most notably the mandibular septum and the orbital retaining septum.[32,24]

The prezygomatic space

The prezygomatic space is a glide plane space overlying the body of the zygoma, deep to the orbicularis oculi and the suborbicularis fat (see Fig. 1.8).[33] Its floor is formed by a fascial layer covering the body of the zygoma and the lip elevator muscle (namely the zygomaticus major, zygomaticus minor, and the levator labii superioris). This fascial layer extends caudally over the muscles, gradually becoming thinner and allowing the muscle to be more discernible. The superior

boundary of the prezygomatic space is the orbicularis retaining ligament, which separates it from the preseptal space. The more rigid inferior boundary is formed by the reflection of the fascia covering the floor as it curves superficially to blend with the fascia on the undersurface of the orbicularis oculi. This inferior boundary is further reinforced by the zygomatic retaining ligaments. Medially, the space is closed by the origins of the levator labii and the orbicularis oculi muscle from the medial orbital rim. Finally, the lateral boundary is formed superiorly by the LOT over the frontal process of the zygoma and more inferiorly by the zygomatic ligaments.[34] The facial nerve branches cross in the roof of (i.e., superficial to) this space. The only structure traversing the prezygomatic space is the zygomatic branch of the facial nerve, emerging from its foramen located just caudal to the ORL.

The malar fat pad and the subcutaneous fat compartments of the face

Rohrich and Pessa, in an extensive study of the facial subcutaneous fat, found the cheek to be partitioned into multiple, independent anatomical compartments superficial to the superficial fascia.[35] These subcutaneous fat compartments (also referred to as fat pads) are separated by distinct facial condensations that arise from the superficial fascia and insert into the dermis of the skin.[36–38] These superficial fat pads include the nasolabial, jowl, malar, or cheek (subdivided into medial, middle, and lateral-temporal compartments); periorbital (subdivided into inferior, superior, and lateral compartments); and forehead (subdivided into central and medial compartments).[36] This anatomy is important because elements of facial aging may be characterized by how these compartments change relatively in both position and volume with time.[38] Elevation of the malar fat pad, which is triangular in shape with its base at the nasolabial crease and its apex more laterally towards the body of the zygoma, is important for facial rejuvenation and in facial palsy.[39] During facelift dissection, septal transition zones between these superficial fat compartments are regions of potential injury to deeper structures, including branches of the facial nerve as well as the greater auricular nerve.[38]

The buccal fat pad

The buccal fat pad is an underappreciated factor in post-traumatic facial deformities and senile aging and is frequently overlooked as a flap or graft donor site.[40,41] Senile laxity of the fascia allows the fat to prolapse laterally, contributing to the square appearance of the face.[42] With many traumatic injuries the fat herniates, either superficially, towards the oral mucosa, or even into the maxillary sinus.[25,43–45] This fat is anatomically and histologically distinct from the subcutaneous fat. It is voluminous in infants to prevent indrawing of the cheek during suckling, and gradually decreases in size with age.[46] It functions to fill the glide planes between the muscles of mastication.

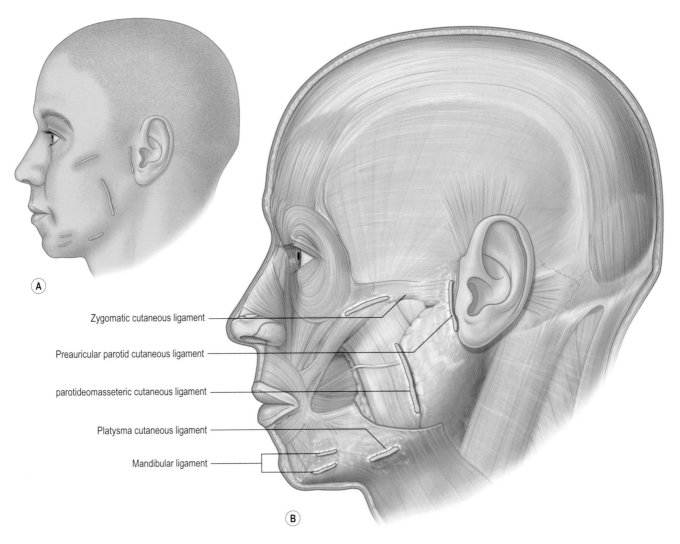

Zygomatic cutaneous ligament

Preauricular parotid cutaneous ligament

parotideomasseteric cutaneous ligament

Platysma cutaneous ligament

Mandibular ligament

Fig. 1.9 The retaining ligaments of the face. *(Reproduced with permission from Gray's Anatomy 40e, Standring S (ed), Churchill Livingstone, London, 2008.)*

It is usually described as being formed of a central body and four extensions, the buccal, pterygoid, and superficial and deep temporal. The body is located on the periosteum of the posterior maxilla (surrounding the branches of the internal maxillary artery) overlying the buccinator muscle and extends forwards in the vestibule of the mouth to the level of the maxillary second molar. The buccal extension is the most superficial, extending along the anterior border of the masseter around the parotid duct. Both the body and the buccal extension are superficial to the buccinator and deep to the deep facial fascia (parotideomasseteric fascia) and are intimately related to the facial nerve branches and the parotid duct. The buccal extension is in the same plane as the facial artery, which marks its anterior boundary. The pterygoid extension passes backwards and downwards deep to the mandibular ramus to surround the pterygoid muscles. The deep temporal extension passes superiorly between the temporalis and the zygomatic arch. The superficial temporal extension is actually totally separate from the main body and lies between the two layers of the temporal fascia above the zygomatic arch.[47]

The facial nerve

During most facial plastic surgeries, whether congenital, reconstructive, or aesthetic, there are one or more branches of the facial nerve that are at risk for injury. Although there is abundant literature on the anatomy of the facial nerve branches, the majority of publications describe two-dimensional anatomy, depicting the trajectory of the nerve and its surface anatomy in relation to anatomic landpoints (see Fig. 1.3).[9,16,48–55] However, it is the third dimension, the depth of the facial nerve in relation to the layers of the face, that is most relevant to the practicing surgeon. In spite of the significant variability in the branching patterns, the facial nerve consistently passes in defined planes, crossing from one plane to another in certain zones.[1] It is in these "danger zones" that dissection should be avoided or done carefully. In the rest of the face, the dissection can proceed relatively quickly by adhering to a certain plane, either superficial or deep to the plane of the nerve.

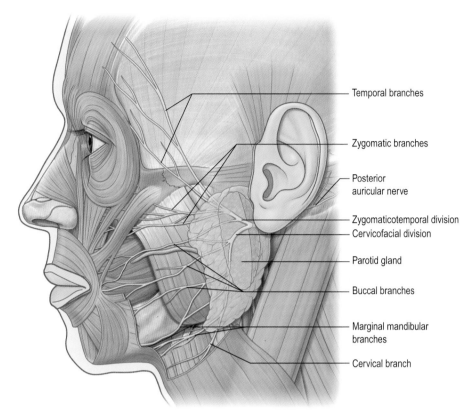

Temporal branches

Zygomatic branches

Posterior
auricular nerve

Zygomaticotemporal division
Cervicofacial division

Parotid gland

Buccal branches

Marginal mandibular
branches

Cervical branch

Fig. 1.10 The facial nerve.

The facial nerve nucleus lies in the lower pons and is responsible for motor innervation to all the muscles derived from the second branchial arch. A few sensory fibers originating in the tractus solitarius join the facial nerve to supply the skin of the external acoustic meatus. The nerve emerges from the lower border of the pons, passes laterally in the cerebellopontine angle, and enters the internal acoustic meatus. The facial nerve then traverses the temporal bone (being liable to injury in temporal bone fractures) to exit the skull through the stylomastoid foramen. Just after its exit it is enveloped by a thick layer of fascia that is continuous with the skull periosteum and is surrounded by a small aggregation of fat and usually crossed by a small blood vessel. This makes its identification in this area a challenging task. Several methods for identification of the facial nerve trunk have been described:

1. If the tragal cartilage is followed to its deep end, it terminates in a point. The nerve is 1 cm deep and inferior to this "tragal pointer". There is an avascular plane anterior to the surface of the tragus that allows a safe and quick dissection to this tragal pointer.
2. By following the posterior belly of the digastric posteriorly, the nerve is found passing laterally immediately deep to the upper border of the posterior end of the muscle.
3. If the anterior border of the mastoid process is traced superiorly, it forms an angle with the tympanic bone. The nerve bisects the angle formed between these two bones (at the tympanomastoid suture).
4. By feeling the styloid process in between the mastoid bone and the posterior border of the mandible. The nerve is just lateral to this process.

5. By following the terminal branches of the nerve proximally.

The nerve passes forwards and downwards to pierce the parotid gland. In the parotid gland the nerve divides into the zygomaticotemporal and the cervicofacial divisions, which in turn divide into the five terminal branches of the facial nerve: frontal, zygomatic, buccal, marginal mandibular, and cervical (Fig. 1.10). However, the zygomatic and buccal branches show significant variability in their location and branching patterns, as well as a significant overlap in the muscles they innervate – they are sometimes grouped together and referred to as "zygomaticobuccal". The temporal and the mandibular branches are perhaps at the highest risk for iatrogenic injury, especially as the muscles they innervate show little if any cross-innervation, making injury to these branches much more noticeable.

Frontal (temporal) branch

This consists of 3–4 branches that innervate the orbicularis oculi muscle, the corrugators and the frontalis muscle. Several anatomic landmarks are used to describe their surface anatomy. The most common description is Pitanguy's line, extending from 0.5 cm below the tragus to a point 1 cm above the lateral edge of the eyebrow (or 1 cm lateral to the lateral canthus).[9,56] Ramirez described the nerve as crossing the zygomatic arch 4 cm behind the lateral canthus.[57] However, other surgeons describe the area spanning the middle two-thirds of the arch as the territory of the nerve. Gosain *et al.* found frontal nerve branches are found at the lower border of the zygomatic arch between 10 mm anterior to the external auditory meatus and 19 mm posterior to the lateral orbital rim.[16] Finally, Zani *et al.* in 300 cadaver dissections reported that the nerve is in a region limited by two straight diverging lines; the first line from the upper tragus border to the most cephalic wrinkle of the frontal region, and the second line from the lower tragus border to the most caudal wrinkle of the frontal region.[51] Although there is no connection between the frontal nerve and other branches of the facial nerve, there are connections within the frontal branches themselves.[16] In addition, the more posterior divisions of the frontal nerve may be less clinically significant than the anterior branches, the injury of which will lead to noticeable brow deformities.[16] A line from the tragus to 1 cm above the lateral eyebrow or 1.5 cm lateral to the lateral canthus seems to be a fairly accurate marking of the largest branch of the frontal nerve.

With this great variation in surface anatomy, it is the plane of the nerve (the depth) that is most important (see Fig. 1.4). After emerging from the parotid gland, the nerve is protected by the deep facial fascia (parotideomasseteric fascia) lying on the masseter muscle. In midfacial procedures (e.g. facelift), dissection is usually *superficial* to the deep facial fascia (which protects the nerve deep to it). In the temporal area, the nerve is on the undersurface of the superficial temporal fascia (see Fig. 1.5). Here dissection is usually *deep* to the nerve, either directly superficial or deep to the deep temporal fascia (or the superficial layer of the deep temporal fascia). However, the crossing of the nerve from deep to superficial in the vicinity of the zygomatic arch is a matter of debate. This is largely because of the confusion regarding the anatomy of the fascia in relation to the arch. Directly over the arch, the facial layers are tightly adherent (with little thickness of tissues from the bone to the skin). While the SMAS is continuous with the temporoparietal fascia across the arch, it is not clear if the deep facial fascia is continuous with the deep temporal fascia or they are separate layers that adhere to the periosteum of the zygomatic arch.[7,8,58,59] At the lower border of the arch, the nerve is very close to the periosteum.[60–63] The nerve is still deep to the SMAS/TPF and deep to the areolar tissue between the TPF and the deep temporal fascia (which, as described above, is sometimes considered as a separate layer of fascia called the parotidotemporal fascia). This deep location of the nerve allows safe transection of the SMAS at the level of the zygomatic arch in facelift surgeries.[13,63,64] The nerve passes from its deep location to the superficial temporal fascia in the region right above the zygomatic arch.[13] In this area, the fascia layers are more tightly adherent, which is a warning sign that the facial nerve is in close proximity. Dissection in this transition zone, extending over the arch and the 2–3 cm above it, should be done carefully (see Fig. 1.3).

Zygomatic and buccal branches

These branches emerge from the parotid and diverge forwards lying over the masseter muscle under the parotideomasseteric (deep facial) fascia. The exact point where they pierce the deep fascia is variable but is in the vicinity of the anterior border of the masseter. The upper branches to the midfacial muscle (zygomatic branches) pierce the deep fascia approximately 4 cm in front of the tragus in close proximity (around 1 cm inferior) to the zygomatic ligaments (see Fig. 1.2C). These branches soon innervate the zygomaticus major muscle through its deep surface. The zygomatic and masseteric

retaining ligaments can aid in identification of these nerve branches. As mentioned previously, the major zygomatic ligament is located around 45 mm in front of the tragus (it might be helpful to mark this location on the skin prior to facelift surgery). Medial to this ligament is the zygomaticus major muscle and the overlying prezygomatic space, and just inferior to this ligament are the upper zygomatic branches of the facial nerve. These branches are deep to the deep facial fascia at this level. The lower zygomatic branches of the facial nerve pass inferior to the upper masseteric ligaments and are closer to the SMAS. Therefore, both the zygomatic and upper masseteric ligaments should be divided close to the SMAS to protect the facial nerve branches.[30] The buccal branches emerge from the parotid in the same plane as the parotid duct (deep to the parotideomasseteric fascia). They pierce the deep fascia at the anterior edge of the masseter, close to the masseteric cutaneous ligaments (see Fig. 1.2C). Together, the zygomatic and buccal branches supply the orbicularis oculi, midfacial muscle, orbicularis oris, and the buccinator. Unlike the marginal mandibular and the frontal divisions, there are a number of communicating branches between the buccal and zygomatic divisions, and injury to a single branch of these nerves is usually unnoticeable. Facial lacerations medial to the level of the lateral canthus are usually not amenable to exploration or repair of the facial nerve.

Marginal mandibular

The marginal mandibular nerve is one of the most commonly encountered branches of the facial nerve and is in jeopardy in multiple operations, including neck dissections, submandibular sialadenectomy, and exposure of the mandible.[65] There are numerous descriptions and variations of both the trajectory of the nerve and its plane (i.e. depth), necessitating care in a wide area of dissection in the lower face and the submandibular triangle.[2,50,66–70] In addition, the nerve can vary between a single branch and up to 3 or 4 branches.[2,67,71,72]

After exiting the parotid gland near its lower border, the nerve loops downward, often below the mandibular border. Whether the nerve crosses the mandibular border into the submandibular triangle in all individuals is a matter of debate.[2,66,73] Although several cadaver studies found the nerve to be more commonly above the mandibular border, clinical experience has shown that it is frequently located in the submandibular triangle, up to 3 or even 4 cm below the mandible.[2,50,66,74–76] This might also vary with the position of the neck, and the surgeon must consider the wide variability of the nerve location in his dissection.[2] The nerve then passes upwards back into the face midway between the angle and mental protuberance. Once the nerve crosses the facial vessels, its major trunk is usually above the border of the mandible, although smaller branches may continue in the neck to supply the platysma.[2]

After exiting the parotid gland, the nerve is initially deep to the parotideomasseteric fascia. In the submandibular triangle, the nerve is usually described as lying between the platysma and the deep cervical fascia. However, it might occasionally be found deep to the deep fascia near the superficial surface of the submandibular gland. The nerve is deep to the platysma and superficial to the facial vessels throughout its course. As the nerve crosses into the lower face, the platysma thins and the nerve can be injured during a subcutaneous dissection.

The marginal mandibular nerve supplies the lower lip muscles, depressor anguli oris, mentalis, and the upper part of the platysma.[67,71] Injury to the marginal mandibular branch usually causes a recognizable deformity,[77–79] and several surgical maneuvers have been advocated to protect the nerve.[80,81] When exposing the mandible, the surgeon can identify the nerve in the usual subplatysmal location. However, it might be safer and faster to go to a deeper plane, elevating the deep fascia and/or the facial vessels and using them to protect the nerve. Dissection above the platysma laterally will also avoid nerve injury.

Cervical branch

The cervical branch of the facial nerve primarily supplies the platysma. It has received little attention in the literature, as injury of this nerve may pass unnoticed. However, such injury may cause weakness of the lower lip depressors, which is often confused with injury to the mandibular nerve (marginal mandibular nerve pseudoparalysis).[82,83] However, mentalis function differentiates the two conditions, as it is preserved in cases of cervical branch injury.

The cervical nerve exits the parotid gland and passes 1–15 mm behind the angle of the mandible. It then passes forwards, in the subplatysmal plane 1–4.5 cm below the border of the mandible.[84] The cervical nerve is often composed of more than one branch. It may communicate with the marginal mandibular nerve (which might explain the lower lip asymmetry after its injury), and consistently communicates with the transverse cervical nerve, although this latter communication is currently of little significance.[66,85]

Connection with sensory nerves

Several authors have noticed connections between the branches of the facial nerve with sensory nerves, including the infraorbital, mental nerves, and transverse cervical nerves.[72,84,86–88] The exact clinical importance of this finding is yet to be seen.

The scalp

The five layers of the scalp are well known by the mnemonic SCALP:

- Skin
- Connective tissue
- Galea Aponeurotica
- Loose areolar tissue
- Pericranium.

The galea aponeurotica is also known as the epicranial aponeurosis and corresponds to the SMAS in the face. Peculiar to the scalp is the tight connection of the skin to the galea by a dense network of connective tissue fibers. This makes separation of the skin from the galea difficult (similar to the palm) and bloody. In addition, this lattice of connective tissue stents the vessels open which, combined with the scalp's rich vascularity, leads to profuse bleeding.

The galea is a dynamic structure, being controlled by the frontalis muscle anteriorly and the occipitalis posteriorly. The skin moves together with the galea due to their tight attachment. This is important in brow rejuvenation where weakening of the brow depressor muscles allows the epicranial aponeurosis to move backwards leading to elevation of the brow.

The loose areolar tissue between the galea and the periosteum is also referred to as the subgaleal fascia. This fascia is loose especially over the vertex of the scalp, allowing a quick dissection with minimal bleeding. It becomes more dense closer to the supra orbital rims. Most surgeons consider this layer as a potential dissection "plane" rather than a discrete "layer".[8,89] However, it has been shown to be a distinct layer that can be elevated independently as a vascularized flap.[90] This is especially possible closer to the zygomatic arch and the supraorbital rims where this layer is more substantial. It is formed histologically of multiple lamina, with most of the vasculature along the superficial and the deep lamina.[33,91,92]

The pericranium is simply the periosteum of the skull bones and is tightly adherent to normal sutures but easily dissected over the flat skull bones. It can be elevated as a separate flap for various uses, although once separated from the skull bones it significantly retracts.[93,94]

Five arteries supply the scalp. From the front, there is the supraorbital artery and the supratrochlear artery (branches of the ophthalmic artery from the internal carotid artery), the superficial temporal artery from the side, and the posterior auricular and the occipital arteries form the back (the latter three arteries arise from the external carotid artery). In general, these vessels run along the galea as they enter the periphery of the scalp. At this level, they give multiple perforating branches to the deeper subgaleal fascia. Closer to the vertex, most of the vessels become more superficial, anastomosing with the contralateral vessels. This explains why scalp flaps (formed of skin and galea with an intact subdermal plexus) can be safely extended across the midline, while pure galeal flaps cannot.[95]

The nerve supply of the anterior part of the scalp is by four branches of the trigeminal nerve: supratrochlear nerve (STN), supraorbital nerve (SON), zygomaticotemporal nerve (ZTN), and the auriculotemporal nerve. The posterior part of the scalp (roughly behind the level of the auricle) is supplied by four branches of the cervical nerves (C2 and C3): the great auricular nerve, the lesser occipital nerve, the greater occipital nerve, and the third occipital nerve.

The musculature

In general, the muscles of the forehead and eyebrow are arranged in three planes: the superficial plane right under the skin formed by the frontalis, procerus, and the orbicularis oculi; the deep plane formed by the corrugators; and an intermediate plane formed by the depressor supercilii (Fig. 1.11).

Frontalis, galeal fat pad, and the glide plane

The frontalis muscle originates from the galea aponeurosis and inserts distally (inferiorly) into the eyebrow skin interdigitating with the procerus, corrugator, and the orbicularis oculi. Just above the nasion, both frontalis muscles are contiguous with each other. At a variable point (1.5–6 cm) above the level of the superior orbital rim, the muscles diverge, with the medial borders becoming connected by an extension of

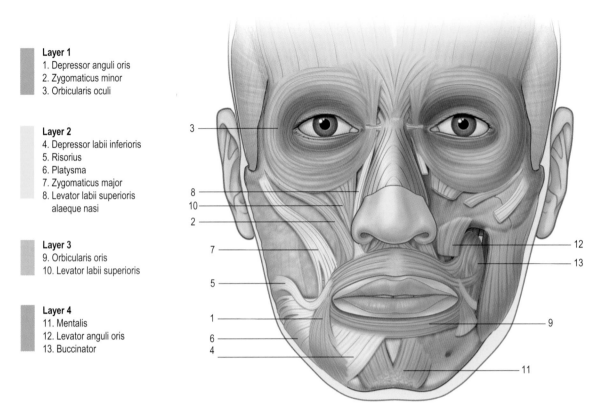

Layer 1
1. Depressor anguli oris
2. Zygomaticus minor
3. Orbicularis oculi

Layer 2
4. Depressor labii inferioris
5. Risorius
6. Platysma
7. Zygomaticus major
8. Levator labii superioris
   alaeque nasi

Layer 3
9. Orbicularis oris
10. Levator labii superioris

Layer 4
11. Mentalis
12. Levator anguli oris
13. Buccinator

Fig. 1.11 Muscles of facial expression.

the galea aponeurotica.[96] This divergence point is higher in females. This is important when injecting botulinum toxin for treatment of forehead rhytides.

Deep to the frontalis at the level of the eyebrows is the galeal fat pad, a band of fibroadipose tissue that is frequently encountered in brow lift procedures.[97] This fat pad extends for 2–2.5 cm above the supraorbital rims being intimately related to the corrugator muscles. Between the galeal fat pad and the periosteum is the glide plane space, which allows mobility of the brow over the underlying bone. Similar to the SMAS in the face, the galea aponeurotica in the scalp seems to split to cover both deep and the superficial surfaces of the frontalis. At the level of the supraorbital rim, the fascia covering the deep surface of the frontalis becomes more adherent to the periosteum, sealing the galeal fat pad and the glide plane space above it from the eyelids. It is possible that the weakness of these attachments may be predisposed to brow ptosis, especially laterally.[98,99]

Corrugators

The anatomy of the corrugators has gained significance recently, with the realization of its role in browlift, migraine surgery and treatment of forehead rhytides. This renewed interest has led to multiple anatomical studies reporting that the muscle is larger than originally described.[100,101] The muscle originates from the supraorbital ridge and passes obliquely upwards and laterally to insert into the skin of the eyebrow. Usually described as being comprised of a transverse and an oblique head, Park *et al.* found that this distinction is not clear

and described the muscle as being formed of three or four parallel muscle groups with loose areolar tissue in between.[100] Janis *et al.* similarly found that both heads are indistinguishable shortly after their origin.[102] In all cases, the muscle fibers blend together laterally and become more superficial. Medial to the SON, the corrugator is clearly separated from the overlying frontalis/orbicularis oculi muscle. However, it becomes more superficial laterally near its insertion blending with the frontalis. This close interdigitation with the orbicularis explains the difference in description of the anatomy in this region between the different authors. Intraoperatively, the corrugator can be recognized by its parallel oblique fibers, darker color, and deeper location, as opposed to the orbicularis oculi which is more superficial and inferior, is lighter in color, and has a circular orientation of the fibers.

The muscle origin is approximately 2.5 cm in width and 1 cm in height, starting a few millimeters lateral to the midline and reaching almost to the level of the SON.[100] The muscle then passes laterally to insert in the skin of the eyebrow, reaching as far as the lateral third of the eyebrow. Janis *et al.* found that the most lateral extension of the muscle is 43 mm from the midline and 7 mm medial to the lateral orbital rim, while the most superior extension is 33 mm cephalad to the level of the nasion.

The nerve supply of the corrugator is probably from both the frontal (temporal) and the zygomatic divisions of the facial nerve.[72,76,102,103] The branch(es) from the frontal nerve enter the muscle from its lateral end, and hence the importance of complete muscle excision lateral to the SON so as not to leave intact innervated muscle. The zygomatic (or upper buccal) division sends a nerve that travels cranially along the side of the nose to innervate the nasalis followed by the procerus and the corrugator.[72,103]

Procerus

This small muscle arises from the nasal bone and the upper lateral cartilages and ascends superiorly to insert into the glabellar skin between the eyebrows, blending with frontalis along the medial ends of the eyebrow.[104] Contraction of the procerus produces transverse glabellar rhytides.

Depressor supercilii

This small muscle lies between the orbicularis oculi and the corrugators, although some authors consider it part of either muscle.[99,105–107] It arises from the frontal process of the maxilla 2–5 mm below the frontomaxillary suture, slightly posterior and superior to the posterior lacrimal crest.[105] Daniel and Landon described it as running vertically between the pale circular orbicularis oculi more superficially and the brownish transverse corrugator lying in a deeper plane.[106] It finally inserts into the dermis of the medial eyebrow.

Midfacial muscles

From lateral to medial, the zygomaticus major, zygomaticus minor, and the levator labii superioris originate from the anterior surface of the maxilla (see Fig. 1.11). Their line of origin is a curved line, convex downwards, with the medial limit higher than the lateral end. These muscles form the floor of the prezygomatic space and are covered by a fascial membrane that is more stout superiorly, being around 2–3 mm thick. This fascial membrane is identified by its pale color and coarse lobulation. The levator labii superioris origin reaches the inferior orbital rim while the zygomaticus major origin is separated from the inferior orbital rim by the front of the body of the zygoma. The three muscles insert into the substance of the upper lip.

The levator labii superioris alaeque nasi originates from the frontal process of the maxilla. Its fibers pass downwards and laterally to insert into the lower lateral cartilage of the nose and the upper lip.

The levator anguli oris arises from the maxilla below the orbital foramen lying deep to the lip elevators. It is one of the few facial muscles innervated on their superficial surface.

The depressor labii inferioris and the depressor anguli oris are continuous with the platysma and draw the lip downwards and laterally.

The mentalis is a thick small muscle that is important in exposure of the mandible and in chin surgery. It arises from the buccal surface of the mandible over the roots of the incisors and inserts into the chin. Repair of the mentalis is vital after buccal incisions to prevent chin ptosis.

Muscles of mastication

The four muscles of mastication, the temporalis, masseter, and lateral and medial pterygoids, are mostly present in the temporal and infratemporal fossae and control mandibular movement during speech and mastication. Being derivatives of the first pharyngeal arch, they are all supplied by the mandibular division of the trigeminal nerve.

The temporalis muscle

The temporalis arises from the bony floor of the temporal fossa, with attachments to the deep surface of the deep temporal fascia. It passes deep to the zygomatic arch to insert into the coronoid process of the mandible and the anterior border of the ramus of the mandible almost down to the third molar tooth. It receives its blood supply from the anterior and posterior deep temporal arteries, arising from the maxillary artery and supplying the muscle through its deep surface.[108] It receives secondary blood supply from the middle temporal artery, which arises from the superficial temporal artery near the zygomatic arch and travels along the deep temporal fascia. Based on its dominant deep pedicle, the muscle's arc of rotation is at the zygomatic arch, and can be rotated as a flap for coverage of the orbit, upper cheek, and ear.[109,110] The muscle is also frequently used for facial reanimation.

The masseter muscle

This strong muscle arises from the lower border and inner surface of the zygomatic arch by two heads: a superficial head from the anterior two-thirds of the arch and a deep head forms the posterior third. The superficial head descends downwards and backwards, while the deep head descends vertically downwards. Both heads then insert together at the lateral and inferior surfaces of the mandible.

The medial pterygoid muscle

The medial pterygoid muscle arises by two heads: a small superficial head from the maxillary tubercle behind the last molar and a deep large head from the medial surface of the medial pterygoid. Both heads run downwards and backwards to insert on the inner surface of the angle of the mandible. In mandibular fractures the action of this muscle is responsible for the upwards and forwards movement of the posterior segment.

The lateral pterygoid muscle

This muscle also has two heads, a smaller upper head from the infratemporal surface and ridge of the greater wing of the sphenoid, and a lower larger head from the lateral surface of the lateral pterygoid plate. The fibers pass backwards to insert into the anterior surface of the neck of the mandible and the capsule of the temporomandibular joint. Some of the fibers pierce the capsule to attach to the intra-articular disc. In condylar fractures, this muscle is responsible for the displacement of the mandibular condyle, while in Le Fort fractures, the muscle pulls the maxillary segment downwards and backwards resulting in premature contact of the molar and resulting in an anterior open bite.

Actions of muscle of mastication

Together, these muscles control most of the movements of the mandible. Elevation of the mandible is achieved by the temporalis and the masseter, while the pterygoids protract the mandible and move it to the contralateral side.

The pterygomasseteric sling

The masseter and the medial pterygoid insert respectively into the lateral and medial surfaces of the lower edge of the mandible near the mandibular angle. These insertions are connected to each other by the pterygomasseteric sling, a fibrous raphe extending around the mandibular border and connecting both insertions.[111] Disruption of this raphe will lead to an unaesthetic upward retraction of the masseter, most visible on clinching the jaws.[112]

The aesthetic importance of the masseter and the temporalis muscle

Atrophy, hypertrophy, or displacement of either the masseter or the temporalis can be aesthetically bothersome. Masseter hypertrophy leads to an increased bigonial angle, although most cases of benign masseteric hypertrophy (BMH) are actually caused by a laterally positioned mandibular ramus and not by a true hypertrophy of the muscle. Deformities of the temporalis muscle are more common, and are usually iatrogenic due to improper resuspension of the origin of the muscle during a coronal incision leading to retraction of the muscle inferiorly. This leads to a visible bulge above the zygoma and a depression near the origin of the muscle. Repair of the atrophy or displacement of the masseter and the temporalis often involves the use of alloplastic implants, as the muscles cannot usually be stretched to their original lengths.

The sensory innervation

The anatomy of the sensory nerves and their relation to the surrounding muscles has gained significant importance with the recognition of their role in the aetiology of migraine headaches.[113,114] Knowledge of the anatomy of these nerves is also important both to avoid iatrogenic injury and for local anesthetic blocks.[115,116] In general, the face is supplied by the three divisions of the trigeminal nerve (through three branches from each division), with the scalp receiving additional supply from the cervical superficial spinal nerves (Fig. 1.12; see Fig. 1.9).

The frontal division of the trigeminal nerve supplies the upper eyelid, forehead, and a large portion of the scalp through three branches: the supraorbital, supratrochlear, and the infratrochlear nerves (Fig. 1.13A; see Fig. 1.12). The first two are particularly important due to their role in triggering frontal migraine and the possibility of their injury during forehead and eyebrow rejuvenation.[114] In addition, successful anesthetic blocks of the SON can effectively anesthetize large areas of the scalp.

The SON exits the orbit through either a notch or foramen located at the level of the medial limbus.[117] There is significant variation in its exit point,[114,117–123] which can be a notch, a foramen, or a canal. This point of emergence is approximately 25–30 mm from the midline. It is usually a few millimeters above the orbital rim but can be up to 19 mm above it.[118–121] The nerve then divides into a superficial (medial) and a deep (lateral) branch. The superficial division passes superficial to the frontalis to supply the forehead skin.[114] The larger deep division, which is more prone to iatrogenic injury, passes cephalad in a more lateral location. As its name suggests, it is in a deeper plane lying between the galea and the periosteum.[122,123] It passes upwards 1 cm medial to the temporal fusion line, and supplies sensation to the frontoparietal scalp. Forehead dissection is safer in the subperiosteal plane as opposed to a subgaleal (subfrontalis) plane which places the deep branch of the SON in risk.[124]

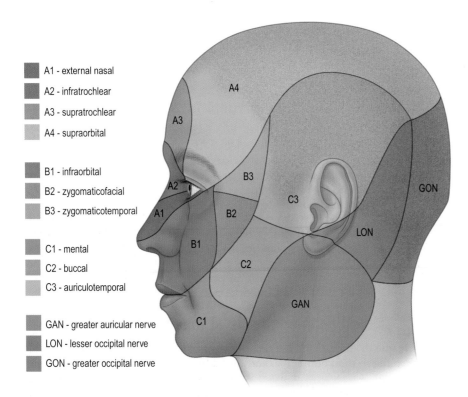

A1 - external nasal
A2 - infratrochlear
A3 - supratrochlear
A4 - supraorbital

B1 - infraorbital
B2 - zygomaticofacial
B3 - zygomaticotemporal

C1 - mental
C2 - buccal
C3 - auriculotemporal

GAN - greater auricular nerve
LON - lesser occipital nerve
GON - greater occipital nerve

Fig. 1.12 The sensory supply of the face.

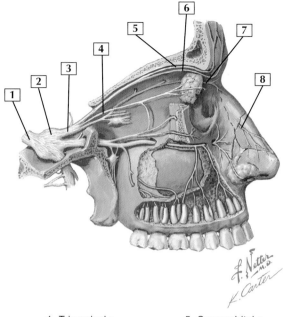

1. Trigeminal n.
2. Trigeminal ganglion
3. Ophthalmic division
4. Lacrimal n.
5. Supraorbital n.
6. Supratrochlear n.
7. Infratrochlear n.
8. External nasal n.

(A)

1. Maxillary division of the trigeminal n.
2. Zygomatic n.
3. Infraorbital n.
4. Zygomaticofacial n.
5. Zygomaticotemporal n.

(B)

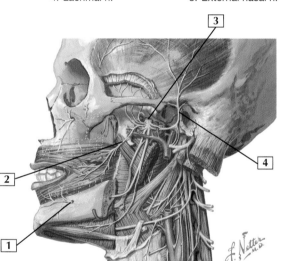

(C)
1. Mental n.
2. Buccal n.
3. Mandibular division of the trigeminal n.
4. Auriculotemporal n.

Fig. 1.13 (A–C) The sensory nerves of the face. *(Reprinted with permission from www.netterimages.com © Elsevier Inc. All rights reserved.)*

The STN emerges from the medial orbit above the trochlea approximately 1 cm from the midline and is usually composed of multiple branches. It supplies the central forehead. The infratrochlear nerve (ITN) is a smaller nerve that supplies the medial eyelid and a small part of the medial upper nose.

The maxillary division contributes three branches to the sensory supply of the head: the zygomaticotemporal, zygomaticofacial, and the infraorbital nerve (Fig. 1.13B; see Fig. 1.12). The ZTN pierces the temporalis muscle and emerges through the deep temporal fascia 17 mm lateral and 7 mm cephalad to the lateral canthus to supply the temporal forehead.[125] It has also been incriminated as a cause of temporal migraine. The zygomaticofacial nerve exits the orbit through a foramen in the zygomatic bone to innervate the skin of the cheek below the zygoma. The infraorbital nerve is the direct continuation of the maxillary nerve and passes to the cheek through a foramen 1 cm below the infraorbital rim lying along in the same vertical plane with the SON and the mental nerves (roughly along the midpupillary line).[121] It supplies the skin of the cheek and the upper lid.

The mandibular division also gives three branches to the face: the auriculotemporal, the buccal, and the mental nerves (Fig. 1.13C; see Fig. 1.12). The mental nerve is at risk for injury in exposures of the mandible. It is the continuation of the inferior alveolar nerve, exiting the mandible through the mental foramen, which is located in line with the mandibular first premolar (or first molar in children). It soon divides into 2–3 branches to innervate the lower lip and the chin.

The auriculotemporal nerve passes around the neck of the mandible and ascends over the posterior root of the zygomatic arch, giving a branch to supply the temporomandibular joint. As its names indicates, it supplies the auricle (and the external acoustic meatus and the tympanic membrane) and the skin of the temple. It also carries parasympathetic postganglionic fibers to the parotid gland, explaining its role in the development of Frey's syndrome (gustatory sweating). The best place for an auriculotemporal nerve block is 10–15 mm anterior to the upper origin of the helix.[118]

The buccal nerve runs in deep plane on the surface of the buccinators. It sends branches to the skin of the cheek before piercing the buccinator to supply the mucous membrane of the cheek.

Of all the cervical cutaneous nerves, the great auricular nerve has the most significance to the plastic surgeon.[126] It supplies the lower two-thirds of the lateral surface of the ear, the posterior and lower cheek, and the skin over the mastoid. It appears around the midpoint of the posterior border of the sternomastoid passing obliquely upwards towards the angle of the jaw. However, along the mid-belly of the muscle, it gently curves changing its direction towards the ear lobe. It passes either superficial or deep to the sternomastoid fascia.[127] It can be consistently found at a point on the mid-belly of the sternomastoid muscle 6.5 cm caudal to the bony external auditory meatus.[126]

Anatomy of the ear

The appearance of the external ear is unique. Its shape and contour follows the cartilaginous framework that is enveloped by a very thin skin and soft tissue. In general, there are three parts of external ear: helix–antihelical complex, conchal complex, and lobule. Each of these complexes has its own convoluted structures forming the surface anatomy with specific landmark nomenclature.[128]

These three divisions of ear are closely related to the embryological development process. The ear arises from the first and second branchial arches, also known as mandibular and hyoid. These arches then continue to develop into hillocks between the 3rd and 6th week of gestation. Located anteriorly, the first branchial arch forms into three hillocks: root of helix, tragus, and superior helix. The second branchial arch, which is located posteriorly, gives rise to the other three hillocks: antihelix, antitragus, and lobule. They become fully formed structures by the 4th gestational month and continue to develop around the external meatus, which will canalize by week 28. The middle ear arises from the first pharyngeal arch during the 4th week and forms into the incus and malleus. The stapes, on the other hand, is formed from the second arch.[128,129]

The component of soft tissue covering the cartilaginous framework is comprised of vestigial intrinsic muscles of the ear, such as helicis major and minor, tragicus and antitragus, and the transverse and oblique muscles. Most of the extrinsic muscle covering is comprised of auricularis muscles (anterior, superior, and posterior). All of these structures are vascularized by the arborization of vessels from superficial temporal and posterior auricular arteries. The majority of the anterior

surface of the ear is supplied by the latter through its perforating branches and over the helical rim. The branches of the superficial temporal artery only supply the superior helical rim and triangular fossa and scapha network. These vasculature networks form an interconnecting system, which allows either of the systems to support the ear.[128–130]

The sensory nerve supply of the ear is derived from a combination of cranial and extracranial branches. The posterior ear and lobule are innervated by the greater auricular nerve (C2, C3) and the lesser occipital nerve (C2). The anterior ear and tragus are supplied by the trigeminal nerve (auriculotemporal branch of V3). The inferior ear and parts of the preauricular area are innervated by the greater auricular nerve (C2,3). The superior portion of the ear and mastoid region are innervated by the lesser occipital nerve (C2).

Anatomy of the eyelids

There is no consensus on the "ideal" aesthetic eyelids, with several factors such as age, ethnicity, and surrounding skeletal structure causing wide variation in what are considered normal eyelids. In general, the palpebral fissure measures 29–32 mm horizontally and 9–12 mm vertically, with the lateral canthus 1–2 mm higher than the medial canthus. The upper eyelid usually covers the upper 1–2 mm of the iris (lying approximately halfway between the edge of the pupil and the limbus), while the lower eyelid rests at roughly the level of the inferior limbus. The highest point of the upper eyelid lies just nasal to the center of the pupil. Ensuring the eyelid lies in normal position is important after periorbital surgery, especially if the canthal tendons are disrupted.

The eyelids can be separated into an anterior lamella, formed of skin and orbicularis oculi muscle, and a posterior lamella, formed by the tarsus and the conjunctiva (Fig. 1.14).

The skin of the eyelids is the thinnest skin of the body, mainly due to its thin dermis, and is relatively more elastic. As the skin crosses over the orbital rims, it abruptly thickens. Incisions in the eyelids usually heal rapidly and with minimal scarring.

The orbicularis oculi lies directly deep to the skin with minimal subcutaneous fat in between, and is divided into pretarsal, preseptal (both lying in the eyelid) and orbital (around the eyelids) portions. The pretarsal muscle arises medially by two heads that surround the lacrimal sac and attach to the anterior and posterior lacrimal crests. The deep head, also known as Horner's muscle, also attaches to the fascia over the lacrimal sac. This peculiar arrangement allows the muscle to play an important role in the lacrimal pump mechanism.[131] The preseptal orbicularis originates from the medial canthal ligament and inserts on the zygoma lateral to the orbital rim. The orbital part of the orbicularis muscle originates from the medial canthal ligament and the adjacent maxillary and frontal bones, and inserts with the preseptal portion into the lateral palpebral raphe (see below).

The tarsi provide support and rigidity to the eyelids. They are formed of collagen, aggregens, and chondroitins. The upper tarsus measures 10–12 mm, while the lower tarsus measures 4–5 mm.[132] The edges of the tarsi are firmly attached to the eyelids margins, while the opposite edge is convex giving the tarsus a semilunar shape. The Meibomian glands are embedded within the tarsus, and their ducts orifices are

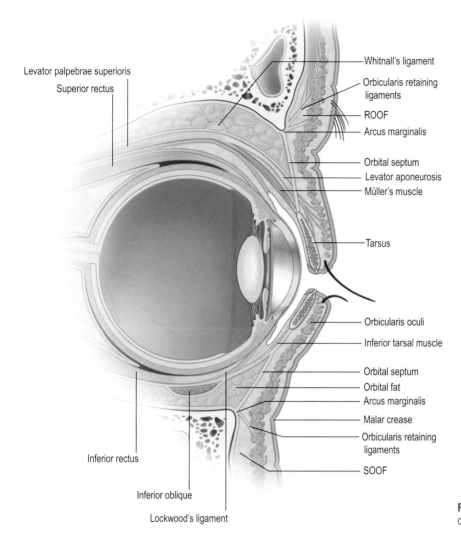

Levator palpebrae superioris

Superior rectus

Whitnall's ligament

Orbicularis retaining ligaments

ROOF

Arcus marginalis

Orbital septum

Levator aponeurosis

Müller's muscle

Tarsus

Orbicularis oculi

Inferior tarsal muscle

Orbital septum

Orbital fat

Arcus marginalis

Malar crease

Orbicularis retaining ligaments

SOOF

Inferior rectus

Inferior oblique

Lockwood's ligament

Fig. 1.14 Sagittal view through the eyelids. ROOF, retro-orbicularis oculi fat; SOOF, suborbicularis oculi fat.

located along the eyelid margin posterior to the eyelashes. Between the dust orifices and the lashes is the "gray line", which can be seen as a faint gray line or groove. This line corresponds to a terminal extension of the orbicularis muscle known as Riolan's muscle.[133] The gray line serves as an important landmark; the plane between the anterior and posterior lamella of the eyelids.

The orbital septum extends from the edges of the tarsi to the orbital rims, attaching to the edge of the rim except inferiorly, where it extends for 1–2 mm on the anterior surface of the inferior orbital rim, sharing a common origin with the orbicularis retaining ligament (see above). Directly deep to the septum is the orbital fat and the retractors of the upper and lower eyelids.

The levator palpebrae superioris is the important upper eyelid retractor; injury or weakness to this muscle leads to eyelid ptosis. Originating from the back of the orbit, its muscular fibers pass forwards above the superior rectus muscle. They then turn into the fibrous levator aponeurosis and curve inferiorly into the upper eyelid. This transition is encircled by the Whitnall's ligament. The Whitnall's ligament sends medial and lateral horns to attach to the zygomatic bone laterally and the medial canthal ligament and the posterior lacrimal crest medially. These attachments maintain the eyelids opposed to

the eyeball with its movement. The levator aponeurosis inserts into the anterior surface of the tarsus, sending fibrous attachments thought the orbital septum and the orbicularis muscle to skin to form the upper eyelid crease. The deep part of the levator muscle is Müller's muscle, which is sympathetically innervated.[134] In hyperthyroidism, sensitization of Müller's muscle leads to upper eyelid retraction and pseudoproptosis. On the other hand, in Horner's syndrome loss of this muscle action leads to ptosis. Müller's muscle also sends a lateral extension surrounding the lacrimal gland and playing a role in tear excretion.[135]

The capsulopalpebral fascia assists in lower eyelid retraction and coordinates it with extraocular movement. It arises as an extension of the inferior rectus muscle and inserts into the lower edge of the lower tarsus and the adjacent orbital septum.[136]

The medial and lateral canthal ligaments are of significant importance due to their role in supporting and shaping the eyelids. The anatomy of the lateral canthal ligament has been controversial in terms of composition, and various terminology has been used to describe this structure.[23,137–141] Gross anatomical and histological studies show that the lateral canthal ligament is a bifurcated structure comprised of a superficial tendinous and deep ligamentous component.[23,141]

The deep stronger ligamentous component connects the lateral ends of the upper and lower tarsus to Whitnall's tubercle, located on the deep surface of the lateral orbital wall, 3 mm behind the rim.[138,141,142] The superficial tendinous component receives contributions from the muscle of Riolan, the pretarsal orbicularis oculi muscle, and the septum orbitale which are fused to the underlying anterior surface of the tarsal plates.[138,141] The superficial portion attaches laterally to the anterior surface of the orbital rim and is continuous with the lateral orbital thickening and adjacent temporalis fascia.[23] The orbicularis oculi muscles, superficial to the tarsi and the ligaments, curve around the eyelids and interlace together forming the lateral orbital raphe, which is superficial to the superficial component of the lateral canthal ligament.[139] Medially, the medial canthal ligaments arise from the medial edge of the upper and lower tarsus, and are similarly formed of anterior and posterior limbs that attach to the anterior and posterior limbs of the lacrimal crest.

Anatomy of the nose

The nose is strategically located in the central portion of the face with three-dimensional projection associated with complex and intricate anatomy. Nose anatomy can be divided into three parts: the outer skin and soft tissue envelope, bony and cartilaginous framework, and inner lining. The intricate relationship between first two components form contour reflections, which forms a unique individual nasal appearance varying from individual to individual.[143–145]

The skin and soft tissue covering of the nose is variable in its thickness, texture, and components. It is relatively thin in the cephalad two-thirds of the nose, especially at the osseo-cartilaginous junction (rhinion). The lower third portion of the nose covering has thicker skin and subcutaneous tissue with varying presence of sebaceous glands, contributing to the nasal tip morphology.[146] The nerves and vasculatures reside within this subcutaneous tissue. The nasalis muscle lies under the subcutaneous tissue and partially covers the bone and cartilages.

The skeletal framework of the nose is structured by nasal bones and cartilages. They determine the individual nose configuration and shape. Starting cephalad, the paired nasal bones bridge the frontal process of the maxilla and frontal bones at the nasofrontal suture. The overlapping region between the inferior portion of the nasal bones with the superior portion of the upper lateral cartilages is called the keystone area. The most caudal portion of the framework is supported by a uniquely shaped lower lateral (alar) cartilage. The inferior medial portion of this cartilage is called the medial crus. As it ascends, it becomes the middle or intermediate crus and continues curving laterally to become the lateral crus. The junction between the middle and lateral crus is called the dome, the most angulated portion of the structure plays an important role in forming nasal tip definition. There are accessory cartilages, which are interspersed in the aponeurosis connecting the lateral crus and piriform aperture.[147–149]

The inner lining of the nose is mostly covered by thin mucosa, providing passage of the airway. Destruction or inappropriate reconstruction of this thin mucosal lining can cause a narrowing of the breathing passage.

The surface anatomy of the nose follows the underlying structural anatomy of its framework in combination with the skin and soft tissue envelope. The most cephalad portion of the nose is called the root or radix of the nose. This continues caudally in the midline as a sloping downward segment called the dorsum of the nose. The tip of the nose has several landmark anatomies. The region just above the tip of the nose is called the supra-tip region or break. It is the surface landmark above the dome (lateral genu) of the lower lateral cartilages. The dome of each lower lateral cartilage marks the tip defining point, and the region caudal to this point forms the infra-tip lobule and columella. The lateral curvature portion of the nose is called the alar lobule, which forms the nostril opening. These surfaces form topographic subunits of the nose that are often used in recognizing the boundaries of light reflections bordering the anatomic landmarks: dorsum, sidewalls, nostril sills, nasal tip, soft triangles, and columella.[150]

The nose is vascularized by dual blood supply. Superiorly, the branches of the ophthalmic, anterior ethmoid, dorsal nasal, and external nasal arteries supply the proximal portion of the nose. The inferior region and tip of the nose is primarily supplied by branches of the facial artery, which include superior labial and angular vessels.[145]

🌐 Access the complete reference list online at   **http://www.expertconsult.com**

2. Baker DC, Conley J. Avoiding facial nerve injuries in rhytidectomy: Anatomical variations and pitfalls. *Plast Reconstr Surg.* 1979;64:781–795.

5. Stuzin JM, Baker TJ, Gordon HL. The relationship of the superficial and deep facial fascias: relevance to rhytidectomy and aging. *Plast Reconstr Surg.* 1992;89:441. *The authors performed cadaveric dissections and made intraoperative observations to clarify the relationships between the muscles of facial expression, the facial nerve, and fascial planes. It is confirmed that the facial nerve branches in the cheek lay deep to the deep facial fascia.*

16. Gosain AK, Sewall SR, Yousif NJ. The temporal branch of the facial nerve: how reliably can we predict its path? *Plast Reconstr Surg.* 1997;99:1224–1236.

21. Moss CJ, Mendelson BC, Taylor GI. Surgical anatomy of the ligamentous attachments in the temple and periorbital regions. *Plast Reconstr Surg.* 2000;105:1475–1490. *The authors report consistent deep attachments of the superficial fascia in the temporal and periorbital regions. The clinical relevance of predictable relationships between neurovascular structures and this connective tissue framework is discussed.*

47. Stuzin JM, Wagstrom L, Kawamoto HK, et al. The anatomy and clinical applications of the buccal fat pad. *Plast Reconstr Surg.* 1990;85:29–37. *The clinical importance of the buccal fat pad is discussed. Anatomical dissection and clinical experience inform recommendations for surgical modification of the structure to maximize aesthetic outcomes.*

64. Barton FE Jr, Hunt J. The high-superficial musculoaponeurotic system technique in facial rejuvenation: an update. *Plast Reconstr Surg.* 2003;112:1910–1917.

83. Ellenbogen R. Pseudo-paralysis of the mandibular branch of the facial nerve after platysmal face-lift operation. *Plast Reconstr Surg.* 1979;63:364–368. *The clinical importance of injury to the cervical*

branch of the facial nerve is addressed. In platysmal facelifts, diminished modiolus retrusion may be secondary to an injury to the cervical, rather than the marginal mandibular, branch of the facial nerve.

94. Wolfe SA. The utility of pericranial flaps. *Ann Plast Surg.* 1978;1:147–153.

106. Daniel RK, Landon B. Endoscopic forehead lift: anatomic basis. *Aesthet Surg J.* 1997;17:97–104. *Forehead anatomy as it relates to endoscopic rejuvenation is discussed.*

113. Mosser SW, Guyuron B, Janis JE, et al. The anatomy of the greater occipital nerve: implications for the etiology of migraine headaches. *Plast Reconstr Surg.* 2004;113:693–700.

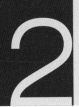

Facial trauma: Soft tissue injuries

Reid V. Mueller

SYNOPSIS

- Look for hidden injuries under the skin.
- Thoroughly cleanse to prevent dirt tattoo.
- Conservative debridement.
- Careful anatomic alignment and suture technique.

Introduction

As humans, we live in a complex social structure that depends not only on the words we use for communication, but the emotive subtext of facial expression that imbues our words with greater meaning. Our faces are able to express a wondrous range of subtle emotions and silent messages. Because the face is so important for negotiating the complex social interactions that are part of our everyday lives, the careful repair and restoration of function is an important task we must not engage in lightly. The achievements of those who have gone before us have given us the knowledge to repair the majority of soft tissue injuries to the face, provided we carefully consider the nature of the injury and craft a well thought out reconstructive plan.

Soft tissue injuries are commonly encountered in the care of traumatized patients. Many of these injuries are simple superficial lacerations that require nothing more than a straightforward closure. Other seemingly uncomplicated wounds harbor injuries to other structures. Recognition of the full nature of the injury and a logical treatment plan will determine whether there will be future aesthetic or functional deformities. All wounds will benefit from cleansing, irrigation, conservative debridement, and minimal tension closure. Some wounds will benefit from local or regional flaps for closure; and a few wounds will need tissue expansion or free tissue transfer for complete restoration of function and appearance.

Access the Historical Perspective section online at
http://www.expertconsult.com

Basic science

The etiology of facial soft tissue trauma varies considerably depending upon age, sex, and geographic location. Many facial soft tissue injuries are relatively minor and are treated by the emergency department without a referral to a specialist. There are little data regarding the etiology of facial trauma that is subsequently referred to a specialist, but it is weighted towards more significant traumas such as road crashes and assaults. The location of facial soft tissue trauma tends to occur in certain areas of the head depending on the causative mechanism. When taking all etiologies of facial trauma into account, the distribution is concentrated in a "T-shaped" area that includes the forehead, nose, lips, and chin. The lateral brows and occiput also have localized frequency increases.[4] These areas are more prone to injury because they primarily overlie bony prominences that are at risk from any blow to the face, whether that be an assault, fall, or accident (Fig. 2.1).

Global considerations

Almost all soft tissue injuries of the head involve the skin in some manner. The skin of the head shows more variety than any other area of the body in terms of thickness, elasticity, mobility, and texture. Consider the profound differences between the thick, inelastic, hair-bearing skin of the scalp compared with the thin, elastic, mobile skin of the eyelids. Consider also, the transitions from external skin of the face to the orbital, nasal, and oral linings. Significant differences in the structure of the facial skin in different areas require different methods for the repair and reconstruction. In addition, many facial structures are layered with an outer skin layer, central cartilaginous support or muscular layer, and an inner mucosal lining or second skin layer (e.g., eyelids, nose, lips, ears).

Anyone who has suffered a cut lip or scalp knows firsthand that the face is well perfused. The dense interconnected network of collateral vessels in the face means that injured tissue with seemingly insufficient blood will in fact survive, whereas the same injury would result in tissue necrosis in another area of the body. The implication is that more (and

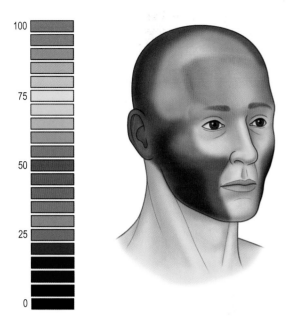

Fig. 2.1 A total of 700 facial soft tissue injuries segregated into the number of injuries for different facial areas, indicated by color. Note the "T" distribution across the forehead, nose, lips, and chin. Also note the concentration of injuries at the lateral brow. *(Data from Hussain K, Wijetunge DB, Grubnic S, et al. A comprehensive analysis of craniofacial trauma. J Trauma. 1994;36:34.)*

potentially invaluable) tissue can be salvaged. This is especially important for areas with little or no excess tissue to sacrifice, or areas that are notoriously difficult to recreate later, for example, the oral commissure. When repairing the face, conservative debridement is usually preferable. If a segment of tissue appears only marginally viable but is indispensable from a reconstructive standpoint, it should be loosely approximated and re-examined in 24–48 h. At that time, a line of demarcation will usually delineate what will survive and what will die. Nonviable tissue may then be debrided during a second look procedure.

Because the face is so well perfused its ability to resist infection is better than other areas of the body. Human bites to the hand treated without antibiotics have approximately a 47% risk of infection,[5] whereas if we inadvertently bite our cheeks, lips, or tongue we almost never develop an infection. The lower risk of infection in the face has practical applications for management of facial soft tissue injuries. Many a medical student has been told that any wound that has been open for 6 hours cannot be closed primarily. This belief is based on tradition rather that good science. While there is no doubt that the longer a wound is open the more likely it is to become contaminated, there is no magical time cut-off for primary closure.[6] Because the face carries such profound cosmetic importance, the small increased risk of infection associated with delayed closure of a wound will be trumped by improved cosmesis associated with primary closure. This author recommends closure of facial wounds at the earliest time possible that will not interfere with the management of other more serious injuries, but do not let time deter you from obtaining primary closure.

Diagnosis and patient presentation

Our attention is often captured by the obvious external manifestations of craniofacial soft tissue injuries because of the alteration in appearance; however, we should not be distracted from a methodical examination for other injuries. Seemingly straightforward wounds often harbor injuries to the facial skeleton, teeth, nerves, parotid duct, eyes, or brain.

Evaluation for immediate life-threatening injuries

Evaluation of an injured patient should always start with establishment of an airway, ventilation, volume resuscitation, control of hemorrhage, and stabilization of other major injuries – the ABCs of an initial trauma assessment. While the plastic surgeon is rarely "on the front lines" of trauma care, neither can the plastic surgeon be complacent and assume that the emergency or trauma physician has completed a trauma assessment.

Once you are satisfied that there are no immediate life-threatening injuries, you should begin your examination. The assessment of facial injuries is guided by the nature of the mechanism of injury. A thermal burn will be approached very differently than a motor vehicle crash. The history of the injury, if known, will often provide some clue as to what other injuries one might expect to find. A child who falls against a coffee table is unlikely to have any associated fractures whereas a soccer player has a 17% chance of having an underlying fracture. Practitioners will have their own style of examination, but one should stick to a routine to decrease the likelihood of forgetting to check something. The author prefers to move from outside to inside, and top to bottom.

Systematic evaluation of the head and neck

Initial observation, inspection and palpation will generally provide most of the information a practitioner will need. Ideally, the examination should be done with adequate anesthesia and sterile technique, as well as good lighting, irrigation, and suction as needed.

Inspection of the skin will reveal abrasions, traumatic tattoos, simple or "clean" lacerations, complex or contusion type lacerations, bites, avulsions, or burns. A careful check for facial symmetry may reveal underlying bone injury. One should systematically palpate the skull, orbital rims, zygomatic arches, maxilla, and mandible feeling for asymmetry, bony step-off, crepitus, or other evidence of underlying facial fracture. Palpation within the wound may identify palpable fractures or foreign bodies. Sensation of the face should be tested with a light touch, and motor activity of the facial nerve should be tested before the administration of local anesthetics. If local anesthetics are administered it is important that the time, location, and composition of the anesthetic is well documented in the chart so that subsequent examinations will not be confounded.

Eye examination

Trauma to the periorbital area or malar prominence should raise concern for associated orbital injury. Having the patient read or count fingers can be used to test gross visual acuity. The presence of a bony step-off, diplopia, restricted ocular movements, enophthalmos, or vertical dystopia may suggest an orbital blowout fracture. Traction on the eyelids can be used to test the integrity of the medial and lateral canthi. The canthi should have a snug and discernible endpoint when traction is applied. Rounding or laxity of the canthi suggests canthal injury or naso-orbital-ethmoidal (NOE) fracture. Any laceration near the medial third of the eye should raise suspicion of a canalicular injury. If there is any suspicion of globe injury, an immediate ophthalmology consultation is needed.

Ear examination

The ears should be inspected for hematomas that will appear as a diffuse swelling under the skin of the auricle (Fig. 2.2). Any lacerations should be noted. Otoscopy should be done to look for lacerations of the auditory canal, tympanic membrane injuries, or hemotympanum.

Nose examination

Inspect the nose for any asymmetry, or deviation to one side or the other. Palpate the nasal bones and cartilage for fracture or crepitus. Examine the internal nose with a speculum and good light to look for mucosal lacerations, exposed cartilage or bone, a deviated or buckled septum, or septal hematoma (a bluish boggy bulge of the septal mucosa).

Cheek examination

Any laceration of the cheek that is near any facial nerve branch or along the course of the parotid duct will need to be investigated. Asking the patient to raise their eyebrows, close their eyes tight, show their teeth or smile, and pucker while looking for asymmetry or lack of movement will reveal any facial nerve injury. An imaginary line connecting the tragus to the central aspect of the philtrum defines the course of the parotid duct (Fig. 2.3). The duct is at risk from any injury in the central third of this line. If you are unsure about a duct injury, Stensen's duct should be cannulated and fluid instilled to see if it leaks out of the wound.

Oral cavity and mouth

Inspect the oral cavity for loose or missing teeth. Any unaccounted for teeth may be loose in the wound, lost at the scene,

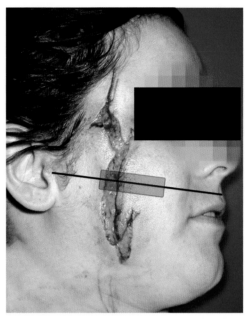

Fig. 2.3 The middle third of a line between the tragus and the middle of the upper lip defines the course of the parotid duct. Evidence of injury to the zygomatic or buccal branches of the facial nerve or lacerations or the cheek near the area shaded in green should raise suspicion for parotid duct injury.

or aspirated. If you cannot account for a missing tooth an X-ray of the head and chest should be done. The oral lining should be inspected for lacerations, and the occlusion should be checked. Palpation of the maxillary buttresses and mandible may reveal fractures. A sublingual hematoma suggests a mandible fracture.

Neck examination

The first priority when evaluating a soft tissue injury to the neck is evaluation of the airway. You should be concerned about the patient's airway if they have garbled speech, dysphonia, hoarseness, persistent oropharyngeal bleeding, or if they appear agitated or struggling for air.[7] Once the airway is secured and the exam shows no compromise, the soft tissue injury should be examined with adequate light and suction to rule out penetration deep to the platysma. If the soft tissue injury penetrates through the platysma then the trauma surgeons must be consulted to evaluate a penetrating neck injury.

Diagnostic studies

Any diagnostic studies are directed towards defining injuries to underlying structures. Most soft tissue injuries in and of themselves do not need any special diagnostic studies, however the search for foreign bodies, missing teeth, or concomitant facial fractures should be followed-up with a radiographic evaluation.

Plain films

Plain films may be helpful in the evaluation of foreign bodies or to elucidate underlying facial fractures. In most institutions, imaging of facial trauma with plain films has largely been supplanted with computed tomography (CT).

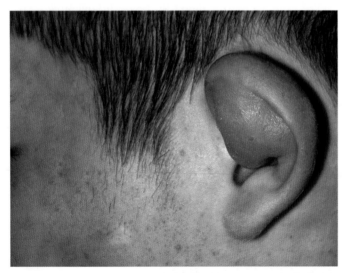

Fig. 2.2 An auricular hematoma after a wrestling injury. The collection of blood must be drained to prevent organization and calcification of the hematoma. Untreated hematomas will result in a "cauliflower ear".

CT

Maxillofacial CT is primarily used to evaluate brain injury and underlying facial fractures, and it may have some utility in identifying or locating foreign bodies within the soft tissues.

Consultation with other providers

Ophthalmology

Any patient with zygomaticomaxillary fractures, naso-orbital-ethmoidal fractures, orbital blowout fracture, canalicular injury, or suggestion of ocular injury should have an evaluation by an ophthalmologist.

Dental/OMFS

Dental injuries are commonly associated with facial soft tissue trauma and are rarely an emergency. A dentist should evaluate dental injuries, such as fractured or missing teeth, once the patient has recovered from their initial injury. If the patient has an avulsed tooth, an urgent consult should be called to replant the tooth if possible.

Treatment and surgical techniques

Anesthesia for treatment

Good anesthesia is often necessary for patient comfort and the cooperation that is needed to complete a comprehensive evaluation. Most soft tissue injuries of the head and neck can be managed with simple infiltration or regional anesthesia blocks. Patients who are uncooperative because of age, intoxication, or head injury may require general anesthesia. Patients with extensive injuries requiring more involved reconstruction, or who would require potentially toxic doses of local anesthetics, will likewise require general anesthesia.

With the exception of cocaine, all of the local anesthetics cause some degree of vasodilatation. Epinephrine is commonly added to anesthetic solutions to counteract this effect, to cause vasoconstriction, to decrease bleeding, and to slow absorption and increase duration of action. Epinephrine should not be used in patients with pheochromocytoma, hyperthyroidism, severe hypertension, or severe peripheral vascular disease or patients taking propranolol. Every medical student has learned that epinephrine should never be injected in the "finger, toes, penis, nose, or ears". This admonition is based on anecdotal reports or simple assumptions. There is very little data to support the notion, and plastic surgeons routinely use epinephrine in the face including the ears and nose with very rare complications.

Topical

Topical anesthetics are well established for the treatment of children with superficial facial wounds and to decrease the pain of injection. The most widely used topical agent is a 5% eutectic mixture of local anesthetics (EMLA) containing lidocaine and prilocaine.[8,9] EMLA has been shown to provide adequate anesthesia for split-thickness skin grafting[10] and minor surgical procedures such as excisional biopsy and electrosurgery.[11] Successful use of EMLA requires 60–90 min of application for adequate anesthesia. The most common mistake leading to failure is not allowing sufficient time for diffusion and anesthesia. Some areas, such as the face, with a thinner stratum corneum may have onset of anesthesia more quickly.

Local infiltration

Local anesthetics are appropriate for the repair of most simple facial soft tissue trauma. Subdermal infiltration will provide rapid onset of anesthesia and control of bleeding if epinephrine has been added. However, injection may distort some facial landmarks needed for alignment and accurate repair (such as the vermilion border of the lip), and, therefore, anatomic landmarks should be noted and marked prior to injection.

Facial field block

Field block of the face can provide anesthesia of a larger area with less discomfort and fewer needle sticks for the patient. A field block may provide better patient tolerance of multiple painful injections of local anesthetic when a local infiltration of an epinephrine-containing solution is needed. Field blocks are more challenging to perform and take time to take effect. Impatient surgeons often fail to wait a sufficient amount of time (at least 10–15 min) for most blocks to take effect.

Forehead, anterior scalp to vertex, upper eyelids, glabella (supraorbital, supratrochlear, infratrochlear nerves)

Anatomy: The supraorbital nerve is located at the superior medial orbital rim about a finger-breadth medial to the mid-pupillary line. The supratrochlear nerve lies about 1.5 cm farther medially near the medial margin of the eyebrow. The infratrochlear nerve is located superior to the medial canthus.

Method: Identify the supraorbital foramen or notch along the superior orbital rim and enter just lateral to that point. Direct the needle medially and advance to just medial of the medial canthus (about 2 cm). Inject 2 cc while withdrawing the needle (Fig. 2.4).[12]

Lateral nose, upper lip, upper teeth, lower eyelid, most of medial cheek (infraorbital nerve)

Anatomy: The infraorbital nerve exits the infraorbital foramen at a point that is medial of the mid-pupillary line and 6–10 mm below the inferior orbital rim.

Method: Identify the infraorbital foramen along the inferior orbital rim by palpation. An intraoral approach is better tolerated and less painful (Fig. 2.5). Place the long finger of the nondominant hand on the foramen and retract the upper lip with thumb and index finger. Insert the needle in the superior gingival buccal sulcus above the canine tooth root and direct the needle towards your long finger while injecting 2 cc. You may also inject percutaneously by identifying the infraorbital foramen about 1 cm below the orbital rim just medial to the mid-pupillary line. Enter perpendicular to the skin, advance the needle to the maxilla, and inject about 2 cc (Fig. 2.6).[12]

Lower lip and chin (mental nerve)

Anatomy: The mental nerve exits the mental foramen about 2 cm inferior to the alveolar ridge below the second premolar.

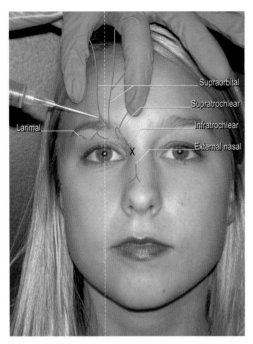

Fig. 2.4 The majority of the forehead, medial upper eyelid, and glabella can be anesthetized with a block of the ophthalmic division of the trigeminal nerve (CN V₁). Identify the supraorbital notch by palpation and enter the skin just lateral to that point near the pupillary midline. Aim for a point just medial to the medial canthus (marked by an X) and advance the needle about 2 cm. Inject 2–3 cc while withdrawing the needle.

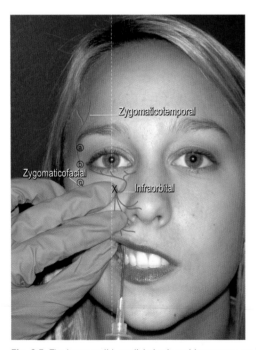

Fig. 2.5 The lower eyelid, medial cheek, and lower nose can be anesthetized with an infraorbital nerve block. The infraorbital foramen may be palpable about 1 cm below the orbital rim just medial to the mid-pupillary line (X). The intraoral approach is less painful and anxiety provoking for most patients. Place the long finger of the nondominant hand on the orbital rim at the infraorbital foramen. Grasp and retract the upper lip. Insert the needle in the superior gingival buccal sulcus above the canine tooth root and direct the needle towards your long finger and the foramen while injecting 2–3 cc.

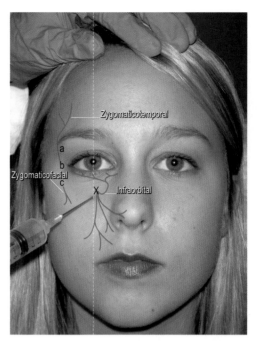

Fig. 2.6 The lower eyelid, medial cheek, and lower nose can be anesthetized with an infraorbital nerve block. The infraorbital foramen may be palpable about 1 cm below the orbital rim just medial to the mid-pupillary line (X). Enter the skin directly over the palpable or anticipated location of the infraorbital foramen and advance to the maxilla. Inject about 2 cc of anesthetic. Anesthesia of the anterior temple area can be achieved with a block of the zygomaticotemporal nerve. Enter just posterior to the lateral orbital rim at a level above the lateral canthus (marked a) and advance towards the chin to a point level with the lateral canthus (b). Inject 2–3 cc while withdrawing the needle. The zygomaticofacial nerve supplies the lateral malar prominence. To block this nerve, enter at a point one finger-breadth inferior and lateral to the intersection of the inferior and lateral orbital rim. Advance the needle to the zygoma and inject 1–2 cc.

The nerve can often be seen under the inferior gingival buccal mucosa when lower lip and cheek are retracted. It branches superiorly and medially to supply the lower lip and chin.

Method: The lower lip is retracted with the thumb and finger of the nondominant hand and the needle inserted at the apex of the second premolar. The needle is advanced 5–8 mm, and 2 cc are injected (Fig. 2.7). When using the percutaneous approach, insert the needle at the mid-point of a line between the oral commissure and inferior mandibular border. Advance the needle to the mandible and inject 2 cc while slightly withdrawing the needle (Fig. 2.8).[12]

Posterior auricle, angle of the jaw, anterior neck (cervical plexus: great auricular, transverse cervical)

Anatomy: Both the great auricular nerve and transverse cervical nerves emerge from the midpoint of the posterior border of the sternocleidomastoid muscle at Erb's point. The great auricular nerve parallels the external jugular vein as it passes up towards the ear. The transverse cervical nerve is located about 1 cm farther inferiorly and passes parallel to the clavicle and then curves towards the chin. Both are in the superficial fascia of the sternocleidomastoid muscle.

Method: Locate Erb's point by having the patient flex against resistance. Mark the posterior border of the sterno-cleidomastoid muscle and locate the midpoint between clavicle and mastoid. Insert the needle about 1 cm superior to Erb's point and inject transversely across the surface of the muscle towards the anterior border. A second more vertically oriented

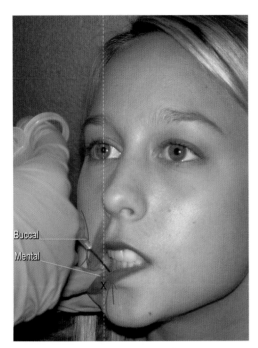

Fig. 2.7 The lower lip and chin can be anesthetized with a block of the mental nerve (CN V₃). Retract the lower lip with the thumb and index finger of the nondominant hand. Many times the mental nerve is visible under the mandibular gingival buccal sulcus near the apex of the second premolar. Insert the needle at the apex of the second premolar and advance the needle 5–8 mm while injecting 2 cc.

injection may be needed to block the transverse cervical nerve.[12]

Ear (auriculotemporal nerve, great auricular nerve, lesser occipital nerve, and auditory branch of the vagus (Arnold's) nerve)

Most ear injuries will not require a total ear block and can be managed with local infiltration of anesthetic. While there is a theoretical concern of tissue necrosis when using epinephrine in any appendage (in medical school we learned "finger, toes, penis, nose, and ears"), there is no good data to support this. Most plastic surgeons routinely use 1:100000 epinephrine in the local anesthetics for ear infiltration. The advantages are prolonged duration of anesthesia and less bleeding. Complications attributed to the anesthetic infiltration are extremely rare.

Anatomy: The anterior half of the ear is supplied by the auriculotemporal nerve that branches from the mandibular division of the trigeminal nerve (CN V₃). The posterior half of the ear is innervated by the great auricular and lesser occipital nerves that are both branches from the cervical plexus (C2, C3). The auditory branch (Arnold's nerve) of the vagus nerve (CN X) supplies a portion of the concha and external auditory canal.

Method: Insert a 1.5 inch needle at the junction of the earlobe and head and advance subcutaneously towards the tragus while infiltrating 2–3 cc of anesthetic (Fig. 2.9). Pull back the needle and redirect posteriorly along the posterior auricular sulcus again injecting 2–3 cc. Reinsert the needle at the superior junction of the ear and the head. Direct the needle along the preauricular sulcus towards the tragus and inject 2–3 cc. Pull back and redirect the needle along the posterior auricular

sulcus while injecting. It may be necessary to insert the needle a third time along the posterior sulcus to complete a ring block. Care should be taken to avoid the temporal artery when directing the needle along the preauricular sulcus. If the artery is inadvertently punctured, apply pressure for 10 min to prevent formation of a hematoma.

If anesthesia of the concha or external auditory canal is needed, local infiltration will be required to anesthetize the auditory branch of the Vagus nerve (Arnold's nerve).

General treatment considerations

The ultimate goal is to restore form and function with minimum morbidity. Function generally takes precedence over form, however the face plays a fundamental role in emotional expression and social interaction, and therefore the separation of facial appearance from function is impossible.

Irrigation and debridement

Once good anesthesia has been obtained, the wound should be cleansed of foreign matter and clearly nonviable tissue removed. This is the process of converting an untidy to a tidy wound. Clean lacerations from a sharp object will result in little collateral tissue damage or contamination, while a wound created by an impact with the asphalt will have significant foreign material and soft tissue damage. The process starts by irrigating the wound with a bulb syringe or a 60 cc syringe with an 18-gauge angiocatheter attached to forcibly irrigate the wound. More contaminated wounds may benefit from pulse lavage systems.

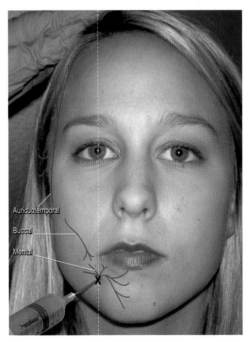

Fig. 2.8 The lower lip and chin can be anesthetized with a block of the mental nerve (CN V₃). The mental foramen is located near the mid-point of a line from the oral commissure and the mandibular border. Enter the skin at this point and advance to the mandible. Inject 2–3 cc while slightly withdrawing the needle. The auriculotemporal nerve emerges deep and posterior to the temporomandibular joint and travels with the temporal vessels to supply the temporal scalp, lateral temple, and anterior auricle. Palpate the temporomandibular joint and base of the zygomatic arch. Enter the skin superior to the zygomatic arch just anterior to the auricle. Aspirate to ensure you are not within the temporal vessels and inject 2–3 cc.

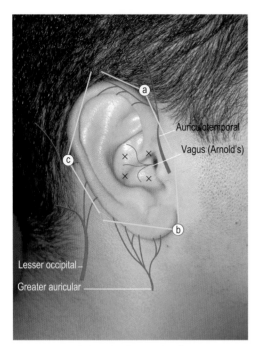

Fig. 2.9 The majority of the external ear can be anesthetized with a ring block. Insert a 1.5-inch needle at the superior junction of the ear and the head at (a). Direct the needle along the preauricular sulcus towards the tragus and inject 2–3 cc. Pull back and redirect the needle along the posterior auricular sulcus while injecting. Reinsert the needle at the junction of the earlobe and head, at (b), and advance subcutaneously towards the tragus while infiltrating 2–3 cc of anesthetic. Pull back the needle, and redirect posteriorly along the posterior auricular sulcus again injecting 2–3 cc. It may be necessary to insert the needle a third time at (c), along the posterior sulcus to complete a ring block. If anesthesia of the concha or external auditory canal is needed, local infiltration (marked with Xs) will be required to anesthetize the auditory branch of the vagus nerve (Arnold's nerve).

After irrigation, hemostasis should be secured to give the surgeon a better opportunity to inspect the wound. The use of epinephrine in the local anesthetic will cause some degree of vasoconstriction and assist in this regard. Electrocautery should be applied at the lowest setting conducive to coagulation and applied to specific vessels. Wholesale indiscriminate application of electrocautery causes unnecessary tissue necrosis. Use electrocautery cautiously when working in areas where important nerves might be located to avoid iatrogenic injury. Remember that nerves often are in proximity to vessels.

Limited sharp debridement should be used to remove clearly nonviable tissue. In areas where there is minimal tissue laxity or irreplaceable structures (e.g., tip of nose, oral commissure), debridement should be kept to a minimum and later scar revision undertaken if needed. Areas such as the cheek or lip have significant tissue mobility debridement and will tolerate more aggressive debridement.

After the preliminary debridement and irrigation, a methodical search for foreign material should be undertaken. Small fragments of automobile glass become embedded through surprisingly small external wounds. They are usually evident on X-ray or CT scan or by careful palpation. Patients thrown from vehicles will often have dirt, pebbles, or plant material embedded in their wounds. Patients who have blast injuries from firearms or fireworks may have paper, wadding, or bullet fragments present. One should not undertake a major dissection for the sake of retrieving a bullet fragment, however one should make sure that other identifiable pieces

of foreign matter are removed. Failure to do so may result in later infection.

Abrasions

Abrasions result from tangential trauma that removes the epithelium and a portion of the dermis leaving a partial-thickness injury that is quite painful. This type of injury is often the result of sliding across pavement or dirt and therefore embeds small particulate debris within the dermis. If dirt and debris are not promptly removed the dermis and epithelium will grow over the particulates and create a traumatic tattoo that is very difficult to manage later. Topical anesthetics, if properly applied and given sufficient time for onset, can give good anesthesia for cleansing of simple abrasions. This can be accomplished with generous irrigation and cleansing with a surgical scrub brush (Fig. 2.10). If more involved debridement is needed, general anesthesia is advisable.

Traumatic tattoo

There are two basic types of traumatic tattoo: those which result from blast injuries and those which result from abrasive injuries. In either case, various particles of dirt, asphalt, sand, carbon, tar, explosives, or other particulate matter are embedded into the dermis.

Abrasive traumatic tattoos are more common. Typically, a person is ejected from a vehicle, or thrown from a bicycle and subsequently grinds their face into the pavement. This causes a simultaneous traumatic dermabrasion of the epidermis and superficial dermis, and embedding of the pigment (dirt). If left untreated, the dermis and epidermis heal over the pigment resulting in a permanent tattoo (Fig. 2.11).

Blast type injuries seen in military casualties and civilian powder burns, as well as firework and bomb mishaps, produce numerous particles of dust, dirt, metal, combustion products, un-ignited gunpowder, and other foreign materials that act like hundreds of small missiles, each penetrating the wound to various depths. The entry wounds collapse behind the particle, trapping them within the dermis.

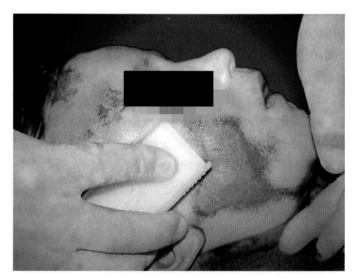

Fig. 2.10 Facial abrasions should be cleansed of any dirt and debris with generous irrigation and gentle scrubbing with a surgical scrub brush.

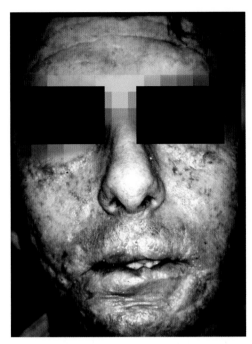

Fig. 2.11 This man has an established traumatic tattoo. The best opportunity to prevent such an outcome is meticulous debridement at the time of injury. Secondary treatment of traumatic tattoo is very difficult and includes dermabrasion, excision, and laser treatments.

Regardless of the mechanism of injury, prompt removal of the particulate matter results in a far better outcome than later removal. Once the skin has healed, the opportunity to remove the particles with simple irrigation and scrubbing is lost. The initial treatment is vigorous scrubbing with a surgical scrub brush or gauze and copious irrigation.[13–17] Wounds treated within 24 hours show substantially better cosmetic outcome than those treated later;[15] however, some improvement has been seen as late as 10 days.[18] Larger particles should be searched for and removed individually with fine forceps or needles, loupe magnification, and generous irrigation.[19] The tedious and time-consuming nature of this procedure may require serial procedures over several days to complete, nonetheless meticulous debridement of the acute injury is the best opportunity for optimal outcome.

The treatment of a traumatic tattoo remains an unresolved problem in plastic surgery, and as such, there are multiplicities of techniques, none of which are perfect. Some of the treatment options include surgical excision and microsurgical planning,[20,21] dermabrasion,[22–25] salabrasion,[26] application of various solvents such as, diethyl ether,[16] cryosurgery, electrosurgery, and laser treatment with carbon dioxide, argon lasers,[13,14,16,27] Q-switched Nd:YAG laser,[28,29] erbium–YAG laser,[30] Q-switched alexandrite laser,[31,32] and Q-switched ruby laser.[33,34] The mechanism for laser removal is not entirely understood but is thought to involve the fragmentation of pigment particles, rupture of pigment-containing cells, and subsequent phagocytosis of the tattoo pigment.[35,36] Laser therapy for pigment tattoos will require slightly higher fluencies than those used for removal of professional tattoos.[34]

A note of caution is in order when treating gunpowder traumatic tattoos. Several authors have noted ignition of retained gunpowder during laser tattoo removal,[25,34] resulting in spreading of the tattoo or creation of significant dermal pits.

If initial laser treatment suggests the presence of un-ignited gunpowder in the dermis, laser removal should be discontinued in favor of other treatments such as dermabrasion or surgical micro-excision of the larger particles.

Simple lacerations

Sharp objects cutting the tissue usually cause simple or "clean" lacerations. Lacerations from window and automobile glass or knife wounds are typical examples (Fig. 2.12). Simple lacerations may be repaired primarily after irrigation and minimal debridement, even if the patient's condition has delayed closure for several days. When immediate closure is not feasible, the wound should be irrigated and kept moist with a saline and gauze dressing. Prior to repair, foreign bodies such as window glass should be removed. Wounds of this type usually require little or no debridement. A few well placed absorbable 4-0 or 5-0 sutures will help align the tissue and relieve tension on the skin closure. The temptation to place numerous dermal sutures should be avoided because excess suture material in the wound will only serve to incite inflammation and impair healing. The skin should be closed with 5-0 or 6-0 nylon interrupted or running sutures; alternatively, 5-0 nylon or monofilament absorbable running subcuticular pullout sutures can be placed. Any suture that traverses the epidermis should be removed from the face in 4–5 days. If sutures are left in place longer than this, epithelization of the suture tracts will lead to permanent suture marks known as "railroad tracks". Sutures of the scalp may be left in place for 7–10 days. Pullout sutures should usually be removed following the same guidelines, however there is less risk of permanent suture marks. It should be noted that fast gut or plain gut sutures may not fall out within a sufficiently brief time period to avoid "railroad track" scars and should be removed in a timely manner if needed.

Complex lacerations

When soft tissue is compressed between a bony prominence and an object, it will burst or fracture resulting in a complex laceration pattern and significant contusion of the tissue. Typical examples of these types of lacerations are a brow laceration sustained when a toddler falls onto a coffee table, or when an occupant is ejected from a vehicle in a crash striking an object (Fig. 2.13). Many wounds on first impression suggest that there is significant tissue loss; however, after irrigation, minimal debridement, and careful replacement of the tissue fragments piece by piece it becomes apparent that most of the tissue is present (Fig. 2.14). Contused and clearly nonviable tissue should be debrided. Tissue that is contused but has potential to survive should usually be returned to anatomic position. Elaborate repositioning of tissue with Z-plasties and the like should usually be reserved for secondary reconstructions after primary healing has finished. Limited undermining may be used to decrease tension and achieve closure; however, wide undermining is rarely indicated. It is probably better to accept a modest area of secondary intention healing and plan for later scar revision rather than risk tissue necrosis from overzealous undermining of already injured tissue.

Avulsions

Many wounds of the face suggest tissue loss upon initial inspection, but closer examination reveals that the tissue has

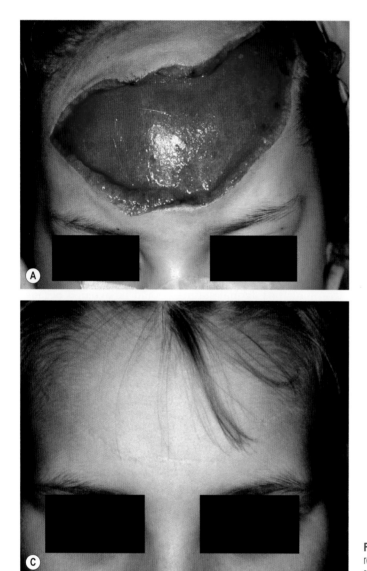

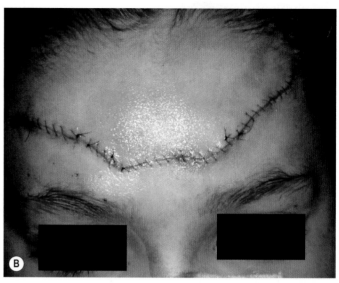

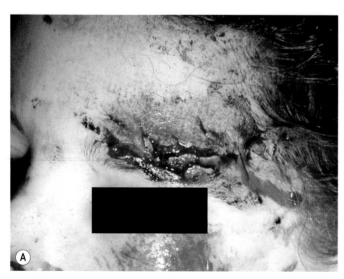

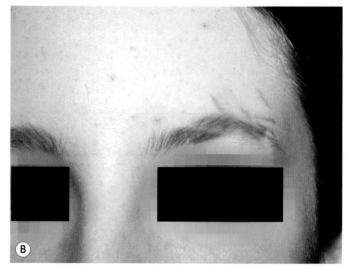

Fig. 2.12 A clean forehead laceration sustained in a motor vehicle crash **(A)** requires nothing more than irrigation and closure **(B).** Several months later, a good result can be expected **(C).**

Fig. 2.13 Initial debridement of eyebrow lacerations should be minimal. Even badly contused tissue will survive and usually lead to a result better than any graft, flap, or hair transplantation.

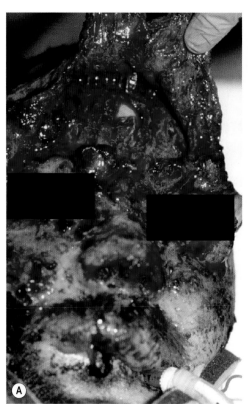
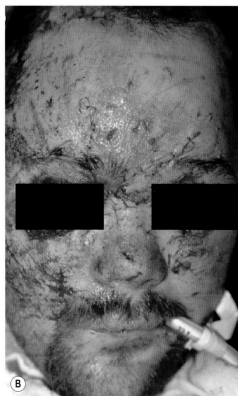

Fig. 2.14 Complex facial laceration after motor vehicle crash **(A)** that gives the impression of significant tissue loss. Irrigation, minimal debridement, and careful repositioning of the tissue fragments – "solving the jigsaw puzzle" – reveals that most of the tissue is present and usable **(B)**.

simply retracted or folded over itself. Avulsive injuries that remain attached by a pedicle will often survive, and the likelihood of survival depends on the relative size of the pedicle to the segment of tissue it must nourish. Fortunately, the remarkably good perfusion of the face allows for survival of avulsed parts on surprisingly small pedicles. If there is any possibility that the avulsed tissue may survive it should be repaired and allowed to declare itself. If venous congestion develops it should be treated with medicinal leeches until the congestion resolves. Reconstruction of a failed reattachment can always be undertaken later, but a discarded part can never be replaced.

Many avulsed and amputated parts are amenable to replantation provided that the patient does not have underlying injuries or medical conditions that would preclude a lengthy operation. Examples of facial parts that have been successfully replanted include scalp, nose, lip, ear, and cheek. Vein grafts are often needed to complete the replantation, and venous congestion is a common complication that can be successfully managed with leeches or bleeding the part.

If tissue is truly missing such that primary repair cannot be accomplished then a more complex repair with an interpolation flap or other reconstruction may be needed. These specific techniques for specific areas are covered elsewhere.

Secondary intention healing

Some wounds with tissue loss may be best treated by secondary intention healing rather than a more complex reconstruction. The advantages of secondary intention treatment are that it is simple, it does not require an operation, the wound contraction can work to the patient's advantage, and in certain situations, the cosmetic result can rival other methods of closure. The best cosmetic results are obtained on concave surfaces of the *N*ose, *E*ye, *E*ar, and *T*emple (NEET areas), whereas those on the convex surfaces of the *N*ose, *O*ral lips, *C*heeks, and chin, and *H*elix of the ear (NOCH areas) often heal with a poor-quality scar. Most wounds can be dressed with a semi-occlusive dressing or petrolatum ointment to prevent desiccation. Common complications include pigmentation changes, unstable scar, excessive granulation, pain, dysesthesias, and wound contracture.[38,39]

Treatment of specific areas

Scalp

Most scalp injuries are the result of blunt force injuries sustained in road crashes, assaults, and falls. Motor vehicle crashes cause most of the avulsive injuries, while complete avulsion of the scalp happens in industrial or farm accidents when the hair becomes entangled around a rotating piece of machinery.

Scalp injuries can generally be evaluated with inspection and palpation of the scalp. One should determine if there is underlying unrecognized skull or frontal sinus fracture by palpation of the wound or X-ray examination.

The thickness of the skin of the scalp ranges from 3 to 8 mm making it some of the thickest on the body.[40] The galea is a strong relatively inelastic layer that is an important structure in repair of scalp wounds. It plays a role in protecting the skull and pericranium from superficial subcutaneous infections, provides a strength layer when suturing, and limits elastic deformation of the scalp, often making closure more difficult.

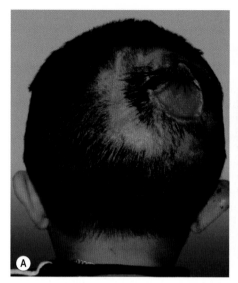
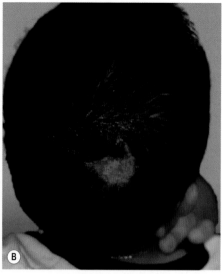
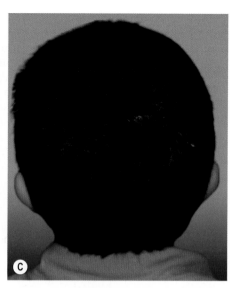

Fig. 2.15 A dog bite scalp avulsion with intact pericranium in a child **(A)**. After 1 month of secondary intention healing with bacitracin ointment and petrolatum gauze dressings the wound has contracted and epithelized markedly **(B)**. Several months later the wound was fully epithelized, and a simple scar excision and primary closure achieved a good cosmetic result **(C)**.

The subgaleal fascia is a thin loose areolar connective tissue that lies between the galea and the pericranium and allows scalp mobility. The emissary veins cross this space as they drain the scalp into the intracranial venous sinuses. This is a potential site of ingress for bacteria contained within a subgaleal abscess leading to meningitis or septic venous sinus thrombosis although the incidence is very low.[41–44]

The treatment of other life-threatening injuries will take precedence over the scalp with the exception of bleeding. The adventitia of scalp arteries is intimately attached to the surrounding dense connective tissue so that the cut ends of vessels do not collapse and tend to remain patent and bleeding. This coupled with the rich blood supply can make the scalp a source of significant and ongoing blood loss.[45] A pressure dressing or rapid mass closure will provide time for treatment of other more urgent injuries with deferred treatment of the scalp up to 24 h later.

Closed scalp injuries such as abrasions and contusions will heal without surgical intervention. Small scalp hematomas are common and do not need to be evacuated acutely. Large hematomas may benefit from evacuation after bleeding has stopped from tamponade and the patient is otherwise stabilized. Large undrained hematomas have the potential to organize into a fibrotic or calcified mass. This is of minimal consequence in the hair-bearing scalp, but may be a cosmetic deformity on the forehead.

Full-thickness scalp wounds with tissue loss may be treated with nonsurgical management as a bridge to later reconstruction. The bone or periosteum must be kept moist at all times, if there is to be any growth of granulation tissue over it or secondary intention healing. If the bone becomes desiccated, it will die. Once a bed of granulation tissue has formed, a skin graft may be applied, or allowed to epithelize from the margins of the wound. Often secondary intention healing will contract the wound such that later excision of the scar and associated alopecia will be easily achieved (Fig. 2.15). Some have advocated a purse-string around the wound to expedite closure of the scalp wound.[46]

The wound should be thoroughly irrigated and hemostasis of major vessels should be completed with electrocautery or suture ligature. All foreign material such as dirt, glass, rocks, hair, plant matter, grease, and small bone fragments should be removed. The wound should be explored for any previously unrecognized skull fractures. There is seldom a need for radical debridement of the scalp due to the rich blood supply. Surprisingly large segments of scalp can survive on relatively small vascular pedicles and therefore it is often preferable to preserve any scalp tissue that has even a remote probability of survival. Shaving of the scalp in nonemergent neurosurgery has not been shown to be of any benefit in reducing wound infections.[47–50] It is reasonable to shave sufficient hair so that clear visualization of the injury is had. There is probably no benefit to shaving the scalp for simple clean lacerations.

In general, scalp closure involves closure of the galea and subcutaneous tissue to control bleeding and provide strength, followed by skin closure. Absorbable 3-0 sutures are used for the galea and subcutaneous tissue in either a running or an interrupted manner. The skin can be closed with staples, or sutures. In children, a rapidly absorbable suture is often used to avoid the need for later removal.

Repair of the scalp will depend on the nature of the injury, whether there is tissue loss, and the condition of the underlying pericranium and bone. Simple cuts from sharp objects require nothing more than simple closure. Blows to the head from assaults, falls, and road crashes often crush the soft tissue against the skull resulting in a jagged bursting of the tissue. In these injuries, the initial impression may be that there has been tissue loss, but after careful inspection, and systematic replacement of tissue (solving the jigsaw puzzle) it becomes apparent that very little tissue is missing. The pieces should be reassembled and any areas of dubious survival should be given time to declare themselves. They often will survive.

Defects of 3 cm or less in diameter can usually be closed with wide undermining of the scalp at the subgaleal level.[51] The scalp is notoriously inelastic and will often require scoring of the galea with multiple incisions perpendicular to the desired direction of stretch. This is best done with electrocautery on low power or a scalpel. Care should be taken to only cut through the galea leaving the subcutaneous tissue and vessels within unharmed (Fig. 2.16). Scalp defects too large for primary closure may be dressed with a damp dressing and closed with other standard scalp reconstruction techniques as described elsewhere in this volume.

Total scalp avulsion is best treated with microsurgical replantation whenever possible (Figs. 2.17, 2.18). Avulsion injuries are most commonly caused when long hair becomes entangled around a rotating piece of industrial or agricultural machinery. The scalp detaches at the subgaleal plane with the skin tearing at the supraorbital, temporal, and auricular areas. Many authors have reported excellent results with scalp replantation, even when only one vein and artery were available for revascularization.[52–74] The scalp will tolerate up to 18 h of cold ischemia. Because the injuries are usually avulsive in nature, the veins and arteries needed for replantation have sustained significant intimal stretch injury. Because of this, vein grafts are frequently needed to bridge the zone of injury. Blood loss can be significant and blood transfusion is common. If possible, the venous anastomoses should be completed before the arteries to minimize unnecessary blood loss.[61] The scalp can survive on a single vessel, however other vessels should be repaired if possible.

Eyebrows

The eyebrows are nimble structures that are an important cosmetic part of the face and serve as nonverbal organs of communication and facial expression.[75–78] Several notable anatomic considerations are important in the treatment of soft tissue injuries in this area. The most conspicuous aspect of the eyebrow is the pattern and direction of the associated hair follicles. The hair bulbs of the eyebrows extend deeply into the subcutaneous fat, placing them at risk if undermining is undertaken too superficially. The hairs grow from an inferior medial to superior lateral direction; therefore, incision placed along the inferior aspect of the brow may inadvertently transect hair bulbs lying inferior to the visual border of the brow. Any incision in the brow should be beveled along an axis parallel to the hair shafts to avoid injury to the hair bulbs or shafts.

Lacerations of the lateral brow area are common and place the temporal branch of the facial nerve at risk. The administration of local anesthetics will cause loss of temporal nerve function and mimic a nerve injury, and therefore temporal branch injury should be tested before the administration of anesthetics. After adequate anesthesia and irrigation, the underlying structures should be inspected and palpated. In particular, the wound should be inspected for possible frontal sinus fracture, orbital rim fractures, and foreign bodies.

Reconstruction of the brow is difficult because the short thick hair of the brows and the unique orientation of the hair shafts are nearly impossible to accurately reproduce. Therefore, every effort should be made to preserve and repair the existing brow tissue with as little distortion as possible. After testing the integrity of the frontal branch of the facial nerve, local infiltration with local anesthetic will provide good anesthesia in most cases. Despite the fact that generations of medical students have heard that the brow should never be shaved for fear that it will not grow back, there is no scientific evidence to support this belief.[79] It is rarely necessary to shave the brow, and in fact shaving the brow may make proper alignment of the eyebrow repair more difficult. If the brow prevents proper visualization, it may be lightly clipped.

After irrigation, the underlying structures should be inspected and palpated. In particular, the wound should be inspected for possible frontal sinus fracture, orbital rim fractures, and foreign bodies. Debridement of the wound should be very conservative. Any tissue that has a potential to survive should be carefully sutured into position. If clearly nonvital tissue must be removed then the incision should be created parallel to the hair shafts to minimize damage to the underlying hair follicles. The closure should not be excessively tight, as constricting sutures may damage hair follicles and cause brow alopecia (see Fig. 2.13).

Most brow wounds are simple lacerations, and as such may be simply closed by approximating the underlying muscular layer with fine resorbable suture and the skin with 5-0 or 6-0 nylon. Areas of full-thickness brow loss (up to 1 cm) with little or no injury to the surrounding area can be repaired primarily with a number of local advancement flaps including a Burow's wedge advancement flap,[80] double-advancement flap,[81] and O-to-Z repair (Fig. 2.19).[82] Primary closure of larger defects may distort the remainder of the brow excessively. The medial half of the brow is thicker and cosmetically more prominent, and therefore the illusion of symmetry is easier to preserve if the medial brow position is not disturbed. For this reason, it is generally better to advance the lateral brow medially to accommodate closure.[80] Small areas of tissue loss not amenable to primary closure should be allowed to heal by secondary intention. The resulting scar or deformity can be revised 6–12 months after the injury when the tissues have softened. Wound contracture and the passage of time may allow for local flap reconstruction that was impossible initially. Larger defects may need to be reconstructed with a variety of scalp pedicle flaps[83–91] or individual hair follicle transplants.[92,93]

Local flap

A variety of local brow advancement flaps have been described for brow reconstruction of smaller defects. The cosmetic focus of the brow is in its medial half where the hair growth is thickest. When possible, it is usually preferable to advance the lateral brow medially, rather than advance the medial brow laterally, to close a defect. This is most important for defects of the medial brow. A Burow's wedge advancement flap is suitable for these defects (see Fig. 2.19). When elevating the flap to be advanced, it is important that the dissection is of sufficient depth that the vulnerable hair follicles are not damaged. Defects of the lateral brow can be closed by advancing tissue from both directions with two advancement flaps (the so-called A-to-T closure), so long as there is no undue distortion of the medial brow.

The double advancement flap method that uses two rectangular flaps for closure affords similar capabilities as the Burow's wedge rotation flap but requires four incisions (see Fig. 2.19). It is important that the margins of the hair-bearing skin are accurately aligned in much the same way as the vermilion border is aligned for lip lacerations. Inaccurate repair will result in an unsightly step-off. Both the Burow's wedge rotation flap and the double advancement flap closures make alignment of the hair-bearing margin relatively easy.

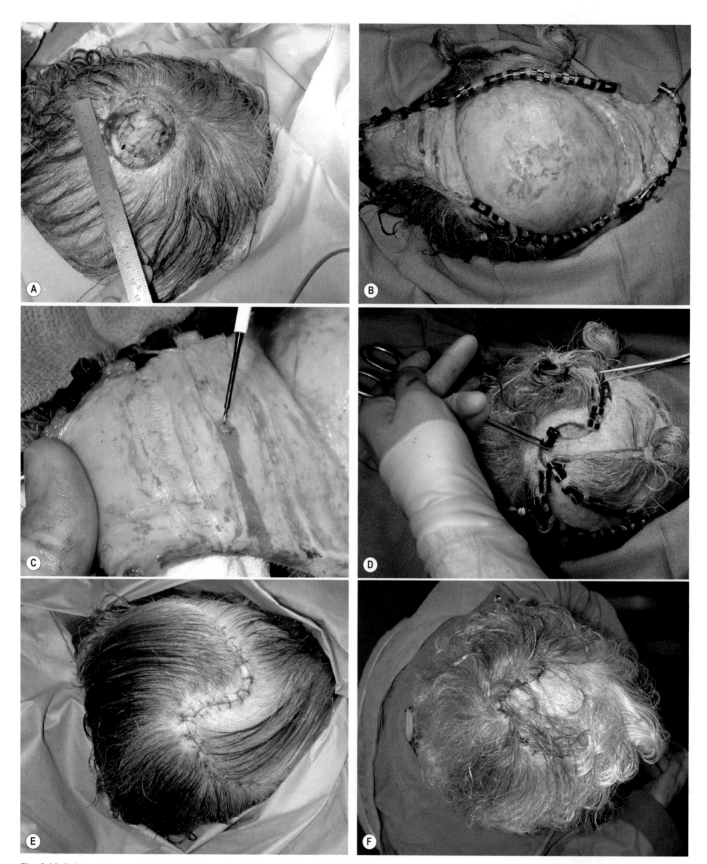

Fig. 2.16 Defects of the scalp of more than 2 cm **(A)** will often require creation of scalp flaps **(B)** for closure. Scoring the galea with electrocautery **(C)** or a scalpel will allow advancement of the flaps **(D)** and wound closure **(E)**. It is not necessary to shave any hair as a matter of routine when repairing scalp wounds unless visualization is impaired. The scalp tends to heal well. Sutures are removed in about 14 days **(F)**.

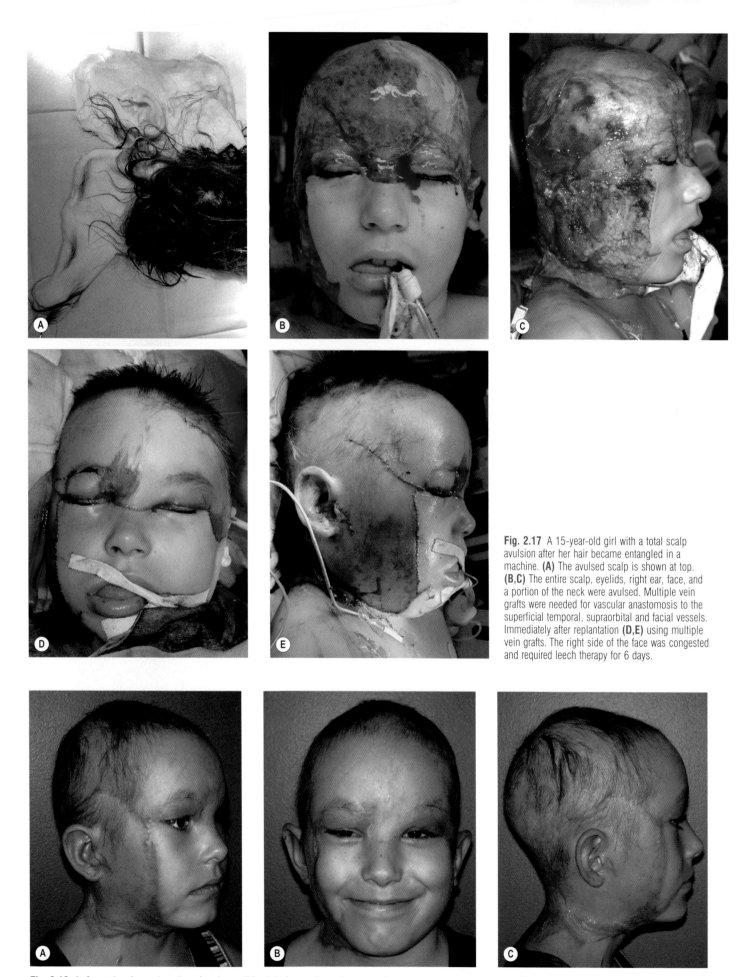

Fig. 2.17 A 15-year-old girl with a total scalp avulsion after her hair became entangled in a machine. (A) The avulsed scalp is shown at top. (B,C) The entire scalp, eyelids, right ear, face, and a portion of the neck were avulsed. Multiple vein grafts were needed for vascular anastomosis to the superficial temporal, supraorbital and facial vessels. Immediately after replantation (D,E) using multiple vein grafts. The right side of the face was congested and required leech therapy for 6 days.

Fig. 2.18 At 2 months after replantation of scalp, eyelids, right face and ear. An area on the posterior neck needed skin grafting.

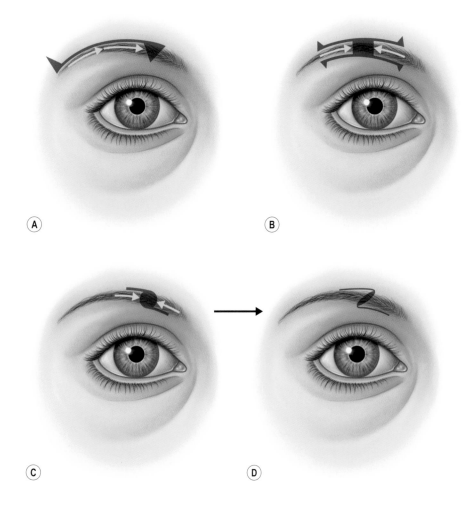

Fig. 2.19 A Burow's wedge triangle closure **(A)** favors movement of the lateral brow medially. It affords easy alignment of the hair-bearing margin and a broad-based flap design. Two opposing rectangular flaps can be advanced with the aid of Burow's wedge triangle excisions **(B)**. This flap also provides easy alignment of the brow margins but has a greater scar burden. The O-to-Z excision **(C)** and closure **(D)** results in some distortion of the eyebrow hair orientation.

Local graft

More significant brow defects will require more involved brow reconstruction with grafts and flaps. These techniques are discussed elsewhere.

Eyelids

Treatment of eyelid injuries is important to preserve the vital functions of the eyelids, namely protection of the globe, prevention of drying, and appearance.

The eyelids are composed of very thin skin, alveolar tissue, orbicularis oculi muscle, tarsus, septum orbitale, tarsal (meibomian) glands, and conjunctiva (Fig. 2.20). At the lid margin, the conjunctiva meets the skin at the gray line. Embedded within the margins of the lids are the hair follicles of the eyelashes. The tarsal plates are dense condensations of connective tissue that support and give form to the eyelids and assist in keeping the conjunctiva in apposition to the globe. It is important to remember that the eyelids are lamellar structures and in general each layer should be individually repaired. A detailed discussion of eyelid anatomy can be found elsewhere.

The eyelids should be inspected for ptosis (suggesting levator apparatus injury) and rounding of the canthi (suggesting canthus injury or NOE fracture). It may be helpful to tug on the lid with fingers or forceps to check the integrity of the canthi. A firm endpoint should be felt (try it on yourself).

Epiphora may be a tip-off for canalicular injury. A search for concomitant globe or facial fractures should be undertaken.

Any injury to the eyelids should raise suspicion to a globe injury. If there is any doubt about ocular injury, an ophthalmology consultation is needed.

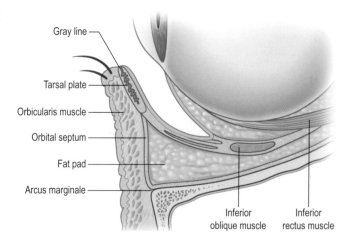

Fig. 2.20 Lower eyelid seen in cross-section shows the lamellar nature of the eyelids. Repair of full-thickness eyelid lacerations should include repair of the conjunctiva, tarsal plate, and skin. The lash line or gray line should be used as an anatomic landmark to ensure proper alignment of the lid margin during repair.

In general, nonsurgical treatment of eyelid injuries or neighboring areas with tissue loss is not advisable because the natural contraction of secondary intention healing may distort the lid and result in lagophthalmos, ectropion, or distortion of the lid architecture (Fig. 2.21). Nonetheless, some wounds are amenable to nonsurgical treatment,[38,39,94] in particular wounds of the medial canthal area that do not involve the lid margin nor lacrimal apparatus tend to do well especially in the elderly, who have greater intrinsic laxity of the skin. In most cases secondary intention nonsurgical treatment should be reserved for those cases where primary closure is not possible due to tissue loss, or where secondary intention healing is preferable to skin grafting or other reconstruction.

Simple lacerations of the eyelid that do not involve the lid margin or deeper structures may be minimally debrided and closed primarily. The eyelid is a layered structure and as such, full-thickness injuries should be repaired in layers. Usually, repair of the conjunctiva, tarsal plate, and skin is sufficient. Small injuries to the conjunctiva do not require closure, but

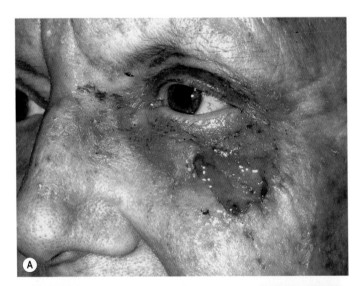

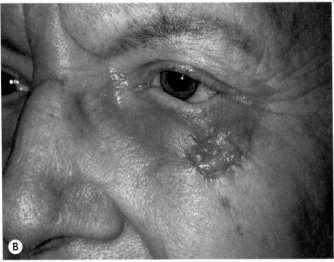

Fig. 2.21 A superficial cheek avulsion injury **(A)** was allowed to heal by secondary intention **(B)** resulting in a cicatricial ectropion. Any injury to the eyelids or on the upper cheek has the potential to distort the eyelid from the normal contractile forces of healing.

larger lacerations should be repaired with 5-0 or 6-0 gut suture. The tarsal plate should be repaired with a 5-0 absorbable suture and the skin with 6-0 nylon.

Lacerations that involve the lid margin require careful closure to avoid lid notching and misalignment. The technique involves placement of several "key sutures" of 6-0 nylon at the lid margin to align the gray line and lash line. These sutures are not initially tied but used as traction and alignment sutures. The conjunctiva and tarsal plate are repaired, and then the "key sutures" may be tied. The sutures are left long. Subsequent skin sutures are placed starting near the lid margin and working away. As each subsequent suture is placed and tied, long ends of the sutures nearer the lid margin are tied under the subsequent sutures to prevent the loose ends from migrating towards the eye and irritating the cornea (Fig. 2.22). Avulsive injuries to the lids that involve only skin may be treated with full-thickness skin grafts from the postauricular region or contralateral upper eyelid. Lid switch pennant flaps are also an option. Injuries that involve full thickness loss of 25% of the lid may be debrided and closed primarily as any other full thickness laceration.[95] Loss of more than 25% of the lid will require more involved eyelid reconstruction covered in other chapters.

Any laceration to the medial third of the eyelids should raise suspicion for a canalicular injury (Fig. 2.23). The canaliculus is a white tubular structure that is more easily seen with ×3 loop magnification. If the proximal end of the canaliculus cannot be found, a lacrimal probe may be inserted into the puncta and passed distally out the cut end of the canaliculus. It is important to remember that the canaliculus travels perpendicular to the lid margin for 2 mm and then turns medially to parallel the lid margin.

The distal end of the inferior canaliculus may be located by placing a pool of saline in the eye while instilling air into the other (intact) canaliculus. Bubbles will reveal the location of the distal canalicular stump. Avoid instilling methylene blue or other tissue dye as it will color all the tissue blue and limit your ability to distinguish the canaliculus from the surrounding tissue. Once identified, the canaliculus is repaired over a small double-ended silastic or polyethylene lacrimal stent with 8-0 absorbable sutures. The stent is left in place for 2–3 months. Unless the physician has specific experience with this procedure, a consultation with ophthalmology is indicated. Most patients with one intact canaliculus will not experience epiphora;[96,97] however, if repair can be accomplished at the time of injury without jeopardizing the intact canaliculus, most authors would repair it. Good results are generally had with repair over a stent.[98,99]

Ears

Traumatic ear injuries may result from mechanical trauma such as motor vehicle crashes, boxing, wrestling, sports, industrial accidents, ear piercing, and animal or human bites. Thermal burns to the ear are seen in over 90% of patients with other head and neck burns.[100] The ears are at particular risk because they are thin and are exposed on two sides.

Anatomy

The skin of the anterior ear is tightly adherent to the underlying auricular fibrocartilage that gives shape to the external ear. The posterior skin is somewhat thicker and more mobile. The

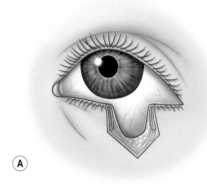

(A)

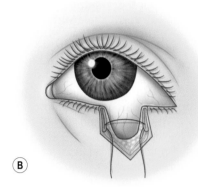

(B)

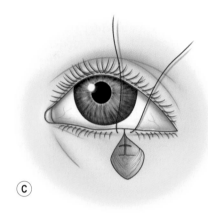

(C)

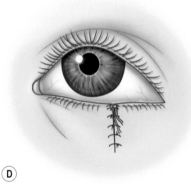

(D)

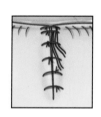

Fig. 2.22 A full-thickness eyelid injury involves skin, tarsal plate, and conjunctiva **(A)**. Repair starts with the conjunctiva and tarsal plate **(B)**; a "key" suture is placed at the lash line to align the eyelid margin and prevent an unsightly step-off **(C)**. The repair progresses from the lid margin outward. The ends of each suture are left long, such that they are captured under the subsequent sutures **(D and inset)**. This prevents the loose suture ends from migrating up and irritating the eye.

anterior surface is rich in topography, while the posterior surface is simple. As with most other areas of the face, the blood supply is rich.

A clinical examination is generally all that is required to diagnose and treat ear trauma. The pinna should be examined to determine if there has been any tissue loss or injury to the auricular cartilage. After blunt trauma or surgical procedure, patients may develop an auricular hematoma, which is an accumulation of blood under the perichondrium that can take several hours to develop. This presents as a painful swelling that obliterates the normal contours of the surface of the ear (see Fig. 2.2).

The goal of treatment is to restore cosmetic appearance of the ear, to maintain a superior auricular sulcus that can accommodate eyeglasses, and to minimize later complications from infection or fibrosis.

Hematoma

The most common complication of blunt trauma to the ear is the development of an auricular hematoma. Blunt trauma may cause a shearing force that separates the cartilage from the overlying soft tissue and perichondrium. Inevitably there is bleeding into the space that further separates the cartilage and perichondrium. The clinical appearance is of a convex ear with loss of the normal contours (see Fig. 2.2). If left untreated the blood will clot and eventually develop into a fibrotic mass that obliterates the normal ear topography. Over time (and with repeated injury), the fibrotic mass may develop into a calcified bumpy irregular mass leading to what is known

as a "cauliflower ear". Ear cartilage is dependent upon the adjacent soft tissue for blood supply, and therefore separation of the cartilage from the perichondrium places the cartilage at risk for necrosis and infection.

The treatment for an ear hematoma is evacuation of the hematoma, control of the bleeding, and pressure to prevent an accumulation of blood and to encourage adherence of the soft tissues to the cartilage. Simple aspiration within a few hours of the injury may evacuate the blood, but without any other treatment hematoma or seroma will reaccumulate.[101,102] Some have advocated using a small liposuction cannula to more effectively evacuate the hematoma.[103] Aspiration with subsequent pressure dressing has been used effectively;[104,105] most authors recommend a surgical approach for more reliable removal of adherent fibrinous material that may delay healing of the soft tissue to the cartilage.[101,104,106–115]

Surgical drainage can be accomplished with an incision placed parallel to the antihelix and just inside of it where the scar can be hidden. The skin and perichondrial flap is gently elevated and a small suction used to evacuate the hematoma. If adherent fibrinous material remains, it should be removed with forceps. After the wound is irrigated, it should be inspected for bleeding that may require cautery for control. There are many different methods of pressure dressing. Some mold saline-soaked cotton behind the ear and then mold more cotton into the anterior contours of the ear.[107] A head wrap dressing follows this. Others have used thermoplastic splints molded to the ear.[116] The author prefers to mold Xeroform (petrolatum jelly, bismuth tribromophenate impregnated)

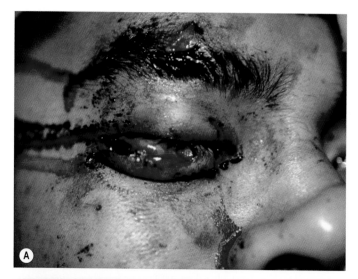

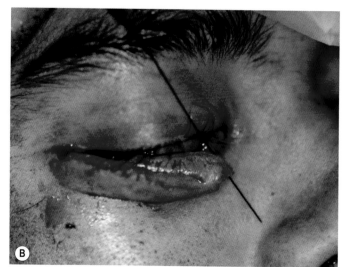

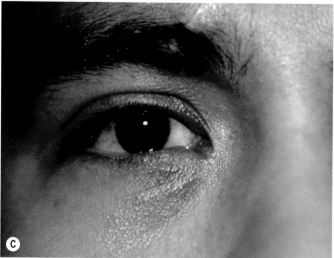

Fig. 2.23 A lower lid laceration involving the medial third of the lid **(A)**. A lacrimal probe is passed through the inferior puncta to identify the proximal end of the canaliculus **(B)**. The canaliculus was repaired over a silastic stent after locating the distal canalicular duct, and the lid repaired in layers **(C)**.

gauze into the ear contours and secure the bolsters with several 3-0 nylon through-and-through mattress sutures (Fig. 2.24). A head wrap dressing is applied and the sutures and bolsters are removed in 1 week.

Lacerations

Simple lacerations should be irrigated and minimally debrided. Like other areas of the face, the blood supply of the ear is robust and will support large portions of the ear on small pedicles (Fig. 2.25). The cartilage is dependent on the perichondrium and soft tissue for its blood supply; as long as one surface of the cartilage is in contact with viable tissue, it should survive. Known landmarks such as the helical rim or antihelix should be approximated with a few "key" sutures. The remainder of the repair is accomplished with 5-0 or 6-0 nylon skin sutures.[112] It is important that the closure be accurate with slight eversion of the wound edges, using vertical mattress sutures if needed. Any inversion will persist after healing and result in unsightly grooves across the ear.[117] It is usually not necessary to place sutures in the cartilage, and most authors prefer to rely on the soft tissue repair alone.[107,114,118–122] There is some concern that suturing the cartilage is detrimental,[123]

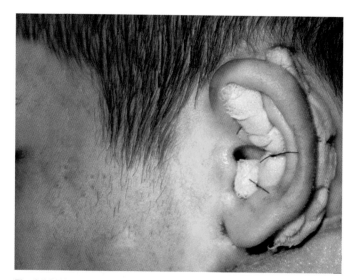

Fig. 2.24 After evacuation of an auricular hematoma, a through-and-through tie-over bolster should be molded and secured to the ear to prevent reaccumulation of the hematoma.

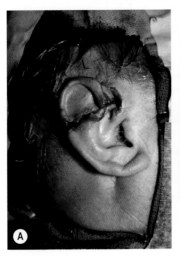 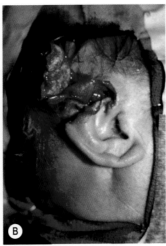 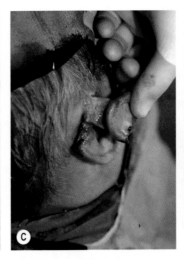 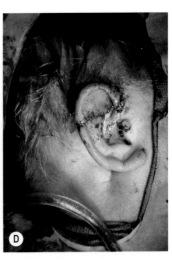

Fig. 2.25 An upper ear laceration from a motor vehicle crash **(A)** is attached by a posterior skin bridge **(B,C)**. The upper auricle survived on this pedicle because of the generous blood supply of the ear. The helical rim was sutured first for alignment and the remainder of the skin closed with 6-0 nylon **(D)**.

leading to necrosis and increased risk of infection. If cartilage must be sutured, an absorbable 5-0 suture is best.[124]

There are no good data regarding the use of postoperative antibiotics following repair of ear lacerations; however, many authors recommend a period of prophylactic antibiotics to prevent suppurative chondritis, especially for larger injuries or those with degloved or poorly perfused cartilage.[125–131] There is no role for postoperative antibiotics after repair of simple lacerations of the ear.

Auditory canal stenosis

When an injury involves the external auditory canal, scarring and contracture may result in stenosis or occlusion of the canal. Canal injuries should be stented to prevent stenosis.[114] If a portion of the canal skin is avulsed out of the bony canal it may be repositioned and stented into place as a full-thickness skin graft.

Partial amputation with a wide pedicle

Fig. 2.25 demonstrates a partial amputation with a wide pedicle relative to the amputated part. Because the pedicle is relatively large it should provide adequate perfusion and venous drainage of the part. The prognosis is excellent after conservative debridement and meticulous repair. Because there is no way to quantitatively assess for the adequacy of venous drainage the ear should be observed over the first 4–6 h for any signs of venous congestion if there is any suspicion that it may not be adequate. If venous congestion develops, leech therapy should be instituted.

If the pedicle is very narrow with inadequate or no perfusion, the avulsed part should be treated like a complete amputation (see below) or the perfusion should be augmented with local flaps.[121,132–139] Many varieties of local or regional flaps have been devised for ear salvage, and all rely on opposing the flap to dermabraded dermis or denuded cartilage. Some have advocated elevating a mastoid skin flap and applying the flap to a dermabraded portion on the lateral[135] or medial[121] surface of the avulsed ear, while others have dermabraded the avulsed part and placed it into a subcutaneous retroauricular pocket. In 2–4 weeks, the ear is removed from the pocket and allowed to spontaneously

epithelize.[114,123,136,140–142] These techniques are simple and provide a period of nutritive support until the wound heals and the ear becomes self-sustaining. It further maintains the delicate relationship between cartilage and dermis, so important in maintaining the subtle folds and architecture that give an ear its shape.

Some authors have recommended similar techniques that remove the entire dermis and then cover denuded cartilage under retroauricular skin,[143] under a cervical flap,[144] or with a tunnel procedure.[145,146] Others have used a temporoparietal fascial flap to cover the denuded cartilage and then cover the temporoparietal fascial flap with a skin graft.[147] Another method involves removing the posterior skin from the avulsed part and fenestrating the remaining cartilage in several areas and then surfacing the posterior part with a mastoid skin flap.[148] The idea behind the cartilage fenestrations is to allow vascular ingrowth from the posterior to the anterior surface and increase the likelihood of survival. One criticism of all of the methods that attempt to cover denuded cartilage is that the subtle architecture of the ears is often lost, resulting in a distorted thick formless disk.[149]

Complete amputation of all or part of the ear with the amputated part available

Amputated ear parts are difficult to reconstruct, and the larger the defect the more challenging and time consuming the reconstruction. Reattaching amputated facial parts as composite grafts has a long history dating back to at least 1551.[150] Contemporary reports describe occasional successes and many failures.[125,136,148–152] A good outcome after simple reattachment of a composite graft is probably the exception rather than the rule. The final outcome is often marred by scar, hyperpigmentation, partial loss, and deformity.[114] Spira and Hardy[153] stated, "if the amputated portion consists of anything more than the lobe or segment of helix, replacement is invariably doomed".

In an effort to salvage the cartilage, many authors have advocated burying the cartilage in a subcutaneous pocket in the abdomen[153–156] or under a postauricular flap.[143] Mladick improved upon these techniques by dermabrading the skin, rather than removing it, prior to placement in a subcutaneous pocket.[123,142,157,158] This has the advantage of preserving the intimate and delicate relationship between the dermis and cartilage that is so important for maintaining the subtle architecture of the ear.

Microsurgical replantation should be considered whenever feasible for patients who do not have concomitant trauma or medical conditions that would preclude a lengthy operation. The ear has fairly low metabolic demands and, as such, will tolerate prolonged periods of ischemia, with successful replantation reported after 33 hours of cold ischemia time.[159] After sharp injuries, the branches from the superficial temporal artery or posterior auricular artery may be identifiable and repairable. In some cases, a leash of superficial temporal artery may be brought down to the ear. In a similar manner, veins may be repaired primarily or with vein grafts. Nerves may be repaired if they can be identified; surprisingly, however, a number of replanted ears without any nerve repair are reported to have had good sensation.[160] A protective dressing is placed that will allow for clinical monitoring for arterial or venous compromise.

Nose

The prominent position of the nose on the face places it at risk for frequent trauma. Many injuries result in nasal fractures without any soft tissue involvement. Failure to treat nasal injuries appropriately at the time of injury may result in distorted appearance or nasal obstruction, whether due to loss of tissue, scarring, or misalignment of normal structures.

The nose is a layered structure that in simple terms can be thought of as an outer soft tissue envelope composed of skin, subcutaneous fat, and nasal muscles; a support structure composed of cartilage and bone to give the envelope shape; and an internal mucosal lining that filters particulates, and exchanges heat and moisture.

When examining the nose, the three primary components (external covering, support structures, and lining) should be considered. The external soft tissue envelope can be quickly assessed for lacerations or tissue loss. The support structures of the nose can be assessed by observation for asymmetry or deviation of the nasal dorsum. Fractures can usually be ascertained with palpation for bony step-off or crepitus. Significant nasal fractures are usually evident from clinical exam; X-rays rarely add significant information. If the lacerations are present, they will provide a window to the underlying structures of the nose. After adequate anesthesia and irrigation, any open wounds should be inspected for evidence of lacerations or fractures of the upper lateral or lower lateral cartilages.

Examination of the internal nose requires a nasal speculum, good lighting, and suction if there is active bleeding. The mucosa should be examined for any evidence of septal hematoma, mucosal laceration, or exposed or fractured septal cartilage. Septal hematoma will appear as a fusiform bluish boggy swelling of the septal mucosa. After adequate anesthesia and irrigation, the full nature of the injury to the support framework of the nose and lining can be appreciated.

Nasal fractures are common and should be suspected after blunt nasal trauma. Plain radiographs rarely add significant information to a thorough clinical exam in most isolated nasal injuries. If there is any suspicion of other facial fractures, or paranasal structures, a facial CT scan should be acquired. The incidence of orbital injuries following major midfacial fractures has been reported to be as high as 59%.[161]

The goal is to restore normal nasal appearance without subsequent nasal obstruction. Less complex nasal injuries can be managed with local anesthesia, while major nasal injuries are best managed with general anesthesia. Laceration of the nose should be repaired primarily when possible. Smaller avulsive injuries of the cephalic third of the nose may be allowed to heal by secondary intention because of the mobility and laxity of the overlying skin in this area. Avulsive injuries to the remainder of the nose, if allowed to heal by secondary intention, will cause distortion of the nasal architecture due to contractile forces during healing.[94]

Abrasions

Nasal abrasions tend to heal rapidly and well due to the rich vascular supply and abundance of skin appendages that allow for rapid epithelization. The skin of the caudal half of the nose is rich in skin appendages that allow for rapid epithelization. Traumatic tattooing is not uncommon after nasal abrasions. Meticulous cleaning of the wound with pulse lavage, loop magnification to remove embedded particles, and very conservative debridement are needed. Occasionally, one is faced with the difficult decision to debride further, thereby creating a full-thickness wound, or leaving some embedded material within the dermis. In general, when faced with such a decision it is best to stop the debridement and proceed with excision and reconstruction later, if needed, for cosmesis.

A septal hematoma should be evacuated to prevent subsequent infection and septic necrosis of the septum, or organization of the clot into a calcified subperichondrial fibrotic mass. If a clot has yet to form within the hematoma, it is possible to aspirate with a large bore needle. Evacuation that is more reliable can be achieved with a small septal incision in the mucosa of the hematoma. The blood and clot is evacuated with a small suction, and a through-and-through running 4-0 chromic gut quilting suture is placed across the septum to close the dead space and prevent reaccumulation of the blood.

Lacerations

In general, the repair of nasal trauma should begin with the nasal lining and then proceed from the inside out, repairing in turn lining, framework, and finally skin.

Lining

The lining of the nose should be repaired with thin absorbable sutures such as 5-0 gut sutures. Because of the confined working space, a needle with a small radius of curvature will facilitate placement of the sutures. The knots should be placed facing into the nasal cavity. Small areas of exposed septal cartilage associated with septal fractures or mucosal lacerations will not pose a significant problem as long as intact mucosa is present on the other side. If lining is missing from both sides a mucosal flap should be created to cover at least one side.

Framework

Fractures of the septum should be reduced, and if the septum has become subluxed off the maxillary ridge, it should be reduced back towards the midline. Lacerations of the upper or lower lateral cartilages should be repaired anatomically if they are structurally significant. Usually 5-0 absorbable or clear nonabsorbable sutures should be used. Displaced bony fragments within the wound should be repositioned anatomically or removed if not needed to maintain the structure or shape of the nose. If loss of important support structures has occurred, then reconstruction of the nasal support must be undertaken within a few days. Delay will result in contraction and collapse of the soft tissues of the nose. Later, reconstruction is almost impossible. Reconstruction of this type will usually involve bone or cartilage grafts. If there is doubt about the viability of lining or coverage over the area where grafted cartilage or bone will be placed, then reconstruction should be delayed for a few days until the survival of the soft tissue coverage is no longer in doubt or secondary soft tissue reconstruction can be accomplished.

Skin covering

After repair of the lining and framework, the skin of the nose can be repaired. Key sutures should be placed at the nasal rim to ensure proper alignment prior to the remainder of the closure with 6-0 nylon sutures. The mobile skin of the cephalic nose is forgiving and can be undermined and mobilized to close small avulsive wounds.[162]

Avulsions

Avulsive injuries are frequently the result of automobile crashes and animal or human bites. They usually involve only skin, but may involve portions of the underlying cartilage. One is frequently faced with the decision to proceed with nasal reconstruction with a local flap or temporary coverage with a skin graft. Smaller defects of the cephalic portion of the dorsum and sidewalls will heal by secondary intention without significant distortion of the anatomy. The skin of the caudal dorsum, tip, and ala is adherent and less mobile and will often defy primary closure. Secondary intention healing will result in contraction and distortion of the nasal anatomy and are best treated with a retroauricular skin graft (Fig. 2.26). Retroauricular full-thickness skin grafts have excellent color and texture match. The healed skin graft limits most wound contraction. If secondary reconstruction is needed, the skin graft can be excised and a local flap reconstruction can be performed later.

Amputation

Small, amputated parts can be reattached as a composite graft;[163,164] however, some authors warn of the risk of poor outcome and infection after reattachment of bite amputations.[162,165] Davis and Shaheen[166] have reported up to 50% failure of composite grafts, even under ideal conditions. They recommend that composite graft be attempted only when the wound edges are cleanly cut; there is little risk of infection; the repair is not delayed; no part of the graft is more than 0.5 cm from viable cut edge of the wound; and when all bleeding is controlled. Others have advocated hyperbaric oxygen

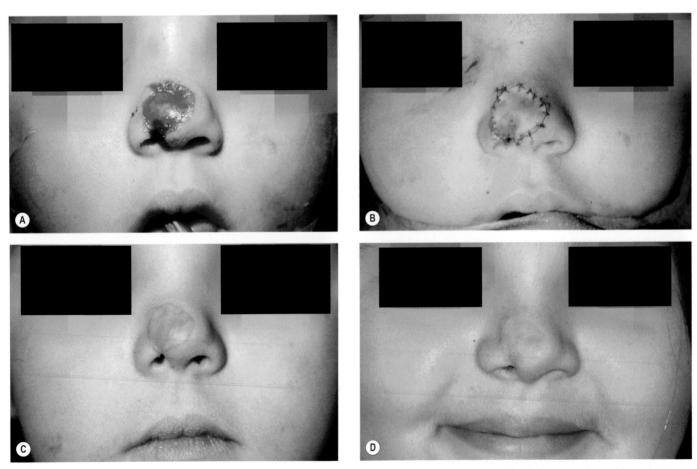

Fig. 2.26 A full-thickness dog bite avulsion injury to the nose **(A)** was treated with a full-thickness retro-auricular skin graft **(B)**. **(C)** At 6 weeks after grafting. **(D)** At 2 years later there is good contour and color match **(D)**.

therapy[163] or cooling[167] to improve tissue survival. Microsurgical replantation may be possible with larger amputated nasal segments[168] or nose and lip composite replantation.[169]

Cheek

When repairing lacerations of the cheek, the primary concern is for injury to the underlying structures, namely facial nerve, facial muscles, parotid duct, and bone.

The blood supply of the cheek is derived primarily from the transverse facial and superficial temporal arteries. Generous collaterals and robust dermal plexus provide reliable perfusion after injury and reconstruction.

The facial nerve exits the stylomastoid foramen. It divides into five main branches within the substance of the parotid gland. The temporal and zygomatic branches run over the zygomatic arch; the buccal branch travels over the masseter along with the parotid duct. The mandibular branch usually loops below the inferior border of the mandible, but rarely more than 2 cm, and then rises above the mandibular border anterior to the facial artery and vein.[170–176] The zygomatic and buccal branches are at particular risk from cheek lacerations. The buccal branches usually have a number of interconnections and therefore a laceration of a single buccal branch may not be clinically apparent.

The parotid gland is a single-lobed gland with superficial and deep portions determined by their relation to the facial nerve running between them. The superficial part of the gland is lateral to the facial nerve and extends anteriorly to the border of the masseter. The parotid duct exits the gland anteriorly and passes over the superficial portion of the masseter, penetrating the buccinator to enter the oral cavity opposite the upper second molar. The course of the parotid may be visualized on the external face by locating the middle-third of a line drawn from the tragus to the middle of the upper lip (see Fig. 2.3). The parotid duct travels adjacent to the buccal branches of the facial nerve. If buccal branch paralysis is noted in conjunction with a cheek laceration, then parotid duct injury should be suspected.

Clinical examination is directed towards identifying underlying injury to bone, facial nerve, or parotid duct. The function of facial nerve branches should be tested prior to administration of local anesthetics. Some patients will exhibit asymmetry in facial movement, simply due to pain and edema not related to any underlying facial nerve injury.

If parotid duct injury is suspected, a 22-gauge catheter may be inserted into Stensen's duct and a small quantity of saline solution can be injected. This can be facilitated with a lacrimal probe; however, care must be taken not to injure the duct with overzealous probing. If egress of the fluid from the wound is noted, the diagnosis of parotid duct injury has been made.

Repair of parotid duct

Laceration to the parotid gland without duct injury may result in a sialocele but will rarely cause any long-term problems. If a gland injury is suspected, the overlying soft tissue should be repaired and a drain left in place. If a sialocele develops, serial aspirations and a pressure dressing should be sufficient (Fig. 2.27).

Facial nerve injury

Facial nerve injuries should be primarily repaired. Surgical exploration and ×3 magnification with good lighting and hemostasis will assist in locating the cut ends of the nerve. Wounds with contused, stellate lacerations will provide greater challenges to finding the nerve ends. A nerve stimulator can be used to locate the distal nerve segments if within 48 hours of injury. After 48 hours, the distal nerve segments will no longer conduct an impulse to the involved facial musculature rendering the simulator useless. If the proximal ends of the facial nerves cannot be located, the uninjured proximal nerve trunk can be located and followed distally to the cut end of the nerve. The nerves should be repaired primarily with 9-0 nylon. If primary repair is not possible, nerve grafts should be placed, or the proximal and distal nerve ends should be tagged with nonabsorbable suture for easy location during later repair.

Mouth and oral cavity

The lips are the predominant feature of the lower third of the face and are important for oral competence, articulation, expression of emotion, kissing, sucking, playing of various

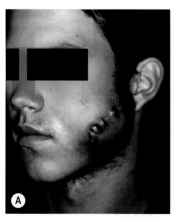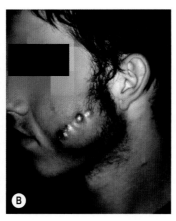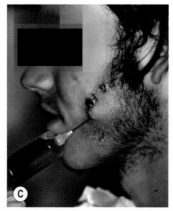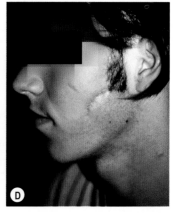

Fig. 2.27 A laceration of the cheek may injure the substance of the parotid gland resulting in an accumulation of saliva under the skin or a sialocele **(A,B)**. If recognized at the time of injury, a drain may be left in place and a pressure dressing applied. When a sialocele presents after initial repair, serial aspirations **(C)** and a pressure dressing will resolve the problem **(D)**.

musical instruments, and as a symbol of beauty. In addition, the lips are important sensory organs that may provide pleasure and protect the oral cavity from ingestion of unacceptably hot or cold materials. The primary function of the lips is sphincteric, and this is accomplished by the action of the orbicularis oris muscle. Other facial muscles are important for facial expression and clearing the gingival sulci but are not important in maintaining oral competence. The oral cavity should be carefully examined for dental, dentoalveolar, oral mucosal, tongue, and palate injuries.

Repair of the lip must provide for oral competence, adequate mouth opening, sensation, complete skin cover, oral lining, and the appearance of vermilion.[177] The restoration of the mental and nasolabial crease lines, philtral columns, and precisely aligned vermilion border are important cosmetic goals. The lip is a laminar structure composed of inner mucosal lining and orbicularis oris muscle, and outer subcutaneous tissue and skin. Closure of lip lacerations should consider repair of each of these structures.

Smaller lacerations of the cheek mucosa or gingiva will heal well without any repair. The exceptions are larger lacerations (>2 cm) where food may become entrapped in the laceration, and those that have a flap of tissue that falls between the occlusal surfaces of the teeth. Small flaps of tissue that fall between the teeth should be debrided.[178]

The majority of lip lacerations can be managed in the outpatient setting after infiltration of local anesthetic with epinephrine. If the laceration involves the white roll or vermilion border, it may be useful to mark this important landmark with a needle dipped in methylene blue prior to infiltration with larger amounts of local anesthetic because subsequent vasoconstriction may obscure the vermilion border.

A good rule of thumb is to work from the inside of the mouth outwards. To this end, urgent dental or dentoalveolar injuries should be treated first so that repaired soft tissue is not disrupted by retraction during repair of deeper structures. The wounds should be gently irrigated to remove any loose particles and debris. In most cases, normal saline applied with a 30 cc syringe and an 18-gauge angiocatheter will be sufficient. If there is evidence of broken teeth, and the fragments are not accounted for, a radiograph should be obtained to make sure the tooth fragments are not embedded within the soft tissues. Dead or clearly nonviable tissue should be debrided: once again, it should be emphasized that tissue of the face, and lips in particular, can survive on small pedicles that would be inadequate on any other part of the body. Fortunately, the lips have sufficient redundancy and elasticity that loss of up to 25–30% of the lip can be closed primarily. This also means that, unlike many other areas of the face, more aggressive debridement may be undertaken.

The oral cavity

The tongue has a rich blood supply, and injuries to the tongue may cause significant blood loss. In addition, subsequent tongue swelling after larger injuries may cause oropharyngeal obstruction. Most tongue lacerations such as those associated with falls and seizures are small, linear, and superficial and do not require any treatment. Larger lacerations or those that gape open or continue to bleed should be repaired. The subsequent edema of the tongue may be profound, and therefore the sutures should be loosely approximated to allow for some edema.

Repair of the tongue can be challenging for the patient and physician alike. Gaining the patient's confidence is important if cooperation is to be had. Topical 4% lidocaine on gauze can be applied to an area of the tongue for 5 min and will provide some anesthesia that will allow for local infiltration of anesthetic or lingual nerve block. General anesthesia is frequently needed when repairing such lacerations in children. The laceration can be closed with an absorbable suture such as 4-0 or 5-0 chromic gut or polyglycolic acid.

Oral mucosa repair

The buccal mucosa can be approximated in a single layered closure using interrupted 4-0 or 5-0 chromic gut or polyglycolic acid sutures. Only the minimal sutures should be placed. Occasionally, large flaps of degloved gingiva will need repair. It can be difficult to suture these wounds because the gingiva does not hold suture well. It can be helpful to attach these flaps of tissue with a suture passed around a nearby tooth.[178]

The lips

Poorly repaired lip lacerations can cause prominent cosmetic defects if not treated in a precise and proper manner. In particular, small misalignments of the white roll or vermilion border are conspicuous to even the casual observer.

Anesthesia of lip wounds is best accomplished with regional nerve blocks and minimal local infiltration. This will prevent distension and distortion of anatomic landmarks critical for accurate repair. An infraorbital nerve block is used for the upper lip and a mental nerve block for the lower.

When repairing simple superficial lip lacerations involving the vermilion border, the first suture should be placed at the vermilion border for alignment. The remainder of the laceration is then closed with 6-0 nonabsorbable sutures. If the laceration extends onto the moist portion of the lip, 5-0 or 6-0 gut sutures are preferred because they are softer when moist and therefore less bothersome for the patient.

Full thickness lip lacerations are repaired in three layers from the inside out. The oral mucosa is repaired first with absorbable suture such as 5-0 chromic or plain gut. If the oral mucosa and gingiva has been avulsed from the alveolus, the soft tissue may be reattached by passing a suture from the soft tissue around the base of a neighboring tooth. In general, proceeding from buccal sulcus towards the lip makes the most sense. The muscle layer is approximated with 4-0 or 5-0 absorbable suture. Failure to approximate the orbicularis oris muscle or later dehiscence will result in an unsightly depression of the scar. It is best to include some of the fibrous tissue surrounding the muscle for more strength when placing these sutures. A key suture of 5-0 or 6-0 nylon is placed at the vermillion border, and then the remainder of the external sutures are placed.

Avulsive wounds of the lip will often survive on surprisingly small pedicles. It is usually advisable to approximate even marginally viable tissue because of the possibility of survival (Figs. 2.28, 2.29).

Neck

The most important consideration in soft tissue injuries of the neck is to exclude penetrating neck trauma deep to the platysma and compromise of the airway. Once those are excluded, closure of neck wounds is generally straightforward. Because

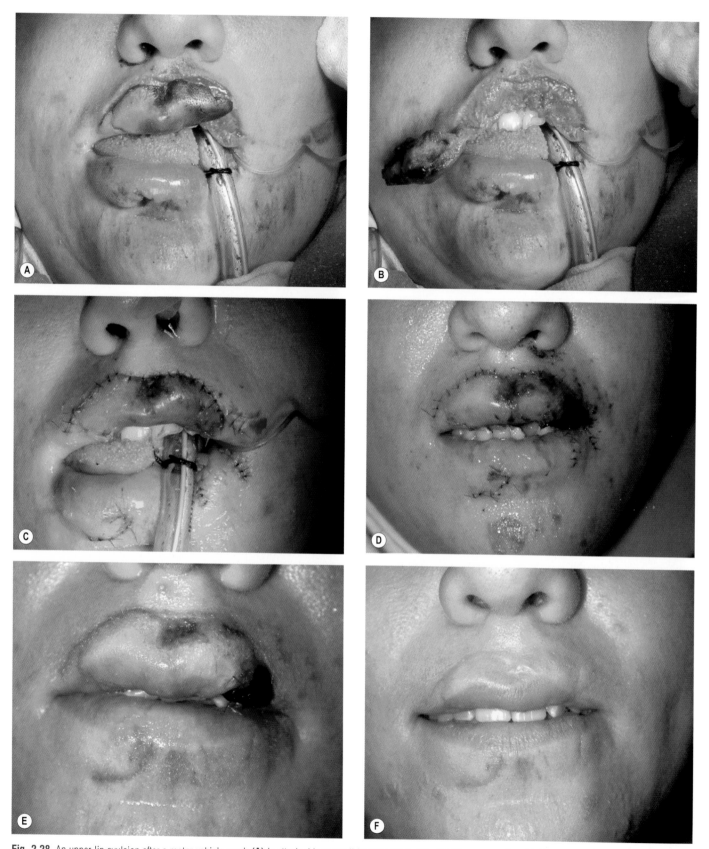

Fig. 2.28 An upper lip avulsion after a motor vehicle crash **(A)** is attached by a small lateral pedicle **(B)**. **(C)** After conservative debridement the landmarks were approximated and the wound closed. **(D)** An area of poor perfusion was present resulting in a small area of necrosis 4 days later. The necrotic area was allowed to heal by secondary intention **(E)** and ultimately resulted in a healed wound **(F)**.

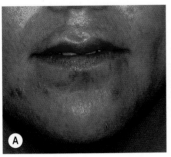 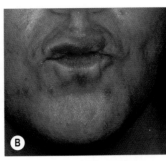 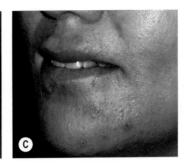 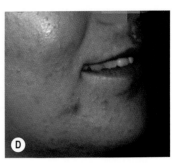

Fig. 2.29 At 3 months after repair of an avulsive lip wound **(A)** there is good orbicularis oris function and oral competence **(B)**, and an acceptable cosmetic result **(C,D)**.

the skin is mobile and has a fair amount of redundancy, neck lacerations can usually be closed primarily. Remember the course of the marginal mandibular branch deep to the platysma just below the mandibular border during the repair.

Conclusion

The repair of facial soft tissue injuries can be very satisfying for the patient and physician alike. Recognition and prompt treatment of underlying injuries will minimize complications for the patient. Meticulous cleansing of particulate matter will spare the patient a lifetime of facial discoloration from traumatic tattoo. Minimal debridement will salvage irreplaceable soft tissue structures. Careful approximation of important landmarks will minimize unsightly visual step-offs. And careful suture technique and timely suture removal will give your patient the best possible cosmetic outcome.

🌐 Access the complete reference list online at   **http://www.expertconsult.com**

4. Hussain K, Wijetunge DB, Grubnic S, Jackson IT. A comprehensive analysis of craniofacial trauma. *J Trauma*. 1994;36:34–47. *Craniofacial soft tissue injuries occur most often on the forehead, nose, lips, and chin in a "T"-shaped zone. There is significant variability in the common causes of craniofacial trauma that can be stratified by sex and age. Falls are the most common cause in children and the elderly. Interpersonal violence and alcohol are associated with the majority of injuries in young men. Sports are a common cause of injury among youth. This article is a detailed review of craniofacial trauma patterns.*

5. Zubowicz VN, Gravier M. Management of early human bites of the hand: a prospective randomized study. *Plast Reconstr Surg*. 1991;88:111–114.

6. Leach J. Proper handling of soft tissue in the acute phase. *Facial Plast Surg*. 2001;17:227–238. *An excellent overview of basic techniques for management of craniofacial soft tissue injuries, starting with initial evaluation, wound preparation, and anesthetic techniques. The management of wound contamination and steps to reduce the risk of infection are discussed. Planning of difficult closures by respecting the resting skin tension lines is discussed. Wound undermining and specific suture techniques are discussed in detail.*

7. Kesser BW, Chance E, Kleiner D, Young JS. Contemporary management of penetrating neck trauma. *Am Surg*. 2009;75:1–10.

8. Friedman PM, Mafong EA, Friedman ES, Geronemus RG. Topical anesthetics update: EMLA and beyond. *Dermatol Surg*. 2001;27:1019–1026.

9. Chen BK, Eichenfield LF. Pediatric anesthesia in dermatologic surgery: when hand-holding is not enough. *Dermatol Surg*. 2001;27:1010–1018.

10. Ohlsen L, Englesson S, Evers H. An anaesthetic lidocaine/prilocaine cream (EMLA) for epicutaneous application tested for cutting split skin grafts. *Scand J Plast Reconstr Surg*. 1985;19:201–209.

11. Gupta AK, Sibbald RG. Eutectic lidocaine/prilocaine 5% cream and patch may provide satisfactory analgesia for excisional biopsy or curettage with electrosurgery of cutaneous lesions. A randomized, controlled, parallel group study. *J Am Acad Dermatol*. 1996;35:419–423.

12. Eaton JS, Grekin RC. Regional anesthesia of the face. *Dermatol Surg*. 2001;27:1006–1009. *Successful regional blocks for facial trauma repair can often provide anesthesia for repair of larger facial wounds and provide initial anesthesia for later widespread infiltration of vasoconstricting agents. Successful regional anesthesia is based on a clear understanding of the anatomy. This article provides a detailed guide for success.*

39. Zitelli JA. Secondary intention healing: an alternative to surgical repair. *Clin Dermatol*. 1984;2:92–106. *This article reminds us that in cases of tissue loss secondary intention healing may produce acceptable outcomes in certain anatomic areas. The best cosmetic results are obtained on concave surfaces of the nose, eye, ear, and temple (NEET areas), while those on the convex surfaces of the nose, oral lips, cheeks and chin, and helix of the ear (NOCH areas) often heal with a poor-quality scar. Most wounds can be dressed with a semi-occlusive dressing or petrolatum ointment to prevent desiccation. Common complications include pigmentation changes, unstable scar, excessive granulation, pain, dysesthesias, and wound contracture.*

3

Facial injuries

Eduardo D. Rodriguez, Amir H. Dorafshar, and Paul N. Manson

SYNOPSIS

- Facial injuries often involve bone and soft tissue, and each must be managed precisely in a timely fashion.
- Soft tissue injuries include contusions, lacerations, hematomas, and avulsions.
- Bone injuries are fractures, and they are classified by anatomic area and are characterized by displacement and comminution.
- Bone injuries are treated with open or closed reductions, and typically rigid fixation is used for stabilization. The thick areas and edges where bones articulate are called "buttresses"; these areas guide application of fixation devices. Fracture stabilization is conducted through aesthetic incisions, which provide access to buttress articulations. The sequence of reduction and the need for exposure of a specific buttress articulation depend upon the level of comminution, displacement, and the presence of adjacent fractures.
- Anatomic closure of incisions, reattaching the soft tissue to its proper location on the bone, provides the soft tissue "reduction" necessary to obtain aesthetic results.
- Finally, a specific sequence of immediate injury management for both the bone and soft tissue is necessary in ballistic or high-energy injuries where bone and soft tissue are badly contused, avulsed and/or missing.

Introduction

Over ten million people are injured in automobile accidents in the US yearly.[1] Statistics on the number of facial injuries vary widely based on social, economic, and geographic differences. The causes of facial injuries in the US include motor vehicle collisions, assaults, altercations, bicycle and motorcycle accidents, home and industrial accidents, domestic violence, athletic injuries, and falls, particularly in the elderly.[2] The automobile is frequently responsible for some of the most devastating facial injuries, and injuries to the head, face, and cervical spine occur in over 50% of all victims.[3,4] Seat belts and airbags have reduced the severity and incidence of facial

injury, but primary and secondary enforcement of the laws vary in effectiveness with ethnicity, education, and geographic location.[5-7]

A unique aspect of facial injury treatment is that the aesthetic result may be the chief indication for treatment. In other cases, injuries may require surgery to restore function, but commonly, both goals are necessary. Although there are few facial emergencies, the literature has underemphasized the advantages of prompt definitive reconstruction and early operative intervention in achieving superior aesthetic and functional results. Economic, sociologic, and psychologic factors in a competitive society make it imperative that an expedient and well-planned surgical correction be executed in order to return the patient to an active and productive life while minimizing disability.

 Access the Historical Perspective section, including Fig. 3.1, online at
http://www.expertconsult.com

Initial assessment

Management begins with an initial physical examination and is followed by a radiologic evaluation accomplished with computerized tomographic (CT) scanning. CT scans visualize soft tissue and bone.[9] It is no longer feasible or economically justifiable to obtain plain radiographs with certain exceptions, such as the panorex mandible examination or dental films. The availability of regional Level I and II trauma centers has provided earlier, safer, and improved trauma care for polytrauma, severely injured patients.

Clinical examination of the face

A careful history and thorough clinical examination forms the basis for the diagnosis of almost all facial injuries. Thorough

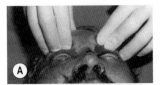

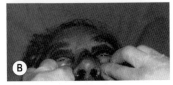

Fig. 3.2 Palpation of the superior and inferior orbital rims. (**A**) The superior orbital rims are palpated with the pads of the fingertips. (**B**) Palpation of the inferior orbital rims. One should feel for discontinuity and level discrepancies in the bone of the rim and evaluate both the anterior and vertical position of the inferior orbital rims, comparing the prominence of the malar eminence of the two sides of the face.

examination of the face is indicated even if the patient has only minor wounds or abrasions.

The clinical examination should begin with the evaluation for symmetry and deformity, inspecting the face and comparing one side with the other. Palpation of all bony surfaces follows in an orderly manner. The forehead, orbital rims, nose, brows; zygomatic arches; malar eminence; and border of the mandible should be evaluated (Fig. 3.2). Careful inspection of the intra-nasal areas should be made using a nasal speculum to detect lacerations or hematomas. A thorough inspection of the intra-oral area should be made to detect lacerations, bleeding, loose teeth, or abnormalities of the dentition (Fig. 3.3). Palpation of the dental arches follows the inspection, noting mobility of dental–alveolar arch segments. The maxillary and mandibular dental arches are carefully visualized and palpated to detect any irregularity of the bone, loose teeth, intra-oral lacerations, bruising, hematoma, swelling, movement, tenderness, or crepitus. Mobility of the midface and mandible should be methodically assessed (Figs. 3.4 & 3.5).

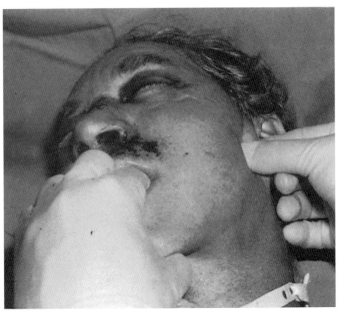

Fig. 3.4 Condylar examination. The mandible is grasped with one hand, and the condyle area is bimanually palpated with one finger in the ear canal and one finger over the head of the condyle. Abnormal movement, or crepitation, indicates a condylar fracture. In the absence of a condylar fracture, a noncrepitant movement of the condylar head should occur synchronously with the anterior mandible. Disruption of the ligaments of the condyle will permit dislocations of the condylar head out of the fossa in the absence of fracture.

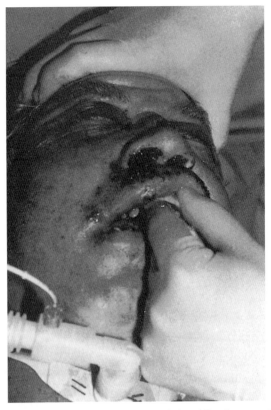

Fig. 3.5 With the head securely grasped, the midface is assessed for movement by grasping the dentition. Loose teeth, dentures, or bridgework should not be confused with mobility of the maxilla. Le Fort fractures demonstrate, as a rule, less mobility if they exist as large fragments, and especially if they are a "single fragment", than do lower Le Fort fractures. More comminuted Le Fort fractures demonstrate extreme mobility ("loose" maxillary fractures).

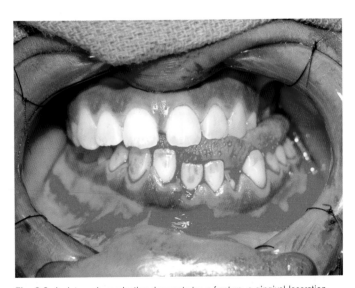

Fig. 3.3 An intraoral examination demonstrates a fracture, a gingival laceration, and a gap in the dentition. These alveolar and gingival lacerations sometimes extend along the floor or roof of the mouth for a considerable distance.

An evaluation of sensory and motor nerve function in the facial area is performed. The presence of hypesthesia or anesthesia in the distribution of the supraorbital, infraorbital, or mental nerves suggests a fracture along the bony path of these sensory nerves (cranial nerve V). Cutaneous branches of these nerves may also have been interrupted by a facial laceration.

Extraocular movements (cranial nerves III, IV, and VI) and the muscles of facial expression (cranial nerve VII) are examined in the conscious, cooperative patient. Pupillary size and symmetry, speed of pupillary reaction, globe turgor, globe excursion, eyelid excursion, double vision, and visual acuity and visual loss are noted. A funduscopic examination and measurements of globe pressure should be performed. The presence of a hyphema, corneal abrasion, visual field defect, visual loss, diplopia, decreased vision, or absent vision should be noted and appropriate consultation requested.

Computerized tomographic scans

The definitive radiographic evaluation is the craniofacial CT scan with axial, coronal, and sagittal sections of bone and soft tissue windows.[10,11] CT evaluation of the face can define bone fractures, whereas the soft tissue views allow for soft tissue definition of the area of the fracture. 3D CT scans[12] allow for comparison of symmetry and volume of the facial bones bilaterally. Specialized views, such as those of the orbital apex, provide a special magnified visualization.

Timing of treatment

Timing is important in optimizing the management of facial injuries. Bone and soft tissue injuries in the facial area should be managed as soon as the patient's general condition permits. Time and time again it has been the authors' impression that early facial injury management decreases permanent facial disfigurement and limits serious functional disturbances.[13,14] This does not mean that one can be cavalier about deciding who might tolerate early operative intervention. Indeed, the facial surgeon must have a complete knowledge of the patient's ancillary injuries as well as those of the face. Classically, facial soft tissue and bone injuries are not acute surgical emergencies, but both the ease of obtaining a good result and the quality of the result are better with early or immediate management. Less soft tissue stripping is required, bones are more easily replaced into their anatomic position, and easier fracture repairs are performed. There are some patients, however, whose injuries cannot be definitively managed early. Exceptions to acute treatment include patients with ongoing or significant blood loss (i.e. pelvic fractures), elevated intracranial pressures, coagulation problems, and abnormal pulmonary ventilation pressures.[15] Under local anesthesia, however, lacerations are debrided and closed, interdental fixation applied, and grossly displaced fractures reduced. Many patients with mild brain injuries or multi-system traumas do not have criteria preventing operative management.[16] These patients may receive facial injury management at the time that other injuries are being stabilized. It is not uncommon, however, in the University of Maryland Shock Trauma Unit for several teams to operate on a patient at the same time in several anatomic areas.

Upper facial fractures

Frontal bone and sinus injury patterns

The frontal sinuses are paired structures that have only an ethmoidal anlage at birth. They have no frontal bone component initially. They begin to be detected at 3 years of age, but significant pneumatic expansion does not begin to occur until approximately age 7 years. The full development of the frontal sinuses is complete by the age of 18 to 20. The frontal sinuses are lined with respiratory epithelium, which consists of a ciliated membrane with mucus secreting glands. A blanket of mucin is essential for normal function, and the cilia beat this mucin in the direction of the nasofrontal outflow tracts (NFOT). The exact function of the paranasal sinuses is still unclear. When injured and obstructed, they serve as a focus for infection, especially when NFOT function is impaired. The nature of the open frontal sinuses and the multiple layers of the skull protect the intracranial contents from injury by absorbing energy.

The predominant form of frontal sinus injury is fracture. Fracture involvement of the frontal sinus has been estimated to occur in 2% to 12% of all cranial fractures, and severe fractures occur in 0.7% to 2% of patients with cranial or cerebral trauma.

Approximately one-third of fractures involve the anterior table alone, and 60% involve the anterior table and posterior table and/or ducts. The remainder (7%) involve the posterior wall alone. Some 40% of frontal sinus fractures have an accompanying dural laceration.

Clinical examination

Lacerations, bruises, hematomas, and contusions constitute the most frequent signs of frontal bone or sinus fractures. The "spectacle hematoma" is a sign of an anterior cranial base fracture, and frontal sinus and skull fractures must be suspected if any of these signs are present. Anesthesia of the supraorbital nerve may be present. Cerebrospinal fluid rhinorrhea may occur. There may or may not be subconjunctival or periorbital ecchymoses with or without air in the orbit or intracranial cavity. In some cases, a depression may be observed over the frontal sinus, but swelling is usually predominant in the first few days after the injury, which may obscure the depression.

Small fractures of the frontal sinus may be difficult to detect, especially if they are nondisplaced. Therefore, the first presentation of a frontal sinus fracture may be an infection or symptom of frontal sinus obstruction, such as mucocele or abscess formation.[17] Infection in the frontal sinus may produce quite serious complications because of its location near the brain and meninges. Infections include meningitis, extradural or intradural abscess, intracranial abscess, osteomyelitis of the frontal bone, or osteitis in devitalized bone fragments.[18–22]

Nasofrontal outflow tract

The development of a frontal sinus mucocele is linked to obstruction of the NFOT, which is involved with fractures in up to 50% of cases of frontal sinus injury. The NFOT passes through the anterior ethmoidal air cells to exit adjacent to the ethmoidal infundibulum. Blockage of the NFOT prevents adequate drainage of the normal mucosal secretions and predisposes to the development of obstructive epithelial lined cysts or mucoceles. Mucoceles may also develop when islands of mucosa are trapped by scar tissue within fracture lines and attempt to grow after the injury, producing a mucus membrane lined obstructed cystic structure.[23]

The sinus is completely obliterated only when it is deprived of its lining and when the bone is burred, eliminating the foramina of Breschet[24] where mucosal ingrowth occurs along veins in the walls of the sinuses. Regrowth of mucosa can also occur from any portion of the frontal sinus, especially if incompletely debrided. The reported average interval between the primary injury and development of frontal sinus mucocele is 7.5 years.

Radiography

Frontal bone and sinus fractures are best demonstrated using CT Scans.[25] Hematomas or air fluid levels in the frontal sinus may be visualized as well as potential injuries to the NFOT. Persisting air-fluid levels imply the absence of NFOT function as do displaced fractures in the medial floor of the frontal sinus.

Surgical treatment

The best technique of exposure in major fractures involving the frontal bone is the coronal incision. This allows a combined intracranial and extracranial approach to the anterior cranial fossa which provides visualization of all areas, including repair of dural tears, debridement of any necrotic sections of frontal lobe, and repair of the bone structures.

Frontal sinus fractures should be characterized by describing both the anatomic location of the fractures and displacement. The indications for surgical intervention in frontal sinus fractures include depression of the anterior table, radiographic demonstration of involvement of the NFOT with presumed future non-function, obstruction of the NFOT with persistent air-fluid levels, mucocele formation, and fractures of the posterior table which may have lacerated the dura.[26,27] Some authors recommend exploration of any posterior table fracture or any fracture in which an air-fluid level is visible. Others have a more selective approach, exploring posterior wall fractures only if their displacement exceeds the width of the posterior table, a distance suggesting simultaneous dural laceration.[28,29] Simple linear fractures of the anterior and posterior sinus walls which are undisplaced are safely observed.

Any depressed frontal sinus fracture of the anterior wall potentially requires exploration and wall replacement to prevent contour deformity. Most of these patients have no compromise of NFOT function; however, those that do will have fractures of the medial floor of the sinus. If sinus drainage is compromised, the sinus should be defunctionalized. The anterior wall of the sinus may be explored by an appropriate local laceration or a coronal incision, or more recently endoscopic drainage and elevation have been recommended for simpler fractures. Anterior wall fragments are elevated and plated into position. If it is desired that the NFOT[30,31] and sinus be obliterated because of involvement, the mucosa is

thoroughly stripped, even into the recesses of the sinus, and the NFOT occluded with well-designed "formed-to-fit" calvarial bone plugs or calvarial bone particulate grafting material (Fig. 3.6). If most of the posterior bony wall is intact, the entire frontal sinus cavity may be filled with cancellous bone. The iliac crest provides a generous source of rich cancellous bone.[32] Formerly, the cavity was left vacant to heal by a slow process called "osteoneogenesis", filling slowly with a combination of bone and fibrous tissue. However, the incidence of infection is higher by comparison to filling the empty cavity with cancellous bone graft.[33]

If the posterior table is missing, grafting may be performed for localized defects, but it is always emphasized that the floor of the anterior cranial fossa should be reconstructed with bone. For large defects, a process called cranialization is selected, where the posterior wall of the frontal sinus is removed, effectively making the frontal sinus a part of the intracranial cavity. The "dead space" may be filled with cancellous bone or left open. Any communication with the nose by the NFOT or with the ethmoid sinuses should be sealed with carefully designed bone grafts or bone graft particulate material after debridement. The orbital roof should be reconstructed primarily by thin bone grafts placed external to the orbital cavity. An intracranial exposure is often preferred for large defect orbital roof reconstruction.

The use of a galeal flap in the treatment of extensive frontal bone defects designed with a pedicle of the supraorbital and supratrochlear artery or with the superficial temporal artery is recommended for vascularized soft tissue obliteration of "dead space".

Complications

Complications of frontal bone and sinus fractures include:

1. CSF fluid rhinorrhea
2. Pneumocephalus and orbital emphysema
3. Absence of orbital roof and pulsating exophthalmos
4. Carotid–cavernous sinus fistula

Orbital fractures

Orbital fractures may occur as isolated fractures of the internal orbit (also called "pure") or may involve both the internal orbit and the orbital rim (also called "impure")[34,35] (Fig. 3.7).

Surgical anatomy of the orbit

The orbits are conceptualized in thirds progressing from anterior to posterior. Anteriorly, the orbital rims consist of thick bone. The middle third of the orbit consists of thin bone, and the bone structure thickens again in the posterior portion of the orbit. The orbital bone structure is thus analogous to a "shock-absorbing" device in which the middle portion of the orbit breaks first, followed by the rim, both absorbing energy and protecting the poster third from displacement and the globe from rupturing.

The optic foramen is situated at the junction of the lateral and medial walls of the orbit posteriorly and is well above the horizontal plane of the orbital floor. The foramen is located 40–45 mm behind the inferior orbital rim.

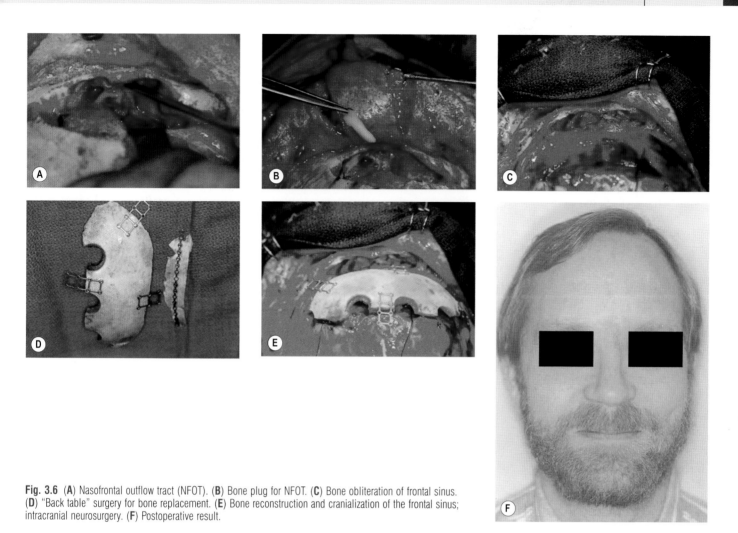

Fig. 3.6 **(A)** Nasofrontal outflow tract (NFOT). **(B)** Bone plug for NFOT. **(C)** Bone obliteration of frontal sinus. **(D)** "Back table" surgery for bone replacement. **(E)** Bone reconstruction and cranialization of the frontal sinus; intracranial neurosurgery. **(F)** Postoperative result.

Orbital physical examination

The most important component of the physical examination is to check the visual acuity in each eye: the patient's ability to read newsprint or an ophthalmic examination card such as the Rosenbaum Pocket card. Visual field examinations should be performed to detect edema, corneal abrasion, globe laceration, contusion, and hematoma. The simultaneous presence of a subconjunctival hematoma and a periorbital hematoma confined to the distribution of the orbital septum (so called "spectacle hematoma") is evidence of a facial fracture involving the orbit until proven by radiographs (Fig. 3.8). Extraocular movements should identify double vision or restricted globe movement. All patients with orbital injuries must be frequently checked for light perception and pupillary afferent defects post-injury, preoperatively and postoperatively. Globe pressure may be assessed by tonometry and should be less than 15 mm. The results of a fundus examination should be recorded. The presence of no light perception generally indicates optic nerve damage or globe rupture.[36] Light perception without usable vision usually indicates optic nerve damage, retinal detachment, hyphema, vitreous hemorrhage, or anterior or posterior chamber injuries. Globe and eye injuries require expert ophthalmologic consultation.

Radiographic evidence of fracture

CT scans performed in the axial, coronal, and sagittal planes, using both bone and soft tissue windows, are essential to define the anatomy of the orbital walls and soft tissue contents, and the relation of the extraocular muscles to the fracture.

Indications for surgical treatment

The indications for surgical treatment include:

1. Double vision caused by incarceration of muscle or the fine ligament system, documented by forced duction examination and suggested by CT scans.
2. Radiographic evidence of extensive fracture, such that enophthalmos would occur.
3. Enophthalmos or exophthalmos (significant globe positional change) produced by an orbital volume change.
4. Visual acuity deficit, increasing and not responsive to medical dose steroids, implying that optic canal decompression may be indicated, although this has become more controversial.[36]

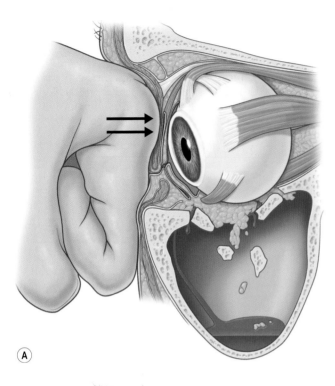

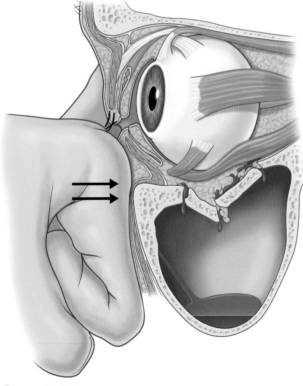

Fig. 3.7 **(A)** Mechanism of blow-out fracture from displacement of the globe itself into the orbital walls. The globe is displaced posteriorly, striking the orbital walls and forcing them outward, causing a "punched out" fracture the size of the globe. **(B)** "Force transmission" fracture of orbital floor.

5. "Blow-in" orbital fractures that involve the medial or lateral walls of the orbit and severely constrict orbital volume, creating increased intraorbital and globe pressure.

Blow-out fractures of the floor of the orbit

A blow-out fracture is caused by the application of a traumatic force to the rim, globe, or soft tissues of the orbit. Blow-out fractures are accompanied by a sudden increase in intraorbital pressure.[37]

Medial orbital wall fractures

Medial orbital wall fractures may be isolated or combined with fractures of the floor.[38] With the loss of the infero-medial orbital strut (connected to the middle turbinate) located between the medial wall and floor, there is increased difficulty achieving the proper shape and volume of the orbital contents. This is an indication for repair with either anatomically contoured calvarial bone grafts or alloplastic implants to reproduce the normal inwardly contoured shape of the orbit. The exposure for reduction of a medial orbital fracture include trans- or retrocaruncular approaches, which can be used in combination with a transconjunctival incision to provide wide exposure to the floor and medial orbit for repair.[39] A coronal incision provides the broadest exposure of the medial orbital wall.

Blow-out fractures in younger individuals

In children, the mechanism of entrapment is more frequently trapdoor than the "blow-out or punched out" fracture seen in adults. As opposed to incarceration of fat adjacent to the

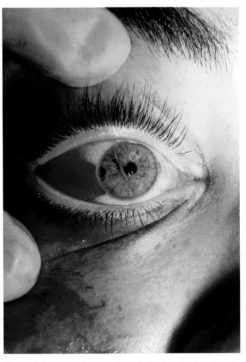

Fig. 3.8 The combination of a palpebral and subconjunctival hematoma is suggestive of a fracture somewhere within the orbit. There is frequently a zygomatic or orbital floor fracture present when these signs are confirmed.

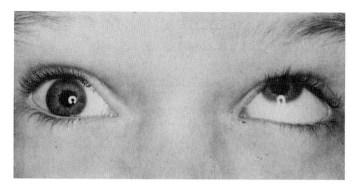

Fig. 3.9 Blow-out fracture in a child produced by a snowball. Note the nearly complete immobility of the ocular globe and the enophthalmos. Such severe loss of motion implies actual muscle incarceration, an injury that is more frequent in children than in adults. This fracture deserves immediate operation with release of the incarcerated extraocular muscle system. It is often accompanied by pain on attempted rotation of the globe and sometimes nausea and vomiting. These symptoms are unusual in orbital floor fractures without true muscle incarceration.

inferior rectus muscle, children more frequently "scissor" or capture the muscle directly in the fracture site, as the springy bone of children recoils faster than the entrapped soft tissue, pinning the muscle. This may be suggested on physical examination with near immobility of the eye when upgaze is attempted on the affected side, pain with attempted eye motion, as well as nausea, vomiting, and presence of an oculocardiac reflex, which consists of nausea, bradycardia, and hypotension (Fig. 3.9). Trapdoor fractures with actual muscle incarceration is an *urgent* situation that demands immediate release of the incarcerated muscle to preserve its perfusion.[40–42] Most practitioners emphasize that a better prognosis occurs if the muscle is released early, although more recently it has been suggested that appropriate surgical technique is more important than the timing of release per se.[43]

Surgical treatment

The surgical treatment of orbital fractures has three goals:

1. Disengage entrapped structures and restore ocular rotatory function.
2. Replace orbital contents into the usual confines of the normal bony orbital cavity, including restoration of both orbital volume and shape.
3. Restore orbital cavity walls, which in effect replaces the tissues into their proper position and dictates the shape into which the soft tissue can scar.

The timing of surgical intervention

In isolated blow-out fractures, it is not necessary to operate immediately unless true muscle incarceration is present. In the presence of significant edema, retrobulbar hemorrhage, optic nerve injury, retinal detachment, or other significant globe injuries, such as hyphema, it is advisable to wait a number of days until stability of ocular condition is confirmed.

Significant orbital fractures are best treated by early surgical intervention. The authors firmly believe that the earlier significant orbital volume change or functional muscle derangement can be corrected, the better the final aesthetic and functional result.

Operative technique for orbital fractures

Endoscopic approaches for orbital floor fractures

Recently, endoscopic approaches through the maxillary sinus have permitted direct visualization of the orbital floor and manipulation of the soft tissue and floor repair with this approach, which avoids an eyelid incision.[44–46]

Cutaneous exposures

A number of incisions have been employed to approach the orbital floor:

1. Inferior lower eyelid incision. These have the least incidence of lower eyelid ectropion of any lid incision location but tend to generate the most noticeable scar and are prone to lymphedema.[47–49]
2. Subciliary skin muscle flap incision. This incision near the upper margin of the lid leaves the least conspicuous scar of any cutaneous incision.[50,51] However, they are prone to have the highest incidence of lid retraction (scleral show and ectropion). The mid-lid variation has less ectropion but more obvious scar if taken lateral to the pupil, and more edema.
3. Transconjunctival incision. A preseptal or retroseptal dissection plane can be established. There is no cutaneous lid scar unless a lateral canthotomy is utilized.

Surgical technique

Generally, a corneal protector is placed over the eye to protect the globe and cornea from instruments, retractors, or rotating drills. The inferior rectus muscle, the orbital fat, and any orbital soft tissue structures should be carefully dissected free from the areas of the blow-out fracture. Intact orbital floor must be located around all the edges of the fracture, and any displaced "blow-out" soft tissue gently released from the fracture.

The fracture may be made larger permitting easier removal of incarcerated soft tissue. The floor must be explored sufficiently posteriorly that intact orbital floor beyond the defect is confirmed. This "ledge" is frequently the orbital process of the palatine bone, 35–38 mm posterior to the rim. Placing a freer into the maxillary sinus, one may locate the back of the sinus and move it superiorly to verify the position of the "ledge" which will be felt as a projection from the back wall of the sinus. The "ledge" may be verified on sagittal CT scan images.[52,53] The "ledges" in fracture treatment are landmarks with which implant material should be aligned to re-establish an anatomic orbital shape and volume.

The forced duction test

Limitation of forced rotation of the eyeball (the "forced duction" test or the "eyeball traction" test) (Fig. 3.10) provides a means of differentiating entrapment of the extraocular muscles from muscle weakness, paralysis, or contusion. The forced duction test should be performed for initial diagnosis, and then 1) before dissection; 2) after dissection; 3) after the insertion of each material used to reconstruct the orbital wall; 4) just prior to closure of the incisions. It is crucial that these

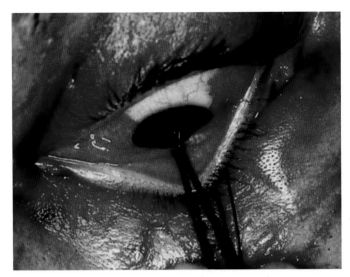

Fig. 3.10 The forced duction test. Forceps grasp the ocular globe at the insertion of the inferior rectus muscle, which is approximately 7–10 mm from the limbus. A drop of local anesthetic instilled into the conjunctival sac precedes the procedure.

measurements all be compared to detect what is causing interference. Reconstructive material must not interfere with globe movement, and a full range of oculo-rotatory movements must accompany restoration of proper eye position.

Restoration of continuity of the orbital floor

The purpose of the orbital floor replacement, whether a bone graft or an inorganic implant, is to re-establish the size and the shape of the orbital cavity. This replaces the orbital soft tissue contents and allows scar tissue remodeling to occur in an anatomic position and proper shape (Fig. 3.11).

Bone grafts for orbital floor reconstruction

Split calvarial, iliac, or split rib bone grafts provide the ideal bone substitute for reconstruction of the internal orbital fractures.[54] It is not known whether bone grafts resist bacterial colonization better than inorganic implants, but that is the presumption. Bone grafts are presumed to survive at the 50–80% level.

Inorganic implants

The inorganic implant offers the reconstruction of the orbital floor without an additional operation for bone graft harvest. Titanium mesh alone or titanium mesh with polyethylene may be easily utilized for larger defects.

The incidence of late infection with any technique is less than two percent, and displacement should not occur if the material has been properly anchored. Rarely, artificial or bone graft materials exposed to the sinus may not re-mucosalize, and may be responsible for recurrent cellulitis.

Postoperative care

Light perception must be confirmed preoperatively and frequently postoperatively. Pupillary reactivity must be assessed before and at least twice daily for the first several days after surgery. Double vision should be noted and compared with

preoperative results. Both double vision and blindness have sometimes occurred after day 1 either in orbital fractures or in postoperative treatment, but these conditions are usually present at the time of injury or acutely following the surgery.

Complications of orbital fractures

Diplopia

Extraocular muscle imbalance and subjective diplopia are usually the result of muscle injury or contusion but can be the result of incarceration of either the muscle or the soft tissue adjacent to the muscles, or the result of nerve damage to the third, fourth, and sixth cranial nerves.[55–59] Traumatic surgical dissection is also a mechanism as is forceful removal of

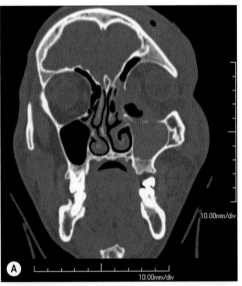

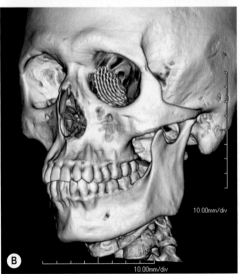

Fig. 3.11 Medial orbital wall fracture. **(A)** Coronal CT scan image illustrating medial orbital wall fracture. **(B)** Postoperative three-dimensional CT scan demonstrating repair of medial orbital wall repair using titanium alloplastic mesh implant.

incarcerated orbital contents from a fracture, where tearing of the muscle occurs.

Enophthalmos

Enophthalmos[60,61] is the second major complication of a blow-out fracture, and the major cause is enlargement of the bony orbit with herniation of the orbital soft tissue structures into a larger space with remodeling of the shape of the soft tissue into a spherical configuration. Displacement of intramuscular cone fat into the extramuscular compartment is another mechanism, initiating a loss of globe position, as is retention of the ocular globe in a backward position by scar tissue. A popular theory was fat atrophy, but computerized volume studies prove that fat atrophy makes a significant contribution in only 10% of orbital fractures.

Retrobulbar hematoma

In severe trauma, retrobulbar hematoma may displace the ocular globe. Retrobulbar hematoma is signaled by globe proptosis and exophthalmos, congestion and prolapse of the edematous conjunctiva. Diagnosis is confirmed by a CT scan image with soft tissue windows. Drainage is not possible as retrobulbar hematomas usually are diffuse. Orbital fracture treatment in the setting of retrobulbar hematoma has increased risk, as volume increase and vascular spasm may affect globe circulation. The reconstruction is best performed when hemorrhage, swelling and congestion have subsided, and vision is stabilized.

Ocular (globe) injuries and blindness

The incidence of ocular injuries following orbital fractures is 14–30%. The incidence depends on the scrutiny of the examination and the recognition of minor injuries, such as corneal abrasion. Ocular globe injury may vary in severity from a corneal abrasion to loss of vision to globe rupture, retinal detachment, vitreous hemorrhage, or a fracture involving the optic canal.[62] Blindness, or loss of an eye, is remarkably infrequent despite the severity of some of the injuries sustained because of the "shock absorber" type construction of the orbit. The incidence of acute visual loss following facial fractures is on average 1.7%,[63] and blindness following facial fracture repair has been estimated to be about 0.2%.[64]

Implant migration, late hemorrhage around implants, and implant fixation

Migration of an implant anteriorly may occur with extrusion if the implant is not secured to the orbital floor or to a plate that attaches to the rim. Spontaneous late proptosis can be caused by hemorrhage from longstanding low-grade infection around orbital implants or from chronic sinus or lacrimal system infection.[65]

Ptosis of the upper lid

True ptosis of the upper lid should be differentiated from "pseudoptosis" resulting from the downward displacement of the eyeball in enophthalmos. True ptosis results from loss of action of the levator palpebrae superioris. Ptosis in the presence of enophthalmos should not be treated until the globe position has been stabilized by enophthalmos correction.

Scleral show, ectropion, and entropion – vertical shortening of the lower eyelid

Vertical shortening of the lower eyelid with exposure of the sclera below the limbus of the iris in the primary position (scleral show) may result from downward and backward displacement of the fractured inferior orbital rim. The septum and lower lid are "fixed length" structures and are therefore dragged downward by their tendency to adhere to the abnormally positioned inferior orbital rim. This can result in scleral show or ectropion if occurring in the "anterior lid lamellae" (skin or orbicularis) or entropion if occurring in the "posterior lid lamellae" (septum, lower lid retractors, and conjunctiva). Only in the actual performance of the operation can the surgeon define the true nature of the problem, release the adhesions, correct the lid shortening, and stabilize the lid position with appropriate grafts into the proper location.[66] Correction procedures generally do not elevate the lower lid by more than 3 mm.

Infraorbital nerve anesthesia

Infraorbital nerve anesthesia is extremely disconcerting to patients who experience it, especially initially. The area of sensory loss usually extends from the lower lid to involve the medial cheek; the lateral portion of the nose, including the ala; and the ipsilateral upper lip. The anterior maxillary teeth may be involved if the branch of the infraorbital nerve in the anterior maxillary wall is involved. Decompression of the infraorbital nerve from pressure of the bony fragments within the infraorbital canal may be indicated either acutely or late after fracture treatment especially if the zygoma demonstrates medial displacement impinging the infraorbital canal with impaction into the nerve.

The "superior orbital fissure" syndrome and the "orbital apex" syndrome

Significant fractures of the orbit extend posteriorly to involve the superior orbital fissure and optic foramen. Involvement of the structures of the superior orbital fissure produces a symptom complex known as the superior orbital fissure syndrome. This consists of partial or complete involvement of the following structures: the two divisions of the cranial nerve III, superior and inferior, producing paralysis of the levator, superior rectus, inferior rectus, and inferior oblique muscles; cranial nerve IV causing paralysis of the superior oblique muscle; cranial nerve VI producing paralysis of the lateral rectus muscle; and the ophthalmic division of the trigeminal nerve (V) causing anesthesia in the brow, medial portion of the upper lid, medial upper nose, and ipsilateral forehead. Symptoms of the superior orbital fissure syndrome may be partial or complete in each of the nerves.[67] When accompanied by visual acuity change or blindness, the injury implies concomitant involvement of the combined superior orbital fissure (CN III, IV, V & VI) and optic foramen (CN II). If involvement of both the optic nerve and superior orbital fissure occur, this symptom complex is called the orbital apex syndrome.

Midfacial fractures

Nasal fractures

Types and locations of nasal fractures

Lateral forces[68] account for the majority of nasal fractures and produce a wide variation of deformities, depending on the age of the patient, intensity and vector of force. Younger patients tend to have fracture dislocations of larger segments, whereas older patients with more dense, brittle bone often exhibit comminution. A direct force of moderate intensity from the lateral side may fracture only one nasal bone with displacement into the nasal cavity (plane I lateral impact). When forces are of increased intensity, some displacement of the contralateral nasal bone occurs and the fracture may be incomplete or greensticked requiring completion of the contralateral fracture to centralize the nasal processes (plane II lateral impact). In more severe (plane III lateral impact) frontal impact injuries, the frontal process of the maxilla may begin to fracture and may be depressed posteriorly on one side. This depression first arises at the pyriform aperture inferiorly and then involves the entire structure of the frontal process of the maxilla, and is in effect the first stage of a hemi-nasoethmoidal fracture, displaced inferiorly and posteriorly (plane III "lateral impact" nasal fractures are identical to "type I" hemi-nasoethmoidal fractures) (Fig. 3.12A–C). These fractures are "greensticked" or almost undisplaced at the internal angular process of the frontal bone. The sidewall of the nose drops on one side, the septum telescopes and displaces, and the nasal airway is effectively closed on the ipsilateral side by the sidewall and turbinate impacting toward the septum blocking the airway. In stronger blows, the septum begins to collapse from an anteroposterior perspective as the comminution increases.

Anteroposterior blows result in posterior displacement of the nose into the nasal cavity and may occur with or without lateral impact. They also occur in three degrees of severity: plane I, where the distal portion of the nasal bones are involved; plane II, where the entire nasal bones and dorsal septum are involved; and Plane III, where the comminution extends beyond the nose into the frontal processes of the maxilla; again, the latter injuries are true nasoethmoidal–orbital fractures. With any nasal fracture of significance, the septum "telescopes", losing height, and the nasal bridge drops. Violent blows result in multiple fractures of the nasal bones, frontal processes of the maxilla, lacrimal bones, septal cartilages, and the ethmoidal areas (i.e. the true nasoethmoidal orbital fracture).

Fractures and dislocations of the nasal septum

Fractures and dislocations of the septum may occur independently or concomitantly with fractures of the distal nasal bone framework. Most commonly, the two injuries occur together, but frontal impact nasal fractures carry the worst prognosis regarding preservation of nasal height with closed reduction techniques (Fig. 3.13). Because of the intimate association of the bones of the nose with the nasal cartilages and bony nasal septum, it is unusual to observe fractures of either structure without damage to the other. In particular, the caudal or cartilaginous portion of the septum is almost always injured in nasal fractures.

The caudal portion of the septum has a degree of flexibility and bends to absorb moderate impact. The first stage of nasal septal injury is fracturing and bending, and the next stage involves overlap between fragments, which reduces nasal height. In mid-level severity injuries, the septum fractures, often initially with a C-shaped or double transverse component in which the septum is fractured and dislocated out of the vomerine groove with or without involvement of the

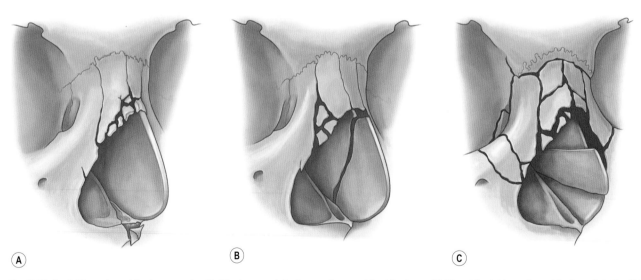

(A) (B) (C)

Fig. 3.12 Frontal impact nasal fractures are classified by degrees of displacement, as are lateral fractures. (**A**) Plane I frontal impact nasal fracture. Only the distal ends of the nasal bones and the septum are injured. (**B**) Plane II frontal impact nasal fracture. The injury is more extensive, involving the entire distal portion of the nasal bones and the frontal process of the maxilla at the piriform aperture. The septum is comminuted and begins to lose height. (**C**) Plane III frontal impact nasal fractures involve one or both frontal processes of the maxilla, and the fracture extends to the frontal bone. These fractures are in reality nasoethmoidal orbital fractures because they involve the lower two-thirds of the medial orbital rim (central fragment of the nasoethmoidal orbital fracture), as well as the bones of the nose.

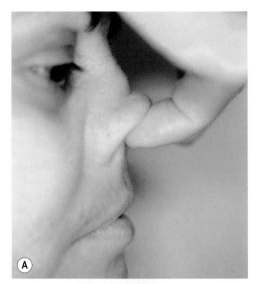

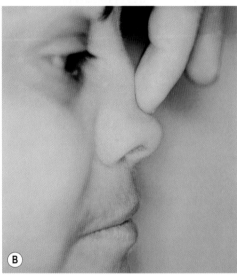

Fig. 3.13 Palpation of the columella (**A**) and dorsum (**B**) detects superior rotation of the septum and lack of dorsal support. There is an absence of columellar support and dorsal septal support.

vomer and anterior nasal spine, where displacement of the fractured segments cause partial obstruction of the nasal airway. Severe fractures of the septum are associated with "telescoping" or overlapping type of displacements, with a "Z-shaped" characteristic deformity,[69] where the septum loses considerable length, obstructing both airways. The septum is severely shortened, giving rise to a retruded appearance in lateral profile: the distal dorsum of the nose slumps posteriorly, and the columella and tip are retruded and upturned.

The treatment of nasal fractures

Most nasal fractures are reduced by closed reduction (Fig. 3.14A–E). In moderate or severe frontal impact fractures where loss of nasal height and length occur (plane II or plane III nasoethmoidal orbital fractures), open reduction and primary bone or cartilage grafting may be the only way to restore the support of the nose and return it to its original volume and shape, filling the soft tissue envelope with new cartilage support and preventing soft tissue contracture[70] (Fig. 3.15).

Open reduction and the use of supporting k wires

In severe nasal injury (i.e. plane II nasal injury), open reduction with bone or cartilage grafting to restore nasal height may be required. Semi-closed reductions[71] with limited incisions using K wires to attempt to stabilize the nasal bones are less effective and accurate.[72] Internal splinting of the septum should be part of the treatment plan (Doyle splints). Some nasal fractures are sufficiently dislocated that they can only be stabilized with an open rhinoplasty reduction and bone or cartilage grafts.[73]

A closed reduction may be best performed before edema prevents accurate palpation and visual inspection to confirm the reduction, and before partial healing or fibrosis limits the effectiveness of reduction. In practice, closed reduction of most nasal fractures is frequently deferred 5–7 days until the edema has partially subsided and the accuracy of the reduction may again be confirmed by visual inspection and palpation. After two weeks, it becomes more difficult to reduce a nasal fracture, as partial healing in malalignment has occurred. The soft tissue shrinks to accommodate the reduced skeletal volume, making anatomic reduction more difficult.

Treatment of fractures and dislocations of the septum

The nasal septum should be straightened and repositioned as soon after the injury as possible. Fractures of the nasal bones and septum frequently occur simultaneously, and it is important to ensure that at the time of reduction the nasal bones and septum fragments can be freely deviated in both lateral directions to ensure completion of partial or "greensticked" fractures. Incomplete fractures create early recurrence of displacement by causing the nasal bones and septum to "spring" back toward their original deviated position. When nasal bones are reduced, their intimate relationship with the upper and lower lateral cartilages tends to reduce the upper septal cartilage as well unless the cartilages are torn or avulsed from their attachments. Displacement of the cartilaginous septum out of the vomerine groove will not be reduced with nasal bone reduction alone and must be done manually with an Asch forcep, and the septal fragments maintained in position with an intranasal (Doyle) splint (see Fig. 3.14). In cases where the septum has been dislocated from the anterior nasal spine, the septum should be reunited by suture or wire fixation to the spine;[74] septal hematomas should be aspirated and minimized by transfixation sutures through and through the mucosa.

When nasal fractures are treated late after the injury, it may not be possible to obtain the desired result with a closed reduction or with a single operation. Healing may make the reduction of the displaced or overlapped fragments impossible without osteotomy at each area of previous fracture by open rhinoplasty, septal resection and repositioning, and/or bone or cartilage grafting. Some advocate acute septal open reductions, where telescoped portions of the septum are resected creating additional mucosal and cartilage injury and causing further loss of nasal height. Septal reconstruction procedures are generally best performed secondarily. All patients with nasal fractures should be warned that a late

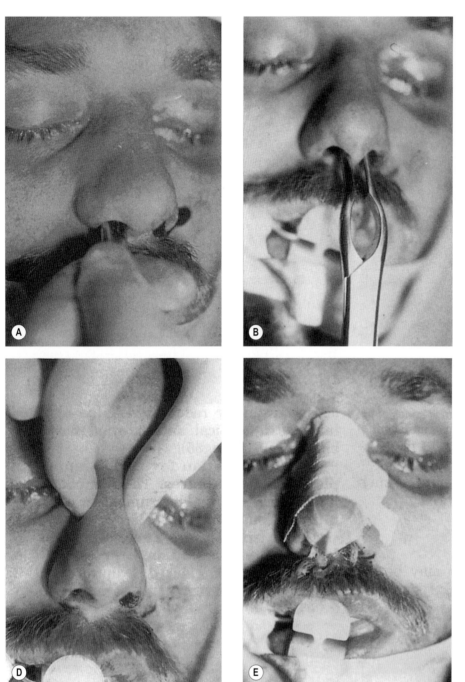

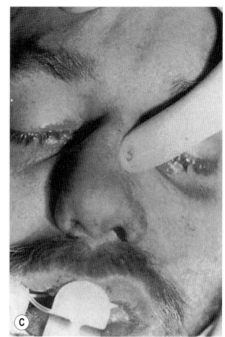

Fig. 3.14 Reduction of a nasal fracture. (**A**) After vasoconstriction of the nasal mucous membrane with pseudoephedrine-soaked pledgets the nasal bones are "outfractured" with a Boies nasal elevator. (**B**) The septum is then straightened with an Asch forceps. Both the nasal bones and the septum should be able to be freely dislocated in each direction (**C**) if the fractures have been completed. If the incomplete fractures have been completed properly, the nasal bones may then be molded back into the midline and remain in reduction (**D**). Care must be taken to avoid placing the reduction instruments into the intracranial space through a fracture or congenital defect in the cribriform plate. (**E**) Steri-Strips and adhesive tape are applied to the nose, and a splint is applied over the tape. Intranasal Doyle splints are placed inside the nose to minimize clot and hematoma in the distal portion of the nose.

rhinoplasty is expected for correcting deviation, irregularity, loss of nasal height, or nasal airway obstruction.

Complications of nasal fractures

Hematomas of the nasal septum, while uncommon, may result in subperichondrial fibrosis and thickening with partial nasal airway obstruction. The septum in these cases may be as thick as 1 cm in areas and may require trimming. In the case of repeated trauma, the cartilages of the septum may be largely replaced with calcified or chondrified material. Submucous resection of thickened portions of the nasal septum

may be required, and in many patients turbinate outfracture, or partial resection of enlarged turbinates, may simultaneously be advisable.

Synechiae may form between the septum and the turbinates in areas where soft tissue lacerations occur and the tissues are in contact. These may be treated by division and placement of a Doyle splint between the cut surfaces for a period of 10–14 days.

Obstruction of the nasal vestibule may occur as a result of malunited fractures of the pyriform margin, especially if displaced and telescoped medially, or from overlap or lateral displacement of the nasal septum into the ipsilateral airway.

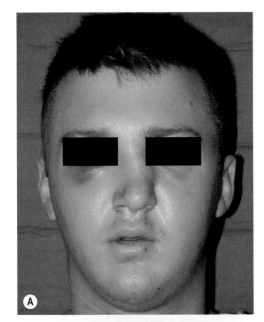

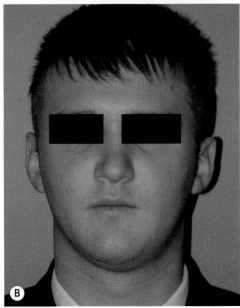

Fig. 3.15 (**A**) Preoperative and (**B**) postoperative images of a 20-year-old male who sustained a nasoethmoidal orbital fracture during a wrestling match.

Osteotomy of the bone fragments can correct displaced fractures; however, contracture due to shrinkage or loss of soft tissue lining may require excision of the scar and replacement with mucosal or composite grafts within the nasal vestibule or in some cases flap reconstruction.

Residual osteitis or infection of the bone or cartilage is occasionally seen in compound fractures of the nose. These conditions are usually treated by repeated conservative debridements until the infected focus is completely removed. Secondary soft tissue grafting may restore absent tissue. Chronic pain is infrequent and usually affects the external nasal branches of the trigeminal nerve.[75]

Malunion of nasal fractures is common after closed reductions, since the exact anatomic position of the bone fragments is difficult to confirm or achieve by palpation alone, and the presence of closed splinting may not prevent recurrent deviation owing to the release of "interlocked stresses" in cartilage.[76,77] Any external or internal deformity of significance may require a corrective rhinoplasty.

Nasoethmoidal orbital fractures

Nasoethmoidal orbital fractures are severe fractures of the central one-third of the upper midfacial skeleton. They comminute the nose, the medial orbital rims, and the pyriform aperture. Nasoethmoidal fractures are isolated in one-third and extended in two-thirds of cases to involve either the frontal bone, zygoma, or maxilla. One-third are unilateral and two-thirds are bilateral.

The central feature characterizing nasoethmoidal orbital fractures is the displacement of the lower two-thirds of the medial orbital rim, which provides the attachment of the medial canthal ligament. Any fractures that separate this part of the frontal process of the maxilla with its canthal-bearing tendon potentially allow canthal displacement.

Surgical pathology

The bones that form the skeletal framework of the nose are projected backward between the orbits when subjected to strong traumatic forces. These bones form the junction between the cranial, orbital, and nasal cavities. A typical cause of a nasoethmoidal orbital fracture is a blunt impact applied over the upper portion of the bridge of the nose producing a crush in the upper central midface. The severity of the impact or penetrating injuries may burst the soft tissues, producing an open, compound, comminuted injury. When displacement of the upper nose and anterior frontal sinus occur, no further resistance is offered by the delicate "matchbox-like" structures of the interorbital space; indeed, these structures "collapse and splinter".

Interorbital space

The term *"interorbital space"* designates an area between the orbits and below the floor of the anterior cranial fossa. The "interorbital space" contains two ethmoidal labyrinths, one on each side, and consists of the ethmoidal cells, the superior and middle turbinates, and a median thick plate of septal bone and the perpendicular plate of the ethmoid.

Traumatic telecanthus and hypertelorism

Traumatic telecanthus is an increase in the distance between the medial canthal ligaments. The patient has a characteristic appearance of telecanthus, where the medial canthal ligaments are further apart than normal. The eyes may appear to be further apart, simulating orbital hypertelorism.[78,79] Traumatic orbital hypertelorism[80] (as opposed to telecanthus) is a deformity characterized by an increase in the distance between the orbits and the ocular globe[81] and requires bilateral laterally displaced zygoma fractures in addition to bilateral nasoethmoidal orbital fractures.

Clinical examination

The appearance of patients who suffer nasoethmoidal orbital fractures is typical. A significant frontal impact nasal fracture is generally present, with the nose flattened and appearing to have been pushed between the eyes. There is a loss of dorsal nasal prominence, and an obtuse angle is noted between the lip and columella. Finger pressure on the nose may document inadequate distal septal or proximal bony support. The medial canthal areas are swollen and distorted with palpebral and subconjunctival hematomas. Ecchymosis and subconjunctival hemorrhage are the usual findings. Crepitus or movement may be palpated when external pressure is deeply applied directly over the canthal ligament. A "bimanual examination" of the medial orbital rim is helpful if the diagnosis is uncertain: it is performed by placing a palpating finger deeply over one medial canthal ligament and placing a clamp inside the nose with its tip directly opposite the pad of the finger. The frontal process of the maxilla may then, if fractured, be moved between the index finger and the clamp, indicating instability and confirming both the diagnosis and the need for an open reduction. The clamp, if placed under the nasal bones too anteriorly (and not at the medial orbital rim to medial canthal ligament attachment), erroneously identifies a nasal fracture as canthal instability.

Radiographs

CT scans are essential to document the injury. The diagnosis of a nasoethmoidal orbital fracture on radiographs requires at a minimum four fractures that isolate the frontal process of the maxilla from adjacent bones. These include (1) fractures of the nose, (2) fractures of the junction of the frontal process of the maxilla with the frontal bone, (3) fractures of the medial orbit (ethmoidal area), and (4) fractures of the inferior orbital rim extending to involve the pyriform aperture and orbital floor. These fracture lines, therefore, define the "central fragment" of bone bearing the medial canthal ligament as "free" and, depending on periosteal integrity, may displace the medial orbital rim.

Classification of nasoethmoidal orbital fractures

Nasoethmoidal fractures are classified according to a pattern established by Markowitz and Manson[82] types I–III, according to the bimanual examination and the CT scan.[83]

Type I is an incomplete fracture, mostly unilateral but occasionally bilateral, which is displaced only inferiorly at the infraorbital rim and piriform margin. Inferior alone approaches (gingival buccal sulcus +/− inferior orbit) are necessary (Fig. 3.16).

Type II nasoethmoidal orbital fractures are comminuted nasoethmoidal fractures with the fractures remaining outside the area of the canthal ligament insertion. The central fragment may be managed as a sizable bony fragment and united to the canthal ligament-bearing fragment of the other side with a transnasal wire reduction. The remainder of the pieces of the nasoethmoidal orbital skeleton are reduced and then stabilized by junctional plate and screw fixation to the frontal bone, the infraorbital rim, and the Le Fort I level of the maxilla. Type II fractures may be unilateral or bilateral (Fig. 3.17).

Type III nasoethmoidal orbital fractures either have avulsion of the canthal ligament (uncommon) or the fractures extend underneath the canthal ligament insertion. The fracture fragments are small enough that a reduction would require that the canthus be detached to accomplish the

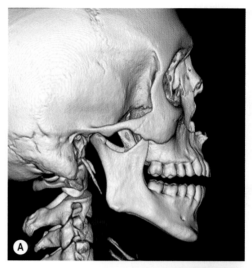

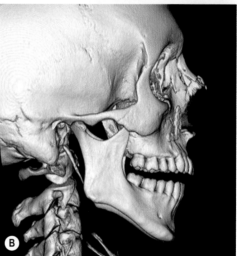

Fig. 3.16 (A,B) Lateral image of 3D craniofacial computer tomography scan of a type 1 nasoethmoidal orbital fracture injury pattern pre- and post-open reduction and internal fixation of midface fractures using the inferior alone approach.

bone reduction. Therefore, canthal ligament reattachment is required as a separate step, accomplished with its own set of transnasal wires for each of the bone of the medial orbital rim and then the canthus. In general, the bony reduction of the intercanthal distance should be 5–7 mm per side less than the desired soft tissue distance (Fig. 3.18).

Treatment of nasoethmoidal orbital fractures

Treatment consists of a thorough exposure of the nasal orbital region by, at most, three incisions: a coronal (or an appropriate laceration or local upper nasal incision (midline or transverse radix), a lower eyelid incision, and a gingival buccal sulcus incision.[84] Nasal and forehead lacerations are common but should not be extended, as the scar deformity from extension is frequently worse than making a separate incision.

The primary principle underlying open treatment of nasoethmoidal orbital fractures involves the preservation of all fragments of bone and their accurate reassembly. Despite even anatomic reassembly of the nasal bone fragments, primary bone grafting is usually necessary to improve the

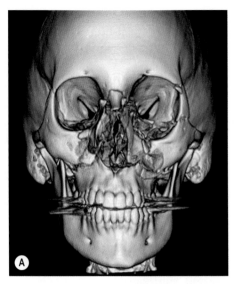 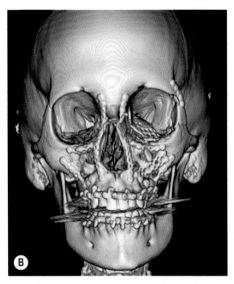 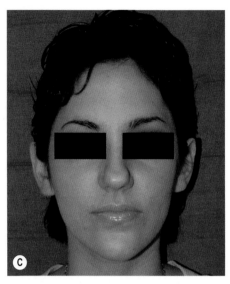

Fig. 3.17 (A) Frontal 3D craniofacial computer tomography scan of a type II nasoethmoidal orbital fracture injury pattern in a 23-year-old female who sustained craniofacial injuries following being struck by a motor vehicle as a pedestrian. **(B)** Pre- and post-open reduction and internal fixation of midface fractures. **(C)** Postoperative frontal photograph view of patient approximately 12 months from surgery.

nasal height and to provide smooth dorsal contour. The bone onto which the canthal ligament is attached (if comminuted) may require replacement with a bone graft.

The importance of the "central fragment" in nasoethmoidal orbital fractures

First, identify and classify what is happening to the bone of the medial orbital rim which bears the medial canthal ligament as there is a direct relationship between surgical techniques, simplicity of surgery, and outcome of the treatment.

The most essential feature of a nasoethmoidal reduction is the transnasal reduction of the medial orbital rims by a wire placed posterior and superior through the bone of the canthal ligament insertion. The medial orbital rim with its attached canthal-bearing segment is first dislocated anteriorly and

laterally and brought clearly into the surgeon's view laterally and next to the nasal bones, where its superficial position allows turning of the fragment; in this position, drilling and wire pass through the "central" fragment. Nasal bone fragments can be temporarily dislocated or removed to permit better exposure of the medial orbital rim segments. Removing the nasal bones is especially helpful in passing a transnasal wire from the posterior and superior aspect of one "central" fragment (medial orbital rim canthal bearing bone fragment) to the other. The medial orbital rims are then replaced in anatomic position and then linked with fine wires to adjacent nasal and frontal bone fragments. Following the placement of two transnasal wires, one should pass one extra wire per side, for soft tissue reapproximation to bone. Junctional plate and screw fixation at the periphery of these reassembled fragments is employed after the initial interfragment wiring is

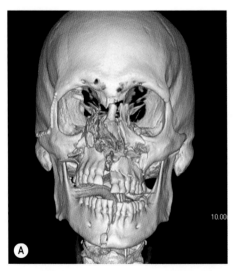 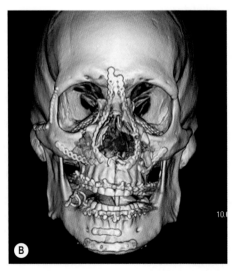 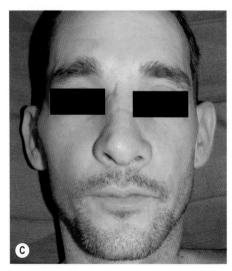

Fig. 3.18 (A) Frontal 3D craniofacial computer tomography scan of type III nasoethmoidal orbital and a Le Fort II type injury pattern in a 33-year-old who sustained craniofacial injuries following being thrown off a motorcycle without a helmet. **(B)** Pre- and post-open reduction and internal fixation of midface and mandibular fractures. **(C)** Postoperative frontal photograph view of patient 6 months from surgery.

tightened. It should be emphasized that the transnasal reduction wires must be passed posterior and superior to the lacrimal fossa in order to provide the proper direction of draping force necessary to create the preinjury bony position and shape of the canthal ligaments. The transnasal reduction is not a "transnasal canthopexy", as it does not involve the canthal ligament per se. It is a reduction only of the "central bony fragment" of the nasoethmoidal orbital fracture.

Canthal reattachment

If the canthal ligament requires reattachment (the canthal tendon is rarely stripped from bone), the canthal tendon[85] may be grasped by one or two passes of 2-0 nonabsorbable suture adjacent to the medial commissure of the eyelids through a 2–3 mm horizontal incision in the skin directly over the canthal ligament.[86] The 2-0 nonabsorbable suture is then passed into the internal aspect of the coronal incision, and the suture is then connected to a separate set of #28 transnasal wires per side that have been passed transnasally superiorly and posteriorly to the expected position of the medial canthus. The transnasal canthal ligament wires are tightened only as the last step after the bone reduction, and after medial orbital and nasal bone grafting are completed. Each set of canthal wires is tightened gently after a manual reduction of the canthus to the bone with forceps is performed, to reduce stress on the ligament by the canthal sutures. Each canthal reduction wire pair is then separately twisted over a screw in the frontal bone.

Lacrimal system injury

Interruption of the continuity of the lacrimal apparatus demands specific action. Most lacrimal system obstruction occurs from bony malposition or damage to the lacrimal sac or duct.[87] The most effective treatment involves initial satisfactory precise repositioning of fracture segments to the bony part of the lacrimal system. If transection of the soft tissue portion of the canalicular lacrimal system has occurred, it should be repaired over fine silicone tubes with magnification.[88]

Complications of nasoethmoidal orbital fractures

The early diagnosis and adequate treatment of nasoethmoidal orbital fractures achieves optimal aesthetic results with the lowest number of late complications. Depending on the quality of initial treatment and the results of healing, further reconstructive surgery may be required in some cases. Late complications, such as frontal sinus obstruction, occur in less than 5% of isolated nasoethmoidal orbital fractures where damage to the anterior frontal sinus walls has not occurred. Deformities and nasal functional impairment are late complications, which can be minimized by early diagnosis and proper early open reduction. The presence of a nasoethmoidal orbital fracture may be obscured by the swelling and escape detection. After several weeks, nasal deformity and enophthalmos are evident.[89]

Fractures of the zygoma

The zygoma is a major buttress of the midfacial skeleton. It forms the malar eminence, giving prominence to the cheek, and forms the lateral and inferior portions of the orbit. The zygomatic bone has a quadrilateral shape with several processes that extend to reach the frontal bone, the maxilla, the temporal bone (zygomatic arch), and orbital processes.

Physical diagnosis and surgical pathology of zygoma fractures

Although the zygoma is a sturdy bone, it is frequently injured because of its prominent location. Moderately severe blows are absorbed at the malar eminence and transferred to its buttresses. Severe blows may cause separation of the zygomatic body at its articulating surfaces; these high-energy injuries dramatically increase the width of the midface. As the zygoma is disrupted, it is usually displaced in a downward, medial, and posterior direction, whereas high-energy injuries displace the zygoma in a posterior and lateral direction because of disruption of the ligaments in addition to the fractures. The direction of displacement varies with the direction of the injuring force and with the pull of the muscles, such as that of the masseter.

Periorbital and subconjunctival hematomas are the most accurate physical signs of the orbital fracture always associated with a complete zygoma fracture. Numbness of the infraorbital nerve is a common symptom as well. The infraorbital nerve runs in a groove in the posterior portion of the orbit and enters a canal in the anterior third of the orbit, behind the infraorbital rim.[90] It may be crushed in a rim fracture with medial displacement, as the fracture occurs in the weak area of bone penetrated by the infraorbital foramen. Direct force to the lateral face may result in isolated fractures of the temporal extension of the zygoma (zygomatic arch) and the zygomatic process of the temporal bone in the absence of a fracture of the remainder of the zygoma and its articulations.

Medial displacement of an isolated arch fracture is usually observed and may impinge against the temporalis muscle and coronoid process of the mandible resulting in restricted mandibular motion. Fractures in the posterior portion of the zygomatic arch may enter the glenoid fossa and produce stiffness or a change in occlusion because of the swelling in the joint or muscles. In high-energy injuries or gunshots, fragments of bone can be driven through the temporal muscle and make contact with the coronoid process and precipitate the formation of a fibrous or bony ankylosis, necessitating excision of the bone of the coronoid process and scar tissue as a secondary procedure.

Fracture dislocation of the zygomatic body with sufficient displacement to impinge on the coronoid process requires considerable backward dislocation of the malar eminence. Level discrepancies or step deformities at the infraorbital margin can usually be palpated in the presence of inferior orbital rim displacement. The lateral and superior walls of the maxillary sinuses are involved in fractures of the zygoma, and torn maxillary sinus lining results in bleeding within the sinus with unilateral epistaxis. The lateral canthal attachment is directed towards Whitnall's tubercle, located approximately 10 mm below the zygomaticofrontal suture, which is a shallow eminence on the internal aspect of the frontal process of the zygoma. When the zygoma is displaced inferiorly, the lateral attachment of the eyelids via the lateral canthal ligament is also displaced inferiorly giving rise to an antimongoloid slant of the palpebral fissure. The globe follows the inferior displacement of the zygoma with a lower (inferior and lateral) position after fracture dislocation. Double vision is usually transient in uncomplicated fractures of the zygoma, which always involve the orbital floor. Diplopia may persist when the fracture is more extensive, especially if a fracture comminutes the inferior orbital floor. Diplopia may result from muscle contusion, incarceration of perimuscular soft tissue or actual muscle incarceration (rare in zygoma fractures), or simply drooping of the muscular sling.

Anterior approaches

The anterior approach may be partial or complete and potentially involves up to three incisions: (1) access to the zygomaticofrontal suture; (2) access to the inferior orbital rim; and (3) access to the zygomaticomaxillary buttress, anterior maxilla, and malar prominence.

Twenty-five percent of complete fractures of the zygoma are undisplaced or have such subtle displacement that they do not benefit from an open reduction. Thirty-five percent of fracture dislocations of the zygoma result in greensticked fractures at the zygomaticofrontal suture, and these may be reduced with a gingivobuccal sulcus incision alone without exposure of the suture. Forty percent of fracture dislocations of the zygoma result in complete separation at the zygomaticofrontal suture, which may be palpable through the skin over the upper lateral margin of the orbit. The latter fractures require exposure through an incision directly over the suture, i.e., the lateral limb alone of an upper lid blepharoplasty. Orbital rim and orbital floor exposures may be necessary based on the fracture patterns visualized on preoperative CT scans.[91]

"Minimalist" approaches for fractures without zygomaticofrontal suture diastasis

In this approach, the gingivobuccal sulcus is opened and the anterior face of the maxilla and zygoma are degloved. The infraorbital rim and infraorbital nerve are visualized from an inferior direction. Palpation with a finger on the rim avoids entry of elevators into the orbit as the maxilla and zygoma are dissected. The infraorbital nerve is protected by the dissection and is immediately seen after detaching the levator anguli oris muscle. The zygoma may often be reduced by placing the tip of an elevator in the lateral aspect of the maxillary sinus directly behind the malar eminence and levering the body of the zygoma first outward and then forward. Alternately, a Carrol–Girard screw (Walter Lorenz Co., Jacksonville, FL) can be placed in the malar eminence through a percutaneous incision and manipulated. In gingival buccal sulcus approaches, after the reduction maneuver has been completed, zygomatic stability depends upon an incomplete fracture at the zygomaticofrontal suture. The floor of the orbit can be inspected with an endoscope through the maxillary sinus. It is also possible to tell from a preoperative CT the degree of orbital floor comminution. Fractures with orbital floor comminution and significant displacement require an additional inferior orbital approach.

Fractures with zygomaticofrontal (Z-F) suture diastasis

If the Z-F suture demonstrates diastasis, direct exposure of the suture permits stabilization through the lateral portion of an upper blepharoplasty incision (<1 cm) which is made directly over the Z-F suture 8–10 mm above the lateral canthus. Palpating the frontal process of the zygoma between the thumb and index finger, the junction of the zygoma with the frontal bone can be marked precisely in eyelid skin. The incision should be short and never progress laterally out of the eyelid skin, as it will scar noticeably. Alternately, the Z-F suture may be approached through a laceration or by superior dissection from a subciliary or conjunctival lower lid incision by canthal detachment. The inferior portion of the orbit may be approached through a midtarsal, subciliary, or conjunctival incision. The conjunctival fornix incision produces the least cutaneous scarring, but the exposure may be restricted by fat prolapse. The treatment of a zygoma fracture has recently become quite specific and directed only at areas that require open reduction for confirmation of alignment or for fixation (Fig. 3.19).

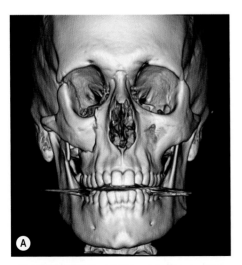
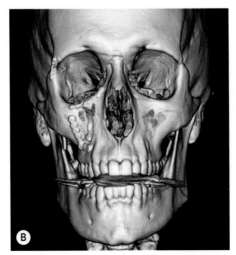
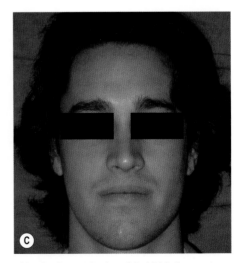

Fig. 3.19 (A,B) Frontal 3D craniofacial computer tomography scan of a right zygomaticomaxillary fracture in a 22-year-old male who sustained craniofacial injuries following a sports-related injury, pre- and post-open reduction and internal fixation of the right zygomaticomaxillary complex and orbital floor fractures. **(C)** Postoperative frontal photograph view of patient 3 months following surgery.

Coronal incisions (posterior approach)

Fractures with extreme posterior displacement and those with lateral displacement of the zygomatic arch often benefit from the addition of a coronal incision. These represent 5% of isolated zygoma fractures. The coronal incision allows exposure of the entire zygomatic arch, roof of the glenoid fossa, the Z-F suture, and the lateral orbital wall, which is the area that confirms proper alignment and medial position of the zygomatic arch (Fig. 3.20).

Treatment of fractures of the zygoma

Closed reduction

Remotely, closed reduction techniques were employed for most zygomatic fractures. In practice, many fractures can be treated reasonably with closed reduction, and especially where cost is an issue, this treatment would have to be considered. Those fractures still amenable to closed reduction

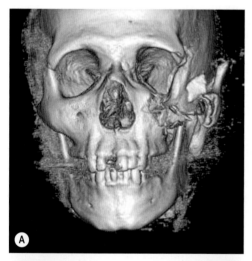

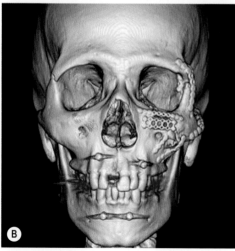

Fig. 3.20 (A) Frontal 3D craniofacial computer tomography scan of a high energy orbito-zygomaticomaxillary complex injury in a 33-year-old who sustained craniofacial injuries following a high speed motor vehicle collision. **(B)** Pre- and post-open reduction and internal fixation of the left orbital and zygomaticomaxillary complex through anterior and posterior (coronal) approaches.

include medial displaced isolated arch fractures and simple large segment or single piece zygoma fractures in which the displacement is medial and posterior, without comminution at the buttresses, and where the fracture at the Z-F suture is incomplete and nondisplaced. An elevator placed beneath the malar eminence allows the zygoma to be "popped" back into position. Palpation is the guide to reduction, such as the inferior orbital rim. The stability of closed reduction depends on the integrity of periosteal attachments and principally "greensticking" at the Z-F suture. The force of contraction of the masseter muscle may act to create postoperative displacement.[92]

Displacement at the Z-F suture[93] comminution of the inferior orbital rim or Z-M buttress and lateral displacement of the zygomatic arch and body are characteristics that were found to predict a poor result from closed reduction.

Buttress articulations and alignment for complete open reduction

Six points of alignment with adjacent bone may be confirmed with complete craniofacial exposures: Z-F suture, infraorbital rim, zygomaticomaxillary buttress, greater wing of the sphenoid, orbital floor, and zygomatic arch. The orbital floor may require reconstruction with bone or artificial materials such as Medpor or titanium mesh.

Methods of reduction

The first step that should be considered in complete open reductions is passing an osteotome through the Z-F suture after exposing it, mobilizing and thoroughly completing all fractures. This step is the most neglected step in open reduction internal fixation (ORIF) of zygomas and routinely simplifies the rest of the reduction.

Reduction through the maxillary sinus

Next, the body of the zygoma is mobilized by displacing it laterally, completing fractures and achieving free displacement and mobility. A Carroll–Girard screw (Walter Lorenzo, Jacksonville, FL) may be utilized percutaneously or from an intraoral approach providing leverage to manipulate the zygoma. This approach is used by persons who do not complete the fractures.

Temporal approach

A temporal approach for the reduction of zygomatic fractures was described by Gilles. An elevator is slipped along the muscle behind the zygomatic arch or under the malar eminence, depending on the areas of reduction required. A small, 2-cm incision placed vertically within the temporal hair heals with an inconspicuous scar. The elevator must be placed deep to the deep temporal fascia, visualizing the temporalis muscle. The bone may be palpated with one hand to document the accuracy of reduction, while the other hand guides the elevator into position and corrects the displacement by force application. Gentle elevation often "clicks" the arch into position. Moving the elevator back and forth with repeated elevation movements may disrupt the periosteum holding arch fragments together, and an open reduction is then required. The approach can also be used for reduction of the zygomatic body.

Fixation required to achieve stability

Several individuals have examined zygomatic stability following open reduction. Rinehart and Marsh[94] studied cadaver heads and used 1, 2, or 3 miniplates and accessed stability of non-comminuted zygoma fractures submitted to static and oscillating loads to simulate the effect of the masticatory apparatus on postoperative displacement. Neither single miniplate nor triple wire fixation was enough to stabilize the zygoma against simulated masseter forces; however, 3 miniplates were sufficient, which stabilized the Z-F, Z-M, and infraorbital rim areas.

Del Santo and Ellis felt that Rinehart and Marsh overestimated the postoperative forces that could be generated by the masseter muscle and suggested that stability with less than 3 plates would be possible, based upon actual human measurements of bite forces after zygomatic fracture treatment.[92]

Surgical techniques for fixation following reduction

The authors' approach varies depending on the complexity of zygoma fracture pattern and the extent of involvement of the orbital floor, which can be assessed using preoperative CT scan.[95]

If there is minimal involvement of the orbital floor and no diastasis at the Z- suture, the zygoma is approached intraorally at the zygomaticomaxillary buttress. It is reduced using one of the techniques described above, and one plate fixation technique is sufficient using an L-shaped plate at the zygomaticomaxillary buttress. If there is diastasis at the Z-F fracture line, then a short (1 cm) upper blepharoplasty incision exposes the Z-F fracture line, a portion of the lateral orbital wall, and the zygomaticosphenoid suture line. Here, the zygoma has its broadest articulation with the greater wing of the sphenoid, and therefore direct visualization may be helpful in confirming anatomical reduction of the zygoma. Since one can only look through one incision at a time, the use of temporary interfragment wire positioning at the Z-F fracture line while holding the zygoma into correct anatomical reduction at the zygomatic–sphenoid fracture line, inferior orbital rim, and zygomaticomaxillary buttress allows relative positioning of the zygoma fracture. The zygomaticomaxillary buttress followed by the Z-F fracture line may then be plated sequentially.

In the authors' experience, the judgment of whether to open the lower lid rests upon whether (1) there is a large orbital floor fracture component of the zygoma fracture that requires replacement, or (2) there remains a significant step-off at a comminuted inferior orbital rim following fracture reduction. A lower eyelid transconjunctival incision without lateral canthoplasty allows reduction and fixation with a low profile inferior orbital rim plate +/− an orbital floor plate. Periosteal resuspension of the lower eyelid and cheek is critically important should eyelid exposure be utilized.[96]

Delayed treatment of fractures of the zygoma

Repositioning after two weeks frequently requires osteotomy of the fracture sites to mobilize the zygoma for reduction. After the bone has been mobilized, an inspection of each fracture site should be conducted to remove any area of fibrous ankylosis or any proliferative bone, which was not present originally, as its presence may prevent proper alignment. Rarely, resorption has occurred requiring bone grafting.

Plate and screw fixation then unites the segments. In fractures treated late, the masseter muscle may require division or mobilization from the inferior surface of the malar eminence and arch in order to allow the bone to be repositioned superiorly. The masseter muscle contracts in the case of the malreduced fracture and may block reduction. Fractures treated with delay are more safely treated with osteotomy than forceful mobilization by blunt forces, which may result in new undesirable fracture lines radiating into the apex of the orbit, with cranial nerve injury (blindness).

Complications of zygomatic fractures

Bleeding and maxillary sinusitis

Bleeding into the maxillary sinus is usually of short duration. It is always prudent to irrigate blood clots from the antrum and to remove bone fragments, which drop from the orbital floor and sequester. Rarely, the ostea of the maxillary sinus will be occluded by the fractures and require endoscopic sinus surgery. In those patients with pre-existing sinus disease, acute exacerbation may be a complicating factor.

Late complications

Late complications of zygomatic fractures include nonunion, malunion, double vision, infraorbital nerve anesthesia or hypesthesia, and chronic maxillary sinusitis. Scarring may result from laceration or malpositioned incisions. Generally, ectropion and scleral show are mild and resolve spontaneously. Gross downward dislocation of the zygoma results in diplopia and orbital dystopia. Usually, more than 5 mm of inferior globe dystopia is required to produce diplopia. Treatment[97] involves zygomatic mobilization by osteotomy with bone grafting to augment the malar eminence when malar projection is deficient. The position of the eye must be restored with intraorbital bone grafts or alloplastic material. Infection is not common, and usually responds to antibiotics and sinus or lacrimal drainage.

Impacted fractures of the zygomatic arch which abut the coronoid process may result in ankylosis. A gunshot wound is especially prone to this problem. If the zygomatic arch cannot be repositioned, coronoidectomy through an intraoral route usually frees the mandible from the ankylosis and permits normal function. It is important that the patient vigorously exercise to preserve and improve the range of motion obtained, which may take 6 months.

Orbital complications

Orbital complications consist of diplopia, visual loss, globe injury, enophthalmos or exophthalmos, and lid position abnormalities.

Numbness

Persistent anesthesia or hypesthesia in the distribution of the infraorbital nerve usually lasts only a short time. If total anesthesia exists for over six months, it is likely that the nerve is severely damaged or perhaps transected. If the nerve is impinged by bone fragments, especially in a medially and posteriorly impacted zygoma fracture, reduction or decompression of the infraorbital canal and neurolysis are sometimes indicated. Bone spurs or constricting portions of the canal should be removed so that the nerve has an adequate opportunity for regeneration and relief of pressure. The nerve must be explored throughout the floor of the orbit so that it is free from any compression by bone fragments, scar tissue, or callus. The functional results of this surgery in terms of pain relief remain unclear.

Anesthesia can be annoying for patients, especially immediately after the injury. Patients generally partially accommodate to the neurological deficit. Some spontaneous reinnervation may occur from adjacent facial regions as well as regrowth of axons through the infraorbital nerve. Usually some vague sensation is then present.

Oral–antral fistula

An oral–antral fistula requires debridement of bone or mucosa, confirmation of maxillary sinus drainage into the nose, and closure with a transposition mucosal flap for cover. A 2-layer closure is required. A bone graft may be placed in between the layers of soft tissue. The buccal fat pad can be mobilized and sewn into the defect prior to the mucosa being closed over it. Rarely, a distant flap is required for difficult persistent fistulae.

Plate complications

Complications include screw loosening or extrusion, plate exposure requiring removal, and tooth root penetration by screws. Prominent plates over the zygomatic arch are directly due to associated soft tissue atrophy (temporalis) and to malreduction of the zygomatic arch laterally. Probably 10% of plates placed at the LeFort I level need to be removed for exposure, non-healing wound, or cold sensitivity. Plate prominence at the Z-F suture are due to inadequate soft tissue closure and poor plate selection.[98]

Midface buttresses

The midface is a system of sinus cavities where certain thicker areas (or buttresses) provide considerable structural support. The important midface supporting skeleton consists of horizontal and vertical structural supports connected by thin plates of bone. In fracture treatment, the thicker pillars are anatomically reconstructed and repositioned to re-establish the preinjury facial bone architecture. The vertical supports consist of the nasal septum in the midline and the nasomaxillary, zygomaticomaxillary, and pterygoid buttresses (Fig. 3.21). The nasomaxillary buttress extends along the pyriform aperture through the frontal process of the maxilla superiorly to the internal angular process of the frontal bone. The zygomaticomaxillary buttress extends through the bony mass of the body of the zygoma and through the frontal process of the zygoma to the external angular process of the frontal bone. Posteriorly, the pterygoid plates provide posterior stabilization of the vertical height of the midface to the skull base.[99] The horizontal buttresses of the midface consist of the inferior orbital rims and the associated orbital floor, the zygomatic arch and the palate at the level of the maxillary alveolus.[100]

Clinical examination

Inspection

Epistaxis, bilateral ecchymosis (periorbital, subconjunctival, scleral), facial edema, and subcutaneous hematoma are sug-

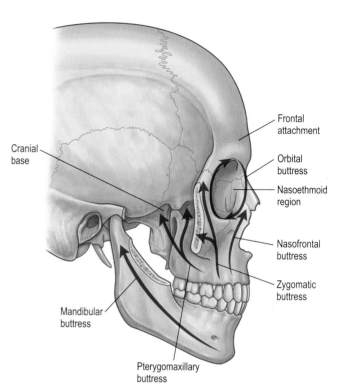

Fig. 3.21 The vertical buttresses of the midfacial skeleton. Anteriorly, the nasofrontal buttress skirts the piriform aperture inferiorly and composes the bone of the medial orbital rim superiorly to reach the frontal bone at its internal angular process. Laterally the zygomaticomaxillary buttress extends from the zygomatic process of the frontal bone through the lateral aspect of the zygoma to reach the maxillary alveolus. A component of the zygomaticomaxillary buttress extends laterally through the zygomatic arch to reach the temporal bone. Posteriorly, the pterygomaxillary buttress is seen. It extends from the posterior portion of the maxilla and the pterygoid fossa to reach the cranial base structures. The mandibular buttress forms a strong structural support for the lower midface in fracture treatment. This support for maxillary fracture reduction must conceptually be achieved by placement of both jaws in intermaxillary fixation. The other "transverse" maxillary buttresses include the palate, the superior orbital rims, and the inferior orbital rims. The superior orbital rims and the lower sections of the frontal sinus are also known in the supraorbital regions as the frontal bar and are technically frontal bone and not part of the maxilla. *(From Manson PN, Hoopes JE, Su CT. Structural pillars of the facial skeleton: an approach to the management of Le Fort fractures. Plast Reconstr Surg. 1980;66:54.)*

gestive of fractures involving the maxillary bone. The swelling is usually moderate to severe indicating the severity of the fracture. Malocclusion with an anterior open bite and rotation of the maxilla suggest a fracture of the maxilla. The maxillary segment is frequently displaced downward and posteriorly, resulting in a class III malocclusion and premature occlusion in the posterior dentition with an anterior open bite. On internal examination, there may be tearing of the soft tissues in the labial vestibule of the lip or the palate, findings that indicate the possibility of an alveolar or palate fracture. Hematomas may be present in the buccal or palatal mucosa. The face, after several days, may have an elongated, retruded appearance, the so-called "donkey-like faces" suggestive of a craniofacial disjunction. An increase in midfacial length is seen.

Palpation

The bone should be palpated with the tips of the fingers both externally through the skin and internally intraorally. Bilateral palpation may reveal step deformities of the zygomaticomaxillary suture, indicating fractures of the inferior orbital rims. These findings suggest a pyramidal fracture of the maxilla and confirm the zygomatic component of a more complicated injury, such as a Le Fort III fracture. Intraoral palpation may reveal fractures of the anterior portion of the maxilla or fractured segments of the alveolar bone.

Digital manipulation

Manipulation of the maxilla may confirm movement in the entire middle third of the face, including the bridge of the nose. This movement is appreciated by holding the head securely with one hand and moving the maxilla with the other hand (see Fig. 3.5). Crepitation may be heard when the maxilla is manipulated in loose fractures. The manipulation test for maxillary mobility is not entirely diagnostic because impacted or greenstick fractures may exhibit no movement but still possess bone displacement and malocclusion.

Malocclusion of the teeth

If the mandible is intact, malocclusion of the teeth is highly suggestive of a maxillary fracture. It is possible, however, that malocclusion relates to a preinjury condition. A thorough study of the patient's dentition and dental models and reference to previous dental records and pictures are helpful.

Cerebral spinal rhinorrhea or otorrhea

Cerebral spinal fluid may leak from the anterior or middle cranial fossa in high Le Fort fractures and is then apparent in the nose or ear canal. A fluid leak signifies the presence of a dural fistula extending from the intracranial subarachnoid space through the skull and into the nose, pharynx or ear.[101] Frequently the drainage is obscured by bloody secretions in the immediate postinjury period.[102,103]

Radiological examination

Maxillary fractures are easily demonstrated in craniofacial CT scans, with the exception that fracture lines in minimally displaced fractures are more difficult to image. The presence of bilateral maxillary sinus fluid should always suggest the possibility of a maxillary fracture.

Treatment of maxillary fractures

Treatment of maxillary fractures is initially oriented toward the establishment of an airway, control of hemorrhage, closure of soft tissue lacerations, and placement of the patient in intermaxillary fixation. The latter manually reduces the fracture, reduces movement and bleeding, and is the single most important step in the treatment of a maxillary fracture. Postoperative intermaxillary fixation may not be necessary after open reduction of large segment maxillary fractures but is increasingly useful for several weeks after comminuted fracture treatment and in panfacial fractures or palatal fractures, where rigid stability is difficult to obtain.[104]

Alveolar fractures

Simple fractures of the portions of the maxilla involving the alveolar process and the teeth can usually be digitally repositioned and held in reduction while an arch bar is applied to these teeth. The position of the teeth may be maintained by ligating the teeth in the fractured segment to adjacent teeth with the use of an arch bar and interdental wiring technique. Fixation of the alveolar segment should be maintained for at least six to twelve weeks, until clinical immobility has been achieved.[105]

Le Fort classification of facial fractures

Le Fort (1901) completed experiments that determined the areas of structural weakness of the maxilla which he designated "lines of weakness" where fractures occurred. Between the lines of weakness were "areas of strength". This classification led to the Le Fort classification of maxillary fractures, which identifies the patterns of midfacial fractures (Fig. 3.22).[106] It should be emphasized that the usual Le Fort fracture consists of combinations of these patterns in that pure bilateral Le Fort I, Le Fort II, or Le Fort III fractures are less common than combination patterns.[107] The level of fracture is frequently higher on one side than the other, and usually the fracture is more comminuted and extensive on the side of the direct injury.

Goals of Le Fort fracture treatment

Goals in the treatment of Le Fort fractures include:

1. Restoration of midfacial height and projection.
2. Achieve proper occlusion.
3. Restore the integrity of the nose and orbit.

The structural supports between the areas of the buttresses and maxillary alveolus are restored to provide proper soft tissue contour.

Transverse (Guerin) fractures or Le Fort I level fractures

Fractures which traverse the maxilla horizontally above the level of the apices of the maxillary teeth section the entire alveolar process of the maxilla, vault of the palate and the inferior ends of the pterygoid processes in a single block from the upper craniofacial skeleton. This type of injury is known as the transverse, Le Fort I, or Guerin fracture. This horizontal fracture extends transversely across the base of the maxillary sinuses and is usually bilateral. The fracture level varies from just beneath the orbital rim of the zygoma to just above the floor of the maxillary sinus and the inferior margin of the pyriform aperture (Fig. 3.23).

Pyramidal fractures or Le Fort II level fractures

Blows to the central maxilla, especially those involving frontal impact, frequently result in fractures with a pyramidally shaped central maxillary segment. This is a Le Fort II "central maxillary segment", and the fracture begins above the level of the apices of the maxillary teeth laterally and posteriorly in the zygomaticomaxillary buttress and extends through the pterygoid plates in the same fashion as the Le Fort I fracture. Fracture lines travel medially and superiorly to pass through the medial portion of the inferior orbital rim and extend across the nose to separate a pyramidally shaped central

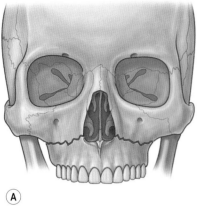
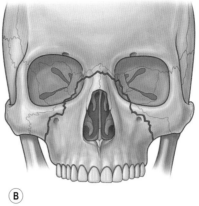
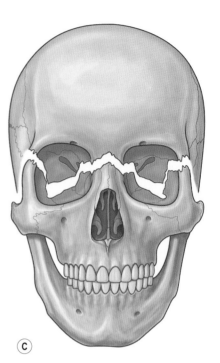

Fig. 3.22 The Le Fort classification of midfacial fractures. (**A**) The Le Fort I (horizontal or transverse) fracture of the maxilla, also known as Guerin fracture. (**B**) The Le Fort II (or pyramidal) fracture of the maxilla. In this fracture, the central maxilla is separated from the zygomatic areas. The fracture line may cross the nose through its cartilages or through the middle nasal bone area, or it may separate the nasal bones from the frontal bone through the junction of the nose and frontal sinus. (**C**) The Le Fort III fracture (or craniofacial disjunction). In this fracture, the entire facial bone mass is separated from the frontal bone by fracture lines traversing the zygoma nasoethmoid, and nasofrontal bone junctions. *(From Kazanjian VH, Converse J. Surgical Treatment of Facial Injuries, 3rd edn. Baltimore MD: Williams & Wilkins; 1974.)*

maxillary segment from the superior cranial and midfacial structures. The fracture line centrally may traverse the nose high through the upper nasal bones or low through the nasal cartilages to separate superior cranial from midfacial structures (Fig. 3.24).

Craniofacial dysjunction or Le Fort III fractures

Craniofacial dysjunction may occur when the fracture extends through the zygomaticofrontal suture and the nasal frontal suture and across the floor of the orbits to effectively separate all midfacial structures from the cranium. In these fractures, the maxilla is usually separated from the zygoma, but occasionally (5% of Le Fort III fractures) the entire midface may be a large single fragment, which is often only minimally displaced and immobile. These fractures present with "black

eyes" and with a subtle malocclusion. The Le Fort III segment may or may not be separated through the nasal structures. In these fractures the entire midfacial skeleton is incompletely detached from the base of the skull (a "greensticked" fracture) (Fig. 3.25).[108] Treatment may be successful with arch bars and elastic traction without open reduction.

Surgical technique

Le Fort I level fractures

In fractures of the Le Fort I type, placing the patient in intermaxillary fixation may occasionally be all that is necessary in the case of a minimally mobile and undisplaced fracture. In most cases, however, the Le Fort I level should be opened through a bilateral gingival buccal sulcus incision and the

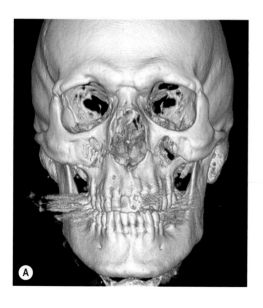
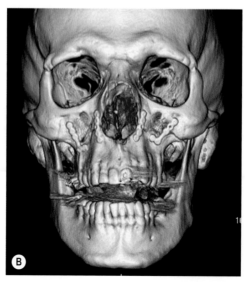

Fig. 3.23 Frontal 3D craniofacial computer tomography scan of a Le Fort I type injury pre- and post-open reduction and internal fixation.

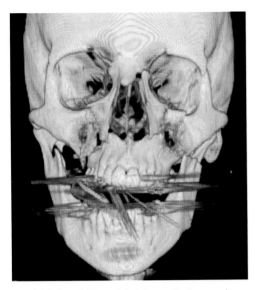

Fig. 3.24 Frontal 3D craniofacial computer tomography scan of a Le Fort II type injury pre- and post-open reduction and internal fixation.

fractures reduced and stabilized with plate and screw fixation at the bilateral nasomaxillary and zygomaticomaxillary buttresses. The primary consideration in Le Fort I fracture treatment is to re-establish normal dental occlusion. Proper lower midfacial height and projection are achieved by open reduction.

Le Fort II level fractures

In the case of a simple Le Fort II level fracture, the patient is first placed in intermaxillary fixation. The fracture should be opened at the Le Fort I level through a gingival buccal sulcus incision and through both lower eyelids to provide reduction and fixation at the orbit, zygomaticomaxillary and nasomaxillary buttresses, and at the inferior orbital rims. The need for opening fractures crossing the nose must be assessed by the CT scan and the displacement at the nasofrontal junction. Lower nasal fractures often do not need this exposure.

Le Fort III fractures

Open reduction of Le Fort III fractures generally involves combining procedures at the Le Fort I, Le Fort II, and zygomatic levels simultaneously for open reduction and fixation in a single operation.

Postoperative care of maxillary fractures

The postoperative management of fractures of the maxilla consists of three times daily dental and oral hygiene, lip lubrication, mouthwashes, skin care (abrasion and laceration cleansing), and lubrication with soaps and antibiotic ointments. Provision of adequate nutrition may be accomplished by a liquid or pureed diet, nasogastric tube, or percutaneous gastrostomy. The liquid or pureed diet is generally possible with intermaxillary fixation (IMF) and a soft diet after the IMF is released.

Cleansing and aspiration of both the nose and mouth is very important. The presence of a fever in patients with facial fractures should always prompt a sinus evaluation if the fever cannot be explained by other sources, especially if air-fluid levels are present. Any foul odor in the nose or on the breath necessitates inspection, cleaning and return to the operating room for drainage and irrigation, and a thorough nasal and oral examination.

Complications of maxillary fractures

Airway

In almost all cases of extensive fractures, the airway is partially compromised by posterior displacement of the fracture fragments and by edema and swelling of the soft tissues in the nose, mouth, throat, and floor of the mouth. In some patients, a nasopharyngeal airway may assist in establishing a route for ventilation. In other patients, intubation or tracheostomy may be indicated.

Bleeding

Hemorrhage may be managed by carefully identifying and ligating vessels in cutaneous lacerations, and by tamponade

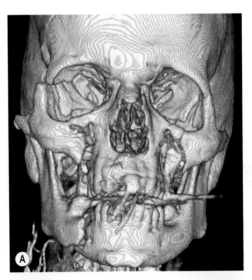

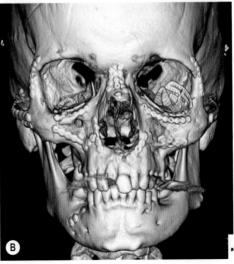

Fig. 3.25 Frontal 3D craniofacial computer tomography scan of a Le Fort III type injury pre- and post-open reduction and internal fixation.

in closed midface injuries with anterior–posterior nasopharyngeal packing, manual reduction of the displaced maxilla and placing the teeth in intermaxillary fixation. Angiographic embolization and the combination of external carotid and superficial temporal artery ligation are rarely necessary.

Infection

Maxillary fracture wounds are less complicated by infection than are mandibular fractures. However, they are contaminated at the time of the injury by entry into adjacent sinuses, fractures of the teeth, and open intraoral wounds. Fractures passing through the sinuses do not usually result in infection unless there has been pre-existing nasal or sinus disease, or in the case of persistent obstruction of the sinus orifice by displaced bone fractures or blood clot. If the maxillary sinuses are obstructed, a nasal–antral window or endoscopic drainage of the maxillary sinus by enlarging the orifice may be required.

Cerebrospinal fluid rhinorrhea

High Le Fort (II & III) level fractures may be associated with fractures of the cranial base or cribriform area, which produce cerebrospinal fluid (CSF) rhinorrhea and/or pneumocephalus and may be associated with death.[109] Antibiotic therapy may be utilized in these fractures at the discretion of the attending surgeon. Although antibiotic prophylaxis in CSF rhinorrhea has been quite widely employed, it is difficult to prove that antibiotics have substantially reduced the incidence of meningitis accompanying cerebrospinal fluid rhinorrhea when administered over a prolonged period. Blowing of the nose and placement of obstructing nasal packing should be avoided, and placement of intranasal tubes should avoid the superior nose.

Blindness

Blindness is a rare complication of any fracture of the orbit and may complicate fractures of the Le Fort II and III levels. It is rare for the optic nerve to be severed by bone fragments. The most common etiology is a traumatic shock to the nerve or swelling of the nerve within the tight portion of the optic canal or interference with the capillary blood supply of the retrobulbar optic nerve by swelling and edema.

Late complications

Specific complications referable to the maxilla include nonunion, malunion, plate exposure, lacrimal system obstruction, infraorbital and lip hypesthesia or anesthesia, and devitalization of teeth. There may be changes in facial appearance due to differences in midfacial height and projection, or the transverse width of the face, and malocclusion.[110]

Nonunion and bone grafting

True nonunion of the maxilla is rare and usually follows failure to provide even the most elementary type of intermaxillary fixation or open reduction. If nonunion occurs, the treatment consists of exposure of the fracture site, resection of the fibrous tissue in the fracture site, reduction of the displaced segments, removal of any proliferative bone edges, placement of bone grafts in all the existing bone gaps, and stabilization by plate and screw fixation.

Malunion

In multiple (complex) panfacial fractures, malunion may result from inadequate diagnosis, inadequate reduction, or inadequate fixation. The period of intermaxillary fixation and observation may need to be longer when the injury is more comminuted.

Malocclusion

If malocclusion is detected, it may respond to elastic traction. Once partial healing has occurred, attempts to re-establish occlusion with elastics may simply extrude or loosen the teeth. Revision of the reduction after removal of the internal fixation devices or a new osteotomy may be necessary. When new (secondary) osteotomies are necessary, generally a Le Fort I osteotomy for repositioning of the tooth-bearing segment of the maxilla is preferred as opposed to a higher level osteotomy. Occasionally, segmental osteotomies of the maxillary arch may be necessary to achieve optimal dental relationships.

Nasolacrimal duct injury

The nasolacrimal duct may be transected or obstructed by the fractures extending across the middle third of the facial skeleton between the Le Fort I and Le Fort III levels. Anatomic repositioning of the fracture fragments of the medial portion of the maxilla and nasoethmoidal orbital area provides the best protection against obstruction. Obstruction of the lacrimal system produces dacryocystitis and may require external drainage.

Lower facial fractures

Mandible fractures

The prominence, position, and anatomic configuration of the mandible are such that it is one of the most frequently injured facial bones. Following automobile accidents, the mandible is the most commonly encountered fracture seen at many major trauma centers. The mandible is a movable, predominantly U-shaped bone, consisting of horizontal and vertical segments. The horizontal segments consist of the body and the symphysis centrally. The vertical segments consist of the angles and rami, which articulate with the skull through the condyles and temporomandibular joints. The mandible is attached to other facial bones by muscles and ligaments and articulates with the maxilla through the occlusion of teeth.

The mandible is a strong bone but has several weak areas that are prone to fracture. The body of the mandible is composed principally of dense cortical bone with a small substantia spongiosa through which blood vessels, lymphatics, and nerves pass. The mandible is thin at the angles where the body joins with the ramus and can be further weakened by the presence of an unerupted third molar or a previous dental extraction.[111]

The mandible is also weak at the condylar neck, cuspid root (the longest root), and mental foramen through which the mental nerve and vessels extend into the soft tissues of the lower lip. The weak areas for fractures are the subcondylar area, angle, distal body, and the mental foramen.[112–114]

Mandibular movements are determined by the action of reciprocally placed muscles attached to the bone. When fractures occur, displacement of the segments is influenced by the pull of the muscles attaching to the segments. The direction of the fracture line may oppose forces created by these muscles.

Dental wiring and fixation techniques

Arch bars

Prefabricated arch bars are ligated to the external surface of the dental arch by passing 24- or 26-gauge steel wires around the arch bar and around the necks of the teeth. The wires are twisted tightly to individual teeth to hold the arch bars in the form of the dental arch. If segments of the teeth are missing, or if anterior support of the arch bar is needed to balance the forces generated by elastic traction anteriorly, the arch bar may be stabilized by additional wires passed from the arch bar to the skeleton (skeletal wires). Suspension wires may be passed through drill holes at the piriform margin or around screws. This is particularly applicable in children where the structure of the teeth tends to render arch bars less stable. The mandibular arch bar may also be stabilized by wires passed to a screw at the lower mandibular border or by circummandibular wiring. It cannot be overemphasized that the stability and alignment of a fracture reduction depends greatly on the alignment of the teeth achieved by this initial application of arch bars.

Newer types of arch bars exist, which utilize fewer points of contact and fixation, or screws passed into the bone as anchor for intermaxillary fixation. They are never better than full arch bars, and commonly achieve less accurate positioning/control of fracture fragments. Postoperatively, IMF may be released if the fracture is stable, and the patient is able to achieve normal occlusion. Our follow-up is at least once a week until complete healing has occurred (6–8 weeks), observing occlusion encouraging range of motion and absence of infection.

IMF screws

This is a rapid method of immobilizing the teeth in occlusion, given good dentition and uncomplicated fracture types.[115] The number and position of the IMF screws is based on the fracture type, fracture location, and surgeon preference. Screws must be positioned superior to the maxillary tooth roots and inferior to the mandibular tooth roots, otherwise transfixation of teeth may occur.[116]

Classification

Mandibular fractures are classified according to location (Fig. 3.26), condition of teeth, direction of fracture and favorability for treatment, presence of compound injury through the skin or mucosa, and anatomical fracture pattern.

Clinical examination and diagnosis

Pain and *tenderness* are usually present upon motion over the fracture and may be noted immediately as a result of injury. Fractures occurring along the course of the inferior alveolar nerve may produce *numbness* in the distribution of the nerve, which represents numbness of the ipsilateral lower lip (mental nerve) and ipsilateral teeth. The patient may be unable to open

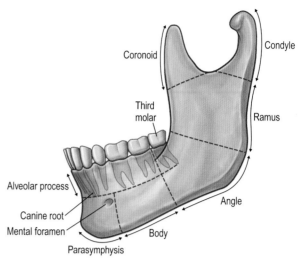

Fig. 3.26 Classification of mandibular fractures.

the mouth or bring the teeth into proper occlusion (*trismus*). The patient may refuse to eat or to brush their teeth, which then causes discomfort and an abnormal, foul-smelling odor (*fetor oris*). Excessive saliva is often produced as a result of local irritation (*drooling*). Small gingival or mucosal *lacerations* or *bleeding* between teeth indicate the possibility of a fracture. These gaps make the fracture compound into the mouth.

Bimanual manipulation of the mandible causes *mobility* or *distraction* at the fracture site, especially when the fracture occurs in the body or parasymphyseal area. One hand should stabilize the ramus, while the other manipulates the symphysis or the body area. The fracture will be demonstrated by abnormal movement, and the condition and the symptom reinforced by the presence of discomfort. The mandible may be pulled forward with one hand while the other hand is placed one finger in the ear canal and one finger over the condylar process (see Fig. 3.4). Abnormal *mobility* or *crepitus* indicates a fracture in the condylar/subcondylar area or ligament laxity, indicating a temporal mandibular joint injury. The most reliable finding in the fractures of the mandible, in dentulous patients, is the presence of a *malocclusion*. Often, the most minute malocclusion caused by the fracture is quite obvious to the patient. The patient may be unable to move the jaw (*dysfunction*) and may request liquid foods that require minimal jaw movement and mastication. Speech is difficult because of pain on motion of the mandible. *Crepitation* may be noticeable by manipulation at the fracture site. Often, the necessary manipulation produces such discomfort that it is not wise to demonstrate this physical sign. *Swelling* is usually quite obvious and frequently associated with ecchymosis and a hematoma. Often, an intraoral laceration is present over fractures in the horizontal portion of the mandible. There is frequently *deviation* to one side or the other, a finding that supports the diagnosis of a fracture. *Tenderness* over the fracture site is present, especially in the region of the temporomandibular joint. Such localized tenderness is highly suggestive of a fracture.

Direction and angulation of the fracture line

Kelsey Frye[117] described fractures as "favorable" or "unfavorable" according to their direction and bevel of displacement

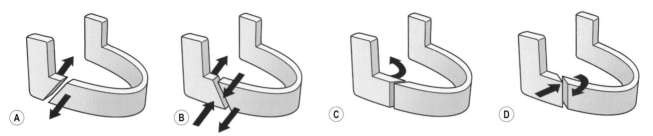

Fig. 3.27 (**A,C**) The direction and bevel of the fracture line does not resist displacement due to muscle action. The arrows indicate the direction of muscle pull. (**B,D**) The bevel and direction of the fracture line resist displacement and oppose muscle action. The direction of the muscle pull in fractures beveled in this direction would tend to impact the fractured bone ends. *(After Fry WK, Shepherd PR, McLeod AC, et al. The Dental Treatment of Maxillofacial Injuries. Oxford: Blackwell Scientific; 1942.)*

(Fig. 3.27). The muscular forces on some fracture fragments are opposed by the direction and bevel of the fracture line. Thus, in some fractures, the muscular force would pull the fragments into a position favorable for healing, whereas in other fractures, the muscular pull is unfavorable and separation of the fracture fragments occurs by action of the muscular forces. Mandibular fractures that are directed downward and forward are classified as horizontally favorable (HF) because the posterior group of muscles and the anterior group of muscles pull in antagonistic directions, favoring stability at the fracture site. Fractures running from above, downward, and posteriorly are classified as horizontally unfavorable (HU). The bevel of the fracture may also influence a displacement medially. If a fracture runs from posteriorly forward and medially, displacement would take place in a medial direction because of the medial pull of the elevator muscles of mastication (vertically unfavorable, or VU). The fracture that passes posteriorly forward and laterally is a favorable fracture because the muscle-pull tends to prevent displacement. It is called a vertically favorable fracture (VF).

Indications for ORIF of mandibular fractures

1. Favorable or unfavorable class I fractures where stability is desired.
2. Class II and class III fractures.
3. Comminuted fractures.
4. Displaced fractures and those subject to rotation.
5. Edentulous fractures.
6. The desire to avoid IMF in the postoperative period.
7. Combined fractures of the upper and lower jaws.
8. Uncooperative (head injured) patients.

Treatment of class I fractures

Class I fractures are those in which there are teeth on each side of the fracture. Although many of these fractures can be managed by intermaxillary fixation (IMF) alone in "favorable" fractures, if function is desired and post-treatment displacement is to be prevented, internal fixation is also preferred. If IMF alone is to be used, the period of fixation is six weeks.[118,119] Many mandibular fractures, even if favorable, are best managed by ORIF. Miniplates may be used for non-comminuted, non-bone gap fractures where impaction of the bone ends bears a significant portion of the load of fracture stabilization (load sharing).[120,121] This technique prevents

displacement and permits light function. ORIF is especially appealing to patients because the teeth do not need to remain wired, which permits intake of soft foods, oral hygiene, and an early return to work. These desirable aspects might not justify open treatment if external incisions are required which would produce permanent scars.[122]

General principles of reduction and fixation

The basic principle underlying all mandibular fracture treatment is superior and inferior border stabilization. The general method of fracture fixation involves arch bar placement and the use of a superior border unicortical non-compression mini plate. The inferior border is aligned and approximated by a stabilization plate. Comminuted fractures (Fig. 3.28) require larger fixation plates and include fractures with "bone loss" and multiple fragments, where the plate itself bears the entire load of fixation across the fracture or missing bone (load bearing).

Treatment of class II fractures

In class II fractures, teeth are present on only one side of the fracture site, and these fractures require open reduction. This type of fracture may occur in any portion of the horizontal mandible but frequently is at the angle. The type and strength of plate needed to control the non-toothbearing fragment and displacement of the fracture will vary according to the direction and bevel of the fracture and the position of the teeth, surrounding muscles, and the absence of comminution.

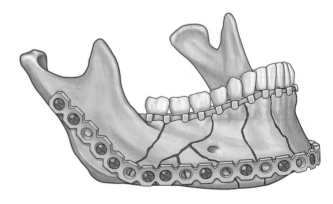

Fig. 3.28 Large reconstruction plate spans fractures of the entire body. *(Courtesy of Synthes Maxillofacial, Paoli, PA.)*

Fractures at the mandibular angle can be treated using a variety of techniques depending on the complexity of the fracture pattern.[123,124] For simple fractures at the mandibular angle, the authors' preferred approach is with a Champy plate placed monocortically on the oblique ridge or superior border of the mandible.

Comminuted fractures

Comminution negatively influences stability and generally increases the degree of fracture displacement. Three to four screws are utilized for fracture stabilization placed in non-fractured bone on each side of the entire fracture defect. Upper and lower border plates are preferred in the horizontal mandible and two plates also in the vertical mandible where possible.

Class III fractures

Class III fractures have no teeth on either side of the fracture. Non-displaced, immobile fractures conceptually may be treated by a soft diet with close follow-up. The majority of class III fractures, however, should be managed with rigid fixation with superior and inferior border fixation.

Extraoral approach to open reduction

The position of an external mandibular incision should always respect the location of the marginal mandibular branch of the facial nerve (Fig. 3.29). The subperiosteal dissection technique also respects neurovascular structures such as the mental nerve. Careful subperiosteal dissection establishes the extent and pattern of the fracture, confirming the impression given from the CT. The fragments at the inferior border of the fracture are aligned with clamps. The occlusal reduction should be checked at this point, and loose arch bar wires on the minor segment are tightened. IMF is then confirmed or established. Usually, a superior border plate is now utilized at the upper border of the mandible and fixated with unicortical screws. The occlusion is again checked, alignment of the fractures re-confirmed, and a lower border plate and screws applied. A larger plate may be utilized. Generally, a large plate is initially "overbent" so that it stands 2–3 mm off the central fracture site. Screw length may be determined by a depth gauge, and bicortical placement is preferred. If a larger plate is used, as the bicortical screws are tightened, the overbent plate flattens itself against the outer border of the mandible and reduces the lingual cortex properly. After the fixation is secure, any initial positioning wires are removed and the

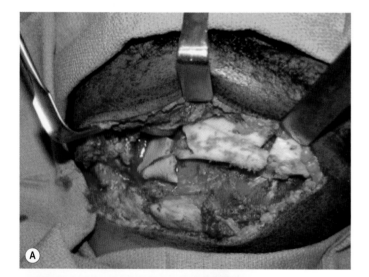

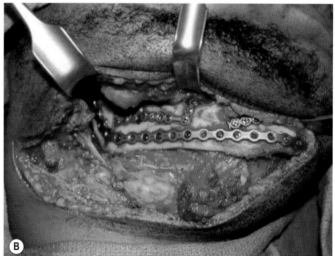

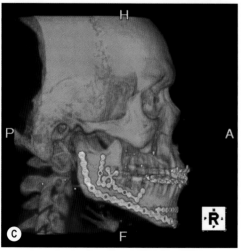

Fig. 3.29 (**A,B**) Intraoperative photograph of comminuted mandibular fracture in a 23-year-old male following attempted homicidal gunshot wound to the face pre- and post-open reduction and internal fixation via the extraoral approach using multiple miniplates. (**C**) Lateral 3D craniofacial computer tomography postoperative scan following open reduction and internal fixation of comminuted mandibular fractures.

musculature repaired. Care must be taken in suture placement to avoid the marginal mandibular branch of the facial nerve, which is located up to 1–2 cm below the inferior edge of the mandible.[125] The platysma muscle and the skin are closed in layers, and a dependent drain placed. The cutaneous wound is closed in layers with subcuticular sutures to avoid suture marks.

Intraoral approach to open reduction

Any fracture in the horizontal or vertical mandible is usually amenable to an intraoral approach.[126]

This is the preferred exposure for any symphysis or para-symphysis fracture and for non-comminuted angle fractures. The body region is also able to be reduced but may require a percutaneous trocar approach for drilling and screw place-ment. In the intraoral approach, the fracture site is exposed through an appropriately placed mucosal incision. The inci-sion is generally brought about a centimeter out of the sulcus on the buccal aspect of the mucosa, and mucosal and muscular layers separately incised.

Selection of internal fixation devices for mandibular fractures: how much fixation is enough

Edward Ellis III[123,127] clarified the issues regarding selection of internal fixation devices for mandibular fractures. Normal bite forces must be initially countered by fixation devices; however, patients who have sustained mandible fractures do not generate normal bite forces for months after the injury. Rigid fixation is defined as internal fixation that is stable enough to prevent motion of the bony fragments under normal function. It has been recognized that absolute rigidity of the bone fragments is not necessary for healing of the fracture to occur under functional loading. Ellis believes "functionally stable fixation" is not "rigid" but satisfies the goals of maintaining fragment alignment and permits healing during limited active use of the bone. Ellis describes "load-bearing" fixation as sufficient strength and rigidity that the device bears the entire loads applied to the mandible seg-ments during functional activities without impaction of the

bone ends. Load-sharing fixation relies on the impaction of the bone on each side of the fracture to bear the majority of the functional load with the small plate holding the bone ends together with force.

Locking plate and screw systems function as "internal external fixators", achieving stability by locking the screw to the plate.[128] The potential advantages of these fixation devices are that precise adaptation of the plate to the underlying bone is not necessary. As the screws are tightened they "lock" to the plate, thus stabilizing the segments without the need to compress the bone to the plate. This makes it impossible for the screw insertion to alter the reduction. This theoretically makes it less important to have good plate bending, as non-locking, large plates must be perfectly adapted to the contour of the bone. Theoretically this hardware should be less prone to inflammatory complications from loosening of hardware since loose hardware propagates an inflammatory response, permits motion, and promotes infection.

Champy or miniplate system

Mandibular fixation by the use of smaller "mini plates", as advocated by Champy, speeded exposure and was more toler-ant for mandibular shape and occlusion versus more rigid plate adaption as the screws were tightened.[129,130] The mal-leable plates minimized malreductions from "plate bending errors" common to stiff larger plates. This technique did not result in maximum rigidity achieved with the large plates but was generally sufficient for required immobilization for many fractures.

Small plates are more "user friendly" than more rigid systems and rose in popularity to surpass the use of rigid plate systems. Champy recommended two plates (upper and lower border) in the anterior (symphysis and parasymphysis) portion of the mandible and a single plate along the superior border in the angle and upper border of the distal ramus (Fig. 3.30). The need for additional fixation must be assessed care-fully, and this technique should be avoided in comminuted fractures and in the multiply fractured mandible. The tech-nique can only be used where the bone at the fracture site is broad enough to be compressed by the plate to bear the

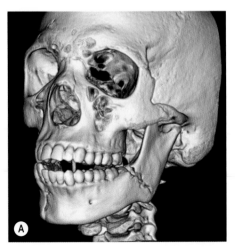
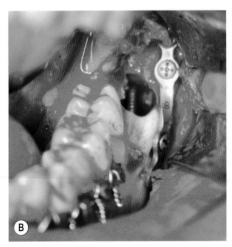
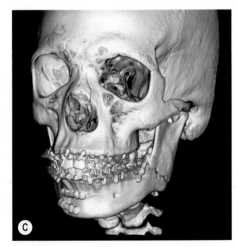

Fig. 3.30 **(A)** Three-quarter view of 3D craniofacial computer tomography preoperative scan on 16-year-old male who sustained a left mandibular angle fracture and right mandibular parasymphyseal fracture following an altercation. **(B)** Intraoperative photograph of open reduction and internal fixation of left mandibular angle fracture using the Champy technique. **(C)** Three-quarter view of 3D craniofacial computer tomography postoperative scan.

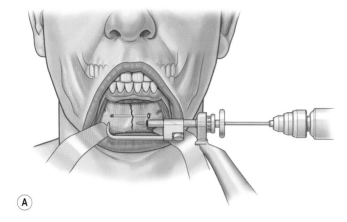

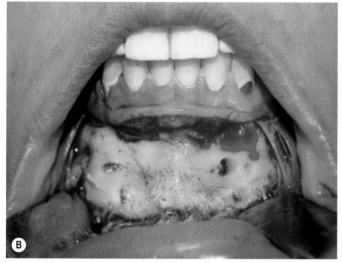

Fig. 3.31 (**A**) Placement of two horizontal lag screws to reduce and stabilize a parasymphysis fracture using a trocar device. (**B**) Intraoperative photograph of open reduction and internal fixation of mandibular symphyseal fracture using lag screws. *(A, Courtesy of Synthes Maxillofacial, Paoli, PA.)*

majority of the "load" of the fracture. The use of a brief initial period of rest in IMF (1 week) is used by some practitioners for soft tissue "rest" and provides an initial period of occlusion where less stress is placed on the fracture and importantly intraoral wounds and the soft tissue.

Lag screw technique

This technique is indicated in non-comminuted parasymphysis or symphysis fractures,[131,132] where a long length of screw can be tolerated (Fig. 3.31). Generally, these screw lengths require 35–45 mm anteriorly. A specific technique is utilized where the first cortex in the bone is over-drilled to the major diameter (thread width) of the screw. The second segment of the screw path is drilled to the minor diameter (core width not including treads) of the screw. Only the screw head will engage bone in the first section of the path, and therefore, as the screw is tightened into the second section of the fracture, the screw head impacts the cortex toward the fracture site. Generally, two lag screws are recommended for each fracture to be stable, for if one becomes loose, the fracture would be unstable by rotation. A sleeve or drill guide is used to protect soft tissue. Oblique body or angle fractures may be lag screwed with 2–3 screws for stability. In screw placement, the angle

between the bone and the direction of the screw should bisect a 90-degree angle from the bone in a plane parallel to the bone.

Third molars in mandibular angle fractures

Extraction of an impacted third molar must be carefully considered. In some circumstances, where the third molar is partially erupted and inflamed, it should be removed at the time of fracture treatment to avoid potential complications (Fig. 3.32).[111]

Otherwise, it makes little sense to remove bone to extract a fully impacted third molar, as this weakens the bone and damages mucosa in the area of the fracture. This can expose the fracture to the intraoral environment, contributing to bone instability and infection and a less stable fracture by third molar removal. The fracture site is less vascularized following third molar removal by virtue of periosteal stripping. Fully impacted third molars which do not prevent fracture reduction by minimal displacement of the tooth can be electively removed when fracture healing is completed.[133–135]

Antibiotic use

Intravenous administration of antibiotics perioperatively is recommended especially in patients undergoing delayed treatment, patients having long operations, patients with badly contused soft tissue, where the fracture treatment is delayed and where the tissues are heavily contaminated, and where multiple intraoral lacerations are present.[136,137] It benefits patients who are medically compromised, have poor nutritional status or systemic illness, or where local conditions of poor dental hygiene, periodontal, or dental infections increase the chance of bacterial complications.

Treatment principles of mandibular fractures

1. Establish proper occlusion.
2. Anatomically reduce the fractured bones into their normal position.

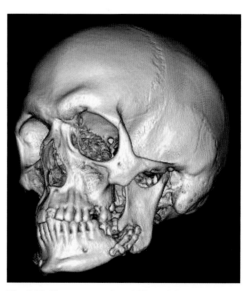

Fig. 3.32 Three-quarter view of 3D craniofacial computer tomography demonstrating malunion and continuity defect of left mandibular angle fracture with tooth in line of fracture.

3. Utilize fixation techniques that hold the fractured bone segments in occlusion and normal position until healing has occurred. Open reduction internal fixation (ORIF) can often permit limited function while healing is occurring.
4. Control infection.

Complications after fracture treatment

Malocclusion

Malocclusion is commonly the result of insufficient or inaccurate initial alignment. Poorly applied or loose IMF is the commonest cause, and inadequate reduction, inadequate plate size, length or strength, contour, or failure (loosening) of fixation. The most common cause of screw loosening is overheating of the bone while drilling. Although subtle malocclusions may sometimes be corrected by elastic traction, grinding the occlusal facets of the teeth or orthodontics, any significant malocclusion requires refracture and/or osteotomy.

Hardware infection and screw migration

Loose hardware generally creates soft tissue irritation, producing a foreign body response and infection requiring hardware removal. Many times the fracture has healed and a repeat osteosynthesis is not necessary. Migration of loose hardware into soft tissue away from the fracture site occasionally occurs.[138]

Increased facial width and rotation of the mandible

Broadening of the distance between mandibular angles is produced by rotation of the lateral mandibular segments lingually at the occlusal surface of the teeth.[139] The distance between the mandibular angles increases as the mandible rotates, and the lower face widens. This rotation (aggravated by tight IMF and the presence of subcondylar fractures) produces a malocclusion (open bite) of the palatal and lingual cusps of the molar dentition (which may only be visible from a lingual location). A characteristic broadening and rounding of the face occurs, which is aesthetically and functionally undesirable. It cannot be treated by orthodontics and requires refracture.[140] The use of a long, strong reconstruction (10–12 hole) plate to keep the mandibular angles unrotated and the width of the mandible at the angles narrow is required.

Non-union

Non-union and pseudoarthrosis are uncommon after plate and screw fixation.[141–143] Their presence may be masked in presence of rigid fixation. Plate removal may unmask a poor union, which requires re-fixation of the fracture after thorough debridement at the site of poor fracture healing and possible bone grafting of the defect.

Osteomyelitis

Soft tissue infection is common after mandibular fracture treatment, but true bone infection, osteomyelitis, is not. Local infection may almost always be managed with drainage and antibiotics. The fixation must be confirmed as adequate and intraoral closure inspected, and any instability in the fracture fixation noted and corrected. Less commonly, devitalized soft tissue and bone fragments that are dead or

exposed must be debrided. Loose or infected teeth should be removed. Fracture stability must be provided by removal of current fixation devices and reapplication of longer, stronger reconstruction plates, whose screw fixation of 3–4 screws in healthy uninvolved bone outside the fracture area can be achieved. In the uncommon persistent infection, the surgeon may wish to convert to external fixation removing all internal fixation devices, but most cases may be stabilized with the debridement and application of a long reconstruction plate. No screws should be placed in an area of questionable bone. Serial debridement of devitalized bone and soft tissue may be required to confirm the absence of infection and adequacy of debridement. Primary or secondary bone grafting is conducted when the soft tissue and local area have been cleared of infection by debridement, drainage, antibiotics, and mucosal closure.[144]

Condylar and subcondylar fractures

One must consider dislocation, angulation between the fractured fragments, fracture override (which translates to ramus vertical length shortening), fracture angulation, and bone gaps between the fragments. In children, growth considerations[145] create a capacity for both regeneration and remodeling which is not present in later years.[146,147] Adults are capable only of partial restitutional remodeling.

High condylar (intracapsular) fractures (head and upper neck) are generally treated with closed reduction with a limited (2 week) period of postoperative IMF, followed by early "controlled" mobilization utilizing elastics for re-establishing occlusion in a rest position. Most neck and low subcondylar fractures with good alignment, reasonable contact of the bone ends, and preservation of ramus vertical height without condylar head dislocation may be treated by IMF for 4–6 weeks, with weekly observation of the occlusion for at least 4 additional weeks after release of fixation in light function or guiding elastics.[148,149] Some shortening of the ramus height is almost inevitable with a closed approach to condylar/subcondylar fracture treatment,[150–152] which may lead to a premature contact in the ipsilateral molar occlusion and a subtle open bite in the contralateral anterior occlusion. Angulation between the fractured fragments in excess of 30 degrees and fracture gap between the bone ends exceeding 4–5 mm, lateral override, and lack of contact of the ends of the fractured fragments should be a consideration for open reduction in mid or low subcondylar fractures types (Fig. 3.33).[153–157]

Edentulous mandible fractures

These fractures represent less than 5% of the mandibular fractures.[158–160] Fractures commonly occur through the most atrophic portions where the bone is thin and weak. The body is a common site for fracture, as compared to the angle and subcondylar region in dentulous patients.[161] Many fractures are bilateral or multiple, and displacement of a bilateral edentulous body fracture is often severe and a challenging condition to treat. The fractures in the horizontal mandible may be closed or open to the oral cavity. Closed fractures demonstrating no displacement may be treated with a soft diet and avoidance of dentures; however, in these cases observation is critical to be sure that healing occurs within several weeks without further displacement. In practice most

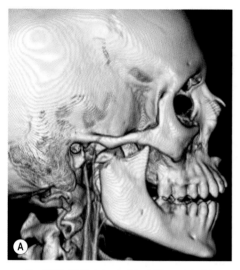 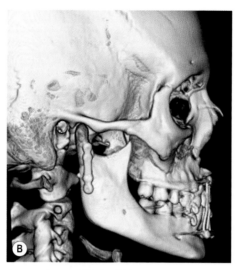 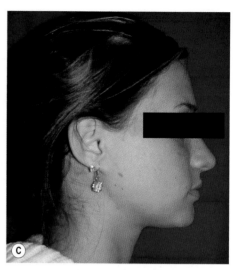

Fig. 3.33 (**A,B**) Lateral view of 3D craniofacial computer tomography on a 20-year-old female involved in a motor vehicle collision who sustained craniofacial injuries, pre- and post-open reduction and internal fixation of a right mandibular subcondylar fracture via a retromandibular extraoral approach. Note that the patient also had a Le Fort II type fracture that was treated with closed reduction and interdental fixation. (**C**) Lateral profile view photograph of patient 1 year postoperatively.

fractures are better treated with a load-bearing plate. The edentulous mandible is characterized by the loss of the alveolar ridge and the teeth.[162] The bone atrophy may be minimal if there is sufficient height (over 20 mm) of the mandibular body to ensure good bone healing. In cases with moderate atrophy, the height of the mandibular body ranges from 10–20 mm, and healing is usually satisfactory but not as certain as if the height were greater than 20 mm. Small plates with few screws often fail, as there is insufficient bone to provide buttressing support for "load-sharing" fracture treatment. The plate must bear the entire load of the fracture, and a large reconstruction ("locking") plate with 3–4 screws per side in healthy bone is recommended (Fig. 3.34). In cases where the mandibular height is less than 10 mm (severe atrophy) one can assume that the patient has a disease of "poor bone healing". Complications following edentulous mandible fractures directly parallel the extent of mandibular atrophy. Obwegeser and Sailer[163] in 1973 documented that 20% of the complications in edentulous mandible fractures were seen in the 10–20 mm mandibular height group, and 80% of the complications (i.e. poor or unsatisfactory bone union) were experienced in cases demonstrating a mandibular height less than 10 mm. Virtually no complications were seen in fractures exceeding 20 mm in height. This experience caused some authors[164,165] to recommend primary bone grafting for the severely atrophic edentulous mandible (*less than* 10 mm in height).

Panfacial injuries

Conceptually, panfacial fractures involve all three areas of the face: frontal bone, midface, and mandible. In practice, when two out of these three areas are involved, the term "panfacial fracture" has been applied.

Treatment of panfacial fractures

The optimal time and the easiest treatment of these injuries is within hours of the accident, before the development of massive edema and soft tissue contamination and rigidity that follow these injuries. Early treatment is possible when other systems are not injured or are evaluated to exclude significant instability. However, no matter how severely the patient is injured, cutaneous wounds can be cleansed and closed, devitalized tissue removed, and the patient placed in intermaxillary fixation. This is the *minimum* urgent treatment of a significant maxillary or mandibular injury and may always be accomplished, despite the condition of the patient.

Presently, a one-stage restoration of the architecture of the craniofacial skeleton is the preferred method of treatment for

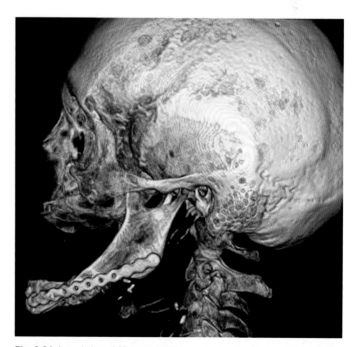

Fig. 3.34 Lateral view of 3D craniofacial computer tomography on a 64-year-old edentulous female, with a history of osteogenesis imperfecta, who was referred for treatment of a malunion of a left mandibular fracture. Postoperative open reduction and internal fixation using a load-bearing mandibular plate and iliac bone grafting via an extra-oral approach.

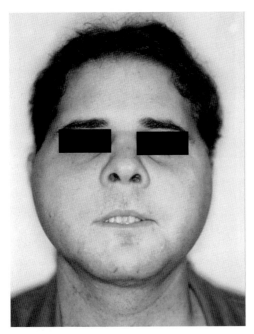

Fig. 3.35 Lack of restoration of the preinjury appearance, even if the underlying bone is finally replaced into its proper anatomic position, is the result of scarring within soft tissue. Examples of soft tissue rigidity accompanying malreduced fractures include the conditions of enophthalmos, medial canthal ligament malposition, short palpebral fissure, rounded canthus, and inferiorly displaced malar soft tissue pad. The lower lip has a disrupted mentalis attachment. Secondary management of any of these conditions is more challenging and less effective than primary reconstruction. A unique opportunity thus exists in immediate fracture management to maintain expansion shape and position of the soft tissue envelope and to determine the geometry of soft tissue fibrosis by providing an anatomically aligned facial skeleton as support. Excellent restoration of appearance results from primary soft tissue positioning.

panfacial injuries, where severe comminution and multiply fractured facial bones characterize the injury.

Open reduction of all fracture sites is performed with plate and screw fixation, adding bone grafts to bone defects. Although local incisions may be useful in selected cases, regional incisions such as the coronal, transconjunctival, and upper and lower gingival buccal sulcus provide complete exposure. An exposure may be avoided when a suitable laceration already exists.

In each subunit of the face, the important dimension to be considered first is facial width. In less severe fractures, correction of facial width is not challenging and an "anterior" approach is sufficient. Control of facial width in more severe injuries requires more complete dissection and alignment of each fracture component utilizing all the peripheral and cranial base landmarks. Reconstructions which emphasize control of facial width are in fact the principle which reciprocally restores facial projection.

The timing and technique of soft tissue reduction are critical. Repositioning of the bone and replacement of the soft tissue onto the bone at its correct anatomical location must be accomplished *before* the soft tissue has developed significant memory (internal scarring) in the pattern of the unreduced bone configuration. Soft tissue replacement requires (1) layered closure of the soft tissues and (2) reattachment of the closed soft tissue to the facial skeleton precisely at several points on the anatomically assembled craniofacial skeleton.

Order of the procedure

Various sequences have been suggested such as "top to bottom", "bottom to top", "outside to inside", or "inside to outside". In reality, it does not make any difference what the order is as long as the order and sequence make logical sense and lead to a reproducible, anatomically accurate bone reconstruction. In our experience, it is more predictable to stabilize the occlusion in comminuted fractures by relating the anatomically aligned maxilla to the mandible than by relating the inferior maxilla to the superior maxilla. The frontal bone is managed first with any brain injury, then the upper midface beginning with the central nasoethmoid area and progressing to the zygoma, emphasizing control of facial width. The mandible is managed next, linking all segments through required exposures with wires temporarily, then achieving mandibular width by relating it to an anatomically reduced and stabilized maxillary dental arch.

Complications of panfacial fractures

Complications of panfacial fractures include complications referable to the bone and the soft tissue. The most common bony facial deformities following midface fracture treatment relate to lack of projection, enophthalmos, malocclusion, and increased facial width (Fig. 3.35).

The most common soft tissue deformities are descent, diastasis, fat atrophy, ectropion, thickening, and rigidity. Lack of periosteal closure over the zygomaticofrontal suture produces the appearance of temporal wasting because of the gap in the temporal aponeurosis with skeletalization of the frontal process of the zygoma (Fig. 3.36). High incisions for arch exposure made higher in the deep temporal fascia require dissection through fat to reach the zygomatic arch and cause fat atrophy by direct fat damage (interference with the middle temporal blood supply).

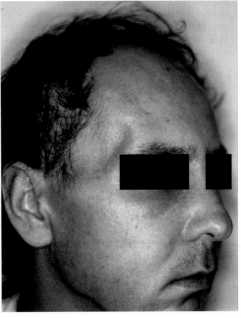

Fig. 3.36 "Skeletonization" of the frontal process of the zygoma from failure to close the temporal fascia to the orbital periosteum over the frontal process.

Postoperative care

Patients with large segment fractures may be adequately stabilized by plate and screw fixation and permit early release of intermaxillary fixation. Patients with comminuted midface or panfacial fractures are best served by varying periods of postoperative intermaxillary fixation of three to four weeks in addition to plate and screw fixation.

Gunshot wounds of the face

While some authors advocate delayed reconstruction of gunshot and shotgun wounds of the face, immediate reconstruction[166,167] and immediate soft tissue closure with serial "second-look" procedures is the current standard of care.[168] Recent experience documents the safety and efficacy of immediate soft tissue closure and bone reconstruction in an anatomically correct position. These two principles prevent soft tissue shrinkage and loss of soft tissue position and provide improved functional and aesthetic results with shorter periods of disability and an improved potential for rehabilitation both functionally and aesthetically. The philosophy of delayed closure of these difficult wounds is no longer appropriate, creates additional soft tissue deformity, and delays effective rehabilitation of the affected individuals, some of whom represent suicide attempts.

Ballistic injuries are classified into low, medium, and high-energy injuries.[169] In formulating a treatment plan for ballistic injuries, it is helpful to identify the entrance and exit wounds and the presumed path of the bullet and to appreciate the mass and velocity of the projectile so that the extent of internal areas of tissue injury can be predicted. Conceptually, the areas of soft tissue and bone injury and areas of soft tissue loss and bone loss must be individually assessed and noted (four separate components) for each injury. The areas of injury and the areas of loss are each precisely outlined, which allows a treatment plan to be developed for early and intermediate treatment for the lower, middle, and upper face.

Low velocity gunshot wounds

Low energy deposit ballistic weapons usually involve projectiles that have a limited mass and travel at speeds of less than 1000 feet per second. In general, low velocity gunshot wounds involve little soft tissue and bone loss and have limited associated soft tissue injury outside the exact path of the bullet. It is thus appropriate that they be treated with immediate definitive stabilization of bone and primary soft tissue closure. Limited debridement of bone and soft tissue are necessary. Small amounts of bone may need to be debrided and replaced with a primary bone graft, which can be performed primarily in the upper face. Because of the lack of significant associated soft tissue injury, little potential for progressive death or progressive necrosis of soft tissue exists, and these injuries may be treated as "facial fractures with overlying lacerations" both conceptually and practically.

Intermediate and high velocity ballistic injuries to the face

Shotgun pellets have a large mass and are considered intermediate energy deposit projectiles. They travel at speeds of approximately 1200 feet per second and when grouped in a close distribution, at close range, are capable of causing massive injury. In civilian practice, many of these injuries represent shotgun wounds or high-energy rifle injuries, and they often result from suicide attempts and assaults. Close range shotgun wounds are characterized by extensive soft tissue and bone destruction.

Intermediate and high velocity ballistic injuries to the face must be managed with a specific treatment plan that involves stabilization of existing bone and soft tissue in anatomic position, and maintenance of this bone and soft tissue stabilization throughout the period of soft tissue contracture and bone and soft tissue reconstruction. Wounds from intermediate and high-energy missiles usually demonstrate areas of both soft tissue and bone loss, as well as areas of soft tissue and bone injury. It is important to reassemble the existing bone and soft tissue as completely as possible, and then serial surgical debridement "second-look" procedures, re-open the soft tissue to define additional areas of soft tissue necrosis, drain hematoma and/or developing fluid collections or infection, and assure bone integrity. These "second-look" procedures are imperative if primary reconstruction is attempted. Thus, the emphasis is on primary soft tissue, "skin to skin" or "skin to mucosa" closures, with stabilization of existing bone fragments in anatomical position. Re-exploration for additional debridements occur at 48-hour intervals, or at an interval determined until soft tissue loss ceases and wound hematoma and fluid collections are controlled. Then, reconstruction proceeds immediately.

In cases where composite tissue loss of bone and soft tissue occur, techniques utilizing free tissue transfer of bone and soft tissue are preferred (Fig. 3.37A–F).[170,171] The use of local tissue advanced over the mismatched cutaneous segment of the free flap ultimately provides the best cutaneous aesthetic result.[172]

Bonus images for this chapter can be found online at
http://www.expertconsult.com

Fig. 3.1 Cutaneous incisions (solid line) available for open reduction and internal fixation of facial fractures. The conjunctival approach (dotted line) also gives access to the orbital floor and anterior aspect of the maxilla, and exposure may be extended by a lateral canthotomy. Intraoral incisions (dotted line) are also indicated for the Le Fort I level of the maxilla and the anterior mandible. The lateral limb of an upper blepharoplasty incision is preferred for isolated zygomaticofrontal suture exposure if a coronal incision is not used. A horizontal incision directly across the nasal radix or vertical incision along the glabellar fold is the one case in which a local incision can be tolerated over the nose. In many instances, a coronal incision is preferable unless the hair is short or the patient is balding.

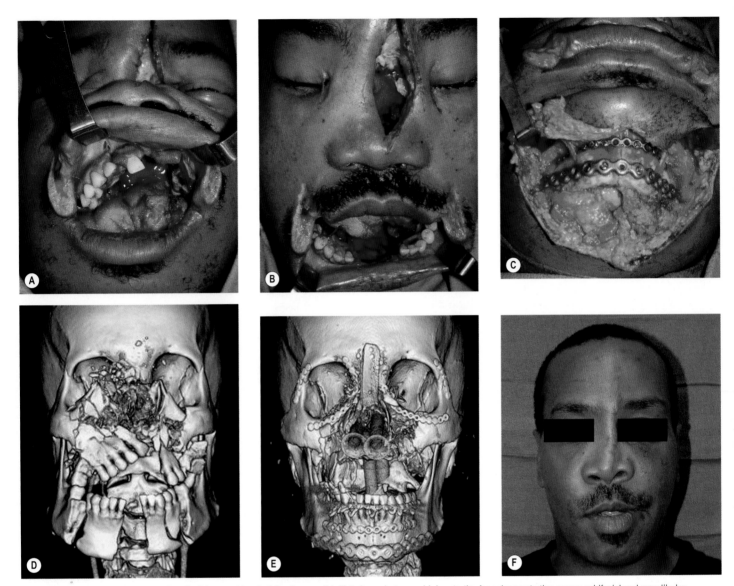

Fig. 3.37 **(A,B)** Frontal photographs of a 34-year-old male following a self-inflicted gunshot wound injury to the face demonstrating severe midfacial and mandibular fractures. **(C)** Intraoperative photographs following open reduction and internal fixation of mandibular fractures using a load-bearing mandibular plate and a monocortical miniplate fixation via an extraoral approach. **(D,E)** Frontal 3D craniofacial computer tomography scan of the patient pre- and post-open reduction and internal fixation of midfacial and mandibular fractures. **(F)** Postoperative photograph 1 year following surgery.

🌐 Access the complete reference list online at   **http://www.expertconsult.com**

33. Rodriguez ED, Stanwix MG, Nam AJ, et al. Twenty-six-year experience treating frontal sinus fractures: a novel algorithm based on anatomical fracture pattern and failure of conventional techniques. *Plast Reconstr Surg.* 2008;122: 1850–1866. *Landmark article describing the longest experience with treating frontal sinus fractures provides an algorithm for its treatment based on their outcomes, to minimize long-term complications.*

59. Iliff N, Manson P, Katz J, et al. Mechanisms of extraocular muscle injury in orbital fractures. *Plast Reconstr Surg.* 1999;103:787–799. *A comprehensive human, cadaveric, and animal study into the effects of orbital fractures on extraocular muscles and their intramuscular vasculature to help understand mechanisms of diplopia and muscle injury.*

64. Girotto J, Gamble B, Robertson B, et al. Blindness following reduction of facial fractures. *Plast Reconstr Surg.* 1998;102: 1821–1834. *Landmark article to define the incidence of blindness following facial fracture repair.*

79. Tessier P, Guiot G, Rougerie J, et al. [Cranio-naso-orbito-facial osteotomies. Hypertelorism]. *Ann Chir Plast.* 1967;12:103–118. *An article by the father of craniofacial surgery describing the possibilities of an intracranial approach for orbital reconstructive surgery.*

82. Markowitz B, Manson P, Sargent L, et al. Management of the medial canthal tendon in nasoethmoid orbital fractures: the importance of the central fragment in treatment and classification. *Plast Reconstr Surg.* 1991;87:843–853. *Landmark article on the classification types of nasoethmoid-orbital region. Knowledge of this fracture pattern classification assists with the treatment of this complex surgical condition.*

100. Manson P, Clark N, Robertson B, et al. Subunit principles in midface fractures: the importance of sagittal buttresses, soft tissue reductions and sequencing treatment of segmental fractures. *Plast Reconstr Surg.* 1999;103:1287–1306. *Landmark article describing the authors' extensive experience in the treatment of midfacial injuries and the importance of correct realignment of bone and soft tissues to improve facial fracture treatment.*

106. LeFort R. Etude experimentale sur les fractures de la machoire superieur. *Rev Chir Paris.* 1901;23:208, 360, 479. *Original article describing the various fracture patterns associated with traumatic craniofacial injury. We associate the author's name to the different types of fracture patterns recognized.*

129. Champy M, Lodde JP, Schmidt R, et al. Mandibular osteosynthesis by miniature screwed plates via a buccal approach. *J Maxillofac Surg.* 1978;6:14–21. *Original article describing the use of monocortical plates for the treatment of mandibular fractures; lines of osteosynthesis are defined.*

4

Surgical treatment of migraine headaches

Ali Totonchi and Bahman Guyuron

SYNOPSIS

- Approximately 30 million Americans suffer from migraine headaches (MH), and lifetime prevalence is estimated to be 11–32%, including 18% of women and 6% of men.
- Medical management is the first line of treatment, but poorly controlled or uncontrolled MH can be treated surgically, specifically since severe migraine could be disabling.
- Before considering a patient for surgical management, they should be evaluated by a neurologist/headache specialist for diagnosis and medical management.
- In the surgical evaluation of patients with MH, the trigger site can be confirmed by botulinum toxin A (BTX-A) injection or nerve block. If the history or computed tomography (CT) scan findings are strongly indicative of a specific trigger site, this step can be bypassed.
- The four major trigger sites are frontal, temporal, occipital, and nasal.
- In the frontal trigger site, the supraorbital and supratrochlear nerves can be irritated by adjacent structures like frowning muscles, vessels, bands over the supra-orbital notch, or bony tunnel, and this area is treated by freeing the nerve from all possible irritating structures and placement of fat graft.
- The temporal trigger site is treated by avulsion/decompression of the zygomaticotemporal branch of trigeminal nerve (ZTBTN) as it emerges from deep temporal fascia.
- The occipital trigger site is located in the posterior part of the neck where the greater occipital nerve is passing through the semispinalis capitis muscle and trapezius fascia and crosses over the occipital artery; treatment includes partial resection of the muscle/fascia, padding the nerve with a subcutaneous fat flap, and resection of the artery adjacent to the nerve.
- Theory behind the rhinogenic trigger point is that nasal mucosa containing a rich nervous supply can be irritated due to contact point or pressure from an entrapped air pocket. Rhinogenic trigger site is treated with septoplasty, elimination of contact points between the turbinate and the septum or nasal side wall, reduction of enlarged turbinates, and removal of concha bullosa.
- Less common trigger sites like the auriculotemporal nerve, lesser occipital nerve, third occipital nerve, or any distal branches of all of

the above mentioned nerves could act as a trigger site often due to irritation by a blood vessel or fascial band.

 Access the Historical Perspective section online at
http://www.expertconsult.com

Introduction

Headaches are the seventh leading presenting complaint in ambulatory medical care in the US.[1] In most neurology clinics, headache, the majority of which is migraine, is the most common chief complaint. Nearly 30 million Americans suffer from MH, and lifetime prevalence is estimated to be 11–32% across several countries. Eighteen percent of women and 6% of men are involved, and two-thirds of these patients do not benefit from over-the-counter medications. In women, MHs are more common than asthma (5%) and diabetes (6%) combined. Many of the available prophylactic medications harbor side effects such as sedation, paresthesia, weight gain, cognitive impairment, and sexual dysfunction. The cost of migraine treatment and loss of time from work associated with MH impose a major economic burden on the patient and society, collectively exceeding $13 billion.[1–11]

Basic science/disease process

The diagnostic criteria of MH are shown in Table 4.1. There are two subtypes of migraine: migraine with aura and migraine without aura. Auras develop over 5–20 min but last for less than 60 min and are followed by a migraine headache. One out of three patients with MH experiences aura. MHs are usually frontotemporal, typically unilateral, and are characterized by recurrent attacks of pulsating, intense pain associated with nausea and photophobia. Traditional, non-surgical treatment of MH can be non-pharmacologic or pharmacologic. Non-pharmacologic treatment of MH consists of avoidance

Table 4.1 The constellation of symptoms that aid in the diagnosis of migraine headache trigger sites

	Frontal	Temporal	Rhinogenic	Occipital
Starting location of pain	Frontal area	Temple area	Behind the eye	At the point of exit of the greater occipital nerve from the semispinalis capitis muscle (3.5 cm caudal to the occipital tuberosity and 1.5 cm off the midline)
Time	Usually in the afternoon	Patient usually wakes up in the morning with pain	Patient commonly wakes up with pain in the morning or at night	Not specific
Exam, observation	Strong corrugator muscle activity causing deep frown lines on animation The points of emergence of the supraorbital and supratrochlear nerves from corrugator muscle or the foramen are tender to the touch Patients usually have eyelid ptosis on the affected side at the time of active pain Pressure on these sites may abort the headache during the initial stages Application of cold or warm compresses on these sites often reduces or stops the pain The pain is usually imploding in nature Stress-related	Sometimes associated with tenderness of the temporalis or masseteric muscle Clenching/grinding Rubbing or pressing the exit point of the zygomaticotemporal branch of the trigeminal nerve from the deep temporal fascia can stop the pain in the beginning Application of cold or warm compresses to this point may reduce or stop the pain The pain is characterized as imploding Stress-related	Commonly triggered by weather changes Rhinorrhea on the affected side Allergy-related Hormone-related, menstrual cycle-related The pain is usually described as exploding	Muscle tightness Heavy exercise-related Compression of this site can stop the pain in the early stage; at the later stage, this point is tender Application of cold or heat at this site may result in some improvement in the pain Stress-related
CT scan			Concha bullosa, septal deviation with contact between the turbinates and the septum, and septa bullosa	

CT, computed tomography.

of triggers, which commonly include artificial sweeteners, monosodium glutamate, and nitrate containing foods or alcohol. Sometimes application of pressure, cold, or heat can mitigate or abort the migraine headaches.

Pharmacologic treatment can be further subdivided into acute abortive and prophylactic treatment:

- Acute abortive treatment consists of simple analgesics like acetaminophen, nonsteroidal anti-inflammatory, or migraine specific abortive medications, which includes Triptan or Ergots. The first-line acute abortive treatment is the use of Triptans or NSAIDs, sometimes together, although intravenous antiemetics and ergotamine can be used as well.
- Preventive treatment consists of antihypertension medications (beta-blockers, Ca++ blockers), antidepressants (tricyclic antidepressants or serotonin-norepinephrine reuptake inhibitors), and antiepileptics (e.g., Topiramate, valproic acid).[12,13]

Opioid-containing analgesics are not recommended in the treatment of migraine. Barbiturate-containing analgesics should be avoided in migraine patients as well. Both of these classes of medications have a very strong potential for causing "medication overuse headache".

Medication overuse headache, which is also sometimes called "rebound" headache, based on the International Headache Society definition, is a headache that occurs more than 15 days per month, developing as consequence of regular use of abortive headache medication. All of the abortive medications, including simple analgesics and migraine-specific medication (Triptan and Ergots), can cause medication overuse headaches if used frequently and generally beyond 3 months.

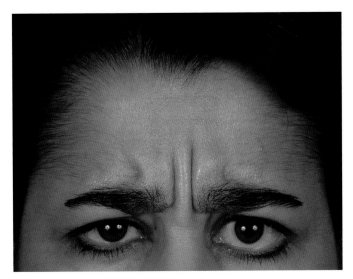

Fig. 4.1 Example of corrugator supercilii muscle hypertrophy.

In practice, opioids and barbiturate-containing analgesics by far are the most common reason for medication overuse headache. The prevalence of medication overuse is reported between 50 and 70% in different tertiary headache clinics. In general, these groups of patients are not ideal candidates for surgical treatment of migraine headache, until they have been off these medications and cleared for surgery by the neurologists or there are clear plans for detoxification after surgery.

Diagnosis and patient presentation

Preoperative history and examination

Surgical treatment of MH should only be considered after the diagnosis of MH is confirmed by a neurologist and more serious causes of headaches have been excluded. The proper surgical candidate is someone whose headaches are not controlled with traditional medical treatment and who has an acceptable surgical risk. Pregnant and nursing women are also typically excluded from surgical consideration. The constellation of symptoms leads the examiner to suspect the potential trigger site (Table 4.1), which is further validated by physical examination.[28,31] The salient piece of information that helps to identify the trigger site is the site from which the pain starts. The patient is asked to complete a migraine form asking a number of critical questions. Keeping a monthly diary of MH prior to the surgery will provide more reliable information than patient recall.

Hypertrophy of the corrugator supercilii muscle with vertical frown lines is a common finding and might be obvious in patients with a frontal trigger site (Fig. 4.1). The nasal exam includes a physical exam with or without endoscopic examination, which must be performed to detect septal deviation and turbinate hypertrophy with contact points between the septum and turbinates, concha bullosa, and septa bullosa, and the findings are confirmed using a CT scan of the septum and sinuses (Fig. 4.2).

Patient selection

Trigger sites

Currently, we have identified four common trigger sites: (1) frontal triggers, where glabellar muscles, vessels, and possible fascial band or bony tunnel in the supraorbital rim compress or irritate the supratrochlear and supraorbital nerves and causes frontal headaches; (2) temporal triggers, where compression of ZTBTN by contraction of the temporalis muscle, fascia, or the artery causes inflammation of the nerve and leads to temporal headaches; (3) occipital triggers, where the semispinalis capitis muscle, trapezius fascia, and occipital artery can irritate the occipital nerve and cause occipital headaches; and (4) septonasal triggers, where intranasal structures compress the trigeminal end branches and cause paranasal and retrobulbar headaches.

There are several less common trigger sites, many of which are at the intersections of nerves and arteries, such as the superficial temporal artery and the auriculotemporal nerve. The lesser occipital nerve and the third occipital nerve can also act as trigger sites.[26,27] In addition to the above-mentioned trigger points, the end branches of the nerve discussed previously could be irritated by a blood vessel, or less commonly by a fascial band, and act as a trigger point.

The role of botulinum toxin injection

BTX-A (Botox, Allergan, Irvine, CA) or abobotulinumtoxin A (Dysport, Medicis Aesthetics, Scottsdale, AZ) blocks the release of acetylcholine at the neuromuscular junction. A deadly neurotoxin produced by *Clostridium botulinum*, its

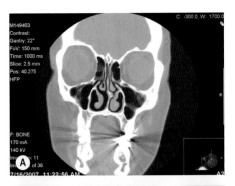

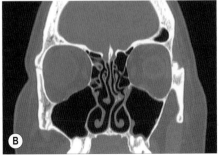

Fig. 4.2 (A) Combination of a large spur protruding into the left inferior turbinate, right middle turbinate concha bullosa, and extensive sinus disease. **(B)** Significant enough deviation of the septum to the left to touch the lateral wall of the nose and the left middle turbinate along with mild maxillary sinus disease. Bilateral concha bullosa of the middle turbinates and Haller's cell.

clinical utility in MH has been gaining popularity over the last two decades.[22,23]

BTX-A was first introduced over three decades ago as a treatment for strabismus[32–35] and since has been used in many neuromuscular conditions, including oromandibular dystonia, laryngeal dystonia, cervical dystonia, writer's cramp, hemifacial spasm, and for aesthetic reasons.[36,37]

Since the original reports regarding the use of BTX-A for treatment of headache[19–21] and subsequent reports for its use in the determination of trigger sites,[23] the review of the neurology literature is contradictory in terms of success rate, possibly because these studies were not specific about the location of the injection.[38–41] Recent practice for prophylactic migraine headache treatment using BTX-A is based on PREEMPT I and PREEMPT II double blind, placebo-controlled randomized trials is profoundly flawed because of lack of focus on the anatomy of the nerve and muscle and using $\frac{1}{2}$ inch length needle for the injection that fails to reach the intended anatomical deep structures.[50,51]

When BTX-A is used to identify trigger sites, the sites are injected systematically, starting with the most common and severe trigger site based on the patient's reported symptoms and physical examination. This is most often the corrugator supercilii muscle. First, 12.5 U BTX-A is injected with a long 30-gauge, 1-inch needle into the glabellar muscle sites through a single deep subcutaneous horizontal injection. Patients then keep a headache diary and refrain from taking prophylactic migraine medication unless contraindicated. Response to the injection over the subsequent 4 weeks will direct the next step. If the headache disappears completely, it means the injected site is likely to be the sole trigger site. If the headaches are improved but not eliminated, it means that the patient has additional trigger sites. If the patient does not respond to the injection, it means that the headaches are not likely to be triggered from the initial injection site (Fig. 4.3). Often the patients will report elimination of the headaches from that trigger site but continuation of headaches in the temporal, retrobulbar, or occipital headaches. The other common trigger sites are injected 1 month apart, up to a maximum of three injections. Those patients with trigger sites that observe at least 50% reduction in intensity or frequency of the headache from baseline are considered for surgical intervention.[28] Nerve

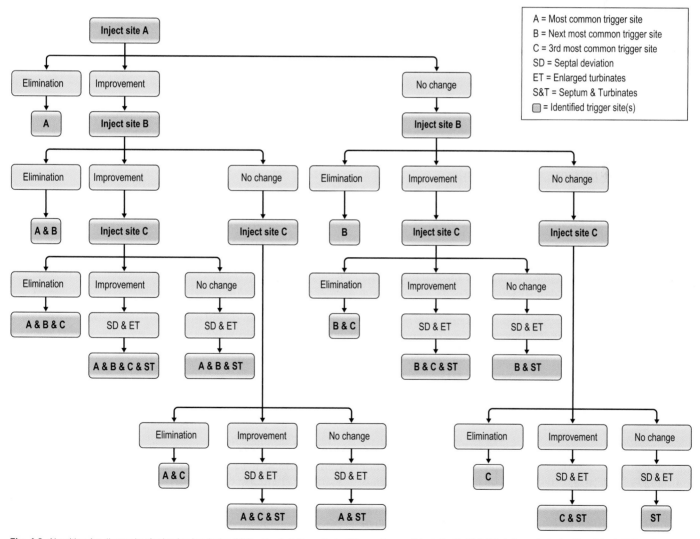

Fig. 4.3 Algorithm for diagnosis of migraine headache (MH) using botulinum toxin. Trigger sites are injected with 12.5 U botulinum toxin A with a 1-inch (2.5-cm) 30-gauge needle. Improvement is operationally defined as a 50% reduction in headache intensity or frequency from the baseline for 4 weeks. *(Redrawn from Guyuron B, Kriegler JS, Davis J, et al. Comprehensive surgical treatment of migraine headaches.* Plast Reconstr Surg *2005;115:1–9.)*

blocks could be used similarly, but the timing of the injections is difficult since it has to be done while the patient has migraine headaches to be meaningful. Lack of positive response to the nerve block or BTX-A does not mean that the patient is not a good candidate for surgery. When the patient has allodynia or the patient has established (centralized) migraine attack the response to the nerve block could be negative.

The primary side effect of BTX-A injected into the temporal area is atrophy of the temporal muscles and related hollowing of the temples and the reported hourglass deformity.[42] This disuse atrophy is temporary, and patients should be counseled appropriately. Eyelid ptosis is the second most common complication. Theoretically, strabismus might happen because of the high dose and deep injection in the temple or brow areas. Some patients have developed antibodies to BTX-A, rendering it relatively ineffective. This has been estimated to occur in 7% of treated patients.[35,43] The use of non-A botulinum toxins for patients resistant to type A is currently being investigated.[35]

While BTX-A had a major role in the detection of the trigger sites and as the prognosticator during the initial phases of the development of this procedure, we currently do not use it routinely due to the cumbersome course of injections which becomes impractical while caring for out-of-the-region patients, increasing cost and delaying potential elimination in patients who otherwise would benefit from the surgery. A nerve block will serve a similar role if it is injected while the patient is in the early stages of the migraine cascade. The constellation of symptoms can serve as reliably as BTX-A in the detection of the trigger sites.[52]

Surgical technique

Deactivation of frontal trigger site

In the frontal trigger site, the supraorbital and supratrochlear nerves are passing through the glabellar muscles, including the corrugator supercilii, depressor supercilii, and procerus. The nerves could be irritated by this group of muscles, vessels traveling with the nerves through bony supraorbital foramen or under the fascial band beneath the supraorbital notch. The goal of surgery is to prevent irritation of the nerves by all of these structures, complete and thorough resection of the muscle is suggested for a favorable outcome.[19] The approach can be either transpalpebral[44,45] or endoscopic. The endoscopic approach is a better choice for those who suffer from MH triggered from both temporal and frontal sites.

Transpalpebral approach

Under intravenous sedation or general anesthesia, the face is prepped and draped. The upper tarsal crease is marked on each eyelid, with an incision length of approximately 1 inch (2.5 cm), unless a concomitant blepharoplasty is planned. For the latter indication, a conventional blepharoplasty incision is utilized. Local anesthesia (0.5% lidocaine with 1 : 100 000 epinephrine) is infiltrated into the eyelid. A skin incision is made with a 10 blade and is extended through the orbicularis muscle. The plane between the orbicularis muscle and the septum is identified, and dissection is continued cephalically with a pair of baby Metzenbaum scissors. The depressor

supercilii muscle comes into view first. This muscle is lighter in color than the corrugator supercilii and it is also less friable. The muscle is then removed as thoroughly as possible. The corrugator supercilii muscle is identified next by its position over the supraorbital rim, as well as its darker color compared with the orbicularis oculi and depressor supercilii muscles. A small communicating vein is often seen between the supraorbital and supratrochlear vessels, deep to the muscle. Almost consistently, a nerve branch can be identified which pierces the muscle. This nerve is followed to its origin in the supraorbital region while the muscle is lifted. The corrugator supercilii muscle is removed in a medial to lateral fashion as thoroughly as possible using electrocautery. Sometimes multi-tooth forceps serve effectively to avulse the muscle completely around the nerve, while the supraorbital and supratrochlear nerves are preserved. Through this approach, supraorbital and supratrochlear vessels are dissected off the nerves, cauterized using a bipolar cautery, and removed. The supraorbital notch also is evaluated for possible compression points by a fascial band or possible presence of bony tunnel. A preoperative peri-nasal CT scan can help with identification and location of the main and the accessory bony tunnel. If present, these are unroofed. If the accessary foramen is very deep, the related branch is removed. Fat is harvested from the medial compartment of the upper eyelid and grafted to the site of the resected muscle. The fat graft serves three purposes: (1) it minimizes contour irregularity resulting from a thorough muscle resection; (2) it protects the exposed nerve branches; and (3) it minimizes the recurrent muscle function. The graft is sutured to the periosteum with 6-0 Monocryl suture, and the skin incision is sutured with 6-0 plain catgut.[44,45]

Postoperatively, the patient is allowed to resume light activities on day 1, regular activities on day 7, and heavy exercise after 3 weeks. Patients observe a reasonable amount of edema and ecchymosis, which usually subside in 10–14 days.

Complications

The most common complication with this approach includes itching of the forehead and frontoparietal scalp, which usually lasts several weeks to several months. Rarely, this may persist for a year or two. Every patient experiences some anesthesia or paresthesia immediately after surgery. This includes the entire forehead and anterior scalp. This paresthesia nearly always resolves if the nerves have been preserved. There is a risk of asymmetry and dynamic imperfections if the muscle is not removed thoroughly and evenly.

Endoscopic approach

For the patients who have optimal or short forehead length and experience migraine headaches in the forehead and temple, an endoscopic approach is preferred. After proper preparation of the face under sedation, the incision sites are marked. There are a total of five or six incisions, each one measuring 1–1.5 cm in length depending on the thickness of the scalp – one or two frontal incisions and two on either temple located 7 and 10 cm from the midline, all placed within the hair-bearing skin. For patients with a normal or short forehead, one midline incision is used. In patients with a borderline long forehead or excessively curved contour, two midline incisions are utilized. Xylocaine containing 1:100 000 epinephrine is injected in the non-hair-bearing skin and Xylocaine containing 1:200 000 epinephrine is injected in the hair-bearing skin. The Endoscopic Access Device (EAD; Applied Medical Technology, Cleveland, OH) is used for hair control and to facilitate insertion of the endoscopic equipment by keeping the wound margin apart. The dissection is performed in the subperiosteal plane down to the supraorbital and lateral orbital rims, and the zygomatic arch. The procedure for ZTBTN resection is described below and requires exposure of the zygomatic arch. For corrugator resection, attention is concentrated in the glabellar area. Once the supraorbital and the supratrochlear nerves and corrugator muscle groups are exposed, the periosteum is then released laterally, leaving the central portion intact over the mid-glabellar area to prevent too much elevation of the medial eyebrows. The corrugator and depressor muscles, along with vessels, are removed as thoroughly as possible while the operating surgeon's non-dominant index finger is compressing the soft tissues against the grasper from the outside. Through this approach, the supraorbital rim is evaluated for any possible compression point and presence of fascial band or bony tunnels which are released using a 2 mm percutaneous osteotome, if present. Fat harvested from the temporal region is delivered to the corrugator site using the technique described by our group.[45,46] To harvest the fat, the junction of the zygomatic arch with the malar body is identified, a small rent in the deep temporal fascia is created cephalad to the arch, and the fat is harvested while the assistant is compressing on the buccal area.

Fascial sutures of 3-0 polydioxanone are placed for suspension of the temple area further laterally and cephalically to achieve some eyebrow lift, if needed. The suture suspends the superficial temporal fascia from the deep temporal fascia. Incisions are repaired with 5-0 polyglactin (Vicryl) and 5-0 plain catgut.[24]

Complications

Alopecia can rarely occur at the port sites. Every patient experiences complete anesthesia immediately after surgery; however, permanent paresthesia or anesthesia is unlikely. Transient itching might happen after surgery. Inadequate resection of muscle may result in recurrence of the symptoms, and dynamic irregularity or dimpling can occur on animation.[47] The temporal branch of the facial nerve can rarely be injured during the dissection. This is exceedingly rare and would result in only a temporary paralysis.

Deactivation of temporal triggers

Temporal headaches are triggered primarily by irritation of the zygomaticotemporal branch of the trigeminal nerve by the muscle, fascia, or the vessels.

After appropriate preparation of the head and face, four 1–1.5-cm incisions are marked – two on each temple, usually 7 and 10 cm from the midline and one in the midline, only if the glabellar trigger site deactivation is also intended. Otherwise, the two most lateral incisions are used. The forehead, temple, and malar regions are then injected with 1% lidocaine with 1:100 000 epinephrine. The hair-bearing scalp is injected with 0.5% lidocaine with 1:200 000 epinephrine.

After the incisions are made with a number 15 scalpel, they are deepened to the deep temporal fascia using the spreading effects of the baby Metzenbaum scissors. The dissection continues using an Obwegeser periosteal elevator, and the EAD is inserted to allow the endoscope to be introduced. The periosteum is raised posteriorly and cephalically. Once dissection is completed on the right side, it is repeated on the left side.

A subperiosteal dissection is then carried out to the supraorbital rim, lateral orbital rim, and zygomatic and malar arches under endoscopic visualization. The dissection is continued immediately superficial to the deep temporal fascia until the Zygomaticotemporal branch is exposed (Fig. 4.4). It is absolutely crucial to the safety and success of this operation to avoid dissection too superficial to the deep temporal fascia. This means that no fat should be left attached to the deep temporal fascia. Grasping forceps or a long hemostat is used to dissect and avulse the nerve. It is important to avulse as much length of the nerve as possible to prevent re-coaptation. Often a segment of the nerve measuring around 2 cm is removed. Any bleeding vessels are coagulated, and the proximal nerve end is allowed to retract into the temporalis muscle to reduce the risk of neuroma formation. In our recent study, the results of nerve decompression have been shown to be the same as nerve avulsion.[53] The decompression will include removing the vessels accompanying the nerve and temporalis fasciotomy around the nerve.

The periosteum and arcus marginalis are released in the lateral orbital and supraorbital regions on patients older than

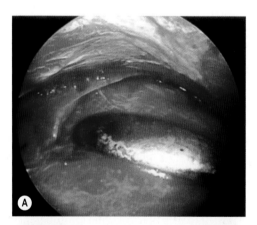

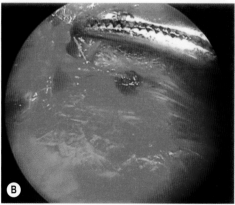

Fig. 4.4 Endoscopic view of the zygomaticotemporal branch of the trigeminal nerve. **(A)** The dissection is performed using a periosteal elevator. **(B)** The nerve can be seen superficial to the deep temporal fascia just under the grasping forceps.

35 to facilitate some rejuvenation.[23] The endoscopic devices are removed, and a single hook is placed on either side of the caudal portion of the incision. A 3-0 PDS suture is used to fix the superficial and intermediate temporal fascia to the deep temporal fascia laterally. Skin incisions are repaired with 5-0 poliglecaprone (Monocryl) and 5-0 plain catgut interrupted stitches.

Patients are allowed to return to light activities the next day, to regular activities within 7 days, and to strenuous exercise within 3 weeks.

Complications

Every patient experiences transient anesthesia and paresthesia in the temple area postoperatively. Permanent anesthesia and paresthesia are rare. Alopecia around the incisions can occur, and often is temporary. Injury to the temporal branch of the facial nerve may rarely cause paralysis of the frontalis muscle. This complication is usually short-lasting as well. A neuroma, although a possibility after the avulsion of the nerve, has not been observed after this surgery.

Deactivation of occipital triggers

A 4-cm midline incision is designed in the hair-bearing caudal occipital region while the patient is seated. After induction of anesthesia, the patient is placed in a prone position with the shoulders raised by a gel roll and the neck stabilized. The area around the incision is shaved to a total width of approximately 3 cm. The incision site is then infiltrated with 1% lidocaine with 1:100000 epinephrine (Fig. 4.5A). The skin incision is made with a number 10 scalpel, and hemostasis is achieved with coagulation cautery. The incision is taken to the midline raphe (Fig. 4.5B), and the trapezius fascia is incised about 0.5 cm lateral to midline (Fig. 4.5C), leaving the midline raphe intact. The trapezius muscle, which rarely reaches the midline, has obliquely oriented fibers and, if encountered, it is divided and retracted laterally; the semispinalis capitus muscle fibers are identified by their vertical orientation and their location directly underneath the fascia. The semispinalis muscle is then further exposed following retraction of the trapezius fascia, and dissection is continued under the fascia with a pair of Metzenbaum scissors. The trunk of the greater occipital nerve is easily located approximately 1.5 cm from the midline and 3 cm caudal to the occipital protuberance (Fig. 4.5D). Munion clamps are used to isolate the nerve. A vessel loop is placed around the nerve for retraction (Fig. 4.5E). A full-thickness, 2.5-cm long piece of the muscle is dissected medial to the nerve and is transected cephalically and caudally using cautery in the coagulation mode. The muscle resection is considered complete when no muscle fibers remain medial to the nerve (Figs. 4.5F & 4.5G). A small portion of the trapezius fascia and muscle immediately overlying the nerve is then removed (Figs. 4. 5H & 4.5I). The nerve is traced laterally ensuring that no fascial bands, which may cause compression, remain superficial to the nerve, similar to carpal tunnel release. Occasionally, the nerve bifurcates within the muscle. In this case, it is necessary to remove muscle fibers between the two branches.

Dissection is continued laterally and superiorly along the direction of the nerve until the nerve reaches the subcutaneous adipose tissue. The occipital artery or its branches that are in contact with the nerve are cauterized using bipolar cautery and removed. A 2 × 2-cm subcutaneous flap, based caudally, is elevated and passed under the nerve to isolate the nerve from muscle (Figs. 4.5J & 4.5K). Usually after incision of the skin and on the way of dissection to the semispinalis muscle, the third occipital nerve is encountered; in this case, the nerve is avulsed on each side and allowed to retract into the muscle.

After completion of the procedure on the opposite side, the two subcutaneous flaps are sutured to the deepest portion of the midline raphe (Figs. 4.5L & 4.5M) using a 5-0 Monocryl suture. A single TLS drain is placed on the left side using a trocar and passed to the right side under the midline raphe (Fig. 4.5N). A total 0.5 mL of a Kenalog 40-mg solution is injected in the perineurium and along the course of the nerves. The wound is irrigated and repaired with 5-0 Monocryl to reattach the subcutaneous tissue to the midline raphe and eliminate the dead space. (Fig. 4.5O). The skin is repaired using 5-0 plain catgut running locked sutures.

Complications

Infection or bleeding is rare after this procedure. Reattaching the skin to the midline raphe reduces the chance of seroma formation. Temporary anesthesia and paresthesia are expected. Permanent anesthesia and paresthesia are unlikely. Every patient experiences a slight depression in the removed muscle site. However, since this is covered with hair, patients are not concerned about this.

Septonasal triggers

Septonasal triggers must be considered when the pain mostly starts from behind the eyes, commonly triggered by weather or hormonal changes, especially when the pain is daily, is worse in the morning, or injection of BTX-A in other trigger sites results in no change or results in improvement without resolution. The main pathologic actors are (1) deviated septum with a spur which is in contact with a turbinate; (2) presence of concha bullosa; and (3) Haller's cell. The main goal of surgery is to eliminate the contact point or decompress the concha bullosa.

The face is prepped and draped after the induction of general anesthesia. The nose is packed with cocaine-soaked gauze and is infiltrated with 0.5% lidocaine with 1:200000 epinephrine initially and 0.5% lidocaine containing 1:100000 epinephrine after a few minutes. An L-shaped incision is made on the left side of the septum, and the mucoperiosteum is elevated. After extending the L shape incision through the quadrangle cartilage, the opposite mucoperiosteum is elevated. The deviated portion of the cartilaginous septum and perpendicular plate of the ethmoid and vomer bone are removed, and the straight portion of the cartilage is placed back in the site. It is crucial to remove any existing spurs and eliminate any contact points between the turbinates and the septum. The mucoperiosteal flap is sutured back into place with 5-0 chromic running sutures. Doyle stents are placed in each side and fixated to the membranous septum with 4-0 Prolene sutures.

The Doyle stents are removed in 3–8 days. The patient may resume light activities on postoperative day 1, heavy activities on postoperative day 7, and strenuous activities in 3 weeks.

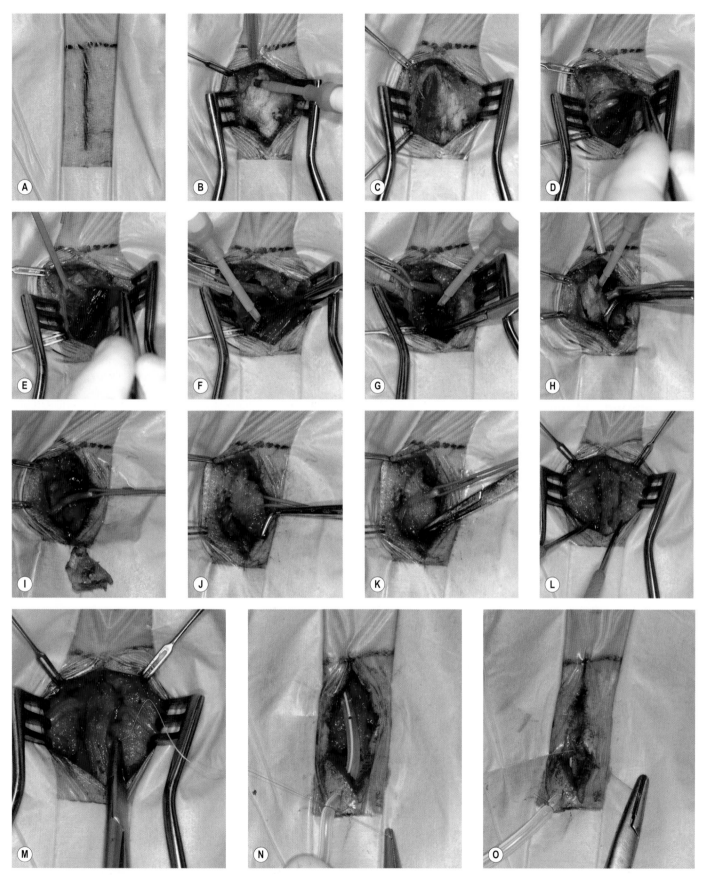

Fig. 4.5 Surgical technique for release of the occipital nerve for occipital migraines. **(A)** The 1.6-inch (4-cm) incision is designed in the caudal occipital region. **(B)** The incision is taken to the midline raphe, and **(C)** the trapezius fascia is incised slightly away from the midline; the semispinalis muscle fibers can be identified by their vertical orientation. **(D)** Dissection continues subfascially and superficial to the muscle, and the trunk of the occipital nerve will be seen approximately 0.6 inch (1.5 cm) lateral to the midline and 1.2 inch (3 cm) caudal to the occipital protuberance. **(E–G)** A 1-inch (2.5-cm) length of muscle is dissected medial to the nerve and transected. **(H–L)** A flap is designed to be placed under the nerve to protect it. **(M)** The flap is sutured to the midline raphe, and **(N)** a drain is placed. **(O)** The incision is closed in layers while attaching the subcutaneous flap to the midline raphe.

In some cases, the inferior turbinates are enlarged or have a contact point with the septum and require reduction. The inferior turbinate is infiltrated with 0.5% lidocaine containing 1:200 000 epinephrine, and 0.5% lidocaine containing 1:100 000 epinephrine after a few minutes. Turbinate scissors are used to resect the inferior turbinates conservatively, leaving normal turbinate size behind. A partial in-fracture is performed and the area is cauterized. A patient who has concha bullosa or significant enlargement of the middle turbinates will require partial or complete resection of the middle turbinates. Using the sharp end of the septal elevator, the mucosa overlying the turbinate is incised and peeled off over the medial half of the turbinate. The medial wall of the concha bullosa is resected, raw margins are cauterized, and Doyle stents are inserted. Turbinate reduction could also be performed using a zero degree scope and 4.3 mm microshaver KPS.

Complications

Temporary dryness of the nose occurs in 12% of our patients. At this time, we have not observed permanent dryness. Synechiae and sinus infection are rare. A small percentage of patients experience postoperative epistaxis, which, if significant enough, is treated with desmopressin (DDAVP) 0.3 microgram/kg of body weight dissolved in 50 cc saline and infused over 45 min without having to pack the nose.[48]

Less common trigger points

The auriculotemporal nerve, lesser occipital nerve, third occipital nerve, and end branches of the other main nerves in the scalp or temporal area could act as trigger sites. Blood vessels are the most common reason for nerve irritation, although fascial bands also can act as trigger sites.

Trigger points in the scalp or lateral temporal area are evaluated by asking the patients to put their fingertip over the pain starting point or maximum tender point. This area is marked, and using a handheld Doppler machine, a vascular signal is almost invariably identified. Having a blood vessel signal over the tender points is suggestive of a close relationship between the peripheral nerve branches with the blood vessels.

These peripheral trigger points could be addressed under local anesthesia. After preparation and draping the area, a small incision is made over the tender point which corresponds to the Doppler signal, dissection is carried down, and usually some type of nerve–vessel crossover could be found in the area. Blood vessels are dissected off the nerve and excised after cauterization. Occasionally, a fascial band is also identified in the area, which could be released. (Fig. 4.6). The small nerve branch is removed to augment the chance of elimination.

Complications

Bleeding and infection are very rare. Temporary anesthesia in the area could happen. Neuroma is very unlikely and, if it occurs, it is excised and the nerve is buried in the muscle.

Conclusion

A patient who presents for surgical treatment for migraine headaches should have a thorough headache evaluation. Trigger sites are then identified by the constellation of the presenting symptoms, CT of the peripheral sinuses, and finding the Doppler signal. For frontal trigger sites, corrugator muscle group resection is performed. For temporal trigger sites, the ZTBTN is avulsed. For occipital trigger sites, the semispinalis capitis muscle medial to the greater occipital nerve is resected. Septoplasty and turbinectomy is performed in patients who have evidence of septal deviation and enlarged turbinates with contact points, and whose clinical profile suggests septal and turbinate related migraine triggers.

⊕ Bonus content for this chapter can be found online at
http://www.expertconsult.com

Box 4.1 Migraine headache diagnostic criteria

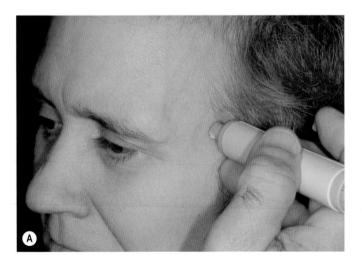
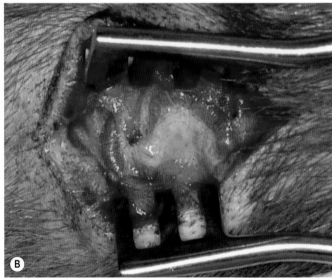

Fig. 4.6 Exploration of peripheral trigger points: **(A)** use of handheld Doppler in tender point, **(B)** artery and nerve relationship,

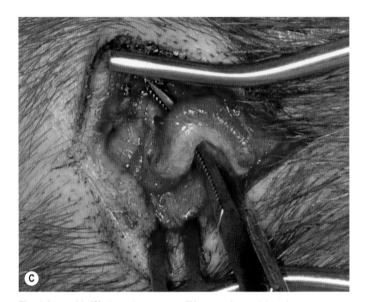 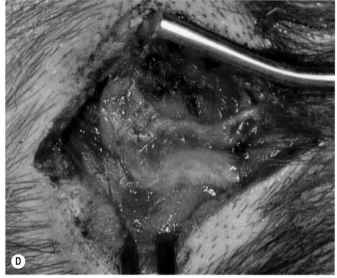

Fig. 4.6, cont'd **(C)** dissection process, **(D)** nerve after excision of artery.

Access the complete reference list online at **http://www.expertconsult.com**

18. Guyuron B, Varghai A, Michelow BJ, et al. Corrugator supercilii muscle resection and migraine headaches. *Plast Reconstr Surg.* 2000;106:429–434, discussion 435–437. *In this retrospective review, migraine headache status was assessed in patients undergoing forehead rejuvenation procedures involving resection of the corrugator supercilii. A strong correlation between corrugator removal and relief of migraine headaches was demonstrated.*

23. Guyuron B, Tucker T, Davis J. Surgical treatment of migraine headaches. *Plast Reconstr Surg.* 2002;109:2183–2189. *This is a prospective trial evaluating a surgical approach (corrugator resection, transection of the zygomaticotemporal branch of the trigeminal nerve, and temple soft-tissue repositioning) to managing migraine headaches. A significant improvement in symptomatology was demonstrated with surgery, and preoperative Botox injection was demonstrated to be useful in predicting this response.*

24. Totonchi A, Pashmini N, Guyuron B. The zygomaticotemporal branch of the trigeminal nerve: an anatomical study. *Plast Reconstr Surg.* 2005;115:273–277.

25. Mosser SW, Guyuron B, Janis JE, et al. The anatomy of the greater occipital nerve: implications for the etiology of migraine headaches. *Plast Reconstr Surg.* 2004;113:693–697, discussion 698–700. *It is theorized that trigger points along the greater occipital nerve may contribute to migraine headache symptomatology. This anatomic study assesses the course of the greater occipital nerve to enhance the efficacy of chemodenervation procedures.*

26. Dash KS, Janis JE, Guyuron B. The lesser and third occipital nerves and migraine headaches. *Plast Reconstr Surg.* 2005;115:1752–1758, discussion 1759–1760.

27. Guyuron B, Kriegler JS, Davis J, et al. Comprehensive surgical treatment of migraine headaches. *Plast Reconstr Surg.* 2005;115:1–9. *In this randomized prospective clinical trial, Botox injections were used to identify migraine headache trigger sites in diagnosed migraine sufferers. Site-specific surgical releases were shown to reduce migraine symptoms significantly compared to controls.*

28. Guyuron B, Reed D, Kriegler JS, et al. A placebo-controlled surgical trial of the treatment of migraine headaches. *Plast Reconstr Surg.* 2009;124:461–468. *This is a double-blind, sham surgery-controlled clinical trial that demonstrates the efficacy of trigger-point-specific surgical management of migraine headaches.*

31. Guyuron B, Tucker T, Kriegler JS. Botulinum toxin A and migraine surgery. *J Plast Reconstr Surg.* 2003;112(suppl):171S–173S, discussion 174S-176S.

5

Scalp and forehead reconstruction

Julian J. Pribaz and Edward J. Caterson

SYNOPSIS

- The scalp and forehead are specialized components of the uppermost part of the head. Although at first glance they appear to be quite different, with the scalp being static hair-bearing tissue and the forehead being hairless with significant mimetic function, they both share a similar layered anatomy remembered by the mnemonic, "SCALP".

- The convexity of the skull results in increased tautness of the overlying soft tissues, which causes increased tension in repairs after injury, and making flap repair more complex.

- There is a rich blood supply from branches of both the external and internal carotid systems, which allows closure of wounds with moderate tension and the safe transfer of flaps as long as the vascularity is respected.

- There are some unique and specific pathological processes as well as other general conditions, both benign and malignant, affecting the scalp and forehead.

- The goal of all reconstruction is to obtain the best possible outcome, which is ideally achieved by using "like" tissue, which is in limited supply. This is feasible for smaller lesions, which can be reconstructed with local tissue transfers. Larger wounds will leave secondary donor defects requiring skin grafting. There are few regional flap options. For very large or complex defects, free tissue transfers are the best solution.

- The subunit principle should be used to design the ideal method of reconstruction to maximize the outcome. The scalp with its hair-bearing feature can be considered as its own extensive subunit, while the forehead is best considered as several different subunits, depending on the location and mobility of the soft tissues.

- In forehead reconstruction, care should be taken to avoid any displacement of the surrounding mimetic or mobile anatomical features, especially the eyebrow, upper eyelid, and glabella at its inferior border.

- Secondary procedures are indicated to maximize the aesthetic outcome for both scalp and forehead reconstruction. For the scalp, this mainly involves restoration of hair-bearing tissue, often performed with the use of serial tissue expansion; for the forehead, this involves restoring any displaced surrounding landmarks, and obtaining a smooth homogeneous surface.

Introduction

The scalp and forehead are a very specialized and unique component of the upper most part of the head and neck. It is dome-shaped and covers the cranium and the underlying brain. Although at first glance, the forehead and scalp looked quite different, mainly due to the hair-bearing character of the scalp, the underlying structures are remarkably similar with some regional difference that impact the approach to reconstruction. Its exposed nature makes it especially vulnerable to all forms of trauma, direct sun exposure with its long-term sequelae, as well as some unique disorders that give rise to pathological conditions that can result in challenging defects that can be difficult to repair. This is due in part to the tautness of tissue compounded by the convexity of the scalp and forehead.

Fortunately, there is a very rich blood supply which permits elevation of hardy flaps that can withstand moderate tension which is typically encountered when covering convex surfaces. Nonetheless, careful analysis of each defect, a sound knowledge of the anatomy, especially the blood supply, and the use of templates and patterns are invaluable in designing appropriate flaps which can result in a satisfactory outcome.

In this chapter we will review the relevant anatomy, disease processes, patient selection, and options for reconstruction with the goal of developing some algorithms to assist in this process. We will consider the overlapping similarities of the scalp and forehead, but then consider the reconstructive options separately.

Basic science/disease process

Anatomy

The scalp and forehead constitute a significant area of the head and neck which is proportionally greater in children than in adults. A thorough understanding of the surgical anatomy of the scalp and forehead is vital to the reconstructive surgeon. This compound unit extends from the superior orbital rims anteriorly to the nuchal line posteriorly. Laterally, it extends from each frontal process of the zygoma and zygomatic arch anteriorly, the ear centrally and mastoid process posteriorly. The most obvious attribute of the scalp is that it is hair-bearing. The forehead is typically the area devoid of hair and is best considered as a separate unit, extending between the side-burns laterally and the supraorbital ridges and glabella inferiorly. Superiorly, the boundary between the forehead and scalp depends on the hairline which is variable with age and gender.

Scalp

The scalp and forehead are often considered as a single unit due to its similar composition of tissue layers, which can be remembered by the mnemonic "SCALP", where S is the skin, C is the subcutaneous tissue, A is the aponeurotic layer, L is the loose areolar tissue, and P is the pericranium. However, there are regional differences in relative tissue composition that impact reconstruction (Fig. 5.1).[1–3]

The outermost layer of the scalp is the skin, containing hair follicles; sebaceous and sweat glands that extend into the dermis and laterally, in the temporal region, are located just superficial to the temporoparietal fascia. There are septa connecting the dermis and deep aponeurotic layer.

The galea aponeurotica is a fibrous aponeurosis that extends and connects the occipitalis muscles posteriorly and the frontalis muscles anteriorly. Laterally, the temporoparietal fascia is an extension of the galea and, anterolaterally, the galea is confluent with the superficial muscular aponeurotic system (SMAS) of the face.[4] The muscles within this layer consist of the paired frontalis muscles anteriorly and occipitalis muscles posteriorly and the auricularis muscles laterally. The frontalis muscles originate from the galea and insert into the dermis of the brow. Contraction of the frontalis causes elevation of the eyebrows producing horizontal wrinkle lines in the forehead. Anteriorly, the frontalis muscles blend with the procerus and corrugator supercilii muscles as well as the upper aspects of the orbicularis oculi muscles. The paired corrugator supercilii muscles arise from the frontal bone near the superomedial orbital rim and then pass superolaterally through the fibers of the orbicularis oculi and the frontalis muscles before inserting into the medial eyebrow skin. The corrugator muscle is the brow depressor pulling the brow medially and inferiorly producing vertical glabella wrinkles. The procerus muscle is a thin muscle that inserts into the glabella and lower mid forehead. It is a brow depressor forming horizontal nasal root creases.[3]

In the posterior scalp, the paired occipitalis muscles take origin from the superior nuchal line and mastoid and insert into the galea. There are also three auricular muscles on each side of the scalp – the anterior, superior, and posterior auricular muscles. They take their origin from the temporalis fascia

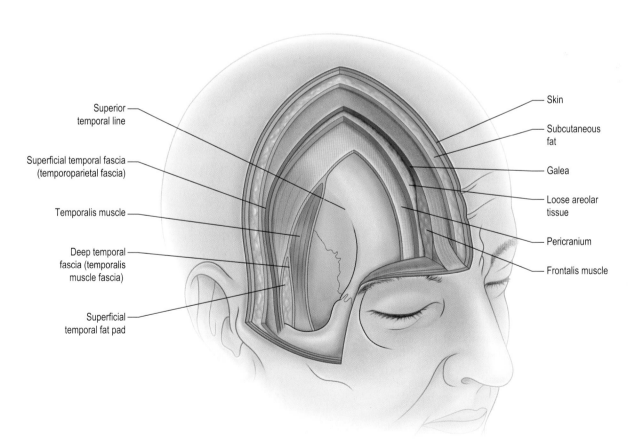

Superior temporal line

Superficial temporal fascia (temporoparietal fascia)

Temporalis muscle

Deep temporal fascia (temporalis muscle fascia)

Superficial temporal fat pad

Skin

Subcutaneous fat

Galea

Loose areolar tissue

Pericranium

Frontalis muscle

Fig. 5.1 Layers of the scalp: S, skin; C, subcutaneous tissue; A, aponeurotic layer; L, loose areolar tissue; and P, pericranium. *(Reproduced from TerKonda RP, Sykes JM. Concepts of scalp and forehead reconstruction.* Otolaryngol Clin North Am. *1997;30:519–539.)*

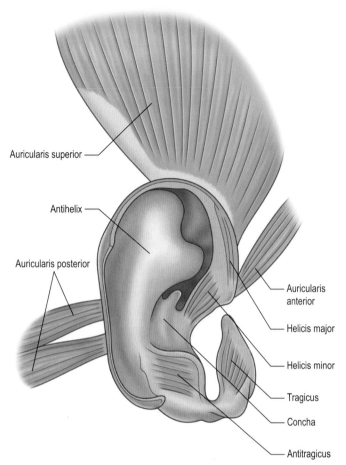

Fig. 5.2 Extrinsic muscles of the ear – anterior auricular, superior auricular, and posterior auricular muscles. *(Reproduced from Agarwal CA, Mendenhall SD, Foreman KB, et al. The course of the frontal branch of the facial nerve in relation to fascial planes: an anatomic study.* Plast Reconstr Surg. *2012;125:532–537.)*

and mastoid bone and insert into of the perichondrium of the external ear (Fig. 5.2).

Beneath the galea is a loose areolar layer that is very thin over the vertex that becomes thicker laterally where it joints the temporoparietal fascia. It is at this level of loose areolar tissue that scalping injuries occur. Historically, scalps were taken as trophies of war, but in modern times similar scalping injuries are produced when hair gets entangled in industrial machinery. The deepest layer of the scalp is the pericranium or periosteum of the cranium. This is a well vascularized layer firmly adherent to the skull in the region of the cranial sutures.

The temporal region of the scalp has additional specialized layers and attributes (Fig. 5.3). The hair-bearing skin typically is the last to lose its hair in cases of male pattern baldness. The temporoparietal fascia (TPF) is an extension of the galea and is closely applied to the skin and the hair follicles and has a rich blood supply which passes on its deep surface. Anteriorly, the frontal branch of the facial nerve passes in this layer. There is a deeper, thin subgaleal fascial layer which can be delaminated from the TPF, which can be useful to expand the width of vascularized fascial coverage as may be required in total ear cartilaginous construct coverage.

Deep to this is the deep temporal fascia which is thick and fuses with the periosteum superiorly above the temporalis

muscle. Its main part overlies the temporalis muscle, and inferiorly it splits into superficial and deep layers. The superficial layer attaches to the anterior aspect of the zygomatic arch, and the deeper layer fuses with medial aspect of the zygomatic arch. This is the plane of dissection for access to the zygomatic arch in cases of zygomatic fractures (Gillies approach) and for raising bicoronal flaps to expose the craniofacial skeleton. Dissection deep to this layer avoids injury to the frontal branch of the facial nerve as it passes over the zygomatic arch within the fascia (Fig. 5.4).

The temporalis muscle is a large strong fan shaped muscle of mastication, which originates from the temporal fascia and skull and inserts into the coronoid process of the mandible. It receives its blood supply from the deep temporal branches of the internal maxillary artery. It is commonly used to provide a moderate sized muscle flap that may be used for orbital, palate, and cheek reconstruction, as well as a functional flap for facial reanimation (which is described in other chapters of this volume).

Forehead

The forehead extends from the superior orbital ridge and glabella inferiorly and is bounded by the hairline laterally and superiorly. The exact height of the forehead depends on the anterior hairline and varies with age and gender. It has a similar SCALP layered composition to the scalp, with some variation in different regions.

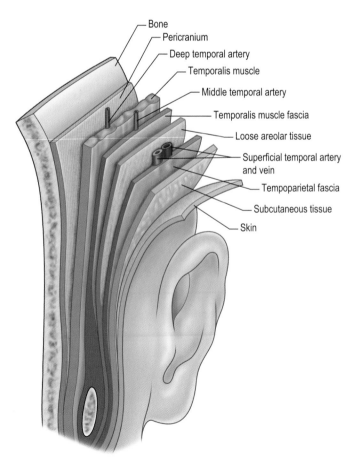

Fig. 5.3 Anatomy of the temporal region.

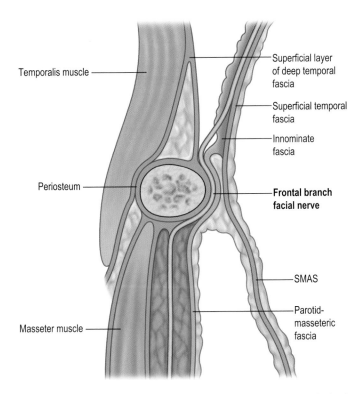

Fig. 5.4 Course of the frontal branch of the facial nerve. Cross section at the level of the zygomatic arch. *(Reproduced from Agawal CA, Mendenhall SD, Foreman KB, et al. The course of the frontal branch of the facial nerve in relation to fascial planes: an anatomic study. Plast Reconstr Surg. 2012;125:532–537.)*

In 1957, Gonzalez-Ulloa proposed the concept of the aesthetic units of the face and in his view, the whole forehead was considered to be a single subunit.[5] Subsequent authors have further modified and refined this concept subdividing the forehead into additional subunits. We believe that the description by Ian Jackson is the best to date.[6] This divides the forehead into a central subunit (which can be further divided into paramedian and lateral components), the supraorbital and glabella subunit, and the temporal subunits (Fig. 5.5). Although the basic anatomy is similar in these different subunits, there are local differences in the thickness and mobility of the tissue layers that allow different reconstructive strategies and flap options in the different subunits, that can enhance the outcomes in forehead reconstruction. The goal of reconstruction is to avoid distortion to the anatomical landmarks and boundaries of the forehead, especially the eyebrow inferiorly and the hairline superiorly and laterally.[7,8]

Blood supply

The blood supply of the scalp and forehead is rich, coming from five paired arteries that form a rich network within the subcutaneous plane. Contributions come from both the internal and external carotid system. Anteriorly, the paired supraorbital and supratrochlear vessels arise from the internal carotid system. Laterally, the superficial temporal and, posteriorly, the posterior auricular and occipital vessels are branches of the external carotid system.

The supraorbital and supratrochlear vessels arise from the ophthalmic artery, which is the first branch of the internal carotid artery, and they enter the forehead at the supraorbital rim and pass through the frontalis muscle at the brow and run in the subcutaneous plane. They anastomose laterally with the anterior branch of the superficial temporal artery.

The superficial temporal artery is the largest of the scalp vessels and is a terminal branch of the external carotid artery. It passes through the superficial lobe of the parotid in front of the ear running with the auriculotemporal nerve. The vessels run within the superficial temporal fascia and divide into anterior and posterior branches. It supplies blood on the temporal and central scalp, anastomosing anteriorly with the supraorbital and supratrochlear and posteriorly with the posterior auricular and occipital vessels.

The occipital artery provides blood supply to the posterior scalp above the nuchal line. It is a branch of the external carotid passing through the vertebral muscles and between trapezius and sternomastoid into the occipitalis muscle and divides into medial and lateral branches. The mastoid and post-auricular region is supplied by the posterior auricular artery, the smallest of the main vessels of the scalp (Fig. 5.6).

The venous drainage of the scalp is by veins that parallel and accompany the main arteries. Venous blood also flows through diploë of the cranium to the dural sinuses by emissary veins. The supratrochlear and supraorbital veins drain into the ophthalmic vein. Laterally, the venous drainage passes through the parotid gland and joins the maxillary vein to form the retromandibular vein. The post-auricular veins join the posterior division of the retromandibular vein to form the external jugular vein. The occipital veins drain into the deep cervical vertebral venous plexus.

Scalp lymphatics are located in the subdermal and subcutaneous layers. There are no lymph nodes in the scalp region. The lymphatic drainage is towards the parotid gland and into the pre- and post-auricular lymph nodes, as well as into the upper cervical and occipital nodes.[9]

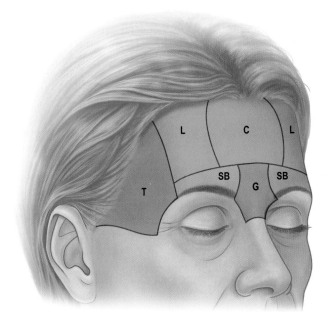

Fig. 5.5 Aesthetic subunits of the forehead region. L=lateral, C=central, SB=suprabrow, G=glabella, T=temporal. *(Redrawn from Jackson IT. In: Local Flaps in Head and Neck Reconstruction, 2nd edn. St. Louis: Quality Medical Publishing; 2007.)*

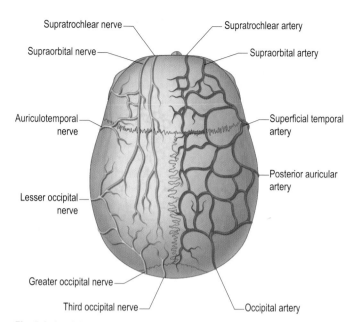

Fig. 5.6 Arterial and nerve supply of the scalp.

Innervation

The motor innervation to the muscles of the forehead comes from the frontal (also called temporal) branch(es) of the facial nerve (VII cranial nerve). There are often several branches, and these emerge from the parotid 2.5 cm anterior to the tragus and pass in the loose areolar plane just deep to the SMAS layer crossing the midportion of the zygomatic arch and then 1.5 cm lateral to the orbital rim to reach the underside of the frontalis muscle.[10] The corrugator muscles are also innervated by the temporal branch of the facial nerve, whereas the procerus muscle is innervated by the deep buccal branch of the facial nerve. The occipitalis muscle is innervated by the posterior auricular branch of the facial nerve. This originates from the facial nerve as it exits the stylomastoid foramen. The temporalis muscle is innervated by two branches from the third or mandibular division of the trigeminal nerve.

The sensory nerve supply to the anterior scalp and forehead comes by the supratrochlear and supraorbital nerves which originate from the ophthalmic or first division of the trigeminal nerve. The supratrochlear nerve exits the orbit between the pulley of the superior oblique and the supraorbital foramen. It passes beneath the corrugator muscles and supplies the medial forehead, the upper eyelid, and conjunctiva. The supraorbital nerve exits the frontal bone through the supraorbital foramen and then divides into a superficial and deep branch. The superficial branch penetrates the frontalis muscle and courses superiorly in the subcutaneous plane to the vertex of the scalp. The deep branch passes laterally between the periosteum and deep aspect of the frontalis muscle to supply the temporoparietal scalp (Fig. 5.7).[11]

The lateral orbit, temple, and scalp are supplied by the zygomaticofacial and zygomaticotemporal nerves which are branches of the maxillary or second division of the trigeminal nerve. The pre-auricular scalp is supplied by the auriculotemporal nerve which is a branch of the mandibular or third division of the trigeminal nerve.

The posterior scalp is supplied by the greater occipital and the third occipital nerve which are branches of the dorsal rami of the cervical spinal nerves. These emerge from the suboccipital triangle, 3 cm below the occipital protuberance and 1.5 cm lateral to the midline and supplies the posterior scalp to the vertex.

Disorders of the scalp and forehead

Scalp and forehead defects may result from a variety of congenital and acquired etiologies. The problems may be acute (lacerations, burns, avulsions, etc.) requiring immediate attention, or more elective, requiring work up and careful planning. The scalp is very vascular and bleeding can be excessive, requiring expeditious wound closure, which is usually the best way to obtain hemostasis.

The defects may be small or extensive, partial or full-thickness loss with possible loss of the underlying bone as well (Box 5.1).

Congenital and neonatal indications

These include aplasia cutis congenita, hemangiomas and vascular malformations, extravasation injuries and other rare conditions.

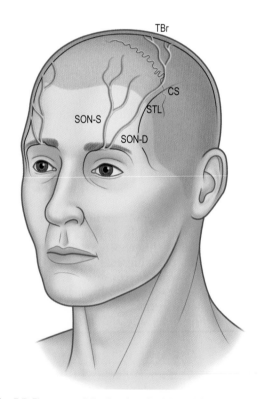

Fig. 5.7 The course of the deep branch of deep (SON-D) and superficial (SON-S) division of the supraorbital nerve. The deep branch superiorly or obliquely across the forehead between the galeal aponeurotica and the periosteum and by the mid-forehead level found between 0.5 and 1 cm medial to the superior temporal crest. It pierces the galea just before the coronal suture (CS). The superficial branch passes through the lower frontalis muscle to run over the surface of the muscle. TBr, terminal branch; STL, superior temporal line of the skull. *(Reproduced from Knize DM. A study of the supraorbital nerve.* Plast Reconstr Surg. *1995;96:564–569.)*

Congenital

A. Aplasia cutis congenita

B. Nevus sebaceous of Jadassohn

C. Nevoid basal cell nevus syndrome

D. Congenital melanoma

E. Dysplastic nevus syndrome

F. Giant hairy nevus

G. Xeroderma pigmentosa

H. En coup de sabre

I. Vascular malformations

J. Autoimmune

K. Scleroderma

Neoplastic

A. Malignant

   1. Basal cell carcinoma

   2. Squamous cell

   3. Malignant melanoma

   4. Sarcoma

B. Benign

   1. Lipoma

   2. Dermatofibroma

   3. Keratoacanthoma

   4. Neurofibroma

   5. Epidermal inclusion cyst

   6. Trichoepithelioma

   7. Hemangioma

   8. Syringoma

Infectious

A. Localized

   1. Bacterial

      a. Folliculitis decalvans

      b. Leprosy

   2. Viral

   3. Fungal

      a. Kerion

      b. Tinea capitis

B. Systemic

Acquired

A. Traumatic

   1. Physical

   2. Burns

      a. Thermal

      b. Chemical

      c. Electrical

      d. Radiation

Aplasia cutis congenita is a rare sporadic congenital deformity of unknown etiology, but it is thought to be a malformation of the neural tube leading to failure of differentiation of the skin in early embryonic life and can present with a range of subtotal to total absence of the skin, underlying fat, skull, dura, and occasionally underlying brain. In most cases it involves the vertex and the ulcers may be single or multiple. At birth, these defects are usually covered with a thin fragile membrane and are generally treated conservatively with dressing changes and allowed to heal by secondary intention, if small. Larger defects with absence of deeper structures are susceptible to infection, meningitis, sagittal sinus thrombosis, and hemorrhage, and may be life threatening and need to be formally closed with a flap. If allowed to heal by secondary intention, an atrophic hairless scar will result, which can be excised when the child is older. These children need to be carefully followed, especially if there is delayed healing with repeated breakdown, as the chronic wound may undergo malignant degeneration many years later, requiring aggressive resection, and complex reconstruction (Fig. 5.8).[12,13,14]

Hemangiomas and vascular malformations may also occur on the scalp and can present very challenging reconstructive problems.[15] The clinical findings and management are described in other chapters.

Intravenous fluid extravasation, especially in a neonate, is also fairly common due to use of scalp veins for fluid administration in the neonate. Generally, these small wounds are treated conservatively.

Traumatic defects

These range from simple lacerations to scalp avulsions and include thermal, electrical, and radiation burn injuries. With lacerations, basic principles of management are followed, obtaining a careful history and physical examination to identify possible associated injuries such as underlying skull fractures. The wound itself is managed by irrigation, debridement, and hemostasis. After debridement, closure may be difficult and it may be necessary to utilize some galeal scoring to achieve primary repair. Smaller defects may be managed conservatively with dressing changes and allowed to heal by secondary intention. However, the best way of achieving hemostasis is with wound closure. Larger defects may require skin grafting or local or distant flaps. Complex local flap reconstruction is best not performed at an acute stage but secondarily.

Partial and total scalp avulsion can be very challenging, but since the advent of microsurgery, the best option is to replant the scalp if at all possible. The level of avulsion is usually in the plane between the galea and the periosteum and may include parts of the forehead, eyebrows, upper lids, and also ears.[16] In 1976, Miller *et al.* reported the first successful total scalp replantation by microvascular anastomosis.[17] Microsurgical replantation should be attempted as this is the only way of restoring "normal"; there is no other way of adequately replacing the very specialized hair-bearing tissue.

Replantation can be very tedious and demanding, and there can be considerable blood loss, especially once the flap is initially revascularized. Blood should be available, and to expedite matters, a two-team approach is used, with one team dissecting the amputated part to identify the arteries (one superficial temporal artery can perfuse the entire scalp), and a second team to prepare the recipient site and vein grafts which are often needed. It can be difficult to identify the collapsed veins in the amputated part, but once the scalp is revascularized, the veins become very apparent with quite profuse bleeding. At least one artery and two veins should be

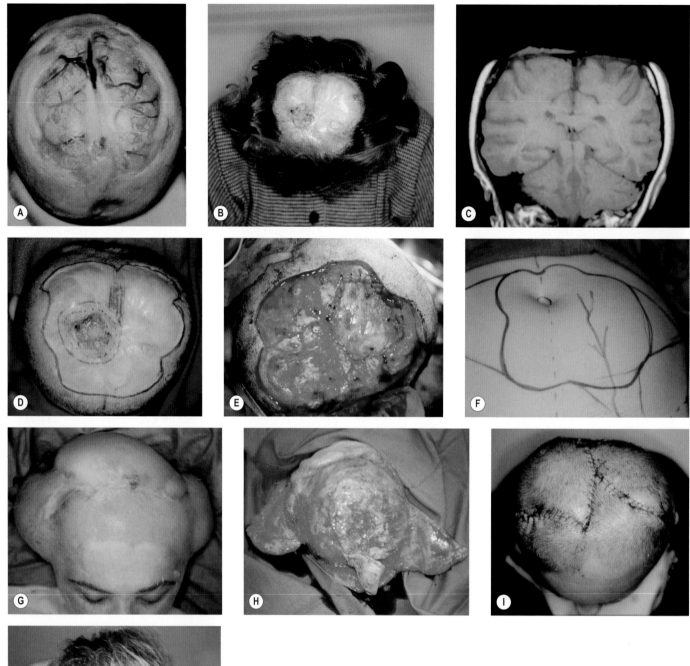

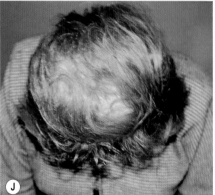

Fig. 5.8 Aplasia cutis congenita: the appearance in the neonatal period **(A)** and 30 years later **(B)**, when a squamous cell cancer developed in the unstable skin. A CT scan shows a lack of scalp and cranium **(C)**. The SCC and unstable skin was excised by neurosurgery **(D)** – it involved the dura and was close to the sagittal sinus. A dural patch was used to repair the dura **(E)** and a free TRAM flap is designed to repair this extensive defect **(F)**. The Free TRAM is well healed and two tissue expanders are in place beneath adjacent normal hair-bearing scalp **(G)**. After expansion, the TRAM flap is de-epithelialized **(H)** and the expanded flaps advanced to cover the central alopecia. The intraoperative **(I)** and later appearance **(J)** with full hair coverage is shown.

repaired and more if suitable.[18] The hair follicles are very susceptible to ischemic injury, and even with successful revascularization, the restoration of hair growth may be delayed (Fig. 5.9 ⊙).

Fig. 5.9 appears online only.

If replantation is not possible, acute management involves wound debridement and local wound care; temporary substitutes such as pigskin, cadaveric allograft, Integra, etc., may be used and followed by delayed skin grafting.

Burns are also common in the scalp and forehead and may be due to thermal, electrical, or radiation causes. Most of the burn injuries are due to thermal damage, but deeper and more severe injuries can result from electrical injuries. In electrical burns, because of the increased resistance to the electric current by the underlying skull, a great deal of local heat is produced increasing the amount of overlying skin damage. Achauer has classified scalp burns according to the extent of the injury as mild (less than 15% of the scalp), moderate, and extensive, without brain involvement and those with full-thickness skull or brain involvement.[19] The treatment options for burn injuries include conservative therapy consisting of early debridement of nonviable tissue and local wound therapy. Tangential excision of the scalp has also been used to debride eschar with an attempt to preserve the deep hair follicles and deeper dermal structures. A burn involving the outer table of the skull may be treated conservatively with moist dressing changes and awaiting granulation, which can arise from the skull emissary veins. Although this may take some time, this may nonetheless be the most appropriate treatment of these patients who have multiple associated injuries. Alternatively, the outer table may be lightly abraded to expedite the formation of granulation tissue which can subsequently be grafted.[20,21,22]

Cicatricial scalp alopecia is commonly seen after burn injury, and this can be managed secondarily either by serial excision of the alopecia if relatively small, or more commonly by the use of tissue expansion of the remaining hair-bearing skin, and subsequent flap advancement (Fig. 5.10A–C).[23]

Injuries to the frontal branch of the facial nerve are common in traumatic lacerations in the lateral portion of the forehead. The frontal branch or branches innervate the thin frontalis muscle on its undersurface and can be found 1.5 to 2.5 cm from the lateral orbital rim. However, the branches take a more variable pattern as they become more distal, and therefore, adequate physical examination should be undertaken in any injury that penetrates the frontalis musculature (Fig. 5.11). Repair of a frontal branch injury is possible, at least until the lateral limbus of the pupil, and the anterior branch of the superficial temporal artery is an excellent guide to the specific location of the distal portions of the frontal branch.

Tumors

Benign and malignant tumors commonly involve the skull and the forehead and can present many challenging defects once resected.

Dysplastic nevus

Dysplastic nevi are compound nevi with cellular and architectural dysplasia. They can be flat or raised and vary in size and have variable pigmentation. They can appear anywhere on the body, but are quite common in the scalp. Atypical moles can be inherited or sporadic. Familial atypical moles may be inherited in an autosomal dominant manner and are referred to as familial atypical multiple mole melanoma syndrome (FAMMM).[24] Melanoma can arise from atypical moles, but this is rare and it is thought that an individual nevus has a 1 in 200 000 chance of becoming malignant. Patients with familial variety (FAMMM) have a higher lifetime risk of malignant degeneration. These patients are followed regularly by their dermatologists with serial photography and changing or suspicious lesions are excised.[25]

Congenital hairy nevi (congenital nevomelanocytic nevi)

As their name suggests, congenital hairy nevi are present at birth and are composed of nevomelanocytes, derived from melanoblasts. They are classified into three groups: small (<1.5 cm), medium (1.5–19.5 cm), and large (>20 cm in adolescents and adults or predicted to reach 20 cm by adulthood). The potential for malignant degeneration of these large nevi is debated in the literature, and the lifetime rate has been estimated from 6–12%. Approximately 40% of melanomas seen in children occur in large congenital nevi, with 50% of malignancies developing by age five, 60% throughout childhood, and 70% by puberty. The onset of malignancy should be suspected with focal growth, pain, bleeding, ulceration, and significant pigmentary changes. Additionally, large giant congenital nevi involving the scalp, back, and neck may also be associated with leptomeningeal melanosis. A magnetic resonance imaging (MRI) scan of the brain should be obtained in these patients.[26]

The mainstay of treatment is prophylactic excision to reduce the likelihood of malignant transformation and to improve the cosmetic appearance, especially when it involves the forehead and periorbital region. This is usually staged, with serial excisions if small, or excision and skin grafting. Very large giant nevi can present major reconstructive challenges and are usually managed with the assistance of tissue expansion and subsequent flap repair.[27]

Nevus sebaceous of Jadassohn

Nevus sebaceous of Jadassohn can occur in the scalp and forehead and appears as a well circumscribed, yellowish, hairless, plaque-like lesion which is present at birth. It grows with the child and, by puberty, it becomes more nodular, secondary to papillomatous hyperplasia of the epidermis. Histologically, it is a hamartoma, consisting of sebaceous glands, abortive hair follicles, and ectopic apocrine glands. The risk of malignant degeneration, mostly to basal cell tumors, has been reported as anywhere from 10–15%, which is an indication for excision of these lesions. There are other benign and malignant tumors that can arise from other cell elements of this hamartoma, with trichoblastoma being the most frequent benign tumor.[28,29]

Epidermal cysts

These are very common and arise from elements of the hair follicle, especially the infundibulum of the hair follicle. They can gradually increase in size, may be multiple, can be annoying when combing hair, and may get infected. They are very easily excised.

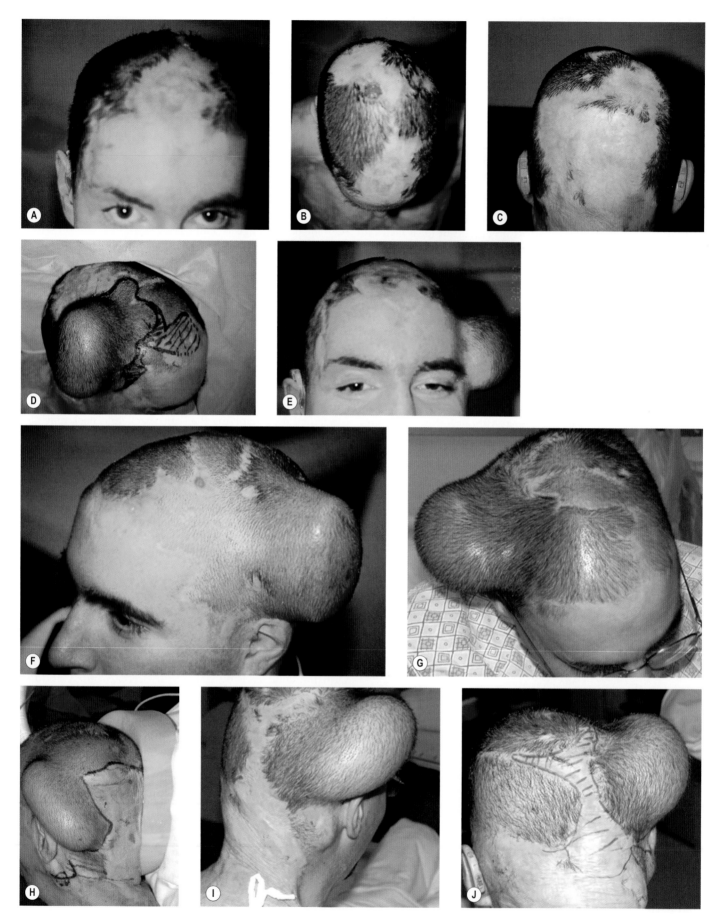

Fig. 5.10 (a) Young male patient with extensive burn alopecia **(A–C)** with first round of expansion with two tissue expanders in right and left anterior temporal regions **(D, E)**. **(b)** Second round of tissue expansion in right and left posterior temporal regions **(F–J)**.

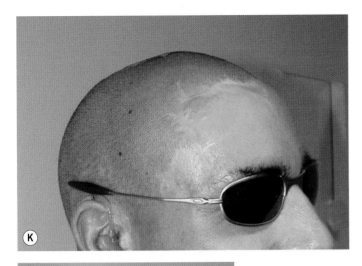

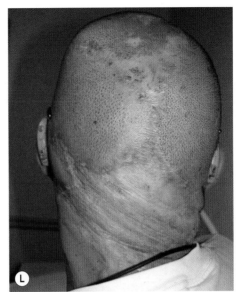

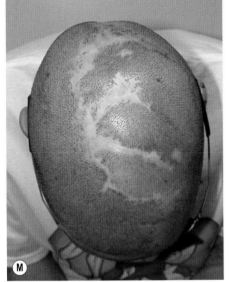

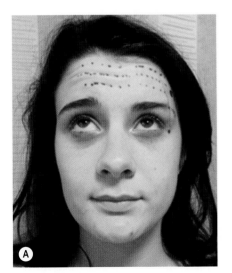

Fig. 5.10, cont'd (c) Postoperative images after advancement of hair-bearing scalp to restore anterior and posterior hairline **(K–M)**.

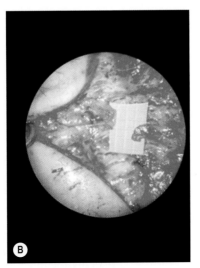

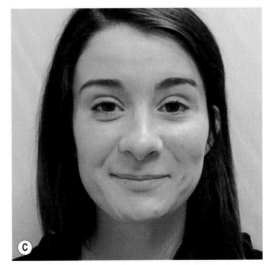

Fig. 5.11 Frontal branch of facial nerve injury **(A)**. Repair and functional recovery **(B, C)**.

Other tumors

Most tumors of the scalp are of epithelial origin and include basal cell[30,31] and squamous cell cancers[32,33] and melanoma.[34,35] The treatment is the same as in other regions of the body, and a detailed description of the pathology is covered in other chapters. Of local importance is a knowledge of the likely lymphatic spread from the scalp malignancies. These are twofold: in the forehead and frontoparietal region, the lymphatics drain to the superficial parotid gland and retromandibular nodes. Posteriorly, the lesions drain to the occipital nodes and occasionally the posterior triangle cervical nodes.

Other primary tumors can arise from adnexal and connective tissue elements and may be benign or malignant. They include sarcomas (fibrosarcoma, dermatofibrosarcoma protuberans, malignant fibrous histiocytoma, leiomyosarcoma, rhabdomyosarcoma), cutaneous T-cell lymphoma, and primary adnexal cancers.

Metastatic tumors to the scalp may also occur due to its rich blood supply. These also occur in the underlying bone and may expand and secondarily involve the skin. Meningiomas also may erode through the bony cortex.

Infections

Both localized and systemic infections can affect the scalp and forehead. These may be due to bacterial, fungal, and viral infections. Local wound care, drainage of abscesses, and appropriate systemic antibiotics are the mainstay of treatment of these conditions. These can all result in secondary scarring and alopecia. The bacterial infections may result in folliculitis which can become chronic, requiring excision and repair. More severe infections including necrotizing fasciitis also occur, though rarely. Appropriate treatment involves extensive debridement, which results in extensive soft tissue deficits requiring complex reconstructions.

Fungal infections, such as kerion and favus, are typically managed by the dermatologist but can result in permanent alopecia, which will be reconstructed by the plastic surgeon. Kerion is the result of the host's reaction to a fungal ringworm infection (dermatophytosis) and appears as a thick mushy area of the scalp, studded with pustules.[36] Favus is a chronic inflammatory dermatophytic (tinea capitis) infection usually caused by *Trichophyton schoenleinii*, which results in the development of a thick yellow crust (scutulum) around the hair follicles. When this is removed, a moist erythematous base results, and, with final healing, extensive scarring and alopecia results.[37]

Linear scleroderma (*en coup de sabre*) – Parry-Romberg syndrome

En coup de sabre is a relatively common deformity seen in the forehead and anterior scalp. It appears as a unilateral, vertically orientated, indented linear atrophic deformity of the skin of the forehead. It may start in childhood or adolescence and is progressive for 3–5 years before it stabilizes. The etiology is not known and is thought to represent an area of localized scleroderma; the most widely accepted theory is that it represents an autoimmune reaction to ectodermal derivatives of the forehead and scalp. This may be associated with

Parry-Romberg syndrome where there is more widespread atrophy involving hemiatrophy of one side of the face and other parts of the body.[38]

If localized, an excision of indented scar, with local tissue advancement, dermis-fat grafting, or structural fat grafting may be used to repair the defect. Not uncommonly, there may be poor "take" of the fat grafts, requiring repeat grafting. Patients with larger deformities, as seen in Parry-Romberg cases, may require free tissue transfers to adequately repair the defect. Treatment is delayed until the condition has stabilized (Fig. 5.12).[39]

Diagnoses and patient presentation

A thorough history and physical examination are critical, and these should include relevant medical factors such as a history of smoking, coronary artery disease, diabetes mellitus, radiation, immunosuppression, and other medical conditions. The etiology of the defect is also important with cases of malignancy, and signs of local infiltration and regional and distal metastasis must be investigated. The wound or defect needs to be carefully analyzed in the context of the particular patient. The surrounding tissues that may be utilized for repair should also be evaluated.

Computed tomography (CT) scans, bone scans, MRI, and positron emission tomography (PET) scans, may all be indicated in selected patients. Incisional or excisional biopsies may also be performed to assist in the diagnosis and planned treatment. Sentinel node mapping of the head and neck may also be indicated in management of patients with malignancy.[40,41] Thus, prior to commencement of treatment, a comprehensive understanding of the cause of the wound or defect, be it malignant or traumatic, is important in predicting intraoperative defect size and to anticipate the natural history of the underlying disease, and surgical management and eventual prognosis for the patient.

Patient selection

There are many factors that need to be considered in developing a treatment plan for reconstructing scalp and forehead defects. Table 5.1, modified from Temple and Ross's original publication, summarizes the factors important in defect analysis.[42]

1. The defect

An assessment of size, shape, orientation, and depth of the defect are all important to consider, as these will determine the amount of tissue needed for closure. The location of the defect is also important. The parietal region of the scalp allows the most advancement of scalp tissue, and defects in this location are more amenable to scalp undermining and primary closure. The occipital region has the least scalp mobility.

In cases of scalp lacerations, the depth of the wound is also an important factor. The lacerations may be down to or through the galea, and often it is the more superficial lacerations with an intact galea that bleed more due to the rich vascularity in the subcutaneous plane which may be stented open by the intact galea. Bleeding can be quite excessive, and this can be corrected by simply closing the wound with a

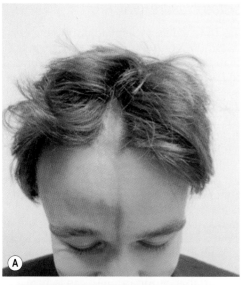
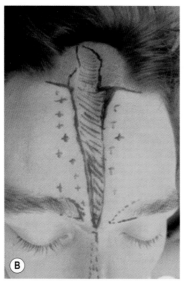
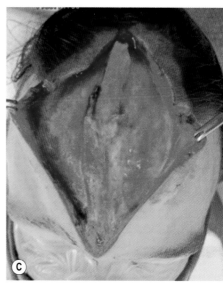
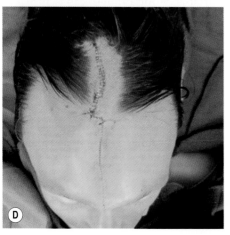
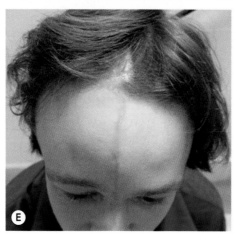

Fig. 5.12 Young man with linear scleroderma of the forehead and scalp **(A)**. Management involved de-epithelialization of depressed scar, leaving the deeper dermal elements, with advancement of adjacent normal forehead and scalp **(B, C)**. The scar at the junction between scalp and forehead is broken up by a z-plasty. The immediate **(D)** and later postoperative appearance **(E)** is shown.

Table 5.1 Consideration in defect analysis	
Wound factors	**Consideration**
Location of the defect	Scalp Forehead Combined
Aesthetic subunits	Median/paramedian/lateral forehead Temporal/parietal/occipital scalp
Exposed structures	Subcutaneous Periosteum Bone Dura Alloplasts
Surrounding soft tissue	Hairline position Eyelids and brows Pattern of baldness Scars/previous procedures Burns Irradiation
Wound size	Small Medium Large
Contour	Dead space

full-thickness suture. If the galea is also lacerated, this is included in the suture.

If skin grafting is contemplated, there has to be an intact pericranium for adequate graft revascularization and take. In defects involving the underlying bone, all exposed devitalized bone needs to be debrided before coverage. Exposed dura usually requires some form of cranioplasty to protect the underlying brain, and then coverage with a well vascularized flap.

When selecting a flap for reconstruction, the size and location of the defect will determine which local, regional, or free flap will be required for initial reconstruction.

Ideally, it is also worth thinking ahead and envisioning the best possible long-term aesthetic outcome. This is best achieved by reconstruction with "like" tissue, as advocated by Millard.[43] In the **scalp**, restoration to "normal" involves re-establishment of a hair-bearing scalp; in the adjacent **forehead**, a natural anterior and temporal hairline, and intact uniform subunit without a "patchwork" effect of different types of tissue reconstruction. With the forehead, it is also important not to distort the surrounding mobile structures such as the brow and eyelids. This may affect the initial flap selection and also set in place staged secondary procedures to maximize the aesthetic outcome.

2. The surrounding tissues

The viability and quality of the surrounding tissues are important. One should note the quality, thickness, and vascularity of the tissues and the presence of scars from previous operations. Prior injury, scars, and radiation damage may diminish the availability of local flaps. All infections should be controlled before attempts at wound closure with flaps or the insertion of tissue expanders. Again, if possible, every attempt should be made to minimize deformity of surrounding critical areas such as the hairline, which can be distorted by excessive undermining and when designing rotation flaps and planning scalp tissue expansion.

For oncological defects, clear margins of malignancy need to be verified before reconstruction is commenced. Local wound care or temporizing reconstruction with allografts, xenografts, or dermal matrices is considered when clear margins cannot be confirmed at the time of tumor excision.

3. Patient factors

Before considering complex reconstruction, it is important to assess the patient's overall health, level of function, compliance, and personal preference. Patients with significant comorbidities may not be candidates for lengthy and multi-staged operative procedures. The oncological patient needs special consideration. Attention should be made to preoperative chemotherapy which may compromise wound healing. Also, the nutritional state of the patient is important.[7,8]

Treatment/surgical technique

A. Reconstructive options – scalp and forehead: common options

We will first consider simpler techniques that are applicable to both scalp and forehead and then more specific local and regional flap reconstructive options for these two sites and, finally, reconstruction of more complex defects that often span both sites, with free tissue transfers.

1. Closure by secondary intention

Small defects may be allowed to heal by secondary intention. In the scalp, this will result in a non-hair-bearing scar. In the forehead, it is preferred to allow residual defects that cannot be closed primarily (e.g., after use of a paramedian forehead flap transfer for nasal reconstruction) to heal by secondary intention. There is consensus that the resulting scar is superior to that that would be obtained by the use of skin grafting. If this method of reconstruction is adopted, daily dressing changes with moist dressing is indicated until the wound heals. Rarely, when the forehead donor site has not yet healed at the completion of nasal reconstruction with a forehead flap, the discarded skin from the pedicle of the forehead flap has been used as a full-thickness graft of the forehead defect, with satisfactory results, which is not surprising as it is a repair with like tissue.[44]

2. Vacuum-assisted closure (VAC)

The VAC system has emerged as a useful adjunct to the treatment of difficult wounds. The wounds are first treated to eliminate infection and all non-viable tissue is also debrided until a clean wound results. The VAC can then be applied. Although cumbersome, its use as a temporary dressing which only needs changing every few days is very well tolerated and appreciated by the patient. The VAC promotes healing and is based on the application of negative pressure to the surface of the wound which helps remove edema, increases the local blood flow, and enhances granulation tissue and wound healing. Intermittent or cyclical treatment appears to be more effective than continuous therapy. The bacterial counts are decreased with the use of a VAC (Fig. 5.13).[45]

The VAC system may be used to completion of healing or as an adjunct to allow a clean granulating wound which can accept a skin graft.[46] However, care must be taken not to use excess pressure which exceeds capillary closing pressure, especially over bony surfaces, as this can result in ischemia of the overlying periosteum. The VAC is also used as a dressing after the application of a skin graft, as it has the benefit of applying even and gentle pressure on the graft. However, ensuring that this pressure is not excessive is again very important to avoid not only graft loss but additional deeper tissue necrosis.[47]

3. Primary closure

Primary closure is possible for scalp defects up to a maximum of 2–3 cm in diameter. Wide undermining of surrounding scalp tissue is needed. Because of the rich vascularity, some degree of tension is allowed. However, the galea is relatively inelastic, and in order to allow primary closure, it is usually necessary to utilize some scoring of the galea, but this should be done carefully to avoid injury to the overlying blood supply. Meticulous hemostasis after incisions of the galea is also necessary.[48]

In the scalp, areas of alopecia may be treated with scalp reduction techniques. This has been popularized by Unger, and involves the excision of an ellipse of non-hair-bearing skin, and wide undermining and advancement of normal hairy scalp with a layered repair that includes the galea, to minimize stretching of the scar.[49,50]

With the forehead, primary closure of defects should not distort the surrounding mobile structures, especially the eyebrows. Thus, for larger defects, it is mainly those that are vertically oriented which can be closed in this manner.

4. Tissue expansion

Tissue expansion is another very useful method of reconstructing the scalp and forehead. This requires a staged reconstruction where a silicon expander is placed beneath adjacent healthy tissue. There is some connecting tubing to an injection port, which is buried remotely from the expander (in children this may be externalized), which is used to inject fluid. Tissue expanders with integrated injection ports have also been introduced recently.[51–55]

A small amount of fluid is injected at the time of insertion of the expander to obliterate the dead space, and after a period of healing which is usually 10–14 days, serial expansion occurs to expand this normal tissue which can subsequently

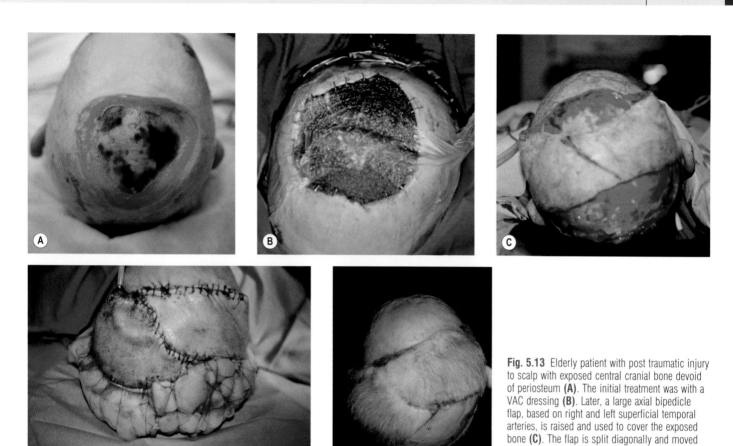

Fig. 5.13 Elderly patient with post traumatic injury to scalp with exposed central cranial bone devoid of periosteum **(A)**. The initial treatment was with a VAC dressing **(B)**. Later, a large axial bipedicle flap, based on right and left superficial temporal arteries, is raised and used to cover the exposed bone **(C)**. The flap is split diagonally and moved sagittally to cover all the exposed ungraftable bone **(D)**. The resulting donor defect if skin grafted. The final appearance is shown **(E)**.

be used to reconstruct adjacent scarred areas. This technique cannot be used acutely, when there are any open wounds or any evidence of infection. The proposed flap design should be mapped out prior to placement of the tissue expander.[55] The best results are obtained with transposition or rotation flaps, rather than simple advancement flaps. It typically takes 2–3 months to expand the tissue sufficiently to perform the reconstruction (Figs. 5.8, 5.10, 5.14).

Tissue expansion of the scalp and forehead is not without its problems. Complication rates as high as 48% have been described. Common complications include hematoma, implant exposure, infection, flap necrosis, alopecia, and widened scars. Prior to cranial suture fusion, pressure from the expander may deform the underlying skull. The simultaneous use of multiple expanders can increase the complication rate via vascular compromise of the skin/scalp envelope. In addition, careful planning of expander position avoiding external pressure when sleeping will decrease the likelihood of extrusion and other complications.[56,57]

4. Skin grafts

Primary split-thickness and full-thickness skin grafting can be used as an expeditious way of closing a wound, especially in a compromised patient. After tumor excision where the risk of recurrence is high, this may also be elected so that the wound could be better monitored. For skin graft to be effective, a vascularized bed is required. If there is exposed bone, this will usually need a flap repair. Alternatively, multiple

drill holes can be done through the outer cortex down to the diploic layer and then await full granulation of tissue to occur.[58] Caution should be used in cases of malignancy, especially in recurred tumors and in irradiated beds, as drilling the outer cortex can potentially implant malignant cells into the bone and dura. The authors have seen this complication and strongly advise against the use of drilling the bone in these cases.

The use of a VAC dressing in these situations assists with the development of the granulation tissue and subsequent wound coverage with the skin graft.

The advantage of skin grafting is that it is fairly simple; however, the disadvantage is that this is not hair-bearing in scalp reconstructions. In the forehead, a skin graft lacks the normal color, texture of the surrounding tissue, and it fails to restore the contour and results in a non-aesthetic patchwork appearance.

The other options of reconstruction, namely local, regional, and free flaps will be discussed separately for the scalp and forehead as there are different options and goals of reconstruction.

B. Reconstructive options – scalp: local and regional flap reconstruction

Leedy *et al.* have developed a very useful algorithm for reconstruction of acquired scalp defects, to achieve not only wound closure but also an aesthetically optimal result.[59]

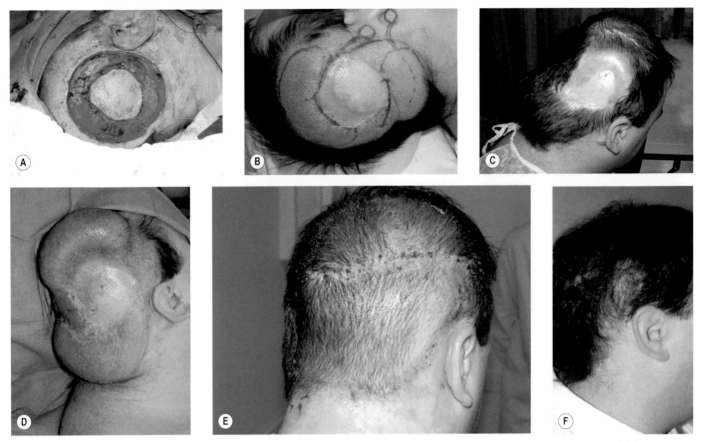

Fig. 5.14 Tissue expansion: patient with prior excision of dermatofibrosarcoma protuberans (DFSP), requiring wider excision and additional skin grafting **(A)**. Two crescentic tissue expanders were inserted **(B)**, slowly inflated over 6 weeks **(C)**, and eventually used to cover the defect after excision of the skin graft **(D, E)**, achieving full hair restoration **(F)**.

Local flaps

Fig. 5.15 concisely illustrates the different local flap options that are commonly used in scalp (and forehead) reconstruction. The immediate surrounding tissue is used for small to medium defects. The flaps move by rotation, transposition, and advancement, and commonly all three elements factor in tissue movement. Small pin wheel flaps (two-flap "ying-yang", and three-flap "Isle-of-Man") are commonly used for small defects (Figs. 5.15–5.17). Larger rotation flaps with judicious back cuts may also be used. For longitudinal defects, bipedicle transposition flaps may be used. Unlike other parts of the body where the secondary defect can generally be closed, this is not the case in the scalp, as usually the curved surface and tautness of tissue make it necessary to skin graft the resulting donor defects (Fig. 5.18 ⊚).

Fig. 5.18 appears online only.

In designing flaps, the possibility of making them axial, with a known dominant vascular pedicle traversing the length of the flap, ensures greater safety and avoids distal tip necrosis (which is usually the most critical part of the flap needed for repair) which can lead to overall failure of the entire reconstruction (Fig. 5.18). The Doppler ultrasound is routinely used to map out the main vascular blood supply. In general, it is safer to use large and longer flaps and to carefully plan the reconstruction to account for the curvature of the scalp. Orticochea was one of the first to propose the use of multiple large flaps, extensively mobilized to close large defects in

the central scalp with hair-bearing flaps. Every attempt is made to make these flaps axial to ensure better perfusion (Fig. 5.19).[60–63]

We find that the use of templates and simulated transfer is invaluable in flap design – this results in a flap that would appear at first glance to be larger than required, but due to the factor of skull curvature, it ends up being just right.

The use of hair-bearing flaps, such as the Juri flap, has been described to reconstruct the anterior hairline.[64,65] This flap is based on the posterior parietal branch of the superficial temporal artery and typically, because long hair-bearing flaps are needed to restore the hairline, it is safer to delay this flap.[66] For very long flaps, two preliminary delay procedures may be required, prior to flap transfer (Figs. 5.20 & 5.21). A disadvantage of the Juri flap is that it alters the natural direction of hair growth, as the hair grows directly upward, whereas normal anterior hair growth is in a downward direction. To correct this, a transfer of the Juri flap as a free flap and anastomosed to the contralateral temporal vessels has been performed to maximize the aesthetic appearance.

Scalp flaps are elevated at the subgaleal level, preserving the underlying periosteum to allow skin grafting of the resulting secondary defect. A dog ear deformity is common at the flap pivot point, again accentuated by the underling rigid skull curvature. It is best not to deal with this acutely as it can impact on the vascularity and typically settles down or can be easily corrected secondarily. It is also important to avoid too much tension, as this can result in alopecia. Alopecia also

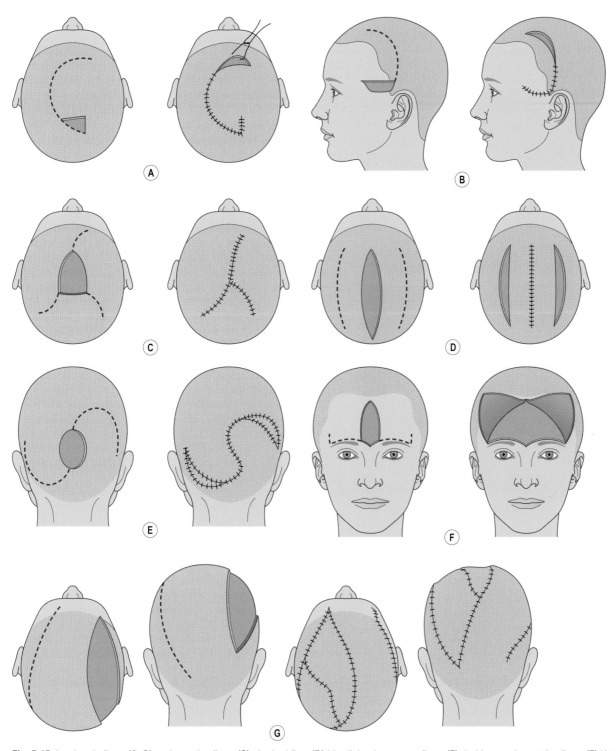

Fig. 5.15 Local scalp flaps. **(A, B)** scalp rotation flaps; **(C)** pinwheel flap; **(D)** bipedicle advancement flaps; **(E)** double opposing rotation flaps; **(F)** Y to T flap; **(G)** bipedicled fronto-occipital flap. *(Reproduced from Marchac D. Deformities of the forehead, scalp, and cranial vault. In: McCarthy JG (ed). Plastic Surgery. Philadelphia: WB Saunders; 1990:1538.)*

occurs along suture lines and may require secondary revision.

Component separation of the scalp, typically with the use of separate galeal flaps for defects created by neurosurgical and craniofacial approaches, is another useful option in the surgeon's armamentarium. This is most commonly used in the frontal area, where the galea and attached frontalis muscle is often used to repair frontal sinus and anterior cranial defects.[67]

The temporoparietal fascial flap based on the superficial temporal vessels has been previously mentioned for its use in ear and orbital reconstruction.[68,69]

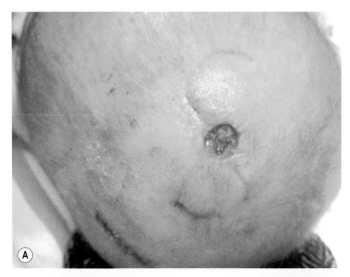

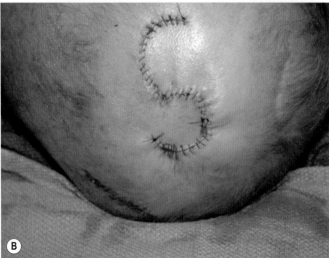

Fig. 5.16 Repair of small scalp defect with exposed bone with "ying-yang" flaps.

Regional flaps

There are very few regional flaps available for scalp reconstruction. One exception is the trapezius myocutaneous flap, based on the transverse or descending branch of the transverse cervical vascular pedicle.[70] This may be considered for post auricular and posterior scalp defects, as the maximum reach is to the upper occipital area. Care must be taken to preserve the accessory nerve supply to the upper part of the muscle to prevent shoulder droop (Fig. 5.22).[71]

The latissimus dorsi, pectoralis myocutaneous, and extended submental platysma myocutaneous pedicle flaps have also been described for repair of defects of the temporal, post auricular, and most peripheral scalp defects but are seldom used, as the most distal parts of these flaps (with the poorest blood supply) are the parts crucial for repair, and failure commonly ensues.[72] The latissimus flap is much more commonly used as a free flap, which is described below.

C. Reconstructive options – forehead: local and regional flap reconstruction

The forehead makes up the upper third of the face and is important for facial aesthetics. Scarring in the uppermost part of the forehead can be partially hidden with appropriate hair styling. In the central and lower forehead, scars that are aligned and parallel to the transverse crease lines (produced by frontalis muscle contraction) fade and become less noticeable with time. In the lower, central part of the forehead, vertically oriented scars also align themselves with the natural creases due to the action of the underlying corrugator and procerus muscles, and with time become less noticeable.

However, wounds and defects can be at many different sites, have different orientations and shapes, and repair results in scars that are not in the "ideal" location. It is far more important that the repair does not distort the mobile structures at the lower border of the forehead and the hairline laterally, as these scars also fade with time and become less noticeable, whereas a displaced landmark will create a persistent deformity. In general, preservation of normal contour and normal landmarks is far more important than the associated scar, and this should be one of the main guiding principles in selecting the most appropriate method of repair of forehead defects.

As discussed earlier, although the forehead appears to be a single subunit, more careful analysis, based firstly on the regional blood supply and secondly on the variations in tissue mobility and the degree of tautness of the different parts, makes it more practical to subdivide the forehead into smaller subunits, as first proposed by Ian Jackson and modified slightly by the current authors. These subdivisions allow a better algorithmic approach in flap selection.

With respect to the blood supply, the forehead has a very rich and unique blood supply with a rich interconnection between branches from the internal carotid and external carotid systems. Centrally, there are two paired, vertically orientated supraorbital and supratrochlear vessels from the internal carotid and, laterally, the transversely running anterior branch of the superficial temporal vessels, from the external carotid system. The resulting rich vascular plexus makes it possible to raise the entire forehead on any of these vessels. This has enabled the forehead to be an extremely useful donor site for reconstructing adjacent tissues **outside** the forehead, especially for nasal reconstruction and less often cheek, eyelid, palate, and intraoral reconstruction. As the focus of the current chapter is forehead reconstruction, we will focus on how best to use similar axial flaps to close various defects **within the forehead**.

With respect of the tissue mobility and tautness, the central part of the forehead is tighter and has less subcutaneous tissue than the tissue in the temporal area and glabella and suprabrow area. The most mobile is the glabella and suprabrow region, where in addition to extra subcutaneous tissue there are also corrugator and procerus muscles, which add to the mobility at these sites. These regional variations help dictate the selection of flaps used for repair. Thus, whereas VY-type advancement flaps work well in the mobile areas of the glabella, suprabrow, and temporal areas, they are not effective in the central forehead and, if used, partial or total necrosis can result.

The following is our algorithmic approach of reconstruction of forehead defects with local flaps:

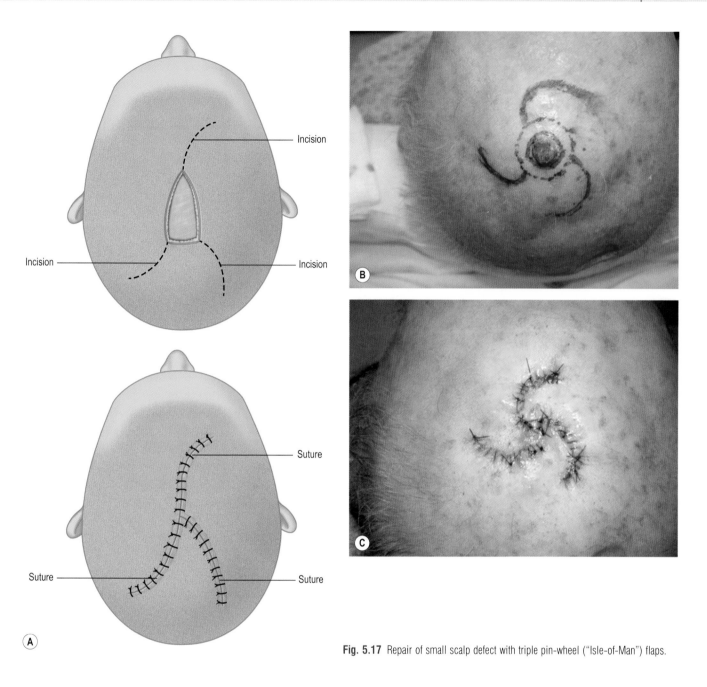

Fig. 5.17 Repair of small scalp defect with triple pin-wheel ("Isle-of-Man") flaps.

1. Temporal subunit

The mobility of tissues in this subunit is due to a relative increase of subcutaneous tissue, and this applies both to the hair-bearing temporal scalp and hairless forehead skin anteriorly that forms the lateral part of the forehead. The blood supply is rich and comes from the superficial temporal vessels. Advancement flaps that do not distort the surrounding tissues work best: VY (Fig. 5.23A,B), extended VY, and double extended VY flaps have all been used effectively (Fig. 5.24).[73] These flaps can be designed to move both hair-bearing and non-hair-bearing tissues as part of the same advancement flap (Fig. 5.25A,B). The advancement is usually in vertical or obliquely upward or forward direction, thus causing minimal distortion of the tissues. When advancing extended type VY flaps, the extended part of the flap moves as a transposition flap on top of the advancement VY component. If this transposition component is hair-bearing, it will result in some alteration in direction of hair growth (Fig. 5.25B). Large transposition, rhomboid, or bilobed flaps tend to distort the natural landmarks and are not recommended.

Fig. 5.25A,B appears online only.

2. Suprabrow and glabella subunits

This tissue is even more mobile than the lateral subunit, and for this reason advancement flaps work very well. Again, it is important not to distort the brow, so the VY flap is designed just above the brow, and it is moved based on its subcutaneous tissue. Double opposing VY flaps can also be used for larger defects (Fig. 5.26 ⊙).

Fig. 5.26 appears online only.

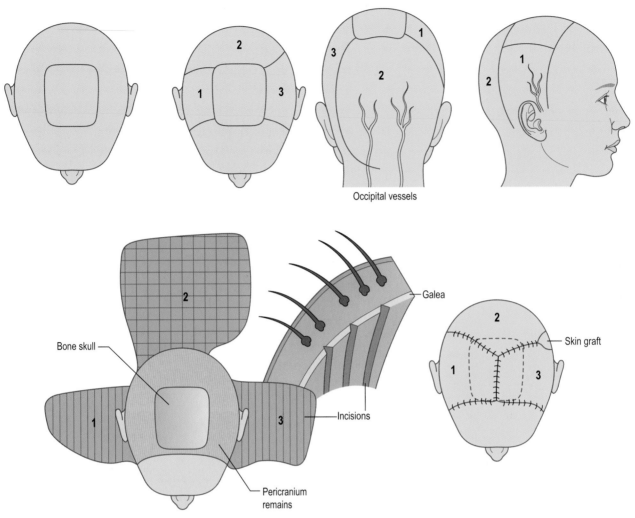

Fig. 5.19 Orticochea three-flap technique. Two flaps based on the superficial temporal artery are used to reconstruct the defect. A posterior-based flap based on the occipital vessels is used to fill the donor defect. *(Reproduced from Arnold PG, Rangarathnam CS. Multiple flap scalp reconstruction: Orticochea revisited. Plast Reconstr Surg. 1982;69:607.)*

Larger defects of the medial suprabrow area require a verti-cally oriented transposition flap, which can be raised from the adjacent glabella. This glabella flap is based on the terminal branches of the angular vessels (Fig. 5.27).

For larger defects where the glabella is missing, a parame-dian forehead flap based on the supratrochlear vessels may be used (Fig. 5.28). All these strategies effectively move "like" tissue into the defect and cause minimal distortion to the brow.

3. General forehead

It is best to divide the main body of the forehead into **(a) central** and **(b) lateral.** The central part is supplied by the supratrochlear and supraorbital vessels, and the lateral part by the watershed area between the temporal and supraorbital vessels.

3(a). Central

Narrow, central, vertically oriented defects, as seen after a paramedian forehead flap transfer, are closed vertically. It is usually very easy to close this inferiorly, but there is more tension superiorly (Fig. 5.28).

Larger vertically oriented defects are repaired by bilateral forehead (+/− and scalp) flap mobilization, with galeal scoring and back cut if needed and results in a central vertical scar (Fig. 5.29).

For central defects that are more transversely orientated, a paramedian transposition flap is used, as any attempt to directly close this would result in an upward pull of the brow (Fig. 5.28). Any smaller areas that cannot be closed after flap transfer can be repaired with a full-thickness skin graft that is harvested as part of a dog ear excision as part of flap mobiliza-tion or allowed to heal by secondary intention. Larger skin grafted areas are cosmetically and functionally suboptimal (Fig. 5.30A). The skin grafted part is depressed, pale, and shiny and potentially liable to breakdown. The skin graft can be excised by serial excision or with the assistance of tissue expansion (Fig. 5.30A,B).

With even larger central defects also involving the glabella area, the repair with local tissue versus free tissue transfer needs to be carefully evaluated. If possible, the use of large

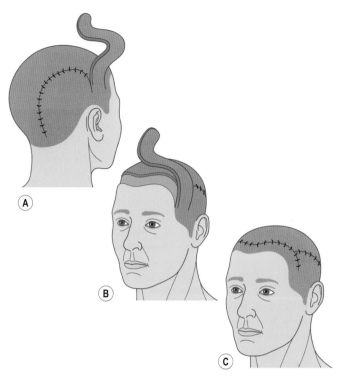

local transposition and advancement flaps is preferred, as the result will have a better color, contour, and texture match than what can be achieved with free tissue transfer. Fig. 5.31 illustrates the use of an extended forehead/scalp flap based on the anterior branch of the superficial temporal artery which is advanced, and the distal part is transposed to close this extensive post Mohs excision of a basal cell carcinoma (BCC). Additionally, a superiorly based nasolabial flap is used to repair the glabella area, with the transfer of part of the beard area which is used to repair the missing medial eyebrow. The postoperative photograph shows the end result after thinning and revision of the nasolabial flap and it also shows good hair growth of the eyebrow reconstruction.

3(b). Lateral

Small defects can be closed by lateral advancement flaps that do not distort the eyebrow and upper eyelid. Larger defects are repaired by large axial rotation/advancement flaps based on the supraorbital and supratrochlear vessels (Fig. 5.32). The resulting secondary defect, although often depicted in line drawings as closing primarily, usually needs a skin graft. This can be later removed serially or with the aid of tissue expansion.

Fig. 5.20 The Juri flap. After two preliminary delay procedures **(A)**, a temporoparieto-occipital flap is elevated **(B)** and used to reconstruct defects in the anterior hairline **(C)**.

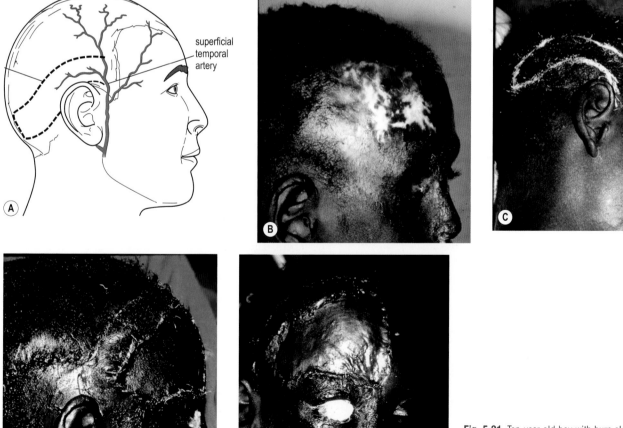

Fig. 5.21 Ten-year-old boy with burn alopecia involving the anterior hairline, repaired with a Juri flap and full-thickness skin graft to the forehead.

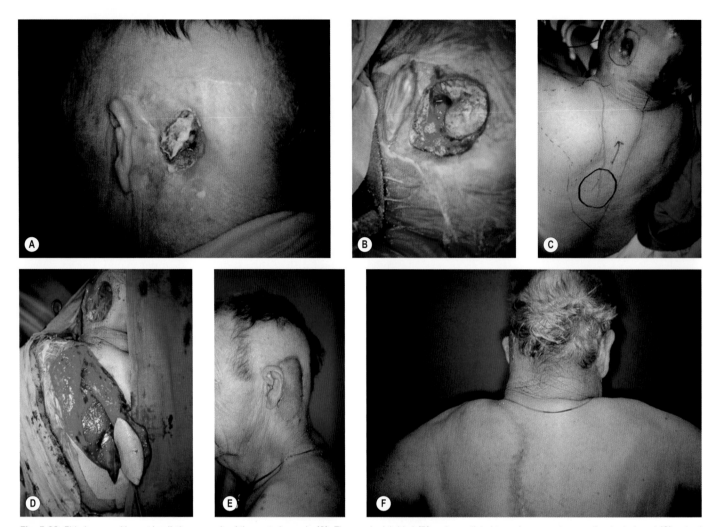

Fig. 5.22 Elderly man with post irradiation necrosis of the posterior scalp **(A)**. The area is debrided **(B)** and a pedicled trapezius myocutaneous flap is designed **(C)**, raised **(D),** and transferred to repair the defect **(E)**. The postoperative appearance and ability to shrug shoulders (due to preservation of the accessory nerve) is shown **(F)**.

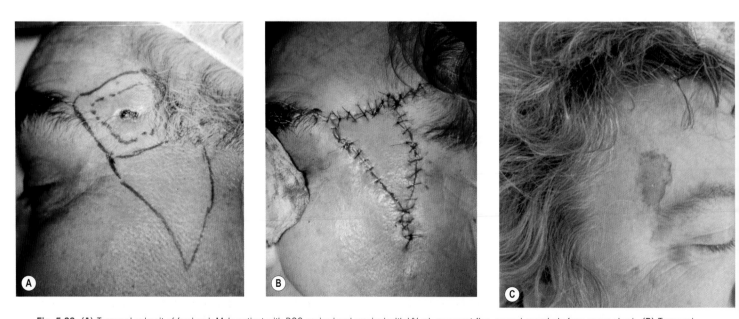

Fig. 5.23 (A) Temporal subunit of forehead: Male patient with BCC excised and repaired with VY advancement flap, moved superiorly from upper cheek. **(B)** Temporal subunit of forehead: VY flap from lateral forehead to repair defect after BCC removed. **(C)** Sixty-one-year-old female with temporal region basal cell carcinoma.

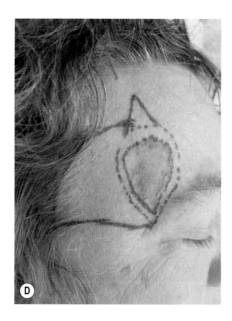

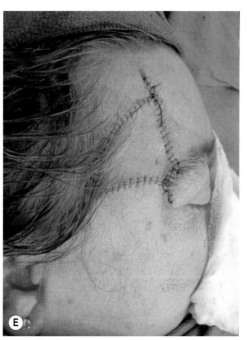

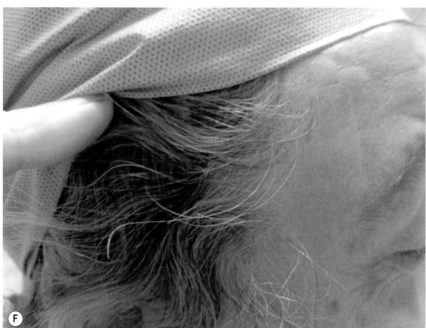

Fig. 5.23, cont'd (D) Design of resection and hairless extended V to Y advancement flap. **(E)** Immediate postoperative result after advancement flap and closure. **(F)** 3 month follow-up after excision and closure of temporal subunit reconstruction.

D. Microsurgical reconstruction with free flaps

Large complex defects, with exposed vital structures, are best repaired with free tissue transfers. The reported success rate, even in debilitated and elderly, is in excess of 95%. Historically, the first described scalp reconstruction with a free flap was by McLean and Buncke who used a free omental flap.[74] This provided a well vascularized bed that covered all vital structures and could accept a skin graft. Free omental flaps are not commonly used for scalp reconstruction today, as they are relatively thin, may not restore the contour, and have greater morbidity as they require an intra-abdominal approach for harvest.[75,76] Also, with the renaissance in the study of the

vascular anatomy of the skin and muscles that followed this early free flap transfer, there are now many more options to the reconstructive surgeon.[77] The focus has shifted from obtaining flap survival using a limited number of flaps, to better flap selection and refinements. Refinements are achieved by careful preoperative and intra-operative assessment of the defect, determining the reconstructive requirements, and then selecting the best donor tissue that gives the best functional and aesthetic result.

The mainstays of free flaps used for **scalp** reconstruction are muscle, musculocutaneous and, to a lesser extent, fasciocutaneous flaps, which are more commonly used for **forehead** reconstructions. Each has its merits and indications, and the choice of a particular method of free flap depends on the

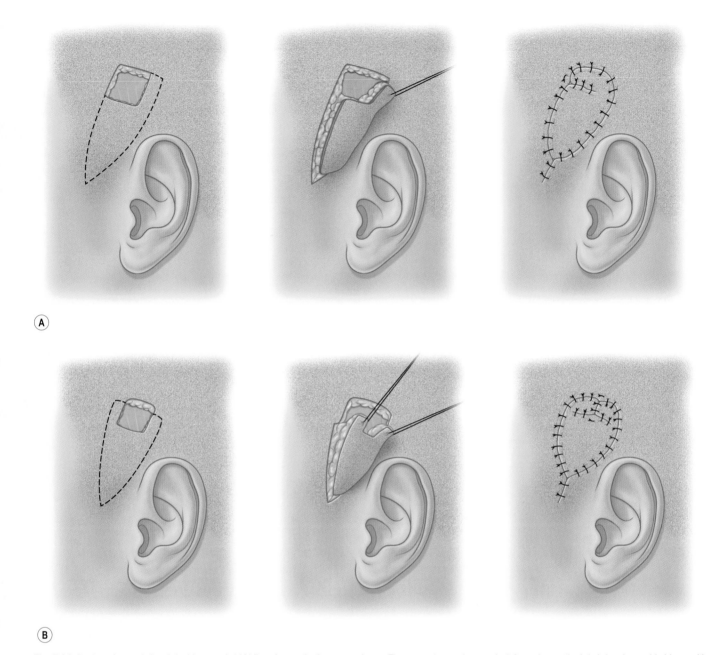

Fig. 5.24 Design of extended and double extended VY flaps for use in the temporal area. These may be used to repair defects that are both hair-bearing and hairless, with appropriate design of the extended part(s) according to hair need, with the goal to preserve the normal hairline. *(Adapted from Pribaz JJ, Chester C, Barrall DT. The extended V-Y Flap. Plast Reconstr Surg. 1992;90:275–80.)*

defect size, wound condition, availability, recipient vessels, as well as surgeon and patient preference (Figs. 5.33 & 5.34).

Recipient vessels

The recipient vessels utilized in both scalp and forehead free flap reconstructions are similar.[78–80]

Ideally, the recipient vessels should be of adequate caliber, be outside of the zone of injury, yet close enough to allow a primary anastomosis. Unfortunately in scalp and forehead reconstruction, there is a paucity of vessels close to the defect, and the next group of available vessels is at a distance which often necessitates the use of vein grafts. The superficial temporal vessels are the only vessels that are close to the scalp and forehead. However, these vessels may be unsatisfactory due to prior injury at the time of ablative surgery or secondary to the effects of irradiation. Although the artery, especially with proximal dissection into the parotid, is usually of adequate caliber, the veins may be small, thin-walled, and fragile. It is best to perform the anastomoses of artery and vein at a similar location to prevent twisting and misalignment of the pedicle. Thus, the surgeon must be prepared to extend the dissection into the neck and isolate other branches of the external carotid system (or the external carotid itself), and adjacent veins which drain into the external or internal jugular systems. The division of the posterior belly of the digastric may facilitate the dissection of the recipient arteries.

In extreme cases, where the neck has had prior radical lymphatic dissection and damaged by irradiation, so that it is "frozen", the choice of recipient vessels becomes more difficult. These patients may already have had a prior free flap, and it may be possible to utilize this flap's pedicle for the new flap.[84–86] Alternatively, to get outside of the zone of injury, the strategies may include the use of vessels on the contralateral neck, or the transverse cervical vessels (branches of the thyrocervical trunk) in the supraclavicular area.[79–81] The use of these distant vascular sources makes the use of long vein grafts or arteriovenous loops mandatory. Rarely, or in salvage situations, where there are no veins, the use of the cephalic vein may be considered. This is located in the deltopectoral groove and dissected down into the arm, and rotated superiorly to the neck.[87]

Flap selection

Appropriate flap selection will depend on the location, size of the defect, desired pedicle length, intraoperative positioning of the patient, initial and final goals of recon-

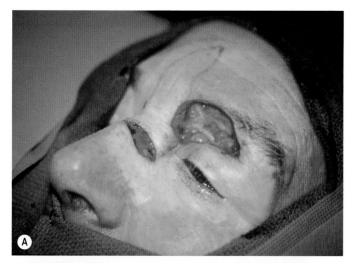

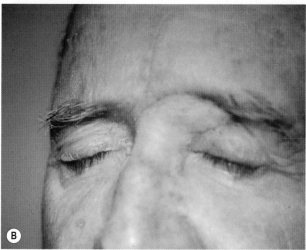

Fig. 5.27 Glabella–suprabrow defect: patient with larger defect in glabella/brow area, repaired with a vertically oriented glabella flap based on the terminal branches of the angular artery to repair a transversely oriented defect.

Although there are more choices of recipient vessels in the neck, the longer distance to the defect is addressed by selection of a flap with a longer pedicle or the use of vein grafts.[81] As both the artery and vein need a bridging graft, the use of an arteriovenous loop is the usual way of resolving this problem.[82] It is best to plan this as part of the reconstruction rather than scrambling after the free flap is detached to minimize ischemia time (Fig. 5.33).

Occasionally, the occipital artery may be utilized as the recipient vessel for reconstruction of posterior scalp defects.

An end-to-end repair of artery and vein is the most common method of repair, although if larger veins, such as the external or internal jugular, are selected as recipient vessels, then an end-to-side repair may be utilized. Some authors believe that the higher negative pressure within the internal jugular vein that occurs because inspiration "sucks" blood out of the flap and decreases the chance of venous thrombosis. Chalian *et al.* compared free flap failures when using the internal jugular versus branches of the external jugular vein and found a reduced thrombosis risk when the internal jugular was used (1% versus 8% in 156 free flaps).[83]

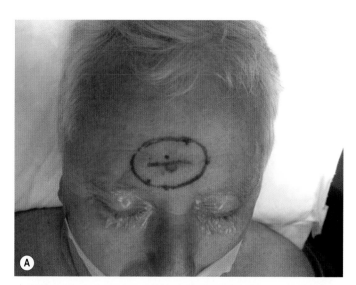

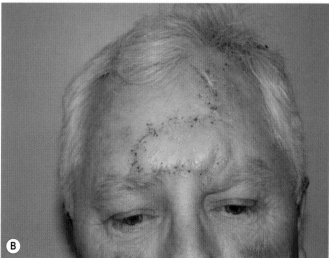

Fig. 5.28 Central forehead: patient with central, transversely oriented forehead defect post melanoma excision and repaired with a vertically oriented paramedian forehead flap which avoids distortion of natural landmarks, like the eyebrows.

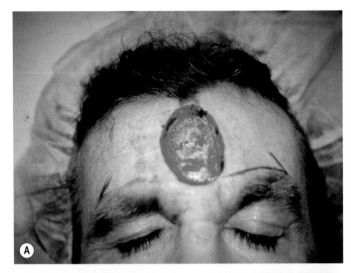

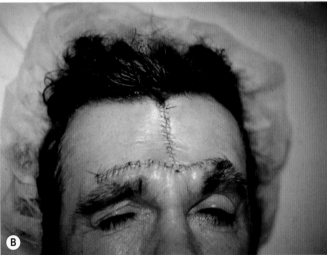

Fig. 5.29 Central forehead: patient with a central, vertically oriented forehead defect post Moh's excision of BCC, repaired with bilateral advancement forehead flaps, with back cuts and galeal scoring.

struction, and surgeon's experience and familiarity with a particular flap.[88–93]

With respect to location, for scalp reconstruction, a muscle or myocutaneous flap is more commonly used; for the forehead, it is preferable to utilize a fasciocutaneous flap.

By far the most common muscle flap used in scalp reconstruction is the **latissimus dorsi muscle** flap, based on the thoracodorsal pedicle. It has the advantages of a relatively long and reliable vascular pedicle, and it is large and can cover extensive scalp defects. The muscle is skin grafted and will undergo atrophy over time, resulting in a soft tissue thickness that closely resembles the native scalp. A fenestrated, unmeshed graft which is typically quilted onto the underlying muscle gives a superior and more uniform appearance than a meshed graft (Fig. 5.33).[94,95]

For smaller defects, a tailored smaller latissimus muscle may be harvested or, alternatively, the lower three or four slips of the **serratus anterior muscle** based on the same (and even longer thoracodorsal) pedicle may be used. The use of only the lower part of the serratus muscle avoids winging of the scapula.

For larger defects, the latissimus dorsi plus the serratus anterior, plus an anterior skin island, (extending beyond the anterior edge of the latissimus dorsi muscle but still based on anterior perforators from the thoracodorsal vessels) may be used. For total scalp defects, bilateral latissimus dorsi muscle free flaps may be required.

In most cases, the authors prefer to take a skin island with the latissimus dorsi flap (i.e., a **myocutaneous latissimus dorsi flap**) for several reasons: the skin island makes it easier to monitor the flap, creates a minimal donor site defect, and minimizes the skin graft requirements. Also, if it is planned to eventually expand the adjacent hair-bearing scalp and restore the hairline, it is preferable to suture the advancing scalp flaps to skin rather than skin grafted muscle. Admittedly, the thickness of the skin island is greater than the thickness of the scalp; this can be easily thinned subsequently or during the scalp hair-restoration phase.

Other muscle and myocutaneous flaps including the **rectus abdominus flap** are also commonly used, due to their ease of elevation remotely from the head and neck, allowing a two-team approach. Although it is a much thicker flap, this may sometimes be indicated in reconstructing compound defects where the calvarium has been removed and additional bulk is need to restore the contour (Fig. 5.8). This flap also has a long pedicle, which can be even longer if elevated as a deep inferior epigastric perforator (DIEP) flap.[96]

Fasciocutaneous flaps are especially indicated for reconstruction of larger forehead defects. If a free flap is contemplated for the forehead, the subunit principle of replacing the entire subunit gives the best cosmetic outcome (Fig. 5.33). Fasciocutaneous flaps may also be considered for scalp reconstruction if the eventual goal is restoration of hair-bearing scalp for, as mentioned above, it is easier to perform staged tissue expansion and suture of hair-bearing scalp flaps to skin rather than skin grafts (Fig. 5.8).

The most commonly used flaps include **radial forearm,**[97,98] **scapular and parascapular,**[99] and **anterolateral thigh (ALT) fasciocutaneous flaps**.[100–104] All these flaps are hardy, easy to raise, and have relatively long vascular pedicles (Figs. 5.33 & 5.34).

Both the radial forearm and ALT have the benefit of being remote from the head and neck facilitating a more expeditious two-team surgery. The approach to the scapula and parascapular flap harvest is similar to the latissimus dorsi and may involve position changes intra-operatively.

Although in the past many have listed numerous potential disadvantages of free tissue transfers, focusing on the length of operation and anesthetic, the fact that it is technically demanding, costly, and has a risk of flap failure, there is no doubt that when indicated this is the best way of solving problems. Also, today, most graduates of our training programs have had an extensive exposure to free tissue transfers and the reported outcomes show, in fact, a high success rate even in patients with advanced disease.[90,91,93,105]

Face transplantation

Despite all the advances that have occurred in reconstructive surgery over the last 30–40 years, the ability to restore severely damaged parts back to "normal" have been elusive. There is no way, for instance, to restore a normal hair-bearing scalp if the entire scalp has been lost and is not available

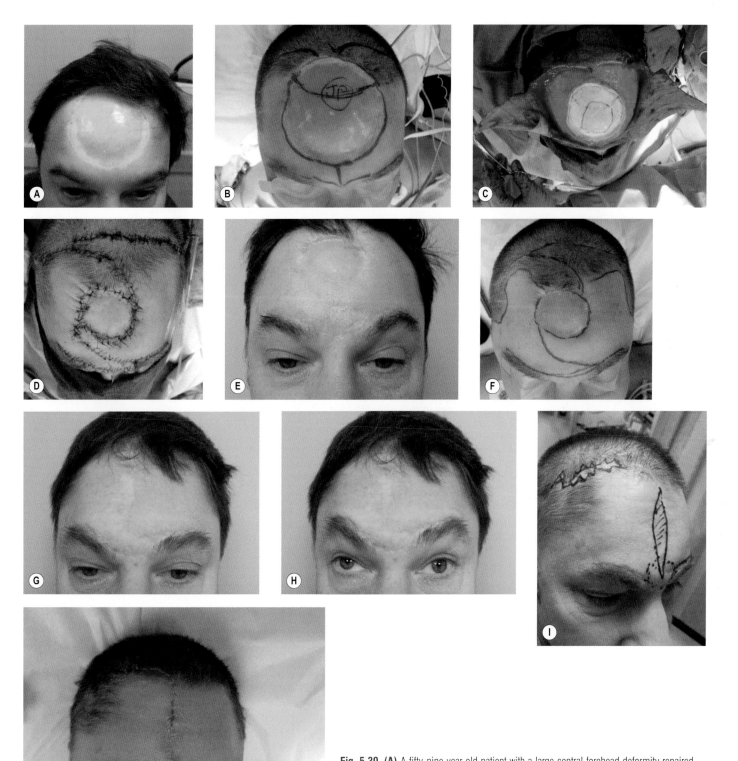

Fig. 5.30 (A) A fifty-nine year old patient with a large central forehead deformity repaired with a skin graft post excision of a DFSP. **(B, C, D)** Preoperative, intraoperative and postoperative pictures of the first stage of serial excision. **(E,F)** 6 months later the remainder of the skin graft was excised. **(G,H)** Early postoperative results showing intact frontalis muscle function after forehead continuity was reestablished. **(I,J)** Again a few months later, a minor scar revision of the forehead and a w-plasty of the scalp were performed to correct an area of scar alopecia.

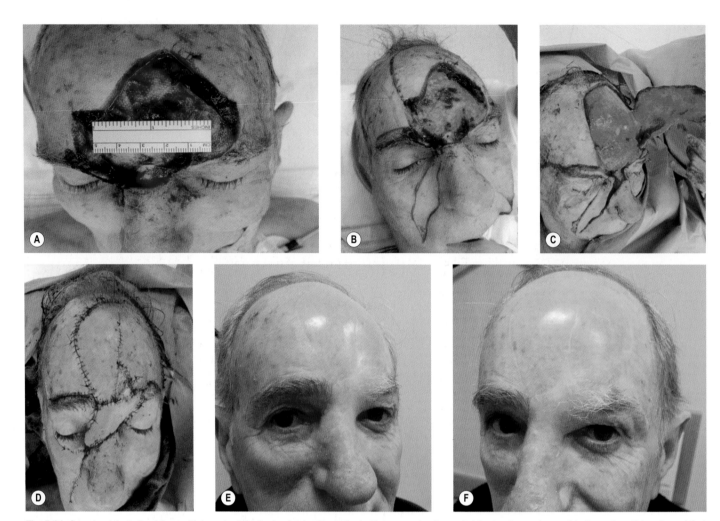

Fig. 5.31 Complex defects involving multiple parts of the forehead subunit: a patient with a very extensive central forehead, suprabrow, glabella, and medial eyebrow defect post Moh's excision of a BCC. The defect was repaired with a large scalp/forehead transposition-advancement flap plus a nasolabial flap (to reconstruct the glabella and eyebrow with hair from the nasolabial area). The final appearance post division, inset, and debulking of the nasolabial flap is shown.

for replantation.[106,107] In recent years, the advent of composite tissue transplantation for management of complex facial deformities has provided a new and exciting option for the ultimate reconstruction of "like" with "like". In fact, it has added a new rung to the reconstructive ladder. With transplantation of the face we have seen a shift in paradigm of repair from the concept of **"reconstruction"** to **"restoration"**.

In our unit, we have successfully performed seven face transplants to date, and four have included the forehead and two of these also included the anterior scalp.[108,109] All of our cases have been transferred based on the facial vessels alone, and yet there was adequate perfusion of the forehead and anterior scalp (as well as the lateral cheek, maxilla, anterior mandible, and neck in our other cases). In our cases, the forehead and anterior scalp did not have a direct axial blood supply but were perfused by connections between the terminal branches of the facial artery and periorbital vessels (Fig. 5.35). The blood supply has been adequate to allow long-term normal appearance and normal hair growth in the transferred scalp. This can be understood by applying Taylor et al.'s angiosome concept, which predicts that one can successfully transfer the next adjoining angiosome to that of the primary axial angiosome.[110] In this case, the axial facial angiosome adequately perfuses the next angiosome – namely forehead, maxilla, mandible, and neck. This has been confirmed in our dissection studies and clinical outcomes in our cases. We do not know how much of the scalp can be successfully transferred based on only the facial blood supply, but certainly the anterior 5–6 cm can. We would predict that the superficial temporal vascular supply would be needed for transfer of larger/total scalp transfers.

Postoperative care

The postoperative management will depend on the condition treated and the type of treatment rendered.

The use of antibiotics also depends on the nature of the problem, but if used prophylactically, they are just administered perioperatively. Patients with infective processes, compromised wounds, exposed dura, or where foreign material and grafts have been used, are treated with a full course of antibiotics.

Defects that are allowed to close by secondary intention will need local wound care until healed.

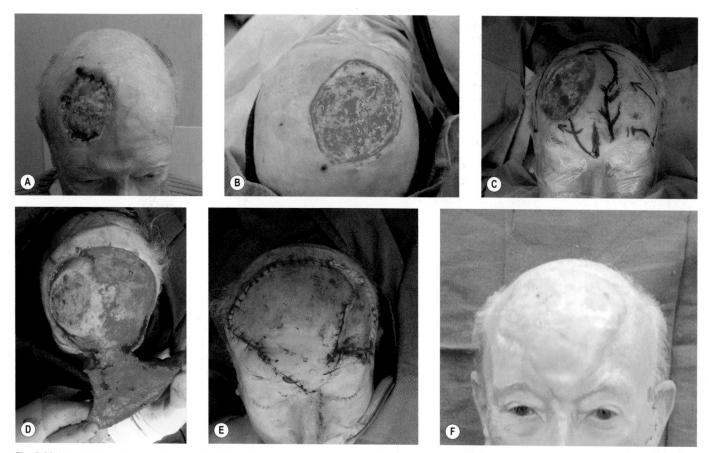

Fig. 5.32 Lateral forehead defect: a 92-year-old patient with a large extensive radionecrotic right forehead/scalp defect post excision of prior BCCs and SCCs. The patient has previously had 11 procedures in attempts to close the wound, including skin grafts, Integra, VAC dressing, hyperbaric oxygen therapy, etc., which all failed. The wound was debrided and margins checked for malignancy. A large axial extended forehead flap, based on the supratrochlear and supraorbital vessels is raised and transferred to repair the defect, and the resulting secondary donor site is skin grafted. The long-term postoperative result is shown.

Skin grafts are immobilized by tie-over bolster dressings or by a VAC device; with both, it is essential that excess pressure is not applied, as this can lead to graft loss and necrosis of underlying previously vascularized tissue, which will result in a wound which will need a more complex method of repair. The bolster or VAC is removed at 5–6 days (Fig. 5.13).

When tissue expanders are used, the expander is partially inflated to obliterate the dead space, and typically a drain is also inserted to avoid seroma due to wide dissection and undermining. The drain is usually removed after a few days. The expansion process begins about 10–14 days later, placing small amounts into the injection port every week or twice weekly as tolerated by patient and the tissues. It typically takes at least 8 weeks until adequate tissue has been recruited. It is important that the injection port is at a distance from the tissue expander so that the expander is not damaged by injections as it expands. An alternative is to have an integrated port, or an exteriorized port, which some surgeons use in pediatric patients, where often the parents are taught to do the expansion.

Local and regional flaps are monitored for their vascularity and protected from direct pressure, which can be difficult in certain locations, especially over the occiput. Occasionally, a temporary halo device may be needed to keep pressure off a vital flap.[111] These patients also have skin-grafted secondary donor site defects which need care as described above.

Free flaps need the same precautions as listed above and, in addition, close monitoring to detect vascular thrombosis. This is done with frequent monitoring of the flap's color and capillary return, the use of an external Doppler and by the use of implantable devices, such as a Cook catheter (Cook Medical) or tissue oximetry using near-infrared spectroscopy (ViOptix).[112] Skin grafted free muscle flaps are frequently used for scalp reconstruction, and these are more difficult to monitor clinically than flaps which also have a skin island, and it is safest to include an implantable Doppler device in these patients.

Outcome, prognosis, and complications

- Wound dehiscence, especially in the setting of tighter closure prevalent in scalp and forehead repairs, can occur following any procedure. These are treated with local wound care, debridement as needed and, once stabilized, secondary repair.
- Postoperative wound infections may also occur, especially when dealing with compromised tissue such as irradiated wounds. However, due to the robust blood supply of the scalp and forehead, infections are relatively less common than in other parts of the body. Antibiotic prophylaxis for problem wounds, and treatment with

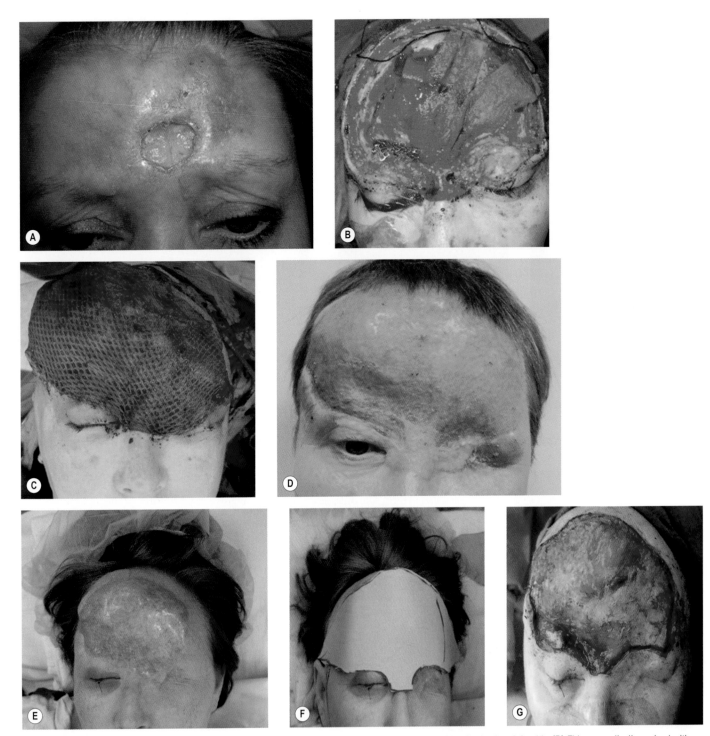

Fig. 5.33 **(A)** This renal transplant patient has an aggressive SCC involving forehead, frontal sinus, inner table of calvarium left orbit. **(B)** This was radically excised with neurosurgery and craniofacial surgery leaving a large frontal bone, orbital roof boney defect and significant soft tissue defect. **(C)** Cranial protection was obtained with titanium mesh for both the orbital roof/skull base and frontal bone deficit and a latissimus dorsi flap with a skin graft was used for soft tissue coverage. **(D)** The healed forehead with skin grafted latissimus flap is shown. **(E)** 6 Months after radiation therapy was completed further surgery to improve the appearance was planned. **(F)** Operative planning involved a template and **(G)** the entire forehead subunit was de-epithelialized in preparation for forehead soft tissue replacement.

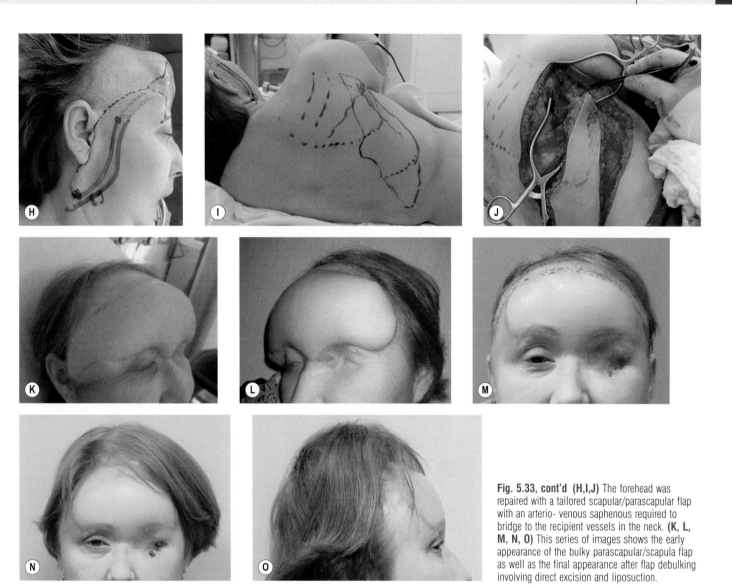

Fig. 5.33, cont'd (H,I,J) The forehead was repaired with a tailored scapular/parascapular flap with an arterio- venous saphenous required to bridge to the recipient vessels in the neck. **(K, L, M, N, O)** This series of images shows the early appearance of the bulky parascapular/scapula flap as well as the final appearance after flap debulking involving direct excision and liposuction.

appropriate antibiotics based on sensitivities, as well as local wound care, usually lead to successful outcomes.

■ In the scalp, all wounds, especially those allowed to heal by secondary intention, will have some degree of alopecia, which may necessitate a secondary revision, with transfer of hair-bearing flaps.

■ When using a VAC device, either for temporary wound management or for immobilization of skin grafts, the avoidance of excessive pressure which can devitalize the underlying periosteal bed is very important.

■ Tissue expansion of highly specialized hair-bearing scalp has become an invaluable method for generating "like" tissue for restoration of the hair, but great care should be taken during the lengthy process of expansion to minimize complications. In some patients, where the tissues are particularly tight or if the tissues are expanded too rapidly, wound dehiscence and expander exposure can occur. If this is minor, local wound care and antibiotics, together with slight deflation of the expander, may allow the process to continue, albeit more slowly. If

this occurs in the later part of the process, the second stage can be expedited, and expander removed and expanded flap transferred. If exposure or infection occurs before adequate expansion has occurred, the expander will need to be removed, antibiotics administered, and the wound allowed to heal for several months before re-expansion can be repeated.

■ Complications tend to be more common if multiple expanders are used, and part of the problem may be related to external pressure effects with sleeping, etc. We typically do not use more than two expanders at the same time.

■ Failure of skin grafts can result from the usual causes such as hematoma, infection, and mechanical effects of sheering, and appropriate measures to minimize these possibilities should be taken. However, in the scalp, probably the commonest cause is a poorly vascularized bed. This can be improved with the initial use of a VAC device to stimulate granulation and other techniques, such as drilling the outer cortex of the skull, and more

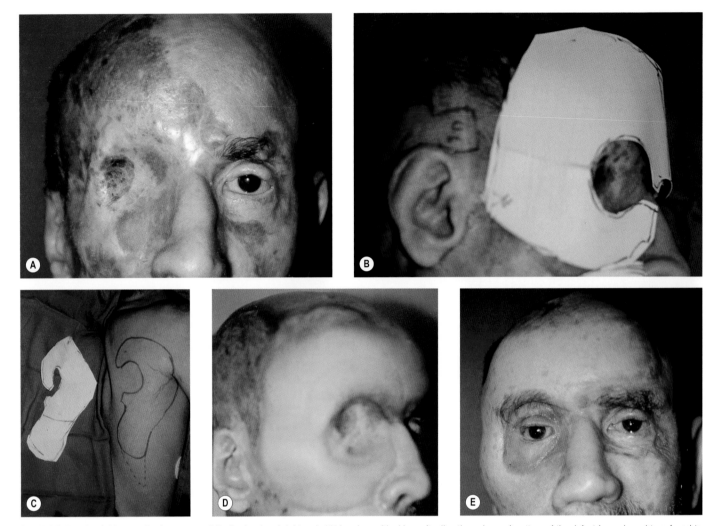

Fig. 5.34 A patient with extensive burn scars of the forehead and right periorbital region, with skin grafts directly on bone. A pattern of the defect is made and transferred to the back where a scapular/parascapular flap is designed and transferred to the upper face. Later, the right eyebrow was reconstructed with follicular hair grafts by Dr. Alfonso Barrera, and a periocular osseointegrated implant by Dr. Elof Eriksson.

elaborate methods such as by using the "crane" principle espoused by Millard have all been used successfully. The "crane" principle involves the temporary transfer of a vascularized flap to a poorly vascularized site, and then after a period of neovascularization, the flap is elevated from the site but leaving behind the deepest part of the flap (which is now vascularized and capable of nourishing a skin graft) and transferred back to its original site. This technique works well for wounds that have not been heavily irradiated – these latter wounds need permanent flap coverage.[113]

■ Common complications following local and regional flap transfers include distal tip necrosis, which can be treated conservatively if vital structures are not exposed. Significant problems following use of local flaps are usually due to errors in judgment and improper flap selection and design. This is especially problematic if the curvature of the scalp is not accounted for in the flap design, as this will cause a tight skin closure, which compromises the distal flap circulation leading to necrosis and dehiscence. It is imperative that the surgeon has a thorough understanding of flap anatomy and adheres to

principles of meticulous technique to minimize these problems.

■ Other complications such as hematoma and seroma can occur, but can be minimized with appropriate technique, the use of drains, etc.

■ Free tissue transfers are lengthy procedures, often undertaken in sick and elderly patients with other co-morbidities, and thus they can have any of the general complications that can arise with any prolonged anesthetic and surgical procedure. To minimize complications, the patient's general health and nutrition should be optimized preoperatively. Complication rates are higher in head and neck free tissue transfers than for elective breast free flap reconstruction.[114] Nonetheless, most centers report a very high success rate for head and neck free flaps, in excess of 95%. Attention to detail at all stages throughout the procedure and especially taking great care with the vascular pedicle to avoid twisting and distortion that can occur with movement of the head, and to assure good flap perfusion before leaving the operating room are key in ensuring a favorable outcome. Postoperatively, careful flap monitoring, especially for the

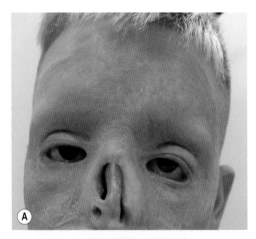

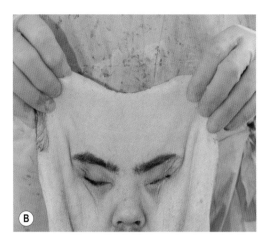

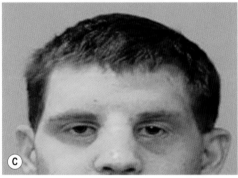

Fig. 5.35 A patient who underwent a total face transplant to reconstruct a major post electrical facial burn, showing the forehead and upper third of the face postoperative result.

first 24 h is mandatory, and any vascular compromise should prompt an emergent return to the operating room to correct the problem. In a large prospective study of microvascular free-flap surgery outcomes by Khouri et al. (in which the authors also participated), salvage rates varied between 54 and 100% depending on the series.[115]

Secondary procedures

Secondary procedures in the scalp and forehead are very often needed to achieve a satisfactory and aesthetic outcome. They may be needed to address complications from wound healing, repositioning of displaced natural landmarks, or as planned second, third (or more) stages of a complex reconstruction, with the goal of restoring to as close to "normal" as possible.

- Repair of widened scars that result from suture under tension, which is common in scalp, and forehead reconstruction may be requested. In the scalp, these scars typically lack hair, and it can be difficult to completely correct alopecia, as hair follicles are very susceptible to tension, and although scar may be narrower, there may still be some alopecia. The use of w-plasty and z-plasty can help break up a long alopecic scar so that it becomes less obvious (Fig. 5.30B). Care must be taken not to injure the hair follicles. Microfollicular hair grafting has also been used although scars are often not the most "fertile" sites to ensure good hair graft take.[116]
- Contour deformities, such as dog-ears at sites of pedicle flap pivot points are fairly easily addressed with simple

excision and repair. Small dog-ears often settle down without revision. Other contour deformities due to bulky flaps are also easily treated with liposuction or direct debulking.
- Depressions and indentations can be corrected with dermis-fat grafting and structural fat grafting. The fat grafting may need to be repeated to restore normal contour.
- Mobile structures such as the eyebrows and upper eyelids can be easily displaced during forehead reconstructions, producing obvious asymmetry. To replace these to their normal location, local tissue rearrangement with z-plasties, full-thickness skin grafting, or the preliminary use of tissue expansion are usually required.
- If skin grafts have been used as part of the initial repair, they will create a large area of alopecia in the scalp and may be unsightly if used on the forehead, due to color mismatch and contour deformity. In the scalp, secondary staged tissue expansion is the commonest way of dealing with the alopecia. In the forehead, attempts to improve the color mismatch and contour abnormality have included dermabrasion of the graft and overgrafting with split-thickness grafts from the scalp. Alternatively, serial excision or tissue expansion can be used.
- Restoration of the hairline, which helps define the subunits, is also a common goal of secondary reconstruction. The temporal sideburn can be replaced with a superiorly based transposition flap from the post auricular region. In males, a VY advancement of lower sideburn and beard area can be used to reconstruct the

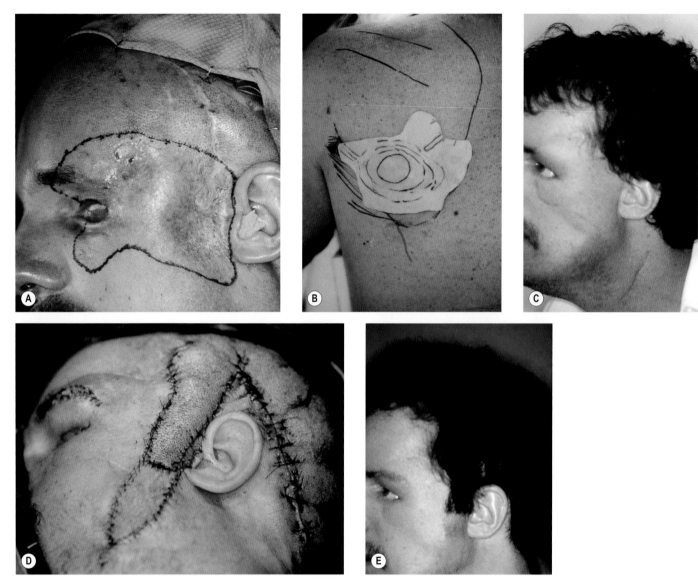

Fig. 5.36 A 25-year-old patient with unstable skin of the forehead and periorbital area due to irradiation for retinoblastoma in infancy. The unstable area was excised and tailored a scapula flap used to resurface the area. Later reconstruction of temporal hairline and sideburn with scalp transposition flap and VY hair-bearing cheek flap, and eyebrow reconstruction with follicular hair grafts.

lower aspect of the sideburn (Fig. 5.36).[117] Sometimes a combination of both the above methods may be used. The anterior hairline can be repaired with a Juri type of transposition flap, although the hair growth will be abnormal.[64–66] Alternatively, it can be restored as part of scalp expansion to correct larger areas of alopecia with serial tissue expansion.

■ Large subunit free tissue transfers may be required to replace the entire forehead if it is unsightly, uneven, and badly scarred from previous reconstructions. For a better color match, flap prefabrication using expanded neovascularized neck skin has been used by the authors.[118]

■ In cases where the cranium has been resected, secondary reconstructions and cranioplasty with bone grafts or alloplastic or synthetic plates may be required. Stable and well-perfused skin coverage over the bony defect is essential for a successful outcome in these cases.

Bonus images for this chapter can be found online at
http://www.expertconsult.com

Fig. 5.9 This series shows a 14-year-old girl who sustained a scalp avulsion injury of the temporal scalp **(A)** due to hair entanglement in a fan **(B)**. The immediate result post replantation is shown **(C)**, as well as a later result with some, but incomplete hair growth **(D)**.

Fig. 5.18 Seventy-year-old man with area of post irradiation necrosis of posterior scalp with exposed bone **(A)**. An axial musculocutaneous flap based on the occipital artery is designed **(B)** and transposed to cover the defect **(C)**. The resulting donor site is skin grafted. The long-term result with good hair growth is shown **(D)**.

Fig. 5.25 (A) Fifty-three-year-old man with defect in hair-bearing temporal region post excision of a chondroid syringoma, repaired with extended VY flap. **(B)** Nineteen-year-old man with a granuloma of the temporal/forehead region, repaired with a hair-bearing extended VY flap. Note the change of direction of hair growth.

Fig. 5.26 Glabella–suprabrow defect: patient with glabella defect post excision of sebaceous hyperplasia, repaired with bilateral VY advancement flaps, without distortion of natural eyebrow landmarks.

⊕ **Access the complete reference list online at** **http://www.expertconsult.com**

1. Seitz IA, Gottlieb LJ. Reconstruction of scalp and forehead defects. *Clin Plast Surg.* 2009;36:355–377. *Techniques in scalp and forehead reconstruction are detailed in this review.*

2. TerKonda RP, Sykes JM. Concepts in scalp and forehead reconstruction. *Otolaryngol Clin North Am.* 1997;30:519–539. *Anatomy and technical versatility are stressed in this primer on scalp reconstruction. The roles of diverse methods in achieving optimal coverage are discussed.*

6. Jackson IT. Forehead Reconstruction. In: *Local Flaps in Head and Neck Reconstruction.* 2nd ed. St Louis: Quality Medical Publishing; 2007. *An extensive summary of local flap options especially for forehead reconstruction by a master surgeon.*

42. Temple CL, Ross DC. Scalp and forehead reconstruction. *Clin Plast Surg.* 2005;32:377–390, vi–vii. *The authors propose an algorithm for scalp reconstruction. Surgical anatomy of the scalp is reviewed.*

44. Angelos PC, Downs BW. Options for the management of forehead and scalp defects. *Facial Plast Surg Clin North Am.* 2009;17:379–393. *This review covers methods in scalp wound management ranging from allowing for secondary healing to performing free tissue transfer.*

59. Leedy JE, Janis JE, Rohrich RJ. Reconstruction of acquired scalp defects: an algorithmic approach. *Plast Reconstr Surg.* 2005;116:54e–72e. *A multifaceted algorithm for scalp reconstruction is presented. The reconstructive surgeon is urged to achieve not only wound closure, but also an aesthetically optimal result.*

73. Pribaz JJ, Chester C, Barrall DT. The extended VY flap. *Plast Reconstr Surg.* 1992;90:275–280. *Details on VY, extended and double extended VY flaps that are very useful in forehead reconstruction.*

106. Pribaz JJ, Caterson EJ. The evolution and limitations of conventional autologous reconstruction of the head and neck: one perspective and a comparison of conventional reconstruction with face transplantation. *J Craniofac Surg.* 2013;24(1):99–107. *A summary of the advances and inadequacies in conventional reconstruction and the implications of the dawn of a new era of allotransplantation.*

117. Ridgway E, Pribaz JJ. The reconstruction of male hair-bearing facial regions. *Plast Reconstr Surg.* 2011;127(1):131–141. *A good summary of options for restoration of the hairline which is important in scalp and forehead reconstruction.*

6

Aesthetic nasal reconstruction

Frederick J. Menick

 Access video content for this chapter online at expertconsult.com

SYNOPSIS

- The field of plastic surgery originated with the first early attempts to reconstruct the face, especially the nose.
- The face tells the world who we are and materially influences what we can become.
- The restoration of a normal appearance and an open airway to allow comfortable breathing remains the goal.
- Treatment choices will depend on an understanding of the deformity and wound healing, missing anatomic layers, available donor tissues, surgical planning, the surgeon's ability to modify them into "like" tissue, and the advantages, disadvantages, and limitations of the technique, and its ability to achieve the desired outcome.

Introduction

The primary functions of the nose are to look normal and allow easy nasal breathing.

The success of reconstruction will depend upon the site, size, and depth of the defect, donor availability and, most importantly, the surgeon's choices in material, method, and approach. An understanding of the deformity, both anatomically and aesthetically, and of wound healing and tissue transfer are required. The advantages, disadvantages, and limitations of each material, technique, and stage must be understood. What is missing must be replaced – external skin which matches adjacent facial skin in color and texture, a midlayer support of soft tissue, bone and cartilage, and internal lining. Covering skin must be thin, conforming, and vascular. Lining must be thin, supple, and vascular, neither occluding the airway nor distorting external nasal shape due to excessive bulk or stiffness. A rigid midlayer must support, shape, and brace the soft tissues against gravity, tension, and scar contraction to prevent collapse and create contour. The surgeon must replace tissues similar in kind to those which are missing. However, although donor tissues may have some characteristics which are similar, all tissues must be modified

– thinned and shaped – to become "like" tissue. Flat forehead skin, ear or rib cartilage, and traditional lining replacements have little similarity to the "normal" nose.

 Access the Historical Perspective section online at **http://www.expertconsult.com**

Basic science/disease process and surgical timing

Nasal deformity may follow congenital malformation, trauma (including burns), and the sequela of skin cancer treatment by excision or radiation, infection, or immune disease.[25]

Often reconstruction is delayed for weeks to years to allow wound stabilization, wound maturation, and verification of disease control.

The extent of the tumor can be estimated visually and an additional margin of normal tissue is excised, based on clinical judgment or published "rules of thumb". Margins can be evaluated by *permanent histologic section or intraoperative frozen sections* to verify the completeness of excision, prior to wound closure. However, large tissue excisions with multiple margins are burdensome for the hospital pathologist, are time-consuming, and disrupt the operative schedule.

To better evaluate peripheral and deep margins, the *Margin Check Technique* can be applied. An en bloc excision is performed, based on physical examination, histology, and clinical judgment. Then, additional 1–2 mm slivers of the entire lateral and deep margins are excised, oriented for the hospital pathologist, and the wound dressed. A delayed primary repair is scheduled 24–72 h later, pending verification of complete tumor excision.

Moh's Histographic Surgery, normally performed in an outpatient setting, utilizes a unique serial horizontal section and mapping technique to maximize cure rate. It is especially useful for difficult tumors – skin cancers greater than 2 cm in size, recurrent, those with poorly defined visible borders, morphea or sclerotic basal cell cancers, and those in difficult locations, such as nose, ear, or eye, where maximum tissue preservation is desirable.

Staged excision with delayed repair is especially advantageous in the more extensive cancer which requires more complex reconstruction. Ideally, the patient is seen prior to tumor excision. The diagnosis is verified, the likely extent of excision and reconstruction is discussed, and the treatment options are outlined. Preoperative medical clearance can be obtained, if necessary. Operative time is scheduled for the future. Excision is performed and a follow-up appointment is made to evaluate the defect after tumor clearance. During the post-excisional consultation, the true extent of the defect is confirmed and anatomic and aesthetic losses are defined. Reconstruction follows within 48–72 h. Because the extent of the defect has been defined prior to repair, the patient understands the requirements of reconstruction and maintains an ongoing informed participant in his/her care.

Such coordinated excision and repair provides an opportunity to think, plan, and discuss options with the patient in a leisurely manner prior to entering the operating room. A surgical plan is developed preoperatively – decreasing patient and surgeon anxiety and ensuring the best result. Because tumor clearance has been confirmed prior to repair, the length of anesthesia and operative times are shortened. Most importantly, disruption of the operative schedule and intraoperative decision making are minimized.

Diagnosis/patient presentation/selection

The preoperative consultation should clarify the diagnosis, define the anatomic and aesthetic deficiencies, ensure a healthy wound and patient, provide patient education, instill confidence and the patient's participation, formulate a surgical plan, and identify donors, methods, and staging. Medical history and physical examination are evaluated with special emphasis on the etiology of the nasal injury, disease remission, or cancer clearance. Facial photographs, combined with calibrated photographs and normative facial measurements, clarify anatomic and aesthetic injury, old scars, landmark malposition, injury to available donor sites, and provide measurements which are useful intraoperatively. In complex three-dimensional (3D) injuries, a facial moulage is obtained preoperatively and a clay model of the desired result designed. This allows the surgeon to intellectually visualize the dimension and contours which require replacement. Prior pathologic exams and old operative reports are examined. Facial X-rays, computed tomography (CT) scans, or magnetic resonance imaging (MRI) are occasionally employed to clarify bony and soft tissue injury to the midface when rebuilding composite defects of the nose and cheek.

Planning an aesthetic nasal reconstruction

The traditional approach

Traditionally,[22,25] the defect determined the repair. Surgeons "filled the hole" to obtain a healed wound. So the design and dimension of a skin graft or flap were determined by the apparent, but often distorted, defect. The emphasis was on tissue transfer (skin graft or flap), blood supply, or the replacement of anatomic layers (cover, lining, support). Scars and additional donor injury were overriding concerns. A comprehensive plan to restore multiple, exact, independent, 3D facial features was rarely envisioned.

This traditional approach failed to appreciate the strong motivation of patients to look as they did before. It followed a "less is more", cautious approach, employing principles with little expectation of restoring the normal.

False principles

Design the flap from a pattern of the defect

Traditionally, skin grafts or flaps are designed to replace the existing defect. But the defect does not reflect what is missing and what needs to be replaced. Fresh wounds are enlarged by edema, local anesthesia, tissue tension, and gravity. Old wounds may be contracted by secondary intention healing or distorted by prior injury or repair.

To restore the normal, the "true" tissue loss must be identified the "true" defect replaced after returning "the normal to its normal position". Then the defect is filled with exactly measured replacements.

Take extra tissue to be safe

Transferring extra tissue for "good measure" or out of fear for vascularity only complicates the reconstruction. If too much tissue is transferred, adjacent landmarks are displaced outward. Additional stages will be needed to excise the extra bulk and restore unit outline.

Make the flap smaller to preserve the donor site

Sharing tissue from an area of excess to one of deficiency is a basic surgical tool but the temptation to cheat the recipient site to preserve the donor site must be avoided.

Central features, such as the nose or lip, have an exact border outline and position. Missing tissues must be replaced in exact quantity to avoid distortion of the size, shape, and position of the nasal subunit by dragging the borders of the defect inward with tissue replacement which is too small.

Employ a tissue expander to conserve the forehead donor site

The nose is an unforgiving facial feature, while the forehead is a forgiving one. Although useful if the hairline is exceptionally low or the forehead is scarred or previously harvested, the routine use of skin expansion is unnecessary. The nose comes first. The forehead donor is of secondary importance. Use an expander only if it will contribute to the overall nasal repair.

Never throw anything away

Surgeons are taught to preserve tissue. However, if skin is transferred to resurface only part of a facial feature, it may appear as a distracting patch, outlined by scars. It is often helpful to alter the defect and discard extra skin prior to repair, even if this makes the defect larger. Discardable tissues may be used for other purposes – hingeover lining, subcutaneous bulk, or shifted to resurface an adjacent injury.

The presence and number of scars determine the final result. Place incisions in existing scars, minimize scars, fear scars

A poor facial repair is identified by incorrect dimension, volume, position, and contour, not by the presence of scars. Scar can be effectively camouflaged by positioning them in the joins between subunits.

Place a supportive framework and debulk excess tissue secondarily after the soft tissues have healed

Traditionally, cover and lining have been replaced without support to avoid the risk of extrusion and infection. Occasionally, flimsy cartilage strips were placed within a prefabricated flap over a skin graft. Months later, bone and cartilage grafts were placed as crude cantilevered grafts to lift the tip and dorsum.

Unfortunately, unsupported soft tissues are rapidly distorted by gravity and tension and become fixed by scar. Late re-expansion with secondary cartilage grafts and soft tissue "thinning" may not be successful.

One hole – one flap – and (often) one operation

It is difficult to reproduce the delicate 3D character of multiple facial units with a single flap. A single flap often fails to supply enough skin to resurface 3D contour. Myofibroblasts within the bed of scar under the flap contracts, drawing the single flap into a dome-like pin cushioned mass. For that reason, it may be preferable to repair individual facial units with separate grafts and flaps of exact dimension and skin quality.

The modern approach to nasal reconstruction

A healed wound, tissue survival, or the replacement of anatomic layers are necessary, but not sufficient, to restore a normal appearance and function. Aesthetic results depend upon the surgeon's and patient's choices.[22,25] The modern approach relies on the visualization of the "normal" to determine what is missing, both anatomically and aesthetically.[27] This regional unit approach emphasizes the judicious choice and modification of recipient and donor tissues to provide for the exact replacement of facial units. The principles of facial reconstruction have switched from a wound perspective (how big, how deep, anatomy, and flap blood supply) to a visual one. The mature surgeon, with training and experience, "sees the future". He or she conceptualizes among available options what will work, while visualizing the desired result. A plan is formulated, principles outlined, and techniques and methods chosen.

Fortunately, although each defect is different, all repairs are simplified because the "normal" is unchanging. The "normal" nose is visually defined by its dimension, volume, position, projection, platform, symmetry, and expected skin quality, border outline, and 3D contour. Major facial landmarks are described as Regional Units – adjacent topographic areas of characteristic quality, outline, and 3D contour. Often, the contralateral normal remains as a visual standard for comparison. If not, the ideal is the guide. A unit approach helps the surgeon conceptualize the goal, define the requirements of repair, balance options, and measure the success of the result. Goals, priorities, stages, materials, and method of

tissue transfer are clearer with the ideal normal in mind (Fig. 6.1, Box 6.1).

In the latter half of the twentieth century, Gonzalez-Ulloa[28] divided the face into regions, based on skin thickness. Millard[29] envisioned major facial landmarks as "units" and recommended replacing them in their entirety with "like" tissue of similar color and texture to avoid a patch-like repair. Burget and Menick[30] divided the nose and face into "subunits", based on skin quality, border outline, and 3D contour.

The concept of peripheral and central facial units

The face can be divided into peripheral and central units areas of characteristic skin quality, border outline, and 3D contour. This regional unit concept guides clinical observation and treatment recommendations.[22,25]

Peripheral units

The forehead and cheek are peripheral facial units. Like a "picture frame", they lie at the periphery of the face and receive secondary intention. Their surfaces are largely flat and expansive and their border outlines variable, according to hairline and eyebrow position. Because their borders are not visible in all views, their borders can only be incompletely compared to the contralateral normal side for symmetry or outline. Because the peripheral units are less exact and constant, their repair is less demanding and of secondary importance. Skin quality, not outline or 3D contour, determines success.

A moderate forehead defect can be allowed to heal secondarily. The resulting shiny, flat scar, supported by the underlying rigid bony platform of the skull, blends into the normal shiny, tight surface of the forehead without significant distortion or malposition of adjacent landmarks. Rarely, a skin graft may be used to replace the entire forehead unit or a lateral subunit, after discarding any residual skin within the unit. The uniform, shiny quality of the skin graft simulates the expected quality and contour of the entire forehead unit or

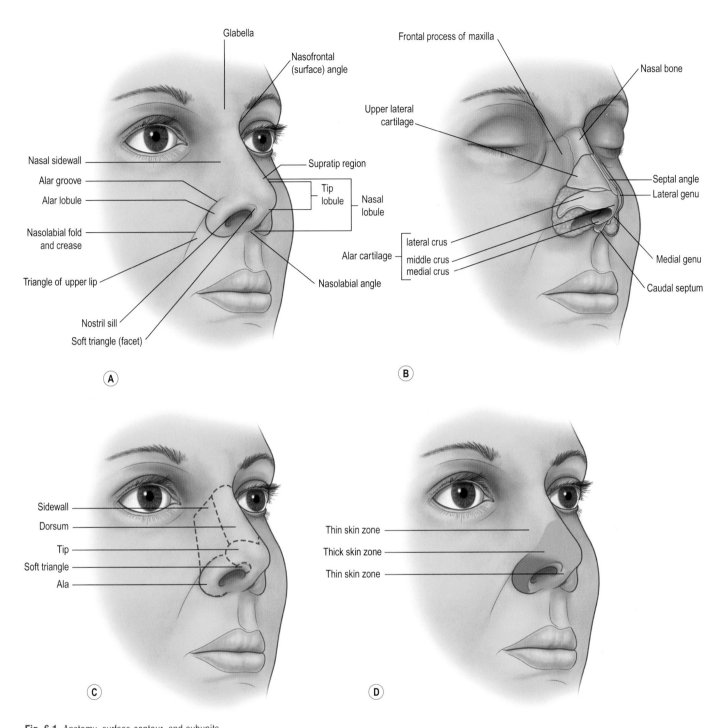

Fig. 6.1 Anatomy, surface contour, and subunits.

subunits and its peripheral scars are masked along the hairline, brow, or contour lines between the lateral and central forehead subunits.

Most often, the lax and excess adjacent skin within the cheek is shared by resurfacing the defect with a non-subunit rotation advancement flap. The Subunit Principle is rarely applied when resurfacing the cheek or forehead. Enlarging the wound so that the entire forehead or cheek

is recovered with one flap is impractical due to the paucity of available donor excess and the unreliability of flap blood supply.

Central units

The central midfacial units of the nose, lip, and eyelids require a different reconstructive approach. The principles of regional unit reconstruction apply primarily to repair central facial defects, not the peripheral units.

The nose has a fixed border outline, a 3D shape, and contralateral symmetry that must be maintained. Although skin quality is important, landmark outline, contour, and symmetry are of greater importance. The central units are seen in primary gaze and demand the highest priority of repair.

The dimension and outline of the nasal wound may be altered by discarding additional residual normal skin within the subunit to resurface the defect as a unit. Large nasal defects are reconstructed with regional transposition flaps of exact dimension and outline to avoid tension, collapse, or distortion of adjacent mobile landmarks. The external skin surface must be shaped in 3D with cartilage grafts for support and contour.

Principles of regional unit repair[25,27]

- Human beings wish to look normal.
- The normal is defined by 3D contour, border outline, and skin quality which describe *Regional Units*. They do not correlate with wrinkle or resting skin tension lines.
- The nasal unit consists of the tip, dorsum, columella, and paired alae, sidewalls, and soft triangle subunits.
- Restore units, do not fill defects.
- If a defect, within part of a central unit, is filled without regard to the unit outline, the tissue replacement may appear as a distracting patch within the subunit. The reconstructive goal must be to restore the character of the unit, rather than simply fill the "hole".
- Alter the wound in site, size, outline, and depth. Discard adjacent normal tissue within convex nasal subunits to improve the result.

When part of a central convex nasal unit is missing, it is often useful to resurface the entire unit or subunit, rather than simply patch the defect. The wound's dimension, outline, or depth may be altered. Subunit resurfacing positions scars so that they are camouflaged within the joins between subunits. More importantly, myofibroblasts lie in the recipient bed under a transferred flap and contract, causing the transposed skin flap to rise above the level of adjacent skin. When an entire convex subunit is resurfaced, the pin cushioned flap shrink-wraps around the underlying cartilage framework, augmenting, rather than distorting, the contour of a convex subunit. Residual tissue within the subunit may be discarded to enlarge the wound. Or the defect may be decreased in size by local advancement rotation flaps, or changed in border outline by a combination of excision and tissue rearrangement.

The subunit principle[22,30]

If a defect of a central convex subunit, such as the tip or ala, is greater than 50% of the subunit, discard adjacent normal tissue within the subunit and resurface the entire subunit, rather than merely "patching the hole".

The consequences of the Subunit Principle are:

1. The defect may be enlarged and the donor requirement increased. A larger defect may preclude closure with local tissue and necessitate a regional flap repair.
2. The number of stages and the complexity of the repair may be increased.

3. The amount of cartilage material required to support the soft tissues may be increased.
4. Patient morbidity may increase if regional flaps or cartilage grafts are needed.

However, when applied appropriately, the final result may be significantly improved. It should be emphasized, however, that a good result does not depend on any one surgical maneuver. It reflects a series of choices, methods, and tissue manipulations that transfer a correctly thinned covering flap which blends into neighboring tissues, establishes a 3D contour, and replaces missing tissues in exact dimension and outline. Resurfacing a facial defect as a unit can be helpful, but it is only a single tool.

Use the contralateral normal or the ideal as a guide

The apparent defect may not reflect the actual tissue loss. Due to edema, tension, gravity, scar, or past repair, the wound may be larger, smaller, or altered in shape. The surgeon must use the contralateral normal – the opposite ala, hemi-tip or hemi nose, and hemilip subunit to design a foil template that reflects the size and shape of the missing subunit. If the contralateral normal is absent, a template can be designed from an ideal clay model, based on a moulage of the patient's face, or a template can be designed from another normal face.

Replace tissues in exact dimensions and outline

If a flap is larger than the defect, its bulk pushes adjacent landmarks outward, creating malposition and asymmetry. Excess skin also obscures the surface details created by the underlying support. If the flap is smaller than the defect, neighboring structures are pulled inward. The tension also collapses underlying cartilage grafts. Exact 3D patterns are designed to fit the needs of the "true" tissue defect, rather than a wound distorted by edema, tension, scar, or prior repair.

Employ templates

An exact foil template of the contralateral normal or ideal is used to design flaps and support grafts. Such templates determine the size of the flap or cartilage graft, the shape of its border and the dimension or the position of facial landmarks (alar base, nasolabial fold, or alar crease).

Choose ideal donor materials and employ an ideal method of tissue transfer

Millard's admonition to use "like for like" applies. Use lip for lip, cheek for cheek, and a forehead or nasolabial flap for nasal resurfacing. Distant tissues are employed for lining, to fill dead space, create a facial platform, or vascularize an ischemic, contaminated, or radiated wound. However, regional skin should be used to replace facial skin because distant skin does not match the facial skin quality.

Understand wound healing and tissue transfer

Traditionally, the method of tissue transfer was chosen based on the vascularity and depth of the defect. Skin grafts were employed to resurface well vascularized superficial defects, when skin and a small amount of subcutaneous tissue are missing. Skin flaps were used to supply bulk to a deep defect or cover a poorly vascularized recipient site, a wound with exposed vital structures, or exposed or restored cartilage and bone.

Postoperatively, skin grafts are typically shiny, atrophic, and hypopigmented or hyperpigmented. Even though a skin graft donor may match the color and texture of the recipient site, the transient ischemia associated with skin graft "take" leads to unpredictable skin color and texture changes, and full-thickness skin grafts shrink modestly but do not trapdoor.

In contrast, a flap maintains its own perfusion and retains the skin quality of its donor site. However, the scar between the flap and the recipient bed contracts, which leads to pin cushioning.

Flaps often develop a convex surface shape. Therefore, skin grafts are best employed to resurface flat or concave recipient sites, such as the nasal side wall, while skin flaps are used to resurface convex surfaces, such as the tip or ala subunits. When an entire convex subunit is resurfaced with a flap as a unit or subunit, wound healing and tissue transfer are harnessed and pin cushioning contributes to the desired contour.

Build on a stable platform

Unfortunately, the lip/cheek platform may shift postoperatively due to resolution of edema, gravity, tension, and scar contraction. The larger and deeper the defect, the greater is the risk. If the lip/cheek platform is unstable and the nose is reconstructed at the same operative procedure, the nose may be dragged inferiorly and laterally over time.

Although a small superficial defect of the nose, cheek, and lip can often be rebuilt during a single stage, large deep defects of the cheek and lip are more reliably reconstructed during a preliminary operation which re-establishes a stable platform. Then the nose is built secondarily at a later stage.

Restore the subcutaneous framework of hard and soft tissue

A nose looks normal because it has a nasal shape. Primary and delayed primary support grafts should be placed to restore missing cartilage and bone which support, shape, and brace cover and lining against collapse and contraction. Although the alar lobule and soft triangle normally contain no cartilage, cartilage must also be placed along the nostril margin. Alar batten grafts brace the alar rim and prevent constriction inward, contraction outward, and airway collapse. Precise soft tissue excision can also add 3D shape by improving overall nasal contour during each surgical stage. Secondary placement of cartilage grafts is less effective, once soft tissues are contracted by scar.

Disregard old scars

To avoid additional incisional scars, bulky flaps are often "thinned" secondarily, during late revision, by elevating the peripheral edges of the flap through its border scar. However, it is frequently preferable to disregard old scars and add additional incisions.

Using accurate templates, based on the contralateral normal or ideal, the desired 3D concavity of the alar crease or nasolabial fold are marked with ink. Once the ideal landmark position is incised and the wound edges on either side of the "new" incision are elevated. Under direct vision, the underlying soft tissue is sculpted in three dimensions to create a flat sidewall, a round ala, a full medial cheek, etc. The overlying skin is then reapproximated to the newly contoured subcuta-

neous bed with quilting sutures. The wound is closed. Although a new incisional scar is created, it lies hidden in the border outline of the newly contoured subunits. Visually, the new scar is hidden within the expected contour depression between units.

Employ surgical staging to advantage

Each surgical stage is an opportunity to recreate the defect, return normal to normal, ensure viability, prepare excess tissue for other uses (hingeover lining flaps, soft tissue bulk, etc.), surgically delay, prefabricate, transfer, and modify tissues by debulking or shaping, add or alter support grafts, or improve imperfections, and treat complications or secondary priorities.

Consider a preliminary operation

Often, the extent of deformity is obscured by secondary healing, prior skin grafts, or flaps. A preliminary operation, prior to formal nasal reconstruction, can be helpful. The defect is recreated and residual tissues returned to their normal position. The dimension and position of the defect and the required tissue replacements are more accurately defined. Although past history, physical examination, old operative reports, or radiographs may provide information, the extent of the true defect may only become apparent after recreating the defect. Excision of scar or soft tissue bulk can open an occluded airway. Residual local tissue or adjacent regional flaps can be positioned for later use or surgically delayed to maximize blood supply, especially when scar lies within the territory or injury to the flap's pedicle is suspected. Ischemic or chronically infected tissue may be debrided. Immature tissues may revascularize, soften, and stabilize. Defects of the lip and cheek may be repaired, establishing a stable platform on which to place the nose at a later date. If indicated, the wound can be biopsied to ensure complete clearance of tumor or immune disease remission.

When a defect is complex, the patient may be anxious and the surgeon uncertain of tissue needs or available options. The diagnosis may need clarification, the wound may need preparation, and the problem may need to be analyzed to prepare a plan.

Classification of defects

Nasal defects are classified into small, superficial, large, deep, or composite defects.[22,25] The difficulty of repair will be determined by the site, size, and depth of injury.

A *"small defect"* is less than 1.5 cm in diameter. A skin graft can be employed to resurface larger defects. But if the defect is larger than 1.5 cm, local flaps are precluded because there is not enough residual skin to "share" over the entire nasal surface without excessive closure tension and landmark distortion.

"Superficial defects" include skin and a small amount of underlying subcutaneous fat and nasalis muscle. Vascularized soft tissue remains in the depth of the wound to revascularize a skin graft or can be resurfaced with a flap. Although a small defect may be allowed to heal secondarily, if periosteum or perichondrium is missing, a skin graft is precluded and a vascularized flap will be required.

"Adversely located defects" are those whose position necessitates a regional flap for cover. If the defect is closer than 0.5 to 1 cm of the nostril margin, local flaps will distort the tip

and nostril rim. Local flaps do not reach the infratip lobule or columella. A regional flap will be needed to resurface adversely located defects, even though the wound is not necessarily large.

"*Large defects*" are greater than 1.5 cm in size. Insufficient skin remains over the residual nose to redistribute with a local flap. Skin must be added by transferring a skin graft or excess cheek or forehead.

"*Deep defects*" are those in which the underlying support or lining is missing.

If a cartilage graft is needed or lining is missing, a skin graft or local flap cannot be employed. Even in the ala which contains no cartilage, if significant alar skin and underlying compact fibro-fatty middle layer are absent, cartilage support must be placed.

A skin graft will not "take" over bare cartilage grafts. And a local flap is precluded because delicate cartilage grafts collapse under the wound tension associated with local flaps which share residual tissue over the nasal surface.

So although a small rim defect can be closed with a composite skin graft, significant full-thickness defects require a vascularized regional flap for cover.

"*Composite defects*"[31] extend from the nose onto the adjacent cheek and upper lip to include individual nose, cheek, and lip units which differ visually, anatomically, and functionally. Quality, outline, and contour are different for each facial unit. The degree of tissue loss varies from unit to unit and the need for cover, lining, support, soft and hard tissue will be different.

The simplest solution is to "fill the hole", replacing missing skin and soft tissue with a single flap. But it is difficult to reproduce the delicate 3D character of a composite defect with a single flap. Geometrically, the shortest distance between two points is a straight line and a single flap often takes a "surgical shortcut" and fails to provide enough skin to restore 3D contours. Scar contraction of a defect which includes multiple units draws a single flap into a domelike mass, outlined by patch-like peripheral scars. Using separate grafts or flaps for each facial unit better positions scars in the expected joins between landmarks and helps control flap pin cushioning.

The repair of nasal defects – treatment options

Although "simple" at first glance, small and superficial defects are difficult to repair. Surgeons and patients fail to appreciate the complexity of nasal contour, the paucity of excess tissue, the difficulty of matching the skin in color and texture, and the risk of distorting the residual mobile tip and nostril margins. The time, trouble, morbidity, donor and recipient scars, number of stages, time to wound maturity, and the cost must be balanced against the likelihood of secondary deformity. Many options are available.

Understanding nasal skin quality

The nose is covered by skin and an underlying layer of subcutaneous fat and nasalis muscle which lay over a rigid bony elastic framework of cartilage and fibrofatty support. However, the quality of the skin is not uniform, unless atrophic due to old age, sun injury, or radiation injury. In the normal nose, it

can be divided into areas of thin smooth skin and thickly pitted skin. Note that the zones of skin quality do not correspond to the nasal units, which are defined by contour.

In the superior half of the nose, dorsal and sidewall skin is thin, smooth, pliable, and mobile. A modest excess of skin is present, which permits primary closure or a local flap to close small defects without distortion of adjacent mobile landmarks. A modest amount of skin can also be recruited from the cheek to resurface a small sidewall or ala defect. Although a simultaneous rhinoplasty, hoping to decrease the size of the nasal skeleton and relatively increase the available skin, has been recommended to ease the closure of small defects in a large nose, it is rarely helpful.

The inferior half of the nose is covered by a zone of tight skin, pitted with sebaceous glands, and adherent to the underlying deep structures. No excess is present. This thick skin zone begins in the alar groove, crosses 5–10 mm above the supratip region, and extends inferiorly towards the caudal borders of the tip and alar subunits. About 2–3 mm above the alar margins and a few millimeters below the outermost point of the tip and onto the columella, the skin thins and loses its sebaceous quality. The lower half of the infratip lobule, including the soft triangle and columella, is covered by thin, but adherent skin fixed to the underlying structures. There is no excess within the inferior nose and the tip and alar margins are mobile and easily distorted by contracting scar or inaccurate tissue replacement.

Restoring nasal cover

Small, superficial defects

Healing by secondary intention

The body responds to injury by epithelialization, granulation tissue, and myofibroblast contraction. The process is simple, inexpensive, somewhat slow, but often satisfactory.

Healing by secondary intention is used for wounds created by a destructive process which preclude primary closure. These include electrodessication and curettage or those associated with wound dehiscence, infection, or necrosis. To avoid further injury due to desiccation or trauma, secondary healing is avoided if vital deep structures are exposed in the base of the wound.

No net gain in tissue occurs with secondary healing. Wound contraction progresses to the degree that adjacent tissue can be pulled into the defect. The residual gap is filled with collagen covered with a shiny adherent, thin layer of epidermis, containing few melanocytes or skin appendages. The result is a pale, shiny, flat, white scar.

Secondary healing is employed for defects which lie within a flat or concave nasal surface, at a distance from mobile landmarks, especially when they lie within sun or radiated injured skin where imperfections of skin quality due to spontaneous healing are less apparent.

A small superficial defect of the flat tight dorsum, sidewall, or deep alar crease may heal satisfactorily by secondary intention. However, imperfections in color or texture or contour depressions are visible in the thicker skin of the tip and ala. The mobile tip and nostril margins are also at risk for distortion due to scar contracture. Despite limitations, almost any wound will heal spontaneously, if medical illness, cost, lifestyle, or patient disinterest precludes a more formal repair initially.

Primary repair

Because a modest excess of skin is present in the more lax upper two-thirds of the nose, primary repair may be possible if the defect is less than 5–6 mm. Because no extra skin is available in the thick adherent skin of the tip and ala, primary closure is avoided to prevent distortion and wide depressed scars.

Skin grafting

Skin grafts have many advantages.[22,25] No new scars are added to the nasal surface, and the amount of locally available tissue is not a limiting factor. Skin grafts are typically harvested from preauricular, postauricular, or supraclavicular donor sites. Forehead grafts are best for the tip and ala.

However, a skin graft must lie on a well vascularized bed to ensure "take" and will not reliably survive when placed on denuded cartilage or a cartilage graft. A skin graft, placed over a narrow primary cartilage graft, may revascularize by the bridging phenomena. The size of the cartilage graft must be limited. Complete or partial skin graft necrosis may occur.

The aesthetic result of skin graft is unpredictable. Because of the transient ischemia which accompanies skin graft transfer, the quality of donor skin deteriorates. Skin grafts often appear pale, smooth, and atrophic. A full-thickness skin graft may blend satisfactorily into the relatively smooth atrophic upper nose within the thin skin of the dorsum and sidewall.

However, traditional skin grafts, within the thick skin zone of the tip and ala, often appear as depressed, shiny, off-colored patches unless the skin of the recipient site is atrophic due to sun injury or radiation.

Preauricular and postauricular skin grafts

Hairless preauricular skin is a good donor site. A strip of skin 2–2.5 cm wide can be harvested. Larger grafts may transfer fine vellus hair in women or bearded skin in men. Postauricular skin can be harvested from the back of the ear and mastoid, across the postauricular crease. In unusual circumstances, the entire posterior surface of the ear can be taken and the donor site skin grafted with more distant skin. Postauricular skin may remain red. The hairless preauricular patch between the tragus and sideburn provides a better match, especially when applied to the dorsum, sidewall, or columella. Supraclavicular skin looks brown and shiny.

The full-thickness forehead skin graft (Figs. 6.2 & 6.3)

Forehead skin is acknowledged as the best match to replace nasal skin. Although not traditionally transferred as a skin graft, forehead skin is useful for resurfacing small superficial defects, especially of the tip and ala. Forehead skin and its underlying compact fibrofatty subcutaneous layer are thicker and stiffer than other donors. Significant amounts of soft tissue can be carried with the graft, permitting the replacement of the deeper soft tissues. Forehead skin grafts revascularize normally, with progressive changes in color from white to blue to pink. A good take is routinely expected. However, when failure seems eminent, unlike grafts harvested from

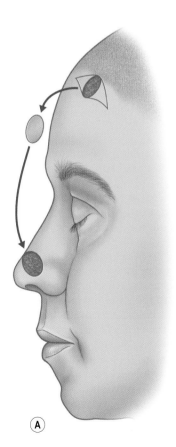

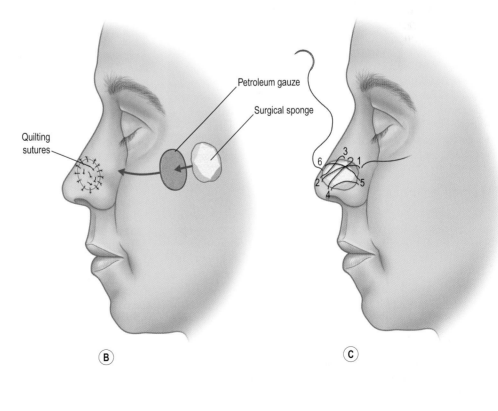

Quilting sutures

Petroleum gauze

Surgical sponge

Ⓐ   Ⓑ   Ⓒ

Fig. 6.2 Forehead skin graft technique.

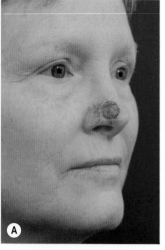

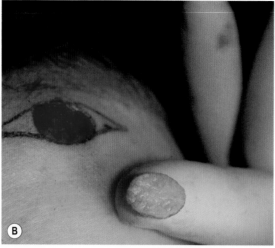

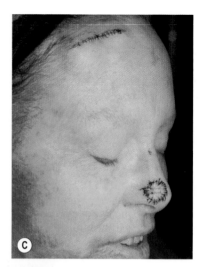

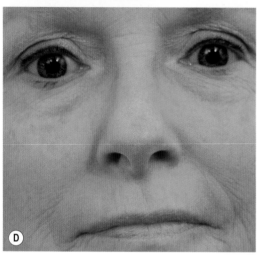

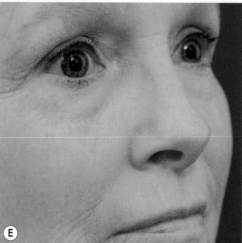

Fig. 6.3 (A–E) Small superficial nasal tip defect resurfaced with full-thickness forehead skin graft.

other sites, early separation does not occur. A hard and tightly adherent eschar develops. It may remain fixed to the underlying tissues for 4–6 weeks. After spontaneous separation, the surgeon often finds that the wound is healed, filled, and the aesthetic result good. One to 1.5 cm of forehead skin is easily harvested below the frontal hairline with primary closure of the donor site. The scar is usually excellent and easily covered by hair.

Skin graft technique

A skin graft must be placed on a vascular bed to ensure "take". It will not survive if tented across the defect or separated by hematoma or seroma. It must be immobile to allow the development of vascular connections to the recipient site.

Because excessive coagulation of the recipient site is avoided, it is often helpful to delay skin grafting for 10–14 days to allow spontaneous separation of burn eschar and allow tissue to granulate. The recipient site is protected from desiccation by daily cleansing with soap and water and antibiotic or petrolatum ointment to prevent drying. The skin graft is then applied as a delayed primary graft, avoiding exposure of the underlying cartilage during preparatory debridement.

A pattern is made of the defect. The margins and base of the wound are freshened to create a clean, sharp, right angle skin edge and a vascular bed, removing old scar or granulation tissue.

The graft is elevated with subcutaneous fat which is removed from its undersurface with curved scissors, but the graft is not necessarily thinned to dermis. The thickness of skin graft and its underlying fat matches the depth of recipient site. The graft is laid on the prepared bed, trimmed, and inset with a single layer of fine sutures, peripherally after placing quilting sutures through the skin graft and into the recipient bed to prevent lateral motion. A layer of antibiotic ointment and fine gauze is applied, followed by a soft foam bolus.

Traditionally, individual bolus tie-over sutures are fixed to the wound edge and tied to each other over the bolus. However, it is more efficient to tie a single 4-0 or 5-0 polypropylene suture about 5–10 mm from the wound edge and then crisscross back and forth across the bolus in a running fashion until tying the suture to itself. The surgeon later clips the suture in one or two areas to easily remove the dressing. The stent dressing immobilizes the skin graft postoperatively and reinforces the quilting sutures. However, it is not a "pressure" dressing and should not be applied to prevent hematoma.

Initially, the skin graft appears white. Over several days, perfusion increases and the graft changes color from blue to visibly pink. Although the bolus can be removed earlier, it is best left in place for 1 week. If the defect is repaired delicately with fine sutures and without tension, suture marks do not occur.

Local flaps

Unlike a skin graft, the quality of the skin transferred as a vascularized flap maintains its original color and texture quality. A skin flap is also thicker than a graft and may better supply missing subcutaneous bulk.

There is no excess within the "thick" skin zone of the tip and ala. But excess skin is present within the more mobile upper "thin" skin zones of the dorsum and sidewall.

Local flaps do not add new skin to the nasal surface. They share the available, but limited, excess within the upper nose.

Guidelines, applicable to nearly all local nasal flaps, should be followed carefully:

- If the defect is larger than 1.5 cm, the remaining skin surface is insufficient to redistribute over the nasal skeleton without excess closure attention and distortion of mobile landmarks.
- Local flaps are used for small superficial defects, greater than 5–10 mm from the nostril margins and above the tip defining points. Commonly described local flaps will not reach into the infratip area.

Unfortunately, hoping to avoid the morbidity or stages required by regional flaps, these rules are often broken, leading to nasal collapse and tip and alar margin malpositions. In such instances, it would be better to allow the wound to heal secondarily or apply a skin graft.

The single lobe transposition flap (Fig. 6.4)

A modest amount of excess mobile and lax skin is available within the superior nose. A single lobe transposition flap, designed as a Banner or Romberg flap, is useful for small defects.[32,33] These flaps transpose skin through an arc of 90°, taking excess from one axis to fill a deficiency in another. Because the skin is relatively mobile, available, and lies at a distance from the nostril margins, these small local flaps are unlikely to distort the tip or alar margin. However, if the flap donor scar crosses the bridge transversely, a depressed scar may become visible on profile view. Single lobed flaps are not useful in the inflexible thick skin of the tip or alar, which shifts poorly. Deforming dog-ears or displacement of adjacent mobile landmarks is common.

The dorsal nasal flap

The dorsal nasal flap elevates skin, subcutaneous tissue, and muscle just above the perichondrium and periosteum and slides excess from the glabella towards the tip. The flap is best applied to defects within the dorsum and superior tip subunit.[34–36] It is vascularized from facial and angular vessels along the sidewall and medial canthus. Closure is facilitated by advancing cheek skin upward onto the nasal sidewall. The dorsal nasal flap can resurface the nasal tip and dorsum and parts of the ala or sidewall with local skin. Unfortunately, it slides thicker glabellar skin and soft tissue downward onto the nasal sidewall near the medial canthus where a mismatch in skin thickness may create an iatrogenic epicanthal fold. The depth of the radix may be obliterated, effacing the nasal root. Recent modifications have eliminated the glabellar extension.

As the dorsal flap slides caudally, a dog-ear is excised inferiorly. Ideally, its borders are planned to lie along the dorsal sidewall junction. The inferior aspect of the flap's border may be visible as a depressed scar crossing the smooth surface of the tip unit. Like all local flaps, the larger the defect and the closer it lies to the nostril margin, the more likely the tip or rim will be distorted by tension or displaced by poor design.

The geometric bilobed flap

The bilobed flap is recommended for defects within the thick, stiff skin of the inferior nose.

The bilobed principle is applied.[37–39] Skin is shifted from an area of excess to an area of deficiency by designing the first lobe adjacent to the tip or alar defect. A second lobe, which lies at a distance in an area of tissue availability within the upper nose, is outlined in continuity. As the primary lobe shifts to repair the defect, the secondary lobe resurfaces the defect from the primary lobe. The tertiary defect from the second lobe is closed primarily, within the area of excess.

Traditionally, bilobed flaps were designed with a 180° rotation. This created large dog-ears. The dog-ear excision subsequently narrowed the flap's vascular base, jeopardizing blood supply. Macgregor, and later Zitelli, developed a geometric design to decrease the flap's rotation to 90–100° and incorporated a dog-ear excision which did not diminish blood supply. It is useful for defects measuring 0.5–1.5 cm in the inferior nose.

The rotation-advancement flap can be oriented anywhere around the defect but the pedicle base must be positioned away from the nostril margin to prevent distortion. The second lobe must also lie within the loose excess skin of the upper sidewall or dorsum. It can be based medially or laterally. The pattern should not extend onto the cheek or lower lid.

Several rules apply:

1.   The pivot point is established at a distance from the defect equal to one half of the defect's diameter. The flap is based laterally for tip defects and medially for defects of the alar lobule. The farther the pivot point is away from the defect, the larger the flap. Sharing the same pivot point, the circumferences of a larger outer and a smaller inner concentric circle are drawn onto the nasal skin. The circumference of the outer circle is outlined at a distance three times the radius of the defect. The second smaller inner circle is marked to equal the distance from the pivot point to the center of the initial defect (the diameter of the defect). Because the nasal surface is round, not flat, a strip of foil or bent paper ruler, rather than a straight ruler, is used as a template which is rotated around the pivot point, until the circumference of both concentric circles are determined.

2.   An exact pattern of the circular nasal defect is positioned immediately adjacent to the defect, along the outer concentric circle. The first lobe should replace the defect exactly, to prevent tip or alar rim distortion on closure. Because the second lobe lies within the more mobile skin of the upper nose, it can be designed slightly smaller than the defect. The secondary defect can be partially closed by recruitment of lax adjacent skin within the upper nose. A dog-ear excision, which

extends lateral to the outer circle, is added to the second lobe.

A dog-ear excision is marked from the defect to the pivot point, creating space for the flap to rotate and advance. The flap rotates less than 100° with a wide base to maintain flap blood supply.

3. The dog-ear extending from the defect of the pivot point is excised. The first and second lobes, including the

distal dog-ear, are elevated above the periosteum. The flap includes skin, subcutaneous fat, and nasalis muscle. Residual normal nasal skin is undermined widely over the perichondrium and periosteum.

4. Significant pin cushioning is infrequent with the bilobed flap, if it is carefully repaired, in layers. The tertiary defect, in the more mobile upper nose, is first closed in layers. This pushes the flap inferiorly, preventing the

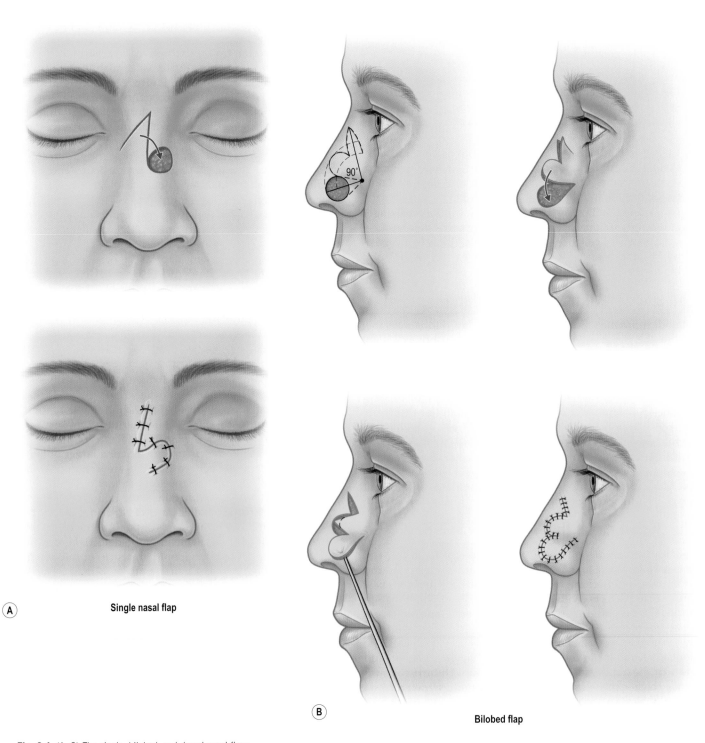

Fig. 6.4 (A–C) The single, bilobed, and dorsal nasal flaps.

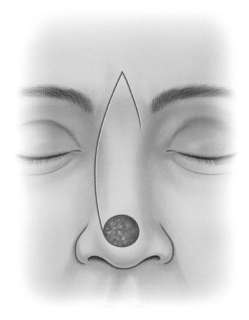

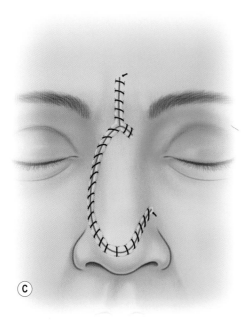

Fig. 6.4, cont'd

tendency of the flap to return to its donor site. The primary lobe, after appropriate "thinning" so that its skin surface will match the level of the adjacent normal skin, is transferred to the primary defect. The secondary lobe is transposed to fill the gap created by the first and its distal dog-ear is excised to fit the secondary defect.

Unfortunately, postoperative tip or nostril distortion is common, especially when the defect lies within the tip or ala.

Although planned as a single-staged repair, it is not uncommon to revise scars, recreate the obliterated alar crease, or reposition the nostril margin.

The geometric bilobed flap is effective, but it should be limited to defects of the tip, which are less than or equal to 1.5 cm in diameter and that lie more than 1 cm away from the nostril margin. This precludes its use for significant alar defects. Despite the relatively small size of these defects, the technique is time-consuming, the dissection extensive, scars multiple, swelling significant, and distortions common.

The one stage nasolabial flap (Fig. 6.5 ⊚)

The one-stage nasolabial flap can resurface defects of the nasal sidewall and ala, up to 2 cm in size.[25] Excess skin of the medial cheek, lateral to the nasolabial fold, is transferred as a random pattern extension of an advancing cheek flap. Unlike local flaps which redistribute residual nasal skin, this technique "adds" regional cheek skin to the nasal surface. This minimizes risk of landmark distortion and permits the use of alar support grafts without fear of collapse due to excessive tension.

Fig. 6.5 appears online only.

1. The sidewall and alar subunits are outlined in ink. Alar subunit excision is not performed but skin, which remains between the defect in the inferior nostril rim, can be excised, enlarging the defect inferiorly to the nostril margin. This positions the scar along the nostril border and improves the flap's blending with the recipient site. The underlying lining is braced with a septal or ear cartilage graft to prevent collapse or retraction of the nostril margin. The ends of the cartilage graft are buried, medially and laterally, in subcutaneous pockets along the rim and fixed with percutaneous 5-0 polypropylene sutures. The cartilage graft is quilted to the underlying lining to fix the support graft and brace the nostril margin.

2. The nasolabial crease is marked and a pattern of the defect is positioned exactly adjacent to the nasolabial fold so that the late cheek scar lies exactly in the nasolabial crease. A dog-ear excision is marked inferiorly, distal to the template. Ensure that the sliding cheek advancement has adequate length to swing and correctly position the nasolabial extension onto the nasal defect. The most important flap dimension is width, which should equal the width of the defect. The distal margin of the flap will be trimmed during wound closure and does not need to be predetermined. The flap is elevated in continuity with the distal dog-ear. The superior lateral incision for the alar or sidewall flap extension should not extend higher than the alar remnant that must be "jumped over" to reach the recipient site. A higher incision is unnecessary and may impair blood supply.

3. The nasolabial skin extension and the cheek flap are undermined, with a few millimeters of subcutaneous fat for 3–5 cm. The cheek is advanced, fixing its underlying raw surface to the deep tissues along the nasal facial groove. This suture fixation advances the cheek flap, closes the donor defect, and restores the nasofacial sulcus. It eliminates lateral and vertical tension on the

nasolabial extension, which travels with a cheek flap to resurface the primary defect. The vascularity of the random extension is good, but can be impaired by tension.

4. Excess subcutaneous fat is excised to match the thickness of the flap to the depth of the recipient bed. Absorbable sutures can be placed to gently fix the deep surface of the flap to the underlying soft tissues at the ideal alar crease if vascularity is maintained. If necessary, the crease can be re-created secondarily. The distal flap is gently laid over the inferior aspect of the nasal wound and trimmed to fit. The incisions are closed in layers.

Final scars blend within the sidewall or lie in the nasolabial fold. Pin cushioning of this non-subunit skin replacement can occur, but is minimized if the ala is supported and braced by primary cartilage grafts to control nostril margin shape and position.

The one stage nasolabial flap is useful for defects of the sidewall and ala, which are not effectively repaired with other local flaps.

It can also be used to resurface the upper lip and nasal sill in a composite defect of the nose, lip, and cheek.[40–42] Often combined with the Millard fat flip flap,[15,16] which hinges over excess subcutaneous fat, from the lateral cheek, to restore missing premaxillary soft tissue bulk.

Large, deep, and adversely located defects

The superiorly based two-stage subunit nasolabial flap (Figs. 6.6, 6.7, 6.8 ⊕)

The two-stage nasolabial flap[22,43] transfers excess skin from the medial cheek, just lateral to the nasolabial fold, supplied by blood vessels which originate from the underlying facial and angular arteries, passing through the underlying subcutaneous tissue, above and below the levator labii muscle. Although the narrow skin pedicle contributes a modest random blood supply, the flap is a subcutaneously based island flap. If the underlying subcutaneous vascular base is intact, the flap is reliable even if skin lateral to the ala is scarred or has been excised. The subcutaneous pedicle permits easy transposition and the narrow skin component eliminates the superior dog-ear and its scar from extending onto the nasal sidewall on wound closure. The flap is designed with its medial border exactly along the nasolabial fold to place the final scar exactly in the nasolabial crease. In young patients or those with a poorly defined fold, the nasolabial crease may be indistinct and should be marked with ink preoperatively, before sedation or general anesthesia.

Figs. 6.7 and 6.8 appear online only.

A two-stage nasolabial flap is best employed to resurface the convex ala as a subunit. Residual skin within the alar subunit is excised so that the entire subunit is resurfaced, rather than just patched.

Stage I

The nasal subunits and nasolabial fold are marked with ink. An exact template is designed, based on the contralateral ala. The template is positioned adjacent to the nasolabial crease at the level of the oral commissure to ensure an adequate arc of rotation. The superior pedicle is tapered to a point lying just at the upper end of the nasolabial crease. A triangular dog-ear excision is designed distally along the nasolabial fold.

Residual skin within the alar subunit is discarded. The contralateral alar template is used to design a cartilage support graft – most often of conchal cartilage – with the correct dimension and nostril margin outline. The graft's medial and lateral ends are buried in subcutaneous pockets with percutaneous sutures within the soft triangle and the alar base. The graft is sutured to the underlying lining.

The skin flap is elevated from distal to proximal with 2–3 mm of fat.

The dissection is deepened superiorly, protecting the flap's base which is dissected in the subcutaneous fat more broadly than the proximal skin pedicle. Restricting subcutaneous fibrous bands are released. Undermining continues until the flap can be comfortably transferred to the defect. The cheek is advanced and the donor site closed in layers, after excision of the distal dog-ear. The flap is inset with a single layer of skin sutures. The exposed raw pedicle is covered with antibiotic ointment.

Stage 2

Three weeks later, the pedicle is divided. Skin is re-elevated with 2–3 mm of fat over the lateral aspect of the alar inset. Underlying subcutaneous fat and scar are excised, sculpting a convex alar contour and a defined alar crease. The flap is re-approximated to the recipient site. The superior aspect of nasolabial cheek scar is re-opened, excess skin and soft tissue is excised, and the cheek is closed.

Practically speaking, the nasolabial flap has a limited role in nasal reconstruction. Because of the limited excess available in the medial cheek, there is only enough nasolabial tissue to resurface a defect of about 2 cm in width. Although a reliable flap, excessive undermining or tension may lead to necrosis. It will not reliably revascularize a skin graft for lining or maintain its blood supply if folded for cover and lining. Its arc of rotation and reach are limited. It can be transposed to the ala, columella, or to resurface the upper lip but it will not safely reach the tip or dorsum. Although a nasolabial flap scar may be hidden in the nasolabial fold, the cheek becomes flattened and may necessitate a contralateral excision of medial cheek tissue to improve symmetry with the opposite cheek. A nasolabial flap routinely transfers beard in the male.

The two-stage nasolabial flap is best employed to resurface the entire ala, as a subunit, or an alar defect which extends a few millimeters above the alar crease onto the nasal sidewall. Although the alar crease will be obliterated if the defect extends into the sidewall, a secondary operation can be performed to restore the alar crease. It can also resurface the columella or a non-nasal defect of the lip or the platform for the nasal base.

The forehead flap

The forehead with its superior color, texture, size, reach, vascularity, lining applications, and forgiving donor site make it the first choice for most nasal repairs. It is multi-laminar, composed of skin, subcutaneous fat, frontalis muscle, and a thin underlying areolar layer which separates it from frontal periosteum. Although forehead *skin* matches the nose in color, texture, and thickness, a forehead *flap* is thicker than nasal

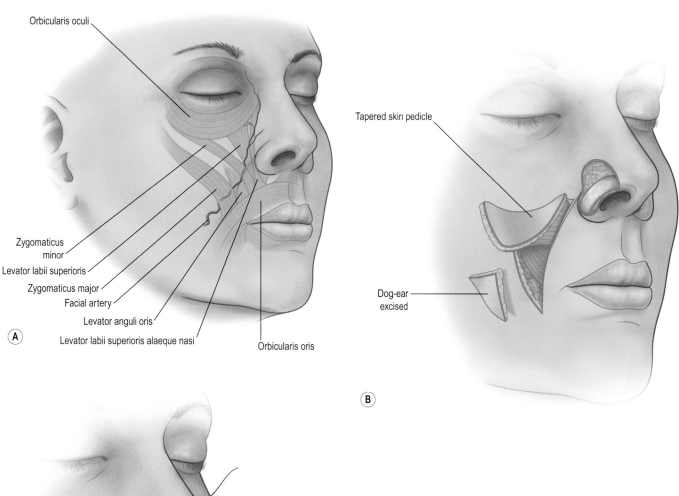

Orbicularis oculi

Zygomaticus minor

Levator labii superioris

Zygomaticus major

Facial artery

Levator anguli oris

Levator labii superioris alaeque nasi

Orbicularis oris

A

Tapered skin pedicle

Dog-ear excised

B

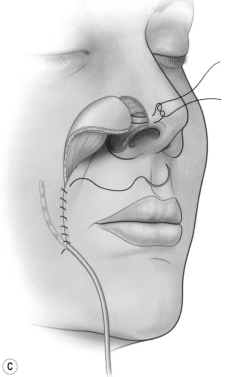

C

Fig. 6.6 (A–D) A two-stage nasolabial flap is employed to resurface the ala as a subunit. Residual normal skin is excised adjacent to the defect and the entire subunit is resurfaced as a subunit at the first stage. The superiorly based two-stage nasolabial flap is perfused by axial vessels which pass through the underlying facial musculature to vascularize the proximal flap base. Primary cartilage must be placed to support and brace the nostril margin. One month later, the proximal pedicle was divided, the alar inset completed after soft tissue sculpturing, and the cheek donor site closed to position the donor scar exactly in the nasal labial fold.
Continued

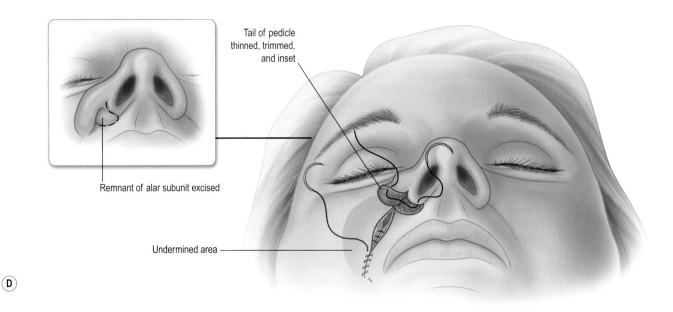

Tail of pedicle
thinned, trimmed,
and inset

Remnant of alar subunit excised

Undermined area

(D)

Fig. 6.6, cont'd

skin. Excess frontalis and subcutaneous fat must be removed to thin the flap to blend into the adjacent facial skin.

The forehead is perfused from the supraorbital, supratrochlear, the superficial temporal and posterior auricular arteries. Flaps can be based on each of these pedicles – the median forehead flap, the horizontal forehead flap, the up and down flap, or the scalping flap.

Today, the paramedian forehead flap is most often used. It transfers central forehead tissue on a unilateral vertical axial blood supply, based on the supratrochlear vessels. Its point of rotation is centered inferiorly towards the medial canthus. The anatomic studies of McCarthy[13] and Reece[14] demonstrate that the paramedian forehead is perfused by an anastomotic arcade from the supratrochlear, supraorbital, infraorbital, dorsal nasal, and angular branches of the facial artery.

The paramedian flap is the first choice for nasal resurfacing because of its vascularity, size, reach, reliability, and relatively minimal morbidity.[22,25,45,46] It takes skin from high on the forehead, under the hairline, with a narrow inferior pedicle base, within or inferior to the medial eyebrow. The inferior aspect of the donor site can be closed primarily. If a gap remains superiorly, it is allowed to heal secondarily. Wound contraction and re-epithelialization close any superior residual defect. Eyebrow distortion does not occur because the gap is away from the mobile brow. Medialization of the eyebrow is not significant because the proximal pedicle is narrow.

A paramedian forehead flap can resurface any nasal defect without significant donor deformity. Its pedicle is based on either the right or left supratrochlear vessels. A central nasal defect can be resurfaced on either pedicle, but a unilateral nasal defect is resurfaced with the ipsilateral pedicle to decrease the distance between its pivot point and the defect, unless precluded by an old scar within its territory. If the hairline is extremely low or the forehead scarred, pre-expansion is employed, but is not routine.[47–50]

The two-stage forehead flap (Figs. 6.9 & 6.10 ⊛)

Anatomically, the supratrochlear vessels pass over the orbital rim, external to the periosteum, sandwiched between the corrugator and frontalis muscles. The vessels then travel vertically upward into the frontalis muscle. At the mid forehead level, they pass through the muscle and lie in a superficial, subdermal position at the hairline.

Figs. 6.9 and 6.10 appear online only.

The flap can be transferred as an island flap[44] in one stage, but excessive bulk of the pedicle, passing under tight glabellar skin, may jeopardize its blood supply or distort the nasal root. Most importantly, the aesthetic nasal result can rarely be obtained in a single stage.

Traditionally, a forehead flap is transferred in two stages.[22] At the first stage, the flap is elevated over the periosteum. Frontalis muscle and subcutaneous fat are excised over the distal 1–2 cm. The distally thinned flap is transferred to the recipient site, perfused proximally through its thick proximal pedicle. During the second stage, 3 or 4 weeks later, when the distal flap has become vascularized by the recipient site, the pedicle is divided. The superior aspect is re-elevated, debulked, and the skin inset is completed.

Unfortunately, excision of muscle and subcutaneous fat, at the time of the initial transfer, removes its myocutaneous blood supply and may diminish vascularity. Although relatively safe, flap necrosis may occur in smokers, if the flap is under tension, or in patients undergoing major nasal repairs which require large flaps and wide initial soft tissue thinning or flaps with multiple narrow extensions for the ala or columella. Most importantly, although tip and alar cartilage support may be placed at the first stage, the skin of the distal nose – the tip and ala – is not re-elevated during pedicle division. Any imperfection in the most aesthetic part of the nose cannot be altered prior to pedicle division.

Although the two-stage forehead flap is routinely applied to heminasal and total nasal defects, aggressive operative debulking is required during both surgical stages. This puts the flap in some jeopardy, leading to occasional flap necrosis, especially in smokers. The two-stage forehead flap may be best limited to small defects of the tip, dorsum, or ala that do not require delicate contour recreation, complex support grafts or lining. It is especially difficult to re-establish the subtle 3D contours of multiple subunits when the defect is large or deep, requiring complex support and lining replacement.

Technique of the two-stage forehead flap (Figs. 6.9 & 6.10 ⊕)

Stage I: flap transfer

The nasal subunits are marked with ink and residual normal skin is excised within the convex tip subunit or ala (the Subunit Principle) but not within the flat dorsum or sidewall. Primary cartilage grafts are positioned, as necessary, over vascularized lining. An exact pattern of the defect, based on the contralateral normal, is outlined under the hairline, directly over the supratrochlear artery, which lies just laterally to the frown crease. It can be identified by Doppler. The proximal pedicle is drawn inferiorly, in continuity with the defect, through the medial brow. Pedicle width at the brow is about 1.2–1.5 cm. The reach of the flap is verified using a simple gauze measure, checking the distance from the pivot point below the eyebrow to the distal end of the flap on the forehead and most inferior aspect of the defect. The flap can be lengthened by extending the design into the hairline or, more often, the pedicle is extended inferiorly across the eyebrow towards the medial canthus.

Figs. 6.9 and 6.10 appear online only.

Frontalis muscle and excess subcutaneous fat are excised within its distal 1.5–2 cm. The skin flap with 2–3 mm of fat distally will be applied to the inferior aspect of the nasal defect. The dissection then passes under the frontalis and over the periosteum, through the medial brow until the flap reaches the defect without tension. It is sutured to the recipient site, from distal to proximal, with a single layer of fine suture. If the flap blanches, stop suturing and let the unsutured lateral flap edges heal secondarily to the recipient site. To avoid excessive oozing and crusting, the raw surface of the pedicle can be skin grafted. The forehead is widely undermined into both temples and closed in layers. The scalp dog-ear is excised superiorly. Any gap, which remains under the hairline, is dressed with petrolatum gauze for one week and allowed to heal secondarily. The scar can be revised later, if needed.

Stage II

Three to 4 weeks later, the pedicle is divided, the proximal aspect of the flap is re-elevated with 2–3 mm of fat, and the underlying excess soft tissue (fat, frontalis, and scar), which is adherent to recipient site, is excised, contouring the superior aspect of the defect. The flap remains well vascularized through its distal inset. The superior inset is completed. The proximal pedicle is untubed and returned to the medial brow as a small inverted "V", discarding any excess (Box 6.2).

The three stage full-thickness forehead flap (Fig. 6.11)

Millard, in the 1970s,[29] and Burget,[26] in the 1990s, added an intermediate operation between transfer and division of the

traditional two-stage forehead flap to improve vascular safety and permit more aggressive soft tissue contouring They thinned the flap distally at transfer but, 3 weeks later, elevated it from its bed over the mid-nose. The proximal pedicle remained intact while the distal inset was left attached over the tip, alar margins, and columella. Underlying fat and muscle over the dorsum and midvault were excised to improve midvault contour.

Although helpful, visualization of the middorsal excision was obstructed by the proximal pedicle and distal inset. Most importantly, once the flap was applied to the ala and tip at the first stage, further soft tissue sculpting or cartilage modification of the distal nose could not be performed.

Menick,[25,71] in the late 1990s, modified the approach by transferring a *full-thickness flap in three stages.* The forehead is multi-laminar and consists of skin, subcutaneous fat, and frontalis muscle. It is perfused with a myofascial, axial, and random blood supply. Initial distal thinning removes the myocutaneous component and creates a wounded soft dermal surface, more prone to contraction and less able to tolerate tension. However, if the flap is transferred with all its layers, maximal vascularity is maintained and the expected induration of wound healing does not occur, even months after transfer, as long as its subcutaneous plane is not injured or the frontalis excised. One month after transfer, the full-thickness flap's blood supply is augmented by surgical delay (its initial peripheral incision, elevation, and transfer). Forehead skin, with 2–3 mm of subcutaneous fat, can be completely elevated off the entire nasal inset, maintaining the proximal pedicle. The underlying excess of subcutaneous forehead fat and frontalis, previously positioned cartilage grafts and lining are rigidly healed together. With complete visualization, the soft tissues are excised and cartilage grafts sculpted, repositioned, or augmented to refine 3D contour. The thin supple forehead skin is then replaced to resurface the nose. Pedicle division is performed one month later.

Although this three-stage approach with a full-thickness flap adds an additional operation prior to pedicle division, it ensures a maximum blood supply at each stage, a thin uniform covering skin flap, unimpeded surgical exposure, controlled soft tissue shaping, and cartilage grafting over the entire nasal surface prior to pedicle division. The surgeon can make intraoperative modifications during each stage and can perform a "revision" before the pedicle is divided. The aesthetic results are improved and the need for late formal revision minimized.

The three-stage full-thickness forehead flap technique, with an intermediate operation, is applied to resurface partial-thickness or full-thickness nasal defects, regardless of defect size or depth. It is especially useful in smokers, when a scar

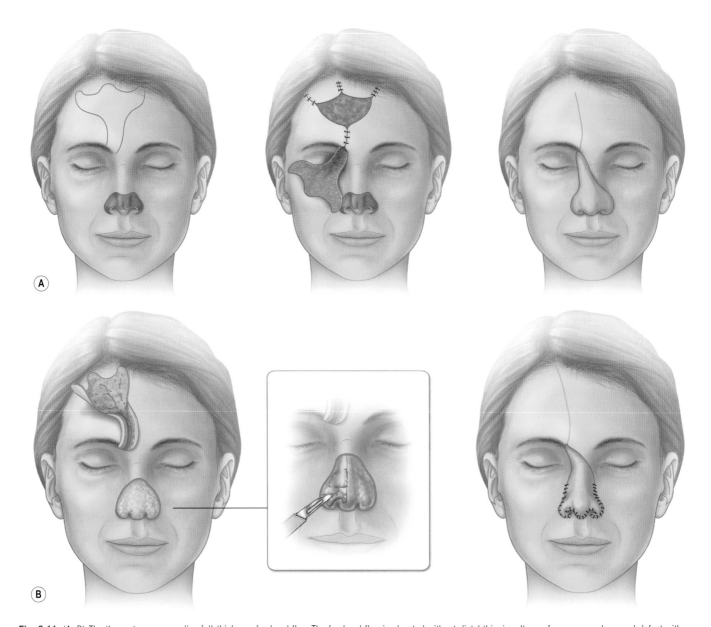

Fig. 6.11 (A–B) The three-stage paramedian full-thickness forehead flap. The forehead flap is elevated without distal thinning. It resurfaces a complex nasal defect with skin, subcutaneous tissue, and frontalis muscle. During the intermediate operation, one month later, the flap is re-elevated completely from the recipient site with 2–3 mm of subcutaneous fat. The excess underlying subcutaneous fat and frontalis muscle is excised to establish the correct 3D contour. Cartilage grafts can be modified by sculpture, repositioning, or augmentation. The skin flap was then returned to the donor site. One month later (2 months after pedicle transfer), the pedicle is divided.

lies within the territory of the flap, or in large nasal defects that require wide thinning of the covering flap, especially with alar and columellar extensions. However, the two-stage flap remains useful for small and superficial defects, such as an isolated alar or tip repair.

Technique of a three-stage full-thickness forehead flap (Figs. 6.12–6.18)

Stage I

The regional units, old scars, and the location of planned vascular pedicles are marked with ink. Residual normal tissue within subunits is excised, when appropriate. An exact template of the nasal surface defect is positioned at the frontal hairline over the supratrochlear pedicle. The more proximal

pedicle, with a 1.2–1.5 cm base, is marked inferiorly through the medial brow. Primary cartilage grafts are placed if vascularized intranasal lining is present or has been restored with intranasal flaps, hingeover flaps, a second flap, or a free flap. If the folded forehead flap or skin graft lining techniques are planned to line a full-thickness defect, primary cartilage grafts are precluded during the first stage but can be positioned in a delayed primary fashion during intermediate operation.

The flap is elevated, with all its layers, above the periosteum. The pedicle is incised through the medial eyebrow towards the medial canthus until the distal flap reaches the defect without tension. Routinely, no frontalis or subcutaneous fat is excised. Frontalis can be trimmed along the nostril margin or distal ala to ease inset if the flap is unusually stiff. The flap is sutured to the recipient site in one layer. The

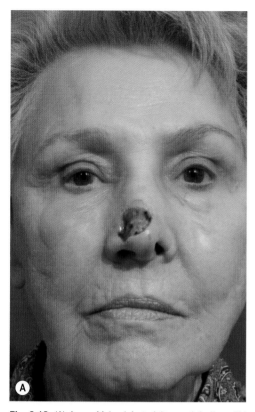

Fig. 6.12 (A) A new Mohs defect of the nasal tip lies within a nose previously reconstructed with skin grafts and a left composite flap for cover and lining. The left rim is retracted.

elevated with 2–3 mm of subcutaneous fat (nasal thinness) over the entire nasal inset. Axial subcutaneous vessels, lying in the subdermal superficial fat, are left adherent to the skin flap and are avoided. The flap is completely re-elevated and placed to the side of the face, maintaining the supratrochlear pedicle.

The underlying excess of subcutaneous fat and frontalis muscle, which remains adherent to the underlying support framework and lining, is now healed together and is a living, rigid structure that bleeds readily. With complete exposure, the entire exposed nasal subsurface is sculpted into a 3D shape, highlighting the dorsal lines, alar crease, and tip contours. Previously placed primary cartilage grafts can be remodeled by sculpting, repositioning, or augmentation. Delayed primary cartilage grafts are placed over lining restored by the folded flap or skin graft techniques. The forehead skin flap is replaced on the recipient bed and fixed with quilting sutures to close the dead space and better conform to the underlying contour.

Although the forehead flap is routinely elevated over the entire inset, it can be left adherent to the columella and nostril margin to maintain a bipedicle blood supply, temporarily hanging from both the brow and the distal inset. This is useful in a heavy smoker, when an old scar lies within the flap's territory; when the flap contains unusually complex extensions; if the defect extends from the columella to high on the radix requiring debulking over an extremely large surface area; or if there is any concern for vascularity at initial transfer. This is rarely necessary. On very rare occasions, it may be helpful to perform two intermediate operations. The flap is re-elevated distally, maintaining the proximal inset into the nasal bridge, to supplement vascularity while the tip and columella are sculpted or delayed primary cartilage grafts placed. In a second intermediate operation, the flap is re-elevated over the mid-bridge and the nasal root, as a bipedicle, while maintaining the columella and rim inset. This approach is useful if there is significant scarring within the proximal flap and the surgeon has a concern for vascularity. The number of stages is unimportant if the final result is good and complications are avoided.

forehead donor site is closed after wide undermining. A superior gap, which cannot be approximated, is allowed to heal secondarily.

Stage II: The intermediate operation

Four weeks later, the forehead flap, now healed to the recipient bed, is physiologically delayed. The forehead skin is

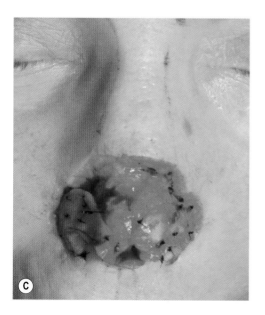

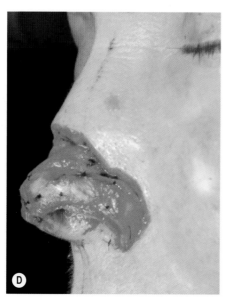

Fig. 6.13 (CD) The subunits of the nose are marked. A subunit excision of the tip and both ala, but not of the dorsum is performed. Skin of the old composite skin graft is hinged over for a left nasal rim lining. Primary cartilage grafts of ear cartilage are placed to support, brace, and shape the lining and future cover.

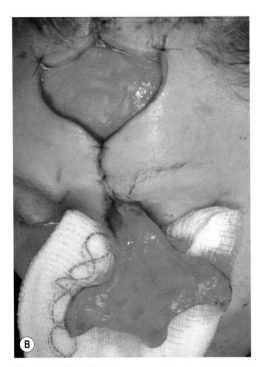

Fig. 6.14 (B) A full-thickness paramedian forehead flap is elevated under the frontalis. The forehead flap contains skin, subcutaneous fat, and all its frontalis layers. It is transferred to resurface the nose without thinning.

Stage III: Pedicle division

Four weeks later (8 weeks after initial flap transfer), the pedicle is divided, the nasal inset completed, and the proximal pedicle returned to the brow as in the two-stage technique (Figs. 6.19–6.22, Box 6.3).

Handling the forehead donor site

Foreheads vary in height and width, laxity, the presence of scars, prior injury, or past forehead flap harvest.

Primary closure of the forehead

The forehead is a forgiving donor site – expansive, highly vascular, self-healing, and lending itself to secondary revision. Preliminary surgical delay or expansion is usually unnecessary.

The paramedian forehead flap, based on the supratrochlear vessels, harvests skin under the hairline. Its narrow 1.2–1.5-cm pedicle width allows primary closure of the inferior forehead, leaving a single line scar above the brow. The eyebrow is not distorted or medialized on return of the proximal pedicle base to the eyebrow. The forehead is closed under moderate tension using several key tacking sutures and a layered closure. The superior dog-ear is excised. If a gap remains superiorly, it is allowed to heal secondarily. A petrolatum bandage is applied to the raw periosteum and fixed temporarily with suture for one week. The open area heals by epithelialization and secondary contraction. The adjacent normal forehead stretches by autoexpansion. Frequently, at the time of pedicle division or during a revision, the area of secondary healing can be excised and the adjacent forehead re-advanced. Occasionally, if the defect extends high onto the radix or extends laterally towards each medial canthus, the inferior forehead donor cannot be closed at the time of initial flap transfer. It is left open or temporarily skin grafted. At pedicle division, the unused proximal pedicle is returned to the donor site, restoring the medial brow and resurfacing the inferior forehead defect. Any defect above it heals secondarily.

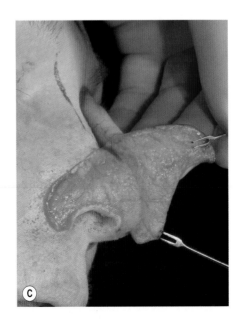

Fig. 6.15 (AC) One month later, forehead skin with 2–3 mm of subcutaneous fat is elevated completely to expose the entire reconstruction. The flap is temporarily placed on the forehead.

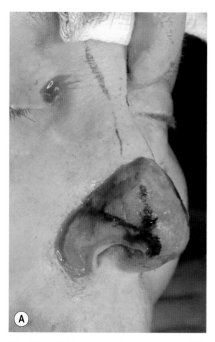

Fig. 6.16 (A) Remaining subcutaneous fat and frontalis are now excised to sculpt a nasal shape. Previous primary cartilage grafts are healed to the underlying lining and can be modified. The uniformly thin forehead flap is returned to the recipient site. It is fixed in place with peripheral sutures and temporarily molded to the contoured surface with percutaneous quilting sutures.

Scars within the forehead territory

If a scar lies within the proposed flap territory, determine its site, direction, depth, and length.

A transverse scar puts the flap at greater risk. Old operative reports may clarify whether the injury extended only superficially, injuring only the random cutaneous blood supply, deeper through the frontalis, or directly to the vascular pedicle. Doppler examination of the supratrochlear vessels may confirm the presence of the supratrochlear artery.

If a scar within the flap's territory is short, vertical, superficial, or the supratrochlear vessels are verified by Doppler, it can be disregarded. Or the surgeon may avoid a scarred area completely by transferring skin from the opposite side of the forehead on the contralateral pedicle. The flap can be surgically delayed to augment its blood supply. The flap can be elevated as a full-thickness flap to maintain all vascular sources. An area of adjacent unscarred skin may be available for expansion, avoiding old scars. In rare instances, when both supratrochlear vessels have been ablated and the inferior forehead is severely scarred, uninjured forehead skin may be transferred on secondary vascular pedicles – a scalping or sickle flap.

Surgical delay of a forehead flap

Surgical delay of a forehead flap should be considered when:

- a significant old scar lies within the proposed flap territory
- the pedicle's named blood supply has been injured
- unusually complex extensions of flap design are required (very uncommon)
- the patient is an end-stage smoker or has a history of high-voltage radiation
- a non-paramedian flap extends across one vascular territory into the territory of another flap (e.g., sickle flap). (Supratrochlear vessels reliably perfuse the forehead and scalp, allowing a paramedian flap to be designed in any size or length without delay)
- the flap's vascularity is in doubt and a preliminary operation is required for other reasons (prefabrication of lining, delay of hingeover flaps).

However, unless needed, delay should be avoided. It adds additional stages, cost, and prolongs the overall reconstruction. It can be difficult to precisely determine the requirements of the defect until the definitive repair. Once incised for delay, the dimension and outline of a delayed flap cannot be altered.

Technique of surgical delay

A template is positioned under the hairline and the proposed flap's outline is incised to periosteum. Two to 4 mm of skin can be left temporarily intact at the columellar and alar tips to ensure vascularity. These skin bridges may be divided subsequently. Because all significant contributions to forehead blood supply arise from peripheral axial vessels, elevation is unnecessary and decreases flap pliability due to scarring of the flap's deep surface. Within 3–4 weeks, vessels at the flap's base enlarge and overall vascularity increases.

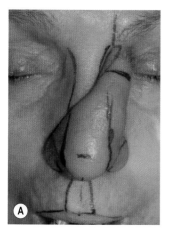
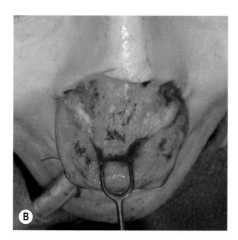
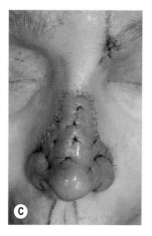

Fig. 6.17 (A–C) One month later (2 months after forehead flap transfer), the pedicle is divided and the distal flap elevated thinly to allow further subcutaneous sculpture of the dorsum, sidewall, and ala.

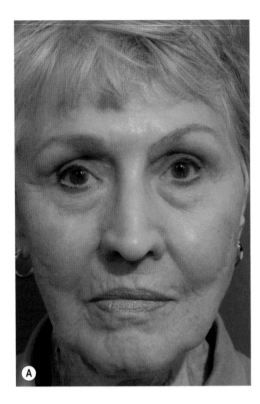

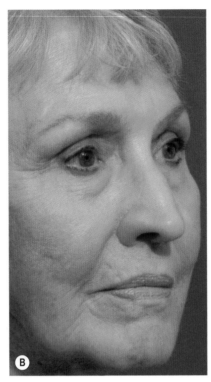

Fig. 6.18 (AB) Postoperative result without revision. The forehead defect healed secondarily.

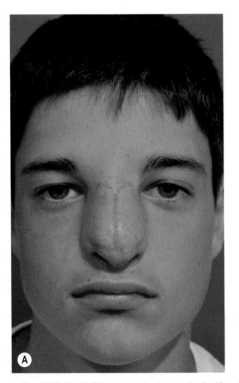

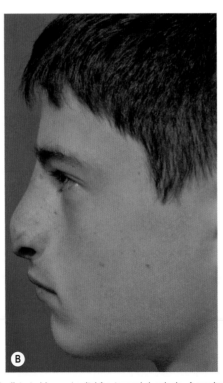

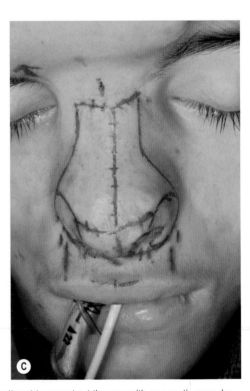

Fig. 6.19 (A–C) This teenage boy's nose is significantly distorted by congenital frontonasal dysplasia. A previous attempt to reconstruct the nose with an osmotic expander and local flaps failed. The nose is bulky and shapeless with inadequate tip support and over projecting radix. His forehead is short.

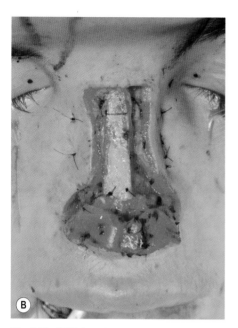

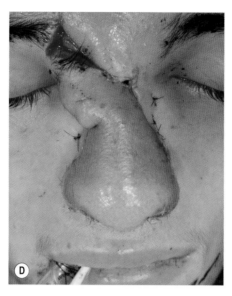

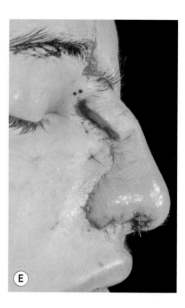

Fig. 6.20 (BDE) A preliminary operation was performed to place a forehead expander and perform an open rhinoplasty to lower the radix, narrow the nasal bones, harvest septal cartilage for a future procedure and advance the old scars onto the nasal subunit. Two months later, the nasal tip and ala were excised as a subunit and all scars excised over the dorsum and sidewall. Lateral skin was advanced almost to the dorsal line to modify the defect. A columellar strut with advancement of the residual medial crura and ear cartilage alar battens supported the tip. A septal cartilage graft shaped the dorsum. A full-thickness forehead flap was transferred to resurface the defect. The position and symmetry of the alar rims seems correct intraoperatively.

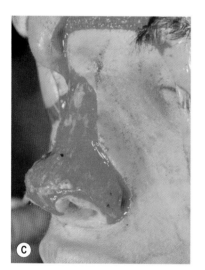

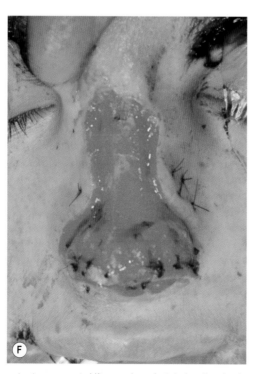

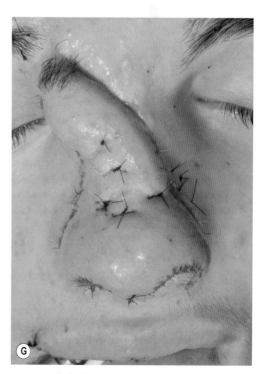

Fig. 6.21 (CFG) One month later, due to scar contracture, support shift, or an imperfect design, the alar rims were asymmetric. During the planned intermediate operation, the forehead skin was elevated with 2–3 mm of subcutaneous fat. The excess underlying subcutaneous fat and frontalis were excised to sculpt an ideal nasal shape. Lining along each rim was released, hinged inferiorly, and positioned with additional delayed primary ear cartilage grafts to reposition the nostril margins inferiorly and in symmetry. The thin forehead flap was returned to the recipient site. The forehead flap pedicle was divided 1 month later.

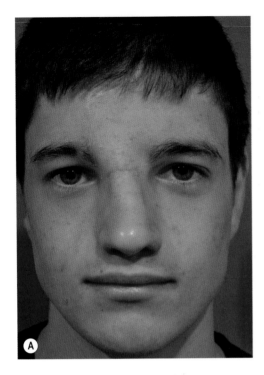

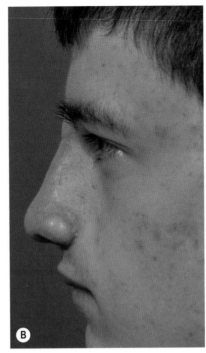

Fig. 6.22 (AB) A normal nose has been restored with symmetrical nostril margins, 10 days after further refinement of the alar creases.

Expansion of the forehead

Pre-expansion, although not routinely helpful, can enlarge the available surface of the forehead for transfer to the nose.

Forehead expansion should be considered:

1. In an especially tight forehead with limited available skin due to scarring or prior forehead flap harvest. Expansion can increase the length and width of available skin within the proposed flap.
2. In the occasional, especially short forehead (less than 3–4 cm in height) to increase flap length and minimize hair transfer to the nose.
3. To expand the donor forehead adjacent to the proposed flap to facilitate closure of the forehead defect after transfer of a non-expanded forehead flap.

However, there are disadvantages to expansion – delay in repair, increased number of operative stages, added expense, more office visits, risk of infection, and extrusion and recoil. Expanded skin, if not rigidly braced with a hard tissue support framework, contracts, leading to retraction and nasal shortening. Expansion does not clinically improve flap blood supply.

Expansion and delay

If scars are present within expanded skin after complete filling, the outline of the proposed forehead flap can be drawn over the dome of the filled expander. Its borders are incised through the skin and subcutaneous tissue to the underlying expander capsule to delay the flap. Subsequently, the flap is transposed and the expander removed.

Technique of forehead expansion

The site for expander placement is outlined in the pedicle's territory. A sub-frontalis pocket is created through a distant radial incision within the scalp or through an old scar. After drain placement, the expander is inserted and modestly filled with saline after closure of the scalp incision. Some weeks later, it is injected weekly over 6–10 weeks. Distance over the expander's dome is measured until the skin is adequate in length and width to resurface the defect. If the vascularity of the flap is in doubt due to past scars, the flap is surgically delayed, in stages, after expansion. At the time of transfer, a template is positioned over the expanded skin. The flap must be elevated across the supraorbital rim, transecting the capsule at the flap's base, to allow transposition and sufficient length. The capsule is excised. Elastic recoil occurs immediately on flap elevation and must be prevented with a strong nasal cartilage framework to avoid retraction and skin contraction.

Guidelines for harvesting multiple forehead flaps

- Check the position and length of old scars.
- Determine the available forehead surface area and compare it to the recipient requirement. Consider use of the contralateral pedicle.
- Use a full-thickness forehead flap to increase vascular safety or delay across old scars.
- Consider tissue expansion of the flap.
- Consider using a non-paramedian forehead flap.
- Expand residual forehead to ease closure of the forehead donor.
- If the donor site cannot be closed primarily under the hairline, allow the gap to heal secondarily.
- If the inferior forehead cannot be closed primarily due to the size and location of the nasal defect, return the unused proximal pedicle to the inferior forehead to facilitate its closure and the appearance of the eyebrow.

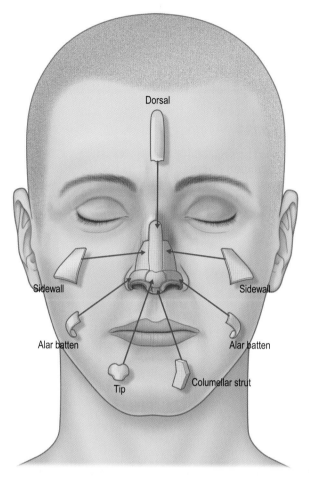

Fig. 6.23 Subunit support. Both cover and lining of the nasal reconstruction must be supported, shaped, and braced against wound contracture, tension, and gravity. The middle architectural layer of the nose must be replaced. Although there is no cartilage within the ala, the nostril margin must be supported during repair. If missing, dorsal, tip, ala, columella, and sidewall grafts of bone or cartilage are designed in the shape and dimension of the normal. When placed under thin supple external skin, they will visually recreate normal surface contour while supporting and maintaining nostril position, shape, and the airway.

- In extreme cases, when the forehead has been extensively destroyed by previous injury or multiple flap harvest, excise scar and residual skin within the forehead and resurface the entire unit with a one-piece, expanded, full-thickness, supraclavicular skin graft.

Restoring nasal contour and support: recreating a subsurface architecture

The 3D contour and landmark outline define a nose as "normal". Incorrect dimension, outline, position, projection, or symmetry describe the "abnormal". Most of these abnormalities reflect a poorly sized, misshapen, or malpositioned skeleton (Fig. 6.23).

The middle plane of the nose, between cover and lining, is composed of two layers. Superficially lies a 3D soft tissue layer of variable thickness composed of fat, nasalis muscle, fibrous ligaments, and areolar tissue. More deeply lies a rigid cartilage and bone framework which includes the nasal bones, upper lateral cartilages, alar cartilages, the columellar and

septal partition, and the compact stiff fibrofatty tissue of the ala. External skin and internal lining impart only minimal stiffness and form to the nose. Bone, cartilage, and the compact fibrofatty soft tissue of the ala determine nasal contour.

It must be remembered that the nose sits on the lip and cheek platform of bone and soft tissue. The reconstructed nose must be positioned and projected in symmetry and proportion to other facial features. So if missing, the facial platform must be restored and the nose built on a stable base, prior to formal nasal reconstruction.

Hard tissue support replacement

If missing, weakened, or distorted, the middle layer of soft and hard tissue must be restored. A complete cartilage and bone framework must extend from the nasal bone, above, to the base of the columella, inferiorly, and from one alar base and sidewall to the other, horizontally. Although the ala normally contains only soft tissue, cartilage support must be added to prevent collapse and retraction. Cartilage grafts support the nose and its airway, shape its external appearance, and brace the repair against gravity, tension, and wound contraction. Unlike the normal, the injured nose is subject to edema, hematoma, tension, and fibrosis and is negatively influenced by unnaturally thick and stiff cover and lining replacements. The framework of the reconstructed nose must be stronger than that of a normal nose.[22,25,51–55]

Timing

Ideally, if the underlying bone or cartilage structure is missing, primary and delayed primary support grafts are placed during flap transfer, the intermediate operation, or at the time of pedicle division. Although, traditionally, support has been replaced secondarily during late revisions, it is difficult to mold cover and lining once contracted by scar.

Design

Each support graft is designed in the shape and dimension of the subunit which it will replace. A template of the contralateral normal or ideal is used to determine the appropriate length, width, and border outline of the cartilage grafts. The grafts are fashioned a few millimeters smaller in all dimensions so when seen through thin, supple cover, they re-establish the 3D contour of the overlying subunit.

When a non-subunit defect is resurfaced, only partial subunit cartilage replacement is necessary (Box 6.4).

Materials

The tissue chosen to restore nasal support is of lesser importance than their shape. But materials must have the correct dimension, bulk, outline, contour, and rigidity to satisfy the needs of the defect.

BOX 6.4 **Functions of a hard tissue framework**

- support cover and lining to create projection and prevent collapse
- shape soft tissue
- brace soft tissue to prevent retraction or contracture

Alloplasts are avoided in reconstructive rhinoplasty to avoid infection and extrusion.

The septum can supply a modest amount (2–3 × 2–3 cm) of thin (2–3 mm), flat, moderately rigid cartilage. It is harvested through a Killian incision or through a dorsal approach, as in an open rhinoplasty. Septal cartilage is especially useful as a single or layered onlay dorsal graft, a tip graft, a sidewall brace, or a columellar strut and can be bent and fixed with sutures to shape anatomic tip grafts or alar batten grafts.

Ear cartilage remains the work course of tip repair. The entire concha can be harvested with little deformity through an anterior or posterior approach. In most instances, the entire concha is removed and the ideal graft is designed with the precise dimension and contour needed to supply the defect, based on a template. Like septal and rib cartilage, ear cartilage can be shaped with horizontal mattress sutures to increase or decrease its convexity. Its cuplike shape can be incorporated into the curve of the alar batten graft or anatomic tip graft. It is more difficult to create a straight columellar, dorsal, or sidewall onlay graft from the ear.

Traditionally, rib cartilage is harvested from the synchondrosis of the sixth, seventh, and eighth ribs, employing Gibson's principles of balanced carving. However, the floating ninth and tenth ribs are excellent donor sites due to their intrinsic length, width, and curvature. The rib is available for a tip graft, columellar strut, a dorsal graft, or alar batten. Osteocartilaginous grafts are especially useful for dorsal replacement. If the dorsal rib graft is 50% bone and 50% cartilage, the risk of late warping is minimized. Unfortunately, the rib donor site is more painful than other options.

Harvest

Based on a subunit template, the graft is examined to determine the ideal area which would best provide the appropriate contour and dimension. Then the exact graft is cut from the harvested material. Leftover graft is replaced in the donor site or banked within a soft tissue pocket under scalp or chest skin.

Graft fixation

Primary and delayed primary grafts are positioned precisely and fixed with sutures to the residual normal skeleton, to each other, and to the underlying lining. Late secondary cartilage grafts can be placed in closed subcutaneous pockets, or after elevation of the flap through peripheral or direct incisions.

It is important to differentiate onlay grafts from cantilever dorsal grafts. If central support remains, an onlay graft in the shape and thickness needed to replace dorsal height is laid over the remaining solid base. If the septum is missing or collapsed, a rigid dorsal graft must be fixed, as a cantilever, with a screw or plate to the radix to support the dorsal profile. If residual septum remains within the pyriform aperture, it may be rotated out of the nose as a septal composite flap, based on its septal vessels, to provide central nasal support. An onlay dorsal graft is added to shape the dorsal subunit.

Soft tissue support and contouring

Normal subcutaneous soft tissue adds shape and a degree of strength to all areas of the nose. It pads the underlying support

and helps contour the external skin. Compact soft tissue is the primary support for the ala and soft triangle, which normally contains no hard tissue.

Staged thinning of a full-thickness forehead flap, soft tissue sculpturing during the intermediate operation, and contouring of the proximal inset at pedicle division contribute significantly to 3D contour.[25]

Restoring nasal lining

It is easy to unappreciate the importance of lining. Nearly as much skin is required to line a nose as is needed to cover its outer surface. Any raw area heals secondarily, distorting the external nasal shape and airway scar contraction (Fig. 6.24).

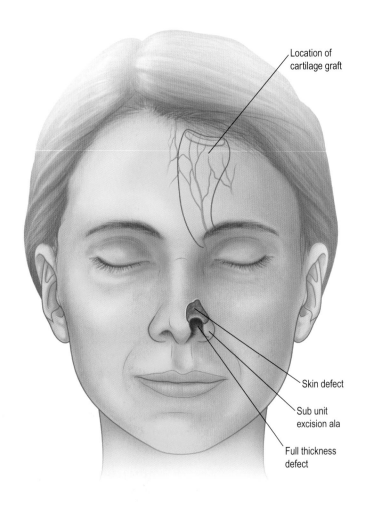

Location of
cartilage graft

Skin defect

Sub unit
excision ala

Full thickness
defect

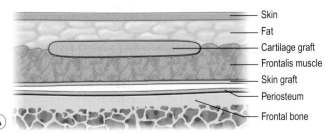

Skin
Fat
Cartilage graft
Frontalis muscle
Skin graft
Periosteum
Frontal bone

(A)

Fig. 6.24 (A–C) Traditional nasal lining options – the prelaminated, hingeover, and nasolabial flaps for lining.

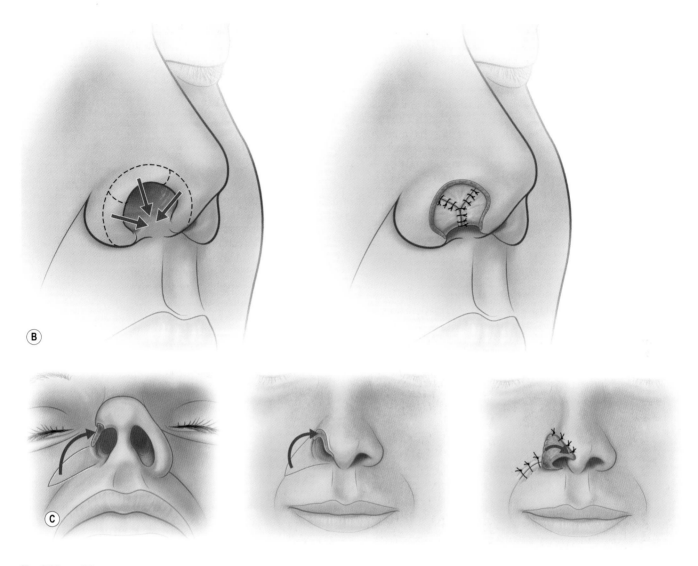

Fig. 6.24, cont'd

It is useful to systematically review all lining options and to make a written list to ensure that no method is overlooked.

Lining can be replaced by:

1. a composite skin graft
2. advancement of residual lining
3. prelamination of a forehead flap
4. folding of the distal forehead flap
5. a second flap (forehead, nasolabial, facial artery myomucosal flap or any available discardable excess local tissue)
6. hingeover lining flaps
7. intranasal lining flaps
8. skin graft for lining
9. microvascular transfer of distant tissue.

Composite skin grafts

Composite skin grafts of skin and cartilage, taken from the ear, can replace small full-thickness defects of skin and carti- lage loss within the soft triangle and nostril margin or isolated defects of the floor or ala.[56,57] Most often, a two- or three- layered sandwich of skin, containing cartilage or fat, is taken from the helical root, helical rim, or lobule. They survive, if placed on a well vascularized recipient, are sutured with care, and immobilized. They are most reliable if less than 1.5 cm in size. Larger grafts have been recommended, with less predict- able results. These larger grafts consist of large full-thickness skin graft component of preauricular skin and a modest distal composite extension for the full-thickness loss along the nostril margin.

The nasal defect and ear are examined. An exact template is created of the proper shape, size, and outline. The area which best matches the contour of the defect is identified. The graft is often harvested from the helical root. If significant coagulative injury is present, the wound is allowed to granu- late for 7–14 days.

The defect is re-created and the graft applied to the clean wound. The repair is performed under local, local anesthesia with sedation, or general anesthesia. The graft is harvested, avoiding pressure injury, and sutured to the recipient site in one layer. The ear defect is repaired by suturing the external skin of the helix to its medial surface or with a local preauricular or postauricular transposition flap, based on a superior or inferior pedicle.

Initially, these grafts appear white. After more than 24–72 h, they become progressively blue and subsequently pink as vascularity improves. Ice cold compresses to decrease the metabolic requirement of the graft in the first 48 h have been recommended, although the clinical significance is questionable.

The "take", color, and textures of composite grafts are unpredictable. However, composite grafts are useful to repair small defects (0.5–1.0 cm) along the nostril margin or within soft triangle due to their simplicity and adequate results. Their shiny atrophic appearance can match defects within the "thin skin zone".

Advancement of residual lining

Occasionally, a superficial defect along the nostril margin is accompanied by a modest lining loss. If minimal, residual vestibular lining can be freed superiorly from its overlying attachment to the alar cartilage and pulled inferiorly, until it reaches the level of the ideal nostril margin. An advancement of 2–3 mm is maintained with a rigid primary cartilage graft to prevent retraction. The external skin loss is replaced with a vascularized cover flap.

The prelaminated forehead flap

In the prelaminated technique (formerly referred to as prefabrication), the nose is "built on the forehead".[58–60,76] During a preliminary operation, a full-thickness skin graft is placed on the deep areolar surface of the forehead's frontalis muscle to supply 1–1.5 cm of distal lining for the alar rims. The flap is elevated only enough to position the skin graft, which is immobilized with a small sponge bolus. A separate cartilage graft is buried in a subcutaneous pocket, placed through an incision along the lateral flap border between the frontalis muscle and overlying skin to support to the future distal nostril margin. If desired, a composite graft from the ear or septum can be used in place of separate skin and cartilage grafts.

Once healed 6 weeks later, the composite forehead is transferred to provide cover, lining, and support as a single unit. Although prelamination adds a preliminary stage, the placement of skin and cartilage grafts and subsequent flap transfer and division are modest procedures and can be performed under light monitored sedation in a sick patient. Prelamination avoids extensive intranasal manipulation.

Traditionally, prelamination has been used to repair significant unilateral or bilateral full-thickness defects and has been combined with hingeover flaps, based on the scar along the border of an old full-thickness defect. The turned-over lining replaced the superior aspect of the defect while the distal aspect was lined with the prelaminated flap. Unfortunately, cartilage grafts, within a prelaminated flap, do not have a nasal shape and are fixed by the scar which forms around them as they heal on the forehead. The limited size, shape, and position of these cartilage strips provide only modest support to the nostril margin. Incompletely braced skin graft lining contracts, retracts the rim, and narrows the nostril aperture.

Prelamination of the forehead flap to repair a full-thickness defect has limited application but may be used for:

- a small-to-moderate defect
- in the elderly or debilitated patients to minimize anesthesia and morbidity
- in salvage cases, when other options are unavailable.

Hingeover lining flaps

When a full-thickness defect is created, whether sutured primarily or allowed to heal secondarily, residual cover and lining become contiguous along the defect margin. Six to 8 weeks later, external skin, an old skin graft previously applied to resurface an adjacent superficial skin loss, or scar adjacent to the healed margin can be hingeover, turning outside cover into inside lining.[15] Although the external skin deficiency is enlarged, the additional skin required to resurface the proximal nose is easily supplied by the proximal pedicle of the forehead flap used for cover.

Turnover flaps are vascularized across the scar at the wound margin. Because of their relative avascularity, they are unreliable if more than 1–1.5 cm in length. Hingeovered scar is less likely to survive. Even a minor hingeover lining loss may lead to infection, especially if cartilage grafts are simultaneously placed for support. To improve their limited vasculariy, a preliminary delay, 3–4 weeks earlier, can be performed. The hingeover flap is incised, elevated inferiorly, and then returned to its bed. However, the usefulness of surgical delay, in this instance, is in doubt. It adds an additional surgical stage, delays the repair, increases fibrosis, and does not definitely improve survival.

Hingeover flaps are thick, stiff, modestly vascularized, and noncompliant. They are less easily shaped by primary cartilage grafts and their bulk may distort external nasal contour.

Indications for hingeover lining flaps

- To line small full-thickness defects after cover and lining have heal together along the wound margin.
- In salvage cases, all layers of the nose may be injured with nasal collapse and retraction. This is most commonly seen after multiple failed rhinoplasties, following intranasal lining necrosis with cartilage infection and collapse (as in the cocaine nose) or after prior failed reconstructions. In these instances, few lining options remain. Because scarred external skin will be replaced with a flap, it can be turned over to line the distorted distal margin, rather than being discarded.
- In pediatric nasal reconstruction, injury to the growth centers of the nose should be avoided until near complete physical maturity. Hingeover flaps of residual skin, which borders the margins of the defect, can provide lining, while avoiding additional intranasal injury in the child.
- Composite skin grafts are another option in the child. The disadvantages of hingeover flaps are:
  - they are not applicable to the repair of a fresh nasal injury and require at least 6–8 weeks to allow the external and internal surface of the nose to heal and establish vascular connections across the scar
  - they are thick, stiff, and less able to be molded by cartilage grafts

- that if the initial defect encompassed most of the circumference of the airway, as the scar contracts, the airway becomes stenotic. Even though the reconstructed nostril margin may appear large after turning over external skin for lining, the internal stenosis cannot be opened initially without jeopardizing the vascular base of the hingeover flap. Late revision to open the constriction deep within the nose is difficult. In such cases, open up the constriction initially, prior to the formal nasal repair. Later adjacent external skin is turned over for lining operation. However, this further postpones formal nasal repair.

Use of a second flap for lining

If the full-thickness defect, external skin can be replaced with a forehead flap and lining replaced with a second flap, with a separate blood supply.

The nasolabial flap

Millard[15] popularized the use of random nasolabial flaps of cheek skin for lining. For large defects, which included the midvault and lower one half of the nose, he hinged over residual skin from the upper nose to line the midvault and rolled over skin and fat within the nasolabial fold to line the distal aspect of the defect. For subtotal nasal defects, bilateral nasolabial flaps were turned inward, after surgical delay, to line each ala and one half of the nasal vault, suturing the distal end of each nasolabial flap together centrally to supply columellar lining.

If employed to line a small defect of the lateral ala, no more than about 1.5 cm in length, they can survive, based only on scar about the pyriform aperture. Longer nasolabial lining flaps should include the angular and facial artery perforators at their base. Unfortunately, these flaps are thick and stiff and cannot be thinned at the time of transfer without jeopardizing blood supply. Primary cartilage grafts are often precluded by the excessive soft tissue bulk and risk of necrosis with infection. Late revision is required to thin the nostril rims, open the airway, and contour the nasal surface. These flaps add scars to the central face and cannot be positioned exactly in the nasolabial fold. The technique is rarely used today.

A second forehead flap[25]

It is possible to line the nose with a second forehead flap based on the opposite supratrochlear or superficial temporal vessels. Whatever forehead skin necessary to rebuild a nose should be harvested. However, forehead skin is best used only for cover. Injury to the remaining forehead skin should be avoided, if possible, to minimize scarring and permit harvesting of a second flap for a second nasal reconstruction needed in the future.

The facial artery myomucosal flap (FAMM flap)

The FAMM flap[61] is an axial oral musculomucosal flap based on the facial artery which can line defects of the mouth and nose. It consists of intraoral mucosa, submucosa, a small amount of buccinator muscle, the deeper plexus of the orbicularis oris muscle, and the facial artery and its venous plexus. Based superiorly at the alar base and centered over the facial artery, oral mucosa and the overlying facial artery are raised,

from distal to proximal, and passed into the nasal cavity at the alar base. The flap is 89 cm long and 1.5–2.0 cm in width and can line an isolated area of lining loss within the middle vault secondary to cocaine injury or Wegener's disease. Its primary advantages are its vascularity and ability to provide intranasal lining without adding visible scars to the external face. Bilateral flaps can be used.

Intranasal lining flaps

Intranasal stratified squamous and nasal mucoperichondrium are perfused by branches of the facial and angular arteries, the septal branch of the superior labial artery, or the anterior ethmoidal vessels.[62–68]

The lateral nose is perfused from branches of the facial and angular artery which supply the ipsilateral alar base and middle vault. The centrally placed septum is perfused inferiorly from bilateral septal branches of the superior labial arteries, which arise from the facial artery. The superior labial artery passes medially through the orbicularis oris muscle along the skin vermilion junction of the upper lip. Its septal branch arises just lateral to the philtral column and moves vertically upward, lateral to the nasal spine, to supply the ipsilateral septal mucoperichondrium. The septal branch is located at the base of the columella within 1.0–1.2 cm of the nasal spine between the anterior plane of the upper lip and the inferior edge of it perform aperture. Each side of the septal mucosa is perfused by its ipsilateral septal branch. The entire septum containing septal cartilage and lined with bilateral mucoperichondrium, is vascularized by both superior labial vessels. The dorsal aspect of the septum is perfused by paired anterior ethmoidal vessels which pass from under the nasal bones to perfuse each side of the septal mucoperichondrium, dorsally (Fig. 6.25 ⊕).

Fig. 6.25 appears online only.

Residual intranasal mucosal can be moved to line a deficiency depending on the defect location and size and the pedicle position, dimension, and reach of each individual lining flap, as described by Burget and Menick.[22,25,69,70] These flaps may be unavailable if prior surgery or traumatic injury has interrupted their named vessels or their mucosal surfaces.

- A bipedicle vestibular skin flap can be employed if residual vestibular skin remains above a marginal defect. It is incised superiorly in the area of the intercartilaginous space, creating a bipedicle flap, based medially on the septum and laterally on the nasal floor. It is perfused, medially by the septal branch of the superior labial artery, and laterally by the branches of the facial angular artery. The flap is pulled inferiorly, like the hem of a skirt, to line the nostril rim. The superior defect, created by advancement of the bipedicle flap, is filled with an ipsilateral septal flap, a skin graft, or with a contralateral mucoperichondrial flap.
  Ipsilateral septal mucoperichondrial flaps, based on the right or left superior labial artery, can be elevated off septal cartilage and transposed laterally and inferiorly to line the vestibule and the lateral sidewall.
- A contralateral mucoperichondrial flap, based on the dorsum of the septum and vascularized from branches of the ipsilateral ethmoidal vessels, can be hinged laterally to line the contralateral midvault. As originally described

by deQuervain, the ipsilateral septal mucosa was discarded, and a flap of cartilage and septal mucous membrane was swung laterally through a large septal fistula. It is more practical to preserve the ipsilateral mucosa, remove the septal cartilage, preserving a septal "L" strut, and pass the flap through a dorsal slit in the ipsilateral septal mucosa, preserving the opposite septal mucosa. The harvested septal cartilage is reapplied to support the mucosal repair after transfer, facilitating its design and positioning. This contralateral dorsal septal flap can line the midvault, an isolated defect of the midvault, the gap above a bipedicle vestibular flap, or above an ipsilateral septal flap transferred to line the inferior nose. It is inadequate in size and reach to line the nostril margin or alar base, inferiorly.

■ A composite septal flap based on paired septal branches of the superior labial artery lying adjacent to close to the nasal spine. The entire septum rotated as an inferior pedicle base out of the pyriform aperture, transposing a "septal sandwich" of support and bilateral lining anterior to the plane of the face to restore basic central support and lining to both vestibules, columella, and the middle vault and dorsum. Its mucoperichondrium lining can be turned to line the lateral nose but is inadequate in length to reach the alar base and must be supplemented laterally, most often with flaps from the residual ala or nasolabial fold.

Intranasal lining flaps may be applied to varied defects, according to their location and dimension:

1. Isolated unilateral defect of the midvault – use contralateral septal mucosal flap.
2. Unilateral defect of the lower one third of the nose – use bipedicle vestibular flap and ipsilateral septal flap.
3. Unilateral defects up to one half of the nose – use bipedicle vestibular flap and contralateral septal flap.
4. Unilateral defects of the vestibule, middle, and upper vaults – use ipsilateral and contralateral septal flaps.
5. Central defect of the dorsum and tip – use septal composite flap.
6. Central defect combined with lateral alar lining loss – use septal composite and turnover alar remnant or nasolabial flaps.

Although significant lining can be provided by intranasal lining flaps, they have no shape and collapse into the nose. However, they are thin, pliable, and vascular which permits the immediate restoration of support with primary cartilage grafts. This combination of intranasal lining flaps and primary cartilage grafts was a significant advance in nasal reconstruction. For the first time, reliable, thin, supple, vascularized lining was available which would not occlude the airway or distort the external shape. And cartilage grafts could be positioned primarily to support, shape, and brace the soft tissues at the initial stage.

However, the limitations of intranasal lining flaps must be understood. Intranasal lining flaps are limited in dimension and availability due to their modest size, limited reach, or prior injury to their blood supply due to trauma or previous

operation. Although highly vascular, they are unpredictable in the smoker or in major repairs when multiple intranasal flaps combined to line large defects. A minor cartilage exposure may lead to serious infection and tissue loss.

They are fragile and should be elevated subperichondrially to protect their blood supply. Their dissection is destructive to the nose and increases the overall morbidity of nasal repair due to temporary bleeding, crusting, and obstruction. Fortunately, the surgical fistula heals spontaneously around its border and becomes self-cleansing. Whistling does not occur because of the fistula's large size. Intranasal flaps are relatively complex and time consuming. The final result may be marred by late retraction, external distortion or narrowing of the airway. The lack of rigidity and limited dimensions of intranasal lining flaps, the relatively unstable cartilage construction with multiple-suture fixated grafts, dead space, and scar contracture limit the final result. Late nostril stenosis may occur. However, intranasal lining flaps remain a valuable tool in the repair of isolated midvault or large unilateral full-thickness defects when other methods are less applicable.

Intranasal lining flap technique (Figs. 6.26–29 ⊕)

Isolated unilateral midvault lining loss

To repair the midvault, the contralateral septal mucoperichondrium is harvested through the full-thickness defect. Or if the ala remains intact but has been malpositioned superiorly by midvault scar or prior excision, a full-thickness incision releases the remaining inferior nose in symmetry to the opposite normal side. The ipsilateral septal mucoperichondrium is incised transversely at the dorsum, exposing septal cartilage. The ipsilateral mucosa is elevated. Preserving 8–10 mm of superior dorsal support, the underlying septal cartilage is incised transversely in line with the anterior dorsal edge and septal cartilage is harvested for graft material. The contralateral mucosa is preserved and the anterior ethmoidal vessels are protected. A dorsally-based flap of contralateral septal mucosa is incised, maintaining its dorsal blood supply. The contralateral flap is then passed through the ipsilateral dorsal slit and pulled laterally to the periphery of the midvault lining loss. The raw surface of ipsilateral flap, which now lies exposed with the contralateral airway, heals spontaneously. Harvested septal cartilage and bone is fashioned into a side-wall brace to support and shape the midvault and prevent the ala from retracting upward postoperatively. Missing external skin is advanced from the cheek or transposed from the forehead to resurface the external skin loss.

Figs. 6.26 and 6.27 appear online only.

If the unilateral defect of the nostril margin is less than 1 cm in height, residual stratified squamous skin remains above the defect. A bipedicle flap of remnant vestibular skin, between the edge of the defect and the internal nasal valve, is moved caudally to line the nostril margin. The dry stratified squamous epithelium of the vestibular flap is less easily traumatized than septal mucosa, which can appear abnormally, secrete mucus, and bleed, if abraded. Medially, the flap is perfused through its connection to the ipsilateral septal lining at the septal angle. Laterally, it is vascularized by multiple branches of the facial angular arteries at the alar base.

A bipedicle flap, 8 mm wide, is designed within the existing lining, just above the defect. The incision of the flap's superior border (similar to the intercartilaginous incision of

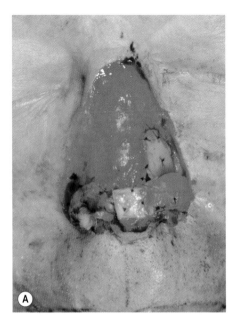

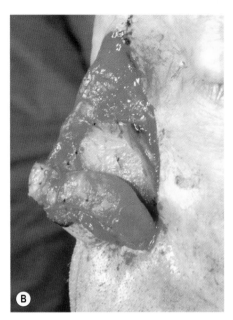

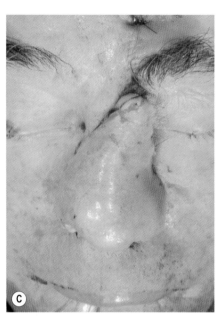

Fig. 6.28 (A–C) Primary ear and septal cartilage grafts are placed to shape, support, and brace the reconstruction. These grafts included a columellar strut, tip graft, bilateral alar margin grafts, and a sidewall brace. The nasal defect with resurfaced as a nasal subunit with a full-thickness forehead flap. An intermediate operation to thin the forehead flap and sculpt the soft tissues and pedicle division were subsequently performed.

an aesthetic rhinoplasty) is carried through the vestibular lining into the overlying soft tissues. The medial crus of the alar cartilage may be divided to mobilize the flap adequately. The flap is separated from the overlying subcutaneous tissues and hinged medially and laterally, as a bipedicle, to the level of the proposed nostril rim. The secondary defect, which remains above after advancement of the bipedicle flap, is filled with an ipsilateral septal flap. The ipsilateral septal flap, which measures up to 3 × 3 cm in width and length, passes

towards the medial canthus about 6–8 mm below the dorsum and then travels posteriorly with a right angle to the nasal floor, proceeding anteriorly back towards the nasal spine. It is incised longitudinally with straight scissors. Its distal end is cut with a right angle scissors. A 1.2 cm soft tissue pedicle is maintained in the vicinity of the nasal spine to maintain the ipsilateral septal branch of the superior labial artery. The mucoperichondrium is elevated off the cartilage and bone of the septum and swung laterally. It is sutured to the superior

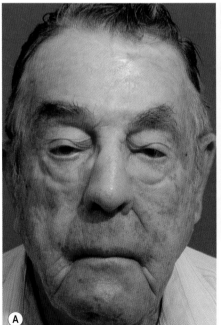

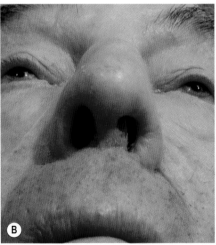

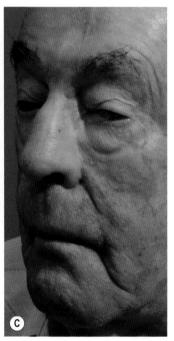

Fig. 6.29 (A–C) Postoperative result. No revision.

aspect of the defect, laterally along the pyriform aperture, and inferiorly to the bipedicle flap to create a complete lining sleeve for a unilateral nasal defect. The size of the flap is primarily limited by the surgeon's ability to incise within the confines of pyriform aperture. The flap can extend up to the medial canthus and inferiorly to the nasal floor. Leaving a strong septal "L", the central septal cartilage is harvested for graft material.

In larger defects, the secondary defect becomes too large to be replaced with an ipsilateral septal flap whose length is limited by the twist of its pedicle. The width of the flap may not be adequate to fill the height of the residual defect. In this instance, the contralateral septal flap is employed. First, the bipedicle flap of vestibular skin and mucosa is swung inferiorly. The ipsilateral septal mucosa is incised below the dorsum and elevated submucosally in line with the nasal bridge. The underlying septal cartilage is incised, protecting the contralateral mucosa. Septal cartilage is harvested, leaving a strong "L" strut. The dorsal mucosa is left intact while two parallel cuts are incised and then connected along the floor of the nose. The flap is pulled to the ipsilateral mucosal slit to line the middle vault in the superior aspect of the vestibule while the bipedicle flap restores the nostril margin. The flaps are sutured to one another and supported by an alar batten and a sidewall brace of primary cartilage graft. The dorsally based, contralateral septal flap can be designed to extend onto the ipsilateral nasal floor, increasing its length and allowing it to reach across the midline to the lateral aspect of the pyriform aperture. A wide flap can be designed along the entire dorsum to insure adequate vertical dimension to fill the height of the defect. However, the contralateral septal flap does not have a length or width to reach inferiorly to the nostril rim. It is only useful for moderate midvault lateral nasal defects.

If the lining defect extends from the nostril margin to the nasal bones, an ipsilateral septal mucosal flap can be used to line the nostril margin inferiorly and a contralateral septal mucosal flap can be swung simultaneously to line the middle and upper vaults. This technique creates a permanent septal fistula, which is usually well tolerated. The mucoperichondrium is dissected off the entire ipsilateral septal, as in an submucous resection (SMR). The flap is swung laterally to expose septal bone and cartilage which is harvested for graft material, maintaining an L-shaped strut of cartilage for dorsal and caudal support. Then a contralateral flap, based the dorsum and anterior ethmoidal vessels, is incised, maintaining its dorsal pedicle and swung laterally to line the midvault. The ipsilateral septal flap is draped laterally towards the alar base to line the vestibule. The contralateral septal flap is passed through the septal fistula and sutured to the lateral edge of the nasal defect and then to the ipsilateral flap. The pedicle of the ipsilateral flap may partially obstruct the airway and need to be divided subsequently to open the airway.

Central lining defects

In superficial dorsal defects, the high, converging medial, and lateral walls of the upper and middle vaults may permit simple side-to-side approximation of lateral sidewall mucosa and medial septum if a modest central defect lies within the superior nose. This may lower the height of the nasal vault but may not significantly diminish nasal function. The height of the nasal bridge is restored with cartilage grafts.

Central deep nasal defects of the inferior nose are classified as subtotal (part of the projecting septum and bones at the radix are preserved) or total (loss of all soft tissue structures, anterior septum and nasal bones flush with the frontal bone of the maxilla). Fortunately, a large part of the anterior septum may remain projecting from the facial plane or lie hidden within the pyriform aperture. Residual septum can be pulled out to provide lining for the projecting parts of the nose and its septal cartilage can be used as a foundation on which to rest a dorsal strut. The loss of the nasal bones is especially significant because they normally provide the fulcrum for a cantilevered dorsal support graft. In these instances, Millard perform a preliminary operation to reconstruct a bony base at the radix using local hingeover lining and a bone graft, covered initially by a median forehead flap. In other cases, he employed a superiorly based, L-shaped, full-thickness septal flap which was hinged out of the pyriform aperture to reestablish limited dorsal and caudal septal support and lining. Later, hinged-over flaps of local tissue and bilateral nasolabial flaps were turned inward to line the midvault, ala, and columella. A cantilever bone graft was anchored to the preplaced fulcrum to establish dorsal support, and a second forehead flap was used for cover. However, such methods are unreliable due to vascularity, bulk, or inadequate support.

The modern septal composite flap, based on both superior labial arteries, mobilizes the entire septum out of the nasal cavity and projects it in front of the face. It positions a vertical sheet of bone and cartilage to support the dorsum of the nose. A dorsal costochondral rib graft can be placed on this hard tissue base and fixed to the residual nasal bones, or with a plate and screw, at the radix. The bilateral excess of septal mucosa is hinged laterally to provide lining for the lateral aspects of the defect.

The full-thickness of the septum is cut superiorly and inferiorly. Distally, it is transected with a right angle scissors. The mucosa is preserved in the region of the nasal spine and upper lip to preserve the right and left septal branches the superior labial arteries within a 1.2-cm soft tissue pedicle. At the base of the flap, mucoperichondrial is separated on each side of the cartilaginous septum to remove a small wedge of bone and cartilage over the nasal spine. This allows the septal composite flap be drawn out of the pyriform aperture on a soft tissue tether. The deep aspect of the flap is anchored to the stumps of the upper lateral cartilage or to the nasal bones with permanent suture or wire. The intranasal donor site is closed by mucosa to mucosa repair where possible. A large permanent septal fistula is created.

If the defect is limited to the superficial upper or midvault, the composite flap restores the central bony platform while the mucosa of the right and left sides of the septum is reflected laterally and sutured to the lateral border of the defect to provide a complete vault lining. Primary subunit cartilage grafts are positioned to support and shape the covering forehead flap. In subtotal or total nasal reconstructions when the tip and ala are also missing, it is safer to mobilize and fix the septal composite flap to the radix or upper lateral cartilages. After insuring vascularity and healing to the residual nasal root, 6–8 weeks later, the exposed dorsal mucosal edge is split at its center and bilateral flaps are turned laterally. Superiorly, the septal mucosa is sufficient to line the upper and middle vaults, however. More inferiorly, it will not reach the alar bases to line the vestibule and ala, laterally. Additional alar lining must be supplied by hingeover flaps, turned up from a residual alar remnant or from a nasolabial flap. Presurgical delay of these local flaps may increase their reliability.

The modified folded forehead flap for lining (Figs. 6.30–6.38 ◉)

Folding the distal end of the forehead flap onto itself to supply external cover and internal lining is a traditional method.[7] Unfortunately, the traditional design made it difficult to position cartilage or bone grafts due to the bulk of soft tissues and limited exposure. The reconstructed nose was thick, shapeless, and the airways were collapsed and occluded. A modified folded approach using a forehead flap in three stages provides an opportunity to combine primary and delayed primary cartilage grafts and subcutaneous soft tissues sculpture. It is an efficient method applicable to many lining defects (Video 6.1 ▶).

Figs. 6.31D, 6.32A,B,D, 6.33B,C, 6.34A,B, and 6.37A,D appear online only.

As described by Menick,[25,71–73] an extension of a full-thickness paramedian forehead flap, based on an exact template of the lining defect, is folded inward. Because the donor site lies within the area of forehead normally discarded as a dog-ear, there is minimal additional injury to the forehead. If the lining template must extend to the hairline, any transferred follicles simulate intranasal vibrissae and can be trimmed, postoperatively.

The flap, as a single cover and lining unit, is elevated from the distal to its proximal base, as a full-thickness flap. The distal lining extension (which can be partially thinned if the full-thickness flap is especially stiff and difficult to turn inward) is folded inward and sutured to the residual mucosal lining of the defect. The more proximal aspect of the flap is folded back onto itself to provide nasal cover, creating a layer of external skin, subcutaneous fat, and frontalis muscle which provides nasal cover resting against an inner layer of frontalis muscle, subcutaneous fat, and skin, which replaces the missing lining.

No primary cartilage support is placed with the folded flap. However, primary cartilage grafts are placed in neighboring areas of more superficial injury over intact vascular lining.

At the second stage four weeks later, the proposed nostril margin is marked with ink, based on templates of the contralateral normal alar rim or the ideal. The nostril margin is incised in the area of folding, separating the proximal covering skin from its distal lining extension. The proximal aspect of the covering flap is re-elevated with 2–3 mm of subcutaneous fat. Because the frontalis muscle was not excised or the subcutaneous plane of the flap injured during transfer, cover and lining skin remain soft, supple, and uncontracted. More importantly, the folded distal extension, which was designed to line the nasal repair, is now healed and integrated into the residual normal lining. It is no longer dependent on the proximal forehead flap and its supratrochlear pedicle for vascularity. The exposed double layer of soft tissue – residual subcutaneous fat and frontalis – is excised to reveal thin, supple, and highly vascular lining. Delayed primary grafts are placed to create a complete alar subunit support framework. The thin, supple, unscarred skin of the proximal flap is returned to the recipient site (Video 6.2 ▶). At the third stage, 4 weeks later (6–8 weeks after beginning the nasal repair), the pedicle is divided.

This modified folded forehead flap lining technique is reliable, efficient, and effective in the repair of full-thickness unilateral and bilateral defects. It is employed to repair of lining defects up to 3.0 cm in size and is useful for all small to moderate full-thickness defects. It avoids complex intranasal manipulation and minimizes the risk of postoperative bleeding or nasal obstruction often associated with intranasal lining flaps. The operative time is shortened, with less intranasal morbidity. If the defect extends from the ala onto the nasal floor, an additional distal extension can be added at right angles to the alar lining extension to line the ala and resurface the nostril sill. The vascularity of a full-thickness forehead flap is illustrated by the safety of such complex skin extensions.

Although all available lining options should be considered for any specific defect, the modified folded forehead lining

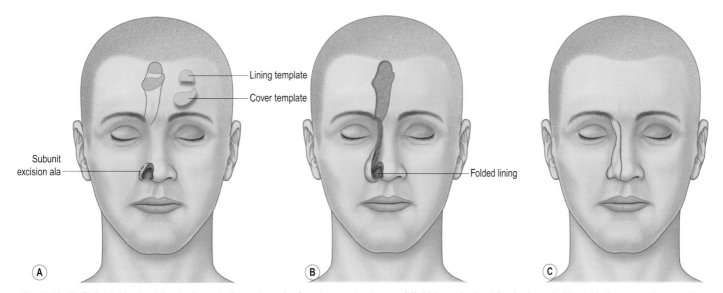

Fig. 6.30 (A–C) Folded forehead flap for lining-design and transfer. Based on exact patterns, a full-thickness forehead flap is elevated without thinning to supply external skin cover with the distal extension which will be folded inward to replace missing nasal lining. No primary cartilage grafts are placed.

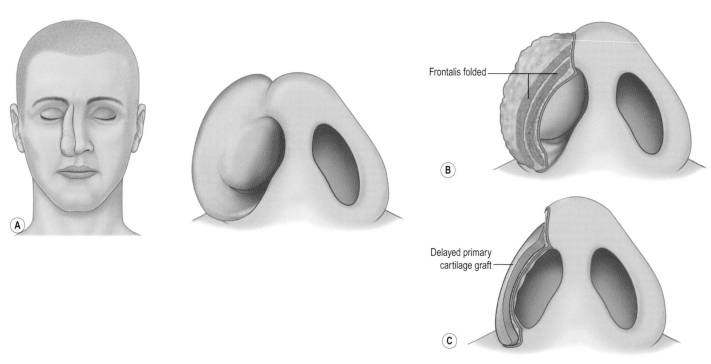

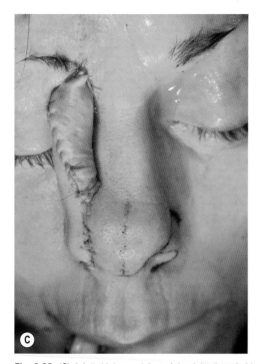

Fig. 6.31 (ABC) The intermediate operation of the modified folded forehead flap. One month later, the folded forehead flap lining extension is healed to the adjacent normal nasal lining and is no longer dependent on the forehead flap for its supratrochlear blood supply. The regional units of the nose an ideal alar margin are marked with ink. The forehead flap is incised between covering lining along the nostril margin and the covering flap was elevated with 2–3 mm of subcutaneous fat. This exposes the underlying unsupported subcutaneous fat and frontalis muscle which is excised from the underlying lining of folded forehead skin. A delayed primary cartilage graft is positioned to support the ala (and sidewall, if needed). The thin forehead flap is returned to the recipient site for nasal cover. One month later (2 months after the initial flap transfer), the proximal pedicle is divided.

Fig. 6.32 (C) A full-thickness defect of the right ala and sidewall is present after Mohs excision. The regional units of the nose and the ideal alar base position are marked with ink based on the template of the contralateral normal upper lip. Templates were designed to replace the missing cover and lining exactly in dimension and border outline. A full-thickness forehead flap is elevated with the distal extension for lining and folded to replace missing nasal lining and the more proximal distal flap is turned back to resurface the defect. No primary cartilage grafts were placed. The raw pedicle of the forehead flap was skin grafted for cleanliness.

technique should be a workhorse in nasal reconstruction. Due to its vascularity, it is safe in the smoker. Due to the shortened operative time and limited and intranasal manipulation, it is useful in the elderly or those with unassociated medical illness. When re-opening a healed defect, the surgeon can define the defect and immediately provide vascularized lining to fit the dimension, position, and outline of the newly created defect, unlike prefabricated or hingeover flaps which require delay or intranasal lining flaps which may be precluded by injury to their vascular base or the position of the defect. It is a simple yet highly effective method.

Skin grafts for lining

Skin grafts have been used to line a forehead flap at the time of transfer. Unfortunately, although a skin graft is thin and pliable, revascularization is unpredictable. More often, a skin graft has been applied to the forehead flap prior to transfer during a preliminary prelamination (prefabrication) 6 weeks before transfer. Later, when "take" was assured, the healed forehead and underlying skin graft were transferred to the recipient site. Graft shrinkage, in these poorly supported noses, was accepted as a part of the technique.

Gillies developed a skin graft inlay method.[16] If the lining and support were lost but the overlying skin remained intact (as in the syphilitic or leprotic saddle nose), internal scar was released on the undersurface of the external skin and a skin graft applied to the raw internal surface. A permanent internal prosthesis, placed through a buccal fistula and fixed to dentures, splinted the graft to maintain airway patency and nasal shape.

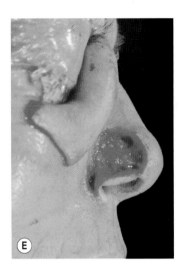

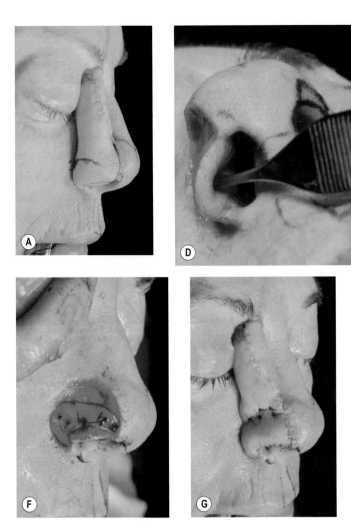

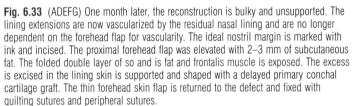

Fig. 6.33 (ADEFG) One month later, the reconstruction is bulky and unsupported. The lining extensions are now vascularized by the residual nasal lining and are no longer dependent on the forehead flap for vascularity. The ideal nostril margin is marked with ink and incised. The proximal forehead flap was elevated with 2–3 mm of subcutaneous fat. The folded double layer of so and is fat and frontalis muscle is exposed. The excess is excised in the lining skin is supported and shaped with a delayed primary conchal cartilage graft. The thin forehead skin flap is returned to the defect and fixed with quilting sutures and peripheral sutures.

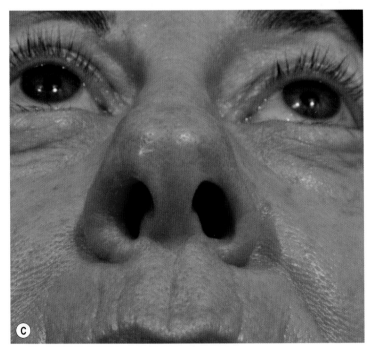

Fig. 6.34 (C) Postoperative result after pedicle division and right alar crease creation.

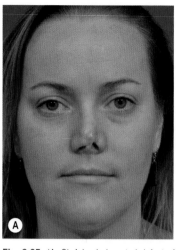
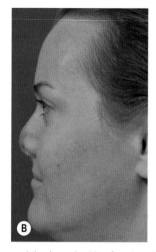
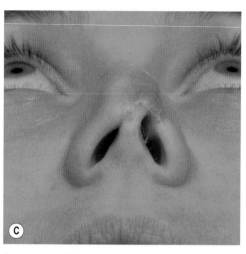

Fig. 6.35 (A–C) A healed central defect of the nasal tip after a dog bite. Covering skin, tip support, and lining for both vestibules is missing.

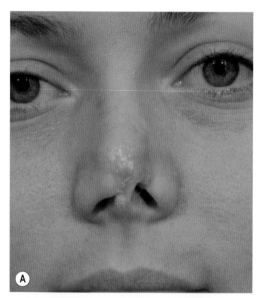
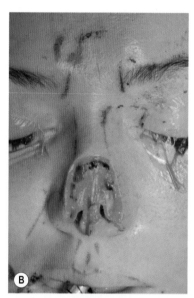
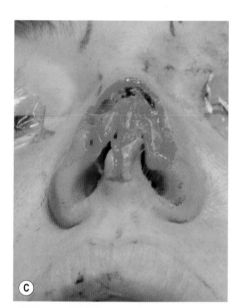

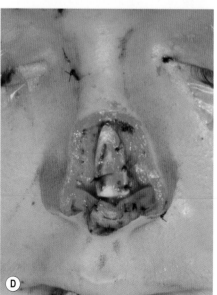
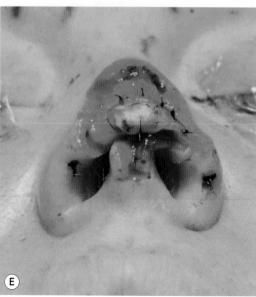

Fig. 6.36 (A–E) The defect is recreated. A subunit excision of the tip, but not of the dorsum, is performed. Tip support was restored with septal cartilage extended, lateral spreader grafts, a columellar strut, and tip graft to lengthen the nose project and shape the tip. Ear cartilage grafts were positioned in subcutaneous pockets within each alar remnant and fixed to the tip repair to shape and support the nostril margins. In lateral defects, unless an expanded forehead flap is employed, primary support of the ala is not positioned at the time of transfer of a folded forehead flap for cover and lining. When the defect is central, the risk of asymmetric rim retraction is significant prior to the intermediate operation and primary cartilage grafts are placed to support the tip and nostril margins at the time of forehead flap transfer. A full-thickness folded forehead flap is designed with bilateral extensions to line the right and left nasal vestibule.

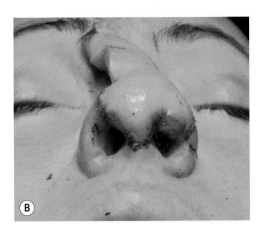

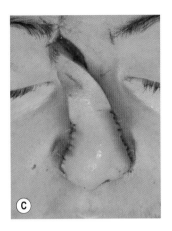

Fig. 6.37 (BC) One month later, the cover and lining flaps are separated along the ideal nostril margin and excess subcutaneous fat and frontalis sculpted to refine the nasal shape. The forehead flap is then returned to the recipient site.

More recently, Burget[22] tunneled a cartilage graft within the subcutaneous fat between the frontalis and the external skin of a forehead flap to repair modest nasal defects of the nostril margin and ala at flap transfer. The cartilage survived within the vascularized soft tissue and supported the nostril margin. A full-thickness postauricular skin graft was sutured to the lining defect, raw surface outward. The deep surface of the frontalis muscle vascularized the underlying skin graft. The buried cartilage graft "stented" the skin grafted lining, much like the Gillies external splint.

In smaller unilateral defects, when significant residual skin remained above the defect, a bipedicle flap of remnant vestibular skin, based on the septum medially and laterally at the alar base, was transposed inferiorly to the level of the proposed alar margin. Because the marginal bipedicle flap had its own blood supply, a primary cartilage graft was fixed to its vascularized external surface. The secondary lining defect above the vestibular flap was repaired with a full-thickness skin graft. No primary cartilage was placed in this area. The forehead flap resurfaced the entire defect and revascularized the lining skin graft. Three to four weeks later, after the skin graft lining was healed and vascularized from adjacent residual lining, the superior ala and sidewall were supported by a delayed primary cartilage graft placed at pedicle division. The forehead flap, maintaining a pedicle from the eyebrow to the distal flap inset along the nostril margin, could also be re-elevated over the mid-vault during an intermediate operation to allow delayed primary support. Scarring in the vicinity of the internal valve, leading to nasal obstruction, occasionally follows and is difficult to correct.

These skin grafts retained most of their original dimensions. Some graft contracture occurs, causing minor distortions. Simplicity is a primary advantage, making it especially useful in an elderly or debilitated patient for whom more complex intranasal dissection should be avoided, when intranasal lining flaps are unavailable, or for the less demanding patient who desires a simple and less delicate repair.

The three-stage full-thickness forehead flap has broadened the applications of skin grafts for lining, based on principles similar to those of the modified folded forehead flap technique.

As described by Menick,[25,74] a full-thickness forehead flap is highly vascular and a skin graft will routinely "take" on its deep raw surface. An exact pattern of the lining defect is

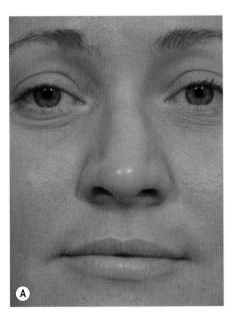

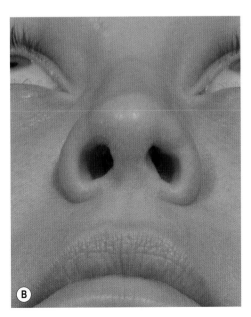

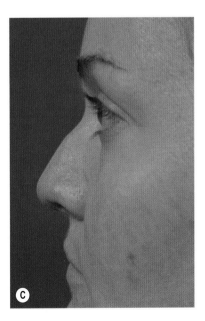

Fig. 6.38 (ABC) Postoperative result without revision.

outlined and a full-thickness postauricular skin graft is sutured to the margins of the lining defect. Primary cartilage grafts are precluded between the skin graft and the undersurface of the flap. But support can be placed over intact lining, adjacent to the full-thickness loss. It provides a vascular bed for lining skin graft which is quilted to the overlying flap and is also splinted with a sponge bolus, placed with the nostril for 3–4 days to immobilize the repair and apply light pressure. The full-thickness flap provides external cover. Support grafts are not placed within soft tissue tunnels within the forehead flap to avoid a thick nostril rim or the initiation of soft tissue injury and scar. It is also difficult to design, position, or fix tunneled cartilage grafts.

Four weeks later, the skin graft is healed to the adjacent normal residual lining and is no longer dependent on the covering flap for its blood supply. At the second stage, covering skin with 2–3 mm of subcutaneous fat is completely elevated from the nose. Excess subcutaneous fat and frontalis, which lie over the skin graft, are excised down to the newly reconstructed lining. The skin graft is thin, relatively supple, and vascularized by the adjacent residual lining. A delayed primary alar margin batten graft is fixed to support the nostril margin and a sidewall brace placed over the mid-vault to prevent upward retraction if the defect extends upward. The thin covering flap is replaced over the delayed primary cartilage grafts and the restored skin graft lining. Four weeks later (8 weeks after forehead flap transfer), the pedicle is divided.

Occasionally, the skin graft fails. If so, the intermediate stage is delayed and the granulating bed on the undersurface of the forehead flap is sharply debrided and a second graft applied. The forehead flap does not need to be re-elevated. The skin graft is simply applied to its raw deep surface. Because frontalis muscle is not excised and injury to the subcutaneous plane of the full-thickness forehead flap spared, fibrosis or contracture does not occur within the covering flap. Although an additional stage is required to replace the skin graft, the overall result is not significantly impaired.

The modified skin graft for lining technique is reliable, efficient, and effective for the repair of small to moderate, full-thickness nasal defects. Scar contracture and secondary distortion are modest and a delicate alar rim can be created. The technique should be limited to lining defects between 0.5–1.5 cm in size. Skin graft "take" is routine, although a second graft may be required in 20–30% of cases. However, an initial skin graft loss delays pedicle division from the expected 8 weeks to 12 weeks. The risk of poor skin graft take and contraction increases as the size of the lining defect increases. The method is especially useful in the elderly or debilitated patient with unassociated medical illness when intranasal lining flaps should be avoided. Overall, as in the folded flap technique for lining, morbidity is minimal.

Because equal or better results can be obtained with the folded forehead flap lining technique, without the risk of skin graft loss, it is preferred to the skin graft lining approach. The folded technique can be applied to larger lining defects up to 3 cm. However, both methods are reliable, less complex, shorten operating time, and are associated with minimal morbidity.

The modified skin graft technique has its most important application in salvage situations when lining is inadequate after forehead flap transfer by any lining technique. Rather than accept an inadequate airway, a lining skin graft can be applied prior to pedicle division to augment the lining surface dimension. If a full-thickness forehead flap has been employed initially, the flap is re-elevated during an intermediate operation; deficient lining at one or both alar bases is cut free. The lining gap is filled with a full-thickness skin graft. The full-thickness flap is reapplied without thinning to revascularize the skin graft. Once healed in place, the forehead flap is re-elevated thinly during a second intermediate operation, excess soft tissue excised, and delayed primary grafts placed to provide permanent support and shape over the augmented skin graft lining, increasing the size of the airway.

Microvascular lining with distant tissue

Especially "difficult" facial wounds are defined by their site, size, depth, and wound character (vascularity, contamination, radiation, immunosuppression, and exposure of vital structures). Such complex and often combined injuries to the adjacent cheek and lip may make local tissues inadequate or unavailable for nasal repair. The volume of missing tissues and the dimensions of the surface requirements must not be underestimated. Large amounts of healthy vascularized tissue will be needed to ensure primary healing. They require the introduction of distant tissue, by microvascular transfer, to re-establish the midface platform or to supply nasal lining.[75] A regional forehead flap can provide covering skin, but distant tissue, transferred as a microvascular flap, is used for lining or facial bulk.

A preliminary operation may be required to first return normal to normal, establish a stable platform, or delay or reposition residual tissues prior to the nasal reconstruction.

Principles of free flap nasal reconstruction

1. If missing, the midface platform must be re-established during a preliminary operation. When in doubt, reconstruct the lip and cheek first and rebuild the nose later. The nose must sit on a stable midface in the correct position and with the correct projection.

2. The septal partition is not restored to avoid excessive intranasal bulk and nasal obstruction. A septal fistula is accepted.

3. Columellar lining is provided only to provide a soft tissue pocket to position cartilage support and "back" the raw surface of the future covering forehead flap. The deeper septum is not restored.

4. The site and dimension of missing nasal lining must be identified. The vault spans from alar base to alar base and from the superior aspect of the defect to the base of the columella. If completely absent, this measures 7–8 cm transversely and 4 cm vertically from the nasal route to the tip with an additional 3 cm for the columella. Re-establishment of vault lining is straightforward because it must simply drape across a central support which prevents its collapse into the pyriform aperture. The *columella* must be long enough to project the nose and narrow enough to maintain patent airways. The *nasal floor* or *sill* is the skin platform onto which the nose must be placed. In many cases, the floor remains intact or has been previously restored during a preliminary operation to build the nasal platform. A floor deficiency may be obvious after

excision or trauma, especially if an open wound is present or, if, by history, the lip has suffered extensive injury. It is less apparent after injury due to cocaine or other intranasal processes. It may also be reconstructed at the time of free flap transfer with local tissue or with part of the free flap. Clinically, the upper lip is drawn back and up, identified by displacement and posterior angulation of the upper aspect of the lip. The tissue deficiency must be released and skin replaced under the future alar and columella inset.

5. The nasal reconstruction is planned in stages. Despite Gillies' admonition to employ "like" tissue, distant skin for lining, bulky rib grafts for support, or a thick, flat forehead flap for external cover are "unlike" the normal. The challenge is to modify these disparate donor materials into "nasal-like tissues" and integrate them together, restoring each anatomic layer to recreate a normal looking and functioning nose. The initial goal is to supply lining for the inner surface of the nose during a preliminary operation. Once in place, the distant lining effectively turns a complex full-thickness defect into a superficial one. Needed support and cover are addressed later using traditional methods using regional tissue.

6. Distant tissue can close dead space, fill a cavity, protect vital structures, create a barrier between the central nervous system and the oral cavity, close a fistula, or build a stable platform. Microvascular distant flaps are used to provide nasal lining and vascularity. Excess is used to refill the wound and provide for other needs – soft tissue cheek bulk, upper lip skin, nasal floor, etc. However, distant tissue always appears as a mismatched, discolored patch when it lies within residual normal facial skin. No free flap has a facial shape. Facial skin flaps, transferred as a forehead flap, must provide matching covering skin with the correct color and texture.

The midfacial defect with an inadequate platform

Often local or regional tissues are insufficient to restore a defect of the nose, lip, and cheek. In smaller composite losses, minor lip and cheek defects may be replaced with local tissues or with extensions of the free lining flap. Distant tissue, often harvested from the trunk, may be needed to provide sufficient soft tissue and skin – a scapular, parascapular, latissimus, or rectus flap – in larger defects.

The immediate goal of surgery is to provide an excess of tissue with adequate bulk and projection, obliterating an open maxillary sinus, if necessary. Both bone and soft tissue can be supplied. The facial platform is restored initially. Nasal reconstruction is delayed until a stable platform is restored.

Restoring nasal lining with a free flap

If the midface platform is stable, the nasal repair is begun.

Defects of the mid-vault alone

If the defect is limited to the nasal vault, only vault lining and preliminary central support are required at the first stage. Because of its thinness and long vascular pedicle, the radial forearm flap is preferred.

If the septum is intact and the defect includes only the mid-vault, the lining defect may be replaced with a free flap, skin inward for lining. Its outer surface is skin grafted. If the residual septum is intact with adequate height, it will temporarily support the lining flap until definitive placement of additional cartilage grafts and a covering forehead flap are placed in the future.

If the septum remains but has been partially resected, it can be swung out of the nasal cavity as an inferiorly based composite septal flap during a preliminary operation. Then the free flap is transferred for lining, once vascularity of the composite flap is assured.

If the majority of the septal partition is missing, it is not reconstructed. Local or distant tissue is too thick to replace the septum without creating airway obstruction. The surgeon only provides lining for the vault and backing for the columella. A permanent septal fistula is accepted. The flap is folded over onto itself along the future nostril margin. This allows placement of an autogenous dorsal cantilever bone graft for immediate central support. Subsequently, during the definitive nasal repair, the external skin graft or folded skin is excised. A complete subunit support framework is placed and the nose is resurfaced with a forehead flap.

Subtotal and total nasal defects: lining for the vault, columella, and nasal floor

Distant tissue has been transferred as cutaneous, composite helical, osteocutaneous, prelaminated, or prefabricated free flaps – with limited application and success.[59,60] The exception is the work of Burget and Walton[26,77–79] that employed multiple, longitudinally oriented forearm skin paddles to repair nasal defects. Two or three separate skin flaps were positioned, skin inward, to individually line the vault, columella, and nasal floor. Each paddle was vascularized by the underlying radial vessel, like a "string of beads". Their external raw surfaces were covered with full-thickness skin grafts, precluding primary soft tissue support. Later, the individual skin paddles were sutured together, thinned, supported with cartilage grafts, and resurfaced with a distally thinned two-stage forehead flap. During a subsequent operation prior to pedicle division, forehead skin was elevated over the mid-vault and soft tissue was excised over the superior two-thirds of the nose, as described by Millard. A second intermediate operation was performed to debulk the airways. Later, the pedicle was divided and a revision performed. Good results were obtained during six or more operations (Fig. 6.39).

However, limitations[9] are apparent. Elevating three separate paddles for the vault, columella, and nasal floor is technically tedious and leaves a short proximal vascular pedicle for anastomosis. Injury to the vascular pedicle during elevation, or kinking during positioning of these multiple paddles, could jeopardize blood flow. The vascular pedicle to each paddle is also exposed to injury during subsequent stages, which may compromise blood supply, already limited by the scars between the skin islands. The cutaneous scars between each paddle may lead to skin contraction and limit the suppleness of the lining. Because primary support cannot be placed under the initial external skin grafts, soft tissue collapse and skin shrinkage occurs. Most importantly, no excess tissue is available to salvage an imperfection in lining design or a complication.

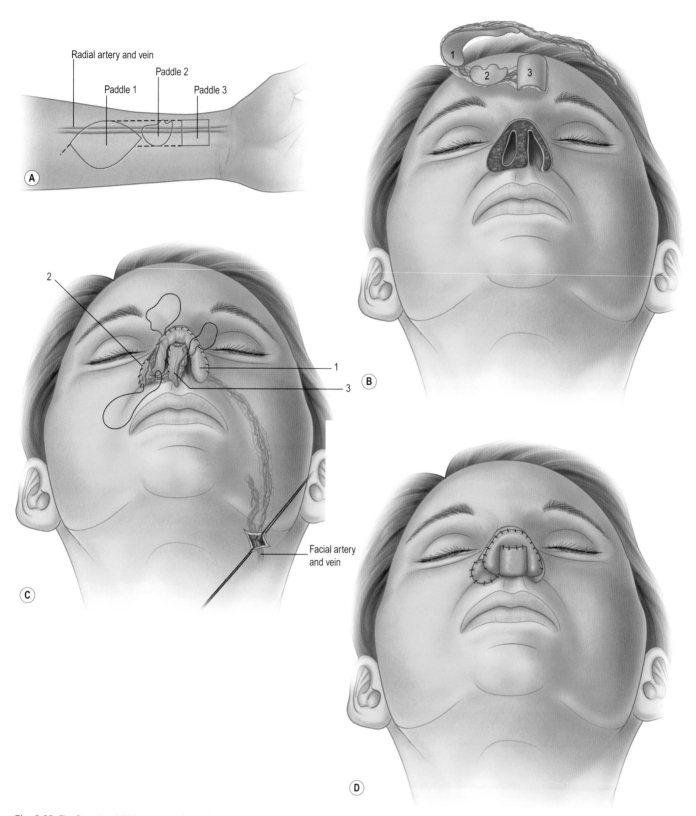

Fig. 6.39 The Burget and Walton approach to microvascular nasal lining. Individual radial forearm flap paddle design to individually replace nasal vault, columellar, and nasal for lining. Islands of skin, each perfused by the radial artery, are designed like a "string of beads" to supply lining for the nasal vault, columellar, and nasal floor. Their unsupported external surfaces are temporarily covered with full-thickness skin grafts. Later, the skin grafts are excised, excess forearm subcutaneous fat excised, individual paddles sutured together to complete the lining, primary cartilage grafts are placed, and the nose resurfaced with a distally thin forehead flap. During an intermediate operation, the flap is elevated over the mid-vault to allow local soft tissue debulking, maintaining the proximal supratrochlear pedicle in the distal inset of the flap to the columella tip and ala.

The use of a two-stage forehead flap, with an intermediate operation, was originally suggested by Millard[66] in 1974. He combined traditional distal thinning of a forehead flap with an additional operation, prior to pedicle division. The forehead flap was elevated over the mid-vault as a bipedicle, maintaining the tip, alar, and columellar inset. The superior two-thirds of the nose was reshaped. However, this forehead flap approach, which combines initial distal thinning of forehead flap and subsequent mid-vault elevation, has several disadvantages. Initial distal excision of frontalis muscle may decrease the overall blood supply to the forehead flap. It is more difficult to create a thin uniform skin flap when the forehead flap is thinned in stages. Precise contouring of the mid-vault is impeded by the bipedicle flap, which limits exposure. Most importantly, the contour of the distal inset – the most aesthetic part of the nose, is fixed. The shape of tip, ala, and columella cannot be altered after initial forehead flap transfer.

Menick and Salibian[80] described a folded single paddle forearm flap approach, combined with a three-stage full-thickness forehead flap for cover, which is a reliable, efficient microvascular design, applicable to varied defects (Figs. 6.40–6.46 ⊕).[14]

Figs. 6.42A,B,C, 6.43B,D, 6.44A,B,F, 6.45B,D,F,H, and 6.46B appear online only.

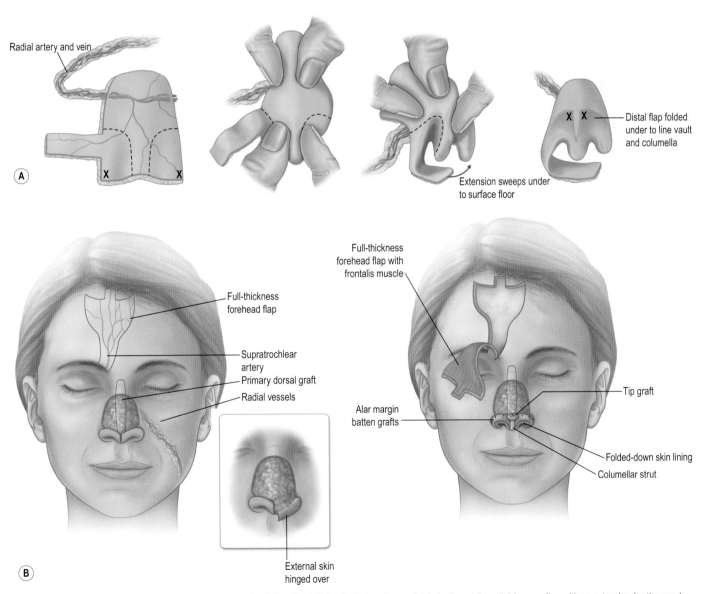

Fig. 6.40 The Menick and Salibian approach to microvascular lining. Nasal lining is designed as a distal single paddle radial forearm flap with an extension for the nasal floor. The flap is folded inward to line the columella and vault, the floor extension spontaneously rotates to resurface the nasal floor. More proximal skin is turned back to provide cover, creating a soft tissue pocket which allows for placement of primary dorsal support at the initial stage. Later, external radial skin can be hinged inferiorly to permit adjustments in the nostril margin of alar base position. Excess radial forearm subcutaneous tissue is excised, maintaining the radial artery pedicle intact. A complete subunit support framework is added to shape the columella, tip alar margins, and sidewalls. The repair is covered with a full-thickness forehead flap. During a subsequent intermediate operation the forehead skin is elevated completely, maintaining the supratrochlear pedicle. The underlying soft tissues are excised to sculpt a 3D shape over the entire nasal surface and permit placement or adjustments of cartilage grafts. The "thinned" flap is returned to the contoured recipient site and the pedicle later divided.

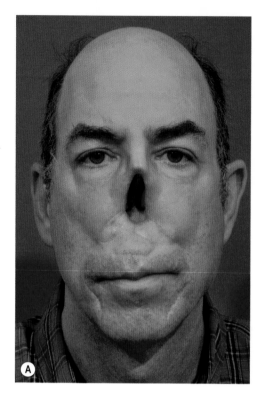

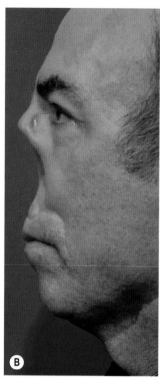

Fig. 6.41 (AB) Subtotal nasal defect after cancer excision and initial bilateral nasolabial flaps to resurface the upper lip.

Operation 1

A pattern of the lining defect is positioned on the forearm and face to verify the flap's size, outline, orientation, pedicle length, area of folding, and the position of the skin extension for the nasal floor.

A single, horizontally oriented paddle of forearm skin (8–10 cm in width and 6–8 cm in height), is outlined on the distal forearm, with or without a proximal extension for the nasal floor.

The flap can be raised as a skin flap, maintaining only fasciocutaneous connections over the radial vessels. However, it is safer to limit primary fascial excision to maintain maximum blood supply. An extension for the nasal floor can be designed vertically, in continuity with the primary flap, just distal to the future site of infolding, if the defect includes the vault, columella, and nasal floor. This positions the extension to resurface the floor when the primary flap is turned inward for lining. Because the single skin paddle is placed distally on

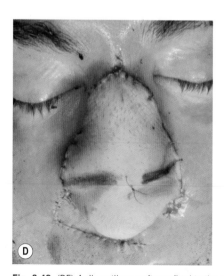

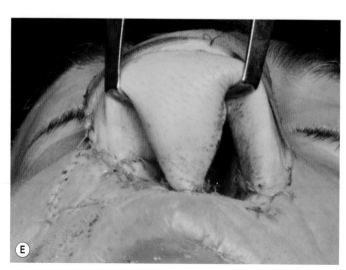

Fig. 6.42 (DE) A rib cartilage graft was fixed to the residual nasal bones to provide primary dorsal support and prevent soft tissue shortening and collapse. Because the missing nasal floor had been repaired with nasolabial flaps, a microvascular radial forearm flap was designed without a distal extension for the nasal floor. Its ulnar border is folded inward to create columella and pulled lining. The skin extension resurfaces the nasal floor. More proximal forearm skin and the radial vessels are turned back to provide temporary cover and permit placement of a primary dorsal osteocartilaginous graft.

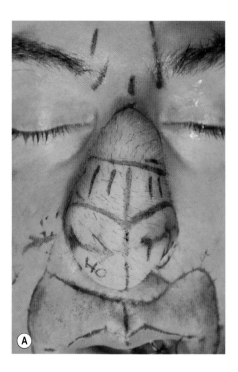

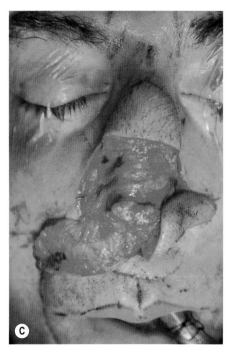

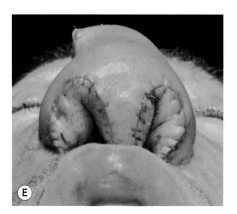

Fig. 6.43 (AC) Two months later, external radial skin is hinged inferiorly. The reconstructed "columella" is split in the midline. The nostril margin and alar base insets are adjusted. The radial vessels are left adherent to the underlying folded lining. Excess forearm soft tissue is excised to thin the lining.

the forearm, a 12–15-cm arterial pedicle and a longer venous pedicle (extended through the communicating vein from the venae comitantes to the cephalic vein) are available. Large high flow recipient vessels may be preferred. The microvascular anastomoses is made to the first branch of the external carotid artery and the internal jugular vein or external jugular vein as recipients. The superficial temporal artery and external jugular vein or facial vessels are used in the short fat neck.

The thin, distal ulnar edge of the forearm flap is pinched together in the midline, suture approximating its posterior raw surface to "manufacture" a skin columella which will later provide a posterior backing for the columellar extension of the forehead flap. The septal partition is not restored.

The distal skin is folded under the more proximal skin flap to line both vaults. The lateral, distal tips of the flap are fixed to the midline of the lining defect and then sutured toward the alar bases, from medial to lateral, completing the inset. The height of the columella and dimension of the vault are adjusted, and slightly exaggerated, by altering the extent of infolding. As the flap folds inward to line the vault, the skin extension spontaneously rotates inward to resurface the floor. The reconstructed columella is inset in the midline to the

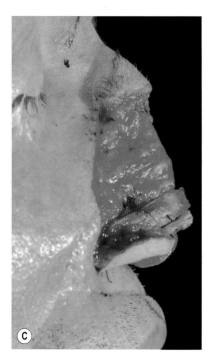

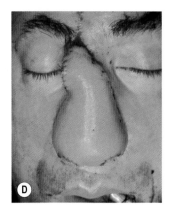

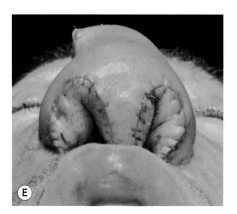

Fig. 6.44 (CDE) Subunit support is completed with a columellar strut, tip graft, and bilateral alar margin rib grafts. The repair is resurfaced with a full-thickness forehead flap.

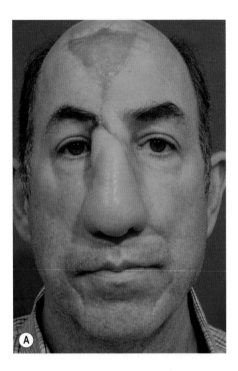

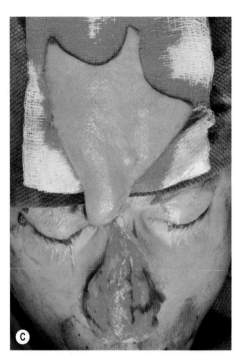

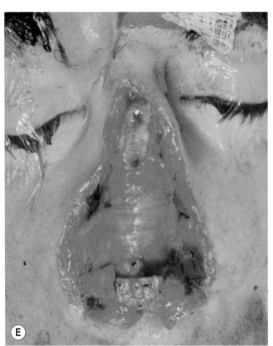

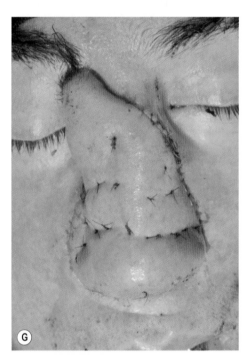

Fig. 6.45 (ACEG) During the subsequent intermediate operation, forehead skin with 2–3 mm of subcutaneous fat is elevated entire nasal inset, maintaining the proximal supratrochlear pedicle. Underlying excess forehead subcutaneous fat and frontalis muscle are excised to sculpt a nasal shape. An additional tip graft is placed. The "thin" forehead skin flap is returned to the recipient site.

residual or resurfaced nasal floor. Tension, tight molding sutures, or aggressive thinning are avoided.

Proximal radial skin, with the vascular pedicle, is turned back over the infolded lining. This places the pedicle externally over the mid-vault, on the outer surface of the repair, out of the airway, and away from the inferior one-third of the nose. The external skin is sutured to the periphery of the nasal defect to provide cover. A smooth, seamless, unscarred arching lining envelope recreates the nasal vault, columella, and nasal floor as needed.

In subtotal and total defects requiring dorsal support, an osteocartilaginous rib graft is fixed to the residual nasal bones or frontal bone with plate or screws. The dorsal graft lies within the soft tissue pocket of external and internal forearm skin. Residual rib cartilage is "banked" on the chest.

Operation 2

Inevitably, errors in flap design, malposition of the folded nostril margin, alar base asymmetry, scar contracture, or a complication, such as rim necrosis or dehiscence, require

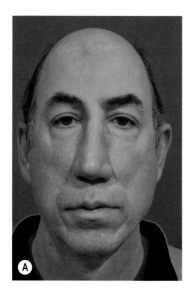

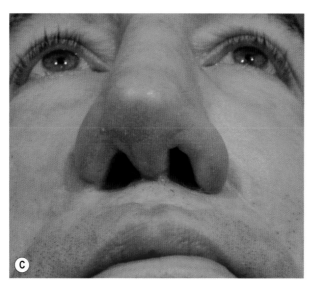

Fig. 6.46 (AC) Postoperative result after pedicle division and subsequent alar crease creation. A nostrils and create nasal shape.

correction. Two months later, excess external skin is discarded or hinged downward to adjust nasal length and modify the nostril rim and the alar base positions in symmetry. External forearm skin, with a few millimeters of subcutaneous fat, is elevated and turned over inferiorly. The hinged-over skin is trimmed to refine or reposition the nostril margins or alar bases, if needed. The external cutaneous surface of the columella is split in the midline. If lining for the columella was not included in the initial vault design or is unavailable due to tissue loss or wound separation with retraction, the external vault excess can be turned over to provide additional columellar or alar lining without delaying the repair or impairing the final result.

The vascular pedicle is not elevated and remains adherent to the underlying lining. The radial vessels, which perfused the folded flap through its external skin surface, are effectively "prelaminated" to the underlying lining. After elevation of external radial skin, the lining remains perfused through the radial pedicle and by its peripheral inset to the recipient site.

Excess subcutaneous fat and fascia, on the exposed surface of the underlying lining, are excised, protecting the radial vessels. This exposes thin, supple, unscarred lining. Delayed primary rib support (a columellar strut, tip graft, alar battens, and sidewall cartilage grafts) are fixed to each other and to the previously positioned dorsal graft to complete the subunit support framework. The base of the columellar strut is sutured to the nasal spine through a buccal incision. A full-thickness forehead flap, with or without expansion and without distal thinning, is transferred for permanent nasal cover.

Operation 3

One month later, the forehead flap is delayed. Forehead skin with 2–3 mm of subcutaneous forehead fat is completely elevated from the recipient site, maintaining an intact supratrochlear pedicle. With complete visualization, the underlying exposed subcutaneous fat and frontalis muscle are artistically excised over the entire nasal surface, including the tip and ala. Previously placed cartilage grafts are sculpted, repositioned, or augmented to shape an ideal 3D support framework. Forehead skin, now with the thinness of nasal skin, is replaced on the recipient site.

Operation 4

One month later, the forehead pedicle is divided.

Further debulking of the airway, by excising excess soft tissue between the lining and cartilage grafts, can be performed through nostril marginal incisions at pedicle division or during a later revision.

Operation 5

Four months later, a revision is performed to improve the forehead scar, define the alar creases by direct incision, add a secondary tip graft, open the airway, or trim the nostril margins or columella.

The result of any reconstruction will be determined by the choice of donor materials, methods of transfer, flap design, and the capacity to modify tissues to the needs of the defect. The ability to adjust the dimension and outline of each anatomic layer, correct imperfections, or salvage complications is vital. This blending of a microvascular distant folded radial forearm lining, timed rib grafts for support, and a three-stage full-thickness forehead flap for cover permits the integration of "unlike" tissues which can restore a nose which looks and functions normally. It is reliable, efficient, and reproducible. Good results – an attractive nose with patent airways – can be obtained in the repair of complex heminasal, subtotal, and total injuries.

The causes of intranasal lining injury:

- Intranasal cocaine
- Wegener's granulomatosis
- Killer "T" cell lymphoma
- Infectious disease – syphilis, leishmaniasis, yaws, leprosy, TB, actinomycosis
- Trauma – s/p septorhinoplasty, nasoethmoid fracture, intranasal cancer excision and radiation, pediatric foreign body insertion, iatrogenic catheterization injury, or corrosive inhalation

Primary intranasal lining injury

Nasal mucous membranes may be injured by immune disease, infection, trauma, or cocaine. The pathophysiology is similar – mucositis, lining necrosis, loss of underlying cartilage and bone followed by scar contraction.

The mucosal damage may be isolated to the septum, creating a septal fistula and subsequent collapse of the dorsum and tip and columellar retraction. It may extend onto the nasal vault and circumferentially onto the floor with destruction of the underlying bone and cartilage, leading to circumferential scar contraction and severe nasal shortening and lip retraction, respectively. Injury to the external skin may progress to full-thickness nasal necrosis, due to devascularization and infection. The process may also extend to the upper lip, hard and soft palate, maxilla, pharynx, and cranial base.

Isolated trauma (iatrogenic intranasal pressure or chemical injury) causes more local destruction.

The clinical deformity is determined by the site, extent, and depth of injury which dictate the technical approach to repair, not by the etiology of the injury. Surgical correction requires an accurate preoperative diagnosis to identify each aesthetic, functional, and anatomic deficiency.

The size of the septal fistula, the extent and strength of the residual dorsal and caudal strut (determined by palpation), the degree of lining contracture and external skin scarring (illustrated by the ability of soft tissues to be repositioned by soft tissue manipulation) and the presence of full-thickness nasal necrosis must be evaluated. Widespread necrosis of lining and subsequent scar contraction, rather than structural compromise of septum, is the primary cause of the severe deformity.

Restoration of central support alone, if vault and floor lining injury are minimal, may restore dorsal contour and tip projection. Extensive vault and floor lining loss require the release of scar contraction, recreation of the lining defect, and replacement of missing vault and/or floor lining with composite grafts, a microvascular flap, or hingeover lining flaps of scarred external skin. A forehead flap may be needed to resurface the nose if the external nasal skin cannot be re-expanded due to scar contraction or is missing. An extensive septal fistula is not repaired due its size and residual mucosal scarring.

Clinically, patients are classified by presentation.

1. Loss of support – Mild saddling, columellar retraction, and lip retrusion are due to a lack of support with otherwise normal cover and lining. The deformity is corrected by support replacement only.

    Onlay dorsal grafting and a columellar strut are sufficient if the residual dorsal and septal strut remain. In more severe cases, a cantilevered rib graft is fixed to the nasal bones and supported by a columellar strut fixed to the nasal spine. This re-establishes a strong septal "L" onto which the residual tip cartilages are advanced and fixed in position with or without an onlay tip graft. Mild retrusion of the upper lip is primarily due to loss of caudal septal support and is corrected by maxillary augmentation.

2. Lining necrosis – As the injury increases in severity and extent, the lining necroses and heals by secondary intention. The injury is often asymmetric. When isolated to the nasal vault, the nose increasingly collapses, shortens, and loses projection and the nostril margins retract. If it extends onto the floor, with circumferential 360° destruction of the airway mucosa, the upper lip is pulled superiorly with retrusion.

    Although loss of support contributes to deformity, release of scar contraction and replacement of the missing lining are paramount.

    If the upper lip deformity is mild and can be corrected by premaxillary grafting alone, the vault lining deficiency can be corrected with a composite skin graft, unilaterally or bilaterally. Simultaneously, a cantilever bone graft and a columellar support are placed through an open rhinoplasty. When the injury involves both nasal vaults and floor, the scar contracture of the nasal floor must also be released to reposition the upper lip. The lining deficit is resurfaced circumferentially with a microvascular radial forearm flap with primary dorsal and columella support grafts.

3. External skin destruction – If severe contraction of the external nasal skin or full-thickness necrosis occurs, all layers must be replaced. Commonly, skin loss is extensive but may be isolated to the columella or ala. Collapse and contraction may lead to nasal obstruction, with or without true stenosis of the nostril margins. Scarred external skin must be discarded and the nose resurfaced with a forehead flap after lining and support replacement.

    If the nostril orifices are adequate in size to permit satisfactory breathing, the nasal shortening is moderate, and the position of the upper lip can be corrected by soft tissue augmentation without lining replacement, hingeover flaps of external nasal skin are turned over along the nostril margin to line the distal nose. Support is restored with reconstructive grafts for the dorsum, columella, and ala. A forehead flap resurfaces the nose in three stages.

    If lining for the vault and floor must be replaced circumferentially or the nostrils are stenotic and must be opened to maintain the airway, the scarred and contracted nose is discarded and a folded forearm flap placed to line both vaults, columella, and the floor. It is turned on itself to temporarily cover the external nose and envelop a primary dorsal bone graft. Subsequently, additional alar and columellar support are placed and the missing external skin replaced with a forehead flap to resurfaces a subtotal nose or an isolated alar or columellar defect.

    Reconstructive methods and materials must be reliable, efficient, and available and minimize facial scarring and complication. Most importantly, the procedure must address each aspect of the patient's specific deformity. Some patients require simple support; others require local or circumferential lining; others need isolated or complete skin cover replacement and the complete array of reconstructive support grafts (Figs. 6.47–6.55 ⊕).
    Figs. 6.48A–C, 6.50A–C, 6.51A–D, 6.52A–C appear online only.

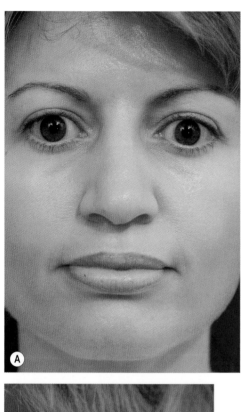

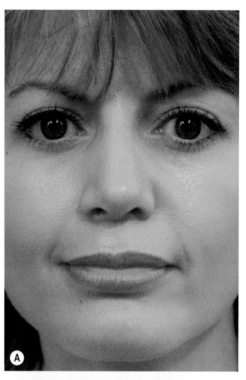

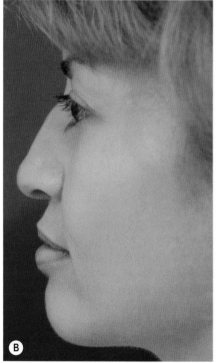

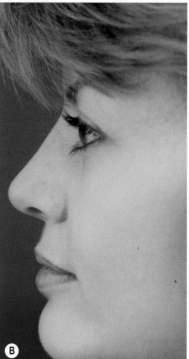

Fig. 6.47 (AB) Primary intranasal lining injury can lead to a septal fistula, loss of nasal support, significant nasal collapse and shortening due to scar contracture, and retrusion of the upper lip. In this case, a large septal fistula, the septum is destroyed and dorsal and tip support missing. The upper lip is retruded. But the injury to vault and floor lining is minimal and the external covering skin normal.

Fig. 6.49 (AB) Postoperative result after restoration of support. The septal fistula remains.

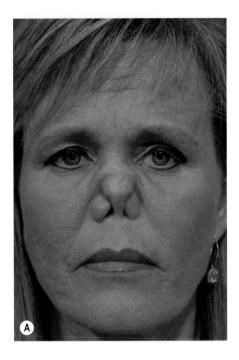

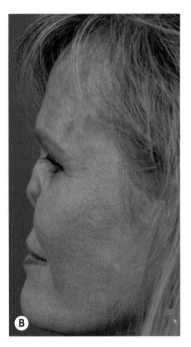

Fig. 6.53 (AB) Severe primary intranasal lining injury to the septum, nasal vault, and floor with subsequent scar contraction has collapsed and shortened the nose. A huge septal fistula is present. The overlying external nasal skin is relatively normal.

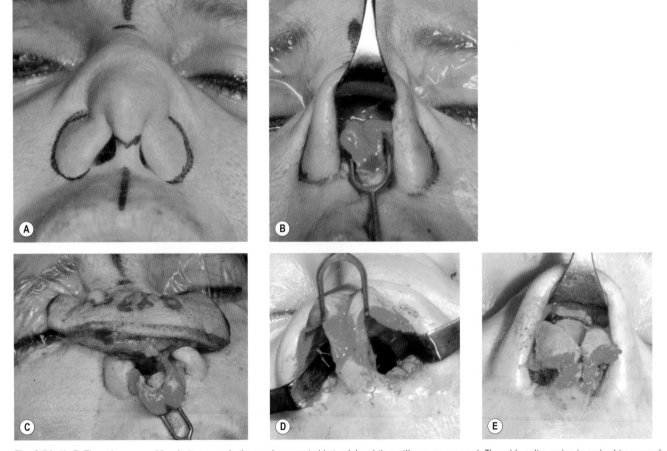

Fig. 6.54 (A–E) Through an open rhinoplasty approach, the poorly supported but uninjured tip cartilages are exposed. The mid-vault scarring is excised transversely at the dorsum, extending laterally along each nasal vault and then along the nasal floor to create a 360° circumferential release of the deformity. A 2.5 × 7 cm microvascular radial forearm flap is positioned to circumferentially replace the missing lining. A primary cantilever dorsal graft and columellar strut are also placed.

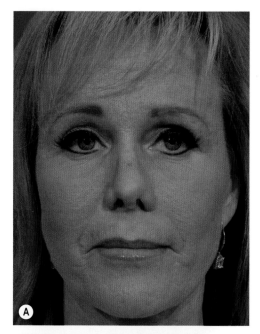

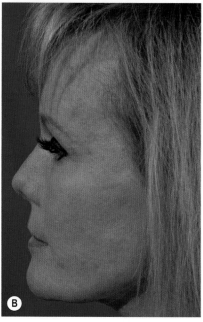

Fig. 6.55 (AB) Postoperative result.

Outcomes, prognosis, and complications

Complications are uncommon.[22,25,81] Fortunately, the abundant blood supply of the face limits ischemia and infection. However, badly scarred tissues, a history of multiple past operations, prior alloplastic implant, or previous infection increase the risk of complication.

If a complication ensues, the repair is almost always salvageable. The rich vascularity of the soft tissues of a full-thickness forehead flap, transferred in three stages, may lessen the risk of complications and allow more reliable treatment. However, a complication is of great concern due the potential loss of the building materials and the emotional stress on the

patient and surgeon. Correction may prolong the reconstruction and increase the number of stages. The patient may have to live with undivided pedicle until the problem is resolved, the tissues have matured, and unplanned procedures are performed. This may require an early reoperation or a postponement of a previously scheduled operation. But the complication must be dealt with. Most importantly, save the repair. If not, limit the damage. Preserve viable donor materials for another day, at the very least. Watchful waiting for the resolution of tissue loss or infection, with or without antibiotic coverage, is rarely successful.

Forehead flap necrosis is uncommon. It may be caused by inadequate flap dimension or aggressive suturing of the flap to the recipient site leading to tension on wound closure, failure to identify a significant old scar within the flap's territory, injury to the vascular pedicle, overzealous thinning at transfer, or excessive re-elevation of the flap from the recipient site at pedicle division. Ensuing cartilage infection is prevented by early local debridement of a significant covering flap necrosis (more than a few millimeters) and immediate resurfacing with a second vascularized flap (often as a subunit). This approach is often preferable to watchful waiting which may lead to progressive cartilage exposure, infection, and late severe soft tissue contraction.

Fulminant acute infection is extremely uncommon but may follow a failure in aseptic technique or lining necrosis. If limited necrosis of lining is identified prior to gross infection, early debridement of the necrotic lining, removal of overlying primary cartilage grafts, and skin grafting of the lining deficit are performed. The forehead flap is replaced. One month later, the skin graft will be revascularized from adjacent lining and the forehead flap can be re-elevated and resupported with delayed primary grafts. If the infection is severe, aggressive debridement of infected and necrotic nasal tissues and return of the forehead flap to the donor site, to preserve it for a later reuse, may be required.

Chronic cartilage infection presents as local redness with purulent discharge several weeks after surgery. It should be treated quickly with limited flap re-elevation and debridement of infected cartilage. It does not respond reliably to simple antibiotic coverage. Once controlled, delayed primary cartilage grafts are placed to resupport the deficient area 6–8 weeks later.

Revision

Complex nasal reconstructions often require a revision to re-establish ideal nasal form and function.[83] Exact templates, based on the contralateral normal or ideal, guide the revision, which is performed under general anesthesia, without local anesthesia, to avoid intraoperative distortion and blanching (Figs. 6.56–6.62).

Revisions can be classified[25,82,83] as:

Minor: Essential quality, outline, and contour are restored with inadequate landmark definition.

Major: Failure of dimension, volume, contour, and symmetry or function.

Redo: Cover and lining are grossly deficient. Normal must be returned to normal and the repair redone with a second regional flap.

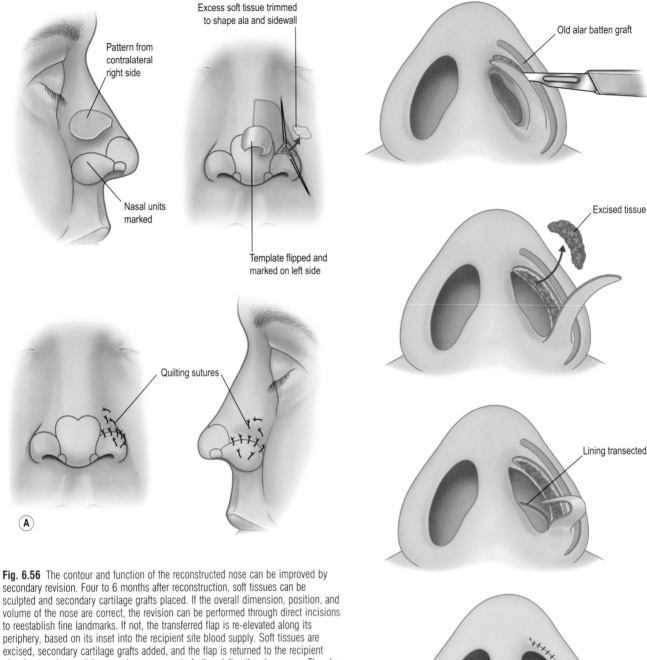

Fig. 6.56 The contour and function of the reconstructed nose can be improved by secondary revision. Four to 6 months after reconstruction, soft tissues can be sculpted and secondary cartilage grafts placed. If the overall dimension, position, and volume of the nose are correct, the revision can be performed through direct incisions to reestablish fine landmarks. If not, the transferred flap is re-elevated along its periphery, based on its inset into the recipient site blood supply. Soft tissues are excised, secondary cartilage grafts added, and the flap is returned to the recipient site. A secondary revision may be necessary to further define the alar crease. The alar crease is re-created by direct incision, based on the contralateral normal or on the ideal. Disregarding old scars, an incision at the ideal alar crease position, thin skin flaps were elevated superiorly and inferiorly a sculptured excision to restore the shape of the convex ala, a crisp alar crease, and a flat sidewall. A thick alar rim and a stenotic nostril can be improved. The ideal alar margin is incised and lining elevated thinly. Excessive subcutaneous bulk is excised between the lining and deep surface of the old alar margin Support grafts to thin the lining and the nostril margin. The stenotic lining is incised at right angles to the nostril margin. Excess skin along the inferior edge of the nostril margin is transferred as a superiorly or inferiorly based skin flap to fill the lining gap and increase the dimension of the nostril.

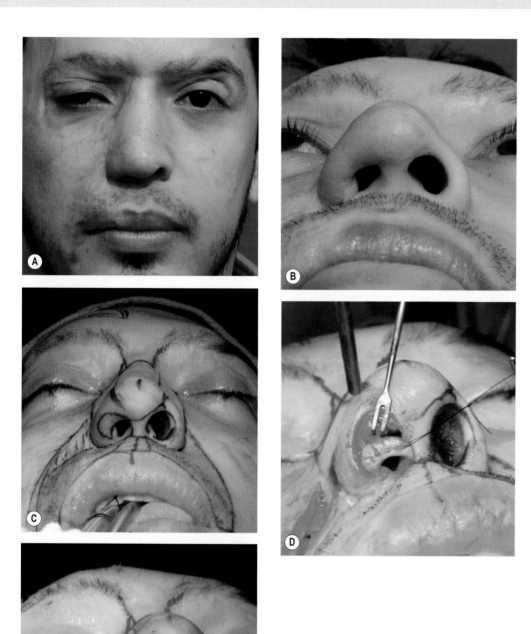

Fig. 6.57 (A–E) After complex facial fractures and soft tissue avulsion of the forehead, cheek, and nose, a full-thickness defect of the right tip and ala was repaired with a cervical tube flap and cartilage grafts. The right alar rim is thick; the nostril small; the nostril margins asymmetric; and the alar crease and nasal labial fold absent. The ideal alar crease, nasal labial fold, and nostril are marked with ink based on pattern to the contralateral normal. The nostril margin is incised and the lining elevated thinly. Excess bulk is excised between the lining and the previously positioned alar margin support graft. The lining was transected laterally at the alar base and excess tissue within the thick nostril margin transposed with inferior base to fill a lining deficiency.

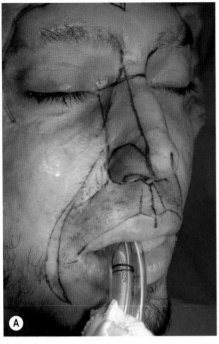
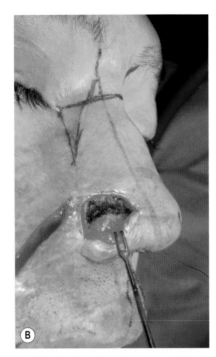
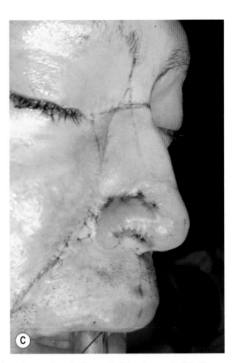

Fig. 6.58 (A–C) At the same time, direct incisions were made within the ideal alar crease and nasal labial fold based on pattern to the contralateral normal. Skin flaps were elevated and soft tissues are excised to sculpt a round ala, flat sidewall, and flat hairless triangle of the upper lip.

The minor revision

When the overall dimension and volume of the nose are correct, "finesse definition" is achieved through direct incisions hidden in the joins between subunits, disregarding old scars. The alar crease or nasolabial fold is defined and secondary support placed. A minor revision can often be accomplished in one stage.

The nostril margin and columella are thick and the airway stenotic. The nostril margin is incised, separating cover and lining. Lining is elevated thinly into the airway. Excess subcutaneous fat and scar are excised between the lining layer and the deep surface of previously positioned support grafts, debulking the airway. The lining is incised in the anterior vestibule and/or nasal floor at right angles to the nostril margin. Skin excess, from the thick reconstructed alar rim and columella or from the lip, inferior to the nostril floor, is transposed, as small flaps, to fill the gap and augment the lining deficiency, opening the airway.

The major revision

When the nose is shapeless and bulky, "gross debulking" is performed through peripheral incisions around the border of the flap. The random blood supply of the old flap permits re-elevation of at least 80% of inset, permitting wide exposure. Underlying soft tissue and support are modified by sculpting excision and secondary cartilage grafting.

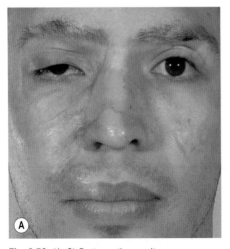
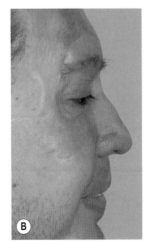
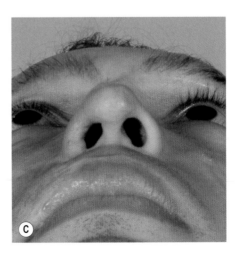

Fig. 6.59 (A–C) Postoperative result.

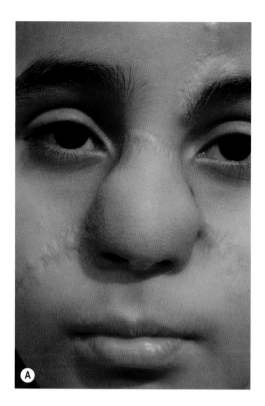

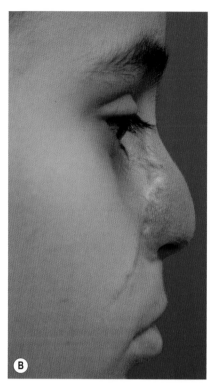

Fig. 6.60 (AB) Some years previously, a congenital nevus of the nose and cheek had been excised in this eight-year-old boy and the nose resurfaced with a two-stage forehead flap. No alar rim support had been placed. The nose remains shapeless and the tip and alar rims collapsed and unsupported.

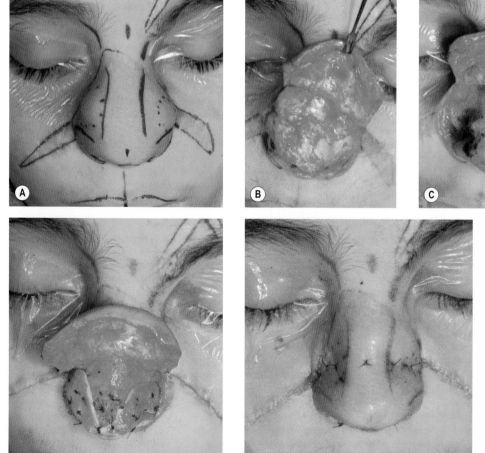

Fig. 6.61 (A–E) The old forehead flap is elevated on a superior base. Approximately 80% of the flaps inset were re-elevated to expose excess bulky soft tissue and inclusion cysts. The soft tissues were excised to sculpt a nasal shape and secondary ear cartilage grafts placed to support the alar rims and projected tip. The forehead flap was then returned to the recipient site with peripheral and quilting sutures.

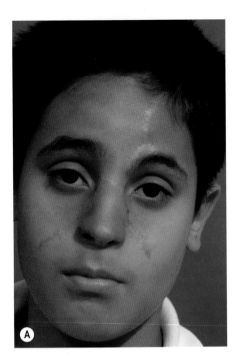

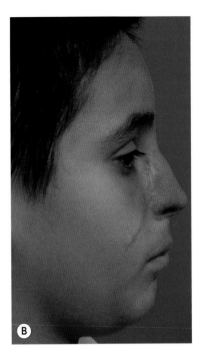

Fig. 6.62 (AB) Postoperative results without revision. An old forehead flap can be extensively re-elevated, underlying soft tissue sculpted, secondary cartilage grafts added. The overlying flap can be resupported and shaped by soft tissue sculpting and secondary cartilage grafts.

When all anatomical layers are fibrotic, the forehead flap is re-elevated with a few millimeters of subcutaneous fat. Scarred soft tissue and poorly designed support are completely excised. After excision of scar, the thinned cover and lining often re-expand and can be reshaped with a new, complete rigid support.

A second finesse revision, through direct incisions, will often be needed to improve landmark definition.

The redo

If tissues are grossly deficient, the repair must be redone using a second regional flap. The defect is recreated, tissues are returned to their normal position, the deficiencies of cover, lining, and support identified and replaced.

🌐 Bonus images for this chapter can be found online at

http://www.expertconsult.com

Fig. 6.5 (A–E) Nasal defect after excision of basal cell carcinoma of the medial ala and tip resurfaced with one stage nasolabial flap. No revision.

Fig. 6.7 (A–E) Subunit reconstruction of left ala with two-stage nasolabial flap. The subunits of the nose are marked with ink. A template of the right contralateral alar subunit will define the dimension and outline of the nasal labial flap and the primary cartilage graft. Residual skin within the left alar subunit is excised. A primary ear cartilage graft is fixed to support the alar lining. A subunit superiorly based axial nasolabial flap was elevated to resurface the alar subunit.

Fig. 6.8 (A–E) One month later, the pedicle is divided, the nasal inset is partially elevated, and the underlying excess soft tissue bulk excised to create a convex alar contour and deep alar crease. Excess skin is excised and the flap inset completed. The cheek is closed to lie exactly within the nasal labial fold. No revision.

Fig. 6.9 (A–E) Two-stage paramedian forehead flap resurfacing of the ala as a subunit. After Mohs excision of a basal cell carcinoma, greater than 50% of the left alar skin is missing. The nasal subunits are marked with ink. Excess skin within the alar subunit is discarded. The lining is supported with a primary ear cartilage graft. A right paramedian forehead flap is designed vertically over the supratrochlear vessels. It is thin distally and transferred to the defect.

Fig. 6.10 (A–F) One month later, the forehead pedicle was divided. Skin within the superior aspect of the recipient site is elevated thinly an underlying the cutaneous fat and primary cartilage graft is excised to sculpt a convex ala and deep alar crease. Excess skin history and in the inset is completed with quilting sutures in a single layer of fine peripheral sutures. No revision.

Fig. 6.12 (B) A new Mohs defect of the nasal tip lies within a nose previously reconstructed with skin grafts and a left composite flap for cover and lining. The left rim is retracted.

Fig. 6.13 (A,B) The subunits of the nose are marked. A subunit excision of the tip and both ala, but not of the dorsum is performed. Skin of the old composite skin graft is hinged over for a left nasal rim lining. Primary cartilage grafts of ear cartilage are placed to support, brace, and shape the lining and future cover.

Fig. 6.14 (A,C,D) A full-thickness paramedian forehead flap is elevated under the frontalis. The forehead flap contains skin, subcutaneous fat, and all its frontalis layers. It is transferred to resurface the nose without thinning.

Fig. 6.15 (B) One month later, forehead skin with 2–3 mm of subcutaneous fat is elevated completely to expose the entire reconstruction. The flap is temporarily placed on the forehead.

Fig. 6.16 (B–D) Remaining subcutaneous fat and frontalis are now excised to sculpt a nasal shape. Previous primary cartilage grafts healed to the underlying lining can be modified. The uniformly thin forehead flap is returned to the recipient site. It is fixed in place with peripheral sutures and temporarily molded to the contoured surface with percutaneous quilting sutures.

Fig. 6.20 (A,C) A preliminary operation was performed to place a forehead expander and perform an open rhinoplasty to lower the radix, narrow the nasal bones, harvest septal cartilage for a future procedure, and advance the old scars onto the nasal subunit. Two months later, the nasal tip and ala were excised as a subunit and all scars excised over the dorsum and sidewall. Lateral skin was advanced almost to the dorsal line to modify the defect. A columellar strut with advancement of the residual medial crura and ear cartilage alar battens supported the tip. A septal cartilage graft shaped the dorsum. A full-thickness forehead flap was transferred to resurface the defect. The position and symmetry of the alar rims seems correct intraoperatively.

Fig. 6.21 (A,B,D,E,H) One month later, due to scar contracture, support shift, or an imperfect design, the alar rims were asymmetric. During the planned intermediate operation, the forehead skin was elevated with 2–3 mm of subcutaneous fat. The excess underlying subcutaneous fat and frontalis were excised to sculpt an ideal nasal shape. Lining along each rim was released, hinged inferiorly, and positioned with additional delayed primary ear cartilage grafts to reposition the nostril margins inferiorly and in symmetry. The thin forehead flap was returned to the recipient site. The forehead flap pedicle was divided 1 month later.

Fig. 6.25 (A–D) Blood supply and design of intranasal lining flaps.

Fig. 6.26 (A,B) Reconstruction of a complex full-thickness nasal defect with a three-stage full-thickness forehead flap and intranasal lining flaps. A large, full-thickness defect is present after skin cancer excision. Skin is missing from the dorsum tip left sidewall and medial cheek. The tip cartilages and left upper lateral cartilage are missing. Lining for the left ala and sidewall are absent. The medial cheek defect was initially repaired with a fat flip-flap and cheek advancement to allow reconstruction on the stable platform. This will be repaired with intranasal lining flaps and a three-stage, full-thickness forehead flap.

Fig. 6.27 (A–C) Six weeks later, the ipsilateral septal mucoperichondrium is elevated off the underlying septal cartilage and a hinged downward and laterally on the septal branch of the left superior labial artery. Cartilage within the exposed septum is harvested, maintaining dorsal and caudal septal support. The contralateral septum is incised maintaining a superior base perfused by the anterior ethmoidal arteries. Ipsilateral septal flap is fixed laterally to line the nostril margin and ala and the contralateral septal flap is transposed to provide lining of the nasal sidewall. Because the defect included part of the right ala, additional skin within the residual right ala was discarded to allow resurfacing of the nose as a subunit.

Fig. 6.31 (D) The intermediate operation of the modified folded forehead flap. One month later, the folded forehead flap lining extension is healed to the adjacent normal nasal lining and is no longer dependent on the forehead flap for its supratrochlear blood supply. The regional units of the nose and ideal alar margin are marked with ink. The forehead flap is incised between covering and lining along the nostril margin and the covering flap was elevated with 2–3 mm of subcutaneous fat. This exposes the underlying unsupported subcutaneous fat and frontalis muscle which is excised from the underlying lining of folded forehead skin. A delayed primary cartilage graft is positioned to support the ala (and sidewall, if needed). The thin forehead flap is returned to the recipient site for nasal cover. One month later (2 months after the initial flap transfer), the proximal pedicle is divided.

Fig. 6.32 (A,B,D) A full-thickness defect of the right ala and sidewall is present after Mohs excision. The regional units of the nose and the ideal alar base position are marked with ink based on the template of the contralateral normal upper lip. Templates were designed to replace the missing cover and lining exactly in dimension and border outline. A full-thickness forehead flap is elevated with the distal extension for lining and folded to replace missing nasal lining and the more proximal distal flap is turned back to resurface the defect. No primary cartilage grafts were placed. The raw pedicle of the forehead flap was skin grafted for cleanliness.

Fig. 6.33 (B,C) One month later, the reconstruction is bulky and unsupported. The lining extensions are now vascularized by the residual nasal lining and are no longer dependent on the forehead flap for vascularity. The ideal nostril margin is marked with ink and incised. The proximal forehead flap was elevated with 2–3 mm of subcutaneous fat. The folded double layer of so and is fat and frontalis muscle is exposed. The excess is excised in the lining skin is supported and shaped with a delayed primary conchal cartilage graft. The thin forehead skin flap is returned to the defect and fixed with quilting sutures and peripheral sutures.

Fig. 6.34 (B,C) Postoperative result after pedicle division and right alar crease creation.

Fig. 6.37 (A,D) One month later, the cover and lining flaps are separated along the ideal nostril margin and excess subcutaneous fat and frontalis sculpted to refine the nasal shape. The forehead flap is then returned to the recipient site.

Fig. 6.42 (A–C) A rib cartilage graft was fixed to the residual nasal bones to provide primary dorsal support and prevent soft tissue shortening and collapse. Because the missing nasal floor had been repaired with nasolabial flaps, a microvascular radial forearm flap was designed without a distal extension for the nasal floor. Its ulnar border is folded inward to create columella and pulled lining. The skin extension resurfaces the nasal floor. More proximal forearm skin and the radial vessels are turned back to provide temporary cover and permit placement of a primary dorsal osteocartilaginous graft.

Fig. 6.43 (B,D) Two months later, external radial skin is hinged inferiorly. The reconstructed "columella" is split in the midline. The nostril margin and alar base insets are adjusted. The radial vessels are left adherent to the underlying folded lining. Excess forearm soft tissue is excised to thin the lining.

Fig. 6.44 (A,B,F) Subunit support is completed with a columellar strut, tip graft, and bilateral alar margin rib grafts. The repair is resurfaced with a full-thickness forehead flap.

Fig. 6.45 (B,D,F,H) During the subsequent intermediate operation, forehead skin with 2–3 mm of subcutaneous fat is elevated entire nasal inset, maintaining the proximal supratrochlear pedicle. Underlying excess forehead subcutaneous fat and frontalis muscle are excised to sculpt a nasal shape. An additional tip graft is placed. The "thin" forehead skin flap is returned to the recipient site.

Fig. 6.46 (B) Postoperative result after pedicle division and subsequent alar crease creation. A nostrils and create nasal shape.

Fig. 6.48 (A–C) Through an open rhinoplasty approach, the external nasal skin is elevated, a cantilever rib cartilage graft placed to support the bridge and combination with a columellar strut which is fixed to the nasal spine through buccal incision. The retruded upper lip is augmented with rib cartilage.

Fig. 6.50 (A–C) Due to intranasal lining injury, the septum has been destroyed and the nasal bridge and tip are unsupported. A relatively localized injury to the nasal floor and vault lining with significant scar contraction on the left has caused significant nostril collapse and retraction.

Fig. 6.51 (A–D) An open rhinoplasty is performed. The nose is resupported with a cantilever dorsal rib graft and columellar strut. The residual tip cartilages are advanced onto the columellar strut. The lining defect within the left ala is simultaneously recreated by incision of scar and the defect filled with a 2 × 2 cm composite skin graft.

Fig. 6.52 (A–C) Postoperative result without further surgery. The airway is open and the nasal shape normal.

🌐 Access the complete reference list online at **http://www.expertconsult.com**

1. McDowell F. *The Source Book of Plastic Surgery*. Baltimore: Williams & Wilkins; 1977. *The modern surgeon differs from his ancient predecessors because of the knowledge that developed over time. This book combines reproductions of the early literature in plastic surgery with biographies and modern commentary. The origins of skin grafting, rhinoplasty, cleft lip, and palate, cross lip flaps, otoplasty, and facial fractures contributors are provided. Such history provides perspective and insight.*

8. Gillies HD. *Plastic Surgery of the Face*. London: Oxford Medical Publishers; 1920. *Gillies, the modern father of plastic surgery, clearly describes his experience caring for the massive facial injuries which followed the trench warfare of WW1. The modern principles of facial reconstruction developed and are presented through clear case analysis with excellent photography. His results are superior. Historical but pertinent today.*

16. Gillies HD, Millard DR. *The Principles and Art of Plastic Surgery*. Boston: Little Brown; 1957. *Gillies and his student, Millard, present a comprehensive overview of principle and treatments between WW1 and WW2 into the early 1950s. Core principles and ingenious solutions remain pertinent to any surgeon interested in facial reconstruction.*

22. Burget G, Menick F. *Aesthetic Reconstruction of the Nose*. St. Louis: Mosby; 1993. *The first modern text dedicated to nasal reconstruction. The principles of facial repair are presented with in depth details of varied cases and solutions for small and superficial defects and large deep defects. The indications and use of local and regional flaps, intranasal lining, and primary support are illustrated. The treatment of complications and secondary late revision are detailed. This book is comprehensive, yet useful, as an atlas for the surgeon looking for a solution to a specific clinical problem.*

23. Burget G, Menick F. *Nasal support and lining: the marriage of beauty and blood supply*. Plast Reconstr Surg. 1989;84:189. *The use of thin supple intranasal lining, combined with primary cartilage grafts, and subunit resurfacing with a two-stage forehead flap revolutionized nasal reconstruction in the 1980s. This paper illustrates the technique with superb clinical case presentations.*

25. Menick FJ. *Nasal Reconstruction: Art and Practice*. Philadelphia: Saunders–Elsevier; 2008. *This text complements and expands the fundamental principles and approaches described in Burget and Menick's Aesthetic Reconstruction of the Nose. Analysis, principles, materials, and recently introduced techniques are presented to repair simple or the most complex defects to with both traditional and more recently developed techniques. The use of the full-thickness forehead flap for nasal resurfacing of more difficult defects, the modified folded flap lining and skin graft lining techniques, the treatment of complications, and late surgical revision are presented in depth. The "table of cases", (a compendium of patient photographs repaired by case example within the text) provides a quick reference to specific problems and their solutions within the text to help the reader find the information needed to treat their patient's presenting defect.*

29. Millard DR. *Principalization of Plastic Surgery*. Boston: Little Brown; 1986. *Millard outlines an approach to both cosmetic and reconstruction based on principles. Every clinical problem or defect is different. Principles provide a tool to analyze the difficult problem and guide repair. Millard describes his approach, based on these principles, with wide and varied case examples that can be applied to clinical problems and how to live life in general.*

78. Menick FJ. *Optimal use of microvascular free flaps, cartilage grafts, and a paramedian forehead flap for aesthetic reconstruction of the nose and adjacent facial units*. Plast Reconstr Surg. 2007;120:1171. *Composite defects of the midface are those which combine nasal, cheek, and lip. Their repair is especially difficult due to the complex aesthetics and tissue requirements. The basic principles of repair and current approaches are presented to satisfy the unique needs of these defects.*

82. Menick F, Salibian A. *Primary intranasal lining injury – Cause, deformity and treatment plan*. Plast Reconstr Surg. 2014;134:1045. *Nasal mucous membranes may be injured by immune disease, infection, trauma, or cocaine. The pathophysiology is similar – mucositis, lining necrosis, loss of underlying cartilage and bone, followed by scar contraction.*
The mucosal damage may be isolated to the septum, creating a septal fistula, or may extend onto the nasal vault and floor, leading to circumferential scar contraction and severe nasal shortening and lip retraction. External skin injury may progress to full-thickness nasal necrosis. The clinical deformity is determined by the site, extent, and depth of injury which dictate the technical approach to repair.

83. Menick F. *An Approach to the Late Revision of a Failed Nasal Reconstruction*. Plast Reconstr Surg. 2012;129:92e. *Many nasal repairs with local and regional tissues require a late revision to improve appearance and function. "Minor" deformities, in which the overall dimension and position are correct, require finesse landmark recreation and airway debulking. "Major" deformities fail to restore the basic nasal character due to significant bulk and contour inadequacies. Revisions are performed employing peripheral border scars, new incisions, soft tissue sculpting excision, secondary cartilage grafts, and local lining replacement to open the airway.*

7

Auricular construction

Akira Yamada and Toshinobu Harada

Access video content for this chapter online at expertconsult.com

SYNOPSIS

- The commonest acquired ear deformity presenting for reconstruction is the partial ear defect.
- Apart from acquired ear deformities, microtia is one of the commonest and most complex conditions that present for reconstruction.
- Patients with microtia may have associated anomalies.
- Reconstruction is usually a staged procedure.
- Creation of an adequate cartilage framework is key to the success of reconstruction.

Introduction

What is the goal of ear reconstruction? "Creating a natural-looking auricle". The auricle is located at the lateral aspect of the face and is far away from the facial triangle (eye-nose-eye), where the attention of others is mostly focused. Therefore, the ideal auricle is smooth, natural-looking, quiet, and does not draw too much attention from others. Deformities (e.g., excessive protrusion, cauliflower ear, unnatural curve of helix, and dislocation), on the other hand, may draw the attention of others. Prominent ears may need surgery because they are likely to draw attention. If people do not notice that the constructed auricle is man-made, the goal of the reconstructive surgeon is achieved. If your patient continues to hide the constructed auricle longer than the wound healing period, that is most likely due to failure to achieve the goal mentioned above. The question is how we can construct a natural-looking auricle with balance and harmony. The aim of this chapter is to describe the strategy to achieve that goal.

Five characteristics of the ear

Tolleth[1] states "a proper ear requires five characteristics to have a satisfactory appearance: A posteriorly inclined axis, a

0.6:1 ratio of width to height, and three curved lines that outline its shape, suggest tragus, antitragus, and concha, and indicate a helix with its root beginning in the concha". This thought process may be interpreted as 1) Axis, 2) Ratio, 3) Key line, and 4) Detail (Fig. 7.1).

Anatomy

The auricle is difficult to reproduce surgically because it is made up of a complexly convoluted frame of delicate elastic cartilage surrounded by a thin skin envelope (Fig. 7.2). Like the inner ear, the external ear also has a spiral architecture (Fig. 7.3), connecting the basal layer to the top layer. The auricle's rich vascular supply comes from the superficial temporal artery (STA) anteriorly and posterior auricular vessels posteriorly. The author observes frequently that microtia patients with hemifacial microsomia have STA course anomaly. The sensory supply to the auricle is mainly derived from the inferiorly coursing greater auricular nerve. Upper portions of the auricle are supplied by lesser occipital and auriculotemporal nerves, whereas the concha region is supplied by a branch of vagal nerve. An understanding of the anatomy facilitates nerve block of the auricle with local anesthetic solution. First, the great auricular nerve is blocked by injecting a wheal underneath the lobule. After awaiting its effect, one continues injecting upward along the auriculocephalic sulcus, around the top of the ear, and down to the tragus. Finally, the vagal branch can be anesthetized without discomfort by traversing the conchal cartilage, placing the needle through the already anesthetized auriculocephalic sulcus to raise a skin wheal just behind the canal.

Embryology of the normal ear

The middle ear and external ear are derived from the first (mandibular) and second (hyoid) branchial arches. The auricle itself is formed from six "hillocks" of tissue that lie along

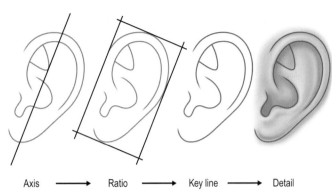

Axis ⟶ Ratio ⟶ Key line ⟶ Detail

Fig. 7.1 A proper ear requires five characteristics to have a satisfactory appearance: A posteriorly inclined axis, a 0.6 : 1 ratio of width to height, and three curved lines that outline its shape, suggest tragus, antitragus, and concha, and indicate a helix with its root beginning in the concha.

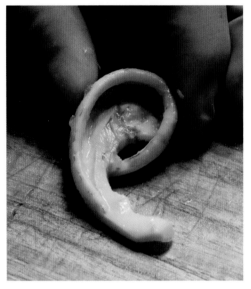

Fig. 7.3 Created ear framework shows that the helix connects to the bottom of the base frame (first level), climbing like a spiral staircase to the top of the frame (second level).

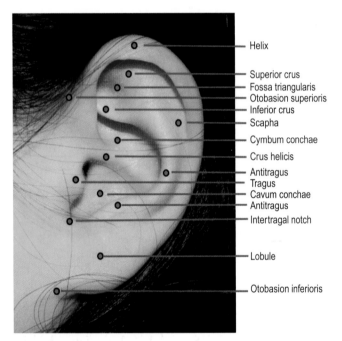

Helix

Superior crus
Fossa triangularis
Otobasion superioris
Inferior crus
Scapha

Cymbum conchae

Crus helicis

Antitragus
Tragus
Cavum conchae
Antitragus

Intertragal notch

Lobule

Otobasion inferioris

Fig. 7.2 Normal anatomy of the auricle.

these arches and can be seen in the five-week-old embryo (Fig. 7.4). Many microtia patients have atresia of the auditory meatus and tympanic membrane with variable deformities of the middle ear ossicles. Microtia patients may present with vestige and a patent or stenotic auditory meatus. Rarely, especially microtia in hemifacial microsomia, patients may present with anterior–inferior dislocated vestige and ear canal (Fig. 7.5).

Classification of congenital ear anomalies

Using a system that correlates with embryological development, Tanzer[2] classifies congenital ear defects according to the approach necessary for their surgical correction (Box 7.1).

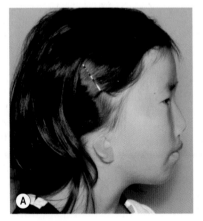
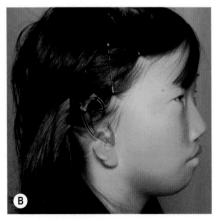
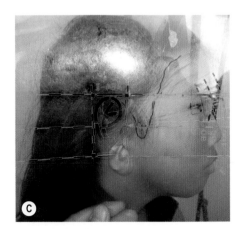

Fig. 7.5 Microtia in hemifacial microsomia; **(A)** vestige skin/incomplete ear canal are dislocated inferiorly. **(B)** Proper ear location is mostly covered with hairs. **(C)** Thirteen sessions of laser treatment eliminated hairs completely from proper ear location.

Microtia

Clinical characteristics

Microtia varies from complete absence auricular tissue (anotia) to a small ear with an ear canal. Nagata classifies microtia into three types: lobule type, small concha type, and concha type.[3-5] Microtia is nearly twice as frequent in males as in females, and the right–left–bilateral ratio is roughly 6:3:1. Approximately one-third to one-half of the patients exhibit characteristics of craniofacial microsomia. Brent found that 15% of his 1000 patients had paresis of the facial nerve.[6] Dellon has shown that the palatal muscles are rarely spared in this syndrome.[7]

Timing of surgery

The timing of auricular construction is governed by both psychological and physical considerations. From a psychological perspective, it would be ideal to begin construction before the child enters school, but autogenous construction should be postponed until rib growth provides substantial cartilage to permit the fabrication of a quality framework. Brent[6] begins ear construction at age six, when the normal ear has grown to within 6–7 mm of its full vertical height, and the amount of cartilage is enough for Brent-type framework. Nagata begins auricular construction at the age of 10, and chest circumference grows over 60 cm, at the xiphoid level.[3-5] These two different timings could be explained by the difference of the amount of cartilage required: Nagata-type 3D framework needs larger amount of 6–9 rib cartilage. In other words, surgeons are less likely to be able to fabricate Nagata-type framework at the age of six.

Epidemiology and genetics of microtia

Microtia (= small ear) is a congenital condition with unknown cause. Prevalence of microtia varies significantly among ethnic groups (0.83 to 17.4 per 10 000 births),[8] and is higher in Asian countries for unknown reasons. Eighty to 90% of microtia is unilateral, and 10–20% is bilateral. There are more than 18 different microtia-associated syndromes with single-gene or chromosomal aberrations; however, there is no causal genetic mutation confirmed to date.[9] Relatively common syndromes associated with microtia are hemifacial microso-mia and Treacher–Collins. Isolated microtia rarely runs in the family. Treacher–Collins Syndrome, inherited in an autosomal dominant fashion, often presents with bilateral microtia.

Middle ear problems

Treatments of microtia ideally involves reconstruction of the external ear and the restoration of normal hearing.[9] Hearing impairment in microtia is related to abnormal auditory canal, tympanic membrane, and middle ear. The problem is conduction. Typically, microtia patients have a hearing threshold of 40–60 dB on the affected side. By comparison, normal function allows us to hear sounds between 0 and 20 dB.

Regarding hearing restoration, most surgeons presently feel that potential gains from middle ear surgery in unilateral microtia are outweighed by the potential risks and complications, and this procedure should be reserved for bilateral cases.[6] Careful selection of the atresia surgery candidate is of paramount importance to achieve optimal outcomes and, more importantly, to avoid unnecessary surgery and its complications. The Jahrsdoerfer criteria[10] are widely accepted guidelines to select the atresia surgery candidate. Fig. 7.6 shows a patient for whom simultaneous framework implantation and atresia surgery was performed at the first-stage of auricular construction. V-shaped skin incision was the employed approach both for microtia construction and atresia surgery. Once the skin flap was prepared, subperiosteal dissection was performed to obtain access to the middle ear through the microtia skin incision. While the ear, nose, and throat (ENT) surgeon was doing atresia surgery under the microscope, the plastic surgeon was performing auricular framework fabrication at the back table.

The bone-anchored hearing aid (BAHA; Cochlear, Möln-lycke, Sweden; and Ponto; Oticon, Kongebakken, Denmark) has been used since 1977, which does not need a functioning middle ear or patent canal.[11] In microtia patients, BAHA was initially used for bilateral microtia with bilateral conducting hearing loss: unilateral BAHA is usually placed because a single aid will stimulate both cochleae simultaneously. Although traditional teaching was that hearing on a single side is sufficient for speech development and education, the evidence indicates both audiological and subjective benefits when treating unilateral conductive hearing with BAHA.[12-14] Indications are evolving, and reconstructive surgeons and otologists should work together to achieve long-term success in hearing restoration and auricular construction.

History of autogenous ear reconstruction

Sushruta (6 BC) was probably the earliest surgeon who performed auricular construction: repairing the ear lobe with a cheek flap. Tagliacozzi described repair of ear deformities with retroauricular flaps.[15] In 1845, Dieffenbach reported the repair of the middle third of the ear with an advancement flap.[16] This technique may have applications today (Fig. 7.7). Early surgical attention focused mainly on traumatic deformities. However, by the end of the nineteenth century, surgeons began to address congenital defects, in particular prominent ears (Ely, 1881).[17] The concept of microtia repair began in 1920, when Gillies buried carved costal cartilage under masts skin,

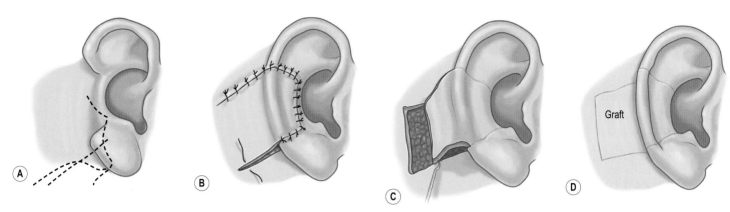

Fig. 7.7 Dieffenbach's technique for reconstruction of the middle third of the auricle, drawn from his description (1829–1834). **(A)** The defect and outline of the flap. **(B)** The flap advanced over the defect. **(C, D)** In a second stage, the base of the flap is divided and the flap is folded around the posteromedial aspect of the auricle. A skin graft covers the scalp donor site.

and elevated it with a cervical flap.[18] Gillies (1937)[19] also used maternal ear cartilage for more than 30 microtic ears; these were found to have progressively resorbed. Peer, in 1948,[20] diced autogenous rib cartilage and place it in a Vitallium ear mold beneath the abdomen. After 5 months, he retrieved the banked mold, opened it, and harvested the ear framework for microtia repair. Steffensen, in 1955,[21] attempted to use preserved cartilage, which resulted in progressive resorption of the grafted cartilage.

Tanzer is considered to be the father of modern auricular construction. Tanzer's excellent results in 1959[22] determined the dominance of autogenous construction with rib cartilage in reconstructive surgery. Surgeons from around the world visited Dartmouth–Hitchcock Medical Center, and autogenous construction spread with them. In the United States, Brent succeeded Tanzer in the early 1970s, and Brent's artistry[23] has influenced reconstructive surgeons for over 40 years and to this day (Fig. 7.8).[6] Nagata in Japan, a student of Fukuda (Fukuda visited Tanzer in 1963), emerged in the 1990s, and the Nagata (two-stage) method[3–5] gradually gained popularity and became the strongest alternative to the Brent (four-stage) method. To date, autogenous cartilage remains the most reliable material that produces satisfactory results with the least complications.

Alloplastic implants

Although silicon breast implants survive until today, the silicon ear framework is seldom used. The silicon framework, introduced by Cronin in 1966,[24] like any other types of synthetic materials, extrudes, causes infection, and loses definition in the long term. PPE framework, a newer synthetic material, was first introduced by Reinisch[25] in 1991. The advantage of PPE over autogenous construction is that it can be applied to younger children whose costal cartilage is less mature and not ready for autogenous reconstruction. The disadvantage of Medpore frameworks include: use of temporoparietal fascial flap, long-term risk of alloplastic implant exposure or loss, and compromise of any future autogenous options.[9] Although Reinisch reported a low complication rate, Firmin (European champion ear maker), Ortiz-Monasterio, and Brent[6] are strongly opposed to PPE framework because

of secondary referrals after PPE framework complications: The PPE frame may become stone-hard over time. Once extrusion occurred, the salvage would become difficult because the temporoparietal fascia was already used during the primary surgery.

Prostheses

Controversies remain regarding appropriate treatment selection for patients with major ear deformities.[9] This is especially true for severe trauma cases, such as extensive third degree facial burns. As the author described in the secondary construction section, natural-looking autogenous construction is possible even with severe burn injuries if you follow the principles of secondary construction.[26] On the other hand, osseointegrated auricular prosthetic reconstruction is complementary to other approaches and provides a reasonable alternative for poor autogenous options and poor autogenous outcomes. The disadvantages of prosthesis include intermittent soft-tissue problems, long-term maintenance, prosthetic remakes every 2–5 years, ongoing cost, possible compromise of future autogenous options, and the need for a compliant patient.[9] Fig. 7.9 shows a patient with 95% loss of his auricle due to third-degree burn. For this particular patient, many surgeons may assume that prosthesis would be the primary choice for this patient, but the author performed autogenous construction which is well maintained 8 years after construction.[27]

Total auricular construction in microtia

Author's method

Patient assessment

Twenty to 60% of children with microtia have associated anomalies or an identifiable syndrome; therefore, individuals with microtia should be examined for other dysmorphic features. Microtia is a common feature of craniofacial microsomia, mandibular dysostoses (e.g., Treacher–Collins and Nager syndrome) and Townes–Brocks syndrome; these conditions

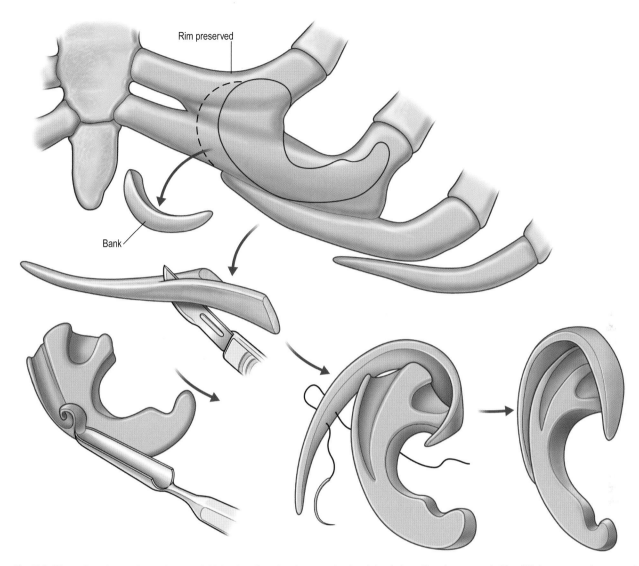

Fig. 7.8 Rib cartilage harvest for ear framework fabrication. Note that the upper border of the sixth cartilage is preserved; this will help prevent subsequent chest deformity as the child grows. The entire he upting cartilagethe sixth cartilage is preserved; this will help prevent subsequent chest deformity as the child grows. t covers thberately warped in a favorable direction by thinning it on its outer, convex surface. The thinned helix is affixed to the main sculptural block with horizontal mattress sutures of 4-0 clear nylon; the knots are placed on the framework on its undersurface.

should be considered among the differential diagnoses when evaluating an individual with microtia.[8]

Facial symmetry

Asymmetry of the face will make it complicated to locate the ear position. The location of vestige skin is sometimes misleading, and it influences the decision-making of surgeons. Even for expert surgeons, it is attempting to make the auricle based on the current location of the vestige skin, so the surgeon could apply their typical techniques right away. It is not uncommon that reconstructive surgeons create the auricle in the wrong location in hemifacial microsomia patients. The discussion continues whether we should correct the skeleton first or microtia first. The author prefers to address skeletal correction first; the majority agrees, because it may make it easier to identify the optimal auricular location (Fig. 7.10).

Skin envelope

Assessment of the available soft, elastic skin is critical, since it will determine the volume, dimension, and size of the 3D structure of the ear framework needed. If the amount of available elastic skin envelope is limited, you may not be able to place the framework with the size matched to the normal side. Imbalance between the skin envelope and framework may make definition of the auricle poor. Surgeons also need to check if there is any scar around the auricle site and inside the hair. Scar interferes with the normal stretching of the supple skin envelope, and may prevent good definition of the auricle.[28-29] Scar along the course of the STA could be the sign of a severed STA, the pedicle of the temporoparietal flap, which is a workhorse and important salvage tool for auricular reconstruction.[30] This is especially important for microtia patients with craniofacial deformities,

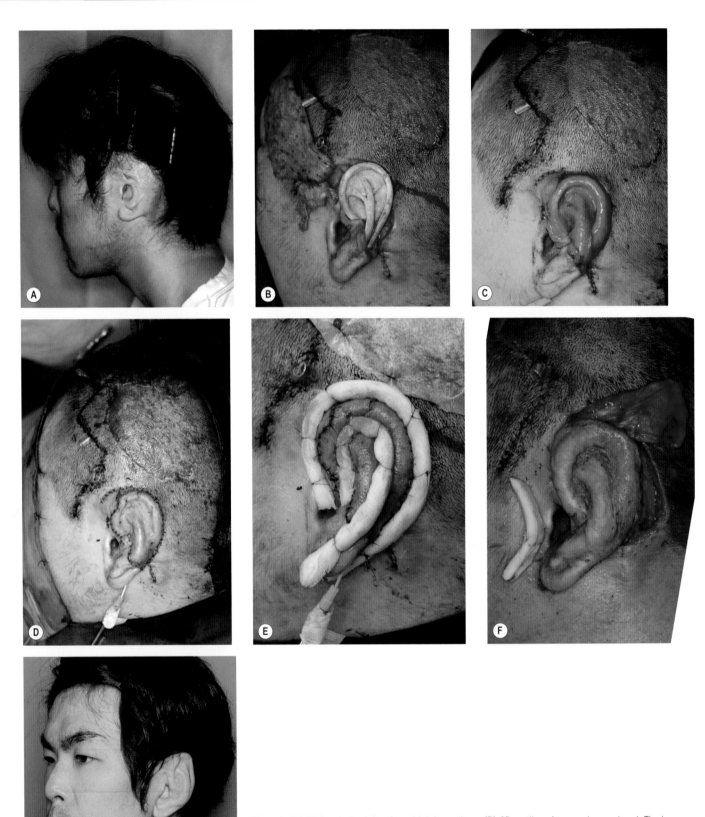

Fig. 7.9 **(A)** 95% auricular defect from third degree burn. **(B)** 3D cartilage framework was placed. The lower one third of the framework was covered with a local skin flap. **(C)** The upper two-thirds of the cartilage framework was covered with a temporoparietal fascia flap. **(D)** Split scalp skin was grafted over temporoparietal fascia flap. **(E)** Bolster sutures were placed to prevent hematoma formation. The temporary suction drain was then removed. **(F)** View of the second stage (elevation). To cover the posterior aspect of the ear, after placement of the rib cartilage block, a deep temporal fascia flap was used. **(G)** Eight years postoperative view of the patient.

such as Treacher–Collins syndrome. These patients may have a bicoronal scar due to previous skeletal reconstruction (Fig. 7.11). Surgeons should be aware of the past medical history, such as atopic dermatitis or sensitive skin, since the barrier of skin may be weaker with atopic dermatitis, and that would be the potential source of perioperative infection, especially with methicillin-resistant *Staphylococcus aureus* (MRSA).

Vestige skin

Since microtia has inherent skin envelope deficiency, how surgeons utilize vestige skin strongly influences the definition of the new auricle. The first thing surgeons need to evaluate is the location, shape, and volume of the vestige. These factors will influence the design of skin incision, and surgical strategy. If the vestige skin is located inside or near the auricular rectangle, the vestige skin is ready to be utilized for auricular construction. If the vestige is located far away from auricular rectangle, staged transposition of vestige skin may be necessary prior to framework placement procedure. The volume of vestige skin will influence the volume and the size of cartilage framework; if the volume/size of vestige is extremely small, the conchal cavity will be shallow no matter how deep you create the auricular framework. If the volume/size of vestige is relatively large, you will have more chance to create a deep concha by using the lobule splitting technique.[3]

Hairline

Surgeons need to recognize the presence of a low hairline at the time of initial evaluation to formulate surgical strategy (Fig. 7.12). The extent of low hairline influences the choice of surgical procedures. If the low hairline exceeds beyond the upper one-third of the auricular framework, either preoperative laser hair removal or intra-operative fascia flap coverage of the framework after hair-bearing skin removal may be necessary. The author routinely uses photographic analysis for surgical planning (Fig. 7.13); it helps locate the proper new ear location (auricular rectangle) and its relation to the surrounding anatomical structures. Photographic analysis tells us the presence of low hairline, the location of the vestige, and its relation to the ear, all of which will strongly influence the choice of surgical treatment. If the extent of low hairline is mild (Fig. 7.14) and hair covers down to scapula fossa, hair can be removed during second-stage surgery (ear elevation).[31,103] Fig. 7.5 shows an 11-year-old hemifacial microtia patient with over 70% low hairline. Laser hair removal[6] was performed prior to cartilage framework implantation. Fig. 7.15 shows a 100% low hairline patient with Pruzansky type 2A HFM. Low hairline microtia cases in severe HFM may develop shrinking of the new auricle after extensive reconstruction.[32]

Trapezium-space behind sideburn

The sideburn is not uncommonly missing in microtia patients. A missing sideburn may be the initial sign of hemifacial microsomia. If the patient has normal sideburn, it is an anatomical landmark useful for locating the proper new ear position. Anthropological study shows that the auricle is normally located approximately 20 mm behind the sideburn (Fig. 7.16A).[33] There is a trapezium-shaped, non-hair-bearing skin space between the sideburn and the auricle in normal anatomy (Fig. 7.16B). Avoiding placement of the ear frame-

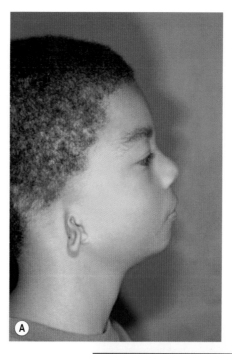

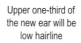

Upper one-third of the new ear will be low hairline

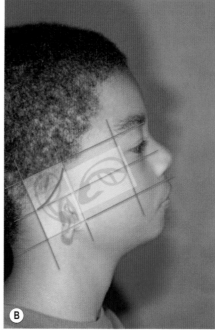

Fig. 7.13 Photographic analysis and surgical planning for a child with microtia. **(A)** Profile view of a child with microtia associated with hemifacial microsomia. **(B)** Photographic analysis revealed that the child has a low hairline and low-set vestige.

work in this trapezium is important to prevent anterior inclination of the auricle (Fig. 7.17). Surgeons tend to avoid the hairline at upper lateral pole, and ear framework tends to be placed inside the trapezium-shape space, which results in anterior inclination of the new auricle.

Location of the normal auricle

Leonardo Da Vinci is known to have analyzed the face, including the location of the auricle. Da Vinci analyzed the facial proportions in similar ways as anthropologists do today. To recognize the normal location of the auricle is critically

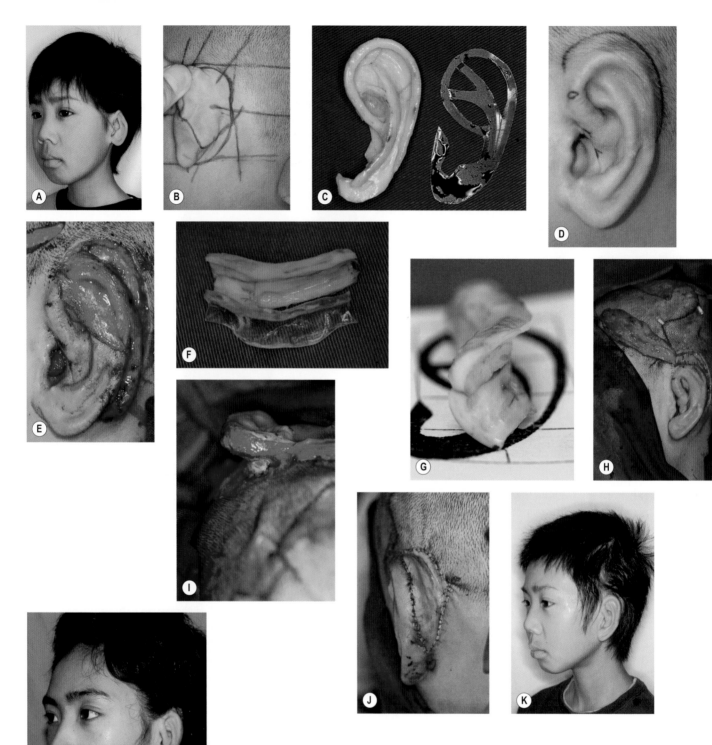

Fig. 7.14 Surgical sequence of two-stage total auricular construction for concha type microtia.[103] **(A)** Preoperative view. **(B)** V-shape posterior skin incision. **(C)** 3D framework with Nagata-type template. **(D)** View prior to second stage (elevation). Upper helix is covered with hair-bearing skin. **(E)** Intraoperative hair removal was performed. TPF was sandwiched between extremely thin skin and framework. **(F, G)** Intraoperative impression and fabricated cartilage block for elevation. **(H)** Second stage intraoperative view. **(I)** Temporoparietal fascia flap was raised. **(J)** Immediate postoperative posterior view. **(K)** One year after surgery. **(L)** Eight years after surgery. *(Reproduced with permission from Yamada A, Ueda K, Harada T. Surgical techniques in microtia reconstruction. (PEPARS 2012; 63:77–94 (in Japanese).)*

and dimension); only a few articles focus on the auricular curve itself. Harada and Yamada developed an auricular shape classification based on the curve ratio analysis study (Fig. 7.20).[36,37] They identified two key lines in ear shape: helix-lobule curve and concha outline curve. There are three major types of helix-lobule curve, types A, B, and C, and two major types of concha outline curve, Type 1 and Type 2. 3 × 2 makes six types of major auricular shapes. Normal ear shape may be classified into six groups based on this analysis (Fig. 7.21). Based on this classification, six types of auricular framework templates were developed as a guide for creating ear frameworks from autogenous rib cartilage (Fig. 7.20). Interestingly,

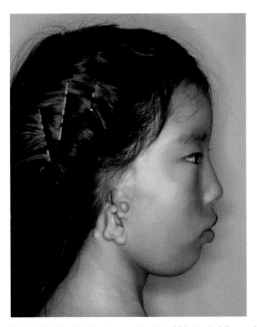

Fig. 7.15 Hemifacial microsomia with 100% low hairline and low set vestige.

important for surgeons to avoid the misplacement of the new auricle. A study showed that a misplaced auricle gives a less attractive impression to others.[34] The normal auricle is located immediately behind the face mask. Surgeons should avoid placing the new auricle inside the face mask, especially in hemifacial macrosomia.[32]

Auricular rectangle

A critical step in preoperative planning is to identify the "auricular rectangle," within which the auricular framework will be placed (Fig. 7.18). Placing the beautiful auricle in the wrong place is something that surgeons should avoid. The ear positioning template[31,33,35] is a tool to identify the auricular rectangle, which the author developed with Nagata (Fig. 7.19). Identifying the auricular rectangle is more challenging for microtia in hemifacial microsomia patients. Once the auricular rectangle is identified, the next step is evaluating the relationship between the auricular rectangle and the vestige skin. A decision has to be made on whether vestige skin can be utilized or not. If the child has a low set vestige in severe hemifacial microsomia, additional surgical procedures to transpose the vestige skin to make it useable may be necessary prior to framework placement.

Ear positioning template (EPT)

The ear positioning template (EPT) is especially helpful for secondary auricular construction, where many landmarks are missing and identification of the proper location of the auricle is likely to be difficult. Harada and Yamada modified the EPT in 2011; more anthropological references were added to the template, and the new template is made of an acrylic plate that facilitates surgical marking. EPT may be used to visualize the extent of low hairline (Figs. 7.12 & 7.5).

Auricular curve analysis

There are numerous articles on auricular morphology, almost all based on anthropological analysis (e.g., angle, proportion,

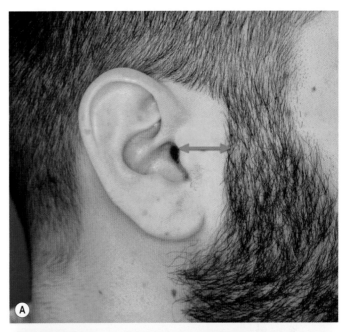

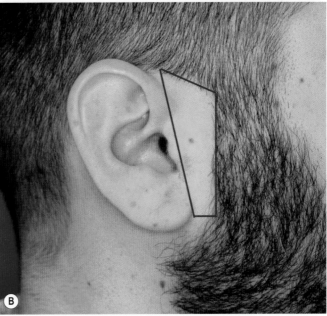

Fig. 7.16 Topographic relationship between hairline and the auricle. **(A)** The distance between sideburn and tragion (upper end of tragus) is approximately 20 mm. **(B)** The trapezium-shape non-hair-bearing skin exists between the sideburn and the auricle.

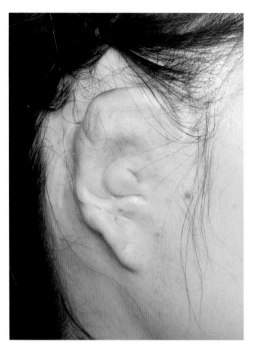

Fig. 7.17 Anteriorly inclined auricle that touches the sideburn.

Harada found that both the Brent framework and the latest Nagata template are similar to Type A-1 framework, based on the curve analysis (Fig. 7.22).[36,37]

Auricular template

When surgeons plan for auricular reconstruction, most surgeons use some kind of template as a guide for fabricating ear framework. The most widely used method has been tracing

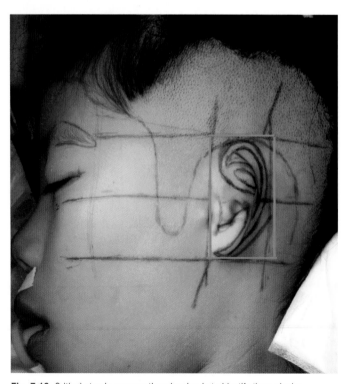

Fig. 7.18 Critical step in preoperative planning is to identify the auricular rectangle, within which the auricular framework will be placed.

the normal auricle with transparent film.[38] The author found that manual tracing looks easy, but it may not be easy to capture the delicate curves of the auricle unless surgeons have background skills in art. The manual tracing tends to be too big and too wide; such an ear frame template may result in poor definition due to skin deficiency. The other disadvantage of manual tracing is that the normal side is not always normal. Minor deformities, such as helix–antihelix adhesion, can disrupt the smooth curve of the helix; in such a case, the contralateral side is not the ideal template for the new auricle. Nagata[2,3,4,31] developed a single ideal ear template for all types of auricular construction. It is based on both anthropometric analysis[39] and Nagata's clinical experiences. Nagata slightly changed his single template twice (Fig. 7.23).[31] From curve analysis point, Nagata changed from uncategorized to Type B-1, and finally Type A-1. The author previously used the Nagata template (Type B-1) for the first 10 years of practice, then switched to the six types of templates which Harada and Yamada developed in 2009.[36,37] These templates are based on the analysis of normal auricular curves (Fig. 7.20). The aim of the six templates is to express the subtle, individual difference of the auricular shape as opposed to applying a single ideal template for auricular construction. The author applies the new templates to various ethnic groups, and believes these templates allow us to cope with individual normal ear shape differences.

A. First-stage of total auricular construction (Video 7.1 ●)

Markings

After the induction of general anesthesia, the author performs preoperative marking with permanent marker before the surgical preparation. The author uses the ear positioning template as a guide for markings (Fig. 7.19).

Patient position

The author uses semi-lateral position to facilitate simultaneous auricle site and cartilage harvesting. Since the duration of surgery will be 5–7 h, preventive measures of pressure sores are mandatory. Keeping the neck in neutral position is crucial to prevent C1, C2 rotary subluxation.[40]

1. Skin flap preparation

Lobule splitting technique for lobule type microtia

Nagata solved the problem of skin shortage in typical lobule type microtia. Creating a deep concha bowl may be achieved by splitting the lobule into two flaps (Fig. 7.24). The skin flap is more likely to create a deeper concha bowl than skin grafting or a composite skin/cartilage graft. Nagata described lobule splitting techniques in 1994,[3] and the techniques remain misunderstood by many surgeons. Contrary to Tanzer/Brent (full-thickness)[2,6] lobule rotation, splitting the lobule creates two flaps: anterior and posterior flaps. Lobule splitting technique is considered to be a modified z-plasty or application of Masson principle.[41] The author uses a #15 scalpel, with blade facing upward, and splits the lobule with a stabbing scalpel motion. Splitting continues down to the fascia level. After completion of the lobule split, the anterior lobule flap will be transposed backward to cover the anterior lobule portion of the framework. The posterior flap will be

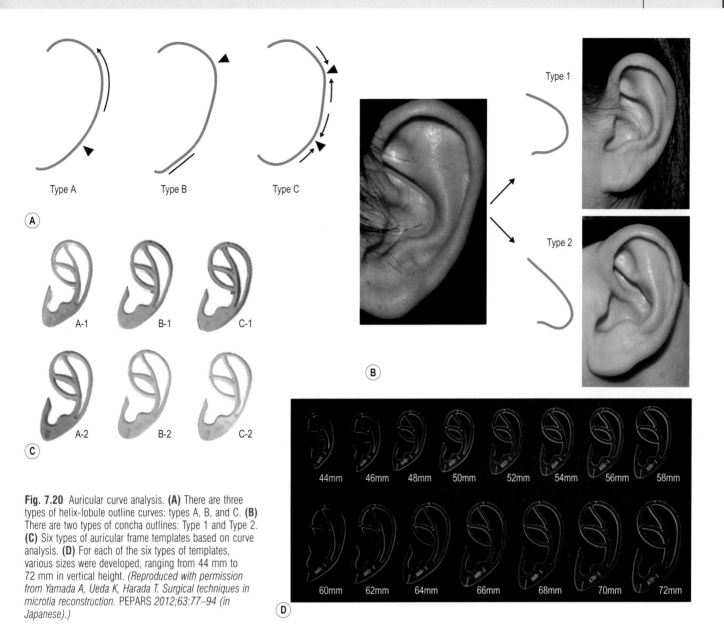

Fig. 7.20 Auricular curve analysis. **(A)** There are three types of helix-lobule outline curves: types A, B, and C. **(B)** There are two types of concha outlines: Type 1 and Type 2. **(C)** Six types of auricular frame templates based on curve analysis. **(D)** For each of the six types of templates, various sizes were developed, ranging from 44 mm to 72 mm in vertical height. *(Reproduced with permission from Yamada A, Ueda K, Harada T. Surgical techniques in microtia reconstruction. PEPARS 2012;63:77–94 (in Japanese).)*

transposed anteriorly to cover the posterior aspect of the tragus and concha cavity. Subcutaneous pedicle is preserved for the posterior skin flap to secure the vascular supply.[2] Firmin argued with Nagata that this subcutaneous pedicle is unnecessary.[42] Studies showed that the subcutaneous pedicle in Nagata's W flaps does increase the vascularity and decrease skin flap necrosis.[43,44] The author prefers to keep the subcutaneous pedicle because the pedicle will keep the posterior flap sticking down to the concha cavity; thus a deep concha bowl is more likely to be achieved with subcutaneous pedicle preservation (Figs. 7.25 & 7.26).

Skin incision for small concha type microtia

Nagata defines small concha type as the presence of a small indentation in the concha region (Fig. 7.12).[4] The skin incision is made along the margin of the small indentation, which is the difference from lobule type microtia skin incision (Fig. 7.27). The indentation is turned inside out to form an inverted cone pocket to cover the framework. The rest of the surgical procedure is similar to lobule type microtia.[31]

Skin incision design for concha-type microtia

Nagata originally (in 1994) described the skin incision as a z-plasty type incision with posterior V-shape design (Fig. 7.14).[3] Recently Nagata changed from V-shape to W-shape incisions (Figs. 7.28 & 7.29)[31] at the posterior aspect of the lobule. There was no explanation why Nagata changed the shape of the incision from V-shape to W-shape for concha type microtia. However, the author found that concha type presents with a higher location of vestige than normal lobule location. A W-shape incision has better freedom to transpose the lobule in the optimal location.

2. Removing vestige auricular cartilage

Lobule type and concha type is slightly different in the way to remove vestige cartilage. The author removes all of the remnant auricular cartilage in lobule type microtia for two reasons: vestige cartilage will not contribute to the auricular framework, and the vestige cartilage obstructs the smooth expansion of the skin envelope. Further, removing the vestige

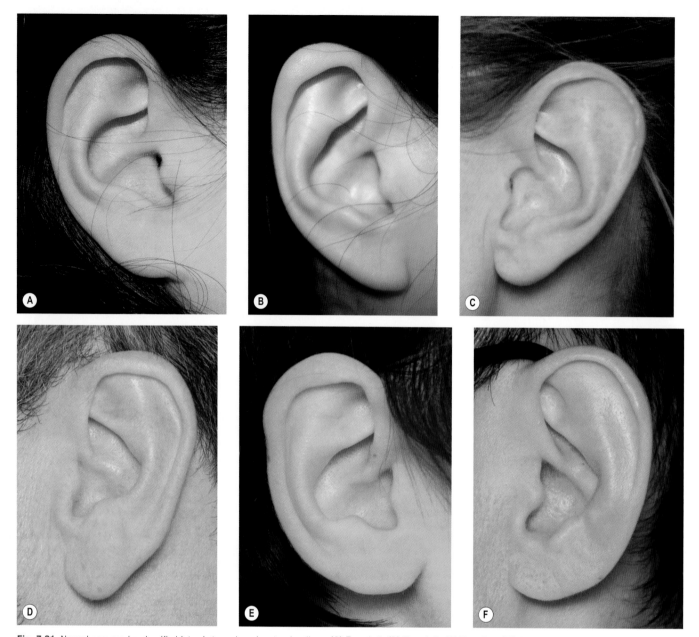

Fig. 7.21 Normal ears can be classified into six types based on two key lines. **(A)** Type A-1, **(B)** Type A-2, **(C)** Type B-1, **(D)** Type B-2, **(E)** Type C-1, **(F)** Type C-2.

cartilage will create a space to accommodate a new framework. In contrast, in concha type microtia, the remnant concha cartilage should be preserved as a cuff to facilitate the smooth transition of the concha cavity. The other important technical tip is that when you remove vestige cartilages, especially from anterior aspect of the auricle, you must preserve as much soft tissue as possible: anterior skin is extremely thin, therefore dissection of the vestige cartilage must be very delicate, and sharp dissection to remove only cartilage is essential, otherwise the chance of skin flap congestion/necrosis may be high. The author's preferred instrument for removal of the vestige cartilage is converse scissors.

3. Skin pocket dissection

The author uses small straight blunt scissors, aiming to create a 2-mm-thick skin flap (Fig. 7.30). The author does not use epinephrine injection for hemostasis purposes because

injection of fluids makes dissection less accurate, and it may cause vascular compromise of the delicate skin flaps. The extent of skin pocket dissection usually goes beyond the hairline border, up to 1 cm beyond the hair line. The author usually dissects hair-bearing skin again with 2-mm thickness. Because hair-bearing skin has more dense fibrous tissue than non-hair-bearing skin, dissection underneath hairs needs more effort. But, at the same time, surgeons must be careful not to dissect too much, and not to make the skin flap too thin, otherwise you may have vascular compromise of the skin flap. The author does not violate trapezium-shaped space in front of the new auricle (Fig. 7.16B) to prevent anterior inclination.

4. Instrumentation

Framework fabrication requires specific types of instruments: a carving knife and 38G double-armed stainless wires are

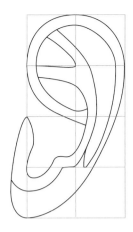

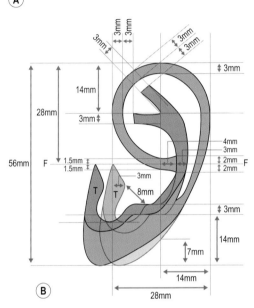

(A)

(B)

Fig. 7.23 Evolution of Nagata ear template; from curve analysis point, Nagata changed from uncategorized to Type B-1A, and finally to Type A-1B.

special instrumentation for Nagata-type framework fabrication. The author uses round, curved 2-mm, 3-mm, 4.5-mm, and 6-mm width wood carving knives (Mikisho Company, Hyogo, Japan). Because of a recent trend of restriction against wood-handle surgical instrumentation, carving knives with disposable blades (2-mm, 3-mm, 4.5-mm, and 6-mm) were developed (KLS Martin, USA). A 38G double-armed microtia wire (Medicon, Tuttlingen, Germany; Bear Medic Co., Tokyo, Japan) allows surgeons more delicate fixation of each cartilage parts compared with conventional 32 or 34G wire.

5. Harvesting costal cartilage

Simultaneous harvesting of costal cartilage and skin dissection in the auricle site is beneficial to shorten the length of surgery as well as lessen the fatigue of the surgeons. Brent harvests costal cartilage himself by attaching perichondrium to the cartilage. Firmin keeps the anterior portion of perichondrium to the rib cartilage and leaves the rest of perichondrium to the donor site, stating that the "deformation at the donor site is minimal".[45]

Nagata let the second surgeon harvest rib cartilage, leaving the entire perichondrium to the donor site (Fig. 7.31). Harvest-

ing rib cartilage without perichondrium attached is a safer technique than harvesting cartilage with perichondrium, in terms of pneumothorax risk. Preserving perichondrium at the donor site and adding leftover diced cartilage into the perichondrium sleeve is proven to boost regeneration of the cartilage/bone matrix (Fig. 7.31). This technique may cause less chest deformity.[46,47] The author uses a transverse 4–5 cm skin incision that usually has better scar quality than an oblique skin incision. After completion of rib cartilage harvest, the author routinely asks the anesthesiologist for manual inflation up to 25–30 cm H_2O to determine if any bubbles come up. Small tears can be repaired by direct closure. If there is any clinical suspicion of pneumothorax, a portable chest X-ray, while under general anesthesia, should be taken for possible chest tube placement.

6. Auricular framework

Creating the auricular framework is a fascinating, fun procedure, if you are properly trained. There are several simulation-type training modules available (Figs. 7.32–7.34),[48–52] which may be helpful prior to starting clinical cases. The architecture of the auricular framework is a critical component to create the complex and delicate definition of the auricle (Fig. 7.35). It is important to remember that the skin envelope to cover the framework is as critical as auricular framework itself: the balance between 3D framework and skin envelope is the key to achieving optimal definition of the auricle. Nagata-type 3D framework is distinct from previous 2D framework: the helix connects to the bottom of the base frame (first level), climbing as a spiral staircase, to the top of the frame (second level) (Fig. 7.3). The tragus component is also unique to the Nagata-type 3D framework, which is covered by the posterior W-shaped skin flap, created by lobule split technique.

Bolster sutures

Nagata uses classic bolster sutures for postoperative dressings that were popularized by Tanzer.[2] Brent uses suction drain postoperatively. At the first stage of total auricular construction, the author uses suction only temporarily during the

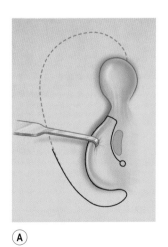

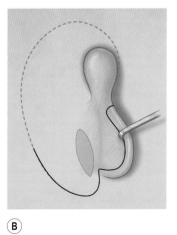

(A)   (B)

Fig. 7.27 (A) The skin incision is made along the margin of small indentation that is the difference from lobule type microtia skin incision. **(B)** The indentation is turned inside out to form an inverted cone pocket to cover the framework. The rest of the surgical procedure is similar to lobule type microtia.

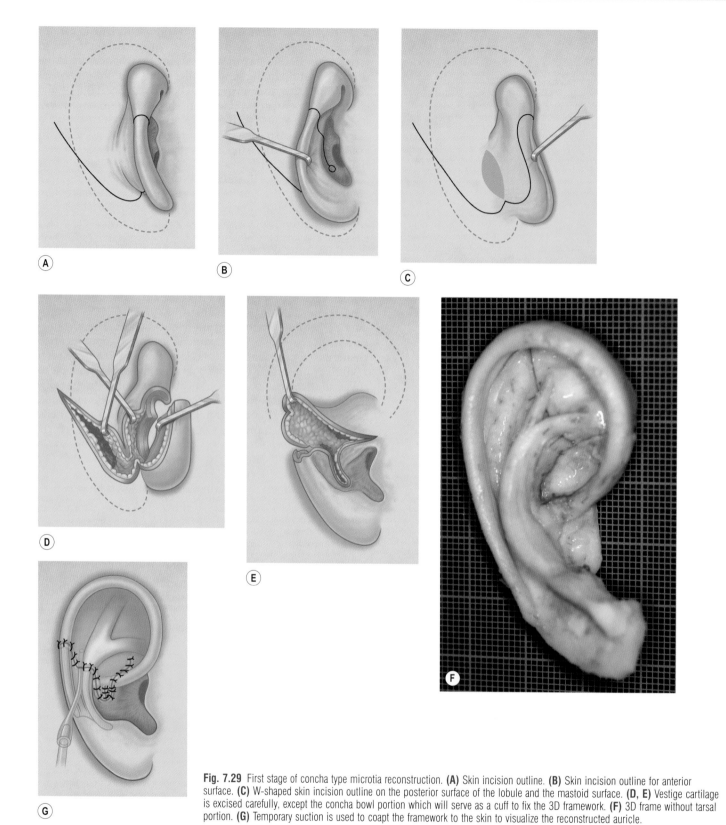

Fig. 7.29 First stage of concha type microtia reconstruction. **(A)** Skin incision outline. **(B)** Skin incision outline for anterior surface. **(C)** W-shaped skin incision outline on the posterior surface of the lobule and the mastoid surface. **(D, E)** Vestige cartilage is excised carefully, except the concha bowl portion which will serve as a cuff to fix the 3D framework. **(F)** 3D frame without tarsal portion. **(G)** Temporary suction is used to coapt the framework to the skin to visualize the reconstructed auricle.

surgery to visualize optimal skin adaptation to the framework. After completion of bolster sutures, the author removes the temporary suction. Based on the author's experiences, bolster sutures cause minimum hematoma formation. The author uses Xeroform with plenty of Vaseline-based ointment to make a roll of bolster, and uses 4-0 Prolene (SH-2 needle,

double-armed, Ethicon) for fixation. Dense roll and too-tight fixation may be the cause of pressure sores underneath the bolster. If you see tightness or discoloration of skin in the postoperative period, especially POD #2–3, surgeons may cut one or two sutures and keep the bolster in place, usually for 10–14 days.

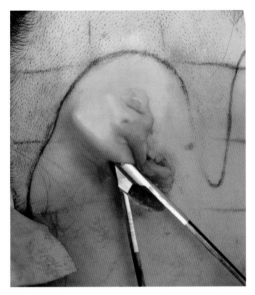

Fig. 7.30 View of skin pocket dissection. Small, straight, blunt scissors are used to create a 2-mm-thick skin flap. The contour of scissors can be seen from outside.

B. Second-stage of total auricular construction (Auricular elevation)

The difficulty of auricular elevation is often underestimated. Normal auricle is separated from mastoid area by supporting cartilage. The simplest way to divide the auricle from the head is to place a skin graft in between the head and auricle without skeletal support. Since the resultant defect after division of the auricle from the head is relatively large, a popular choice of a skin donor site has been the groin area. The disadvantage of auricular division with groin skin grafting includes less optimal elevation, persistent edema of the auricle, pubic hair growth, mismatched skin color, and difficult skin cleaning. To overcome the disadvantages described above, Nagata proposed a more complex auricular elevation that the author routinely performs (Figs. 7.36 & 7.14).[31,53]

1. Raising temporoparietal fascia flap (TPF)

The author uses a TPF to cover the entire posterior aspect of the auricle, not just the cartilage block for elevation. Nagata states that placing TPF has two benefits: to cover the cartilage

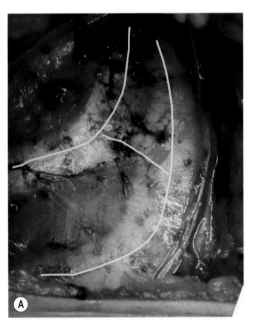

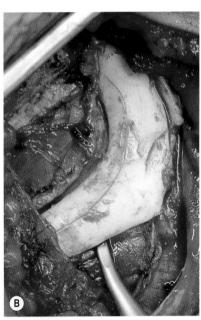

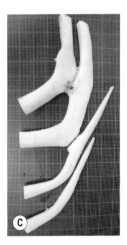

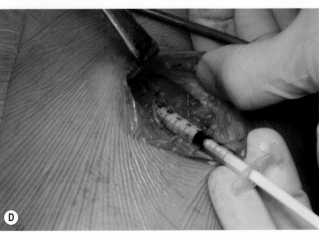

Fig. 7.31 Harvesting rib cartilage technique (usually from ipsilateral side) without perichondrium. **(A)** Incision outline (yellow) to preserve entire perichondrium for sixth and seventh rib cartilage. **(B)** Intraoperative view showing the seventh rib cartilage exposed after peeling off the perichondrium. **(C)** Sixth to ninth rib cartilage without perichondrium. Entire cartilage is white in color which is the sign that they are without perichondrium. **(D)** At the donor site, a perichondrium sleeve was created, and leftover cartilage was diced and injected into the space inside perichondrium sleeve.

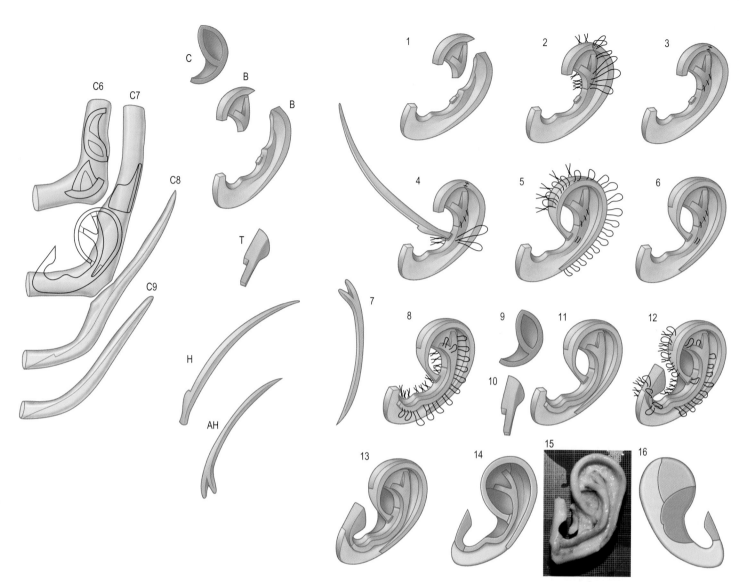

Fig. 7.35 Fabrication of 3D framework. C6-C9, Harvested rib cartilage from sixth to ninth rib. C, conchal bowl unit. This can be fabricated either as one unit or as two separate units. B, Base frame from sixth and seventh. T, tarsal portion; H, helix unit; AH, antihelix unit. 4, Helix is attached to the posterior surface of the base frame. 11 Helix and antihelix are attached to the base frame, prior to tragus and concealed in bowl unit. 13,14,15, Anterior view of completed 3D framework. 16, Posterior view of completed 3D framework.

block and to augment the posterior vascular supply to the auricle that was lost at the time of separation of the auricle from the head.[53] If low hairline is mild (hairs cover helix and scapha fossa), TPF enables surgeons to perform intra-operative hair removal (Fig. 7.14). Since superficial temporal artery (pedicle of TPF) may run an atypical course in hemifacial microsomia, the author routinely uses Doppler ultrasound to plot the course of STA on the temporal skin. If TPF is not available, either deep temporal fascia flap (Figs. 7.37 & 7.9F), or fascia flap based on posterior vasculature (Fig. 7.11) is the second option. If a local fascia flap is not available, the third option may be a free vascularized fascia flap.[23,54–56]

Alopecia has been reported as a complication of TPF harvest. The author uses a zig-zag temporal skin incision, raising the skin flap via sharp dissection with a #15 scalpel to dissect between fat tissue and TPF. Since the majority of hair follicles are located very close to TPF, monopolar electrodissection may cause alopecia (Fig. 7.38).

2. Harvesting scalp split-thickness skin

The author does not use groin skin for auricular elevation because of its poor skin color match and potential pubic hair growth. Nagata proposed the use of split-thickness scalp skin, which has better a color match with auricular skin. Nagata harvests split-thickness scalp manually with a #15 scalpel. The author uses either a #15 scalpel or electronic dermatome with thickness of 0.4 mm (Aesculap, Germany).

3. Cartilage block for elevation

Many agree that without placing a block underneath the ear framework, the ear is not practically elevated from the head

(Fig. 7.39). Placing a cartilage block behind the framework has two purposes: elevating the auricle and creating the auriculocephalic sulcus. Nagata and Yamada studied the normal shape of the auriculocephalic sulcus, and based on that study, a 2D template was developed. The author routinely makes an intra-operative impression to make a 3D template for fabrication of a cartilage block for sulcus construction (Fig. 7.14).

Hemifacial microsomia (craniofacial microsomia)

Auricular construction in hemifacial microsomia (HFM) is complex and challenging.[32] Even in mild forms in terms of mandibular underdevelopment (e.g., Pruzansky Type 1), vestige skin tends to be located in the anterior and lower face, and may accompany low hair line, low set ear canal, and vascular anomalies (Fig. 7.5). If surgeons simply apply the standard formula of auricular construction (place the auricle where vestige is located), the new auricle tends to be located in the face mask, which may be aesthetically unacceptable. Surgeons should avoid placing the new auricle inside the face mask. It is not uncommon to place the new auricle in an anterior–inferior location, trying to avoid the low hairline in HFM. Compromising the location of the auricle to some extent may be necessary; otherwise, the location of the new auricle will be too far back in the occipital area.

In HFM, skeletal correction prior to ear construction may help to place the auricle in proper location (Fig. 7.10).[102] It is notable that laser hair removal works best for black hairs, with multiple sessions (could be more than 10 sessions to complete), but it is currently not effective against blond hairs (Fig. 7.7). The author found that in the microtia patient with severe HFM there is a higher risk of ear shrinkage after complex total auricular construction.[32]

Treacher–Collins syndrome

The patient with Treacher–Collins syndrome has distinctive facial features: high nose, deficient lateral orbit/zygoma, small chin, and overall facial size is small. Placing a large auricle in such a face may be disproportional and unnatural. The size of the new auricle, therefore, needs to be smaller than average. The author usually selects the auricle size 45–50 mm in length, to balance with the rest of the face (Figs. 7.11, 7.40 & 7.41). It is not uncommon that microtia in Treacher–Collins syndrome accompanies a low hairline. To eliminate hairs from the auricle, laser hair removal is one option, and the other is that the local fascia flap such as the temporoparietal fascia or fascia flap based on posterior vascular pedicle may be applied to cover the upper third of the framework, after surgical hair removal.[57]

Tissue expander

The idea to expand the skin to create extra soft, elastic, thin skin to cover the ear framework is a tempting one, and boomed in the 1990s, but the popularity of tissue expander use in microtia reconstruction[58,59] has decreased. Soft-tissue expanders also have been used to expand under a temporo-parietal fascia flap and scalp skin graft to provide coverage in challenging cases of anotia, failed autogenous reconstructions, and post-traumatic cases.[60] The potential for complications including skin necrosis and the added surgical stage are the major concerns with the use of soft-tissue expanders in ear reconstruction.[61,62] Since the skin of the auricular site is thin, the amount of expanded skin may not be enough to eliminate the hairs in the auricle. Even after skin expansion, the constructed auricle still may include hair-bearing skin at the helical rim (Fig. 7.42).

Unsatisfactory outcome

The cause of unsatisfactory outcomes are multifactorial:[26] improper evaluation of the deformities, improper selection of the surgical procedures, non-recognition of the facial asymmetry, improper assessment of low hairline, improper selection of the new auricular location, improper inclination of the auricle, improper timing of the surgery, insufficient amount of costal cartilage, improper cartilage harvesting techniques, improper thickness of skin pocket dissection, failure to utilize lobule spiriting techniques, improper shape, volume, size, and width of framework, and finally improper postoperative care. Thus, secondary construction is a challenge, and must reverse all of the above-mentioned setbacks (see secondary construction section).

Complications

The overall complication incidence in ear reconstruction is reported to be 16.2% in average with a range of 0–72.9%.[63] Probably the most serious complication in total auricular construction is cartilage infection, leading to the entire extrusion of the ear framework. To prevent this disaster, even small skin necrosis has to be addressed immediately. Skin necrosis along the helical rim may be repaired with a local skin flap, but skin necrosis in a medial portion, such as concha bowl, usually requires a local fascia flap to salvage it.[57] Long-term complications include the collapse of the ear framework and extrusion of wires. Total auricular construction in HFM has higher frequency of complications, such as malposition of the new auricle and shrinkage of the auricle.[32]

Secondary construction

Secondary construction is challenging, but it is not impossible. In many unsatisfactory outcomes, patients have lost supple skin, and have developed many scars and disintegrated frameworks. To create a smooth, natural-looking auricle in such situations, surgeons should take an aggressive approach: discard all scar tissue, deformed framework, and the damaged skin envelope, then replace it with a well-vascularized, supple, and thin skin envelope and a well-planned framework.[23,26,31] In secondary cases, the temporoparietal fascia flap is a powerful workhorse to provide a thin envelope to cover the framework (Figs. 7.9 & 7.42).[30] If the local fascia flap is not available, a distant free fascia flap may be the option. Brent described the use of contralateral TPF plus hair-bearing skin to restore the temporal hair line plus auricular construct.[6] If the recipient vessels are not available near the auricle, a vascularized free

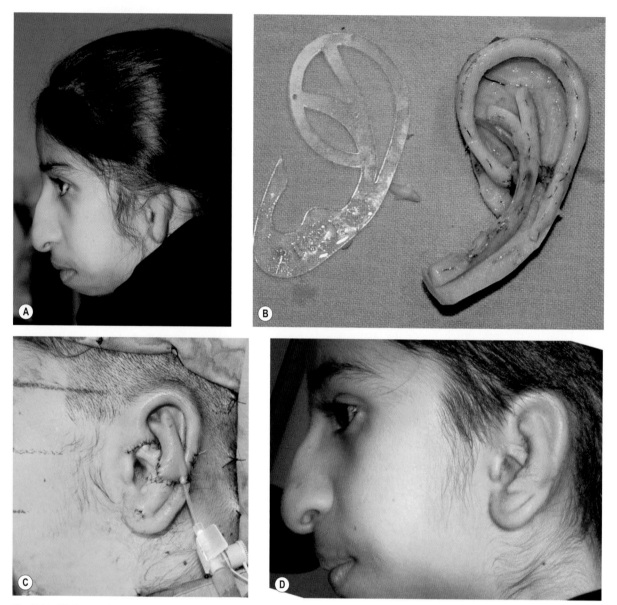

Fig. 7.41 **(A)** Preoperative view of a patient with microtia in Treacher–Collins syndrome. **(B)** Type B-2 template and 3D framework. **(C)** Immediate postoperative view, prior to placing bolster suture. **(D)** Postoperative profile.

fascia flap with a long vascular pedicle, such as serratus fascia[54–56] may be an advantageous option, although it has the disadvantage of creating a long scar at the lateral thoracic donor site.

Role of deep temporal fascia (DTF)

Role of deep temporal fascia in complex ear reconstruction has been advocated by Nagata, but still many surgeons believe that the temporoparietal fascia flap is the last resort as a local fascia flap. Deep fascia is based on the branch of the middle temporal artery, which usually runs a similar course to the STA, one layer underneath it (Fig. 7.37).[64] If the TPF was already used for anterior surface coverage of the ear framework, then at the second stage of ear elevation, DTF can cover the posterior aspect of the auricle (Fig. 7.9).

Constricted ear

Constricted ear is a concept proposed by Tanzer in 1975.[65] In constricted ear, helix and scapha fossa are hooded, and crura of antihelix is flattened in various degrees. One gains an impression that the rim of the helix has been tightened. Constricted ear is often referred to as cup or lop ear. Tanzer classified constricted ear into three groups based on the severity of defect/deformities.

Group 1

Group 1 constricted ear is defined by mild deformities of the helix, often called lop ear (Fig. 7.43). The defect involves helical cartilage with minimum skin defect. The Musgrave (1966)[66] technique is a useful method to expand the helix.

Through either an anterior or posterior skin incision, multiple cuts are made to the curled cartilage, fan upward and backward, fixed to the curved strut made of concha cartilage graft. The skin is then re-draped across the reconstructed framework. For milder constricted ear (groups 1 and 2A), focusing surgical correction to the constructed helical curve is the reasonable option while keeping original elastic cartilage framework and avoiding hard rib cartilage framework. When superior crus is deficient, partial helix plus superior crus frame from rib cartilage[67] can normalize the deformity.

Group 2B

Constricted ear group 2B has both skin and cartilage defects in the upper third of the auricle. The loss of folding may involve antihelical crura, and hooding is more pronounced. The height of the ear is sharply reduced. Park, in 2009,[68] proposed a versatile solution for group 2B constricted ear. For helical skin defect, Park modified the Grotting flap[69] (post-auricular flap), creating both skin flap and fascia flap with the same pedicle. Since width of skin flap is limited by the hairline

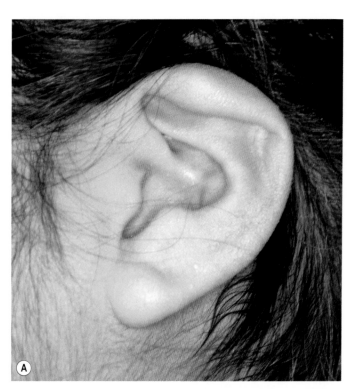

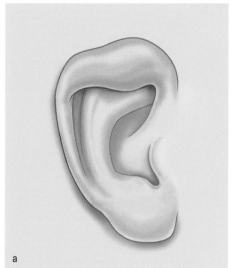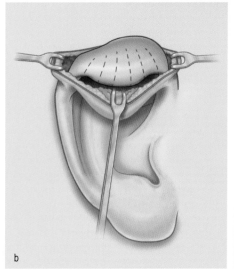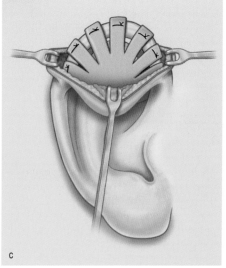

Fig. 7.43 Constricted ear group 1 ear. **(A)** Preoperative view. **(B)** Musgrave technique for correction of cup ear: (a) The deformity, (b) the folded cartilage is exposed through posterior incision, (c) cartilage fingers are elevated and fixed to a strut of conchal cartilage.

Continued

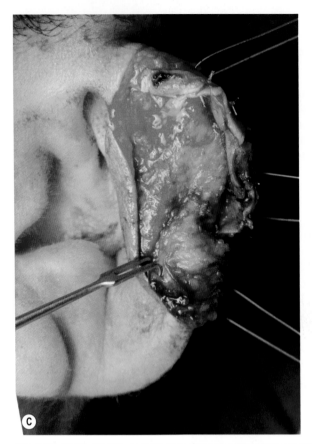

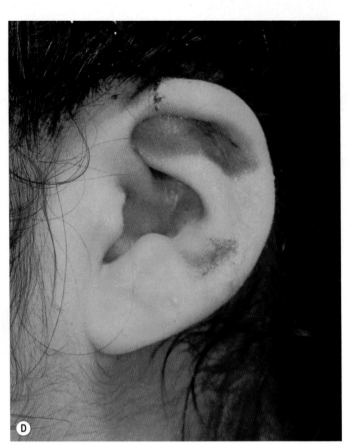

Fig. 7.43, cont'd **(C)** Intra-operative view. Conchal cartilage strut was fixed to the cartilage fingers. **(D)** Postoperative view.

(10–13 mm), a fascia flap can provide additional coverage of the helix, if needed. The distal half of the skin flap can be thinned to facilitate better definition of helix/scapha, with proximal half of skin flap including a fascia layer to boost blood supply. For helical cartilage defect, eighth rib cartilage is harvested, the helix is fabricated, and the entire length of the helix is constructed (Fig. 7.44). Bilateral constricted ear can be operated with single eighth rib cartilage, split into two strips for bilateral helical rim construction. Otoplasty techniques such as the Mustardé sutures[70,71] may be combined with the Park technique to correct excessive ear projection.

Group 3

Tanzer defined group 3 as the most severe cupping: failure of migration.

Brent recommends treating severe constricted ear as if it is a form of microtia, when the construction is severe enough to produce a height difference of 1.5 cm.[6] Nagata recommends treating severe constricted ear as a concha type microtia, to replace the defective framework with a full rib cartilage framework.[72]

Cryptotia

Cryptotia is a congenital ear deformity in which the upper pole of the ear cartilage is buried underneath the scalp.

The superior auriculocephalic sulcus is absent, but can be demonstrated when you pull up the helical pole. Various surgical corrections are reported from Japan, due to the high prevalence of cryptotia as frequently as 1 : 400.[73] Non-surgical, ear molding treatment may be applied if the child is an early neonate.[73–75] The goal of surgical treatment is to create the retroauricular sulcus by skin grafts, Z-plasty, V-Y advancement, or rotation flap (Fig. 7.45)[105]. A common cartilage deformity associated with cryptotia is helix-scapha adhesion, which may be addressed by cartilage remodeling techniques.[76]

Stahl ear

In 1989, Binder[77] described a rare congenital auricular deformity as Stahl ear, named after Dr. Stahl. Stahl ear is characterized by the third crus extending toward the helical rim. Stahl ear is classified into three types. Type 1 has obtuse-angled bifurcation, and it looks like the superior crus is missing. Type 2 has trifurcation (Fig. 7.46). Type 3 has broad superior crus and broad third crus (Fig. 7.47). Ear molding may work well if in early infancy (Fig. 7.47). Surgical treatment is broadly categorized into two types: cartilage/skin excision[78,79] and cartilage alteration.[80] Cartilage/skin excision-type techniques (Fig. 7.46) seem to work better than cartilage alteration techniques in the literature. Type 1 Stahl ear needs special attention to reconstruct the missing superior crus by utilizing the excised third crus[78] or a rib cartilage graft.

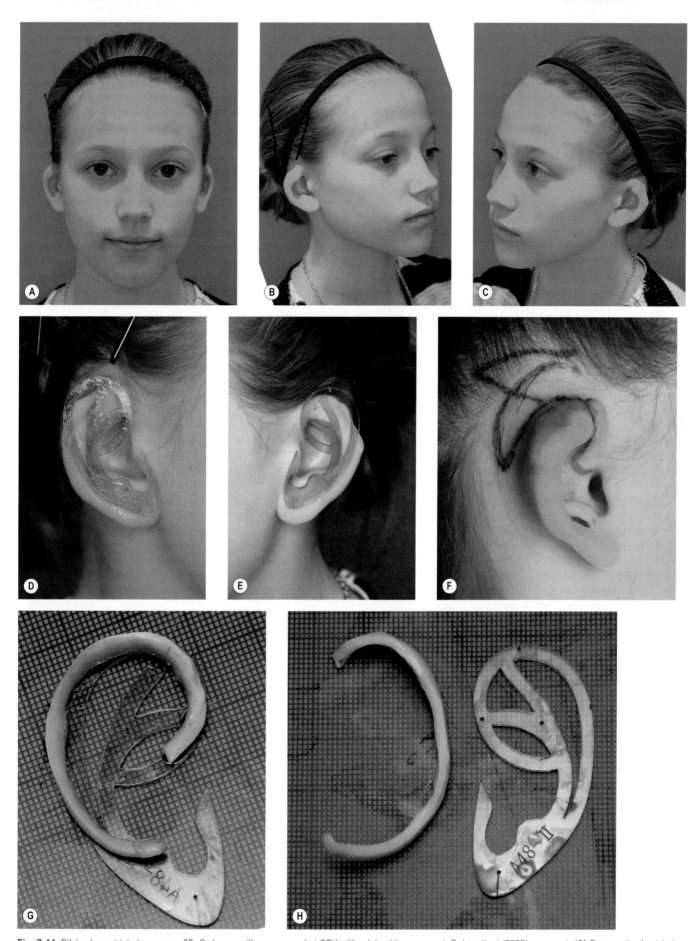

Fig. 7.44 Bilateral constricted ear group 2B. Cadaver cartilage was used at OSH with minimal improvement. Park method (2009) was used. **(A)** Preoperative frontal view. **(B)** Preoperative view of right ear. **(C)** Preoperative view of left ear. **(D)** Evaluating the defect of right ear with 46-mm Type A-1 template. Upper helical pole skin and cartilage are missing. **(E)** Left side has more defect than right side, based on evaluation with 46-mm Type A-1 template. **(F)** Right side surgical marking with modified Grotting flap, combined skin flap and fascia flap based on the same pedicle. **(G)** Split eighth rib cartilage was fabricated for right helix construction. **(H)** Other half of split eighth rib cartilage was used for left ear.

Continued

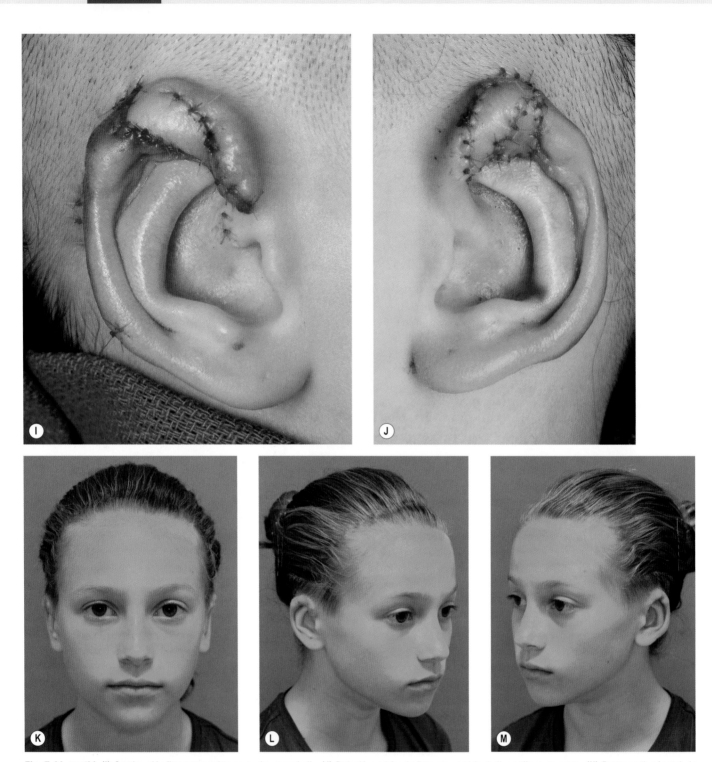

Fig. 7.44, cont'd (I) Grotting skin flap was used to cover the upper helix. **(J)** Park skin and fascia flap was used for helix cartilage coverage. **(K)** Postoperative frontal view. **(L)** Postoperative view of right ear. **(M)** Postoperative view of left ear.

Anotia

Anotia is classified as Tanzer Type 1 ear deformity. There is no vestige skin present, and ear site is completely flat. Anotia is frequently associated with hemifacial microsomia. Anotia is a true reconstructive challenge, and it is extremely difficult to achieve optimal outcomes.

Hypoplasia of middle third of ear

Hypoplasia of the middle third of the auricle is a rare type of ear deformity, classified as Tanzer Type 3.[1] Literally, the middle third is hypoplastic, but the upper and lower thirds have normal anatomical architecture, although the width and the ear dimensions (ratio) are abnormal. Tanzer used staged

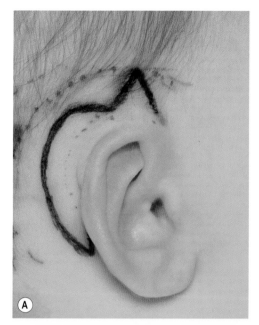

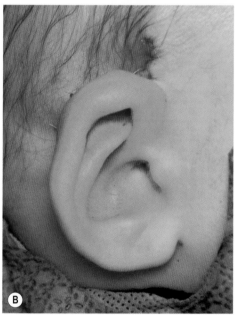

Fig. 7.45 (A) Preoperative marking for cryptotia (buried upper helix pole). V-Y advancement method proposed by Yanai[105] was used to correct the deformities. **(B)** Postoperative view.

reconstruction,[81] starting by dividing the superior and inferior components, obtaining the normal vertical height, and the resultant conchal defect is closed using a retroauricular flap. Later, partial ear framework is transplanted to build up the lower helix and posterior conchal wall. Nagata employs his two-stage approach and treats it as if it is a concha type microtia construction.

Ear molding

Matsuo, who first reported ear molding treatment for congenital ear deformities in 1984,[74] states that when the ear deformities are not hypoplastic, nonsurgical correction is easy and reliable. Lop ear and Stahl's ear respond well to nonsurgical correction only during the neonatal period, while protruding ears and cryptotia respond until approximately 6 months of age (Fig. 7.47).[73] It is widely believed that the early initiation of molding is more effective, because maternal estrogen in the neonate keeps ear cartilage soft and elastic. Although there are a few reports with successful ear molding after 3 months of age, most agree that if ear molding is started after 3 months of age, the response tends to be poor.[75] Helix–antihelix adhesion responds poorly to ear molding treatment and may not be an indication of ear molding (Fig. 7.48). There are minimal complications reported in ear molding; skin irritation is probably the most frequent complication, possibly due to tape or adhesive. Transient edema of helical skin is sometimes observed during ear molding for unknown reasons.

Lobule reconstruction

The lobule is a unique anatomical component of the auricle: there is no skeletal support in the lobule, and it is hanging down from the ear framework. Because the lateral portion of the lobule is composed of free margin, even small surgical alterations can change its shape. In an elliptical excision of a small tumor, if the long axis is perpendicular to the lobule rim, or a piercing scar healed perpendicular to the lobule margin, it may create a square-shape lobule (Fig. 7.49)[82]. If you design the long axis of the ellipse parallel to the lobule margin, the lobule deformity may be preventable. In cleft ear cases, the author routinely uses six types of ear framework templates[36,37,81] as a guide to create a smooth transition of the curve from helix to the lobule (Fig. 7.50). Construction of earlobe is rarely required in congenital microtia, as the lobe is formed by repositioning of auricular remnants. In total auricular construction, the Nagata-type framework always creates skeletal support in the lobule portion. By placing the framework in the lobule, the transition from helix curve to lobule curve becomes smooth. Brent, like Tanzer, switches back full thickness vestige lobule, which allows ear-piercing for children. For traumatic lobule defects, numerous effective techniques have been introduced to repair earlobes with local flap tissues.[83–85]

Trauma of the auricle

Assessing the extent of defect and tissue damage around the auricle is the first step. Doppler ultrasound is a sensitive tool to check the continuity of STA from the beginning to the periphery of the temporal scalp. Because the cartilaginous framework is difficult to produce, the salvage of amputated auricular cartilage is recommended by numerous surgeons. The skin may be removed and the cartilage is buried in an abdominal pocket, in a cervical pocket, or in a retroauricular area;[86] Brent states that this procedure is futile, as the flimsy ear cartilage almost invariably flattens beneath the snug. The author prefers rib cartilage construction in traumatic ear amputation. The amputated cartilage segment was buried underneath a temporal skin pocket at another institution, and it created poor auricular definition. Therefore, rib cartilage framework was constructed and connected with existing residue of frame, and a mastoid skin flap was coapted to the framework. Fig. 7.51 shows a patient with total amputation

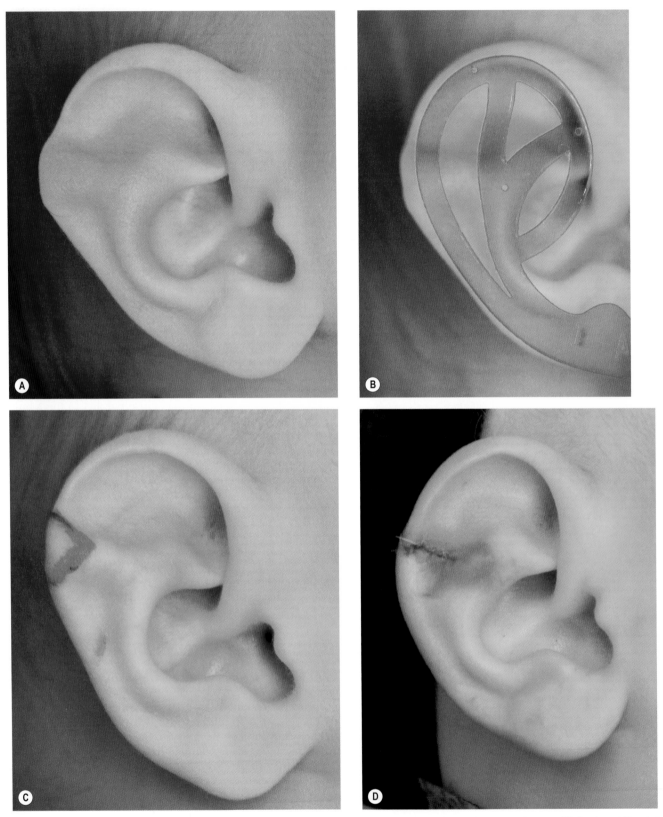

Fig. 7.46 Surgical correction of Stahl ear. **(A)** Preoperative view of Type 2 Stahl ear. Extra crus connects between helix and superior crus. **(B)** Overlapped Type A-1 template demonstrated the curve change at third crus. **(C)** Wedge resection of skin/cartilage was planned, based on the helix curve analysis. **(D)** Immediate postoperative view.

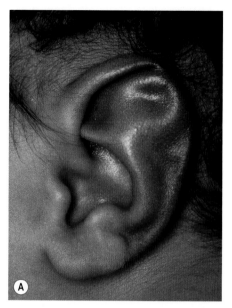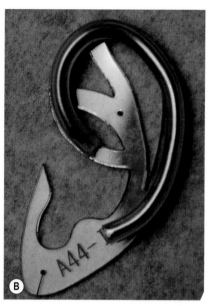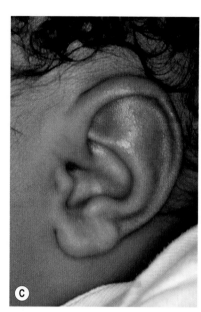

Fig. 7.47 Non-surgical correction of Stahl ear **(A)** Pretreatment view of Type 3 Stahl ear of a one-month-old female. **(B)** Ear splint was shaped according to Type A-2 template. Splint was fixed to the ear with tape. **(C)** View after 5 weeks of ear molding treatment.

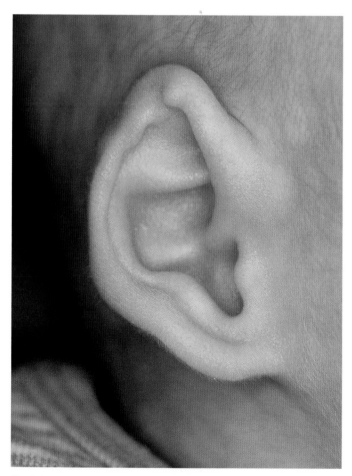

Fig. 7.48 Helix-scapha adhesion causes pointed look of the auricle. This deformity may not be a good indication for ear molding. Park reported effective surgical correction.

of the left auricle with associated vascular injuries. Since the amputated auricle was severely damaged, initial emergency surgery was performed to restore the superficial temporal artery/vein for future auricular construction.[87] At the second stage, total auricular construction was performed with rib cartilage framework; the upper two-thirds of the frame were covered with TPF flap, and the lower third was covered with local skin flaps. To create a deep concha bowl, a Nagata-type posterior lobule flap was transposed.

Burns

Burns may cause extensive injuries to the auricle and surrounding tissues. In severe burn auricular defects, there have been numerous debates on the choice between prosthesis versus autogenous construction. In severe burns, local skin usually does not provide an adequate skin envelope for the entire ear framework. Expanding scarred skin also may not work well. The temporoparietal fascia flap[30] is a powerful tool to cover the framework. Identifying the course of the STA with Doppler ultrasound will determine if TPF will be available for coverage of the ear framework. If scalp hairs are present in the entire temporal area, the STA is likely to be present at the periphery. Fig. 7.9 shows an example of autogenous construction after severe burn amputation of the auricle. A large TPF was used to cover the upper two-thirds of the framework. The lower one-third of the frame was covered with an anterior lobule flap, and a retroauricular island flap was used to construct concha bowl.[27]

Partial ear reconstruction

The key to partial ear reconstruction is how you connect the new parts smoothly to the existing anatomical architecture. Defects involving the helical rim especially need careful

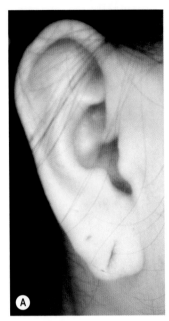
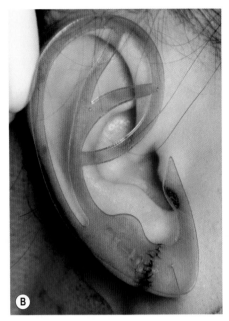
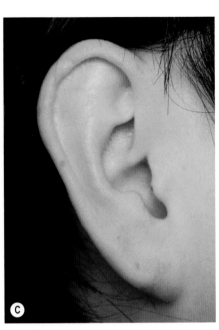

Fig. 7.49 (A) Square shape lobule deformity caused by wound closure perpendicular to the lobule margin. **(B)** Type A-2 template was used as a guide to correct square shape lobule deformity. **(C)** Postoperative view.

planning for a smooth curve transition between old and new. Pure helical rim defects are best closed by advancing the helix in both directions, as described by Antia and Buch (Fig. 7.52).[88] These techniques may also be applied to correct asymmetry of ear size (make a larger auricle small) for otoplasty.[89] Major middle-third auricular defects are classically repaired with a cartilage graft which is either covered by an adjacent skin flap (Fig. 7.7)[16] or inserted via Converse' tunnel procedure (Fig. 7.53).[90] Pearl, in 2011,[91] applied the two-stage total ear reconstruction principle to the partial amputation of the auricle. He created a partial ear framework made of rib cartilage, then attached it to the remaining framework and covered it with

a posterior-based skin flap. Fig. 7.54 shows the partial ear amputation of the middle portion due to trauma, for which the author performed a one-stage partial ear construction. The normal left auricle shape was Type A-1. A partial auricular framework was constructed based on a Type A-1 template, and the frame was sutured to the remaining frame and then covered with a TPF. A split scalp skin graft was placed on top of the TPF. Fig. 7.55 shows a three-year-old who is a victim of a dog bite, and the amputated ear piece was lost. One-stage auricular reconstruction was performed the next day, with the rib cartilage framework covered with a temporoparietal fascia flap and a scalp skin graft.

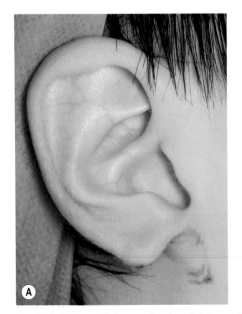
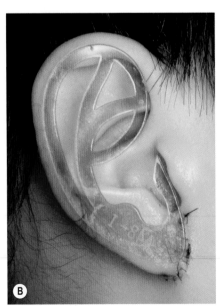
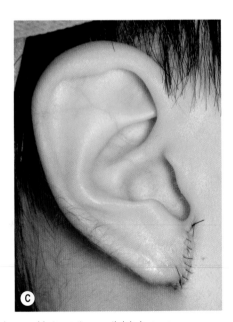

Fig. 7.50 Cleft ear. **(A)** Preoperative view of cleft ear, with rectangular shape lobule. **(B)** Type A template was used as a guide to create smooth lobule curve. **(C)** Postoperative view. *(Reproduced with permission from Yamada A. Cosmetic surgery of the ear. In: Pu LLQ, Chen Y-R, Li Q-F, et al. Special Considerations in Cosmetic Surgery of the Asian Ear. Aesthetic Plastic Surgery in Asians: Principles and Techniques. Boca Raton: CRC Press; 2015.)*

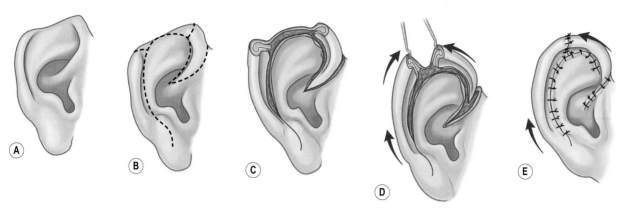

Fig. 7.52 Helical defect repaired by advancement of auricular skin cartilage. **(A)** Defect of the upper portion of the auricle. **(B)** Lines of incisions through skin and cartilage. **(C)** The incisions completed: note the downward extension into the earlobe. **(D)** The skin–cartilage flaps mobilized. **(E)** The repair completed. *(Modified from Antia NH, Buch VI. Chondrocutaneous advancement of flap for the marginal defect of the ear. Plast Reconstr Surg. 1967;39:472.Copyright © 1967, The Williams & Wilkins Company, Baltimore.)*

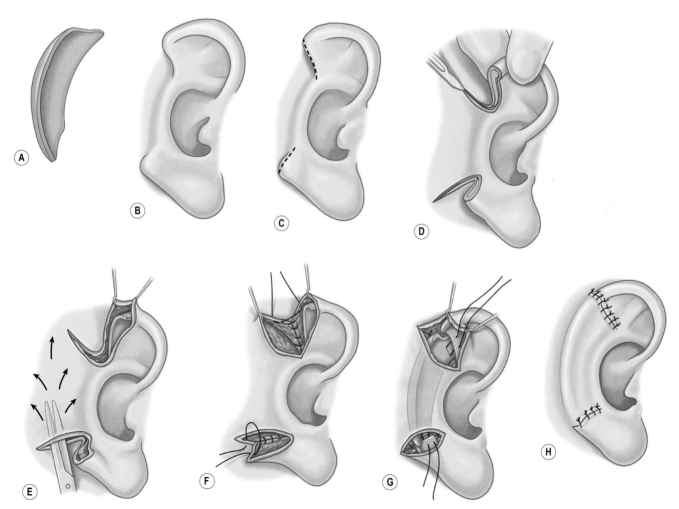

Fig. 7.53 Repair of a defect of the middle third of the auricle: the tunnel procedure. **(A)** Carved costal cartilage graft. **(B)** The defect. **(C)** Incisions through the margins of the defect. **(D)** Incisions through the edge of the defect are extended backward through the skin of the mastoid area. **(E)** The skin of the mastoid area is undermined between the two incisions. **(F)** The medial edge of the incision at the border of the auricular defect is sutured to the edge of the postauricular incision. A similar type of suture is placed at the lower edge of the defect. **(G)** The cartilage graft is placed under the skin of the mastoid area and anchored to the auricular cartilage with sutures. **(H)** Suture of the skin incision. *(Reproduced from Converse JM. Reconstruction of the auricle. Plast Reconstr Surg. 1958;22:150, 230.Copyright ©1958, The Williams & Wilkins Company, Baltimore.)*

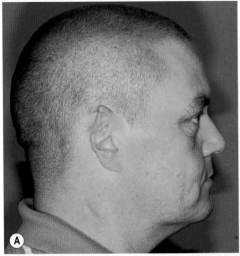

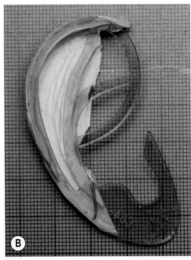

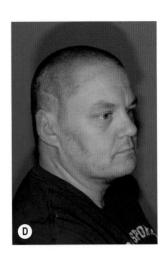

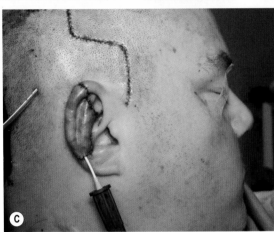

Fig. 7.54 Traumatic partial amputation of the auricle. **(A)** Preoperative profile. **(B)** Preoperative planning to identify the extent of cartilage defect. **(C)** Immediate postoperative view after one stage of surgery. **(D)** Postoperative view.

Learning to create ear framework

Three-steps training method

Surgical simulation is not a new concept. Sushuruta (600 BC) used vegetables for surgical simulation. Since microtia patients have only one primary chance to obtain the best outcome, surgeons must train well before they actually perform surgery on patients, otherwise the surgeon may create an unsatisfactory auricle. Although experienced surgeons can salvage a difficult secondary auricular construction, the secondary cases are still unlikely to be as good as the primary cases even in expert hands. Since we cannot practice on patients, surgeons should perform hands-on training prior to become ear makers.

First step

Brent uses vegetables for ear carving practice. The author uses a potato as the first step in training. The potato is cheap, and readily available.[50] In step 1 training, acrylic 2D template and 3D framework models are used as a guide for curving practice; a #15 scalpel and carving knife are the main instruments used.

Surgeons carve the auricular framework from the potato block, like a sculpture. This is the practice of pure carving to grasp and understand the three dimensional structure of the framework (Fig. 7.32).

Second step

Once surgeons become comfortable sculpting the framework out of a potato, the next step is the carrot framework. The carrot is a bit more solid and flexible than the potato, and it is suitable for making each part of the framework, which are then assembled together. Surgeons can create a base frame, helix, antihelix, tragus, and concha cap. The ear parts model developed by Wilkes may be used as a guide.[9] The carrot has a longitudinal fiber along the long axis in the inner cortex; it allows surgeons to practice carving the helical portion. By thinning the helical rim portion little by little, surgeons can experience the moment when the helix suddenly becomes flexible. The best portion for helix practice is just medial to the outer skin. The outer skin itself is not the best portion, since it has many creases, and it is easily fractured at a crease when you try to bend it. The final portion of the practice is to assemble each part of the frame with 38G double-armed stainless wires as surgeons do in clinical cases (Fig. 7.33).

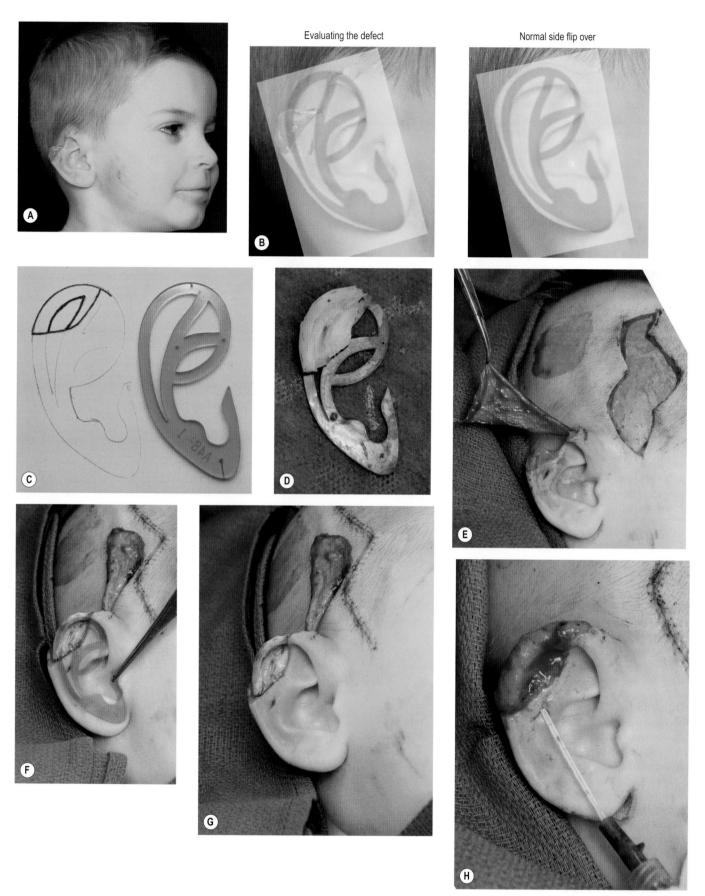

Evaluating the defect

Normal side flip over

Fig. 7.55 A three-year-old male with partial amputation of the auricle due to dog bite. **(A)** Preoperative view. **(B)** Photographic analysis to identify the cartilage defect. **(C)** Simulated cartilage defect. **(D)** Partial cartilage framework and Type A-1 46-mm template. **(E)** Temporoparietal fascia flap was tunneled to the ear defect. **(F)** Partial cartilage framework was fixed to the remaining framework. **(G)** Continuation of helix curve was confirmed with Type A-1 template. **(H)** TPF was coated to the framework.

Continued

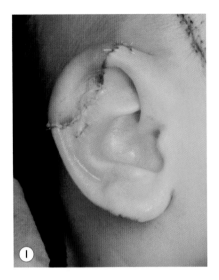
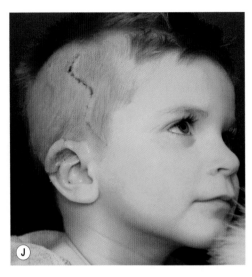

Fig. 7.55, cont'd (I) Split scalp skin was placed over TPF. **(J)** Postoperative view.

Third step

The final step is to transform costal cartilage into an auricular framework. Wilkes is the first to develop a rib cartilage model from dental impression materials.[51] The author modified the shape, creating a more precise rib cartilage copy.[49] With the rib cartilage model, surgeons can simulate the framework fabrication in a very realistic way. Exactly the same instrumentation as the clinical setting is used, and surgeons perform carving, cutting, assembling, and adjusting of the cartilage framework (Fig. 7.34).

Prominent ear

Background

Protruding ears are the most frequent congenital deformity of the head and neck area, affecting 5% of the general public. Ear deformities affect both genders equally and may be unilateral or bilateral. In many cases protruding ears result in an abnormal appearance. Although hearing may be normal, the individual may suffer significantly from peer ridicule and lowered self-esteem.

Evaluation

The first step in assessing the patient for otoplasty is determining the anatomic causes of protrusion of the ear. The most common causes of protrusion of the external ear are (1) underdevelopment or effacement of the antihelix, (2) overdevelopment of the deep concha, or (3) a combination of both of these features.

Auricular protrusion may be one element of a more complex auricular deformity such as a constricted ear, Stahl ear (third crus), macrotia, or syndromic facial deformity. Chronic otitis media, otitis externa, or conditions such as scalp infections or acne must be treated well in advance of surgery. A simple surgical wound infection can lead to an ear-threatening chondritis.

Goal of otoplasty

As the author described in the microtia section, the auricle should not be the anatomical part to draw attention of others. A protruding auricle is more likely to draw attention. As for the shape of the auricle, the goal is to restore soft, smooth, and natural auricles. Therefore, surgeons must choose surgical techniques that are simple, reliable, and least likely to cause complications. Surgeons must delicately execute anterior scoring technique because if surgeons did excessive scoring, it may create sharp edges and an unnatural, unsmooth contour of the auricle.

Timing of surgery

There is no absolute rule on timing of otoplasty.[92–94] Otoplasty may be performed in children or adults, although the procedure is more common in children. Surgery is often recommended near an age when ear growth is nearly complete, such as 5–7, when a child's ear cartilage is stable enough for correction. At this point, the child can cooperate with their care, and the social and psychological problems associated with peer ridicule are avoided at a critical time in their social development. Almost all young children require general anesthesia for the procedure.

Surgical techniques

It is important to remember that symmetry is crucial in treating the prominent ear, because asymmetry is more likely to draw attention. A unilateral case may be more difficult for achieving symmetry. As part of the basic goals of otoplasty, McDowell described the normal distance from skull to the helix: the upper third of the helix, 10–12 mm; the middle third, 16–18 mm; and the lobule, 20–22 mm from the mastoid.[95] Each case has a different combination of the deformities; therefore, surgeons must combine the surgical options as well. Surgeons should direct their efforts toward correcting the specific problem areas of each individual ear rather than following a recipe. If the upper third of the ear protrudes because of an absent or weak antihelix, an antihelix must be formed. If the middle third is too prominent, the concha must be recessed by either cartilage excision or suture fixation. Lastly, if the lobule protrudes, the surgeon should either resect or retroposition the cauda helicis' cartilaginous tail and/or excise retrolobular skin.[96]

1. Antihelical fold alteration

Scapha-conchal suture

Mustardé[70,71] created the antihelix by inserting permanent mattress sutures through the cartilage without using any cartilage incisions. This technique is particularly useful in the soft auricular cartilage of young children (Fig. 7.56), but it also can be applied to adult patients (Fig. 7.57).

Anterior cartilage alteration

Chongchet[97] scored the anterior scapha cartilage with multiple cartilage cuts to roll it back and form an antihelix. While Chongchet performed this technique under direct vision using a scalpel, Stenstrom[98] produced the same effect by using a short-tined rasp instrument to score the antihelical region through a posterior stab incision near the cauda helicis.

Restore antihelical fold by excision

Luckett[99] restored the antihelical fold by excising a crescent of anterior skin and cartilage. The majority of subsequent reports have focused on creating a smoother antihelix than Luckett's sharp cartilage-breaking technique.

2. Conchal alteration

Dieffenbach[16] is credited with the first otoplastic attempt in 1845. This consisted of excising skin from the auriculocephalic sulcus and then suturing conchal cartilage to the mastoid periosteum. In addition to narrowing the auriculocephalic sulcus, Ely[17] and others excised a strip of conchal wall, a procedure that is attributed to Morestin.[100] This method of tacking back the concha to the mastoid periosteum has been revived through the years. The wide concha can be corrected by excising a cartilaginous ellipse beneath the antihelix.

Future direction

As a part of a facial allotransplant, composite auricular allotransplantation may be an option in the near future. Tissue engineered-autogenous elastic cartilage has been in progress[99–101,104], but the issue of skin envelope deficiency has not been completely solved yet.

Man-made skin flaps are not as thin as natural skin; currently only hard cartilage can create the definition of the auricle. When both ear cartilage and thin skin regeneration are achieved simultaneously, we will see the new era of auricular construction.

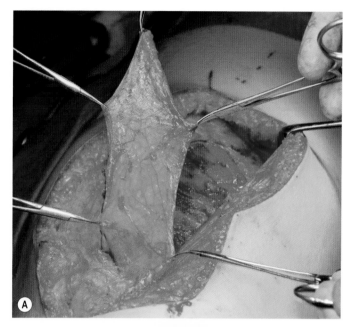
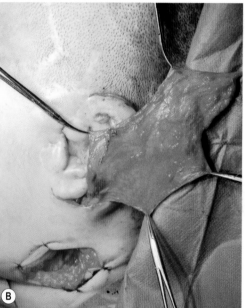

Fig. 7.57 Free serratus fascia flap. **(A)** Elevation of fascia flap. **(B)** Fascia flap was used to cover the posterior half of the auricle. Vascular pedicle was anastomosed to neck vessels.

Bonus images for this chapter can be found in online at

http://www.expertconsult.com

Fig. 7.4 Development of the auricle in a 5-week human embryo: 1–6, elevations (hillocks) on the mandibular and hyoid arches; ov, otic vesicle; af, auricular fold. (Modified from Arey LB. *Developmental Anatomy*, 7th edn. Philadelphia: WB Saunders; 1974.)

Fig. 7.6 Combined microtia/atresia surgery was performed as a first stage reconstruction. Atresia surgery was performed by Dr. Shinichi Haginomori. **(A)** Preoperative view of a 10-year-old male with concha type microtia. **(B)** Concha type skin incision was used both for microtia construction and atresia surgery. **(C)** Canal wall up mastoidectomy was performed. The malleus (M) and incus (I) formed the complex. EAC, external auditory canal; Ma, mastoid cavity. **(D)** The malleus-incus complex was removed. Mobility of the stapes (S) was good. MM, manubrium of the malleus; CT, chorda tympani nerve; EAC, external auditory canal; Ma, mastoid cavity. **(E)** The columella (3 mm in length) was made from the cortical bone. **(F)** The columella (C) was inserted between the manubrium of the malleus (MM) and stapes (S). **(G)** Audiological finding, one year post; the patient is able to hear whisper voice with affected side. **(H)** One year postoperative appearance.

Fig. 7.10 Microtia patient with hemifacial microsomia. First, mandibular distraction osteogenesis was performed, then microtia reconstruction was done. **(A)** Preoperative view. **(B)** 3D CT reconstruction demonstrates new bone generation of the mandible between distraction pins. **(C)** Frontal view of the patient after mandibular distraction osteogenesis. Tilt of the commissure is corrected. **(D)** Profile view of the patient prior to total auricular construction. **(E)** Type A-2 template and 3D framework **(F)** Immediate postoperative view. **(G)** View of the patient 2 years after total auricular construction.

Fig. 7.11 Treacher–Collins patient with bilateral microtia. The patient had bicoronal scar, and TPF was not available. **(A)** Preoperative view of the left side. **(B)** Left side view after two-stage auricular construction. **(C)** Intraoperative view of right microtia. Posterior pedicle fascia was used for ear elevation. Surgery was performed with Dr. Satoru Nagata. **(D)** Immediate postoperative view of the right side.

Fig. 7.12 (A) A seven-year-old male with small concha type microtia. **(B)** 30% low hairline was demonstrated by ear positioning template.

Fig. 7.19 The ear positioning template is a tool to identify the tauricular rectangle, within which the auricular framework will be placed.

Fig. 7.22 Type A-1 auricular construction was performed for lobule type microtia. **(A)** Preoperative view. **(B)** Type A-1 rib cartilage framework. **(C)** Postoperative view.

Fig. 7.24 First stage surgery for lobule type microtia **(A)** Skin incision outline for anterior surface of the lobule. **(B)** W-shaped skin incision outline on the posterior surface of the lobule and the mastoid surface. **(C)** Undermining the mastoid area to create 2-mm thick skin flap, using straight blunt scissors. Skin pocket extends 1 cm beyond the ear outline. **(D)** 3D frame is inserted from tarsal portion by rotating around the subcutaneous pedicle. **(E)** Under temporary suction, skin flap is coapted to 3D frame, and excessive skin is trimmed.

Fig. 7.25 Lobule type microtia. **(A)** Preoperative profile. **(B)** One year after surgery. **(C)** Eight years after surgery.

Fig. 7.26 Lobule type microtia. **(A)** Preoperative profile of an 11-year-old female. **(B)** Topographic marking and skin incision outline (red). **(C)** 3D framework and Nagata type template. **(D)** Intra-operative view; anterior lobule flap and posterior W-shaped flap are seen.

Fig. 7.28 Concha type microtia for which W-shaped posterior incision was used. **(A)** Preoperative profile. **(B)** Type A-1 52-mm template is overlapped onto the normal ear to confirm the needed size and shape of template needed. **(C)** W-shaped posterior lobule skin incision (red). **(D)** Type A-1 52-mm template and 3D framework. **(E)** One year after surgery.

Fig. 7.32 The author's training method of creating 3D framework: Step 1; practice by using potato. **(A)** Type C-2 template was placed on a potato. **(B)** Type C-2 template was printed on a flat potato surface. **(C)** Relief of 3D framework carved out from potato. **(D)** Completed potato 3D frame.

Fig. 7.33 Step 2: practice on a carrot 3D framework **(A)** Type A-1 template was printed on flat surface of carrot. **(B)** Five parts of 3D framework are created from carrots. **(C)** Five parts are assembled to create a carrot Type A-1 3D framework.

Fig. 7.34 Step 3: practice to create a 3D framework from precise rib cartilage copy. **(A)** Type A-2 template is placed on 6–7 rib cartilage model. **(B)** Five parts of 3D framework are created from a rib cartilage model. **(C)** Completed 3D framework from rib cartilage model; anterior surface. **(D)** Posterior surface of 3D framework.

Fig. 7.36 Second stage of surgery (ear elevation). **(A, B)** Framework is separated from head. **(C, D)** Fabricated cartilage is wedged, and then the entire posterior surface is covered with temporoparietal fascia flap. **(E)** Split scalp is harvested and grafted over TPF.

Fig. 7.37 The nutrient vessel for deep temporal fascia can be seen one layer below temporoparietal fascia flap. The course of the branch of the middle temporal artery (yellow arrows) is similar to the temporal branch of STA.

Fig. 7.38 Unsatisfactory auricular construction; poor definition, exposed auditory canal, hairs on helix, and pubic hairs grow from groin skin graft.

Fig. 7.39 Ear separation by skin grafting without cartilage support; helix is touching the head. The patient has difficulty cleaning the back of the auricle.

Fig. 7.40 (A) Preoperative view of a patient with microtia in Treacher–Collins syndrome. **(B)** Postoperative view. Small ear was created to balance the face.

Fig. 7.42 Secondary auricular construction, after unsatisfactory tissue expander ear reconstruction. **(A)** Preoperative profile. **(B)** Size and shape of normal side are confirmed with Type A-1 56-mm template. **(C)** Preoperative markings; proper location of the auricle, skin flaps for lower third of the auricle, and zig-zag temporal incision for harvesting TPF. **(D)** Previous framework was removed. **(E)** Type A-1 3D framework. **(F)** Lower third of 3D framework is covered with local skin flaps. **(G)** Upper two-thirds of framework was covered with TPF. **(H)** The fascia was covered with split scalp skin. **(I)** One year after surgery.

Fig. 7.51 Total amputation of the auricle associated with multiple injuries. **(A)** View at the time of initial evaluation. **(B)** STA and STV were reconnected, and skin coverage was performed using amputated skin. **(C)** Profile view prior to total auricular construction. **(D)** Since rib cartilage was partially calcified, helix portion was harvested peripheral to the base frame unit. **(E)** Completed 3D framework with Nagata type paper template. **(F)** Lower portion of 3D framework was covered with skin flaps, and upper two-thirds were covered with temporoparietal fascia flap (STA/STV was reconstructed at the initial surgery). **(G)** Split scalp skin was placed over TPF. **(H)** Postoperative view.

Fig. 7.56 Unilateral protrusion of the auricle. **(A)** Preoperative frontal view. **(B)** Preoperative posterior view. **(C)** Postoperative frontal view. **(D)** Postoperative posterior view.

Access the complete reference list online at **http://www.expertconsult.com**

6. Brent BD. Reconstruction of the ear. In: Neligan PC, ed. *Plastic Surgery*. 3rd ed. Philadelphia: Elsevier Saunders; 2013:187.

9. Wilkes GH, Wong JW, Guilfoyle R. Microtia reconstruction. *Plast Reconstr Surg*. 2014;134(3):464e–479e.

46. Wallace CG, Mao HY, Wang CJ, et al. Three-dimensional computed tomography reveals different donor-site deformities in adult and growing microtia patients despite total subperichondrial costal cartilage harvest and donor-site reconstruction. *Plast Reconstr Surg*. 2014;133(3):640–651.

63. Long X, Yu N, Huang J, Wang X. Complication rate of autologous cartilage microtia reconstruction: a systematic review. *Plast Reconstr Surg Glob Open*. 2013;1(7):e57.

64. Yano T, Okazaki M, Yamaguchi K, Akita K. Anatomy of the middle temporal vein: implications for skull-base and craniofacial reconstruction using free flaps. *Plast Reconstr Surg*. 2014;134(1):92e–101e.

67. Kon M, van Wijk MP. T-bar reconstruction of constricted ears and a new classification. *J Plast Reconstr Aesthet Surg*. 2014;67(3):358–361.

75. Doft MA, Goodkind AB, Diamond S, et al. The newborn butterfly project: a shortened treatment protocol for ear molding. *Plast Reconstr Surg*. 2015;135(3):577e–583e.

81. Yamada A. Cosmetic surgery of the ear. In: Pu LLQ, Chen Y-R, Li Q-F, eds. *Special Considerations in Cosmetic Surgery of the Asian Ear: Aesthetic Plastic Surgery in Asians: Principles and Techniques*. Boca Raton: CRC Press; 2015.

88. Sinno S, Chang JB, Thorne CH. Precision in otoplasty: combining reduction otoplasty with traditional otoplasty. *Plast Reconstr Surg*. 2015;135(5):1342–1348.

104. Liao HT, Zheng R, Liu W, Zhang WJ, Cao Y, Zhou G. Prefabricated, ear-shaped cartilage tissue engineering by scaffold-free porcine chondrocyte membrane. *Plast Reconstr Surg*. 2015;135(2):313e–321e.

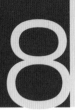

Acquired cranial and facial bone deformities

Blake D. Murphy, Craig Rowin, and S. Anthony Wolfe

 Access video content for this chapter online at expertconsult.com

SYNOPSIS

- Treatment of acquired cranial and facial bone deformities begins with a thorough physical examination prior to radiologic studies.
- Access incisions must allow visualization and exposure of the entire defect.
- Surgical treatment must follow Tessier's principles of subperiosteal exposure, judicious use of autogenous bone grafts, and rigid fixation.
- Alloplastic materials are to be avoided if possible.
- Late presentation of acquired deformities may require an osteotomy through the defect site prior to reduction.
- Additional details regarding facial fractures can be found in Section 1, Chapter 3: Facial injuries.
- Additional details regarding mandibular and maxillary reconstruction can be found in Section 2, Chapter 10.1: Midface reconstruction introduction and Chapter 11: Oral cavity, tongue, and mandibular reconstructions.

Introduction

The various causes of acquired deformities of the facial skeleton include trauma, infection, and surgical or radiotherapeutic treatment of neoplasia. The surgical treatment of these acquired deformities has changed radically during the past three decades as a result of advances in the subspecialty of craniofacial surgery. Craniofacial surgery developed almost entirely from the work of Paul Tessier, who revolutionized facial skeletal surgery with his seminal work regarding treatment of congenital malformations, such as Crouzon disease,[1] Apert syndrome,[2] Treacher Collins–Franceschetti syndrome, vertical orbital dystopias, and orbital hypertelorism.[3–8] The basic principles Tessier stressed when operating on the facial skeleton include the following:[9]

Key points

- Complete subperiosteal exposure of the areas of interest through coronal, lower eyelid, or intraoral incisions.
- Repositioning misaligned segments of the craniofacial skeleton with rigid fixation and interposed autogenous bone grafts to provide consolidation of the structure.[10] Onlay "camouflage" grafts are to be avoided because they do not provide a three-dimensional (3D) correction of the entire deformity.
- Utilizing only fresh, autogenous bone grafts, obtainable from the ribs, anterior and posterior ilium, tibia, and the skull.[11,12] There is little place for bone substitutes, whether alloplastic materials or cadaver bone, in craniofacial reconstruction.[13]
- If a structure is not present to be repositioned, it can be constructed *in situ* or constructed and then moved to the proper location.
- The once forbidden boundary zone between the cranial cavity and the midface can safely be transgressed if proper care is taken in its reconstruction. Regular and frequent collaboration between the plastic surgical and neurosurgical members of a craniofacial team decreases the risks associated with a transcranial approach.
- Other members of a craniofacial team, such as ophthalmologists and orthodontists, will need to be involved in the treatment of acquired deformities, just as for congenital malformations.

Basic science/disease process

Access incisions

Access to the facial skeleton is provided through coronal, lower eyelid, and intraoral incisions. The following paragraphs describe the proper techniques to be used when making these incisions. Further detail regarding surgical approaches to the craniofacial skeleton can be found elsewhere.[14] In addition, a thorough knowledge of the craniofacial anatomy is essential and is detailed in Part 1, Chapter 1: Anatomy of the head and neck in this volume.

Coronal incisions

Coronal incisions (not *bicoronal* as it is often mistakenly referred to) should be made at least 3 cm behind the anterior hairline, almost at the vertex. The incision is carried to a point just above the anterior attachment of the ear, where a small cutback of 8–10 mm is made in the direction of the lateral canthus, allowing the coronal flap to be turned forward without tension. Incisions close to or along the anterior hairline can be noticeable and difficult to improve in areas of scarring alopecia. The dissection is carried out in a supraperiosteal plane to the level of the supraorbital ridge, where it then becomes subperiosteal. The superficial temporal fascia (STF) is generally divided, exposing the deeper temporal fascia upon approaching the zygomatic arch and malar region. The temporalis muscle should be elevated separately from the scalp and re-sutured to the lateral orbital rim, anterior temporal crest, and posterior portion of the coronal incision, maintaining its original tension upon closure of the incision. The STF should also be resuspended at the time of closure. After the temporal muscle has been sutured back into position under proper tension, a suture is taken from near the lateral canthal raphe and passed through the temporal aponeurosis to reposition the lateral canthus properly (Fig. 8.1).

Once a coronal incision has been made, the same incision should be used for any future surgeries, as a scalp with multiple scars may greatly complicate later reconstruction. Additionally, previously described incisions, such as the hemicoronal incision with an extension on to the forehead, are relics of the past, and have no place in modern day craniofacial surgery.

Lower eyelid incisions

The lower eyelid, inferior orbital rim, and orbital floor can be accessed through either the conjunctiva or the lower eyelid. If a cutaneous approach is used, it should be lower in the eyelid, beneath the tarsal plate, rather than in the immediate subciliary area in order to minimize postoperative ectropion.[15,16]

Intraoral incisions

Upper buccal sulcus incisions should have an adequate inferior mucosal cuff for subsequent closure. The infraorbital nerve should be protected and the buccal fat pad avoided during dissection. The entire mandible up to the sigmoid notch and 1 cm inferior to the coronoid process and condyle are accessible through a lower buccal sulcus incision.[17]

Bone grafts

The key element to success in repositioning or replacing portions of the facial skeleton lies in the liberal and exclusive use of fresh autogenous bone grafts. Cranial bone is the preferred donor site, given the ease of harvest, quality, and quantity of the bone, and proximity to the operating field.

The preferred donor area for cranial grafts is the right parietal area in right-handed patients.[18] When large grafts are required, the craniotomy can be extended anteriorly beyond the coronal suture and posteriorly into the occipital region. If additional bone is required, the opposite parietal region may be utilized. The harvested bone should be slightly larger in dimension than the area to be corrected. Each graft can be split through the diploic space to give two segments of equal dimensions. The inner table is replaced in the donor area with one of the segments. A defect several millimeters in width will be present, varying with the thickness of the craniotome blade. This defect is placed posteriorly and filled in with small bone chips, slivers, and bone dust and covered with a pericranial flap.[19] The bone graft for the defect is tailored exactly to the defect (Fig. 8.2). On occasion, it is good to enlarge the defect slightly by burring back to healthy bone. Fixation with wires is preferred over miniplates for reasons of cost and ease of use.

Although cranial bone is the preferential donor site in craniofacial cases, iliac bone provides an excellent graft for the orbital floor because of the thin cortical floor with malleable cancellous bone that is rigid enough to support the globe. Also, iliac bone is an excellent choice when large amounts of cancellous bone are required, such as for obliterating a frontal sinus (Fig. 8.3). Rib is often used when other donor sites are not available or advisable and are best suited for areas of the hair-bearing scalp when contour irregularities are less conspicuous.

Soft-tissue cover

The success of free bone grafts depends on the intimate contact of well-vascularized soft tissues both above and below the grafts. This means that areas between bone grafts must be filled in with other graft material and hematoma formation

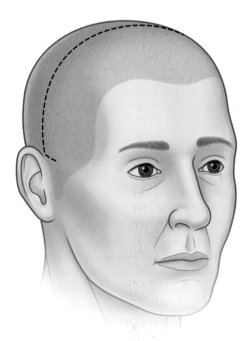

Fig. 8.1 Coronal incision.

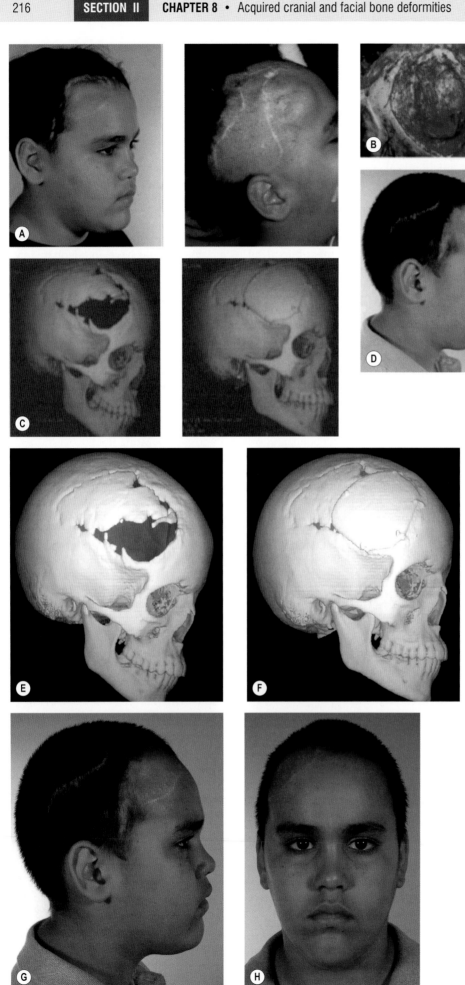

Fig. 8.2 This 12-year-old boy was in an automobile accident in Cuba and sustained an open right frontal fracture. The original laceration is apparently the sweeping scar from near the midpoint of the anterior hairline to a point above the right sideburn. A subsequent neurosurgical procedure was performed through an incision just along the right anterior hairline, and yet another procedure was performed through a more posterior incision **(A,B).** Through one of these incisions, an attempt was made to correct the cranial defect with an alloplastic material that had to be removed because of infection. The cranial defect was approached through an anterior hairline incision that extended into a more posterior coronal incision on the left side. A left parietal craniotomy of a slightly larger dimension than the measurements of the right frontal cranial defect was performed, and the cranial flap was split (*ex vivo*) into two segments through the diploic space. The outer table segment was used for the frontal defect after precise trimming, and the inner table segment was placed back in the donor area **(C,D). (E,F)** A postoperative 3D computed tomography scan displays the precise repair of the cranial defect with the split calvarial graft. **(G,H)** Healing was uneventful. There are two important lessons to be learned from this patient. First, use a posterior coronal incision, and use it for all subsequent procedures. Second, use autogenous cranial bone for cranioplasties whenever possible.

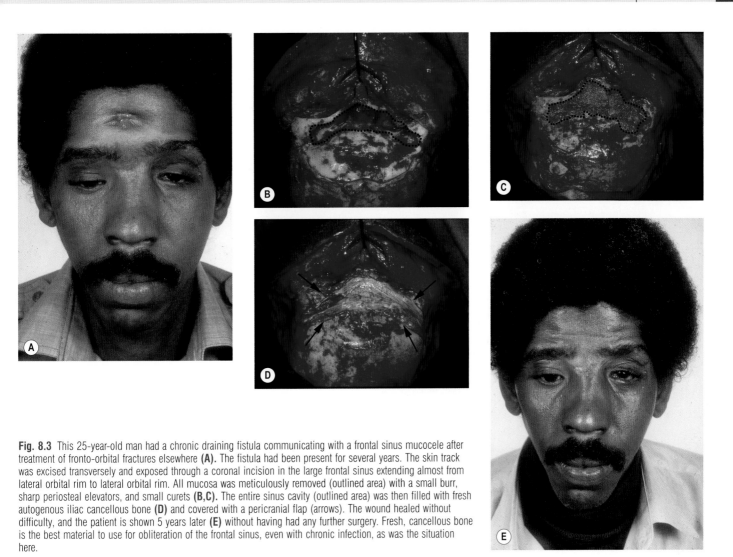

Fig. 8.3 This 25-year-old man had a chronic draining fistula communicating with a frontal sinus mucocele after treatment of fronto-orbital fractures elsewhere **(A)**. The fistula had been present for several years. The skin track was excised transversely and exposed through a coronal incision in the large frontal sinus extending almost from lateral orbital rim to lateral orbital rim. All mucosa was meticulously removed (outlined area) with a small burr, sharp periosteal elevators, and small curets **(B,C)**. The entire sinus cavity (outlined area) was then filled with fresh autogenous iliac cancellous bone **(D)** and covered with a pericranial flap (arrows). The wound healed without difficulty, and the patient is shown 5 years later **(E)** without having had any further surgery. Fresh, cancellous bone is the best material to use for obliteration of the frontal sinus, even with chronic infection, as was the situation here.

prevented by fastidious hemostasis and adequate postoperative drainage. When soft tissues are inadequate because of the original trauma or radiotherapy, they must be replaced with good soft tissue before bone grafts can survive. This includes filling the dead space under planned autogenous cranioplasty (Fig. 8.4). Given adequate exposure, an acceptable amount of autogenous bone grafts, and the means to provide rigid fixation, the correction of deformities in various areas of the facial skeleton should proceed smoothly.

Treatment/surgical technique

Treatment of specific defects

Acquired defects of the cranium and facial skeleton can be divided into two groups: those resulting from displaced fractures and those resulting from a loss of substance. We will discuss each specific area of the cranial and facial bone defects and their treatment.

Cranium

Cranial defects greater than half the thickness of the skull in patients older than 2 years of age should be repaired. In children younger than 2 years of age, they often spontaneously ossify and do not require treatment. Cranial bone is the material of choice for most cranioplasties due both to the quality of bone and proximity to the field of operation (Figs. 8.2, 8.4, 8.5).[20,21] In the authors' experience, the youngest patient with a cranial bone that can be successfully split *ex vivo* is between 3 and 4 years of age. Good results can also be obtained with split rib (Fig. 8.6). Rib grafts can be used from the age of 4–5 years, depending on the size of the patient.

Alloplastic materials should not be used in children as a primary reconstructive option. If the cranial defect has been corrected with autogenous bone grafts and all reconstructive work is complete, for minor surface irregularities present after 1 year, small amounts of alloplastic material such as Norian (Synthes Inc., West Chester, PA, USA), BoneSource (Stryker Inc., Kalamazoo, MI, USA), or hydroxyapatite may be utilized. In adults, small defects remote from the frontal sinus may also be primarily corrected with these materials.

Near the frontal sinus, only autogenous bone should be used due to the proximity to the sinuses and elevated risk of infection.[22] If there is a full-thickness cranial defect near the frontal sinus, the sinus should be cranialized; if the posterior wall of the sinus is intact and the nasofrontal duct appears to be blocked, all mucosa should be removed and the sinus filled with autogenous cancellous grafts (Fig. 8.3).[23, 24]

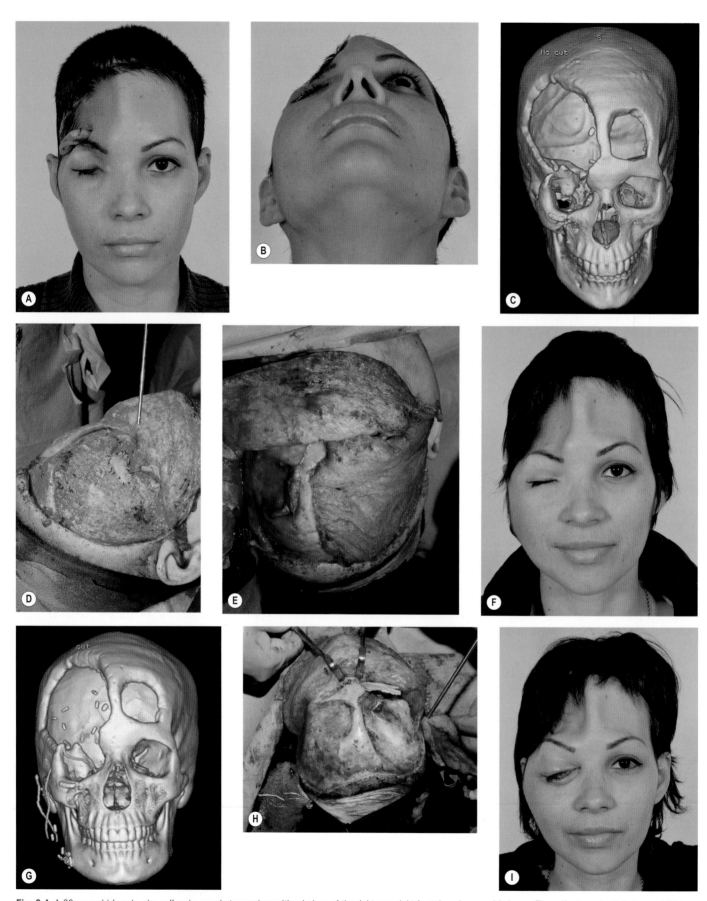

Fig. 8.4 A 28-year-old female who suffered a gunshot wound, resulting in loss of the right eye, right frontal, and supraorbital area. The patient was treated at an outside institution with debridement and craniectomy, right orbital exenteration, and attempt at frontal sinus obliteration. She is seen at presentation with Penrose drain in place (A,B,C). The patient underwent excision of draining fistula tract, dural patch (D), and obliteration of dead space with free latissimus dorsi flap (E). Photographs and CT postoperatively (F,G). She then underwent reconstruction of the right supraorbital area with iliac bone graft (H) and is seen postoperatively in photographs (I) and CT (J).

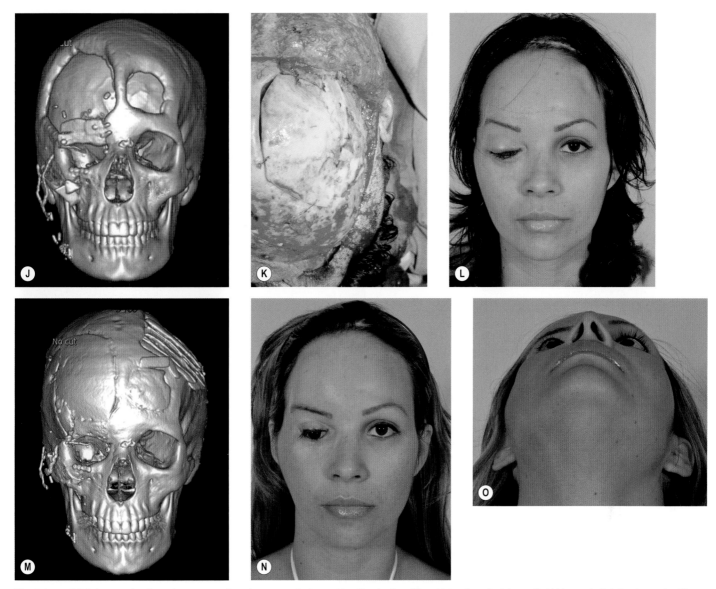

Fig. 8.4, cont'd Subsequently, she underwent staged autologous cranioplasty with split calvarium (K) and later rib graft of donor site hidden under hair bearing scalp. She is seen postoperatively in photographs (L) and CT (M). Current clinical photographs (N,O) with soft tissue revisions planned for right periorbital area surrounding her ocular prosthesis.

Nose

This region involves the nasal bones, cartilaginous and bony septum, and the upper lateral cartilages. Minimally displaced fractures can often be treated with closed reduction and placement of nasal splints. Comminuted fractures require an open rhinoplasty approach and usually require placement of an autogenous bone graft.[25–28] This approach makes it possible to separate the alar cartilages and then replace them over the nasal bone graft. Bone grafts for a depressed dorsum are simply placed into an appropriate pocket after dissection of the skin alone. In general, the bone graft is not rigidly fixed in place; care must be taken that the posterior portion of the bone graft is flat to avoid shifting of the graft. Making bilateral nasal vestibular incisions also helps provide an appropriate pocket so that the graft will remain in the center of the nose. If a graft does shift in the postoperative period, it can often

be repositioned and maintained with a percutaneous K-wire, placed under local anesthesia, and maintained in position until consolidation of the bone graft occurs (Fig. 8.7).

If substantial lengthening (>1 cm) of the nose is required, such as in Binder syndrome[29] or post-traumatic nasal foreshortening, dissection of the skin alone is not sufficient. The lining needs to be lengthened as well. Tessier *et al.* have shown that considerable lengthening can be obtained, even in congenitally short noses, by dissecting the lining from beneath the nasal bones all the way back to the pharynx.[30] Another approach is purposely to section the lining (and bone) at the nasofrontal area, as in a Le Fort III osteotomy (Fig. 8.8).[31]

The undersurface of the bone graft may be exposed to the nasal cavity, but healing proceeds uneventfully, as it does in a Le Fort III over bone grafts exposed to the maxillary sinus. This type of procedure would not be applicable to the contracted, foreshortened nose that is associated with sustained

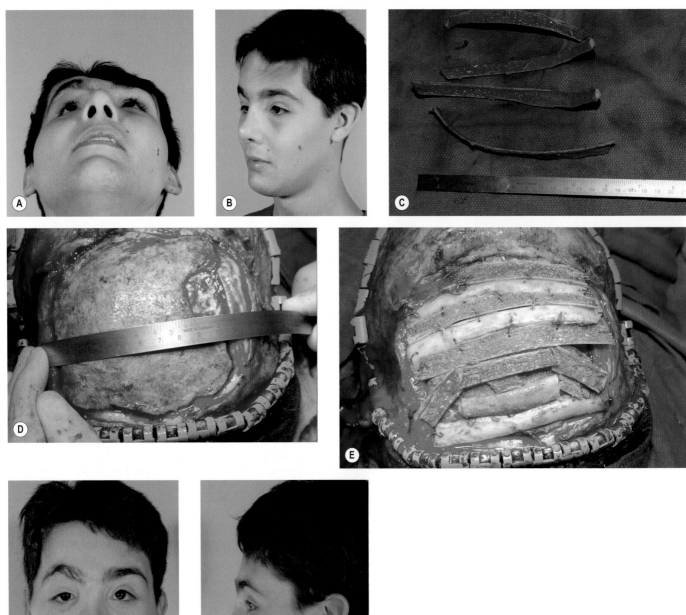

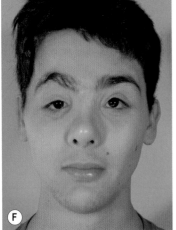

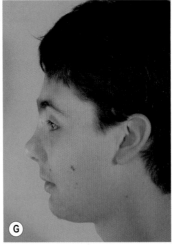

Fig. 8.6 This 22-year-old man had multiple facial and cranial fractures following a motor vehicle accident. He had a craniotomy for an acute epidural hematoma and subsequently developed a retrofrontal mucopyocele, necessitating removal of the infected frontal bone flap **(A,B)**. Six months later, the frontal defect was repaired with split-rib grafts **(C–E)**. He is shown 8 months after surgery with improved contour of the previous defect **(F,G)**.

cocaine use. Here, the lining is either altogether absent or chronically granulating and infected. Before a nasal bone graft can be added, nasal lining must be provided by local and regional flaps such as nasolabial, forehead, or buccal sulcus flaps. Alternatively, free flaps such as the radial forearm can be utilized for severely deficient tissue.[32]

Nasoethmoid area

Fractures in this region are often referred to as naso-orbital–ethmoid fractures, although the ethmoidal involvement,

by definition, involves the orbit. Telecanthus, as a result of lateral displacement of the medial orbital walls and nasal foreshortening, is commonly seen after these fractures. One must resist the temptation to treat this conservatively with packing alone, as this pushes the structures further in, adding to the nasal foreshortening. A coronal incision should be used for adequate exposure unless a large facial laceration provides excellent exposure. Correction of telecanthus secondary to displaced bone fragments with the medial canthal tendons still attached can often be accomplished by anatomic reduction of the bone segments, without having

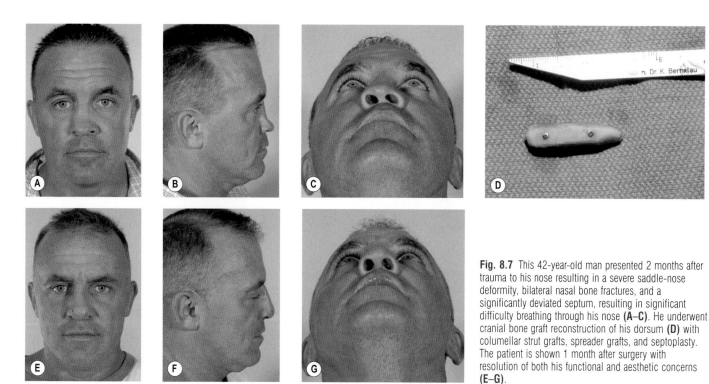

Fig. 8.7 This 42-year-old man presented 2 months after trauma to his nose resulting in a severe saddle-nose deformity, bilateral nasal bone fractures, and a significantly deviated septum, resulting in significant difficulty breathing through his nose (**A–C**). He underwent cranial bone graft reconstruction of his dorsum (**D**) with columellar strut grafts, spreader grafts, and septoplasty. The patient is shown 1 month after surgery with resolution of both his functional and aesthetic concerns (**E–G**).

to detach the tendons and perform a transnasal medial canthopexy.[33,34]

If the medial canthal tendon has been detached, a transnasal canthopexy must be performed. Some overcorrection of the medial wall segments is desirable, as in the correction of orbital hypertelorism. If there is significant loss of substance in the medial orbital wall, it may be necessary to perform a primary bone graft and medial canthopexy. The nasal dorsum will usually require a bone graft to repair the foreshortening resulting from the fracture (Fig. 8.9).

Late reconstructions may pose an even greater challenge if the bones have consolidated in malposition. In such cases, the dissection must be extensive, often involving coronal, lower eyelid, and buccal sulcus incisions. The displaced segments must be delineated and osteotomized in order to return to their proper position. Plate and screw fixation is used to stabilize the segments.[35] A nasal bone graft is frequently necessary for dorsal support and soft tissue may be needed to keep in conjunction with the principle of aesthetic subunits.

Orbitozygomatic region (Video 8.1 ◉)

Acute, isolated fractures of the zygomatic arch require an open approach if they cannot be reduced percutaneously. A coronal incision gives access for reduction and plating of the fracture or harvesting of bone grafts, if necessary.

Isolated orbital floor fractures are seen more commonly in younger patients, where the infraorbital rim is more elastic in comparison to adult patients (Fig. 8.10). It appears that the causative force strikes the rim, which bends and then springs back to its original position. These actions can cause a fracture in the thin orbital floor. These injuries have the highest incidence of entrapment, diplopia, and inferior rectus damage which requires prompt intraoperative release.

Orbitozygomatic fractures vary considerably in their presentation, depending on the vector and force of the causative injury. Lesser injuries may result in nondisplaced fractures of the zygoma with minimal disruption of the orbital floor. In this instance, no treatment other than follow-up observation is necessary. If one has underappreciated the extent of the orbital floor fracture, late enophthalmos is a possible sequela;[36] however, one certainly does not have to operate on questionable fractures simply because of this possibility. Some advocated this approach when it was thought that enophthalmos could not be corrected.[37,38]

Greater forces cause greater disruption, and because of the elastic nature of bone, the extent of bone displacement during the injury may be much greater than the displacement seen when the patient first presents. Again, late enophthalmos may develop if these injuries are not repaired properly (Fig. 8.11). If one puts the orbital framework into proper position with rigid fixation and repairs the internal orbital defects with autogenous bone grafts, enophthalmos will not result. Examination of the orbital floor and globe position must be reassessed after reduction, followed by a forced duction test to ensure unrestricted movement of the globe.

Reduction of an orbitozygomatic fracture in which the zygomatic body has been displaced away from the globe can usually be accomplished in the first week after the fracture simply by removing callus in the fracture lines and grasping solid segments of bone with bone clamps. When the zygoma has been displaced by the injury toward the globe, proptosis or at least lack of enophthalmos may be present when the patient is first seen. In some instances, it may not be possible to reduce the fracture. In these instances, one must be prepared to perform an osteotomy through the fracture lines in order to reduce the fracture adequately.

Most fractures that are seen after a delay of 3 weeks or more will have consolidated and will require osteotomy and

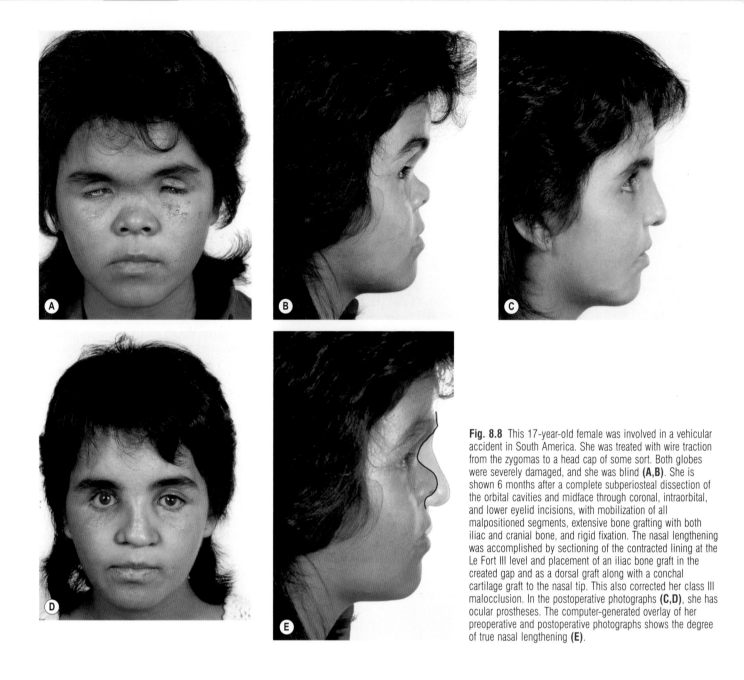

Fig. 8.8 This 17-year-old female was involved in a vehicular accident in South America. She was treated with wire traction from the zygomas to a head cap of some sort. Both globes were severely damaged, and she was blind **(A,B)**. She is shown 6 months after a complete subperiosteal dissection of the orbital cavities and midface through coronal, intraorbital, and lower eyelid incisions, with mobilization of all malpositioned segments, extensive bone grafting with both iliac and cranial bone, and rigid fixation. The nasal lengthening was accomplished by sectioning of the contracted lining at the Le Fort III level and placement of an iliac bone graft in the created gap and as a dorsal graft along with a conchal cartilage graft to the nasal tip. This also corrected her class III malocclusion. In the postoperative photographs **(C,D)**, she has ocular prostheses. The computer-generated overlay of her preoperative and postoperative photographs shows the degree of true nasal lengthening **(E)**.

repositioning. Coronal, lower eyelid, and buccal sulcus incisions are used in most of these patients to provide good access for the osteotomies and also to allow the surgeon to appreciate the internal orbital anatomy fully, both of the medial orbital wall and of the lateral orbital wall. The sphenoidal portion of the lateral orbital wall should be perfectly aligned and is an excellent starting point to ensure proper reduction and correction of rotational deformity. A positioning wire is then placed through the frontozygomatic suture, and finally the inferior orbital rim is aligned. A wire is usually all that is needed for the frontozygomatic suture, and a small plate is placed to stabilize the inferior orbital rim. The zygomatic buttresses[39] should be checked through the upper sulcus incision and fixed in proper position with a larger plate. Finally, the zygomatic arch is plated, and one should have exposure of the normal side to check the exact shape of the normal zygomatic arch. If the arches are fractured on both sides, recall that they should be fairly straight, and not bowed, in order to provide proper projection of the midface.

Post-traumatic enophthalmos

Post-traumatic enophthalmos can result either from isolated defects of the orbital floor and medial orbital wall, in which there is herniation of orbital contents into the maxillary and ethmoidal sinuses, or from displaced orbitozygomatic fractures, in which there is herniation of orbital contents into the paranasal sinuses.[40] If there is even a slight displacement of the zygoma from its proper position, it should be osteotomized and properly positioned. Autogenous bone grafts are used to replace missing or displaced portions of the internal orbit.[41,42] In the presence of a seeing eye, post-traumatic enophthalmos can be completely corrected in most instances if the bony orbit is completely reconstructed and all of the

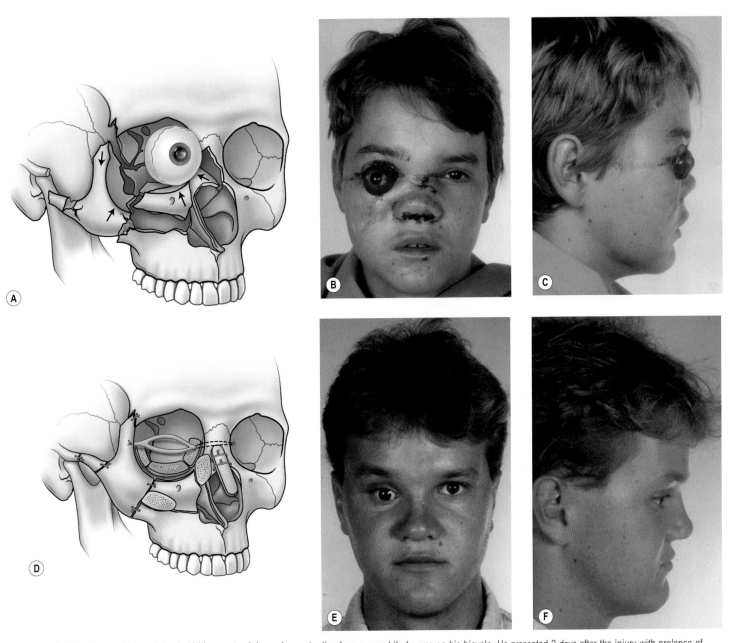

Fig. 8.9 This 13-year-old boy, living in Haiti, was struck by a pipe protruding from a car while he was on his bicycle. He presented 2 days after the injury with prolapse of the right globe and loss of vision, even though some extraocular motions were still present **(A–C)**. Additionally, avulsion of the right medial rectus was noted. Fractures of the right orbit and nasoethmoid region were present, as well as right telecanthus **(A)**. Treatment consisted of exposure of the fractures through coronal, right lower eyelid, and upper buccal sulcus incisions. Fractures were reduced and wire osteosynthesis placed. Replacement of the right globe into the orbital cavity required making multiple scoring incisions of the periorbitum. Iliac bone grafts to the nose, orbital floor, medial orbital wall, and anterior maxilla were placed, and a transnasal medial canthopexy through the medial orbital wall bone graft was performed **(D)**. He is shown 5 years postoperatively with a cosmetic cover shell over the right eye and good maintenance of nasal contour with the bone graft **(E,F)**.

orbital contents are returned to the orbital cavity.[43] Overcorrection by several millimeters in both the vertical and sagittal directions should be performed to compensate for operative swelling.

In patients with inadequate late correction of enophthalmos, even if it is mild, a coronal and sagittal computed tomographic (CT) scan will show a few areas where further bone grafting can provide a complete correction. When one is performing secondary bone grafting such as this, it is important to bear in mind that the orbital cavity may not have any areas of egress because all of the communications into the

paranasal sinuses have been closed off with bone grafts. Bringing a small drain (such as a TLS drain) from the orbital floor out through the sideburn area will lessen the possibility of a volume and pressure increase due to hematoma (Figs. 8.12 & 8.13).[44]

The irradiated orbit

Irradiation of the orbit in early childhood, such as for retinoblastoma, will result in a small orbit and often restriction of growth of the temporal fossa. If a seeing eye is still

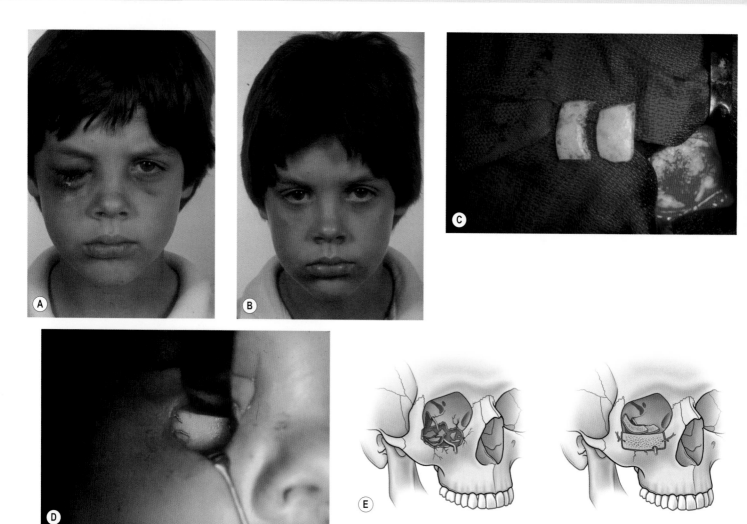

Fig. 8.10 This 9-year-old boy was kicked in the face by a horse. Ophthalmologic examination showed no damage to the eye itself. There was considerable ecchymosis and swelling of the eyelids, and, even with that, some enophthalmos was present **(A)**. There was a palpable depression of the infraorbital rim. A computed tomography scan showed comminution of the infraorbital rim and anterior maxilla with a large defect of the orbital floor. The malar bone, however, was not otherwise displaced. Treatment consisted of a lower lid incision, removal of multiple small comminuted bone fragments of the infraorbital rim, exploration of the orbital floor, with retrieval of orbital contents from the antrum, and placement of cranial bone grafts on the orbital floor and infraorbital rim/anterior maxilla **(C–E)**. His postoperative appearance at 1 year shows no evidence of enophthalmos **(B)**.

present, one can deal with the temporal fossa defect with a soft-tissue flap, most efficiently by composite tissue transplantation. The orbit itself should not be altered. If the eye is absent and the orbit small, an orbital expansion can be performed to give an orbit of normal dimensions.[45] This is followed by socket reconstruction and placement of an ocular prosthesis.

Primary and secondary facial bones reconstruction

The overall approach for secondary correction of displaced facial bone segments is the same as for primary correction: obtain adequate exposure, place the segments into proper position, utilize rigid fixation, and liberally use autogenous bone grafts for any residual bone defects. The main difference is that the soft-tissue dissection is often much more difficult because of scarring and contraction of the soft-tissue envelope over the malpositioned facial bone segments. The buccal fat pad and other soft-tissue elements of the midface may have

prolapsed into the maxillary sinus through defects in the anterior maxillary wall, and these must be completely retrieved. Autogenous bone grafts are used to recreate the anterior maxillary wall and to keep the soft tissues in their proper place. As noted previously, the dissected midfacial tissues are suspended to the temporal aponeurosis, and a lateral canthopexy is performed.

Maxillary fractures

When evaluating fractures of the maxilla, one must remember the importance of the maxillary buttresses, as described by Gruss and Mackinnon[46] and Manson et al.[39] These thickenings of bone conduct masticatory and other forces through the midface to the thicker bones of the skull and are divided into four categories:

1. Central: septo-vomerine-ethmoidal-frontal
2. Medial/paracentral: maxillo-naso-frontal
3. Lateral: maxillo-malar-frontal
4. Posterior: maxillo-pterygoid.

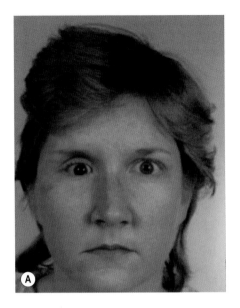

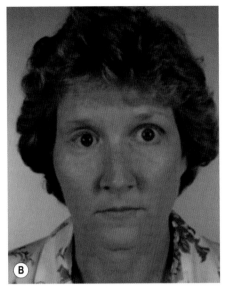

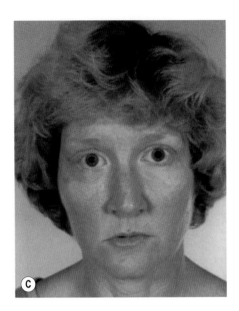

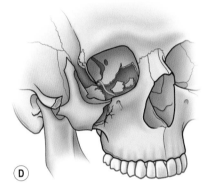

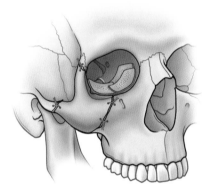

Fig. 8.11 This woman was 32 years old when an osteotomy and repositioning of the right zygoma were performed along with an iliac bone graft **(A)**. An undercorrection was noted 6 years later **(B)**. A computed tomographic evaluation showed a persistent small defect in the posteromedial orbital wall as well as an enlargement of the inferior orbital fissure; the addition of a small amount of cranial bone corrected the persistent enophthalmos completely, as seen in her photo 4 years after her second surgery **(C)**. **(D)** Illustration showing the repositioning of the right zygoma.

When any of the maxillary buttresses is fractured transversely in only one place, but is otherwise intact, treatment consists of reducing the fracture to a proper occlusal relationship with the mandible, followed by rigid fixation across the fracture line. The use of intermaxillary fixation depends on the stability of the osteosynthesis. If the buttresses are comminuted with a loss of facial height, treatment must include reconstitution of the bony deficiencies with primary bone grafts. It is not uncommon for a Le Fort I fracture to be treated by intermaxillary fixation with a satisfactory occlusal result but a shortened midface. This occurs if the maxillary buttresses have all been fractured and the maxilla is displaced upward until bone contact occurs.[47] This deformity can be prevented if a primary reconstruction of the buttresses is carried out at the initial repair.[48,49]

If maxillary fractures have not been adequately reduced in the primary operation, they may require late treatment. This requires sectioning of the maxilla at the Le Fort I level, mobilization of the maxilla, and intermaxillary fixation. If the maxilla–mandible complex in intermaxillary fixation is allowed to find its own position in the lightly anesthetized, unparalyzed patient, this position represents the degree of lengthening desired. The two sides of the sectioned maxilla can now be plated in this position. Again, adequate amounts of autogenous bone grafts are essential to the consolidation of the maxilla in its new position.

Maxillary reconstruction

The same dissection previously described for traumatic deformities can be employed for either primary or secondary reconstruction of maxillary defects subsequent to removal of maxillary tumors, including use of the temporalis muscle.[50] A portion of the temporalis is mobilized through the coronal incision and the arch of the zygoma is removed to allow passage to the oral cavity. A hemimaxillary defect can easily be closed with this muscle flap. The muscle does not need to be covered by mucosa or skin grafted because it is rapidly covered by mucosa naturally. An alveolar defect, either lateral or anterior, must be present to bring in the muscle flap easily. If the alveolar ridge is intact, it is difficult to bring in a muscle flap because it involves making a hole through the anterior maxillary wall or bringing the muscle behind the maxillary tuberosity (Fig. 8.14). For large central palatal defects that cannot be closed by local palatal flaps, a microsurgical solution is preferred with preference for the radial forearm flap.[51] After complete healing of the soft-tissue palatal repair, a bony alveolar ridge can be reconstructed with iliac bone grafts or

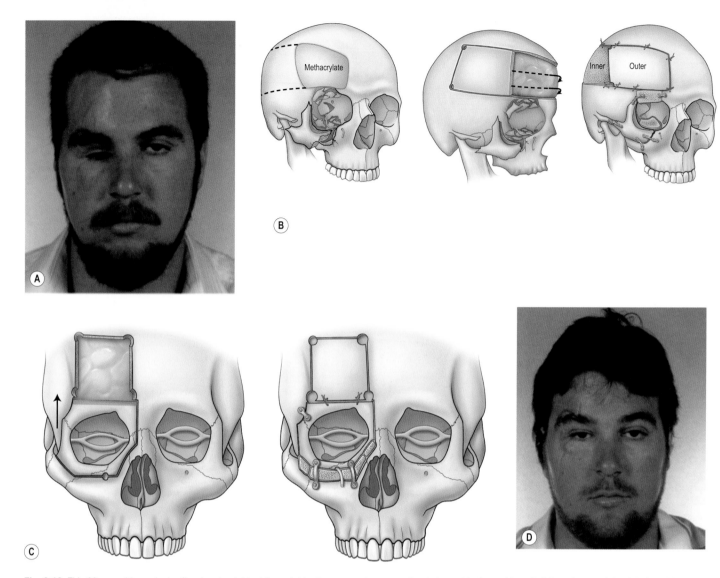

Fig. 8.12 This 23-year-old man had suffered major right orbitocranial fractures several years previously in a vehicular accident. A defect of most of the right frontal bone had been reconstructed with methyl methylmethacrylate. There was profound enophthalmos and hypoglobus of the right eye, which still retained some vision **(A)**. In the initial operation, the alloplastic material was removed, and the frontal defect was reconstructed with split cranial bone **(B)**. Major reconstructive orbital surgery is not recommended if there is any alloplastic material in the region of the periorbital sinuses. At the same time, refracture and repositioning of the right zygoma were performed along with cranial bone grafting of the medial orbital wall and orbital floor defects. This corrected the enophthalmos, but the patient was left with a considerable persistent hypoglobus. This was treated as a true vertical orbital dystopia, with an intracranial elevation of the entire – now intact – orbital cavity **(C)**. The medial canthal tendon was left attached to bone and was elevated with the orbit. The patient is shown 3 years after the second operation **(D)**.

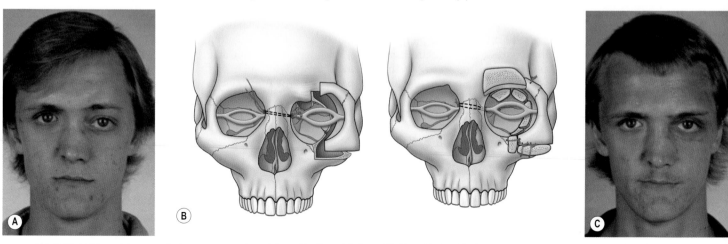

Fig. 8.13 In this post-trauma patient, one can see a hypoglobus without enophthalmos **(A)**. The orbital roof had been pushed into the orbital cavity, resulting in a slight proptosis. The globe was elevated by an osteotomy and repositioning of the zygoma, elevation of the orbital roof, and bone grafting of the orbital floor along with a transnasal medial canthopexy **(B)**. The canthopexy shows that the canthal tendon is brought through a drill hole in the medial orbital wall just above and posterior to the lacrimal fossa and tied over a toggle on the contralateral side. He is shown operatively with correction of his hypoglobus **(C)**.

microvascular osseous flaps (fibula or parascapular flaps are the most common).[52] After the bone repair is well consolidated, osseointegrated implants can be placed to accept a denture and finish the reconstruction.

Mandible fractures

When evaluating a patient with a suspected mandibular fracture, the diagnosis can often be made by physical examination alone. Common findings include malocclusion, a step in the occlusal plane, a change in the axial inclination of the teeth, mental nerve paresthesias, ecchymosis or a tear in the buccal mucosa overlying the fracture, and localized pain on palpation and movement at the fracture site. To locate the fracture and any associated fractures precisely, a Panorex or CT scan should be performed.[53]

Treatment of nondisplaced mandibular fractures in compliant patients may consist of a soft diet and careful observation alone with repeat radiological studies over 4–6 weeks. If the patient is noncompliant, he or she may be best served with 4–6 weeks of intermaxillary fixation.

Displaced fractures of the mandibular symphysis, body, or ascending angle are usually associated with malocclusion and require treatment with open reduction and internal fixation. In 1976, Spiessl[54] described the concept of the "tension band" in the treatment of displaced mandibular fractures. He described the use of one fixed point of osteosynthesis as a fulcrum in order to achieve greater compression of the bone fragments and, therefore, more stability and primary bone healing. Two levels of fixation, along the upper and lower border of the mandible, are required. In the non-tooth-bearing regions (ascending ramus and angle), two plates may be used. In the tooth-bearing regions, an arch bar will provide stability for the upper border and a plate may be used along the lower border. In the symphysis and parasymphyseal regions, two plates can be placed in the space below the roots of the incisors and the lower border. Miniplates can be used with this approach, unless there have been significant comminution and fragmentation of the mandible.[55] In such cases involving comminution of the fracture, larger mandibular plates are required. When significant loss of mandibular substance occurs, a large reconstruction plate is necessary.

The edentulous state results in loss of alveolar bone, leaving a mandible that can be 1 cm or less in vertical height along the body. The thickness of the symphysis and structure of the vertical ramus change little, which accounts for the majority of fractures in edentulous mandibles occurring at the parasymphyseal area and body. These patients may have difficulty with fracture healing even with the use of rigid fixation, due to lack of bone stock. In select cases, primary bone grafting should be done to reinforce the fracture site.

Much debate remains as to the treatment of condylar fractures. In children under 12 years of age, no operative treatment is almost always indicated due to the tremendous potential of the condyle to remodel and regenerate.[56] In teenagers and adults, definite indications for operative treatment include the following: displacement of the condyle in the middle cranial fossa, bilateral fractures with an anterior open bite, multiple other maxillary and mandibular fractures where mandibular stability is important to maintaining facial height, and the situation in which the patient cannot be brought into occlusion with less invasive measures.[57] If the patient has sustained a subcondylar fracture with the condyle in the glenoid fossa and no malocclusion, treatment consists of application of arch bars with elastics or wire fixation, soft diet, and occlusal splint for 4–6 weeks, followed by aggressive physical therapy. If, however, the condyle is out of the fossa, the debate continues as to whether open or closed treatment is best.[58]

Mandibular reconstruction

Incontinuity defects of the mandible less than 3–4 cm in length covered by healthy soft tissue can be corrected with free bone grafts (iliac and cranial represent the bone grafts of choice) and rigid fixation with miniplates.[59,60] An adequate amount should be present (20 mm or more) in the vertical dimension in tooth-bearing areas for placement of osseointegrated implants. If defects involve the alveolus alone, either in the maxilla or in the mandible, getting enough bone for implants to take as a free graft may be difficult. If enough bone is present to permit a horizontal osteotomy, distraction osteogenesis will provide the best result because the gingiva will come up with the distracted bone and one can easily overcorrect the bone defect. Overcorrection may cause premature contact at the apex of the (now overcorrected) deficiency, with overeruption of the posterior molar teeth.

Although incontinuity defects of the mandible longer than 5 cm can be dealt with by free non-vascularized bone grafts, these larger defects are better corrected with microvascular transplantation of osseous flaps, particularly when the overlying soft tissues are less than optimal in condition or have been irradiated.[59] The fibular free flap is ideal for longer defects because it can be repeatedly osteotomized and fabricated to any desired shape, while the iliac free flap is well suited for anterior defects. The lesser amount of bone available in the radial forearm and scapular free flaps makes them less desirable choices.[61]

Chin

The most common reason for osseous procedures on the chin for acquired deformities has been an unfortunate outcome from a chin implant. Many of the patients have indeed had a number of chin implants, with removal, replacement, and often removal again, for reasons of infection and displacement.[62] Under these circumstances, an osseous genioplasty[63] should be performed, rather than trying again with an alloplastic material.[64] The capsule that forms around the implant should be removed to allow the osseous expansion to keep the soft-tissue envelope properly stretched. In some patients, a proper diagnosis had not been made in the first place, and the corrective procedure may need to provide proper correction of the original deformity, such as lengthening the chin for a congenital shortness (Fig. 8.15). Rarely, if the chin has had many previous operations and there is not adequate bone stock for an osseous genioplasty, a microvascular osteocutaneous free flap may provide the only solution (Fig. 8.16).

Postoperative care

With the exception of isolated orbital or nasal bone fractures, all patients will be placed on a liquid or soft diet for 2 weeks after surgery. Nasal splints can be removed after 1 week, and interdental fixation is usually removed within 4–6 weeks. All suture material on the face should be removed within 7 days.

Outcomes, prognosis, and complications

It is advisable to obtain postoperative radiographic images to assess the adequacy of reduction achieved. If the fractures are not adequately reduced on imaging, the surgeon must plan to return the patient to the operating room for proper correction of the defects. Inadequacy of reduction of facial fractures can lead to enophthalmos, malocclusion, and loss of proper facial proportions.

Secondary procedures

If a secondary operation is required more than 1 week after the initial operation, it is best to perform osteotomies to recreate the defect. This is almost certainly to be followed by the use of bone grafts to restore facial harmony.

Bonus images for this chapter can be found online at http://www.expertconsult.com

Fig. 8.5 This 23-year-old was shot through the right frontal region and has extensive debridement of the left frontal bone, supraorbital ridge, and orbital roof **(A,D,E)**. He is shown after a split cranial bone cranioplasty **(B,C)**, reconstruction of the orbital roof and supraorbital ridge, and subsequent ptosis correction by reattachment of the levator muscle to the tarsal plate **(F)**.

Fig. 8.14 This 29-year-old woman had undergone a hemimaxillectomy and postoperative irradiation for a neuroesthesioblastoma **(A)**. She was left with a large palatal defect **(B)**, as shown in her post-resection computed tomography scans **(C,D)**. Shortly after the initial preoperative photograph was taken, her right eye spontaneously perforated and she underwent an evisceration (removal of all of the orbital contents down to periosteum). Reconstruction of her maxilla was performed using a temporalis muscle flap to close the palatal defect **(E)**. The radiation-damaged skin of the lower eyelid and cheek was resected and a skin graft placed over the temporalis muscle. At a subsequent operation, an iliac bone graft was placed from alveolar ridge to pterygoid region **(F)**, well nourished by the underlying temporalis muscle; the lower eyelid was reconstructed with a forehead flap. Osseointegrated implants have been placed in the maxillary bone graft, and this portion of her reconstruction has been completed **(G)**. A second forehead flap was required for the lower eyelid reconstruction and her final postoperative result is shown **(H)**.

Fig. 8.15 This 30-year-old man had had five different chin implants **(A,B)**, the last one being a long "wrap-around" model placed below the lower border of his mandible. As with the others, he was displeased with the result of this one. He is shown after removal of the implant and a "jumping genioplasty" **(C,D)**. If he wished further projection of the chin, after an interval of 6 months or so, a sliding advancement genioplasty could be done through the previous genioplasty. Chin implants are appropriate for mild degrees of retrogenia, but severe retrogenia, chins requiring vertical or lateral alteration, and failures of previous chin implants should be treated with osseous genioplasties.

Fig. 8.16 This 67-year-old woman stated that she had undergone some sort of jaw injury as a child (perhaps condylar fractures) and had been treated, among others, by Dr. Robert Ivy in Philadelphia and Dr. Varaztad Kazanjian in Boston. In total, she had undergone more than 26 operations in attempts to construct a chin. Segments of block hydroxyapatite had been successfully placed along the mandibular body, but all of the chin implants had to be removed because of infection or intraoral exposure **(A,B)**. She had only a thin segment of bone connecting the parasymphyseal areas, and the intraoral soft tissues were thin and scarred; it was thought that they would not provide adequate coverage for any type of conventional genioplasty. After considerable explanation to the patient and her husband, the decision was made to go ahead with the only method that could most likely provide her with a chin: microsurgical reconstruction with use of an iliac osteocutaneous free flap. The U-shaped segment of iliac bone was attached to the inferior border of what remained of her native symphysis and a skin paddle and soft-tissue attachments were transferred with the bone segment **(C)**. She is shown a month after the operation, with the skin paddle in place **(D)**, and a year after the original operation, following defatting of the pedicle and removal of the skin island **(E,F)**.

Access the complete reference list online at   http://www.expertconsult.com

9. Wolfe SA. The influence of Paul Tessier on our current treatment of facial trauma, both in primary care and in the management of late sequelae. *Clin Plast Surg.* 1997;24:515–518. *This article reviews the principles of facial skeletal surgery taught by Paul Tessier, the father of craniofacial surgery. His principles, such as obtaining complete subperiosteal exposure and the use of autogenous bone grafts, have withstood the test of time and remain critical for the education of all craniofacial surgeons.*

11. Wolfe SA. Autogenous bone grafts versus alloplastic materials. In: Wolfe SA, Berkowitz S, eds. *Plastic Surgery of the Facial Skeleton.* Boston: Little, Brown; 1989:25–38.

14. Ellis IIIE, Zide MF. *Surgical approaches to the facial skeleton.* 2nd ed. Baltimore: Lippincott Williams & Wilkins; 2006.

23. Rodriguez ED, Stanwix MG, Nam AJ, et al. Twenty-six-year experience treating frontal sinus fractures: a novel algorithm based on anatomical fracture pattern and failure of conventional techniques. *Plast Reconstr Surg.* 2008;122(6):1850–1866.

31. Wolfe SA. Lengthening the nose: a lesson from craniofacial surgery applied to post-traumatic and congenital deformities. *Plast Reconstr Surg.* 1994;94:78. *This article describes a variety of causes of nasal hypoplasias, from traumatic to congenital and the author's treatment strategies. The article stresses the liberal use of bone and cartilage grafts in rebuilding the nose.*

36. Wolfe SA. Application of craniofacial surgical precepts in orbital reconstruction following trauma and tumor removal. *J Maxillofac Surg.* 1982;10:212. *This article describes the principles of craniofacial surgery, as described by Paul Tessier, in working with the orbit and their application to management of the reconstructive or trauma patient. These include the use of subperiosteal exposure and liberal use of autogenous bone grafts when reconstruction of the floor is necessary to prevent enophthalmos.*

39. Manson PN, Hoopes JE, Su CT. Structural pillars of the facial skeleton: an approach to the management of Le Fort fractures. *Plast Reconstr Surg.* 1980;66:54. *This landmark article describes the facial buttresses and their relationship to facial structure. It describes the importance of these relationships in treating Le Fort fractures.*

46. Gruss JS, Mackinnon SE. Complex maxillary fractures: role of buttress reconstruction and immediate bone grafts. *Plast Reconstr Surg.* 1986;78:9.

47. Wolfe SA, Baker S. Fractures of the Maxilla. In: Wolfe SA, Baker S, eds. *Operative Techniques in Plastic Surgery: Facial Fractures.* New York: Thieme Medical Publishers; 1993:61–71.

64. Cohen SR, Mardach OL, Kawamoto HK Jr. Chin disfigurement following removal of alloplastic chin implants. *Plast Reconstr Surg.* 1991;88:62, discussion 67. *This article describes the risks involved with the use of alloplastic chin implants, particularly the associated changes in the mandible. It advocates the use of the osseous genioplasty.*

9.1

Computerized surgical planning: Introduction

Eduardo D. Rodriguez

Introduction to computerized surgical planning

In an era of exponential technological progress, it is fitting that, for the first time in *Plastic Surgery*, two chapters on the topic of computerized surgical planning have been selected for publication. The first chapter is the perspective of the craniofacial orthodontist, an inseparable collaborator of the multidisciplinary craniofacial team. Outlining the transition from traditional two-dimensional (2D) craniofacial planning to current three-dimensional (3D) techniques, a step-by-step guide details the process of digital component creation for synthesis of an operative orthognathic surgical plan. State of the art software has enhanced our understanding of 3D craniofacial deformities, allowing for more meticulous design of pre-surgical guides, ultimately fashioning osteotomies with more precision and ease in reproducibility while minimizing errors. This technology is undeniably here to stay, and familiarizing oneself with the concepts is essential for today's modern reconstructive surgeon.

The second chapter describes a handful of computerized surgical planning applications in head and neck reconstruc-

tion. The authors chronicle their evolving experience and emphasize important considerations based on anatomical location and mechanism of injury. A summary of the planning process – from imaging studies and web meetings with engineers to the design and 3D printing of patient-specific anatomical models and positioning and osteotomy guides – provides a complete overview of the resources available to reconstructive surgeons. Redefining the true sense of the surgeon's armamentarium, this chapter details the planning and streamlined execution of increasingly complex reconstructions with reduced operative times and consistent outcomes. The future of *Plastic Surgery* is rooted in the discovery of techniques for tomorrow.

Both installments embody the collaborative spirit of plastic surgeons: a multidisciplinary approach that involves engineers, orthodontists, and ablative surgeons. This has led to remarkable synergy and unprecedented outcomes. The early adoption of these advances reminds us of the dynamic and innovative nature of our specialty. In an age of mobile smartphones, tablets, and 3D printers, one can only imagine how rapidly this will be available when evaluating the patient at the bedside. Far from a path to stagnation, new technologies seem to spark our creativity and inspire us to push the envelope even further.

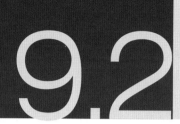

Computerized surgical planning in orthognathic surgery

Pradip R. Shetye

SYNOPSIS

- Recent advances in imaging technology have significantly changed the practice of surgical treatment planning for patients undergoing orthognathic surgery. With improvements in imaging technology, such as computed tomography (CT), cone beam computed tomography (CBCT), 3D photography, and 3D intraoral dental scanners, the ability of the clinician to evaluate and treat facial dysmorphology has been revolutionized.

- Advancements in 3D surgical planning software, 3D printing of stereolithography models, cutting guides, positioning guides, and surgical splints using computer-aided design/computer-aided manufacturing (CAD/CAM) technology enable surgeons to significantly improve surgical treatment planning in terms of accuracy, efficiency, and time.

- This chapter will focus on the step-by-step process of computerized surgical planning in orthognathic surgery, from image acquisition to surgical plan execution in the operating room, using this 3D technology.

Introduction

A well-planned and executed orthognathic surgical treatment plan can consistently deliver predictable and successful clinical results. Over the past few years, efforts have been made to better identify and understand patient expectations of orthognathic surgery and to consistently deliver the planned skeletal correction in the most efficient and predictable manner possible. Traditionally, orthognathic surgical treatment planning was based on the two-dimensional (2D) records of patients, i.e., photographs and radiographs (lateral and postero-anterior cephalograms). The surgical splints used to position the maxilla or mandible was fabricated by performing model surgery in a laboratory on plaster dental study models mounted on a semi-adjustable articulator. This process did not allow the surgeon to visualize the direct changes in the skeleton in real time or the secondary changes

to the unoperated jaw when the position of one jaw was altered. This traditional technique of surgical planning also has several opportunities for error.[1] There could be error in obtaining accurate facebow registration and transferring the patient's maxillary and mandibular jaw relationship to the semi-adjustable articulator through a facebow transfer. Patients with facial asymmetry may also have postero-anterior and vertical discrepancy with the position of the ears and eyes, and achieving a facebow transfer in these patients is difficult (Fig. 9.2.1). Planning surgery on plaster dental study models, constructing surgical splints, and then transferring the plan to the operating room can all lead to inaccuracies if there was an error in recording the facebow transfer. This process is also time-consuming in both the clinical setting and the laboratory.

3D imaging and computer-aided design/computer-aided manufacturing (CAD/CAM) have revolutionized the surgical treatment planning process for patients undergoing orthognathic surgery. The advent of computed tomography (CT and CBCT), 3D photography, 3D dental model scanners, 3D surgical planning software, and 3D printing of models allow for clinically significant improvements in surgical treatment planning, leading to greater accuracy and efficiency.[2] 3D technology and surgical planning software enable the orthodontist and the surgeons to develop a virtual treatment plan and simulate complex orthognathic surgeries on a personal computer with the visualization necessary to deliver predictable and optimal end results.

3D imaging not only helps the surgeon to better understand the complex craniofacial deformity and plan the surgery but also helps to generate patient-specific cutting guides, position guides, and surgical splint for orthognathic surgery. CAD/CAM technology allows 3D designing and printing of cutting guides, positioning guides, intermediate and final splints, and templates to harvest bone grafts, if needed. This technology also eliminates the need for facebow transfer to register the maxillary and mandibular jaw relationships and for mounting dental study models on an articulator for model surgery and splint construction.

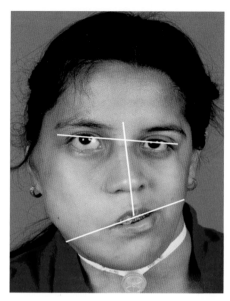

Fig. 9.2.1 A patient with significant facial asymmetry, including eye dystopia and discrepancy with the position of her ears. This poses a challenge to obtain an accurate facebow transfer and mount dental study models on an articulator to accurately represent the orientation of the model to the craniofacial skeleton.

In orthognathic surgery, surgeons are often faced with complex skeletal malformations in such syndromes as craniofacial microsomia, Treacher–Collins syndrome, syndromic craniosynostosis, and hypertelorism, which have a variable amount of skeletal and soft tissue deficiency. To correct these skeletal deformities, surgical treatment often involves complex osteotomies with intricate movements and repositioning of multiple skeletal components in relation to one another. There may also be a need for an autogenous bone graft to reconstruct the deficient craniofacial skeleton. In patients with asymmetric skeletal deformities, the osteotomized bony segments need to be repositioned in all three spatial planes to correct the anteroposterior, vertical, and transverse deformities and re-establish facial symmetry. In addition to the linear movement, the patient will need some angular change in the pitch, roll, and yaw to correct occlusal plane, cant rotation, and arch rotation, respectively (Fig. 9.2.2). The 3D pre-surgical

planning technology then becomes an invaluable tool for the surgeon by allowing for more precise three-dimensional control over the osteotomized segment. Another advantage of 3D technology is that the surgeon and the patient can visualize the postsurgical treatment predicted changes in facial appearance in 3D prior to surgery.

The 3D technology does not affect the importance of detailed pre-surgical clinical examination findings of the patient, which primarily drive the surgical treatment plan. 3D technology has replaced the traditional 2D cephalometric analysis and prediction, 2D photographic prediction, facebow transfer, dental study model surgery, and laboratory surgical splint construction. Surgical planning simulation software efficiently integrates a patient's 3D CT/CBCT data, 3D photograph, and dental occlusal relationship, and reconstructs a virtual 3D patient. This allows for complete visualization of the patient's soft tissue surface contours, craniofacial skeletal deformity, and dental occlusion as a reconstructed 3D image on a personal computer. The surgeon can then use this data to plan the orthognathic surgery and design various patient-specific cutting and position guides and splints (intermediate and/or final) to execute the orthognathic surgical treatment plan.

Presurgical orthodontics preparation

Orthodontic treatment for a patient requiring orthognathic surgery must be closely coordinated with the surgeon. The orthodontic treatment can be divided into three phases: the pre-surgical, perioperative, and post-surgical periods (Fig. 9.2.3). The pre-surgical orthodontic treatment plan to prepare a patient for jaw surgery is to decompensate dental malocclusion and coordinate the patient's maxillary and mandibular dentitions through orthodontic tooth movement with fixed orthodontic appliances.[3] In this phase of orthodontic treatment, the maxillary and mandibular dental arches are coordinated so they fit optimally in an occlusion after surgical skeletal correction. Decompensation of the maxillary and mandibular dentitions is necessary prior to orthognathic surgery because dental compensation of skeletal malocclusion can occur naturally with growth, and the position of the teeth might have been compensated through orthodontic intervention during the early teenage years (Fig. 9.2.4). Decompensation of malocclusion is also necessary to optimize the position of the jaws with surgery and to achieve the best possible final facial aesthetic results. This pre-surgical orthodontic phase

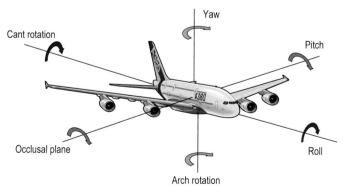

Fig. 9.2.2 In addition to AP, transverse and vertical changes in the osteotomized bony segment may have to be corrected for yaw, pitch, and roll to change the occlusal plane, cant rotation, and arch rotation, respectively, in patients with craniofacial asymmetry.

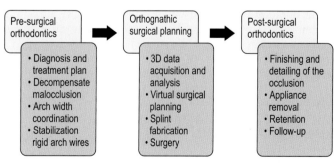

Fig. 9.2.3 The coordination of orthodontic treatment pre-, peri- and post-orthognathic surgery to achieve an optimal result.

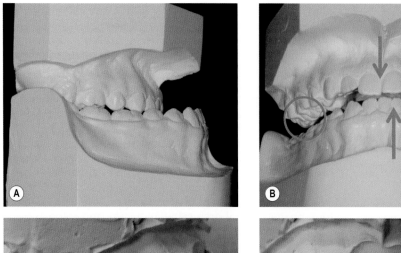

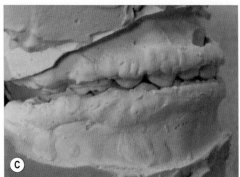

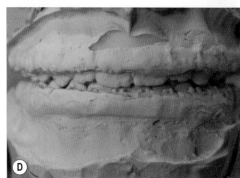

Fig. 9.2.4 (A) Pre-orthodontic study models. **(B)** Posterior transverse and anterior midline discrepancies after hand articulation of pre-orthodontic treatment study models in the anticipated post-surgical position. **(C,D)** After completion of pre-surgical orthodontic treatment with the extraction of the maxillary right and left first premolars and decompensation of malocclusion. Note the coordination of the posterior dental arch width and the maxillary and mandibular midlines.

can take between 4 and 18 months depending on the severity of the malocclusion. After surgery, the post-orthodontic treatment phase can vary from 6 to 12 months. Recently, there has been keen interest in performing surgery first and initiating orthodontic treatment to decompensate for malocclusion after the orthognathic surgery. It is believed that orthodontic tooth movement immediately after surgery is accelerated due to increasing cellular activity.[4] This method may work very well in patients with a simple, straightforward orthognathic surgery treatment; however, a patient who requires complex jaw correction in all the three spatial planes may have a better outcome if pre-surgical orthodontic treatment goals are completed before surgery. Most patients with these types of craniofacial conditions have multiple missing teeth, unerupted teeth, or a significant transverse discrepancy and will have a stable and predictable postsurgical dental occlusion if they undergo pre-surgical orthodontic treatment. 3D technology can also be applied in pre-surgical and post-surgical orthodontic treatments to accurately plan for the position of the teeth. The orthodontic tooth position can be controlled using 3D technology and robotic wire bending created by Suresmile Technology.[5] This helps to achieve optimal pre-surgical dental occlusion before orthognathic surgery.

Goals of pre-surgical orthodontics

The goals of pre-surgical orthodontic treatment in preparing the patient for orthognathic surgery include:

1) Coordinating tooth size and dental alveolar arch length discrepancy. If there is a significant discrepancy between tooth size and dental arch length and the patient

exhibits crowding of teeth, permanent premolars may have to be extracted to correct this discrepancy.

2) Coordinating the anteroposterior inclination of the maxillary and mandible anterior teeth. Correction of the anteroposterior inclination of the maxillary and mandibular dentitions will allow for optimal skeletal jaw movement for the best facial aesthetic results. In a Class III skeletal malocclusion, the dental compensation occurs in the maxillary arch by proclination of the maxillary teeth, and teeth in the mandibular arch tend to be retroclined. By contrast, in a Class II skeletal malocclusion, the mandibular dentition is compensated by excess proclination.

3) Coordinating the transverse anteroposterior dental relationship. The posterior arch width needs to be coordinated so that when the maxillary and mandibular dentitions are brought into the predicted final occlusion, the teeth have the best intercuspation. This allows for better dental function and long-term stability of the occlusion.

4) Coordinating the vertical dental relationship. The maxillary and mandibular arches need to be leveled by either extrusion or intrusion of the anterior or posterior teeth. This will allow better post-treatment occlusion with little interference and greater stability of surgical correction.

Progress toward the pre-surgical orthodontic treatment goals must be closely monitored with periodic orthodontic study models. These study models must be hand articulated in the anticipated postsurgical occlusion and checked for arch width coordination and any premature interference with opposing teeth.

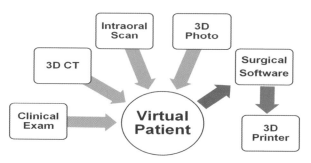

Fig. 9.2.5. A schematic diagram of 3D data acquisition to create a virtual patient for virtual surgical planning and simulation.

After the completion of pre-surgical tooth movement goals, the orthodontist must fit the patient with heavy, rectangular, stainless steel archwires with surgical hooks in preparation for the pre-surgical evaluations. It is preferred that wires be secured with stainless steel ties in all orthodontic brackets. If any of the orthodontic brackets accidentally become debonded in the operating room, the bracket will remain on the orthodontic archwire.

Constructing a 3D virtual patient for virtual surgical planning

After the patient has completed the pre-surgical orthodontic preparation, he or she will be ready for updated pre-surgical evaluations to construct a 3D virtual patient for surgical planning. The data that are usually required to create a virtual patient using virtual planning software are a clinical examination, 3D CT scan, intraoral dental scan, and 3D photographs (Fig. 9.2.5).

The data that are usually acquired for 3D computerized surgical planning include:

1) A 3D image acquisition of the craniofacial skeleton

A 3D skeletal image can be acquired using medical-grade 3D CT or CBCT. The medical-grade CT is usually obtained with the patient lying in the supine position. This position will require an extra step to reposition the patient's head in the virtual space during computerized surgical planning. A CBCT is normally obtained with the patient standing upright with a natural head position. This position will not require an additional step to reposition the patient's head in the virtual space (Fig. 9.2.5). The most common CT file format is Digital Imaging and Communications in Medicine (DICOM). This format is the standard for handling, storing, printing, and transmitting information in medical imaging. Individual DICOM files with voxel orientation must be requested if the patient is referred to an outside facility for imaging. The CT slices must be less than 1 mm; CBCT slices must be less than 0.4 mm.

One important consideration before obtaining 3D images is the patient's dental occlusion relationship. If the patient does not have any functional shift, it is acceptable to obtain a scan with the teeth in maximum intercuspation. However, if the patient has a significant functional shift from centric relation (CR) to centric occlusion (CO), the scan should be obtained with the patient in centric relation (Fig. 9.2.6). This can be

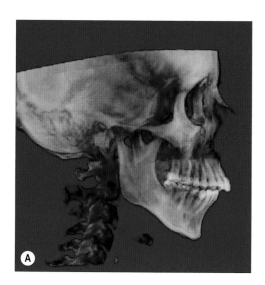

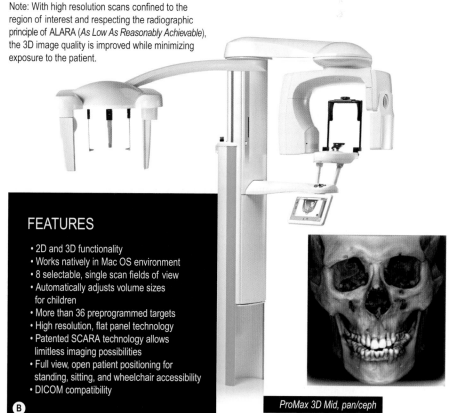

Note: With high resolution scans confined to the region of interest and respecting the radiographic principle of ALARA (As Low As Reasonably Achievable), the 3D image quality is improved while minimizing exposure to the patient.

FEATURES

- 2D and 3D functionality
- Works natively in Mac OS environment
- 8 selectable, single scan fields of view
- Automatically adjusts volume sizes for children
- More than 36 preprogrammed targets
- High resolution, flat panel technology
- Patented SCARA technology allows limitless imaging possibilities
- Full view, open patient positioning for standing, sitting, and wheelchair accessibility
- DICOM compatibility

ProMax 3D Mid, pan/ceph

Fig. 9.2.6 **(A)** A 3D cone beam computed tomography (CBCT) image (DICOM file format). **(B)** Image taken with an in-office CBCT machine with the patient in an upright standing position with a natural head position. *(Planmeca Group.)*

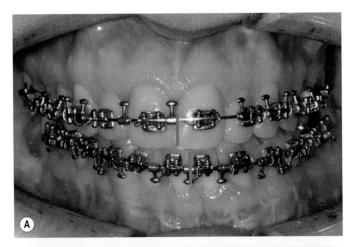

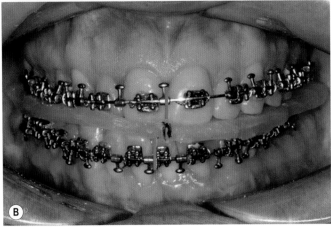

Fig. 9.2.7 (A) A patient in centric occlusion (maximum intercuspation). Note the mandibular midline to the left of the maxillary midline. **(B)** A patient photograph taken with the mandible in centric relation (condyles in centric relation in the condylar fossa).

achieved by using wax with the condyle in CR. This is important in the operating room if the mandible is to be used as a reference to reposition the maxilla during fixation with a split. If there are significant CR and CO discrepancies, after surgery the actual position of the maxilla can differ from the planned position. To overcome this, mandibular surgery can be performed first or position guides can be used to position the maxilla independent of the mandible. This is discussed in more detail later in this chapter.

2) 3D dental scan or dental study models

Currently, CT/CBCT imaging data do not provide enough dentition detail to make precise CAD/CAM splints. CT/CBCT data are volume data rather than surface data. The 3D volume is reconstructed by registering and integrating multiple slices that are 1 mm or less apart with the help of software. The details of the teeth and occlusion are not captured with high accuracy in these slices. Therefore, acquiring 3D surface data of the teeth with the help of a 3D surface dental scanner is recommended (Fig. 9.2.7). This can be obtained directly using an intraoral dental scanner or indirectly by making a dental impression of the teeth and scanning the impression or the dental stone models. This allows for the fabrication of

splints from these 3D dental study models that will fit the teeth accurately during surgery.

The typical file format for 3D dental scans is stereolithography (STL). This file format is native to the stereolithography CAD/CAM software used to create it. STL is also known as standard tessellation language and is used for rapid prototyping and computer-aided manufacturing. STL files describe only the surface geometry of a three-dimensional object without any representation of color, texture, or other common CAD model attributes.

3) 3D craniofacial photograph or 2D photographs

The 3D photograph is not absolutely necessary for virtual surgical planning; however, it does help in evaluating the post-surgical simulation changes (Fig. 9.2.8). As CT data does not include skin color, superimposing the soft tissue with surface skin color does give a better visualization of the surgical prediction. This also helps in patient education and in understanding patient expectations.

The common file format for 3D photography is obj, which holds 3D object files created with computer drawing software. These files contain texture maps, 3D coordinates, and other 3D object data (Fig. 9.2.9). Another file format is BMP, also known as a bitmap image file, a device independent bitmap (DIB) file, or simply a bitmap. This is a raster graphics image file format that is used to store bitmap digital images independent of the display device (such as a graphics adapter).

4) Patient interview and clinical exam

The patient's primary complaints and the clinical examination are important factors in making a decision on repositioning the jaw to accomplish optimal functional and facial aesthetic results. It is important to understand and discuss what the patient expects from the surgery so that the surgeon is better prepared to address the patient's primary complaints at the time of surgical planning.

The clinical exam should focus on capturing dynamic data that are not easily captured on a patient's static radiographic, or photographic images. One of the important facial aesthetic features is the amount of incisor show at rest and smiling. It is important to maintain approximately 3.5–4 mm of incisor show at rest after surgery. The mandibular rest position and path closing from the rest position to habitual occlusion must also be evaluated. These can be important considerations when obtaining pre-surgical records and using the mandible to reposition and fixate the maxilla after osteotomy with an intermediate splint. If centric relation and centric occlusion discrepancies are not detected, the post-surgical outcome may be compromised. If the patient has a CR–CO discrepancy, it is important that all pre-surgical records be obtained in CR.[8] The path of opening and closing must also be assessed from the rest position to maximum occlusion. Temporo-mandibular joint (TMJ) pain and dysfunction, if observed, should be well documented in the patient's record. If the patient complains of persistent TMJ pain or progressive condition, it is recommended that the TMJ symptoms be addressed prior to orthognathic surgery. It is important to remember that CT scans, dental study models, and photographs are all static

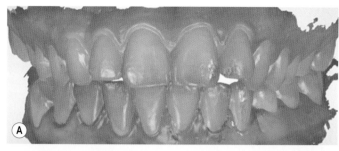

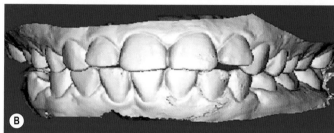

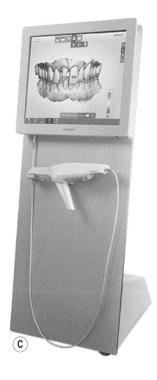

Fig. 9.2.8 (A–B) A 3D intraoral dental scan (STL file format) acquired with a **(C)** Trios intraoral scanner from 3Shape. *(3Shape A/S.)*

data, and soft tissue, which captures the dynamic data, is the key element driving the orthognathic surgical plan.

Surgical planning software

To perform surgical planning, surgical planning software is needed. Software using CAD/CAM technology is used for processing images; registering all 3D data sets (CT, dental cast, and 3D photograph); performing the surgical simulation; and designing cutting guides, positioning guides, and surgical splints. Currently, two popular software programs are commonly used in the US: Proplan CMF by Materialise and 3D Surgery by Dolphin Imaging. Several third-party

companies offer services to assist surgeons and orthodontists in surgical planning via web meeting using one of these software packages. Surgical planning software is becoming user-friendly, and in the near future, the surgeon will be able to perform in-office surgical planning independent of these third parties.

The orientation of 3D craniofacial volume in space

Unlike traditional 2D lateral cephalograms, which are obtained with the patient's head either in a natural head

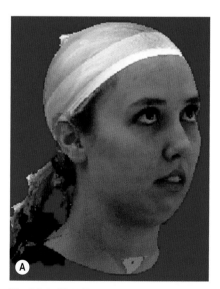

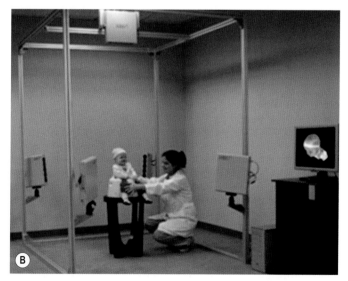

Fig. 9.2.9 (A) A 3D photograph (obj file format) of the face and **(B)** cranium using 3DMd equipment.

position or in a Frankfort horizontal plane parallel to the floor, 3D medical-grade CT images are acquired with the patient lying in the supine position. The orientation of the 3D volume in the virtual space becomes a challenge because improper head orientation will adversely affect the surgical outcome. For a patient with facial asymmetry (including orbital dystopia) or torticollis, transferring a natural head posture to the digital world is critical. Xia *et al.* have described a novel method of recording head posture with a help of a gyroscope and transferring the registration to the 3D digital volume to orient the patient's head in space if the CT was obtained with the patient in the supine position.[6] Another method is obtaining a 3D facial photograph in a natural head position and then registering the 3D CT volume to a 3D soft tissue facial photograph.[7]

Head orientation is not an issue with CBCT technology because CBCT images are obtained with the patient standing or sitting upright. At the time the CBCT image is obtained, the patient can be asked to look straight ahead to document the patient's NHP (natural head position) or to use a Frankfort horizontal plane parallel to floor, depending upon user preference. This process will eliminate the need for the external registration methods that are required for medical-grade CT. Before confirming the head position in the virtual space, clinical findings, such as the skeletal midline, dental midline, and occlusal cant, need to corroborate with the patient CT in virtual space. The skeletal midline and the patient's horizontal plane will be the primary reference planes to perform all skeletal movements during computerized surgical planning.

Processing and registering 3D data to create a virtual patient for surgical simulation

The next step involves processing and registering all 3D CT data. The 3D images need to be processed to remove artifacts and scatter. Once the images are processed and cleaned, the registration between the patient's 3D scan and the study models is initiated. The superimposition can be performed manually by selecting corresponding anatomical points on the CT and the dental study models, or the automatic superimposition feature in the software program can be used in some cases. Registration may need fine tuning by manual manipulation for the best final fit. The final superimposition for a 3D photograph can be accomplished by importing the 3D patient photographs and superimposing the 3D CT volume (Fig. 9.2.10).

Generation of 2-dimensional images

The 3D CT scan allows one to generate traditional radiographs, such as a panoramic radiograph, lateral cephalogram, postero-anterior cephalogram, and TMJ sections. Generating 2D images from 3D images may sound redundant; however, 2D images may need to be generated because of a lack of age-based 3D cephalometric norms. Using traditional cephalometric measurements is a good way to start.

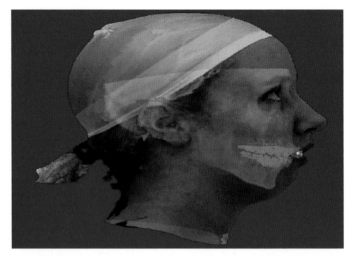

Fig. 9.2.10 A 3D virtual patient created by the registration of a 3D cone beam computed tomography (CBCT) image, 3D dental scan, and 3D photographs.

Three-dimensional identification of hard and soft tissue landmarks

The 3D CT provides a greater understanding of the craniofacial deformity, which cannot be visualized on 2D films, particularly in patients with facial asymmetry. 3D images eliminate any magnification distortion observed in 2D images, and the right and left sides of the craniofacial skeleton can be examined and measured independently. The mirroring effect on the non-affected side can also be used to define the skeletal discrepancy.

Three-dimensional surgical simulations for skeletal correction

3D surgical simulation takes the guesswork out of 2D surgical planning. Surgical simulation was traditionally performed using 2D lateral cephalograms and photographs, and the surgical plan was later transferred to study models that were mounted on a semi-adjustable articulator using facebow transfer. The model surgery was then performed to create surgical splints. This multistep transfer left many opportunities for errors in splint construction and in transferring the surgical plan to the operating room.

In a 3D surgical simulation, there is no need to perform a facebow transfer, which eliminates the step of transferring the surgical plan from the lateral cephalogram to the study models. As the dental occlusion and CT are superimposed as one unit, the changes performed on the skeleton are transferred directly to the dental occlusion. CAD/CAM technology can generate the intermediate and final surgical splints by 3D printing.

In two-jaw surgery, an additional advantage of 3D simulation software is that the surgeon has the freedom to perform either the maxillary or mandibular surgery first. This does not affect the final outcome of surgery. The software can also generate surgical cutting guides and splints to make precise osteotomy cuts and place rigid internal fixation accurately.

For single-jaw surgery, virtual surgical planning is not of great benefit regardless of whether the maxilla or mandible is to be operated on. Once the surgeon determines which jaw is in the normal position, the abnormal jaw can be corrected to the normal jaw position.

Step-by-step surgical simulation planning for two-jaw surgery

After completion of a thorough diagnosis and a tentative surgical treatment plan, the next step is to simulate the treatment plan on the virtual patient using a personal computer. The orientation of the virtual patient should match the patient's natural head position. The skeletal facial midline has to be established before any skeletal movement is performed. The condyle needs to be confirmed to be in the correct relation to the condylar fossa. The next step involves making appropriate osteotomies to simulate the surgical treatment plan. The surgeon can define the path of the osteotomy for an individual patient. For maxillary surgery, there are multiple options, from a single-piece Le Fort I osteotomy to a four-piece asymmetric osteotomy. The specific path of the osteotomy can be user-defined. Once the osteotomy is defined based on the needs of the patient, the segments can then be moved to the desired end position. The first step is to correct all maxillary asymmetry. This will involve correcting the maxillary dental midline to coincide with the patient's skeletal facial midline in the transverse plane. This step should be followed by the correction of the maxillary occlusal cant (roll). Depending on the severity of the occlusal cant, this can be achieved by differentially impacting one side and disimpacting the opposite side or by unilateral disimpaction or impaction to level the canted occlusal plane. Finally, the maxillary arch rotation (yaw) is corrected to make the maxilla more symmetric. As these movements are carried out, the actual changes can be recorded in millimeters by the software.

After correction of maxillary asymmetry, the mandible is then brought into occlusion with the maxilla. For a mandibular osteotomy, several options are available, including a bilateral sagittal split osteotomy, inverted L osteotomy, and vertical ramus osteotomy. Once the osteotomy is completed, the mandibular distal segment can be moved. The mandibular skeletal component is coordinated with the maxilla based on the preset final dental occlusion. This is accomplished by importing the preset, hand-articulated final occlusion models and superimposing them on the maxillary dentition and by superimposing the mandibular skeleton on the mandibular dental cast dentition.

Once the maxillary and mandibular skeletal components are coordinated in the final occlusion, the next step involves moving the maxillary and mandibular skeletal components as one unit to the final desired position. In this step, two additional variables that need to be corrected are the amount of maxillary impaction and the amount of maxillary and mandibular advancement. These will be determined by the initial skeletal deformity and the desired final facial aesthetic results. The last skeletal correction that can be accomplished is the correction of the occlusal plane (pitch). The normal occlusal plane angle to the Frankfort horizontal plane is approximately 9°, with a range of 2° to 17°. The patient's occlusal plane can be corrected by moving the maxillary and mandibular skeletal components in a clockwise (steeping occlusal plane) or counterclockwise (flattening occlusal plane) movement. This will have a significant impact on the chin projection and ANS (anterior nasal spine) position. Clockwise changes in the occlusal plane will increase maxillary projection and decrease mandibular projection, and counterclockwise changes will have the opposite effect.

After completion of the desired skeletal movements based on the treatment plan, bony overlaps or bony gaps need to be evaluated. This will inform the surgeon whether bone needs to be removed or whether the patient will need a bone graft to augment the bone in the area of the large bony defect. In the mandible, the relationship of the proximal and distal segments can be evaluated. As the maxillary and mandibular skeletal components are moved, the x, y, and z coordinates of displacement for each identified skeletal landmark can be viewed in real time and modified as needed. If soft tissue was added to the CT data, soft tissue changes can also be evaluated (Figs. 9.2.11 & 9.2.12).

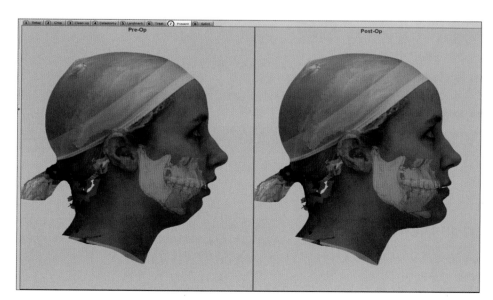

Fig. 9.2.11 Pre- and post-surgical simulation prediction of a patient who will undergo two-jaw surgery.

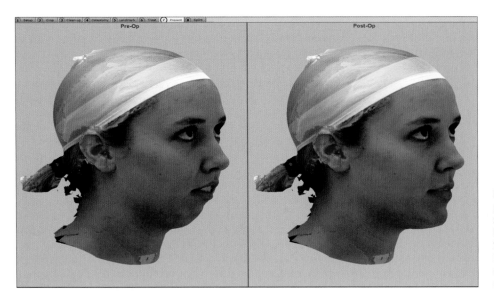

Fig. 9.2.12 Pre- and post-surgical simulation prediction for a patient who will to undergo two-jaw surgery. In this image, the 3D photograph's opacity has been changed, and the cone beam computed tomography (CBCT) data and 3D dental scan are invisible. This is simulation is used for patient education and for understanding the patient's expectations from surgery.

Decision of whether to perform maxillary or mandibular surgery first

Virtual surgical planning technology allows surgeons to easily plan mandibular surgery first, followed by maxillary surgery. This was very difficult with traditional facebow transfer and model surgery. Mandibular surgery may be performed first if the patient exhibits a significant mandibular deviation from rest position to habitual occlusion. This is most commonly seen in patients with asymmetrical mandibular morphology and facial asymmetry. If maxillary surgery is performed first with planned cant correction, the mandible has to be opened for splint construction, and it would be difficult to predict the path of the opening of the mandible in the virtual patient. This may lead to an improper position of the maxilla. In such situations, performing mandibular surgery first makes more sense (Figs. 9.2.13A & 9.2.13B). An alternate option would be to use skeletal-based positioning guides to position the maxilla

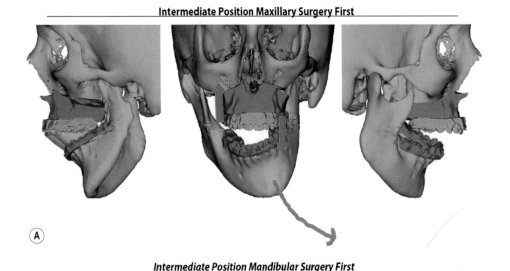

Fig. 9.2.13 (A) The displacement of the mandible inferiorly when the maxillary surgical plan involved correction of the occlusal cant by moving the left side of the maxilla down and the right side superiorly. The patient's clinical exam had demonstrated that the path of the opening of the mandible was deviated to the left side from habitual occlusion to the maximum opening. This would have been difficult to simulate, and it would have been a challenge to accurately position the maxilla with the intermediate splint. **(B)** The design of the intermediate splint if the mandible was operated on first. This would provide a more predictable postsurgical result.

during skeletal fixation. There are several designs of the position guides, and each guide can be customized based on the surgeon's preference.

Cutting guides, positioning guides, bone graft templates, and splints

Guides, templates, and splints are key armamentaria for 3D computerized surgical planning. The guides help the surgeon to precisely transfer the surgical plan from the virtual patient on a personal computer (PC) to the operating table. Significant improvements have been made over the years to develop more sophisticated guides to accurately transfer the surgical plan to the operating table. Guides can be divided into two types: bone borne and tooth borne.

In most patients, an intermediate split to position the maxilla and a final splint to position the mandible is a very efficient process. During maxillary fixation with the intermediate splint after intermaxillary fixation, the variables that the surgeon has to control are the vertical position of the maxilla and the proper position of condyles in the condylar fossa (Fig. 9.2.14 A-I).

Cutting guides help to make osteotomies in the planned locations. They also help to remove overlapping bony interference more accurately while maintaining good bone-to-bone contact for bone plating during fixation. Position guides are helpful for repositioning the osteotomized Le Fort I bone to the desired final position independent of the mandible. This eliminates the concern of a CR–CO discrepancy affecting the final position of the Le Fort I segment. It also takes the guesswork out of the position of the condyle in the condylar fossa at the time of Le Fort I fixation. Position guides can be custom designed based on the surgeon's need. One important factor that needs to be considered in designing positioning guides is that they must be rigid enough to allow the position of the osteotomized bony segment and at the same time allow enough room for plate fixation. One such design is the Orthognathic Positioning System (OPS), which is used to transfer the virtual surgical plan to the operating table during orthognathic surgery.[9] The system comes with a maxillary splint with two sets of removal attachments. The first set is used to establish the register of the unoperated maxilla to the rest of the skeleton with a drill hole, and the second is used to reposition the maxilla at the time of fixation.

For genioplasty surgery for asymmetric chin position, the guide becomes very important to accurately position the chin during fixation. There have been many designs of chin positioning guides. Some are tooth borne and some are bone borne, and they may be connected to the dental splint. For patients who will receive autogenous bone grafts, virtual surgical planning helps to design a template for the harvest that will fit perfectly in the bony defect. The template saves significant time in the operating room.

A recently completed prospective study using a computer-aided surgical simulation protocol showed that a computerized plan can be transferred accurately and consistently to the patient to position the maxilla and mandible at the time of surgery.[10]

Conclusion

Virtual surgical planning has significant benefits for patient needing orthognathic surgery. With the acceptance and advancement of new in-office CBCT machines, user-friendly surgical treatment planning software, and in-office 3D printers, the technology will become more accessible as the benefits become more apparent to the growing number of surgeons performing orthognathic surgery using 3D virtual surgical planning. In addition, many new technologies continue to be developed to assist surgeons in planning orthognathic surgery more accurately. CAD/CAM-designed surgical cutting guides, positioning guides, and splints allow for clinically significant improvements in accuracy and efficiency and a reduction in surgical error, all of which benefit both the patient and the surgeon. Prediction of surgical outcome can only be enhanced by better pre-surgical diagnosis and treatment planning using the information from a clinical exam. Continued improvements in state-of-the-art software applications that enable enhanced planning give orthodontists and surgeons the vision necessary to deliver the desired results while providing excellent communication between clinicians as well as with the patient.

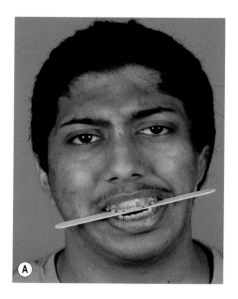
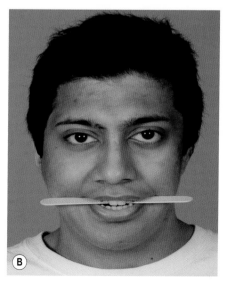

Fig. 9.2.14 (A–F) Pre- and post- frontal, profile, and smiling photographs after the patient underwent two-jaw surgery using virtual surgical planning and simulation. *Continued*

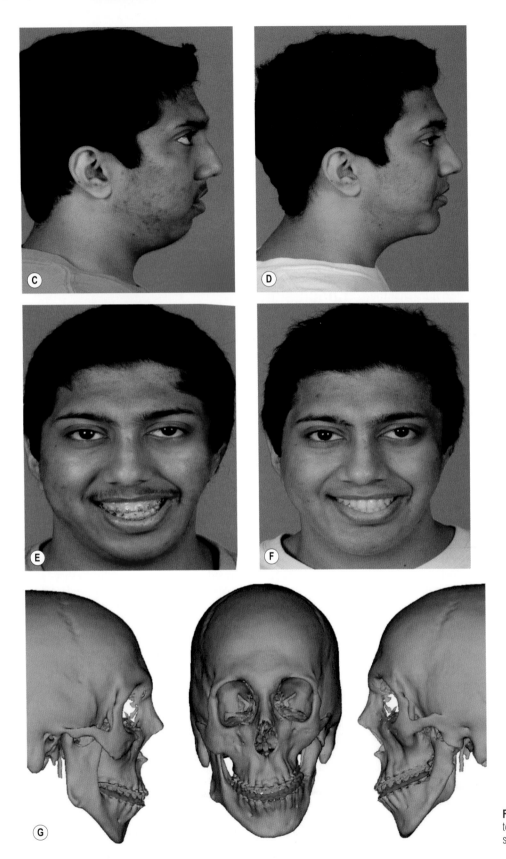

Fig. 9.2.14, cont'd (G–I) Pretreatment computed tomography (CT) and after completion of maxillary surgery and mandibular surgery simulation.

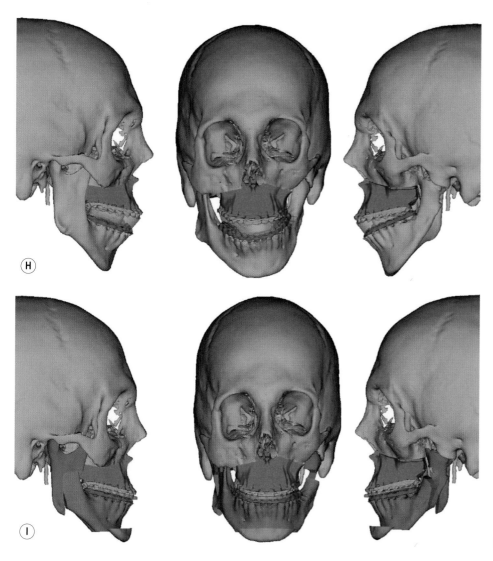

Fig. 9.2.14, cont'd

References

1. Ellis EIII. The accuracy of model surgery: evaluation of an old technique and introduction of a new one. *J Oral Maxillofac Surg.* 1990;48(11):1161–1167.

2. Kwon TG, Choi JW, Kyung HM, Park H-S. Accuracy of maxillary repositioning in two-jaw surgery with conventional articulator model surgery versus virtual model surgery. *Int J Oral Maxillofac Surg.* 2014;43(6):732–738.

3. Proffit WR, White RP Jr. Combined surgical-orthodontic treatment: How did it evolve and what are the best practices now? *Am J Orthod Dentofacial Orthop.* 2015;147(5 sup):S205–S215.

4. Liou EJ, Chen PH, Wang YC, et al. Surgery-first accelerated orthognathic surgery: orthodontic guidelines and setup for model surgery. *J Oral Maxillofac Surg.* 2011;69(3):771–780.

5. Mah J, Sachdeva R. Computer-assisted orthodontic treatment: the SureSmile process. *Am J Orthod Dentofacial Orthop.* 2001;120(1):85–87.

6. Xia JJ, McGrory JK, Gateno J, et al. A new method to orient 3-dimensional computed tomography models to the natural head position: a clinical feasibility study. *J Oral Maxillofac Surg.* 2011;69(3):584–591.

7. Xia JJ, Gateno J, Teichgraeber JF. New clinical protocol to evaluate craniomaxillofacial deformity and plan surgical correction. *J Oral Maxillofac Surg.* 2009;67(10):2093–2106.

8. Cordray FE. Three-dimensional analysis of models articulated in the seated condylar position from a deprogrammed asymptomatic population: a prospective study. Part 1. *Am J Orthod Dentofacial Orthop.* 2006;129(5):619–630.

9. Polley JW, Figueroa AA. Orthognathic positioning system: intraoperative system to transfer virtual surgical plan to operating field during orthognathic surgery. *J Oral Maxillofac Surg.* 2013;71(5):911–920.

10. Hsu SS, Gateno J, Bell RB, Hirsch DL, Markiewicz MR, Teichgraeber JF, Zhou X, Xia JJ. Accuracy of a computer-aided surgical simulation protocol for orthognathic surgery: a prospective multicenter study. *J Oral Maxillofac Surg.* 2013;71(1):128–142.

9.3

Computerized surgical planning in head and neck reconstruction

Jamie P. Levine and David L. Hirsch

SYNOPSIS

- When planning a resection, the computed tomography (CT) scan should be relatively close in time to the planning session and the surgery. The modeling team should outline the tumor and generous margins should be planned. It is best to do this with the ablative team directly to avoid any discrepancy in the plan. If there is a question about margin safety and need for further intraoperative resection, an alternate guide can be made to accommodate for these potential changes.

- Take into account your soft tissue needs when planning these procedures. Take as much skin as you need from your primary flap or plan in alternative flaps, especially if a complex resection is planned and there is a large intra- and extra-oral soft tissue demand.

- In cases with significant tissue loss or lack of tissue flexibility, such as in radiation injury, the bony reconstruction can be designed to minimize the strain on the remaining soft tissue and decrease the complexity of the reconstruction.

- All specialties involved in the surgical and peri-operative treatment should be invited and try to attend the virtual planning session. The involvement of the team will allow for fewer critical errors in the planning process. Also, each team should evaluate the plan that is reconstructed by the engineers after this meeting and sign off before the plans are considered final.

- As the reconstruction becomes more complex and may have multiple segments, predesigned plates can play an important role in obtaining very precise reconstruction results.

- Consider primary osteointegrated implants in benign cases.

- In free flap reconstruction, plan bone segments to remain at least 2 cm in length to maintain appropriate circulation.

- Use virtual planning to appropriately position your bone segments. With appropriate scanning, perforators can even be noted in which to assist in the soft tissue design. Make sure to maintain a sufficient proximal and distal osteotomy so that knee and ankle stability is not affected.

- When bone loss or malposition is part of the deformity, reposition the bone with the assistance of imaging technology. This can be planned using mirror-imaging techniques, etc. Plan the repositioning of the bone segments along with any grafts or flaps that will be taken.

- When using multi-segmental repositioning, or complex rotational segments where alignment is critical such as in implant placement, make intermediary splint devices to help confirm the position of the reconstruction as you advance through each step.

Introduction

Craniofacial, maxillofacial, and head and neck surgery started long before the advent of three-dimensional (3D) imaging. Historically, the field of head and neck reconstruction did not exist. This lack of head and neck reconstruction truly limited the surgeon's ability to perform any type of head and neck ablative, trauma, and congenital surgery. The advances first in pedicled flap surgery and then in microsurgery techniques forever changed the field of head and neck oncologic surgery. The ability to now reconstruct larger and larger composite defects gave significant freedom to the ablative surgeon. Similarly, over the last generation, advances made in imaging technology have been a quantum advance for the reconstructive surgeon. Radiographic techniques, such as computed tomography (CT) imaging, suddenly allowed the surgeon to assess a defect or injury and helped them to plan a more precise and strategic reconstruction. New approaches and operative techniques were developed because of these advances. Even with this advancement in imaging technology, the surgeon still only had a two-dimensional (2D) representation of a 3D problem. There was no physical translation that could be made between the images and the patient. The information obtained from imaging was best translated through anatomic knowledge and increased experience from the surgeon. Teaching of these reconstructive techniques is also difficult. In repairing the three dimensional bony architecture of the craniofacial skeleton, one is visually limited by access and the inability to gain complete 3D exposure of the desired surgical sites. Also, because of the very 3D nature of the craniofacial skeleton, even small degrees of error can lead to poor outcomes. Traditional reconstructive techniques require a large learning curve and can lead to inconsistent results, especially with less experienced surgeons. Surgical experience and an innate sense of 3D anatomy has been important in obtaining better outcomes, but not all surgeons have the same skill set or experience, so outcomes become more variable. With advances made over the last decade in computer modeling and virtual surgery, we are now able to translate the information received from radiographic imaging studies to actual intraoperative tools that can help us overcome the complex 3D anatomy of the head and neck (Fig. 9.3.1). This has led to more predictable and, we believe, more functional outcomes for the patient. As these techniques improve along with guidance technology, the accuracy and outcomes should continue to improve. It also allows the less experienced surgeon to potentially obtain similar outcomes to the more experienced ones.

At our institution, we have been utilizing 3D facial analysis and virtual surgical planning (VSP) in all of our craniomaxillofacial reconstructive and ablative cases. Over the past 8 years, many cases have been planned, modeled, and executed in this manner and have led to more reliable and predictable outcomes. Over this time, we have been continuously refining these techniques, and this approach has truly revolutionized the way we diagnose, treat, and reconstruct head and neck diseases and defects. In our modern computer era, digital

planning has been the standard in architectural design and biomedical fabrication. In all aspects of surgery, proper planning facilitates more predictable operative results, but prior to the use of virtual planning, much of this relied on 2D imaging and surgical trial-and-error. It has been our goal to make all forms of reconstructive surgical procedures, including oncologic, traumatic, congenital, and aesthetic, treatable with this methodology. These techniques are teachable, have a shallow learning curve, allow for precise and anatomic bony reconstruction, and ultimately decrease surgical time. In specific cases, we have married the virtual planning with navigation guidance technology to allow for even more accuracy in both ablative and reconstructive procedures when indicated (Fig. 9.3.2).

The goal of this chapter is to illustrate how virtual surgery and computer assisted design can be utilized by the surgeon to decrease operative time and create accurate postoperative results when compared to traditional craniomaxillofacial surgical treatment planning. We will review our methodology in approaching some of these problems and illustrate application of these techniques. This will only be a small representation of the types of cases to which we have applied these techniques and we feel the applications will broaden as surgeons find the ease in which their operations can be planned and executed. We have reliably achieved excellent results in both malignant and benign head and neck oncologic surgery and reconstruction, orthognathic surgery, maxillofacial trauma, temporomandibular joint reconstruction (TMJ), and skull base surgery. These techniques have become our preferred method for complex craniomaxillofacial surgery and reconstruction.

Techniques

The evolution of our current technique initially involved the use of stereolithographic models as templates (Fig. 9.3.3). These models were printed directly from the CT scan, and we would use them to preoperatively bend plates around the presumed bony resection, to develop plates to work around exophytic lesions, and for intraoperative reference to help us to navigate these operations. We first utilized this technique and these models for mandibular reconstruction after tumor resection. This was an area where we felt there was great variability in outcome based off of how well all the bony segments were reconstructed. Although helpful, this technique was still quite labor intensive, and there was still often "guesswork" and room for error both in performing osteotomies of the mandible and fibula correctly, aligning the released jaw segments, and in setting of the fibula into the resection site. The current evolution of our technique involves preplanning each phase of the operation including the osteotomies on the mandible and the lower extremity by using staged cutting guides. Currently, these techniques allow for surgically efficient and highly predictable outcomes as far as bone and soft tissue positioning. We continue to refine these techniques as far as cutting guide design and surgical planning, including placement of permanent implants, dentures, and ideal bone positioning. We will describe the basic process of planning and using computer-aided design/computer-aided manufacturing (CAD-CAM) technology for reconstruction.

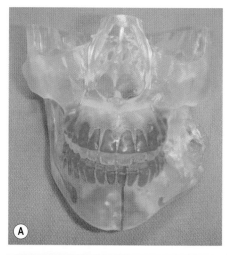

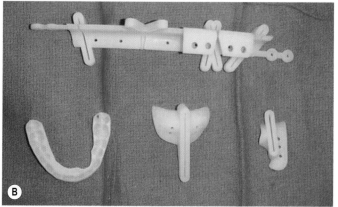

Fig. 9.3.1 (A) A stereolithographic model of the skull with the tumor and virtual cuts colored. **(B)** The cutting guide specific to the patient's fibula and mandible are noted along with an occlusal splint.

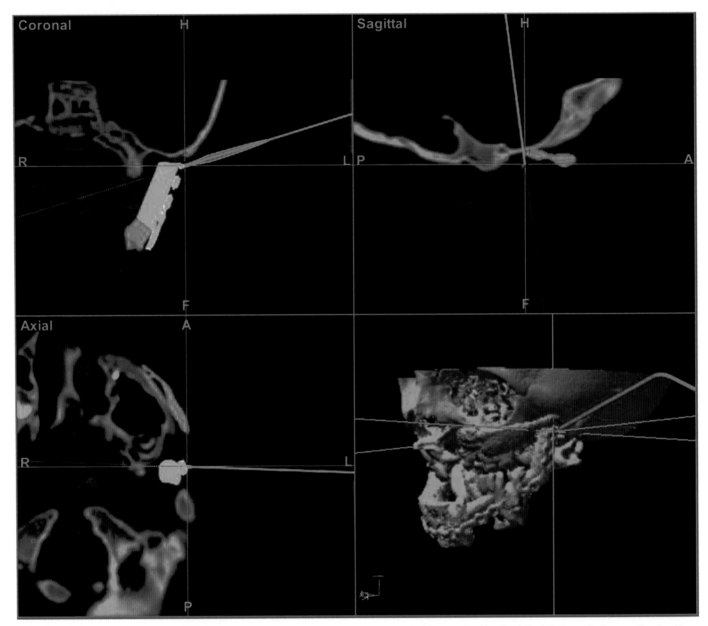

Fig. 9.3.2 Guidance technology showing intraoperative positioning of the reconstructed segments; in this case, checking the desired fibula positioning near the glenoid fossa.

Computer-aided surgical modeling

Head and neck reconstruction

Evolution:

Hidalgo first published the use of the free fibula flap for mandibular reconstruction in 1989.[1] The advantages of this flap for mandibular reconstruction soon became apparent. It has the ability to provide a long segment of bone (up to 25 cm), along with the surrounding soft tissue, and has a donor site with a relatively low morbidity. Perhaps the most important aspect of the fibula is the unmatched ability for 3D contouring permitted by a reliable periosteal blood supply and multiple osteotomies.[2] The free fibula flap has ultimately evolved into the gold standard for mandible reconstruction.[3]

Today, the free fibula flap is almost universally the first choice for oromandibular reconstruction in patients with both benign and malignant disease. The introduction of key technologies has refined the surgery. Initially, the reconstruction relied on intraoperative evaluation of the post-ablative defect. The surgeon would then employ any number of imperfect and tedious manipulations to re-sculpt the bony gap. This increased operative times with often imperfect results.

The introduction of CT-based stereolithographic models allowed for an element of pre-operative planning. The ability to simulate defects on these printed 3D models allowed us to pre-operatively plan the reconstruction and contour of the reconstruction plate, etc. This was catapulted to the next level with software using the CT data for 3D virtual surgery.[4]

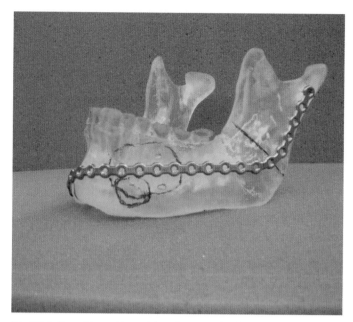

Fig. 9.3.3 Stereolithographic model used as a template for plate bending. The plate can then be used for the intraoperative reconstruction and bone alignment.

Computer- aided design technology uses this information to recreate a virtual representation of the diseased mandible and donor fibula. In this virtual environment, 3D resection of the mandible can be simulated on the computer model. The computer generated fibula is then transposed to the virtual mandible and recontoured with simulated osteotomies in multiple orthogonal planes. Complimentary osteotomies are virtually created to ensure bony apposition (Fig. 9.3.4). The simulated osteotomies are then translated to pre-manufactured cutting guides. This ensures that the VSP is precisely translated to the intraoperative environment.[5]

The anatomic recreation of the bony mandible is unmatched using this technique. Bony apposition is maximized with a superior aesthetic result. From an orthognathic perspective it has also revolutionized function. Optimal restoration of oromandibular function involves mastication, deglutition, and the management of oral secretions. A critical component of re-introducing these functions is dental rehabilitation. VSP has revolutionized the reconstructive surgeons ability to accomplish this (Fig. 9.3.5).[6]

While this technology has been extensively reported in the literature, we have continued to add technical refinements that are unique.[7] Today, we routinely perform complex reconstructions that involve several of these elements in each surgery. Some of these technical improvements include precise placement of primary endosteal implants, double barreling techniques to improve the bony contour, customized reconstruction plate fabrication, implants with a dental prosthesis

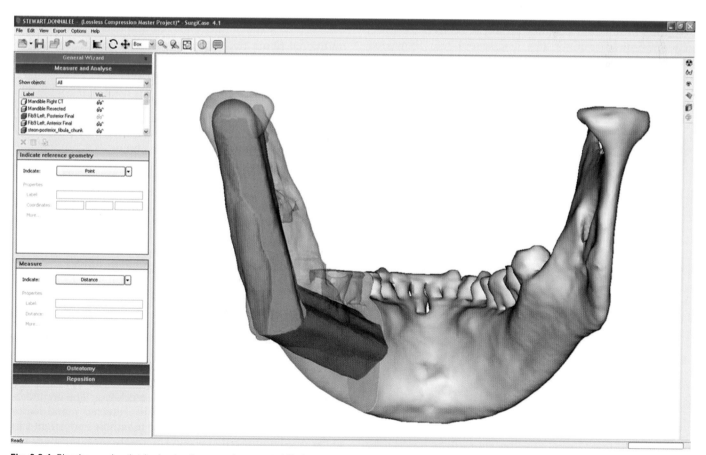

Fig. 9.3.4 Planning session that is showing the computer generated fibula transposed to the virtual mandible, after the resection, and recontoured with simulated osteotomies in multiple orthogonal planes. Complimentary osteotomies are virtually created to ensure bony apposition.

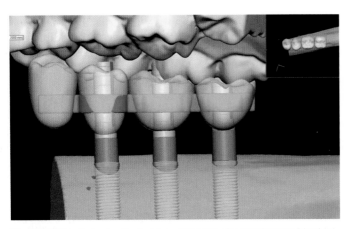

Fig. 9.3.5 Virtual planning for dental reconstruction. The osteointegrated implant position is optimally planned as well as the precisely positioned denture.

in a single stage, and free flap placement along with complex orthognathic repositioning (Fig. 9.3.6).[8] Anecdotally, these technical refinements have allowed for even more efficient and predictable reconstructive outcomes.

Technical aspects:

Computer-aided mandibular ablation and reconstruction involves four distinct phases: planning, modeling, surgical, and evaluative. It has only been with the evaluative phase that we have been able to continually refine our techniques and improve our surgical outcomes. Planning begins with a high-resolution CT scan of the patient's craniofacial skeleton according to standard scanning protocols. Scans of the lower extremities or other donor sites (iliac, scapula, etc.), if needed, are obtained to have an exact understanding of the vascular and bony anatomy. These images are then forwarded to the

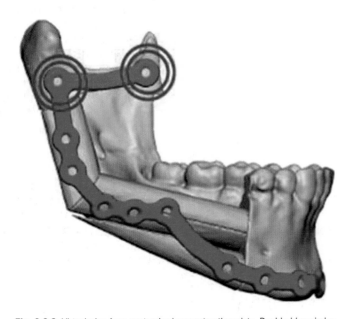

Fig. 9.3.6 Virtual plan for a customized reconstruction plate. Double blue circles represent predictive holes that will be placed into the mandibular cutting guides. These predictive holes are placed in the mandibular cutting guides and will correspond exactly to holes in the customized reconstruction plate. This allows for a very precise reconstructive outcome overall.

desired modeling company (we have primarily worked with and evolved our techniques with 3D Systems Medical Modeling Inc., Golden, CO, USA). The scans are converted into 3D reconstructions of the craniomaxillofacial skeleton and the donor site. The donor site is not always required, but we normally obtain this since our reconstructions have become more complex and precise over time. It is helpful for us to see the 3D variability in the donor site, which can be important, especially when planning implants and multiple segments, and the associated vasculature and perforator anatomy. We will obtain this using CT angiography. A web meeting is then held with biomedical engineers from the modeling company and the surgical team. The key parameters of the planning phase for mandibular reconstruction (or any type of head and neck surgery) are the margins of resection, repositioning of any malpositioned tissue, and the location of fibula placement in relation to the remaining mandible and craniofacial skeleton (Fig. 9.3.7). For traumatic injuries the goal is relocation of the displaced bony fragments and planning of bone grafts and/or permanent implants. In orthognathic surgery, the staged movement of the jaws for the desired endpoint is also planned. These inputs are determined by the surgeon and marked during the web meeting by the modeling engineer on the 3D reconstruction image (Fig. 9.3.8). Control of the mouse pointer can be transitioned between both teams, and real-time cephalometric, volumetric, and linear analysis can be extrapolated as bony segments are being virtually manipulated.

A good example of the power and precision of virtual planning is for fibula reconstruction of mandibular and maxillary defects. These were the first reconstructions that we approached with complete virtual planning. We were able to overcome many of the challenges that we faced in utilizing traditional fibula free flap reconstructive methods once we began fully utilizing CAD-CAM technology. Communication between the ablative, reconstructive, and engineering teams is necessary in maximally translating the surgical resection and reconstruction into a virtual model that can then be used to create personalized cutting guides and templates that allow us to create seamless fibula–mandible continuity. By incorporating the engineers into the surgical planning, they understand the importance and reality of tissue positioning, including bone segments, soft tissue, and vascular pedicles. The virtual resection of the mandible is completed first. The cutting paths are chosen at the desired margins of the diseased mandible, and the segment is virtually removed. The 3D reconstructed fibula image is then superimposed on the mandibular defect in its desired vascular and soft tissue orientation (Fig. 9.3.7). Virtual fibular osteotomies are created to fit the idealized reconstruction. The first osteotomy is designed to precisely fit the proximal angle of resection on the native mandible. Additional osteotomies are created, as needed, to recreate the shape of the resected portion of the native mandible. Although any shape and bend can be created using this technique, it is the reconstructive surgeons job to keep the reconstruction realistic with appropriate sized segments (usually 2 cm or greater) and to respect the limits of the blood supply. Simple is sometimes better, even with virtual modeling. The engineers can use the geometry of the virtually resected mandible or mirror the contralateral disease-free mandible and orient this to the overlying maxilla in order to create ideal orthognathic relationships. The shape of the plate and the number and lengths of fibula segments can be modified to optimize the

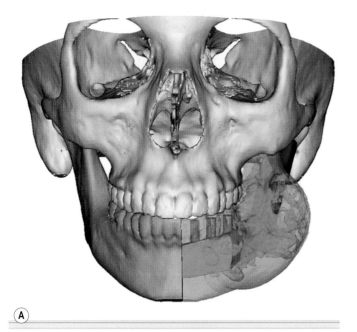

(A)

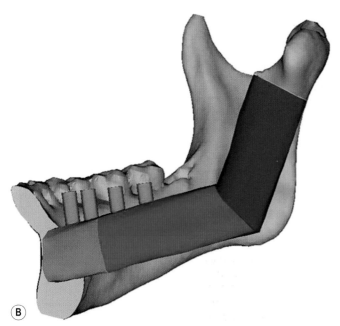

(B)

Fig. 9.3.7 Figure shows a complete virtual planning session prior to plate placement. **(A)** The margins of resection are noted around the tumor, and within this area the fibula is planned. You can also see the positioning of implants in red. These are being aligned to the overlying dentition and arranged within the fibula placement. The location of fibula placement in relation to the remaining mandible is shown **(B)**.

shape of the neomandible, maintain well-vascularized segments of fibula, provide appropriate bone-to-plate relationships for positioning of implants, provide seamless bony approximation, and maintain a perfect occlusal arrangement. The virtual osteotomies in both the mandible and fibula are planned to optimize bone apposition for subsequent bony union and to ease positioning and placement intraoperatively. Bone positioning is seamless between the osteotomies created on the mandible for the resection and the osteotomies created on the fibula for the reconstruction. Currently, for

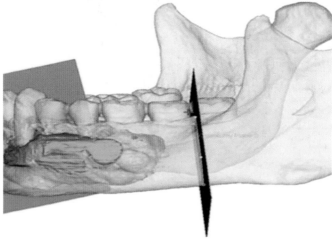

Fig. 9.3.8 This shows margins of resection around the tumor and the location that the fibula will ultimately be placed into.

most benign cases, we will also plan precise dental endosseous implant placement by choosing the desired position to obtain appropriate postoperative prosthetic occlusion (Fig. 9.3.9).

The modeling phase involves stereolithographic manufacturing of the planned components. This includes a model of the native craniofacial skeleton for intraoperative reference and to augment the education of residents, surgeons, and the patient. Next, sterilizable cutting guides are produced that fit flush onto the native mandible and fibula and allow the osteotomies to precisely match those created during the planning phase. A reconstruction plate template is then designed that facilitates pre-bending of the titanium plate preoperatively and is made to match the plate design of the desired plating company. The challenge of determining the fibula

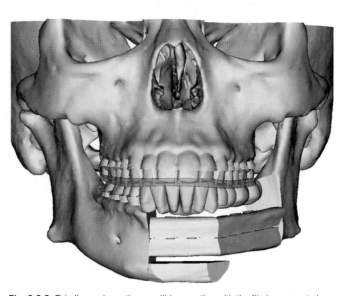

Fig. 9.3.9 This figure shows the mandible resection with the fibula segments in place. Fibula segments can be modified to optimize the shape of the neomandible, including a central double barrel segment. The planning provides seamless bony approximation and maintains a perfect occlusal arrangement. The planned dental prosthesis is also noted in appropriate occlusal position.

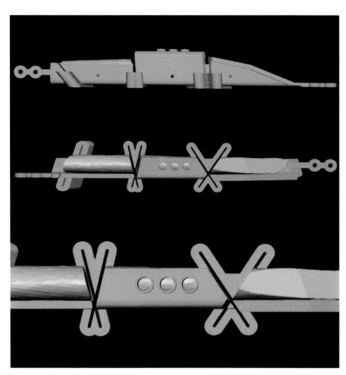

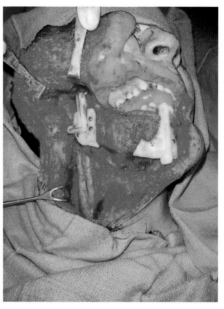

Fig. 9.3.12 Mandibular cutting guides in place. The cutting guides enable an exact duplication of the angles of osteotomy that were planned during the web meeting.

Fig. 9.3.10 The fibula lengths and intersection angles are made simple and reliable with the fibula cutting guides which are created to fit on the fibula precisely and create seamless ostomies. These cutting guides facilitate the osteotomy process and provide precise integration between the mandibular and fibular portions of the reconstruction.

lengths and intersection angles is made simple and reliable. These cutting guides facilitate the osteotomy process and provide seamless integration between the mandibular and fibular portions of the reconstruction (Figs. 9.3.10 & 9.3.11). A linearized cutting guide is fabricated from the cut pieces of the virtual fibula, with cutting slots that are located at the appropriate lengths along the fibula and at the proper angles

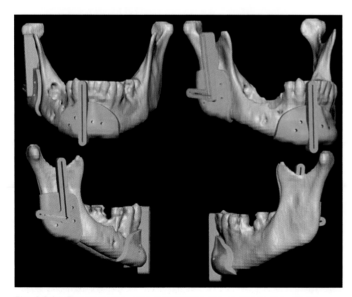

Fig. 9.3.11 This figure shows the mandibular cutting guides in place. These cutting guides facilitate the osteotomy process and provide precise integration between the mandibular and fibular portions of the reconstruction.

to recreate the desired shape without any intraoperative measuring. The learning curve that is required to perform the appropriate osteotomies is removed, and we believe the results obtained from using these techniques are consistently better than any other.

Next is the surgical phase of the reconstruction.[6,9] Access to the mandible is based on location and severity of tumor or pathology. After access to the mandible is obtained, we use the techniques described by Marchetti *et al.* for maintenance of maxillomandibular relationships.[10] The mandibular cutting guides, after sterilization, are then introduced into the field and secured to the mandible with bone screws. The cutting guides enable an exact duplication of the angles of osteotomy that were planned during the web meeting (Fig. 9.3.12). A saw is introduced into the slots of the cutting guides, and the osteotomies are performed. Once the mandible is resected, the definitive reconstruction plate is placed on the mandible in the predetermined position and holes drilled at the appropriate locations. The mandibular cutting guides are often designed with predictive holes so that we use the same screw holes as the reconstruction plate to provide a precise anatomic reference in hardware positioning. With these predictive holes, precise plate placement and exacting bone orientation is always maintained. We prefer to do the fibula shaping with the pedicle intact and perfusion uninterrupted (Fig. 9.3.13). The fibula cutting guide is used to replicate the cuts for both the end and closing wedge osteotomies that were planned previously. We now take the fibula segment straight up to the mandible, never losing control of the mandibular segments (Fig. 9.3.14). This has also allowed us to perform minimal incision approaches for even very large resections (Fig. 9.3.15).

The evaluation phase usually includes a CT scan and/or X-rays along with standard postoperative follow up. The CT scan is used as the ultimate comparison to the operative plan that was virtually generated. This allows critical analysis of accuracy and can help refine the techniques for the future. In

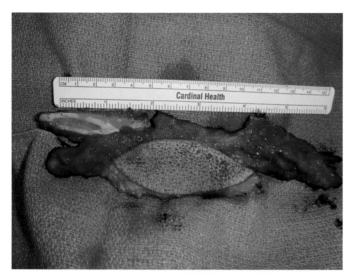

Fig. 9.3.13 Fibula after the osteotomies are completed and the device is removed. Fibula shaping we perform with the pedicle intact and perfusion uninterrupted. This can also be done off the field but this will increase the ischemic time accordingly. Note in the picture a beveled double barrel osteotomy segment and planned skin paddle for intraoral lining.

general, accuracy is excellent and is within 1–5 mm (Fig. 9.3.16). The main source of error is probably due to the hand bending of the reconstruction plate. With the newer types of modeled plates even this has been significantly improved allowing us greater accuracy in the reconstruction. These pre-modeled titanium plates not only help the accuracy of the outcome but shorten the length of the case.

For most benign pathology cases, we virtually plan and then place dental implants and, in some cases, the dental prosthesis intraoperatively (Figs. 9.3.17 & 9.3.18). Most

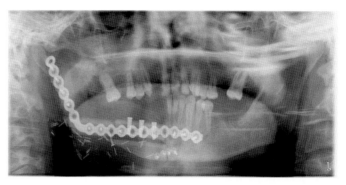

Fig. 9.3.15 Postoperative X-ray showing precise position of the fibula segments and osteo-integrated implants are also noted to be in the appropriate position.

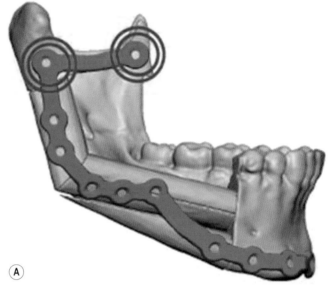

(A)

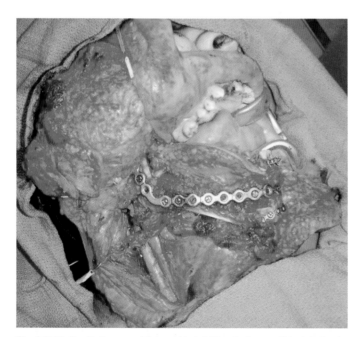

Fig. 9.3.14 The fibula segment is brought straight up to the mandible defect and is placed directly into position below the prepositioned plate. Control of the mandibular segments is never lost during the procedure. The double barrel segment in this patient is plated with a separate miniplate and lag screw. New preplanned plates can be designed to engage all of these segments with a single plate.

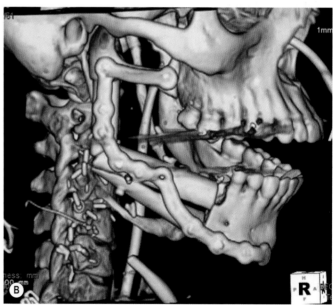

(B)

Fig. 9.3.16 (A,B) Images show the preplanned reconstruction along with predictive holes for the plate placement. The 3D CT scan is noted with the postoperative result showing a very close appearance to the operative plan that was virtually generated. Also note the plate design which was preplanned and is placed around the mental foramen and incorporates a screw hole to also engage the double barrel segment.

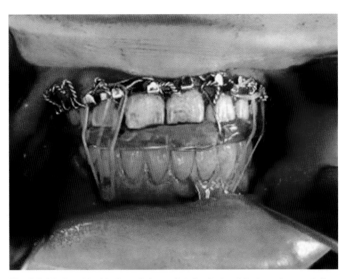

Fig. 9.3.17 Noted in this figure is immediate implant and denture placement. For most benign pathology cases, we virtually plan and then place dental implants and, in some cases, the dental prosthesis.

patients advance to complete dental rehabilitation within the first year postoperatively. We believe, even if not placed intraoperatively, placement of dental implants and prosthetic dental reconstruction is facilitated by the precise alignment and positioning of the fibula we obtain from virtual planning.

Maxillofacial trauma

Treating complex multi-segment maxillofacial trauma is a challenge even to the most experienced surgeons because of anatomic distortion, bony displacement, etc. When treatment planning surgical correction of a traumatic injury, many factors must be considered including status of the dentition and pre-existing occlusal relationship, facial widths, facial heights, and bone segment continuity. Restoration of normal facial width, facial height, and antero-posterior projection is not only difficult to achieve but is extremely difficult to teach. Historically, no single approach guarantees a satisfactory outcome.[11–16] Post-operative deformities from these injuries is common and often impossible to correct.[17] We have successfully and very accurately utilized 3D virtual surgery and modeling techniques for the treatment of these type of complex injuries.[18] Each injury is approached individually. The modeling allows us to optimally reposition the craniofacial skeletal fragments, provide splints to assist in and confirm alignment, and provides templates for bone replacement or augmentation if necessary.

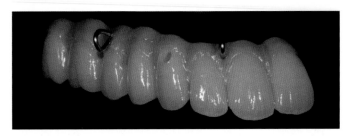

Fig. 9.3.18 Another example of a dental prosthesis for immediate placement.

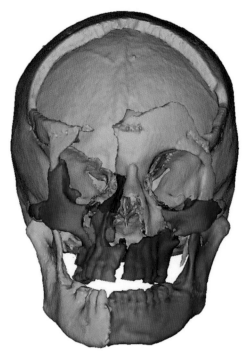

Fig. 9.3.19 This figure shows a reformatted 3D CT scan of a pan-facial fracture. Different colors represent the larger fracture segments.

Unfortunately, many complex traumatic injuries involve avulsion of teeth and bony comminution making accurate reduction of these fractures technically difficult intraoperatively. This is where computer-assisted virtual surgery is extremely beneficial. A CT scan of the facial skeleton is acquired, along with dental casts of the maxilla and mandible if possible. These techniques are also utilized in virtual orthognathic surgery. The casts are laser scanned by the modeling company and virtually integrated into the image data. The use of CAD-CAM based occlusal splints has gained popularity in recent years, and we have also found similar benefit in using them for these cases of complex facial trauma, particularly where tooth-bearing bony segments are comminuted, or there is loss of dentoalveolar hard tissue.[19–22]

Planning of the surgery always starts with a virtual web meeting. In the meeting, the fractured segments are virtually reduced to optimize bony alignment (Figs. 9.3.19 & 9.3.20). This "virtual reduction" reduces the trial and error that is normally required for open reduction. The bony injuries are analyzed in all planes and virtual reduction of the fractures is carried out to the surgeon's preference depending on the planned surgical approach. Volumetric analysis of the reduced segments can be easily computed by the virtual software to aid in establishing symmetry. Occlusal splints are fabricated for the tooth-bearing segments based on the desired maxillary and mandibular reduction. Templates for non-tooth-bearing facial bones can also be created to allow for proper restoration of facial width and projection. Although virtual surgery helps the surgeon determine how to best restore anatomic alignment preoperatively, the true benefit of this technology has been its intraoperative application and the personalized device design (Fig. 9.3.21). Using the 3D models finalized from the VSP, surgical guides are then designed and manufactured and used intraoperatively for more accurate

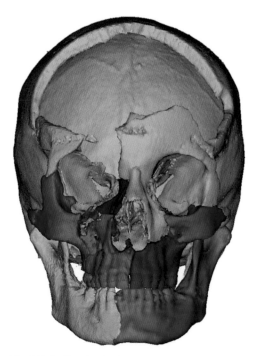

Fig. 9.3.20 Planning for the surgery starts with a virtual web meeting. In the meeting, the fractured segments (colored) are virtually reduced to optimize bony alignment.

model to guarantee appropriate bone position and facial width. The guide can be used at the time of surgery to help reduce these segments relative to the non-injured cranial region. The fragments can be built off each other and the position checked and confirmed with each bone segment that is reduced and plated.

In addition to the intraoperative guides that allow for optimal reduction, virtual surgery affords the opportunity for the design of precise permanent implants. This can be either autologous tissue (bone graft) or alloplastic implants (titanium mesh, acrylic, reconstruction plates, customized poly-etheretherketone (PEEK)) depending on the operative need. Virtual 3D surgery can be used to create a template of the defect to guide preoperative or intraoperative creation of the graft or plate as well as creating custom milled prefabricated facial implants.

In the surgical phase, all of the fractures are exposed and the operation is carried out as planned, using the prefabricated templates and guides to ensure correct positioning of the fracture segments (Fig. 9.3.21). The guides are secured with screws and are designed to not interfere with placement of osteosynthesis plates. We have also utilized guidance technology, in very complex and multifragment cases, that integrates between our preoperative scan and our desired reconstruction to help guarantee bony repositioning.

Frontal sinus

A representative area where modeling has significant benefit is the frontal sinus.[23] In either tumors or fractures, this technique allows an elegant and safe approach to this hidden area (Fig. 9.3.22). The frontal sinus represents an area that is somewhat hidden anatomically, and the approach to it usually requires a much larger surgical dissection than the problem may warrant. Because of potential injury to the dura and the brain, traditional approaches usually require a craniotomy for a direct anterior approach. In very select problems in this area,

alignment of the bony segments. The guides are fixated to the maxillofacial bones with bone screws and provide precise reference points for bony reduction and reconstruction and prove to be very useful for re-establishing proper facial width. In cases where there is significant comminution and associated facial widening, guides can be manufactured from the

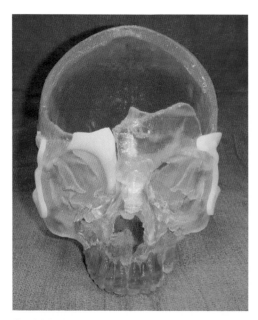

Fig. 9.3.21 Printed stereolithographic skull model showing the desired bony reduction. There are individualized surgical devices which are noted in white on the zygoma and help to precisely guide the fracture reduction intraoperatively. Also noted in white in the right supraorbital region is a template to help create a bone graft intraoperatively for missing bone. In the surgical phase, all of the fractures are exposed and reduced and the prefabricated templates and guides are used to ensure correct positioning of the fracture segments.

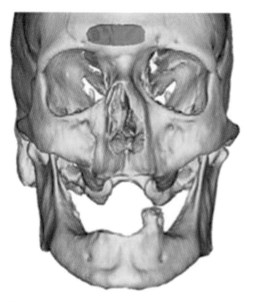

Fig. 9.3.22 The frontal sinus represents an area that is hidden anatomically from an anterior approach. This figure shows a planning session where the frontal sinus position is precisely shown anteriorly.

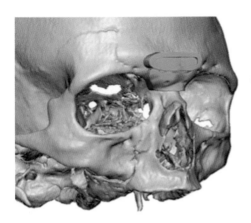
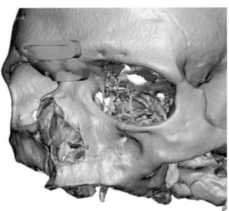

Fig. 9.3.23 On the anterior table of the frontal sinus a planned cutting guide is shown which will allow for the widest possible access to the sinus with minimal risk of injury. Options for the cutting guide can be customized to fit very precisely for the planned exposure and help minimize the incision for access.

or even in other confined locations, the surgery can be planned virtually and guides can be created to position the surgeon safely and directly into the area of the defect without a full intracranial dissection (Fig. 9.3.23).

The incidence of frontal sinus fractures ranges from 10% to 15% of all facial fractures, and they often occur in combination with other facial fractures, such as orbital walls and nasal bones.[24] Diagnosis can be made clinically in cases where the frontal table is severely involved; however, CT scanning has become the standard for both diagnosis and planning of surgery.[25] Uniquely, the frontal bone has both an anterior and posterior table, which, in addition to the nasofrontal duct, can be variably involved in the injury pattern. Fracture of the anterior wall poses mostly a cosmetic concern. The involvement of the nasofrontal duct or posterior table is another important factor in determining treatment of frontal sinus factures.

It has been shown that surgical planning and using CAD-CAM technology for craniofacial reconstruction allow for surgically efficient and highly predictable outcomes in both bony and soft tissue reconstructions.[9] Planning begins with a high-resolution CT scan of the patient's craniofacial skeleton according to standard scanning protocols. A web meeting is then held. During this meeting, the surgeons can precisely outline where the borders of the frontal sinus are located. In cases of fractures, bony segments are being virtually manipulated. A cutting guide for the surgeon can be designed and created that allows for safe and rapid access to the entire frontal sinus while maximizing the size of the available bone segments and minimizing further fracture dislocation. Most importantly, in cases of minimal or no fracture of the anterior table of the frontal sinus, the guide allows the widest possible access to the sinus with minimal risk of injury (Fig. 9.3.23).

The modeling phase involves stereolithographic manufacturing of the planned guides and a model of the involved craniofacial skeleton for intraoperative reference. The cutting guides facilitate the osteotomy process and provide seamless transition between the frontal bone and entrance through the bone of the anterior table.

The precision and speed in performing these complex osteotomies are greatly improved by utilizing this technique. During the surgical phase, the cutting guide is placed and secured to the craniofacial skeleton with monocortical depth screws into the frontal bone. These are designed not to interfere with the placement of osteosynthesis plates. This use of guidance technology, which integrates between the preoperative scan and the desired reconstruction, helps to guarantee bony alignment by preplanning plate and osteotomy positioning. The planning and guide fabrication allows for a safe osteotomy and access directly into the frontal sinus for fracture repair, tumor removal, etc.

Temporomandibular joint/skull base

The key to a successful operation involving the TMJs or base of skull is exposure and access. Because of the density of vital structures in this area, care must be taken to avoid inadvertently damaging these when manipulating the area of interest. Precise positioning of autograft or allografts in reconstructing the TMJ is essential to restoring mandibular and occlusal function. Traditionally, reconstructing a TMJ has been carried out as a two-stage operation. Initially, a gap arthroplasty is performed and postoperative CT is acquired to aid in the custom fabrication of a TMJ prosthesis. Once fabricated, a second operation is required for adaptation of the custom joint prosthesis. Recently, intraoperative navigation has been utilized to prevent injury in the middle cranial fossa.[26] By combining techniques of virtual planning and intraoperative navigation, this can be a safe single-stage operation, and the virtual plan can be confirmed intraoperatively.

The CT scan and the maxillomandibular dental casts are sent to the modeling company and uploaded into the virtual software. 3D rendering is completed and stereolithographic models are fabricated. Surgical resections are designed via web meeting, and reconstruction of the joint can be virtually created using a stock TMJ prosthesis or any other desired methodology and merged into the virtual 3D rendering. By manipulating the osteotomies and ramal and glenoid fossa components in the software, ideal positioning of the joint replacement is possible. This allows for a one-stage ablative and reconstructive operation without compromising the functional outcome. These techniques have also been used in microvascular free flap reconstruction of the TMJs. Just as previously described in reconstruction of head and neck defects with microvascular free fibula flaps, imaging of the proposed donor site is sent to the modeling company in order to properly plan the reconstruction.

Conclusion/future directions

VSP and model design has given us the ability to visualize the surgery before it happens, design the desired outcome, provide guides for performing the surgery, and furnish tools for confirming the match between the planned and desired outcome. The techniques we describe in this chapter have been evolving and represent a portion of the type of cases that this technology can be used for. This has become a team project between the ablative surgeons, reconstructive surgeons, and the engineers.[27] As the software improves and surgeon's experience with it increases, communication with the engineer may not always be necessary, but currently, they play an integral role in VSP and creating the stereolithographic models, guides, and templates. With the recent addition of customized plate fabrication, another potential source of error has been addressed and optimized. Our results and creativity have improved because of this addition.

Intraoperative guidance will likely be utilized more commonly in the future to help double-check bone position against the virtual plan in very complex cases. As the software improves and techniques are further developed, integration of various technologic elements will continue to evolve. For now, the greatest utility of this technology has been for bone reconstruction and repositioning, but in the future we will be able to accurately plan and predict the soft tissue outcome as well. Lastly, and most importantly, the learning curve associated with these techniques is less steep. A surgeon's experience will not be the major obstacle in obtaining the desired outcome. Based on our experiences and results, virtual planning for correction of all forms of acquired and congenital craniofacial deformities has great benefit and can produce more desirable results than traditional methods. Operative time and operative access can often be minimized due to preoperative planning and the accuracy inherent in these techniques. We have been able to increase the complexity of our reconstructions adding multiple elements into a single reconstruction. We commonly have multiple bone segment reconstructions including layered double barrel segments and very precise endosseous implant placement. We have also had success in placing implant-retained dental prostheses intraoperatively to provide an unparalled single stage reconstruction. The options and opportunities created by VSP are only limited by the surgeons imagination and desired outcome.

Access the complete reference list online at   **http://www.expertconsult.com**

1. Hidalgo D. Fibula free flap: a new method of mandible reconstruction. *Plast Reconstr Surg*. 1989;84:71–79.

2. Wallace C, Chang Y, Tsai C, Wei FC. Harnessing the potential of the free fibula osteoseptocutaneous flap in mandible reconstruction. *Plast Reconstr Surg*. 2010;125:305–314.

3. Hidalgo D, Rekow A. A review of 60 consecutive fibula free flap mandible reconstructions. *Plast Reconstr Surg*. 1995;96:585–596.

4. Hidalgo D. Aesthetic improvements in free-flap mandible reconstruction. *Plast Reconstr Surg*. 1991;88(4):574–585.

5. Tepper O, Hirsch DL, Levine JP, Garfein ES. The new age of three-dimensional virtual surgical planning in reconstructive plastic surgery. *Plast Reconstr Surg*. 2012;130:192e–194e, author reply 194e–195e.

6. Hirsch DL, Garfein ES, Christensen AM, et al. Use of computer-aided design and computer-aided manufacturing to produce orthognathically ideal surgical outcomes: a paradigm shift in head and neck reconstruction. *J Oral Maxillofac Surg*. 2009;67:2115–2122.

7. Haddock N, Monaco C, Weimer K, et al. Increasing bony contact and overlap with computer-designed offset cuts in free fibula mandible reconstruction. *J Craniofac Surg*. 2012;23(6):1592–1595.

8. Levine JP, Bae JS, Soares M, et al. Jaw in a day: total maxillofacial reconstruction using digital technology. *Plast Reconstr Surg*. 2013;131(6):1386–1391.

9. Sharaf B, Levine JP, Hirsch DL, et al. Importance of computer-aided design and manufacturing technology in the multidisciplinary approach to head and neck reconstruction. *J Craniofac Surg*. 2010;21:1277–1280.

10. Marchetti C, Bianchi A, Mazzoni S, et al. Oromandibular reconstruction using a fibula osteocutaneous free flap: four different "preplating" techniques. *Plast Reconstr Surg*. 2006;118:643–651.

10.1

Introduction to midface reconstruction

Eduardo D. Rodriguez

The reconstruction of composite midface defects remains a challenge to even the most experienced surgeons. Advances in microsurgery and craniofacial surgery have transformed the approach to midface reconstruction by increasing surgical options, which have improved functional outcomes and aesthetic results. The list of available techniques and applicable flaps for complex head and neck reconstruction continues to expand, and without convincing evidence that a single reconstructive option is superior to another, surgeon preference remains the dominant factor determining treatment choice for craniofacial defects. Harnessing and implementing technological advances has enhanced surgical planning and precision in execution of surgical plans. Ultimately, this precision creates optimal conditions for long-term oral rehabilitation. Interestingly, these innovations have served to reinforce the age-old surgical principles that have guided facial reconstruction for the past century.

A new feature of this fourth edition of *Plastic Surgery* are two chapters dedicated to midface reconstruction. For the first time, the reconstructive approaches at the M.D. Anderson Cancer Center and the Memorial Sloan Kettering Cancer Center are showcased side by side to provide readers with successful yet different philosophies adopted at two world-renowned academic oncologic healthcare institutions. In addition to their vast operative experience, the scholarly contributions of the participating authors have helped define these institutions as the core of reconstructive innovation and education. Therefore, it is with enthusiasm and academic fervor that the new chapters of this new edition be released to serve a discerning audience in nuanced perspectives on such a complex reconstructive problem.

10.2

Midface and cheek reconstruction: The Memorial Sloan Kettering approach

Leila Jazayeri, Constance M. Chen and Peter G. Cordeiro

SYNOPSIS

Reconstructive goals for midface and maxillary defects:

- Wound closure
- Obliterate the maxillectomy defect
- Restore barrier between sinonasal cavity and anterior cranial fossa
- Separate oral and sinonasal cavities
- Support orbital contents/maintenance of ocular globe position
- Speech
- Mastication
- Maintain patent nasal airway
- Facial contour

Reconstructive goals for cheek defects:

- Wound closure
- Obtain good color and texture match
- Use local and regional flaps when possible
- Avoid ectropion and complications secondary to undue tension

Midface and maxillary reconstruction

Introduction/general principles

Reconstruction of the midface starts through a clear understanding of the complex three-dimensional (3D) anatomy of the maxilla.[1] In the most basic terms, the maxilla may be thought of as a six-walled geometric box that includes the roof, which is made up by the orbital floor; the floor of the box, which is made up by each half of the anterior hard palate and alveolar ridge; and the medial wall of the box, which forms the lateral walls of the nasal passage (Fig. 10.2.1). The maxillary antrum is contained within the central portion of the maxilla. The cranial base overlies the posterior pterygoid region of the maxilla. The two horizontal and three vertical buttresses produce facial width, height, and projection. The overlying soft tissues, including the muscles of facial expression and mastication, insert on the maxilla and are responsible for individual facial appearance and function.

The goals of reconstruction are functional and aesthetic. Most extensive midface defects require free flaps for reconstruction, with the flap selection dependent on the amount of resected skin, soft tissue, and bone.[2–7] Complex structures such as lips, eyelids, and the nose should be reconstructed separately, usually with local flaps, without incorporating free tissue transfer.[8–12] By following an algorithm based on a clearly delineated classification system of midfacial defects, even patients with very large, complex defects can be restored to good function. The author's algorithm is described below (Fig. 10.2.2).[1,13]

The goal of midface reconstruction is not necessarily to reconstruct all the walls of the maxilla that have been resected. Rather, successful midface reconstruction should:

1. Close the wound.
2. Obliterate the maxillectomy defect.
3. Support the globe if preserved or fill the orbital cavity if the globe is exenterated.
4. Maintain a barrier between the nasal sinuses and the anterior cranial fossa.
5. Restore facial shape.
6. Reconstruct the palate.

Diagnosis and treatment

The algorithm we use to reconstruct complex midface defects is based on the extent to which the maxillary bone has been resected. Once the bony defect is assessed, we address the soft tissue defects, including skin, muscle, palate, and mucosal lining of the cheek. Finally, important structures such as the palate, oral commissure, nasal airway, and eyelids are dealt with in an attempt to restore function.

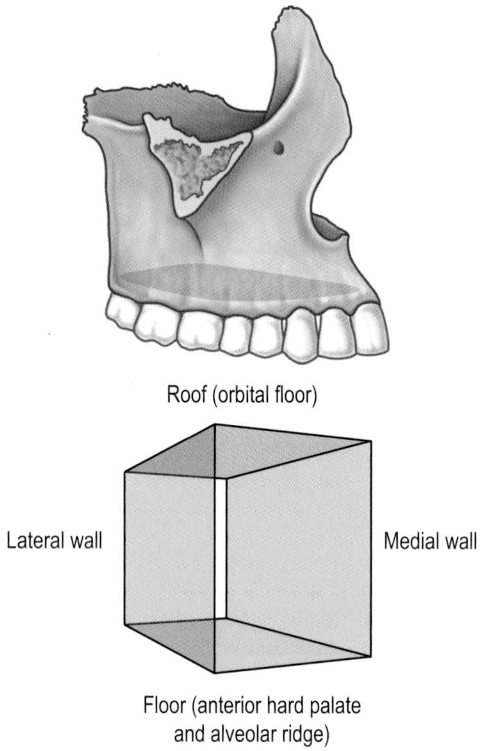

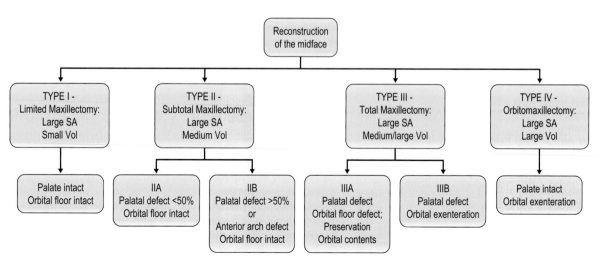

Fig. 10.2.1 The maxilla may be thought of as a six-walled geometric box that includes the roof, which is made up by the orbital floor; the floor of the box, which is made up by each half of the anterior hard palate and alveolar ridge; and the medial wall of the box, which forms the lateral walls of the nasal passage.

Type I: limited maxillectomy defects

Type I, or partial, maxillectomy defects are those that involve one or two walls of the maxilla, most commonly the anterior and medial walls (Fig. 10.2.3). Both the palate and the orbital floor are intact. The resection will often include the soft tissue and skin of the cheek, and even the lips, nose, and eyelids. Occasionally, the orbital rim will be resected and non-vascularized bone grafts will be necessary for reconstruction. Type I maxillectomy defects are small-volume deficiencies with large surface area requirements, often needing one or two skin islands. Our flap of choice is the radial forearm free flap, as it provides good external skin coverage and minimal bulk while allowing multiple skin islands that can be de-epithelialized to improve contour, wraparound bone grafts, and supply lining for the nasal cavity (Fig. 10.2.4).

Type II: subtotal maxillectomy defects

Type II, or subtotal, maxillectomies are those that involve resection of the lower five walls of the maxilla, including the palate, but leave the orbital floor intact (Fig. 10.2.5). These defects may be further subdivided into type IIA defects, which include <50% of the transverse palate, or type IIB defects, which include >50% of the transverse palate and/or the anterior arch of the maxilla. Both type IIA and type IIB maxillectomy defects are moderate-volume deficiencies with large surface area requirements, which usually need one skin island.

For type IIA defects, which involve <50% of the transverse palate, reconstruction may proceed with either a microvascular free flap or a skin graft and an obturator, depending on patient and surgeon preference. If a free flap is selected to avoid the inconvenience and maintenance of a palatal obturator, our flap of choice is the radial forearm fasciocutaneous free flap (Fig. 10.2.6). The skin inset is critical, and the skin paddle must be equal to or smaller than the original defect to keep the soft palate taut and recreate the buccal sulcus. Without a taut inset, the skin paddle can prolapse into the oral cavity. If adequate teeth or bone stock remain, dentures or even osseointegrated dental implants may be used.

For type IIB defects, which involve >50% of the transverse palate or a significant portion of the anterior arch, an osteocutaneous free flap is needed. These defects require bone for structural support as well as skin lining of the neopalate

Fig. 10.2.2 By following an algorithm based on a clearly delineated classification system of midfacial defects, even patients with very large, complex defects can be restored to good function.

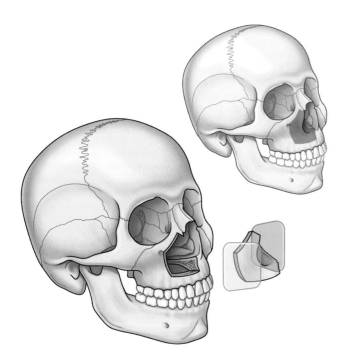

Fig. 10.2.3 Type I, or partial, maxillectomy defects are those that involve one or two walls of the maxilla, most commonly the anterior and medial walls.

and nasal floor. A prosthesis is inadequate, because bone is needed to provide support to the upper lip. Our flap of choice is the radial forearm osteocutaneous "sandwich" flap (Fig. 10.2.7).[14] The bone segment can be shaped to recreate the maxillary alveolar arch and support the upper lip, and the thin pliable skin can be wrapped around the bone like a sandwich to replace the lining of the palate and nose. If adequate bone is harvested, osseointegrated dental implants

or conventional dentures may also be used to recreate teeth.

Type III: total maxillectomy defects

Type III defects are total maxillectomies that involve resection of all six walls of the maxilla. Type III defects can be further subdivided into resections that exclude (type IIIA) or include (type IIIB) the orbital contents. Both type IIIA and type IIIB maxillectomy defects are moderate-to-large-volume deficiencies with large surface area requirements, which usually need at least one skin island.

For type IIIA defects, which involve resection of all six walls of the maxilla, including the palate and orbital floor, but preserve the orbital contents (Fig. 10.2.8), a bone graft is needed to reconstruct the orbital floor and a free flap with one or more skin paddles is needed to recreate the palate, nasal lining, and/or the cheek. The goals are to support the globe, obliterate any communication between the orbit and nasopharynx, and reconstruct the palatal surface. For bony support, we have used split calvarium, iliac crest, or less commonly, split ribs to reconstruct both the maxillary prominence and the orbital floor. For mucosal and skin lining, our flap of choice is the rectus abdominis myocutaneous flap, which may be wrapped around the bone graft to separate the orbital contents from the oral cavity (Fig. 10.2.9A). The bulk of the rectus can also fill the dead space of the antrum and use of this can provide a water-tight closure of the palate. In patients who are not candidates for free tissue transfer, a temporalis flap may be used to cover the orbital floor bone graft and provide some volume to fill the midfacial defect (Fig. 10.2.9B). Reconstruction with a temporalis flap, however, requires simultaneous use of a palatal obturator.

The type IIIB defect, which involves resection of the entire maxilla including the orbital contents, is also known as an extended maxillectomy (Fig. 10.2.10). The reconstructive goals for these extensive, large-volume defects are to close the

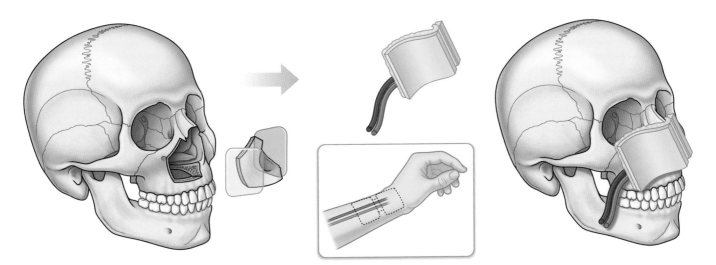

Fig. 10.2.4 For type I defects, our flap of choice is the radial forearm free flap, as it provides good external skin coverage and minimal bulk allowing multiple skin islands to be de-epithelialized to improve contour, wraparound bone grafts, and supply lining for the nasal cavity.

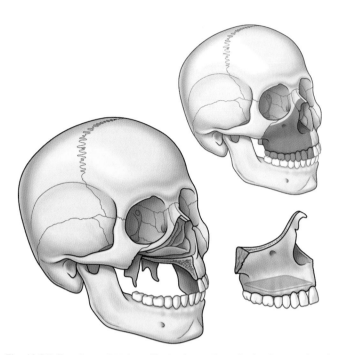

Fig. 10.2.5 Type II, or subtotal, maxillectomies are those that involve resection of the lower five walls of the maxilla, including the palate, but leave the orbital floor intact.

palate, restore the nasal lining, and reconstruct the eyelids, cheek, and lip as necessary. If the anterior cranial base is exposed, the brain must also be covered. Our flap of choice is a rectus abdominis myocutaneous free flap with one or more skin islands used to recreate the palate, lateral nasal wall, and any cutaneous deficits (Figs. 10.2.11 & 10.2.12). The latissimus dorsi flap may also provide adequate soft tissue bulk and pedicle length, but it is not as versatile with regard to providing multiple skin island coverage.

Type IV: orbitomaxillectomy defects

Type IV defects involve resection of the upper five walls of the maxilla and will usually include resection of the orbital contents, leaving the dura and brain exposed; the palate is usually left intact (Fig. 10.2.13). These are large-volume defects with large surface area requirements. Our flap of choice is the rectus abdominis flap, with one or more skin islands used for external skin and/or nasal lining (Fig. 10.2.14).

Functional and aesthetic outcomes

Speech

In 44 patients who underwent resection of the palate, speech was rated as normal in 22 patients (50%), near normal in 15 patients (34.1%), intelligible in six patients (13.6%), and unintelligible in one patient (2.3%). Speech results by maxillectomy classification are presented in Table 10.2.1.

Diet

After midface reconstruction with palatal resection, 26 patients (52%) were able to eat an unrestricted diet, 21 patients (42%) could manage a soft diet, three patients (6%) were only able to tolerate liquids, and one patient (2%) required tube feeding (Table 10.2.1).

Globe position and function

Of the 42 patients who underwent resection of the orbital floor with preservation of the orbital contents, 21 patients were assessed. All patients maintained vision. Mild vertical dystopia developed in one patient (4.8%), but no treatment was necessary. Mild horizontal diplopia developed in four patients (19%), which did not cause functional problems. Enophthalmos developed in one patient (4.8%). Lower eyelid ectropion developed in 10 patients (47.6%), which was rated as mild in four patients (19%), moderate in three patients (14.3%), and

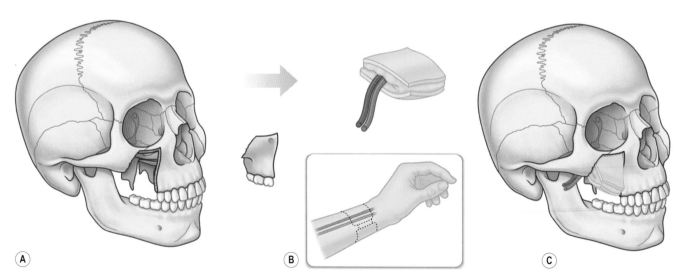

Fig. 10.2.6 (A) For Type IIA defects, which involve <50% of the transverse palate, reconstruction may proceed with either a microvascular free flap or a skin graft and an obturator, depending on patient and surgeon preference. If a free flap is selected to avoid the inconvenience and maintenance of a palatal obturator, our flap of choice is the radial forearm fasciocutaneous free flap. **(B)** Radial forearm free flap is prepared. **(C)** Inset of the free flap.

Table 10.2.1 Functional and aesthetic outcomes

Maxillectomy defect	Type I (n = 20)	Type IIA (n = 8)	Type IIB (n = 8)	Type IIIA (n = 22)	Type IIIB (n = 23)	Type IV (n = 19)	Total (n = 100)
Speech	N/A = 18	N/A = 2	N/A = 3	N/A = 8	N/A = 8	N/A = 17	n = 44
Normal	2	3	2	8	5	2	22 (50%)
Near normal		2	1	5	7		15 (34.1%)
Intelligible		1	2	1	2		6 (13.6%)
Unintelligible					1		1 (2.3%)
Diet	N/A = 18	N/A = 1		N/A = 6	N/A = 7	N/A = 17	n = 50
Unrestricted	1	4	3	9	7	2	26 (52%)
Soft		3	4	7	7		21 (42%)
Liquids			1		2		3 (6%)
Feeding tube	1						1 (2%)
Eyeglobe position and function	N/A = 16	N/A = 8	N/A = 8	N/A = 4	N/A = 23	N/A = 19	n = 21
Normal	1			4			5 (23.8%)
Dystopia				1			1 (4.8%)
Diplopia				4			4 (19%)
Enophthalmos	1						1 (4.8%)
Ectropion	1			9			10 (47.6%)
Mild				4			4 (19%)
Moderate				3			3 (14.3%)
Severe	1			2			3 (14.3%)
Oral competence	N/A = 20	N/A = 6	N/A = 6	N/A = 21	N/A = 17	N/A = 18	n = 12
Yes		2	2	1	5	1	11 (91.7%)
No					1		1 (8.3%)
Microstomia	N/A = 20	N/A = 6	N/A = 6	N/A = 21	N/A = 21	N/A = 14	n = 12
Yes			1		1	1	3 (25%)
No		2	1	1	1	4	9 (75%)
Aesthetic result	N/A = 8	N/A = 1		N/A = 5	N/A = 9	N/A = 7	n = 70
Excellent	6	6	5	12	5	7	41 (58.6%)
Good	5	1	1	4	9	5	25 (35.7%)
Fair	1		2	1			4 (5.7%)
Poor							0 (0%)

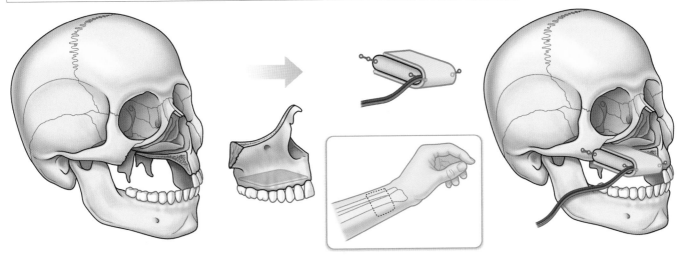

Fig. 10.2.7 For type IIB defects, which involve >50% of the transverse palate or a significant portion of the anterior arch, an osteocutaneous free flap is needed. These defects require bone for structural support as well as skin lining of the neopalate and nasal floor. A prosthesis is inadequate, because bone is needed to provide support to the upper lip. Our flap of choice is the radial forearm osteocutaneous "sandwich" flap.

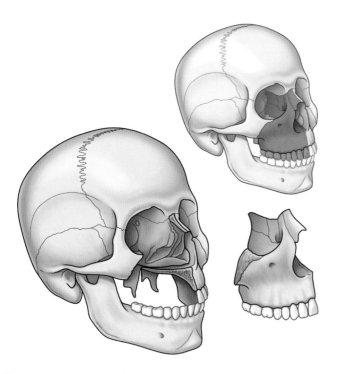

Fig. 10.2.8 For type IIIA defects, which involve resection of all six walls of the maxilla including the palate and orbital floor, but preserve the orbital contents, a bone graft is needed to reconstruct the orbital floor and a free flap with one or more skin paddles is needed to recreate the palate, nasal lining and/or the cheek.

severe in three patients (14.3%). None of the patients with ectropion underwent additional procedures (Table 10.2.1).

Oral competence

Of the 12 patients who underwent resection and reconstruction of the oral commissure, 11 patients (91.7%) had good to excellent oral competence within 1 month postoperatively. After radiation therapy, three patients (25%) developed mild

microstomia. No treatment was needed. Oral competence is described in Table 10.2.1.

Aesthetic results

Out of 70 patients who underwent evaluation of aesthetic outcomes, 41 patients had aesthetic results that were judged as excellent (58.6%), 25 patients had results judged as good (35.7%), and four patients had results judged as fair (5.7%). Although none of the patients were rated with poor results, it was most difficult to obtain a positive aesthetic result in patients who underwent skin, eyelid, or lip resections. Aesthetic results by maxillectomy classification are detailed in Table 10.2.1.

Cheek reconstruction

Introduction/general principles

The reconstructive goals and algorithm associated with maxillectomy defects should be prioritized in midface reconstruction. Once these have been addressed, or in isolated cheek reconstruction, the principles associated with cheek reconstruction should be considered. The cheek is composed of an external skin layer, muscles of facial expression, fat, and oral mucosa. The cheek is a relatively flat and expansive surface. As a peripheral unit of the face, the cheek cannot be fully compared to the contralateral cheek in any one view. As such, exact symmetry and precise subunit reconstruction will optimize the aesthetic results; however, it is not critical, especially compared to reconstruction of central subunits (nose, lip, and eyelid).[15,16] The more critical concept in cheek reconstruction is restoring the skin color and texture. Local tissues provide tissue of like texture, color, and hair growth. Thus, whenever possible, local tissue is the first choice in reconstructing the cheek.

Many cheek defects can be closed primarily. The best results are achieved by hiding the final scar along resting skin tension or contour lines. When treating subtotal facial defects

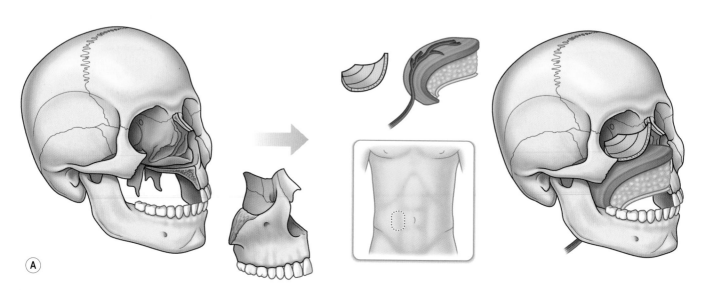

Fig. 10.2.9 Type IIIA defect reconstructed with bone graft for floor of orbit. **(A)** Rectus abdominus free flap for closure of palate and coverage of bone graft.

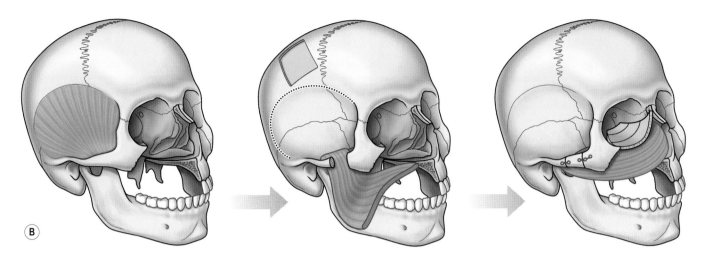

Fig. 10.2.9, cont'd (B) Temporalis flap for coverage of bone graft.

of the cheek skin, split- and full-thickness skin grafts should be avoided. Their unpredictable color and shiny texture violates the important principle of restoring cheek color and texture and creates a patch-like effect in the cheek.[17] Skin grafts are suitable for the reconstruction of the lower eyelid or the preauricular/temporal region.

Diagnosis and treatment

Local flaps

Local flaps provide skin that is similar to that of the face in terms of color and texture and are used for medium-sized

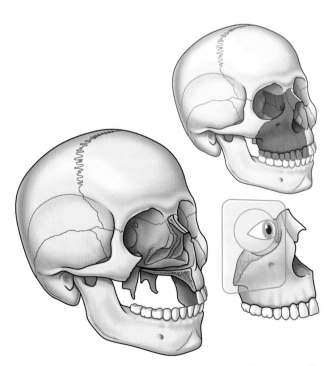

Fig. 10.2.10 The type IIIB defect, which involves resection of the entire maxilla including the orbital contents, is also known as an extended maxillectomy.

cheek defects. Any described local flaps can be used in the cheek with two principles in mind: (1) incisions should be kept parallel to relaxed skin tension lines, and (2) avoid any tension on other facial structures to prevent secondary deformities such as ectropion on the lower eyelid or distortion of the nose or lip.

Cheek rotation advancement flap

Mobilized cervicofacial flaps and myocutaneous flaps from the chest are workhorse options for reconstruction of external defects of the cheek and, at times, can be used for full-thickness defects. These flaps can be based anteriorly or posteriorly (Fig. 10.2.15). Anterior based flaps, described by Juri and Juri,[18,19] are useful for posterior and large anterior defects. The author's preferred flap is the anteriorly based cervicofacial flap (Fig. 10.2.16). The flap is based on the facial and submental arteries and elevated in the subcutaneous plane to the clavicle. The residual cheek skin is shifted forward and the neck upward to close the donor site. The dog-ear is then removed, ideally in the nasolabial fold, immediately or in a delayed fashion, depending on the vascular supply after elevation and inset. For larger defects, the anterior based cheek rotation flap can be extended down to the chest to move neck and chest skin to the face.[20–22] The flap incision should be carried down into the neck behind the trapezius, lateral to the acromioclavicular joint and deltopectoral groove, crossing the chest medially in the third to fourth intercostal space in a male with a back-cut, if needed in the parasternal area. Inferiorly, the flap is elevated with the platysmal muscle and with the deltoid and pectoral fasciae.

Posteriorly based flaps, described by Stark and Kaplan, are used for small and moderate-sized anterior cheek defects or larger posterior defects.[23] These flaps allow for transfer of the jowls and submental area into the face. Posteriorly based flaps can also be extended into the neck and chest for increased reach.[24–26]

Ectropion is an important complication to consider in the use of cervicofacial flaps. These flaps are designed to abut the lower eyelid and thus pull down on the delicate lower eyelid skin. To avoid this, the flap should be designed to avoid any tension in this region and should be suspended to the

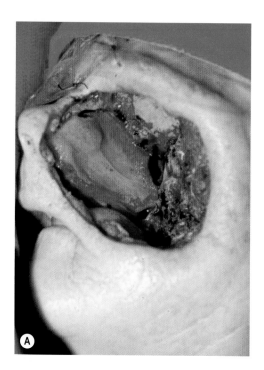

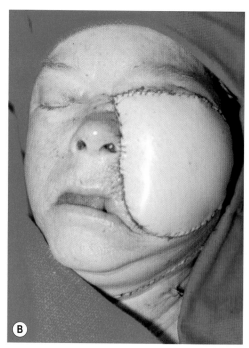

Fig. 10.2.11 Type IIIB defects involve resection of the upper five walls of the maxilla and will usually include resection of the orbital contents, leaving the dura and brain exposed. The palate is usually left intact. **(A)** Intraoperative photograph of type IIIB maxillectomy defect. **(B)** Postoperative photograph of type IIIB maxillectomy defect.

underlying periosteum or bone.[27,28] Another drawback of this flap is its unpredictable blood supply. The risk of ischemic complications is high in radiated patients, smokers, and flaps placed under tension.

Free tissue transfer

There are disadvantages to regional flaps that should be considered. The main disadvantage of regional flaps is a vascular supply that is not always reliable. When turned over on its self for full-thickness defects, regional flaps can get too bulky, leading to the creation of a cheek that has poor functional and aesthetic results. Skin grafts are usually necessary to address the donor site. Finally, regional flaps are occasionally not able to reliably reach the midface. For large defects involving the external skin, intraoral lining, or both, microvascular free flaps are generally indicated; however, color and texture match is more difficult to achieve.

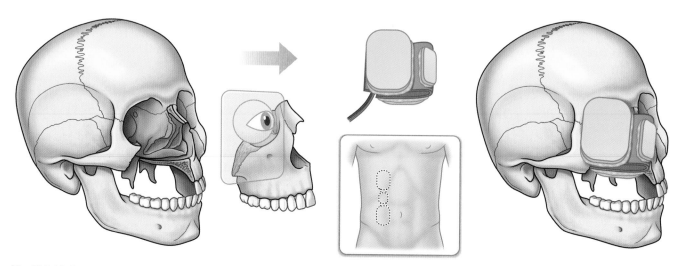

Fig. 10.2.12 For type IIIB defects, our flap of choice is a rectus abdominis myocutaneous free flap with one or more skin islands used to recreate the palate, lateral nasal wall, and any cutaneous deficits.

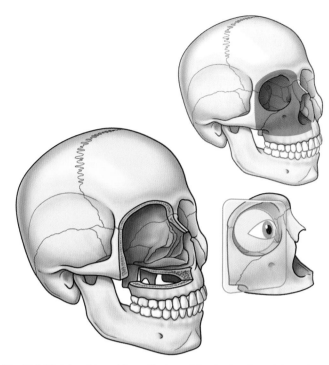

Large external defects require a significant amount of pliable skin with minimal underlying soft tissue. The radial forearm fasciocutaneous flap is ideal for these situations because it provides an adequate quantity of skin with minimal bulk (Fig. 10.2.17). Depending on the amount of soft tissue bulk required, the lateral arm flap, anterolateral thigh flap, and scapular flap are satisfactory options.

Intraoral lining defects that span the maxillary and mandibular sulci require a microvascular free flap. A radial forearm free flap provides thin pliable skin to resurface this area. The flap may also be neurotized to enhance recovery of sensation in this tissue by anastomosing the lateral antebrachial cutaneous nerve to a sensory nerve in the recipient area.

Full-thickness defects of the cheek require at least two skin islands to resurface the inner lining and provide external coverage. The folded radial forearm fasciocutaneous flap is the first choice for small through-and-through defects. Larger resections of the cheek associated with segmental mandibulectomy, as well as partial maxillectomy/orbitectomy, are best reconstructed by using the rectus abdominis free flap with multiple skin islands. If the commissure is resected, it should be reconstructed with a local switch procedure from the intact opposite lip and not with a portion of the free flap. The free flap should be reserved for reconstruction of the intraoral and external skin defects.

Fig. 10.2.13 A type IV or orbitomaxillectomy defect involves loss of the orbital contents and upper walls of the maxilla, leaving the palate intact.

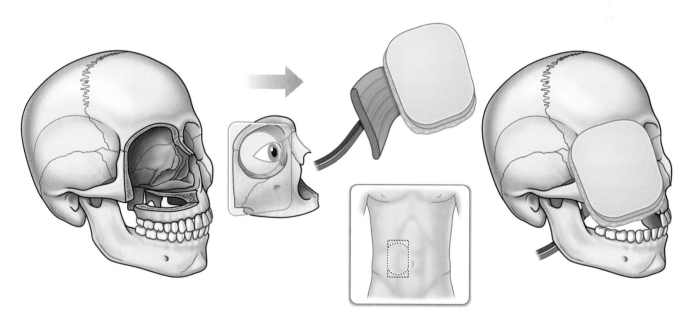

Fig. 10.2.14 For type IV defects, our flap of choice is the rectus abdominis flap, with one or more skin islands used for external skin and/or nasal lining.

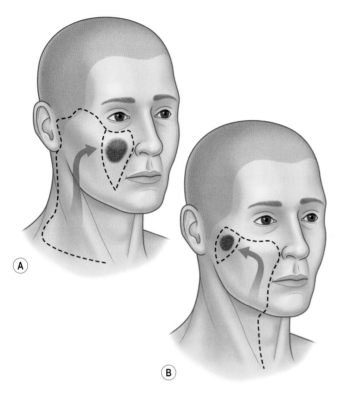

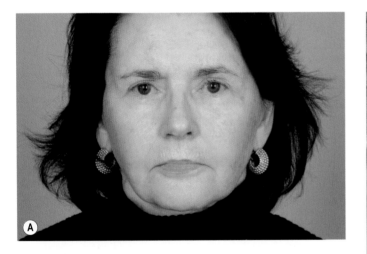

Fig. 10.2.15 The cheek rotation advancement flap. **(A)** Anteriorly based cheek rotation advancement flap is the local flap of choice for partial thickness cheek defects. **(B)** Posteriorly based cheek rotation advancement flap is an alternative design for coverage of posterior or small anterior cheek defects.

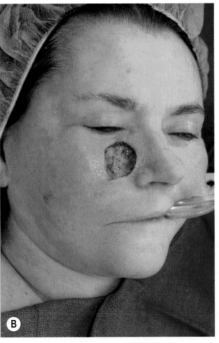

Fig. 10.2.16 The cheek rotation advancement flap is our local flap of choice for partial thickness cheek defects. **(A)** Preoperative view of anterior cheek lesion. **(B)** Partial thickness moderate sized anterior cheek defect.

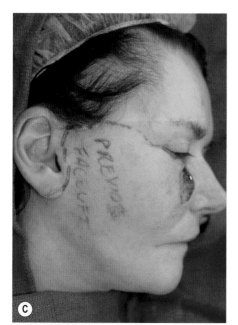

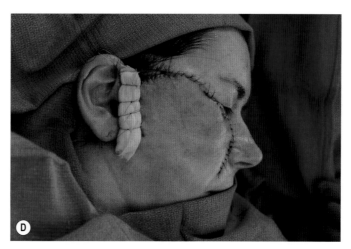

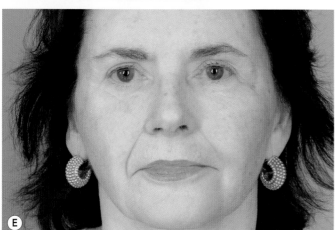

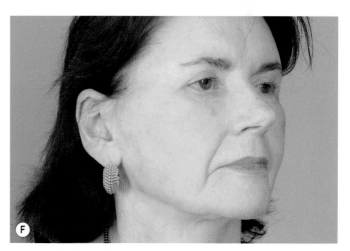

Fig. 10.2.16, cont'd **(C)** Cheek rotation advancement flap design. **(D)** Cheek rotation advancement flap inset with suspending periosteal sutures to avoid ectropion and skin grafting of preauricular donor site. **(E,F)** Postoperative view showing good color and texture match as well as lack of ectropion.

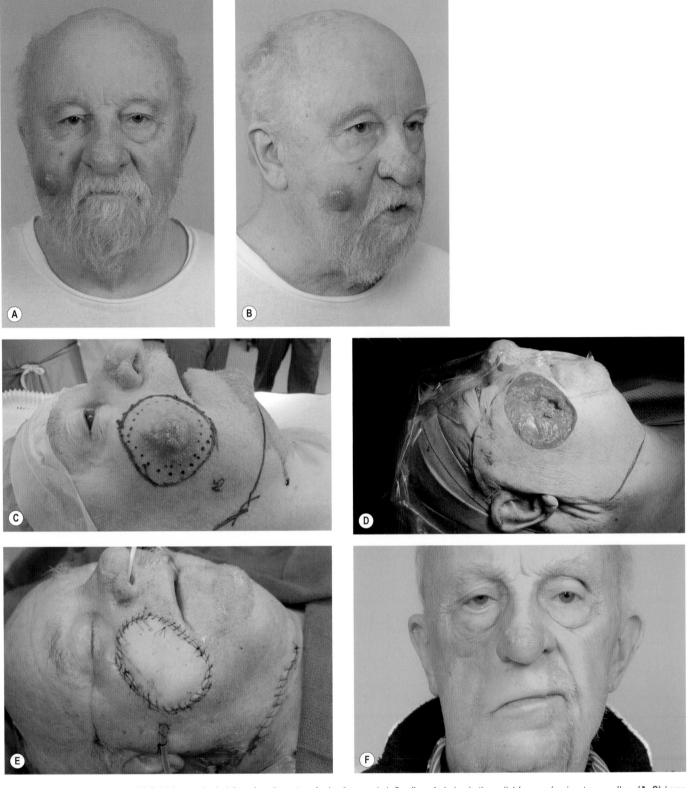

Fig. 10.2.17 For large partial and full thickness cheek defects free tissue transfer is often needed. Our flap of choice is the radial forearm fasciocutaneous flap. **(A–C)** Large anterior cheek lesion. **(D)** Large partial thickness anterior cheek defect. **(E)** Reconstruction with radial forearm fasciocutaneous flap to facial artery and vein. **(F)** Postoperative view of large partial thickness cheek reconstruction with radial forearm flap; color match is acceptable, yet inferior to that obtained using local/regional tissue.

Access the complete reference list online at **http://www.expertconsult.com**

3. Dalgorf D, Higgins K. Reconstruction of the midface and maxilla. *Curr Opin Otolaryngol Head Neck Surg.* 2008;16(4):303–311.

4. Foster RD, Anthony JP, Singer MI, Kaplan MJ, Pogrel MA, Mathes SJ. Reconstruction of complex midfacial defects. *Plast Reconstr Surg.* 1997;99(6):1555–1565. *A series of 26 consecutive midface reconstructions over 5 years was assessed. An algorithm for free flap selection in this setting is advanced based on this experience.*

6. Wells MD, Luce EA. Reconstruction of midfacial defects after surgical resection of malignancies. *Clin Plast Surg.* 1995;22(1):79–89. *Oncologic resections of the midface generate devastating deformities. Local reconstructions are preferred when sufficient support is available for osseointegrated implants; otherwise, osteocutaneous tissue transfer should be considered.*

7. Zhang B, Li DZ, Xu ZG, Tang PZ. Deep inferior epigastric artery perforator free flaps in head and neck reconstruction. *Oral Oncol.* 2009;45(2):116–120. *The DIEP flap is described as a reliable means of head and neck reconstruction with reduced donor site morbidity.*

8. Cordeiro PG, Disa JJ. Challenges in midface reconstruction. *Semin Surg Oncol.* 2000;19(3):218–225.

9. Herford AS, Cicciu M, Clark A. Traumatic eyelid defects: a review of reconstructive options. *J Oral Maxillofac Surg.* 2009;67(1):3–9.

10. Kakudo N, Ogawa Y, Kusumoto K. Success of the orbicularis oculi myocutaneous vertical V-Y advancement flap for upper eyelid reconstruction. *Plast Reconstr Surg.* 2009;123(3):107e.

13. Cordeiro PG, Santamaria E. A classification system and algorithm for reconstruction of maxillectomy and midfacial defects. *Plast Reconstr Surg.* 2000;105(7):2331–2346, discussion 47-8. *Maxillary defects are classified, based on a series of 60 patients presenting for reconstruction after oncologic resection. Free flap selection is discussed in this context.*

14. Cordeiro PG, Bacilious N, Schantz S, Spiro R. The radial forearm osteocutaneous "sandwich" free flap for reconstruction of the bilateral subtotal maxillectomy defect. *Ann Plast Surg.* 1998; 40(4):397–402. *Advantages of the osteocutaneous radial forearm free flap in maxillary reconstruction are discussed. "Sandwiching" the osseous component between the skin paddles provides for nasal and palatal lining as well as support for osteointegrated implants.*

16. Menick FJ. Reconstruction of the cheek. *Plast Reconstr Surg.* 2001;108(2):496–505.

10.3

Midface reconstruction: The M. D. Anderson approach

Matthew M. Hanasono and Roman Skoracki

 Access video lecture content for this chapter online at expertconsult.com

Introduction

Options for treating oncologic midfacial defects include use of prosthetic obturators, pedicled flaps, and free flaps, sometimes combined with grafts or alloplasts. While the popularity of pedicled flaps has declined due to limited reach and volume, prosthetic obturators remain a good solution for patients with limited palatal defects. However, for extensive defects, obturators may be difficult or impossible to retain, particularly in edentulous patients. Furthermore, obturators are usually inappropriate for defects that involve resection of the skull base and orbital floor. Finally, some patients may not like the inconvenience of an obturator, which must be removed and cleaned regularly and periodically adjusted or replaced for fit.

For midfacial reconstructions in which obturators are not an option or not desired by the patient, a variety of bony and soft tissue free flaps have been utilized and flap selection is a subject of debate. The challenge of reconstructing the midface is that resections are highly variable and patient specific, and no one technique is ideal for every defect.[1,2] Successful outcomes in midfacial reconstruction require mastery of a range of soft tissue and bony free flaps as well familiarity with traditional craniofacial techniques such as plating and grafting.

Reconstructive approach

Although there are several important considerations in midface reconstruction, the palate should be considered first (Fig. 10.3.1).[3] The extent of hard and soft palate resected, if any, as well as the defect location and plans for dental restoration, will dictate whether a prosthetic obturator is indicated or a bony or soft tissue free flap should be performed. Accurate reconstruction of the orbital floor, if resected, is mandatory for proper orbital position and eye function (Fig. 10.3.2). Following orbital exenteration (removal of orbital contents), a

pedicled or free flap may serve to line the orbit. If an extended orbital exenteration (removal of orbital contents and one or more orbital walls) or orbitomaxillectomy (orbital exenteration combined with a maxillectomy) is performed, a free flap is indicated to separate the orbit from the nasal cavity and sinuses. Our reconstructive algorithm[4] is presented in Fig. 10.3.3, and a detailed explanation follows.

Unilateral posterior palatomaxillectomy

While any number of palatoalveolar defects are possible, Okay *et al.*[3] recommend distinguishing defects based on whether function can be satisfactorily restored with an obturator or if a flap is required. Palatoalveolar defects that spare both canine teeth can often be successfully treated with an obturator. In these cases, cantilever forces resulting in unstable prosthetic retention are minimized because of the favorable root morphology of the canine adjacent to the obturator and the generous arch length provided by the remaining alveolus. Thus, defects including unilateral posterior palatomaxillary defects can usually be obturated and should be considered separately from those that cannot, including defects that involve half the palate and those that involve the entire anterior arch or whole palate.

As mentioned above, some patients even with unilateral posterior defects will still prefer or require autologous reconstruction. In these patients, we reconstruct posterior palatomaxillary defects with soft tissue rather than bony free flaps. Restoration of posterior maxillary dentition, which is not easily visible even when smiling, is not a priority to many patients.

The anterolateral thigh (ALT) or rectus abdominis myocutaneous (RAM) free flaps are usually well suited to providing the appropriate amount of tissue for posterior palatomaxillary reconstruction (Fig. 10.3.4). These flaps tend to be thicker in Western patients and will fill the maxillary sinus. The radial forearm fasciocutaneous (RFF) free flap can be used on more obese individuals or for small defects in which bulk is not needed to provide cheek projection.

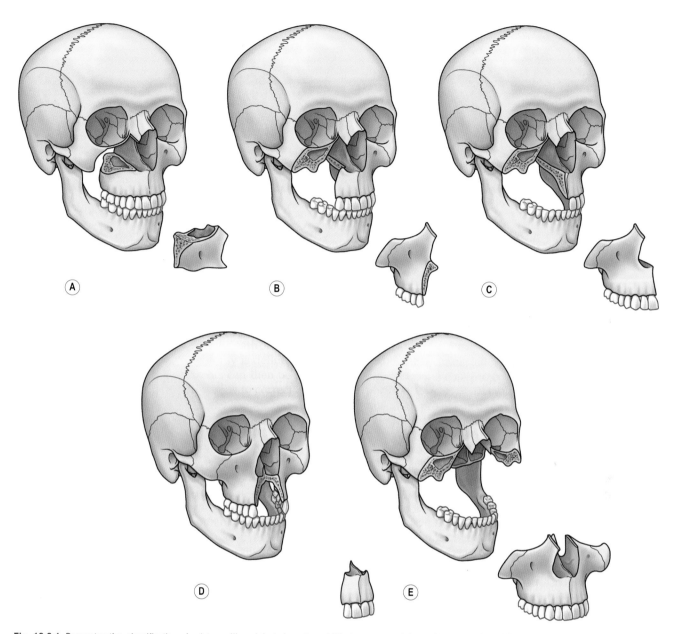

Fig. 10.3.1 Reconstructive classification of palatomaxillary defects based on ability to accommodate an obturator and need for bony or soft tissue reconstruction. Maxillectomy types include **(A)** superstructure maxillectomy (orbital floor removed, palate intact), **(B)** posterior palatomaxillectomy (hard palate and alveolus posterior to the canine tooth removed), **(C)** hemipalatomaxillectomy, **(D)** premaxillary resection, and **(E)** bilateral palatomaxillectomy (hard palate and anterior alveolus, including at least the canine teeth removed).

Unilateral hemipalatomaxillectomy

Unlike unilateral posterior palatomaxillary defects, defects of the palate and alveolus extending anterior to the canine tooth defects are difficult to obturate because of the greater cantilever forces acting on the prosthesis.[5] Free flap selection for these defects is somewhat controversial. Soft tissue free flaps are more straightforward surgically. However, they do not provide a rigid skeletal framework, which can result in a loss of anterior maxillary projection on the side of the defect, and cannot accept osseointegrated implants for dental restoration. To accommodate a dental prosthesis, the soft tissue flap must

not prolapse into the oral cavity. Creating a concave palatal reconstruction with soft tissue flaps can be technically challenging. This may be possible by ensuring the flap is not redundant and, if necessary, suspending the flap to the zygomatic periosteum with sutures.

We favor the use of osteocutaneous free flaps for hemipalatomaxillectomy defects in highly functional patients with a reasonable oncologic prognosis (Fig. 10.3.5). Besides providing better anterior projection, osteocutaneous free flaps offer the possibility of osseointegrated implants for dental restoration. Postoperative radiation therapy increases the risk of failed implant osseointegration, which should play a role in

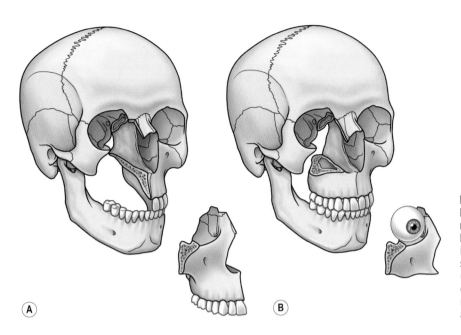

Fig. 10.3.2 (A) Maxillectomy with orbital floor resection. In this case, a hemipalatomaxillectomy is performed with resection of the orbital floor, termed a "total maxillectomy" by some, although others use this term to include defects in which the orbital floor is spared. To avoid confusion, the status of the orbital floor should be mentioned separately. **(B)** Maxillectomy with orbital exenteration. In this case, orbital exenteration is combined with a superstructure maxillectomy, termed an orbitomaxillectomy by some authors.

the timing of osseous-containing free flap reconstruction. Recommendations for free flap selection and shaping with osteotomies are discussed below.

Bilateral (anterior) palatomaxillectomy

Because both canine teeth are preserved, premaxillary defects may be amenable to obturation or reconstruction with a soft tissue free flap combined with a dental prosthesis that clasps to the remaining teeth to maintain midfacial projection and support the upper lip and nose. Otherwise, for these and more extensive anterior palatomaxillectomy defects, bony reconstruction is indicated to maintain midfacial height, width, and projection.[6,7] Extensive bilateral defects cannot usually be obturated due to the lack of teeth to support a heavy prosthesis.

The fibula free flap is our preferred flap for bony hemi- and bilateral palatomaxillectomy reconstruction.[8,9] The lateral surface of the fibula is used to restore the vertical maxillary height, measured from the orbital rim to the occlusal plane of the hard palate, by orienting it to face anteriorly (Figs. 10.3.6 & 10.3.7). The leg that is ipsilateral to the side of the planned microvascular anastomosis is selected for fibula osteocutaneous free flap harvest so that the skin paddle can be used to restore the palate. Vein grafts are used when pedicle length is inadequate to reach the recipient vessels.

After the resection is complete, osteotomies are made in the fibula such that the flap takes on a shape similar to the Greek letter "omega" in the transverse plane. We have found the use of CAD-CAM and three-dimensional (3D) models, when available, useful for shaping the fibula flap in maxillary reconstruction. The fibula is rigidly fixed to the zygomatic bones laterally. When reconstructing bilateral maxillectomy defects, the lateral portions of the "omega" recreate the malar regions. The central portion of the fibula free flap restores the maxillary alveolus. A slight downward angulation of the portion of the fibula used to recreate the anterior maxillae is usually needed to fully restore vertical facial height. For unilateral (see **hemipalatomaxillectomy**, above) or less than

complete bilateral defects, a shorter segment of bone is used and one or more segments can be omitted.

Orbital floor defects

Our experience suggests that, when supported by a soft tissue free flap, the orbital floor can be successfully reconstructed with bone grafts or alloplasts, such as titanium mesh (Fig. 10.3.8).[3] Many surgeons, however, feel that bone grafts are more resistant to radiation-associated complications than alloplasts are. On the other hand, bone grafts are more difficult to shape accurately, which may result in malpositioning of the globe. When using the fibula free flap for reconstructing hemipalatomaxillectomy and bilateral palatomaxillectomy defects that include resection of the orbital floor, we include some flexor hallucis longus muscle to support the bone graft or alloplastic orbital floor reconstruction.

Orbital exenteration defects

The primary goal of reconstruction following orbital exenteration is to line the orbital cavity with durable tissue. The patient's desire for an orbital prosthetic should also be considered when planning the reconstruction. A deep orbital cavity facilitates prosthetic fit while a shallow orbital cavity, or an orbital reconstruction that sits flush with the face, may not securely hold a prosthesis without osseointegrated implants. This also causes unsightly and unnatural appearing protrusion of the prosthesis.[10]

When postoperative radiation is able to be avoided, healing by secondary intention or split-thickness skin grafting, even on bare bone, are usually successful methods for addressing the standard orbital exenteration wound. If the orbital cavity is to be irradiated after surgery, better vascularized reconstruction of the orbital cavity with a soft tissue flap, such as

Text continued on p. 276

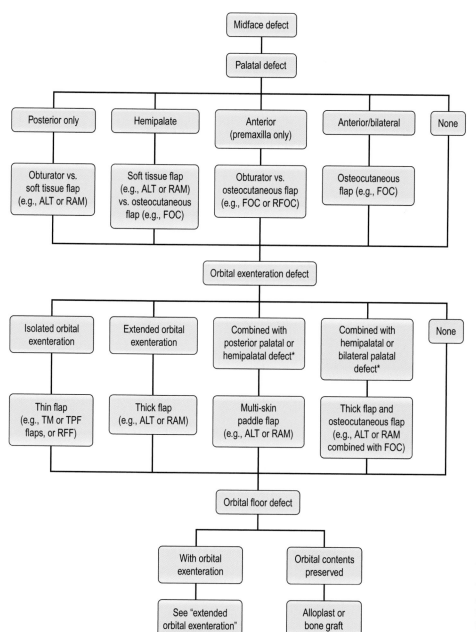

Fig. 10.3.3 Midfacial reconstructive algorithm. ALT, anterolateral thigh; FOC, fibula osteocutaneous; RAM, rectus abdominis myocutaneous; RFF, radial forearm fasciocutaneous; RFOC, radial forearm osteocutaneous; TM, temporalis muscle; TPF, temporoparietal fascia. *We favor osteocutaneous free flap reconstruction for hemipalatal defects (i.e., entire left or right palate) in suitable candidates with a good functional status and favorable prognosis.

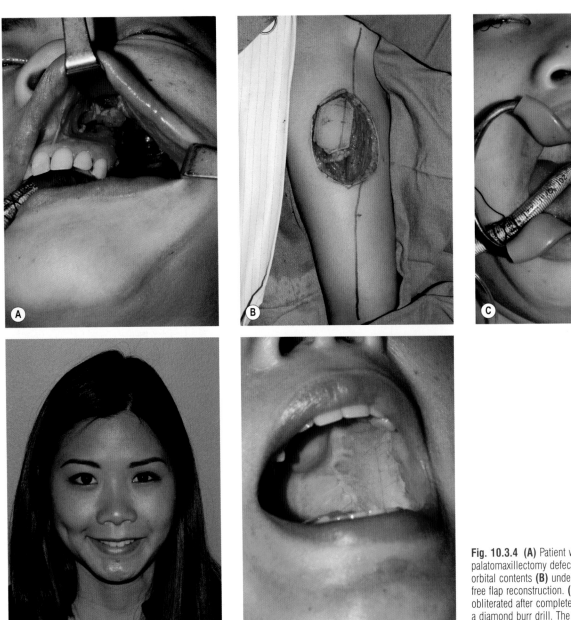

Fig. 10.3.4 **(A)** Patient with a posterior palatomaxillectomy defect sparing the orbital floor and orbital contents **(B)** undergoing an anterolateral thigh free flap reconstruction. **(C)** The maxillary sinus is obliterated after complete removal of the mucosa with a diamond burr drill. The flap is inset so that it does not hang into the oral cavity. **(D–E)** Postoperative external and intraoral appearance.

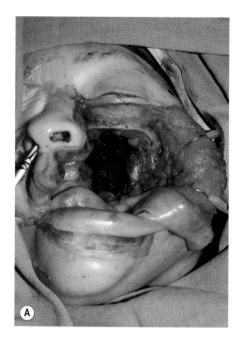

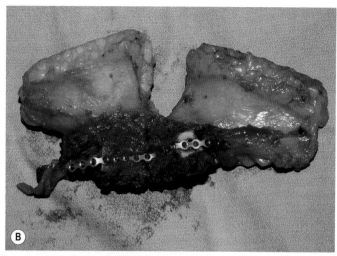

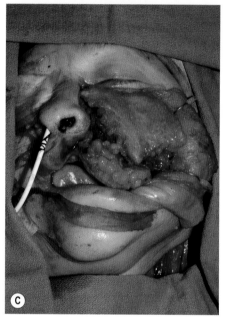

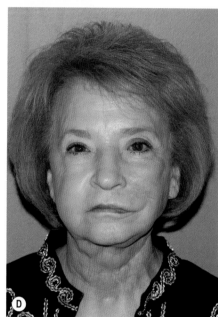

Fig. 10.3.5 (A) Patient with a **unilateral hemipalatomaxillectomy** defect sparing the orbital floor and orbital contents. **(B)** A fibula osteocutaneous free flap was performed with two skin paddles. **(C)** One skin paddle was used to reconstruct the palatal defect and the other was de-epithelialized to give soft tissue bulk to the cheek. **(D)** Postoperative appearance.

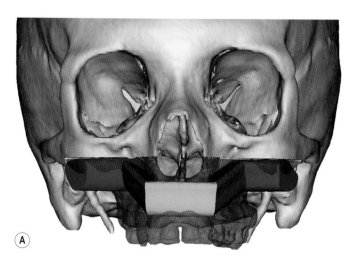

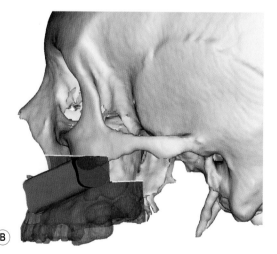

Fig. 10.3.6 (A,B) "Omega-shaped" fibula free flap configuration. The fibula is osteotomized to resemble the Greek letter omega in the horizontal plane.

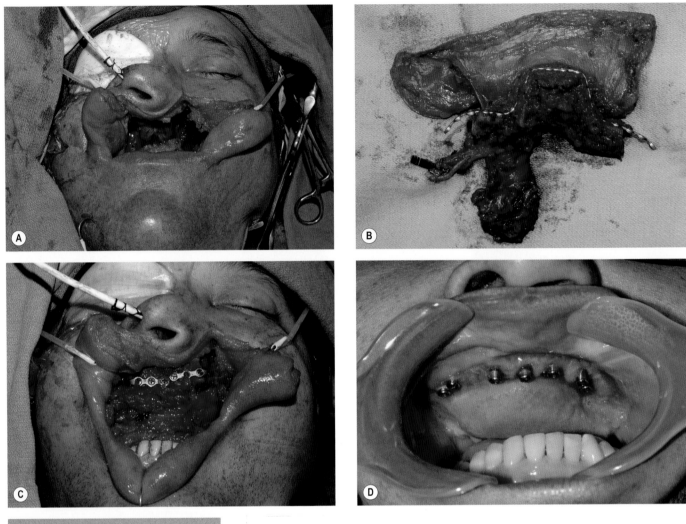

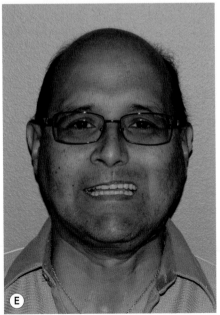

Fig. 10.3.7 (A) Patient with a **bilateral palatomaxillectomy** defect sparing the orbital floors and orbital contents. **(B)** An "omega-shaped" fibula osteocutaneous free flap was used to restore midfacial height, width, and projection. **(C)** Flap inset. **(D)** Osseointegrated implants were placed approximately 6 months after the initial reconstruction for dental restoration. **(E)** Postoperative appearance with a dental prosthesis.

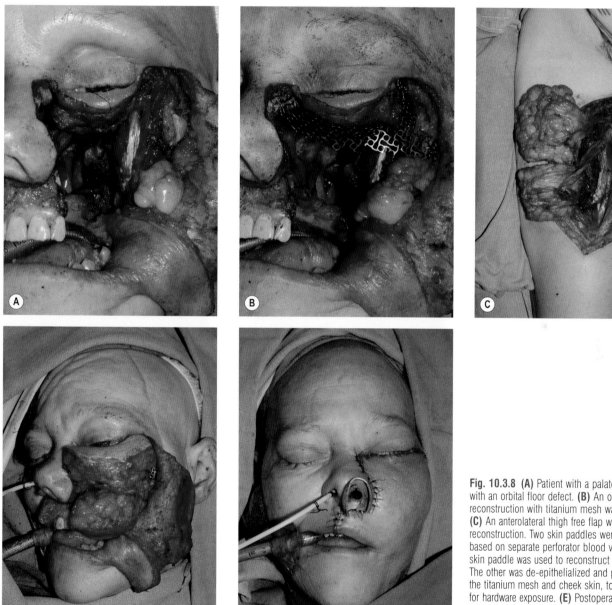

Fig. 10.3.8 (A) Patient with a palatomaxillectomy with an orbital floor defect. **(B)** An orbital floor reconstruction with titanium mesh was performed. **(C)** An anterolateral thigh free flap was harvested for reconstruction. Two skin paddles were dissected, based on separate perforator blood vessels. **(D)** One skin paddle was used to reconstruct the palatal defect. The other was de-epithelialized and placed between the titanium mesh and cheek skin, to minimize the risk for hardware exposure. **(E)** Postoperative appearance with slight intentional volume overcorrection in anticipation of shrinkage following adjuvant radiation therapy.

the temporalis muscle or temporoparietal fascia flaps (combined with a skin graft), is necessary to avoid chronic bone exposure.

In extended orbital exenterations and orbitomaxillectomies, the reconstructive goals are also to separate the orbit from the nasal or sinus cavities and from the dura and brain if the orbital roof has been removed. In extended orbital exenteration, our preference is to reconstruct the cavity with an RFF free flap in cases where the bony resection is limited. This flap

is usually thin, which helps to retain an orbital prosthetic. When the bony resection is more extensive, such as in orbitomaxillectomy, a larger volume flap is preferred. RAM or ALT free flaps are good choices in this situation, although creating a concave orbit needed for a prosthesis may be more difficult to achieve (Fig. 10.3.9). When there is also a palatal defect, the RAM and ALT free flaps can be designed with multiple skin paddles to reconstruct both the orbit and the palate (Fig. 10.3.10).

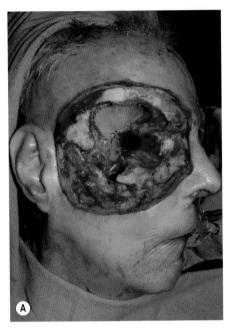
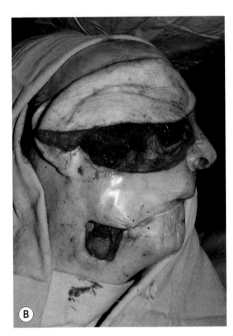
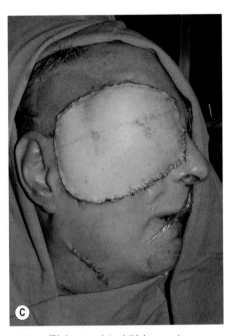

Fig. 10.3.9 **(A)** Patient with an extended orbital exenteration defect, including resection of the roof of the orbit and frontal dura. **(B)** An anterolateral thigh myocutaneous free flap was used to reconstruct the defect, with a portion of the vastus lateralis muscle placed against the dural repair and also used to obliterate the frontal sinus. **(C)** Immediate postoperative appearance.

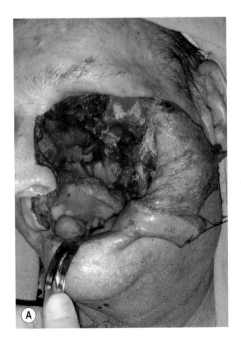
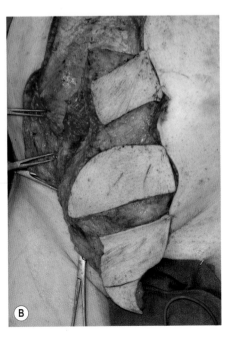

Fig. 10.3.10 **(A)** Patient with an orbitomaxillectomy defect, including resection of the posterior hard palate. **(B)** A rectus abdominis myocutaneous free flap was designed to close the orbital, nasal lining, and palatal defects with separate skin paddles based on separate perforating blood vessels.

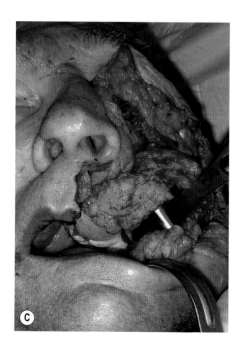 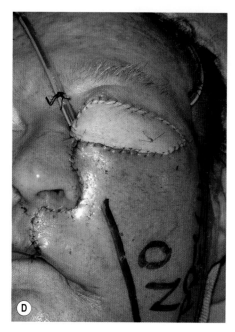

Fig. 10.3.10, cont'd (C) Insetting of the flap.
(D) Completed reconstruction.

References

1. Brown JS, Shaw RJ. Reconstruction of the maxilla and midface: introducing a new classification. *Lancet Oncol.* 2010;11:1001–1008.

2. Cordeiro PG, Santamaria E. A classification system and algorithm for reconstruction of maxillectomy and midfacial defects. *Plast Reconstr Surg.* 2000;105:2331–2346.

3. Okay DJ, Genden E, Buchbinder D, Urken M. Prosthodontic guideline for surgical reconstruction of the maxilla: a classification system of defects. *J Prosthet Dent.* 2001;86:352–363.

4. Hanasono MM, Silva AK, Yu P, Skoracki RJ. A comprehensive algorithm for oncologic maxillary reconstruction. *Plast Reconstr Surg.* 2013;131:47–60.

5. Moreno MA, Skoracki RJ, Hanna EY, Hanasono MM. Microvascular free flap reconstruction versus palatal obturation for maxillectomy defects. *Head Neck.* 2010;32:860–868.

6. Hanasono MM, Skoracki RJ. The omega-shaped fibula osteocutaneous free flap for reconstruction of extensive midfacial defects. *Plast Reconstr Surg.* 2010;125(4):160e–162e.

7. Hanasono MM, Jacob RF, Bidaut L, Robb GL, Skoracki RJ. Midfacial reconstruction using virtual planning, rapid prototype modeling, and stereotactic navigation. *Plast Reconstr Surg.* 2010;126:2002–2006.

8. Chang YM, Coskunfirat OK, Wei FC, Tsai CY, Lin HN. Maxillary reconstruction with fibula osteoseptocutaneous free flap and simultaneous insertion of osseointegrated dental implants. *Plast Reconstr Surg.* 2004;113(4):1140–1145.

9. Rodriguez ED, Martin M, Bluebond-Langner R, et al. Microsurgical reconstruction of posttraumatic high-energy maxillary defects: establishing the effectiveness of early reconstruction. *Plast Reconstr Surg.* 2007;120:103S–117S.

10. Hanasono MM, Lee JC, Yang JS, et al. An algorithmic approach to reconstructive surgery and prosthetic rehabilitation after orbital exenteration. *Plast Reconstr Surg.* 2009;123:98–105.

11

Oral cavity, tongue, and mandibular reconstructions

Ming-Huei Cheng and Jung-Ju Huang

SYNOPSIS

- A comprehensive review of the oral cavity, tongue, and mandibular defect, the patient's disease status, and prognosis are equally important to achieve optimal reconstruction and minimize complications. Evaluation of the defect size, shape, geometry and relationship to the adjacent structures should be performed. A strategic approach to flap selection and flap design restores the defect in the best way possible.

- Patient risk factors, defect characteristics, donor flap selection, and surgical technique should be considered in mandibular reconstruction. The use of different tissue components to achieve composite reconstruction is essential for successful functional reconstruction. An understanding of the anatomical characteristics of all the available osteocutaneous flaps may increase the likelihood of selecting the appropriate donor flap for mandibular reconstruction.

- For reconstruction of type III mandibular defects, several options exist, including the use of a soft-tissue flap with a reconstruction plate, one osteocutaneous flap with one pedicled flap, double free flaps, chimeric flaps such as a composite scapular flap, and a composite osteomusculocutaneous peroneal artery combined (OPAC) flap. The evolution of the fibular flap from a bone-only flap to an osteoseptocutaneous (OSC) flap and an OPAC flap may increase the clinical applications of this flap for type III mandibular defects. Due to the triangular profile of the fibula, the placement of plates and screws on the lateral aspect of the fibula reduces the incidence of injury to its pedicle and septocutaneous perforators.

- Recently, the idea of computer-assisted 3D simulation is emerging. The use of 3D plating and guidance of osteotomy can be applied to ease the surgery and enhance the reconstructive result.

Introduction

Reconstruction of the oral cavity and mandible can be challenging with regard to both functional and aesthetic outcomes. The oral cavity is composed of different structures that integrate with each other to serve with their best functions in speech, swallowing, and facial expression. Any defect involving one of the functional unit can destroy the function of others. An ideal reconstruction should mimic the missing tissue with regard to structure, geometry, and tissue character. A three-dimensional consideration of the defect is required to facilitate the best reconstruction.

The tongue is the most commonly involved organ of primary oral cavity squamous cell carcinoma in the US, while the buccal mucosa is the number one involved structure in Asia where betel nut chewing presents as the most prevalent cause of buccal cancer. Tongue reconstruction may be challenging and deserves special attention as its role in articulation, deglutition, and airway protection makes it irreplaceable. Reconstruction attempts fall into restoring the mobility of the tongue after partial resection and providing bulk when free tongue movement will not be possible after total tongue resection. A well-performed buccal mucosa reconstruction maintains limitless mouth opening, maximizes quality of life, and preserves cosmesis of the facial profile.

When the resection of cancer inevitably involves the mandible, bony reconstruction should be carefully planned or converted to plating and soft-tissue coverage depending on the patient's general and disease status. The cause of mandibulectomy can be for oncologic etiology, treatment of osteoradionecrosis, or a traumatic result from gunshot. Typically a very advanced cancer stage or gunshot trauma can result in severe tissue defects, involving not only the mandible itself but also the surrounding soft tissues like the oral mucosa, oral lining, floor of the mouth, tongue, and external cheek skin. These defects require delicate reconstruction to restore function, cosmesis, and dead space left from resection of the masticator muscle, buccal fat pad, and parotid gland, which indicates soft-tissue obliteration to prevent fluid accumulation and infection.[1]

Basic anatomy/disease process

The oral cavity is bounded by the lip anteriorly, the oropharynx posteriorly, the hard and soft palates superiorly, the tongue and mouth floor inferiorly and the cheeks laterally. Between the cheek skin and oral mucosa lie muscles that act to facilitate facial expression, mouth movement, and oral competence. The skeletal structures, namely the mandible and maxilla, maintain the appearance of the lower and middle face.

Squamous cell carcinoma is the most common cancer of the oral cavity, accounting for 86% oral cavity malignancy. The other pathological causes include verrucous carcinoma, sarcoma, melanoma, lymphoma, and other rare cancers. Trauma, complications from cancer treatment, and benign causes, such as submucosal fibrosis, account for a few reconstruction demands. The mean age-adjusted incidence of oral cavity and pharyngeal cancer is 11.9 per 100 000 from 1975 to 2008 in the US. The incidence is even higher in countries where betel nut chewing is a social problem.[2] In 2008, head and neck cancers comprised 2–3% of all cancers and accounted for 1–2% of all cancer deaths in the US.[3–4] Most patients with head and neck cancer have metastatic disease at the time of diagnosis (with regional nodal involvement in 43% and distant metastasis in 10%). Moreover, patients with head and neck cancer often develop second primary tumors at an annual rate of 3–7%.[4–6] The male-to-female ratio is currently 3:1 for the incidence of oral cavity and pharyngeal cancers.[3]

Statistical analysis of a 10-year period revealed a trend toward earlier diagnosis of head and neck cancer. Surgical treatment with or without radiation and chemotherapy remains the standard of care.[5] Early diagnosis, however, provides a better tissue/organ-preserving surgery and better postoperative cosmesis and functional preservation with a better prognosis. Since the first introduction of the free intestinal flap in 1959[7] and the first fasciocutaneous free flap for head and neck reconstruction in 1976, free-flap transfer has become the gold standard for reconstruction due to its high flap survival rate, improved cosmetic and functional results, and acceptable level of donor site morbidity.[8–9] These techniques also facilitate resection of even more advanced but localized tumors.

Inadequate oral hygiene and contamination may increase the risk of infection and also compromise the survival of any inadequately vascularized tissue.[10–14] Irradiation produces detrimental acute and chronic effects not only in the periosteum and the marrow of the mandible but also in the oral mucosa and surrounding soft tissue.[11–14] With chronic hypoxia, cellular and vascular damage lead to skin atrophy and increase the susceptibility to wound breakdown and decreased healing potential following minor trauma. Vascular changes initially occur in the microcirculation; however, with progression, larger blood vessels can be affected as well. Many of these issues are addressed by the transplantation of well-vascularized tissue with bone and skin components. Vascularized bone resists infection well, does not resorb, and is not dependent on the recipient bed vascularity for survival.[15]

Diagnosis/patient presentation

The most common first sign of the oral cavity is an unhealed ulceration or a growing mass with touch bleeding. Most of the patients experience pain to a variable degree. Cuffari and colleagues demonstrated a positive correlation between the pain character and TNM staging of the tongue and mouth floor.[16] A thorough physical examination, radiographic study of the tumor, and histology with TNM staging should be performed by both surgical oncologists and reconstructive surgeons prior to surgery. Any history of gunshot trauma, X-rays, and three-dimensional computed tomography (CT) scans of the defect should also be considered during preoperative planning. In soft-tissue-involved cancer, such as buccal or lingual, MRI provides better images for soft-tissue evaluation. Whole body PET scan provides an opportunity to identify distant metastasis in patients with more advanced cancer staging. In addition to classical TNM staging,[17] gene expression[18–20] and profiling provide a subclassification based on DNA repair genes. This subclassification plays a role in predicting the clinical outcome after radiotherapy.[18] Liao et al. addressed that upregulation of centromere protein H is correlated with poor prognosis and progression in tongue cancer patients.[21] Chronic ulcer, leukoplakia, and tumor growth are regularly seen at specialized centers.[22] Visual-loss as an initial symptom of squamous cell carcinoma of the tongue had been published by Foroozan.[23] It is important to keep in mind that rare constellations of symptoms may require differential diagnosis: a tumor or abscess of the tongue could also be a sign of atypical metastasis of lung cancer.[24,25] Recently, a rare schwannoma of the tongue was reported by Cohen and Wang.[26] Malignant fibrous histiocytoma of the tongue was reported by Rapidis et al.[27]

Patient selection and decision-making

A comprehensive assessment of the defects, the patient's general condition, and the availability of donor tissue are important before reconstruction. A thorough understanding of the missing tissue, including its geometrical relation to each structure inside the oral cavity, will elucidate the functional and aesthetic requirements of reconstruction and facilitate the selection of an optimal reconstructive method (Tables 11.1–11.3).

Patient factors (Table 11.4)

Many oral cavity cancer patients have a history of smoking and alcohol consumption, which increases the risk of perioperative pulmonary and overall complications. These factors also affect the patency of microvascular anastomoses in a free-flap transfer.[28,29] Diabetes mellitus is a risk factor for peripheral vasculopathy and is associated with a higher incidence of postoperative infection. A patient with end-stage renal disease undergoing a prolonged operation is at greater risk of developing postoperative fluid overload and other associated complications. Patients with Child's class B or C cirrhosis had more complications, including pulmonary complications, acute renal failure, and sepsis, than those with class A cirrhosis (80% versus 19.1%).[30] Advanced age is not an absolute contraindication for microsurgery. However, medical problems associated with chronological age, such as cardiopulmonary disease, atherosclerosis, and previous stroke, indicate a higher incidence of postoperative medical complications.[28] These advanced oromandibular cancer patients are often malnourished, which has an impact on normal wound healing, pulmonary function, and postoperative recovery.[31] Smoking should be ceased 2 weeks before a long operation to

Table 11.1 Comparisons of soft-tissue flaps for buccal mucosa and tongue reconstruction

Flap type / Flap character	Skin or mucosa	Flap dimension	Flap thickness	Pedicle size	Pedicle length	Dissection difficulty
Local/regional flap						
Nasolabial flap	++	+	++	–	–	–
Buccal fat pad flap	–	+	+	–	–	–
Facial artery musculomucosal flap	++	+	++	–	–	–
Submental flap	+++	+++	++	–	–	–
Deltopectoral flap	++	+++	+++	–	–	–
Pectoralis major myocutaneous flap	++++	++++	++++	–	–	–
Free flap						
Radial forearm flap	++++	++++	++	+++	++++	++++
Ulnar forearm flap	++++	++++	++	+++	++++	++++
Lateral arm flap	+++	++	++	++	+	+++
Rectus abdominis musculocutaneous flap	++++	+++	++++	++++	+++	++++
Anterolateral thigh						
fasciocutaneous flap	++++	++++	+++	++++	++++	+
musculocutaneous flap	++++	++++	++++	++++	+++	+
Thoracodorsal artery perforator flap	++++	+++	+++	+++	+++	++
Medial sural artery perforator	++++	+++	++	+++	++++	++

Flap character rates as follows: ++++, excellent; +++, good; ++, fair; +, poor; –, not applicable. Dissection difficulty rates as follows: ++++, not difficult; +++, mild difficulty; ++, moderate difficulty; +, most difficult.

Table 11.2 Selection of soft-tissue flaps for buccal mucosa reconstruction

Flap type / Flap character	Small mucosa defect	Large mucosa defect	Mucosa trigon	Through and through	Mucosa and partial maxilla	Mucosa and marginal mandibulectomy
Local/regional flap						
Nasolabial flap	+	–	–	–	–	–
Buccal fat pad flap	++	++	–	–	–	–
Submental flap	++	++	–	–	–	–
Facial artery musculomucosal flap	++	–	–	–	–	–
Deltopectoral flap	–	+++	++	+++	++	+++
Pectoralis major myocutaneous flap	–	++++	++	+++	++	++++
Free flap						
Radial forearm flap	–	++++	++	+	+	+
Ulnar forearm flap	–	++++	++	+	+	+
Lateral arm flap	–	++	++	+	+	+
Rectus abdominis musculocutaneous flap	–	++	++	+++	++++	++++
Anterolateral thigh						
fasciocutaneous flap	–	+++	+++	+++	++	+++
musculocutaneous flap	–	++	+++	++++	++++	++++
Thoracodorsal artery perforator flap	–	++++	++++	++	++	+++
Medial sural artery perforator	–	+++	++	+	+	+

Recommendation rates as follows: ++++, excellent; +++, good; ++, fair; +, poor; –, not applicable.

Table 11.3 Tongue defects and available reconstructive options

Class	Tongue defect	Considerations	Preferred options	Alternatives
I	Hemi or less	Thin, pliable skin flap, motility	Radial forearm flap/ulnar forearm flap	Medial sural artery perforator flap Anterolateral thigh fasciocutaneous flap
IIa	Two-thirds	Bulky skin flap	Anterolateral thigh perforator flap	Profunda artery perforator flap, Rectus abdominis musculocutaneous flap
IIb	Three-quarters	Bulky musculocutaneous flap	Anterolateral thigh musculocutaneous flap	Tensor fascia lata musculocutaneous flap Rectus abdominis musculocutaneous flap
III	Total	Large musculocutaneous flap with adequate volume for swallowing	Pentagonal anterolateral thigh musculocutaneous flap	Tensor fascia lata musculocutaneous flap Rectus abdominis musculocutaneous flap

reduce pulmonary complications. For a malnourished patient, a short period of tube feeding before surgery improves malnutrition in an effort to optimize wound healing and general recovery after surgery.

Defect factors (see Table 11.4)

As dictated by the principles of reconstruction, it is necessary to replace tissue with like tissue. A complete assessment of the defect is just as important as a careful evaluation of the patient's medical history. However, when a severe medical comorbidity precludes advanced reconstruction, the surgeon should not hesitate to downgrade along the reconstruction ladder. The assessment of the defects should include the size, volume, and components of the involved soft tissue, the length and location of the mandible defect, the available recipient vessels, and the quality of the external skin.

Skin graft

The environment of the oral cavity is not conducive to survival of the skin graft. Its clinical application here has largely been replaced by the use of pedicled and free flaps. The progression of scar contracture from a skin graft often limits the mobility of the oral mucosa and tongue, which worsens the postoperative oral cavity function.

Local/regional flap

Before the development of free tissue transfer, local and regional flaps were the treatment of choice. Today, the applications of pedicled flaps are limited to the reconstruction of small defects or in patients where free tissue transfer is not indicated.

Free tissue transfer

The advent of microsurgical free tissue transfer has significantly increased reconstructive alternatives through the ability to use larger flaps and the increased versatility to ensure a better fit of the defect. The use of free tissue transfer for composite reconstruction has allowed restoration of increasingly complex defects in a single stage with better functional and aesthetic outcomes.

Different decision-making processes for the most common oral conditions will be discussed below.

Requirement of tracheostomy

Making the decision to perform a tracheostomy should not be delayed in elderly patients that will undergo total tongue resection or advanced tongue resection involving the base of the tongue or pre-epiglottis area, small defects involving the base of the tongue or extending to the pre-epiglottis area, resection of mouth floor cancer and involving the genioglossus muscles that may cause tongue drop, and large flap

Table 11.4 Considerations in mandibular reconstruction.

	Consideration	Details
1	Patient's risk factors	• Smoking, old age, diabetes, malnutrition, cardiovascular disease, liver cirrhosis, nutrition • Local advanced disease, distal metastasis, recurrent or second primary cancer, postoperative radiation
2	Defects	• Length and location of bone defects • Size, volume, and components of soft tissue • Radiated skin and vessels, previous scarring, cosmesis
3	Recipient vessels	• Ipsilateral or contralateral
4	Selection of donor flaps	• See Table 11.6.
5	Technique considerations	
	Plating	• Reconstruction plate or miniplates, preoperative 3D CT plating before or after pedicle division • Occlusion with intermaxillary wiring
	Osteotomy	• Lengths and number of segments • Before or after pedicle division
	Flap inset	• Before vs. after anastomosis • Bone inset first, then mucosa or external skin
	Microsurgical anastomosis	• Artery first or vein first
	Osseointegration	• Immediate/delayed • Number of dental implants

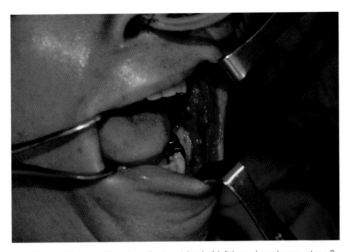

Fig. 11.1 A 55- year-old male patient sustained of left buccal carcinoma, stage 2. A left buccal mucosa defect remained after tumor resection with a left modified radical neck dissection.

reconstruction that subsequently with swelling may accidentally obstruct the airway and require an elective tracheostomy. The tracheostomy can be kept in place for one week or longer and removed whenever the patient's general status becomes stable and the wound heals without the requirement for debridement (requirement for anesthesia).

Decision-making for buccal reconstruction (see Table 11.2)

Reconstruction is relatively straightforward if the defect involves only the buccal mucosa. The size/shape of the defect should be measured with the mouth open at maximum. A retractor can be applied between the upper and lower teeth to facilitate maximal exposure. A sizeable flap for adequate resurfacing is necessary to prevent irreversible trismus and facilitate satisfactory result. The pliability of a soft-tissue flap allows for easier flap inset to fit the contour of the defect. A better functional restoration with regard to postoperative mouth movement, eating, speech, and facial expression can be provided (Figs. 11.1–11.5).

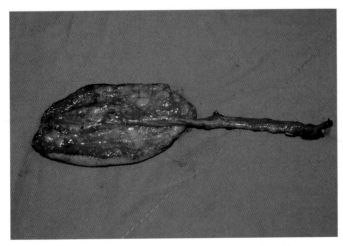

Fig. 11.2 A radial forearm flap sized 10 × 7 cm was harvested from his non-dominant left hand.

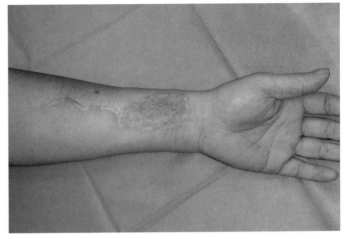

Fig. 11.3 At the 3-year follow-up, the patient was satisfied with the donor site with split-thickness skin graft.

The sulcus should be carefully recreated if the buccal–gingival sulcus is involved in the resection. The sulcus functions as a food reservoir during mastication and helps in directing the saliva and food toward the oropharynx during deglutition. In such cases, a slight folding of the flap is required

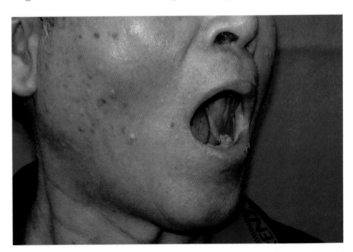

Fig. 11.4 Result of the radial forearm flap for buccal reconstruction showed good functional recovery with flap color match and appropriate thickness and with adequate mouth opening.

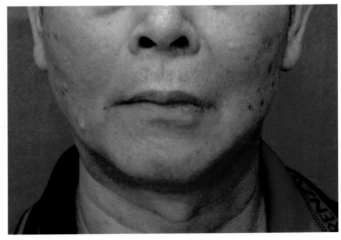

Fig. 11.5 The face looks symmetric after surgery at 3-year follow-up.

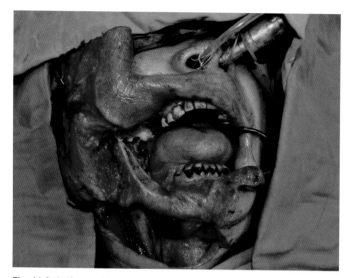

Fig. 11.6 A 46-year-old male patient suffered from buccal carcinoma, stage 1. Right buccal mucosa defect with marginal mandibulectomy was presented post tumor ablation surgery. *(Courtesy of Dr. Chih Wei Wu.)*

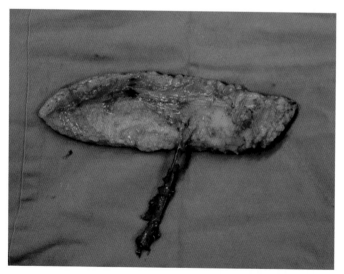

Fig. 11.8 Several myocutaneous perforators were identified with blue arrows. *(Courtesy of Dr. Chih Wei Wu.)*

to form the shape of the sulcus. It is also common that the inner surface of the lower and/or upper lip is involved. Although the wound between the edge of the lip and the lower gum can usually be closed primarily, direct closure results in an unnatural appearance and impacts postoperative function.

If the defect extends from the buccal mucosa to the trigone region, the mandible is often exposed. Such defects commonly involve the posterior tongue. Although the tissues in this area are relatively loose, making primary wound closure possible in some cases, direct wound closure distorts the natural anatomy of the tonsillar pillar and tethers the tongue. An anatomical change can result in food regurgitation into the nasal cavity. Tongue tethering also limits function with regard to eating and speaking.

Flap selection for pure buccal mucosa reconstruction depends on the thickness of the flap required. According to

the authors' experience, a free radial forearm or ulnar forearm flap is usually adequate (see Figs. 11.1–11.5). A anterolateral thigh (ALT) perforator flap is required for a thicker defect. A medial sural artery perforator (MSAP) flap or deep profunda artery perforator flap (PAP) is a feasible alternative[32,33] (Figs. 11.6–11.10). In severe trauma or in advanced cancer resection, the defect can extend from the mucosa to the external skin (through-and-through defect), often requiring a bulky myocutaneous flap or a thick fasciocutaneous flap with chimeric flap design or de-epithelialization of the central flap to facilitate reconstruction (Figs. 11.11–11.14). Each of the skin paddles can be customized according to the defect, preventing distortion of the mouth angle.

If the resection is accompanied by marginal mandibulectomy, sufficient coverage of the exposed mandible bone with a thick fasciocutaneous flap or myocutaneous flap prevents tethering of tongue movement after reconstruction and

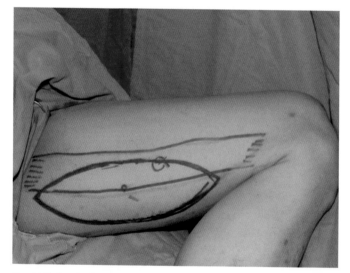

Fig. 11.7 A profunda artery perforator flap 7 × 21 cm was designed on his left medial thigh with the assistance of hand-held Doppler to map the myocutaneous perforators, along the posterior border of the gracilis muscle. *(Courtesy of Dr. Chih Wei Wu.)*

Fig. 11.9 The profunda artery perforator flap was harvested and based on only one myocutaneous perforator with intramuscular dissection. *(Courtesy of Dr. Chih Wei Wu.)*

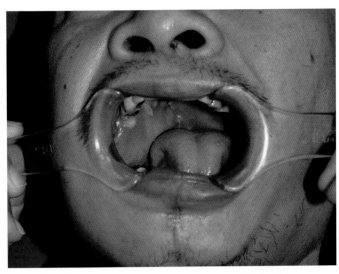

Fig. 11.10 At the 12- month follow-up, the patient was satisfied with the functional result. *(Courtesy of Dr. Chih Wei Wu.)*

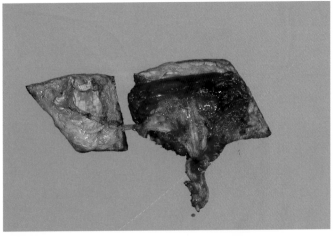

Fig. 11.13 The chimeric flap included one fasciocutaneous skin paddle for cheek skin reconstruction and one myocutaneous flap for buccal mucosa reconstruction and covering the exposed mandible bone with volume replacement after marginal mandibulectomy.

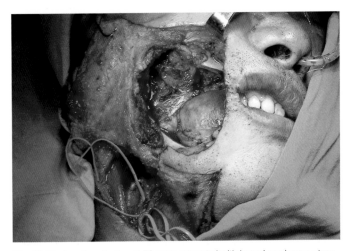

Fig. 11.11 A male patient aged 59 years presented with buccal carcinoma, stage 4. Tumor resection involved his right buccal mucosa, mandible with marginal mandibulectomy, and cheek skin, resulting in a through-and-through defect.

rebuilds the symmetric bulk of the face. An ALT flap with or without the vastus lateralis muscle is the preferred choice for reconstruction.

Sometimes an inferior maxillectomy is part of an advanced buccal mucosal tumor resection, which leaves a dead space in the inferior maxillary area that requires soft-tissue obliteration to avoid fluid accumulation and postoperative infection. It is not uncommon that part of the soft or hard palate is involved in the resection. Few of the palatal wounds can be closed primarily; inadequate tissue resurfacing can result in development of an oronasal fistula and causes food regurgitation and hypernasality. A myocutaneous flap provides sufficient muscle to obliterate the dead space while providing buccal and palatal resurfacing. An ALT flap with vastus lateralis muscle is used most frequently in the authors' experience. A free transverse rectus abdominis myocutaneous (TRAM) or vertical rectus abdominis myocutaneous (VRAM) flap can alternatively be used.

Table 11.1 summarizes the characteristics of each available flap and its clinical applications in buccal mucosa reconstruction. Table 11.2 provides guidelines for flap selection for variable buccal defects.

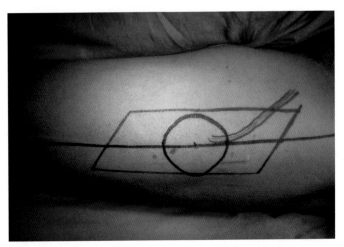

Fig. 11.12 By mapping the perforators with pencil Doppler, a chimeric anterolateral thigh flap 17 × 7 cm was designed on his left thigh based on separate perforators.

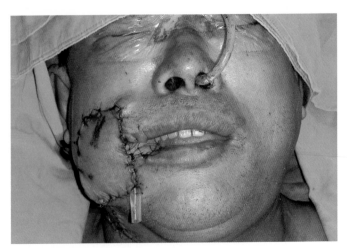

Fig. 11.14 Result of immediate reconstruction.

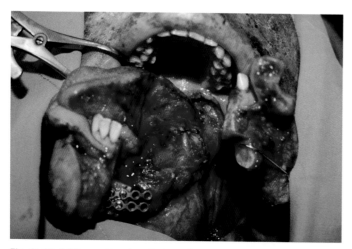

Fig. 11.15 A 27-year-old male patient sustained a hemi-tongue defect after cancer resection.

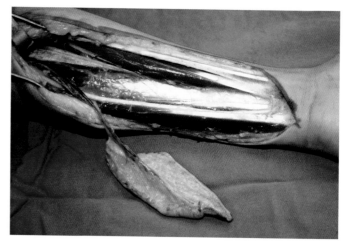

Fig. 11.16 An ulnar forearm flap, 6 × 10 cm, with well-preserved ulnar and all partendons of the flexors, was raised from his left forearm.

Decision-making for tongue reconstruction (see Table 11.3)

The tongue's multifunctional role in articulation, deglutition, and airway protection makes reconstruction difficult. Various flap designs and inset techniques have been introduced for tongue reconstruction, such as creation of omega-shaped profile with radial forearm flap, mushroom flap design for total tongue reconstruction, use of rectangular template to provide simple design with dynamic reconstruction, and combination of native tongue tip rotation and wedge de-epithelialization optimized tongue tip sensation and reduce pooling on the mouth floor.[33–37] Chiu and Burd[38] further expanded on this technique by describing their semicircular design with wedge de-epithelialization or resection to increase tongue elevation and deepening of the tongue floor at the mouth sulcus. Very little has been reported regarding the refinement of total tongue reconstruction, probably due to the mistaken notion that such reconstructions serve no purpose other than volume restoration.[39,40]

Re-innervation of the skin flap to enhance the sensitivity of the reconstructed tongue has been introduced. However, the final result of re-innervation of the skin flap seems to fail to provide better sensation function after reconstruction.[41] The result of re-innervation is also not constant, since many patients will require postoperative radiotherapy and the nerve may possibly be damaged.

Most authors would classify tongue defects after tongue resection as hemiglossectomy, subtotal, and total glossectomy defects.[33,34,42–46] A goal-directed classification for tongue defects should not only provide descriptions but also facilitate precise judgment with therapeutic consequences. Cheng's modified classification (I, IIa, IIb, III) separates tongue defects into three major groups, which dictate the type of donor flap chosen and is useful for preoperative planning (Table 11.3).[47]

Current strategies for tongue reconstruction should either maintain mobility or provide bulk of the tongue depending on the defect. Flaps that maintain mobility are usually thin, such as the infrahyoid myofascial flap,[48–50] MSAP flap,[51,52] radial forearm flap,[33,43–46,53] and ulnar forearm flap.[54,55] Flaps that provide bulk include the rectus abdominis myocutaneous

flap, latissimus dorsi myocutaneous flap,[39] pectoralis major (PM) myocutaneous flap,[56] and trapezius island flap.[57] The ALT flap has emerged in recent decades as a popular option for head and neck reconstruction due to its reliability, long pedicle, and acceptable donor morbidity. Due to its versatility, this flap has been used both to provide bulk and to ensure mobility.[34,45,46,58–61] Most publications have reported only the use of a single flap to reconstruct a limited range of tongue defects while others compared two flaps but generally gave little or no information for why one flap was selected over another. Based on various clinical experiences, there is not one preferred flap over another for tongue reconstruction. Only defect evaluation and proper flap selection based on the defect make a successful reconstruction. For Class I patients (defects ≤50%), a forearm flap, basing on the radial or ulnar artery, which is thin and pliable with a long pedicle is recommended (Figs. 11.15–11.17); an ALT perforator flap can be used alternatively in thin patients. Class II describes defects where up to 75% of the tongue is removed. In this classification system, a distinction is made between defects of less than 66% (IIa) and up to than 75% (IIb). The additional division between

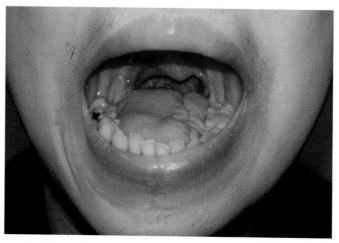

Fig. 11.17 The patient was satisfied with the good functional result as well as cosmesis.

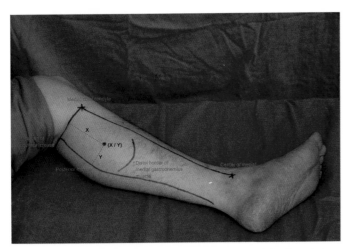

Fig. 11.18 The design of a medial sural artery perforator flap. A line is made from the midpoint of popliteal crease to the Achilles tendon. The distal border of the medial gastrocnemius muscle is also marked. The major myocutaneous perforator is located on the line parallel to the first line and 6 cm from the popliteal crease. *(Courtesy of Dr. Hung-Kai Kao; Plast Reconstr Surg. 2010;125:1. Fig. 1.)*

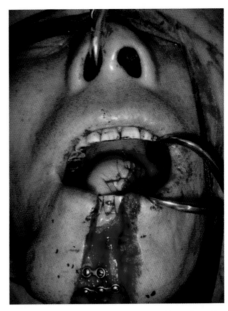

Fig. 11.20 The reconstructed tongue showed good projection and adequate volume by the chimeric medial sural artery perforator flap. *(Courtesy of Dr. Hung-Kai Kao.)*

Class IIa (greater than 50% to 66% resected) and IIb (greater than 66% to 75% resected) permits further refinements in flap selection. For Class IIa patients, an ALT flap is preferred over the radial forearm flap due to the larger flap size available, especially when encountering any accompanying mouth floor or buccal defects. Flaps other than ALT flap can be used as an alternative. Free MSAP with the inclusion of a piece of gastrocnemius can be a good choice (Figs. 11.18–11.21). For Class IIb defects, the small amount of remaining tongue (about 25%) probably has no functional role, but it likely plays an important role in maintaining the anatomical integrity of the base of the tongue, the retromolar trigone, or one side of the pterygoid fossa, depending on its location. The thickness of the subcutaneous tissue in the ALT myocutaneous flap provides a better neotongue profile for defects crossing the midline in Class IIa and IIb. In total glossectomy defects (Class III), a specially designed pentagonal-shaped ALT myocutaneous flap facilitates better flap inset, provides adequate volume, and gives an aesthetically pleasing neotongue tip (see Fig. 11.22). The "V" shape of the pentagon posteriorly allows a greater sloping profile when viewed in cross-section as well as an increasing posterior-to-anterior tongue projection. Such a design yields a well-shaped tissue bulk that resembles a normal tongue more closely in its lateral and frontal views. The anterior "I" shape allows increased elevation and freeing of the neotongue tip and also creates a gingival sulcus that prevents saliva pooling and subsequent drooling. Most of these patients provide ratings of "good" and above for diet or

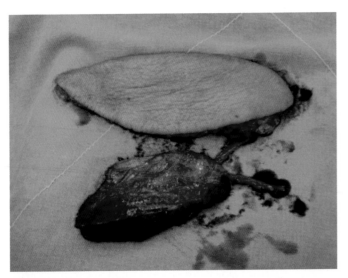

Fig. 11.19 A medial sural artery perforator flap with chimeric partial gastrocnemius muscle was harvested for reconstruction. *(Courtesy of Dr. Hung-Kai Kao.)*

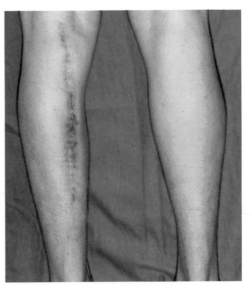

Fig. 11.21 The donor site scar was acceptable by the patient. *(Courtesy of Dr. Hung-Kai Kao.)*

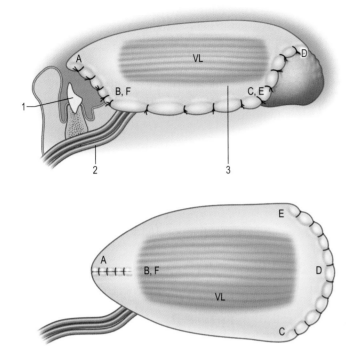

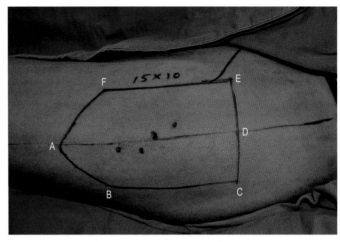

Fig. 11.24 A pentagonal-shape anterolateral thigh myocutaneous flap measured 10 × 15 cm was designed on left thigh.

Fig. 11.22 A pentagonal anterolateral thigh musculocutaneous flap sized 10 × 15 cm with a segment of vastus lateralis is used to reconstruct a total tongue defect. The distance from B to F is 10 cm and from A to D is 15 cm. The vastus lateralis is 5 × 10 cm. B and F are sutured to form the floor of the mouth, and A becomes the tip of the neotongue. The margins between B and C and E and F are repaired to the gingival mucosa of the mandible. The distance between C, D, and E forms the base of the tongue and trigone. The pedicle is placed anteriorly to reach the recipient vessels in the neck. A, tongue tip; B and F, floor of mouth; C and E, trigone; D, base of tongue; VL, vastus lateralis muscle; 1, teeth; 2, lateral circumflex femoral vessel; 3, anterolateral thigh musculocutaneous flap.

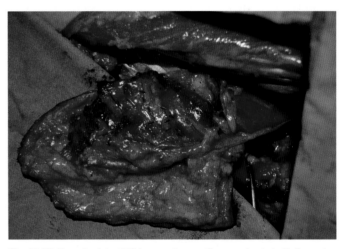

Fig. 11.25 The anterolateral thigh myocutaneous flap was elevated with the vastus lateralis muscle 8 × 6 cm to augment neotongue volume.

cosmetic appearance following reconstruction using this method (Figs. 11.22–11.26).[47]

In both Class IIb and III, an ALT musculocutaneous flap rather than a fasciocutaneous flap should be used for reconstruction to provide more bulk to augment the base of the tongue. The bulk at the base of the tongue is important to close

off the oropharynx during swallowing with the assistance of the movement of hyoid bone. The rectus abdominis myocutaneous flap[62] and the latissimus dorsi myocutaneous flap[39,47] are alternative flap options for near-total or total tongue reconstruction, but with more significant donor site morbidity.

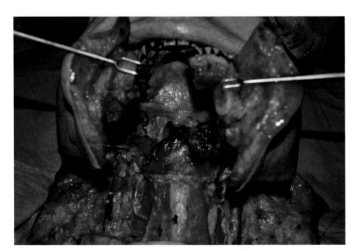

Fig. 11.23 A 52-year-old male patient with tongue cancer cT4aN0M0 stage 4 who has undergone total tongue resection which resulted in total tongue defect.

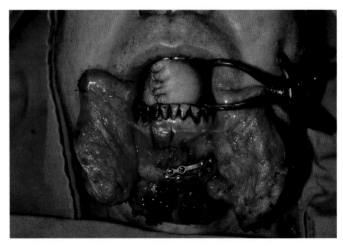

Fig. 11.26 This neotongue flap showed good projection and shape.

Clinical experiences

Table 11.3 addresses the clinical experience of tongue reconstruction by the authors. The review echoes our strategic approaches of tongue reconstruction with the defect-oriented flap selection and inset. More of the defects were reconstructed with recommended flaps while other reconstructions were performed using the alternative flaps for individual reasons. Flap selection should be based on the defect as well as the patient's own character. For example, a defect post tumor recurrence with the previously recommended flap being used before or a positive Allen test in the forearm can drive the surgeon to choose flaps other than recommended ones. With our strategies, the overall complications are acceptable with high success rates. More and more skin flaps are now being explored in tongue reconstruction, all with satisfactory results. There is a trend of using ulnar forearm flaps more often instead of the radial forearm flap, which in our experience, have achieved good results. Advantages of this flap include minimal donor site morbidity creating a less conspicuous scar and offering more sizable perforators. For bulkier flaps, the ALT flap remains our first choice and the authors have also used other flaps, such as anteromedial thigh (AMT) and PAP flaps.

Decision-making for mandibular reconstruction

Daniel categorized lower-jaw defects as isolated, compound, composite, extensive composite, or *en bloc*.[63,64] Isolated defects include any single bone tissue resection; compound defects refer to those involving two tissue layers, such as bone and oral lining or bone and external skin. Composite defects

indicate a three-layer-defect involving the mucosal lining, bone, and external skin; finally, extended composite or *en bloc* defects also include loss of soft tissue. Jewer *et al.* classified mandibular defects of the bone as central, lateral, or hemimandibular.[65] The classification system was further modified by Urken *et al.* to consider associated soft-tissue defects[66] and by Boyd *et al.* to recognize subcategories such as mucosa, skin, or a combination of both.[67] Schultz and colleagues classified the mandibular defect based on the bone defect and the availability regarding ipsilateral recipient vessels.[68] These classifications were based on the availability of reconstructive options. With the development of microsurgical techniques and better understanding of the perforator flap concept, more reconstructive alternatives became available. A modified mandibular defect classification is given here by the authors to define in advance the components involved in the mandibular defect. The modification aims to include the missing tissue in detail and helps with decision-making and choosing the most optimal flaps for reconstruction. This is outlined in Table 11.5 with the integration of different classifications from the literature. The available flaps and their characters are listed in Table 11.6. In Table 11.7, the reader can find the subclassification of Cheng's classification III and recommended reconstruction options.

Clinical experiences

Table 11.5 lists the variable classifications of mandible defects, and Cheng's modified classifications indicate the defects with the orientation of missing bone, inner, and outer layers of soft tissues. By using the classification as a clinical indicator for flap selection, the authors completed 190 cases of mandible reconstructions with fibula-based bone-carrying flaps and

Table 11.5 Variable classifications of mandibular defects

Cheng's classification	Daniel's classification	Jewer's and Boyd's classification	Defects	Available management	Examples
Ia	Isolated	Central (C)	Bone only	Plating, bone graft, bone flap	Benign tumor, trauma
Ib	Isolated	Lateral (L)	Bone only	Plating, bone graft, bone flap	Benign tumor, trauma
Ic	Isolated	Hemimandibulectomy (H)	Bone only	Plating, bone graft, bone flap	Benign tumor, trauma
IIa	Compound	HCL + mucosal (m)	Bone and intraoral mucosa	Osteocutaneous flap	Stage 3–4 oromandibular cancer
IIb	Compound	HCL + skin (s)	Bone and external skin	Osteocutaneous flap	Osteoradionecrosis of mandible
IIc	Compound	–	Bone, external skin, and extended soft tissue	Osteocutaneous flap, OPAC flap	Osteoradionecrosis of mandible
IIIa	Composite	HCL + mucosa and skin (ms)	Composite 3 layers	Options in Table 11.7	Stage 4 oromandibular cancer, gunshot wound
IIIb	Extensive composite	–	Composite 3 layers and partial tongue	Options in Table 11.7	Stage 4 oromandibular cancer, gunshot wound
IIIc	Extensive composite	–	Composite 3 layers and partial maxilla	Options in Table 11.7	Stage 4 oromandibular cancer, gunshot wound

Table 11.6 Comparisons of osteocutaneous flaps for mandibular reconstructions

	Bone			Skin		Muscle availability	Pedicle length	Donor site morbidity	Disadvantages
	Height	Firmness	Length	Reliability	Pliability				
Fibula	++	++++	++++ (25 cm)	++++	++++	++++, soleus	+++	++++	Flap inset
Iliac	++++	++++	+++	+	+	–	+	++	Donor site morbidity, partial skin paddle loss
Scapula	+	+	++ (7 cm)	++++	+++	++++, latissimus dorsi	++	+++	Intraoperative change of position
Radius	+	++	+ (10–12 cm)	++++	++++	–	++++	+	Radius fracture
Rib	++	++	++ (8–10 cm)	++	++	++, pectoralis major, serratus anterior	++	+++	Tenuous periosteal perfusion
Second metatarsal	+	++++	+ (6 cm)	++++	++++	–	+++	++	Donor-site morbidity

turned in an overall flap success rate of 98.95%. The classification system classifies defects, provides recommendations regarding flap selection, and reflects surgical complexity. Class I defect refers to those with only bone missing and is the most straightforward situation for reconstruction. It reached 100% success rate without any flap-related complications or donor site morbidities. Class II defect, being the most common, bears a re-exploration rate of 17.82% in IIa and 12.5% in IIb in our experience. However, with careful surgical planning and early intervention for re-exploration,

Table 11.7 Reconstructive options for mandibular defect Type III in Cheng's classification.

Cheng's classification	Defect	Option 1 Soft-tissue flap with reconstruction plate	Option 2 One free flap, one pedicled flap	Option 3 Double free flaps	Option 4 Chimeric flap – LCFA	Option 5 Composite flap – scapula	Option 6 Composite flap – OPAC
IIIa	Bone	Reconstruction plate	Fibula	Fibula	Iliac	Scapula	Fibula
	Mucosa	ALT flap or RA flap	Fibular skin	Fibular skin	ALT flap	Scapula/ parascapular skin	Fibular skin
	Soft tissue	Vastus lateralis, rectus abdominis	Pectoralis major, deltopectoral	Vastus lateralis, rectus abdominis	Vastus lateralis	LD	Soleus
	External skin	ALT flap or RA flap	Pectoralis major, deltopectoral	Radial forearm or ALT, RA	Groin skin	Scapula/ parascapular skin	Fibular skin
IIIb	Tongue	ALT flap or RA flap	Fibular skin	Fibular skin	ALT flap	Scapula/ parascapular skin	Fibular skin
IIIc	Maxilla	Vastus lateralis, rectus abdominis	Pectoralis major, deltopectoral	Vastus lateralis, rectus abdominis	Vastus lateralis	LD	Soleus

ALT, anterolateral thigh perforator (fasciocutaneous) or musculocutaneous; LCFA, lateral circumflex femoral artery; LD, latissimus dorsi; OPAC, osteomyocutaneous peroneal artery combined; RA, rectus abdominis musculocutaneous.

the overall success rate remains. Class III defines defects involving three layers and requires larger soft-tissue volume than usual. Because of the extended lesion, skin and soleus muscles are both required for reconstruction, in need of resurfacing as well as volume re-establishment. It is understandable that higher incidence of skin/muscle partial necrosis can be developed. But a careful planning and early action of re-exploration maintain our surgical success rate to be as high as expected.

Treatment/surgical technique

Part I: Soft tissue flaps

Local flaps

Submental flap

The submental flap, as indicated by the name, is located in the submental area. Because of its location, it is a soft-tissue flap that can be transferred as a pedicled or free flap to the oral cavity.

Its blood supply derives from the submental artery, which is a continuous branch of the facial artery, located 5–6.5 cm away from the origin of the facial artery. This branch penetrates deep to the submandibular gland through the mylohyoid muscle below the mandible angle, extending medially deep to the anterior belly of the digastric muscle. As the vessel travels along the mandible margin, it sends off cutaneous perforators through the platysma muscle to the skin. The anatomy is constant, and the flow it provides to the submental skin is reliable.[69–72]

Flap design is initiated by marking the inferior mandible border as the upper flap margin. The flap length extends from the ipsilateral mandible angle to the contralateral mandible angle. The flap width depends on the laxity of the skin: usually a width of 5 cm can be obtained and can be even wider in patients with loose skin. The flap can be elevated as an axial flap or a perforator flap. An easier surgical technique involves lifting the tissue as an axial flap without perforator dissection. Incision can be started from either the inferior or superior margin flap directly through the platysma muscle. Then, the dissection is carried out with division of the anterior belly of the digastric muscle, which is included in the flap to ensure inclusion of the submental pedicle. When the pedicle is identified, its branches to the submandibular gland should be ligated carefully. Finally, when reaching the inferior border of the mandible, care should be taken not to injure the marginal mandibular nerve. The pedicle is then skeletonized and the flap is ready to be transferred. If the flap is going to be transferred as a free flap, dissection of the pedicle can be continued to the facial vessels to obtain a better size and length for anastomosis.

The arc of the submental flap is used for rotating it to the lower third of the face and the entire oral cavity, making it a suitable pedicle flap for oral cavity reconstruction.[69–72] The only drawback is that many oral cavity reconstructions are performed during cancer ablation surgery, during which neck lymph node dissection is often required. After a neck lymph node dissection, the continuity of the submental skin and its main pedicle are usually disrupted.

Regional flaps

Deltopectoral flap

The deltopectoral flap was popularized around 1965 by Bakamjian.[73] Based on the internal mammary perforators emerging from the second and third intercostal spaces, the flap extends from the central chest wall to the deltoid region.

The flap can be designed around the perforators mapped with a pencil Doppler. The flap base is situated in the anterior chest wall, and the flap extends superolaterally to the deltoid region. The exact flap required should be measured to ensure its ability to reach the defect. For an oral cavity reconstruction, a lengthier flap is usually required. However, the distal flap is a random flap with an uncertain blood supply. To obtain a longer flap, a prefabrication or a delayed procedure is usually required to reduce the risk of distal flap necrosis.[74]

The disadvantages of the deltopectoral flap include the unattractive donor site scar, the requirement of a second surgery for flap division, and the possibility of a delayed procedure to lengthen the available flap. Today, the deltopectoral flap has been largely replaced by the PM myocutaneous flap and surgeons are encouraged to reserve it as a salvage procedure.

Pectoralis major myocutaneous flap

Since its introduction by Ariyan in 1979, the PM flap has gained in popularity with a reliable blood supply and large skin paddle with sufficient flap bulk.[75] The PM flap can reach the neck and lower third of the face, making it practical for intraoral and external cheek reconstruction. Today, the PM flap is useful for salvage procedures and in a vessel-depleted neck where a free-flap transfer is not possible.

The PM flap is a myocutaneous flap comprising the PM muscle and its overlying skin with blood supply coming from the thoracoacromial artery and parasternal perforators. The lateral thoracic artery runs along the lateral edge of the PM muscle and sends off branches to augment the circulation of the PM muscle. The thoracoacromial artery runs inferiorly at the midpoint of the clavicle and this can be used as a pivot point when designing the flap.

The cosmesis of the donor site is a major concern, with scarring over the anterior chest wall, especially in women. An alternative design is a nipple-sparing crescent-shaped skin paddle from the parasternal area to the inframammary region. However, care should be taken when designing the flap like this because the inframammary region is less reliable in terms of blood supply.

Flap elevation is started from a lateral incision to expose the lateral border of the PM. Dissection is then carried out under the PM muscle to include the thoracoacromial vessel. Once the muscle has been identified and the location of the vessel is confirmed, the medial border of skin edge can be incised. The muscle is then detached medially and laterally, and the flap is elevated toward the pedicle. The pedicle is divided after 2–3 weeks. The PM flap can also be elevated as an island flap with skeletonizing of the pedicle. The muscle part of the flap can be buried under the neck skin, precluding the need for a second operation to divide the pedicle. The PM flap is a good alternative in head and neck reconstruction when a free-flap transfer is not possible.

Free fasciocutaneous or musculocutaneous flaps

Radial forearm flap

Introduced by Yang in 1981, the free radial forearm flap is currently one of the most commonly used flaps in head and neck reconstruction.[76] The radial forearm flap has become a popular flap due to its large skin paddle, lengthy and sizeable pedicle, and ease of flap harvest. Its thinness and pliability also make it the first choice in most cases of thin buccal mucosa reconstruction and small tongue defects (see Figs. 11.1–11.5).[76]

The radial forearm flap is a type C fasciocutaneous flap derived from the radial artery. Before flap harvest, an Allen test should be performed to confirm the dominance of the ulnar artery. One or two of the concomitant veins are usually adequate for venous drainage.[77] Some authors harvest the cephalic vein for another source of venous drainage. The cephalic vein is larger in diameter than the radial vein; therefore, venous anastomosis is easier. The flap is innervated by the lateral antebrachial cutaneous nerves, which can be incorporated if a sensate flap is desired.

Flap design is initiated by locating the radial artery by palpation. The borders of the skin paddle are designed with the radial artery axis centered, but not extending beyond the anterior radial border of the forearm for cosmetic concern. Under tourniquet, the flap dissection is carried out from the radial edge of the flap in the suprafascial plane.[78] A suprafascial dissection keeps the paratendons and lateral antebrachial cutaneous nerve intact, thus reducing the donor site morbidity. After dividing the distal pedicle at the wrist, the dissection is then continued from distal to proximal by carefully preserving the deep fascia and conjoined tendon between the flexor carpi radialis and brachioradialis muscles. After flap dissection is finished, the tourniquet is released to perfuse the flap for 15 minutes. Circulation of the hand should be re-evaluated. Usually, sacrificing the radial artery does not cause any significant change in hand perfusion. However, an interposition vein graft for vascular reconstruction can be indicated if the distal fingers are not well perfused.[79]

The major drawbacks of the radial forearm flap are donor site morbidities and poor donor site cosmesis. Although the donor site morbidity can be reduced dramatically by a suprafascia dissection, the grafted donor site remains unsightly.

Ulnar forearm flap

Located in the ulnar aspect of the forearm, the ulnar forearm flap has similar advantages as the radial forearm flap with a relatively less noticeable donor site scar. It is used much less frequently than the radial forearm flap, probably because dissection of the ulnar nerve is required during flap elevation.

The ulnar forearm flap is based on the ulnar vessels under the flexor carpi ulnaris (FCU) tendon. Similar to the radial forearm flap, this approach requires an Allen test to confirm well perfusion from the radial artery before surgery. The ulnar artery and veins run underneath the FCU tendon and give several sizeable septocutaneous perforators to the skin paddle.[55] The venae comitantes are adequate for venous drainage although some prefer the basilic vein as a backup.

Flap design is started by marking the ulnar artery underneath the FCU tendon. The skin paddle, based on septocuta-neous perforators, is designed with the ulnar vessels centered. The flap dissection is performed under tourniquet. An incision is made in the radial border of the flap and a suprafascial dissection is then carried out until the tendons of the flexor digitorum superficialis are reached. Several septocutaneous perforators can be seen entering the undersurface of the flap. The fascia is then incised and the vascular pedicle is dissected out under the FCU tendon. The entire skin flap can be nourished by these perforators, or split into two skin paddles based on separate perforators in a chimeric fashion. The flap design can therefore be more versatile and sophisticated. After the ulnar vessels are divided and separated away from the ulnar nerve, another skin incision is made on the ulnar side of the flap edge, and dissection is continued until the entire flap is elevated.

The ulnar forearm flap is an alternative to the radial forearm flap when the Allen test demonstrates codominant or dominant perfusion to the hand by the radial artery. The donor scar is also more favorable because of its location on the medial surface of the forearm. Although dissection of the ulnar nerve requires some technical training, flap dissection is straightforward and easy once the surgeon is familiar with the technique. It has been applied in oral cavity and tongue reconstruction with favorable results (see Figs. 11.15–11.17). The authors recommend clinical application of this flap for defects such as thin oral mucosal defects and Class I tongue defects (hemiglossectomy) (see Table 11.3).

Lateral arm flap

The lateral arm flap is perfused by the cutaneous branch of the posterior radial collateral artery, which is within the lateral intermuscular septum of the upper arm. The vascular pedicle provides four to seven branches to the overlying skin.[80]

The flap is designed by drawing a line between the deltoid tuberosity and the lateral epicondyle of the humerus. The septocutaneous perforators are located along the lower part of this line. After the flap is outlined, dissection from the posterior to the anterior aspect is performed to explore the intermuscular septum. Most of the perforators can thus be identified, and the main pedicle can be traced proximally. The lateral arm flap was once commonly used in head and neck reconstruction. However, the vascular pedicle is short and the pedicle vessels are usually small. With the introduction of more soft-tissue flaps, the use of the lateral arm flap in oral cavity reconstruction has been substantially reduced.

Rectus abdominis musculocutaneous flap

The rectus abdominis musculocutaneous (RAM) flap can be designed transversely or vertically depending on the skin paddle required. By applying a perforator dissection technique, a free deep inferior epigastric perforator (DIEP) flap can be harvested from the same donor site without sacrificing the rectus abdominis muscle.

The RAM flap has two vascular supplies: the deep inferior epigastric vessel and the superior epigastric vessel. When transferred as a free flap, the flap is based on the deep inferior epigastric vessel to obtain a better blood supply. The RAM flap has an adequate skin paddle with flap bulk for reconstruction of large head and neck defects. It had been used commonly in buccal mucosa reconstruction (especially when marginal mandibulectomy is present) and in total tongue reconstruction. It is a reliable flap with a sizeable pedicle for the anastomosis. The only drawback of this flap is the potential abdominal wall weakness after surgery. Careful repair of the fascia and use of mesh to repair large fascial defects can decrease the incidence of abdominal bulge or hernia postoperatively.

Anterolateral thigh fasciocutaneous or musculocutaneous flap

The ALT flap was first introduced by Song et al. in 1984.[81] It gradually gained popularity when reconstructive surgeons found it to be a reliable flap with a long and sizeable pedicle that can be harvested with a large skin paddle and additional muscle for the reconstruction of moderate to large oromandibular defects (see Figs. 11.11–11.14).[82–88]

The pedicle of the ALT flap is usually the descending branch of the lateral circumflex femoral artery. Sometimes, its perforators may come from the transverse or oblique branch of the lateral circumflex femoral vessel. The pedicle of the ALT flap runs in the muscle septum between the vastus lateralis and rectus femoris muscles. A sizeable perforator can nourish a skin paddle that is 15 cm in diameter. The vastus lateralis muscle is nourished by the same pedicle and therefore can be harvested together with the ALT fasciocutaneous flap if a large flap volume is required. The transverse branch of the lateral circumflex femoral artery also nourishes the tensor fascia lata muscle and fascia. If fascia is required to serve as a sling, the tensor fascia lata can be included in the flap dissection.

The ALT flap usually contains more than one sizeable perforator and can also be designed as a chimeric flap to cover two or more separate defects.[84,87,88] This is useful when there are multiple buccal mucosal defects or when a through-and-through defect is present (see Figs. 11.11–11.14). The ALT flap can also be separated into two or more small independent flaps to replace two or more defects simultaneously.[87,88] The ALT flap has frequently been applied in head and neck reconstruction, especially when the soft-tissue defect is extremely large or when a forearm flap is not fit. The distance between the lower extremity and the head and neck region also allows a two-team approach during the surgery. The thickness of the ALT flap can be thinned to improve its pliability.[58,83] Flap design is initiated by marking a straight line from the anterior superior iliac spine to the lateral border of the patella. Most of the perforators are located within a circle of 3 cm from the midpoint of this axis. A hand-held Doppler can be used to map the perforators.

Flap dissection can be suprafascial or subfascial. The subfascial dissection is suggested for a beginner to minimize the risk of perforator damage. The perforators can either be septocutaneous (13%) or musculocutaneous (87%).[82] The descending branch of the lateral circumflex femoral vessels can be found in the intermuscular septum between the vastus lateralis muscle and rectus femoris muscle. Unroofing of the musculocutaneous perforators and delicate intramuscular dissection of the perforators are the key points for this flap dissection. When the vastus lateralis muscle is harvested along with the skin paddle, the motor nerve can be preserved to avoid possible knee function compromise.[82,83]

Thoracodorsal artery perforator flap

The thoracodorsal artery perforator (TAP) flap is a modification of the traditional latissimus dorsi flap.[89–91] The TAP flap has the advantages of having similar skin color to the facial skin and therefore can be used for facial resurfacing.

The musculocutaneous perforators of the TAP flap are derived from the medial or inferior branches of the thoracodorsal vessels. The perforators can be detected by a pencil Doppler either 4 cm below the scapular spine (medial branch), or 10 cm below the axilla and 2 cm medial to the posterior axillary line (inferior branch). Flap dissection is initiated from the superior border of the flap with an incision directly above the latissimus dorsi muscle. After the perforator is identified, the intramuscular dissection is continued and the main pedicle is dissected. The inferior border of the flap is incised and the flap is elevated off the latissimus dorsi muscle. The TAP flap has a reliable blood supply and leaves a hidden scar on the back. However, the need to change the patient's position during the operation can lengthen the operation time and decrease its clinical application.

Medial sural artery perforator flap

The medial sural artery perforator (MSAP) flap was developed in 2001 by Cavadas et al. and has now been used in head and neck reconstruction with good results.[92] It is a modification of the gastrocnemius muscle flap, which was originally described for lower-extremity reconstruction.[93]

Most of the sizeable perforators of the MSAP flap are located 8–12 cm inferior to the popliteal crease.[32] Flap dissection is started by making the anterior incision and continued through a subfascial dissection to identify the perforators. The MSAP flap is a good alternative for most small buccal defects or moderate-sized buccal defects in obese patients where an ALT flap is too bulky to be used (see Table 11.2). The donor site can be closed primarily when the flap width is less than 5 cm. The major disadvantages include the visible location of the donor site scar and poor intraoperative posture of the surgeon for dissecting the flap (see Figs. 11.18–11.21).

Profunda artery perforator flap

The profunda artery perforator (PAP) flap is also known as posterior thigh flap or adductor magnus perforator flaps.[94–96] The PAP is used for breast reconstruction in recent years, and the authors found it an alternative flap in head and neck reconstruction (see Figs. 11.6–11.10). It comprises skin from the posterior and medial thigh and can be designed transversely or vertically. Transverse flap design places the scar in a well-hidden area while longitudinal flap design includes more and reliable perforators and allows more versatile flap design.[97–99]

The PAP flap is elevated basing on profunda femoris perforators. These perforators are either septocutaneous perforators running in the intermuscular septum between gracilis and adductor magnus or intermuscular septum between the adductor magnus and semimembranous muscles or myocutaneous perforators running through the adductor magnus muscle. A hand-held Doppler is used to map the perforators. Flaps can be designed with elliptical skin paddle transversely or vertically. The patient is placed in a supine frog-leg position during preparation and flap harvest. An incision is first made along the anterior margin of the flap to identify the perforator.

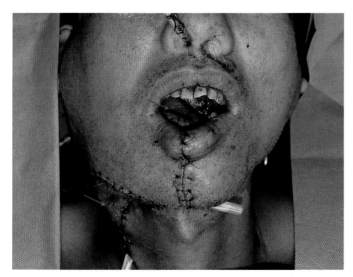

Fig. 11.44 Immediate postoperative result. Red arrows mark two skin paddles.

donor site, and a single set of anastomoses, leading to reduced operative time.

The harvest technique for the free fibular OSC flaps was described by Wei and Cheng.[134,136,137] Fibula bone is marked on the skin. At both the proximal and distal ends, 6 cm in length is preserved for knee and ankle stability (see Figs. 11.30 & 11.41). The septocutaneous perforators to the skin, which are primarily located along the posterior margin of the fibula on the middle and lower third of the leg, are marked preoperatively by a hand-held Doppler. The skin island is centered over the septocutaneous perforators. The skin incision is made to the subcutaneous layer and kept above the fascia through the anterior approach. The flap is partially elevated, and the fascia is incised after passing through the anterior cruciate ligament. The peroneus longus and brevis are elevated off the fibula periosteum. The anterior cruciate ligament is then divided. The periosteum of the fibula at both osteotomy sites is removed, and the bone is osteotomized by an electric saw. The fibula is then retracted posterolaterally to expose the extensor digitorum longus, brevis, and posterior tibialis muscles, which are all elevated off the periosteum. At this time, the posterior skin incision is made with meticulous care to keep the septocutaneous perforators intact inside the posterior cruciate septum. Distal ends of the peroneal vessels, which may be separated from the fibula bone, are ligated and divided. The pedicle is dissected out from the FHL. The FHL is detached with an index finger inserted between the FHL and posterior cruciate ligament, so as to protect the septocutaneous perforators. The residual posterior cruciate septum not containing the perforators is divided. The soleus muscle can be included with the musculocutaneous perforators frequently identified at the proximal third of the peroneal vessels (Figs. 11.31 & 11.42). The soleus muscle can be harvested 6 × 14 cm, even up to half of soleus, without significant donor site morbidity.

Osteotomies

Nowadays, a few surgeons have already shifted from manual-planned osteotomy to computer-aided design (CAD) osteotomies. Here, the authors would like to describe the osteotomy design and procedure using the traditional method for beginners. After division of the proximal peroneal pedicle, further osteotomies are performed with an electric saw according to the tailored paper ruler template displayed on the back table. The skin paddle can be separated into two flaps based on each perforator if two septocutaneous perforators are available (see Figs. 11.31 & 11.42). The pedicle is skeletonized with removal of unnecessary proximal periosteum and bone. Yagi *et al.* highlighted the importance of respecting the geometry of the fibula OSC flap to obtain good outcomes in mandibular reconstruction.[138] Some obstacles may appear during flap shaping and insetting of a fibular OSC flap because of the limited mobility of each integrated tissue component. It is important to protect the vascular pedicle and septocutaneous perforators to the skin paddle during the osteotomies to prevent injury to these structures. Furthermore, the vascularity of the skin paddle can be compromised during flap inset if the septum and its perforators are stretched over the fibula bone and the plate to reach the defect. The minimal recommended bone segment length for osteotomy is 2.5 cm to ensure the adequate inclusion of tiny perforators nourishing the periosteum and subsequently the bone. The more osteotomies are made, the more the decrease of vascularity to the distal segment can be encountered. This is because the proximal bone segments are supplied by periosteal sources as well as nutrient arteries while the distal segments are nourished only by periosteal sources. In addition, when plating is applied on top of the periosteum to fix the bone segments, there is a concern of possible decrease in periosteal vascular flow to the distal bone segments.

Flap inset

The insetting of the OPAC or fibular OSC flap starts with fixing the osteotomized fibular segments that are contoured to fit the reconstruction plate. The authors recommend only a single screw fixation for each bone segment to minimize vascular compromise to the fibula. One skin paddle based on a septocutaneous perforator is then sutured to form the intraoral lining, and a second skin paddle based on a separate septocutaneous perforator from the same pedicle is used for the external cheek if needed.

For certain indications, a piece of soleus muscle of OPAC flap is harvested and placed on top of the fibula and reconstruction plate to improve cosmesis and prevent osteoradionecrosis and plate exposure after postoperative radiation (see Figs. 11.32, 11.33 & 11.43). It is recommended to keep the ischemia time for fibular osteocutaneous flaps to less than 5 hours to reduce partial flap loss and other complication rates.[139]

In an attempt to simplify surgical planning, some surgeons prefer to use the contralateral leg as a donor site for mandibular defects because two teams may work simultaneously without any space conflict. Chang found that the left fibular osteocutaneous flap had a higher vascular complication rate when used for right mandibular reconstructions. This is likely due to the more restricted spatial relationship between the fibular flap inset and the available recipient vessels. An algorithm representing the different factors influencing the inset geometry should include the side from which the flap was harvested, the available recipient vessels, and the need for intraoral or external skin reconstruction. It is recommended

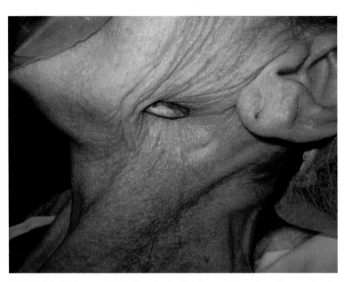

Fig. 11.45 A 61-year-old female patient with left mandible osteoradionecrosis after radiotherapy. The exposed left necrotic mandible bone was presented. *(Courtesy of Dr. Steve Henry.)*

to use an ipsilateral fibular osteocutaneous flap for mandibular reconstruction to decrease the risk of vascular complications. The ipsilateral superior thyroid artery, which is usually preserved by the surgical oncologist, is the preferred recipient artery. The contralateral superior thyroid artery constitutes an equally viable alternative because up to 10–15 cm of the length of the peroneal artery can usually be harvested.

Plating

Intermaxillary fixation with screws or wires can both achieve good occlusion. A titanium reconstruction plate is used to bridge both residual mandibular ends, with at least two screws for each end (see Figs. 11.29 & 11.40). A template using a paper ruler is made to match the contour of the plate. Care must be taken not to injure the pedicle or perforators during plating. Unicortical drilling and screw fixation is recommended with the assistance of normal saline irrigation to prevent overheating injury of the reconstructed bone during platting. The plate can be positioned 1 cm higher than the lower margin of the native mandible to achieve adequate height for occlusion and subsequent osseointegrated

implants. If the height of the transplanted bone is insufficient, the "double-barrel" fibular flap design provides adequate bone height that allows stable fixation for osseointegrated dental implants to be placed.[140,141] Recently, new techniques such as three-dimensional reconstruction images have been introduced to assist the surgeon with complex mandibular reconstruction with good results.[142–147] Furthermore, rapid prototyping technologies can construct physical models from computer-aided designs via three-dimensional printers (Figs. 11.45–11.50).

Computed-aided surgical design in mandible reconstruction

Accurate preoperative three-dimensional planning is very important in mandibular reconstruction. One of the major and rapid evolutions in mandible reconstruction is the involvement of CAD. The earliest CAD can be dated back to 2004, when Warnke *et al.* presented their work on using 3D CT scan to produce scaffolds and incorporated the products with free latissimus dorsi flap for reconstruction.[148] Although it was time-consuming (7 weeks before surgery), the concept and computer-aided technique have inspired reconstructive surgeons. Computer-aided design has fostered tremendous advancement in mandibular reconstruction, and the applications continue to evolve. While clinical application of tissue engineering bone reconstruction remains uncertain, the idea of CAD keeps progressing rapidly, especially in assisting surgery. In general, computer-aided surgery can be applied to preoperative surgical planning as well as patient-specific customized reconstruction plans, guiding mandibulectomy, and guiding osteotomies on bone graft.

The use of CAD helps to provide surgical accuracy, shorten operation time, and minimize surgical morbidities. CAD helps in virtual surgical planning, such as bone resection or osteotomies, and design and manufacturing of customized surgical devices, such as reconstruction plate in mandible reconstruction. With a patient's CT scan data and the incorporation of 3D printing, both the recipient site and donor site can be planned to give more accurate surgical results. CAD with prototyping, patient-specific precontoured reconstruction plate also helps in enhancing surgical results. CAD-guided surgery ends with accurately planned results and is considered more accurate in comparison to manual reconstruction[142–147] (see Figs. 11.45–11.50).

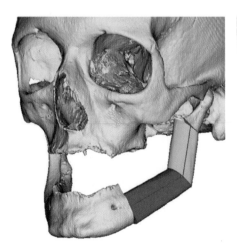
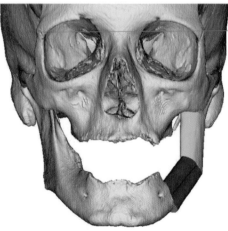

Fig. 11.46 Before surgery, the mandible resection and the reconstruction using fibula osteocutaneous flaps was planned with computer-aided design (CAD). The CAD helped in the planning of fibula osteotomy. *(Courtesy of Dr. Steve Henry.)*

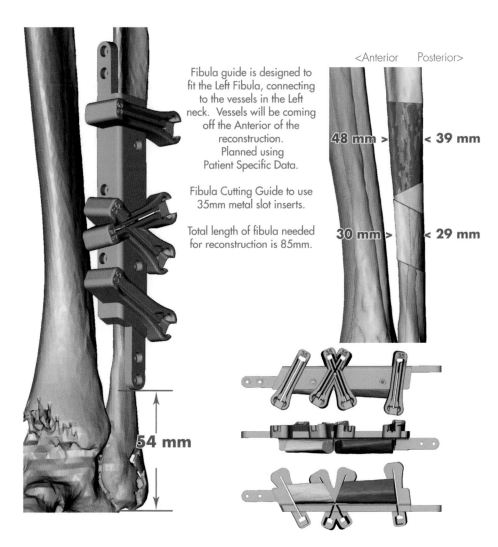

Fibula guide is designed to fit the Left Fibula, connecting to the vessels in the Left neck. Vessels will be coming off the Anterior of the reconstruction. Planned using Patient Specific Data.

Fibula Cutting Guide to use 35mm metal slot inserts.

Total length of fibula needed for reconstruction is 85mm.

<Anterior   Posterior>

48 mm >   < 39 mm

30 mm >   < 29 mm

54 mm

Fig. 11.47 Cutting guide for the fibular osteotomies according to computer-aided design for accurate length and angle of each osteotomy. *(Courtesy of Dr. Steve Henry.)*

Ischemia time

The ischemia time starts at the time of pedicle division and includes the osteotomy, the shaping and inset interval, and ends with the completion of the arterial anastomosis. Several factors determine ischemia time of the fibular flap transfer for mandibular reconstruction: the surgeon's experience; whether the sequence of fibular osteotomies and fixation takes place before or after pedicle division; whether the order of anastomosis is performed before or after flap insetting; and whether the artery or vein is anastomosed first. Partial flap loss has statistically been higher if the ischemia time is greater than 5 hours.[139] Fibula bone survival did not differ significantly with ischemia time. Partial flap loss seems to be primarily a problem of the skin component of the fibular OSC flap, possibly due to kinking, twisting, or too much tension at the septocutaneous perforator during insetting and plating.

Temporomandibular joint reconstruction

Reconstruction of the temporomandibular joint usually yields unfavorable results. If the condyle is not reconstructed, movement of the mandible, which relies only on the contralateral temporomandibular joint, will eventually tilt, causing maloc-clusion and trismus. There are several alternatives to condyle reconstruction, such as avascular bone graft, rounding off the end of the fibula, costochondral graft attached to the fibula end, or titanium condyle prosthesis.[149] The condyle prosthesis has been associated with a higher rate of hardware exposure and even sensorineural hearing loss. The fibular osteocutaneous flap had been reported for temporomandibular joint reconstruction with reasonable functional and cosmetic results.

Dental rehabilitation: osseointegrated dental implants

Dental rehabilitation may enhance functional and cosmetic outcome after mandibular reconstruction. Either permanent prosthesis with osseointegrated dental implants or removable prosthesis can be used for the purpose of dental reconstruction. These procedures are usually performed by the oral surgeons and dentists. Briefly, the vestibuloplasty with split-thickness skin graft or palatal mucosal graft is performed first to obtain lingual and buccal sulci for a vestibule of 1.5 cm in depth. The reconstructed bone stock (10 × 6 mm) is required for the osseointegrated implant. The bone is exposed after elevation of the periosteum and burred to yield a flat surface. Drilling is applied for insertion of the implant at a depth of 5 mm. For a permanent prosthesis, consolidation of the

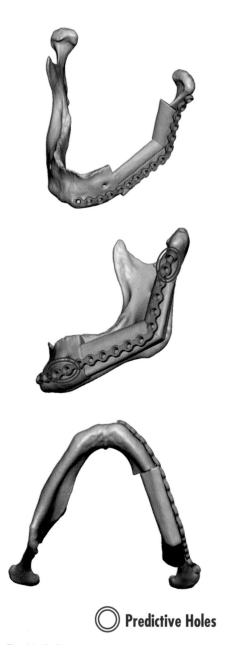

Predictive Holes

Fig. 11.48 The reconstruction plate bending and plating can be performed precisely. From this model a plate was pre-bent; note that the proximal and distal holes in the mandible resection guide ("predictive holes", indicated by the double blue ovals) match the hole pattern in the plate, ensuring that the native mandible, fibula segments, and plate will all fit together as in the computer model, and that the relationship of the two condyles will be perfectly anatomic. *(Courtesy of Dr. Steve Henry.)*

implant requires 3 months. Although the immediate osseointegrated implant was introduced by Chang for benign lesions,[150,151] delayed osseointegration is recommended for cancer patients who may eventually undergo radiotherapy.

Clinical experiences

Table 11.8 provides recommended guidelines for flap and recipient vessel selection in mandibular reconstruction based on the lesion side. Unlike true perforator flaps that allow very versatile flap inset, the unique 3D structure of fibula bone and

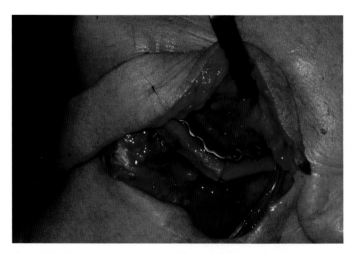

Fig. 11.49 With accurate planning, the osteotomy fit the plate precisely. Photograph of the fibula segments and plate; note the perfect apposition of the fibula segments and neomandibular angle. *(Courtesy of Dr. Steve Henry.)*

the anatomical relationship between the bone, vascular pedicle, and skin paddle have made restrictions to flap inset. An anatomy-based reconstruction plan is required for successful reconstruction with minimized complications. The numbers addressed in Table 11.8 are the authors' experiences using fibula-based bone-carry flaps, either a free fibular OSC flap or an OPAC flap for mandible reconstruction. In our experience, the most important principle in determining skin paddle inset is the pedicle course under minimal tension. This helps to avoid the tension and tethering of the pedicle that would otherwise compromise the perfusion to the skin paddle. As expected, most of the recipient vessels fell into the red-marked recommended ones, helping to place the flap in a well-organized, natural-positioned setting and reduce vascular compromise and its potential complications, such as partial or total necrosis with patent arterial and venous anastomosis. Based on our principles, the incidence of skin flap partial or total necrosis is low and the overall success rate was as high as 98.87%.

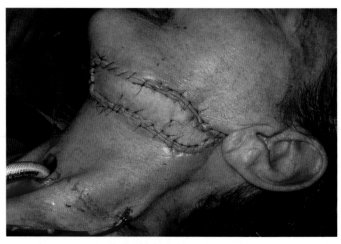

Fig. 11.50 Immediate postoperative appearance with the skin flap used to cover the external defect. *(Courtesy of Dr. Steve Henry.)*

Postoperative care

Patients are transferred to the intensive care unit for postoperative flap monitoring for 3–7 days depending on the patients' condition.

A tracheotomy or an endotracheal tube is required for ventilator support overnight and the patient is usually sedated on postoperative day 1. Restriction of neck motion is sometimes required to prevent traction or avulsion of the vascular anastomosis.

Prophylactic antibiotics for Gram-positive and Gram-negative bacteria are given for 7 days. Due to the length of the operation, a prophylactic proton pump inhibitor is administered for 3 days to prevent stress ulcers. Relative overhydration is preferred in patients without contraindication to maintain adequate perfusion to the flap. Intake and output are carefully monitored. Enteral feeding is started as early as possible to ensure sufficient nutritional support. If enteral feeding is not possible or if nutritional status is already poor before surgery, short-term (3–5 days) partial parenteral nutritional support is recommended.

The flaps are monitored every hour for the first 24 hours and every 2 hours for the next 24 hours, and then every 4 hours starting from postoperative day 3 to the time of discharge. Physical examination of the flap (including color, temperature, capillary refill, and puncture test) is usually adequate. If there is a skin paddle on the outside of the oral cavity, a hand-held Doppler can be used to monitor vascular flow to the flap. Other devices, such as implantable Doppler, laser Doppler, or an O2C machine, can be used as alternatives.

Antithrombotic agents or vasodilation agents such as heparin, low-molecular-weight Fraxiparine, promostan, or dextran are not routinely prescribed. Such medications are given only if the pedicle has a high risk of developing thrombosis inside the vessels or when the surgeons find it necessary.

Patients are given gentle and gradual rehabilitation with regard to mouth opening to prevent postoperative trismus by postoperative day 7.

Outcome, prognosis, and complications

Complications after a flap transfer to the oral cavity are not uncommon. Acute complications often relate to the surgery itself, while chronic complications may result from improper flap design and inset, poor patient self-care, scarring, or complications related to cancer treatment, such as postoperative radiation therapy.

Complications post buccal and tongue reconstructions

Acute complications

The keys for a high success rate of microsurgical free-flap transfers include careful preoperative planning, delicate flap dissection, accurate microsurgical anastomosis, proper flap inset, and careful monitoring of the flap postoperatively. Early re-exploration and management of the complications are also very important. Acute complications include compromised flap circulation that requires re-exploration, poor wound healing, and wound infection.

The rate of re-exploration due to compromised flap circulation was reported at 5–25% of patients. However, the salvage rate for a compromised flap is highly dependent on the time of surgical intervention and the surgeon's experience.[152] Most cases of compromised vascular flow will manifest on the first postoperative day or within the first few days.[152] More than 50% of the vascular compromise cases presented signs of compromise as early as 4 hours postoperatively, and more than 80% of the cases within the first 24 hours.[152] With early intervention, the salvage rate of total flap loss can be greater than 80%. Vascular compromise can result from thrombosis due to poor microsurgical techniques. More frequently, however, it is related to improper flap inset, kinking, or twisting of the vascular pedicle.

Wound infection is a common complication for head and neck reconstruction and accounts for up to 48% of all complications.[153,154] Effective drainage of the neck and obliteration of the dead space are important to decrease postoperative hematoma and subsequent infection. Oral cavity cancer patients are usually malnourished, and this has a negative impact on wound healing. During surgery, a watertight closure is important to prevent saliva leakage from the oral cavity into the neck, which is one of the most common reasons for neck wound infection and delayed wound healing. Although the reported rate of orocutaneous fistula after head and neck reconstruction is only 3%, its presence can threaten the viability of the flap.[155–157] Persistent exposure of the vascular pedicle to oral secretions and oral flora increases the incidence of infection and potential disruption of the anastomosis. This is the most common reason for delayed flap failure after wound infection. Enteral feeding as early as possible can help to reduce malnutrition and other related complications.

Chronic complications

Trismus is the most common long-term complication after oral cavity reconstruction, usually due to scar contracture, inadequate postoperative rehabilitation, and/or postoperative radiotherapy. The size of the free flap will usually shrink to a certain extent after surgery. This condition is exacerbated by radiotherapy. Progressive contraction of the flap can result in a sunken appearance, a condition typically seen in patients with through-and-through defects. Orocutaneous fistulae with persistent saliva leakage from the oral cavity to the neck may result from poor intraoral wound healing, teeth necrosis, or osteoradionecrosis. Patients typically present with nonhealing intraoral and neck wounds with persistent discharge from the neck wound that does not improve despite aggressive wound care and antibiotics. Treatments should include enteral tube feeding and surgical debridement with flap coverage. Occasionally, the fistula is small and cannot be visually identified. A methylene blue-water test or a head and neck computed tomography scan can be performed to help detect the fistulae. Once poor wound healing presents, surgical debridement is frequently required and should not be hesitated. Obtaining tissue around the unhealed region for pathological review is important since some tumor recurrence/residual tumors manifest as poor wound healing.

Complications post mandibular reconstruction

Acute complications

Acute complications appear within 1 week postoperatively, including re-exploration, wound dehiscence, and partial skin paddle loss. Subacute complications occur between 1 week and 1 month postoperatively, consisting of infection, skin flap loss, wound dehiscence, donor site morbidity, and fibula bone loss. Chang reported a success rate of 98.2%, partial skin loss of 29%, and partial bone loss of 3% in a series of 116 mandibular reconstructions using fibular OSC flaps with a mean ischemia time of 3.6 hours.[139]

Chronic complications

Chronic complications beyond the 1-month period include infection, malocclusion, donor site morbidity, skin flap loss, or radiotherapy-related orocutaneous fistula or osteoradionecrosis on the remaining bone or the reconstructed bone. Osteoradionecrosis has been described as hypovascularity, hypocellularity, and local tissue hypoxia.[158] Radiation-related osteoradionecrosis, neck contractures, and wound-healing problems with subsequent plate exposure are frequent in patients undergoing a fibular osteocutaneous flap for mandibular reconstruction.[159,160] Osteoradionecrosis due to obliteration of the inferior alveolar artery and radiated fibrosis of the periosteum was reported to occur in 0.8–37% of cases.[158] Osteoradionecrosis often involves the native residual mandible; this typically occurs in the buccal cortex or the reconstructed bone flap.[159]

Once osteoradionecrosis develops, management should include wide excision of the radionecrotic bone, coverage with a muscle flap, or replacement with another osteocutaneous flap. Hyperbaric oxygen has been used in the treatment of osteoradionecrosis, without significant improvement. Its use should be very careful for cancer patients due to potential local recurrence.

An important concept of preventing osteoradionecrosis is having enough soft-tissue and bone coverage in the irradiated field. The risks of osteoradionecrosis, trismus, and plate exposure were significantly lower in the OPAC flap with soleus (29%) than the traditional fibular OSC flap (53.1%)[161] (option 6 in Table 11.7). Additional soft-tissue coverage of the hardware and bone can also be provided to decrease these complications by means of a double free flap using one fibular osteocutaneous flap and one ALT myocutaneous flap (option 3 in Table 11.7).

Secondary procedures

Common reasons for secondary revisions following oral cavity reconstruction include functional correction and cosmetic improvement. When the tumor resection involves the angle of the mouth, oral incompetence is an issue. The revision improves the drooling, which is an inconvenience in daily life, as well as improving overall aesthetic appearance. If the upper and lower lips are largely preserved, a vermilion advancement flap can usually reach a satisfactory cosmetic result. However, if the lips are inadequate for advancement, a tendon graft (usually the palmaris longus tendon) is required to serve as a sling to reconstruct and restore oral competency, and mucosal flaps such as facial artery musculomucosal (FAMM) flap can be used to restore the appearance of lips.

Scar release with Z-plasty is an easy and effective procedure to reduce scar contracture and to smooth out the flap edges. Another commonly encountered problem is an oversized flap or an inadequate flap volume, which results in an asymmetric lower third of the face. Flap reduction can be achieved by direct excision or liposuction. If inadequate flap volume is present, fat injection can be performed. In selected patients who present with severe soft-tissue insufficiency and bony structure exposure, a second free-flap transfer is another option.[162]

15. Hidalgo DA, Pusic AL. Free-flap mandibular reconstruction: a 10-year follow-up study. *Plast Reconstr Surg.* 2002;110:438–449; discussion 450–431. *One of the earliest references with a single surgeon's experience using bone-carrying free flaps in mandible reconstruction and follow-up of more than 10 years. Excellent results were confirmed with minimal bony resorption, good aesthetic outcome, and well-restored function. Most of the reconstructions were done with free fibula flaps with one exception (Scapula flap). It is one of the signature papers to confirm the applicability of the free fibula flap in mandible reconstruction with long-term follow-up.*

30. Kao HK, Chang KP, Ching WC, et al. Postoperative morbidity and mortality of head and neck cancers in patients with liver cirrhosis undergoing surgical resection followed by microsurgical free tissue transfer. *Ann Surg Oncol.* 2010;17:536–543.

41. Loewen IJ, Boliek CA, Harris J, et al. Oral sensation and function: a comparison of patients with innervated radial forearm free flap reconstruction to healthy matched controls. *Head Neck.* 2010;32:85–95.

47. Engel H, Huang JJ, Lin CY, et al. A strategic approach for tongue reconstruction to achieve predictable and improved functional and aesthetic outcomes. *Plast Reconstr Surg.* 2010;126:1967–1977. *A strategic approach of tongue reconstruction based on the extension of the defects is proposed. Unlike most of the literature that addresses a single flap in all kinds or a specific category of tongue reconstruction, this paper provides comprehensive review of the defects and flap selection based on the defects. There is not a single flap that can fit all the defects. Reconstruction planning and flap selection should be based on the defect and the availability of donor tissue. The information provided is extremely useful and also very helpful for the beginner.*

60. Wei FC, Celik N, Chen HC, et al. Combined anterolateral thigh flap and vascularized fibula osteoseptocutaneous flap in reconstruction of extensive composite mandibular defects. *Plast Reconstr Surg.* 2002;109:45–52. *It is not uncommon that the defect left after tumor resection involves multiple important structures. This paper demonstrates how the reconstructive surgeon can be challenged sometimes by a huge defect and that the reconstruction can be achieved successfully using two different free flaps at the same time to restore both missing soft tissue and bone. It also highlights the importance that reconstruction can actually help to extend the resectability of cancer with the back-up of microsurgical reconstruction.*

68. Schultz BD, Sosin M, Nam A, et al. Classification of mandible defects and algorithm for microvascular reconstruction. *Plast Reconstr Surg.* 2015;135:743e–754e.

134. Cheng MH, Saint-Cyr M, Ali RS, et al. Osteomyocutaneous peroneal artery-based combined flap for reconstruction of composite and en bloc mandibular defects. *Head Neck.* 2009;31:361–370. *One of the major shortcomings of the fibular osteoseptocutaneous flap is the insufficiency of soft tissue to replace soft-tissue deficiency or cover the reconstructed mandible and reconstruction plate, which are both vulnerable to being exposed after radiotherapy. In this paper, Cheng and colleagues modified the free fibula flap with the inclusion of a piece of soleus muscle basing on a pair of separate vessels from the peroneal artery and vein. With the inclusion of the muscle, plate exposure rate was successfully reduced. The soleus muscle designed based on the "chimeric" concept also provides versatility of flap inset. The modification of the fibular flap to the so-called "osteomyocutaneous peroneal artery-based combined flap" expanded the application of the flap to more extensive bone and soft-tissue defect reconstruction following cancer resection. It also minimized long-term complications that may potentially require another free tissue transfer to solve.*

138. Yagi S, Kamei Y, Torii S. Donor side selection in mandibular reconstruction using a free fibular osteocutaneous flap. *Ann Plast Surg.* 2006;56:622–627.

147. Metzler P, Geiger EJ, Alcon A, et al. Three-dimensional virtual surgery accuracy for free fibula mandibular reconstruction: planned versus actual results. *J Oral Maxillofac Surg.* 2014;72:2601–2612. *One of the greatest challenges in performing mandible reconstruction is to reproduce similar contour of the reconstructed mandible and match the symmetry to the contralateral normal mandible. It is experience-dependent. The use of computer-guided preoperative planning provides the possibility to match the defect in maximal strength and improve the reconstruction. It was shown in this paper that preoperative CT planning successfully reproduces the preoperative contour of the mandible and the use of CT-guided surgeries or preoperative planning should be considered the next milestone in mandible reconstruction.*

160. Deutsch M, Kroll SS, Ainsle N, Wang B. Influence of radiation on late complications in patients with free fibular flaps for mandibular reconstruction. *Ann Plast Surg.* 1999;42:662–664.

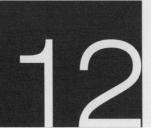

Lip reconstruction

Peter C. Neligan and Lawrence J. Gottlieb

 Access video lecture content for this chapter online at expertconsult.com

SYNOPSIS

- Accurate three-layered closure of lip defects is imperative to preserve function.
- Local tissue should be used whenever possible.
- Small defects can be closed by direct repair:
  - defects up to 25% of the width of the upper lip can be closed; and
  - defects up to 30% of the width of the lower lip can be closed.
- Intermediate defects are best reconstructed with local flaps.
- Total or sub-total lip defects are best reconstructed with free tissue.

Introduction

As the most prominent feature of the lower third of the face, the lips have significant functional, aesthetic, and social importance. Even subtle changes in the appearance of the vermilion border, labial commissures, or Cupid's bow are readily visible to the casual observer, and deformity can have a profound and lasting effect on the patient's self-image and quality of life.

Restoration of the lips is complicated by the fact that they are mobile structures and need to function (aesthetically and mechanically) differently when in repose and when animated since function and aesthetics are inextricably linked in these functional units. In addition, as mobile structures, they are subjected to distortion by gravity, scar, and possibly radiation and denervation. Neuromuscular injury or dysfunction can cause asymmetry at rest and particularly during facial expression. This can lead to distressing functional disability. Loss of labial competence may be characterized by impairment in the ability to articulate, whistle, suck, kiss, and, probably most importantly, to control salivary secretions with consequent drooling. Surgeons have long appreciated the significance of lip function and aesthetics and many creative surgical techniques have been devised to reconstruct various lip defects. These techniques have evolved, and newer procedures have been developed that effectively address small to moderate defects. However, while many of the current techniques work well for small to moderate lip defects, the ultimate reconstructive approach for larger defects of the lip has remained elusive, and currently available methods provide results that are less than optimal.[1]

 Access the Historical Perspective section online at
http://www.expertconsult.com

Anatomic and functional considerations in lip reconstruction

The laminar structure of the lips consists of three layers: mucosa, muscle, and skin. Externally, the cutaneous portion of the lip surrounds and transitions into the mucosal lip. This transition between these two regions is characterized by the mucocutaneous ridge, or vermilion border. At the midline of the upper lip, there is a V-shaped indentation of the mucocutaneous ridge that is known as Cupid's bow. Above Cupid's bow, a vertical groove-shaped depression called the philtrum is bordered on either side by elevations known as philtral ridges or columns (Fig. 12.1). The vermilion forms the major aesthetic feature of the upper and lower lips. The vermilion is composed of modified mucosa that lacks minor salivary glands. The characteristic color of the vermilion stems from a rich blood supply that underlies a very thin epithelial structure. The maxillary and mandibular divisions of the trigeminal nerve provide sensation to both upper and lower lips. The boundaries of the upper lip are defined by the base of the nose centrally and by the nasolabial folds laterally. The inferior margin of the lower lip is defined by the mental crease (labiomental crease) that separates the lip from the chin.[9] The upper and lower lips differ in that the lower lip is composed of a single aesthetic unit while the upper lip has multiple subunits. According to Burget and Menick's description,[10] each side of

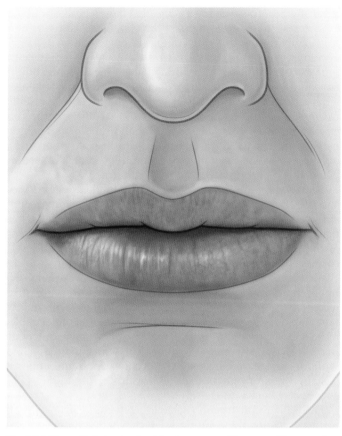

Fig. 12.1 The aesthetic landmarks of the lips are seen. The curve of the upper lip resembles a bow, known as Cupid's bow. The central concavity of the upper lip is the philtrum, bounded on either side by the convex philtral columns. The lateral elements of the upper lip are bounded by the philtral ridge medially, the nasal vestibule and alar base superiorly, and the nasolabial fold laterally. The mental crease separates the lower lip from the aesthetic unit of the chin.

the upper lip has two aesthetic subunits: the medial topographic subunit is one-half the philtrum, whereas the lateral subunit is bordered by the philtrum medially, the nostril sill and alar base superiorly, and the nasolabial fold laterally. Another way to think about the upper lip is that it is composed of three subunits: the philtrum centrally and the lateral lip elements on either side of the philtrum (Fig. 12.1).[11] As we age, multiple rhytids develop on the lips which theoretically and practically divide the lips into many more subunits.

The thickness of the lip largely results from the underlying orbicularis oris muscle, which forms a functional sphincteric ring and is essentially sandwiched between the skin on the outside, and the mucosa on the inside. The orbicularis oris has two functions that, at first, might seem diametrically opposed but that, on reflection, make sense. The superficial fibers of this muscle function to protrude the lips away from the facial plane, whereas the deep and oblique fibers approximate the lips to the alveolar arch.[12] The middle portion of the buccinator muscle extends anteriorly to the corner of the mouth and decussates so that the upper fibers of the mid-buccinator merge with the orbicularis fibers of the lower lip, and the lower fibers merge with the orbicularis fibers of the upper lip.[12] Several muscles elevate the lip. The two most important elevator muscles are the zygomaticus major and the levator anguli oris; the zygomaticus minor and the levator labii

superioris also contribute to this function. The depressor muscles include the depressor anguli oris and the platysma, with minor contributions from the depressor labii inferioris. Variations in the contraction of all of these muscles result in the versatility of movement of this region and the myriad of shapes and expressions that contribute not only to facial aesthetics and animation but also to function. The modiolus is just lateral to the oral commissure. It is a 1 cm-thick fibrovascular region of muscle fiber intersection of the levator muscles and the depressor muscles that attach firmly to the dermis approximately 1.5 cm lateral to the oral commissure. The modiolus can be located by compressing the skin and mucosa of the commissure using bidigital palpation with the thumb and index finger.[13] The appearance of the labial commissures is significantly affected by movement of the modiolus on each side, which results from the summation of opposing contractile forces of the levator muscles (zygomaticus major and levator anguli oris) and the depressor muscles (depressor anguli oris and platysma).[14,15] Sometimes there is a dimple here. When present, the dimple results from a dermal insertion arising from the inferior muscle bundle of a bifid zygomaticus major muscle.[16,17] The elevators and depressors of the lips are innervated by the buccal and mandibular branches of the facial nerve, respectively. Disruption of the musculature that attaches to the modiolar region (or their neural supply) can alter the appearance of the labial commissure at rest and during function secondary to imbalanced muscular contraction. This gives a very abnormal appearance to the mouth and is one of the greatest complaints of patients with facial paralysis. Modiolar motion can be analyzed to measure the success of facial reanimation in these.[18]

The blood supply to the lips comes from the facial arteries, which give rise to the inferior and superior labial arteries. The variability of these vessels, both in terms of course as well as of presence, has been shown by anatomic studies and dissections. The superior labial arteries from each side generally anastomose in the midportion of the upper lip, coursing between the mucosa and orbicularis muscle in some patients and through the muscle in the others.[19] The inferior labial artery, on the other hand, routinely courses between the mucosa of the inner aspect of the lip and the muscle.[19] Two separate cadaveric studies found that the inferior labial artery was absent on one side in 10% and 64%, respectively, of the cadavers evaluated.[19,20] The bilateral presence of inferior labial arteries was not always predictive of an end-to-end anastomosis between these vessels, and other arterial branches from the facial arteries were frequently identified (e.g., labiomental, sublabial arteries).[19,20] Even though the variable arterial distribution of this region could, at least in theory, affect the survival of reconstructive procedures involving the lip, local flap reconstruction has been performed for centuries with predictably excellent survival rates. Although the lips are an important aesthetic feature of the lower face, they also play an important role in facial expression. Oral competence is necessary for eating and drinking, and intact neuromuscular function is essential for speech articulation and other functions such as whistling and sucking. The lower lip functions as a dam that retains saliva and prevents drooling. The upper lip contributes to oral competence by providing opposition to the lower lip to effect closure.[21] Sensation allows the lips to monitor the texture and temperature of substances prior to oral intake.

Lip function

As the principal aesthetic feature of the lower face, an important function of the lips is to facilitate human interaction. This requires the lips to appear normal in repose and animation. In addition to the function of "looking normal", lips facilitate articulating certain sounds; maintenance of oral competence during eating, drinking, sucking, and speaking; as well as the expression of emotions with the ability to smile and kiss. In concert with motion of the mandible, they allow access to the mouth not only for food but also for oral and dental hygiene as well as insertion and removal of dentures. Its mucosal lining keeps its inner surface moist and serves incredibly complex immune functions as a "barrier organ" with the ability to distinguish between commensal and pathogenic microorganisms. Sensation allows the lips to monitor the texture and temperature of substances prior to oral intake.

Patient selection and presentation

Goals of lip reconstruction

The goals of lip reconstruction (Box 12.1) are several. The most important of these is function. No matter how good a reconstructed lip looks, if it cannot maintain oral competence, the reconstruction is a failure. Maintenance of oral competence is vital. Similarly important is maintenance of an adequate oral aperture to facilitate oral hygiene and/or to accommodate removable dentures. The labial vestibule is an important feature of labial anatomy, and its preservation or re-creation is important for oral hygiene, dental care, and denture fitting. In order to achieve these functions, preservation of labial sensation is important, and because of the vital role of the lips in facial aesthetics, maximization of cosmesis is one of the key goals of reconstruction.[22]

In situations where the orbicularis oris muscle has been disrupted, it is vitally important to restore continuity of that muscle if at all possible. Careful re-approximation of muscle edges with intact motor innervation usually results in complete restoration of dynamic orbicularis function. Although some authors contend that the upper lip functions primarily as a curtain that could be replaced with a static flap reconstruction, there is no doubt that a completely intact sphincter with active function and sensation yields the best functional result.[10,23] In cases where reconstruction of a complete circumoral muscular sphincter is not feasible, bridging the gap between the ends of the muscle with an adynamic segment of tendon or fascia, that provides some degree of oral competence, should be pursued. One of the main dangers in

repairing or reconstructing the lips that have significant tissue loss is resulting microstomia. While patients can function reasonably well with a small degree of microstomia, it is very important to minimize it, as it may not only interfere with function but can also hamper oral hygiene and patients should be counseled prior to surgery that denture insertion and removal may be difficult or, quite simply, not possible. Decreases in the shape or depth of the labial vestibule can exacerbate oral incompetence and drooling and may preclude patients from wearing a removable prosthesis. Preservation of labial sensation is vitally important to maximize oral competence and to fulfill its other sensory roles.

Because of the anatomic configuration of the upper lip and, specifically, because of its aesthetic subunit structure, reconstruction of the upper lip presents certain aesthetic challenges that are not of concern during lower lip reconstruction. Loss of the philtral ridges and Cupid's bow creates a noticeable cosmetic deformity that presents a significant reconstructive challenge especially in woman and children. In profile, the upper lip should protrude in front of the lower lip, so a reconstruction that results in excisional tightness with reduction or elimination of this relationship is not only undesirable, but also will certainly result in an inferior aesthetic outcome. In contrast, the lower lip is better able to withstand tissue loss without significant changes in its profile appearance and can sustain a loss of one-third of its breadth before tightness or asymmetry begins to show.

Early lip reconstruction techniques focused primarily on primary closure of the surgical defect, whereas more contemporary techniques attempt to address the importance of an aesthetic, functional result. Reconstruction of the aesthetic subunits as described by Burget and Menick[10] is helpful, and aesthetic features such as Cupid's bow and the philtral columns must be carefully restored. Failure to restore these landmarks results in an abnormal appearance that is instantly detectable. One of the features that is readily picked up by the human eye is asymmetry. Surgery that results in asymmetry is typically more noticeable than symmetric alterations. As an example, rounding of both commissures is less obvious than rounding of one side. Whenever possible, the height, projection, and relationship between upper and lower lips should also be preserved or replicated. This is most easily achieved by using tissue from the adjacent or opposing lip.[24,25]

Patient selection is, arguably, less important than reconstructive choice. In the case of trauma, the damage is already done and the surgeon's task is to repair and reconstruct the lip so that it is as functional and aesthetically pleasing as possible. For patients facing lip resection for disease, the task is no different, i.e., the surgeon must reconstruct the lip to be as functional and aesthetically pleasing as possible. However, in the latter case, the surgeon has the luxury of planning what reconstruction will best suit the patient. The choice depends on multiple factors, such as prognosis, general medical condition, availability of local tissue, history of prior radiation as well as co-morbidities. The lips are somewhat unique, however, in that the need to reconstruct the lips is very different from, as an example, the need to reconstruct a breast. Oral competence is vital for normal eating, articulation, and communication, so the option not to reconstruct the lip is really nonexistent. The algorithm presented later in this chapter (see Fig. 12.17, below) can be used as a guide in selecting the most appropriate procedure for a given defect.

BOX 12.1 **Goals of lip reconstruction**

- Preservation of function.
- Reconstitution of orbicularis oris.
- Three-layered closure.
- Accurate alignment of vermilion.
- Maintenance of relationship between upper and lower lips.
- Optimization of aesthetics in repose and with animation.

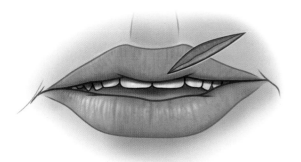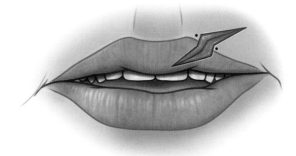

Fig. 12.2 Breaking up the linear scar by introducing a vertical element to an excision will allow for more precise closure as the vermilion borders can be accurately approximated (marked with dots). Furthermore, the resulting scar will not be linear and will therefore be less likely to contract.

Operative technique

Defect-specific reconstruction of the lip

Following injury to the lips or following surgical resection for disease, there are several options for reconstruction of the lips:[12,26] The first choice, of course, is to use the remaining lip segment, and if the defect size allows, this is by far the best option. This choice assumes that there is enough lip to effect the repair while not creating distortion or microstomia. Another consideration is whether or not the defect is full thickness and whether all three elements, skin, muscle, and mucosa, need to be replaced. Regardless of what the defect is, local tissue is the best option because it replaces what has been lost and is the perfect match in terms of color, thickness and composition. Although defects of the upper lip of less than 25% can be closed by direct approximation, it should be noted that direct closure of defects greater than 10% of the upper lip will generally lead to distortion of the philtral column especially in younger patients. For the lower lip, a slightly larger defect, up to 30%, can be closed directly. Once again, care must be taken to ensure accurate closure of all layers. Repair of the orbicularis oris and reconstitution of the circumoral sphincter is the most important aspect of a functional repair.

For through-and-through defects, if there is insufficient lip to effect a direct closure, the next choice becomes flaps from adjacent lip components or the opposite lip. Several lip-switch options are discussed below and fulfill the requirement of providing tissue of like composition and appearance. Sometimes, however, there simply is not enough lip tissue to achieve this, in which case it may become necessary to use tissue from the adjacent cheek, nasolabial region, or neck. A very useful source of tissue that can be used to reconstruct the lip, particularly when a through-and-through reconstruction is not required, is to use tissue from the submental region. For extreme defects, however, there is no other option but to use regional, distant or free flaps.

Defects of the vermilion

There are a few important points of which to be cognizant when repairing a lip. One is the appreciation of the fact that the human eye can detect asymmetry remarkably accurately.

The lips are very symmetrical, and the different elements of the lip blend with each other in a very pleasing and aesthetic way. The junction between vermilion and white lip, for example, is smooth and seamless. When the line of the vermilion is broken or when a segment of vermilion impinges on the white lip, the abnormality is immediately obvious. When dealing with lacerations, there is not a lot, in terms of repair options, that the surgeon can do. However, being precise in repair of the vermilion border and white lip roll will produce a scar that is imperceptible. When resecting a lesion that crossed the vermilion, however, there are some options. As surgeons, we know that scars contract and a straight-line scar that crosses the vermilion will not only contract but may possibly produce a visible deformity. In order to avoid this, breaking up the scar by incorporating a step in the excision may prevent this contraction, make the repair easier and minimize the risk of a visible scar (Fig. 12.2).

Loss or lack of vermilion may be due to injury, denervation, scar, or resection. Vermilionectomy is a procedure that is done to remove very superficial lesions in the vermilion, such as superficial squamous cell carcinoma, or to remove dysplastic tissue with malignant potential such as actinic cheilitis. Following vermilionectomy, a procedure that is also known as a lip-shave, reconstruction is achieved by advancing the buccal mucosa to cover the defect and to re-establish the mucocutaneous junction (Fig. 12.3).[1] If there is any degree of tightness, back-cuts are made to facilitate further advancement of the mucosa. This type of vermilion reconstruction can sometimes result in excessive thinning of the lip from mucosal retraction or scar contraction, and decreased mucosal sensation.[9,27] However, in general, the results of lip-shave are excellent. Other approaches to reconstruction of the vermilion include the mucosal V–Y advancement flap, the cross-lip mucosal flap, and transposition flaps harvested from the buccal mucosa or the ventral surface of the tongue.[9,28] Buccal mucosal flaps tend to be more erythematous than natural vermilion, resulting in a color mismatch with the remaining vermilion.[27] Mucosal tongue flaps require a second procedure 14–21 days later to release and inset the flap. A musculomucosal flap that includes buccal mucosa and buccinator muscle anteriorly pedicled on buccal branches of the facial artery and innervated sensory branches of the infraorbital nerve has been advocated as one option to remedy the loss of sensation in defects that also include loss of orbicularis muscle.[29] A modified Estlander

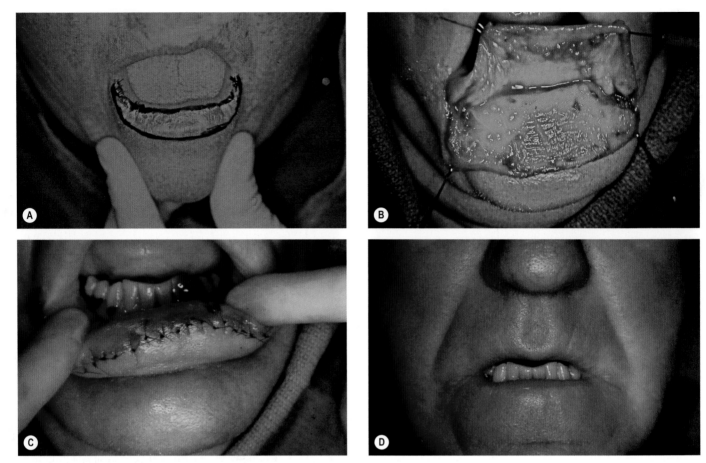

Fig. 12.3 (A) An area of vermilion is marked for excision. **(B)** The vermilion has been excised and a mucosal flap raised from the buccal mucosa. **(C)** The mucosal flap has been advanced and sutured to the white lip to recreate the mucocutaneous junction. **(D)** Postoperative appearance showing good restoration of vermilion.

myomucosal flap transferring vermilion and underlying innervated orbicularis muscle to a denervated atrophic lower lip can be helpful to regain oral competence (Fig. 12.4).

Small defects

Primary closure of defects that involve as much as one-quarter of the upper lip or one-third of the lower lip can be achieved (Box 12.2).[21] A V-shaped wedge design usually permits closure of smaller defects, whereas a W-plasty placed at the base of the V facilitates the closure of larger defects of the lower lip. Furthermore, this modification will generally allow for the scar to be kept above the mental crease. This is particularly important in non-midline excisions. It improves the cosmetic appearance of the repair, as it preserves the integrity of the chin aesthetic subunit (Fig. 12.5). Wedge-shaped defects of the lateral lip should be more obliquely oriented so that the line of closure parallels the relaxed skin tension lines. If a W-plasty is incorporated into a lateral lip defect, the angle formed by the lateral V-shaped subunit of the W should be larger and more obliquely oriented than the medial subunit to properly align the closure.[9,22] Alternatively, rather than using a V or W, resection shape can be dictated by the direction of skin rhytids and relaxed skin tension lines (Fig. 12.6). Careful attention to meticulous approximation of the vermilion border and closure of all three layers will ensure optimal cosmesis and function. Placing a micro-Z-plasty just below the white roll and just

above the mental crease (in situations where the mental crease is violated) helps minimize subsequent contracture and preserves the natural curve of the lip and chin. If actinic cheilitis of the adjacent lip is present, vermilionectomy can also be performed in combination with the wedge excision, using a labial mucosal advancement flap to recreate the vermilion border (Fig. 12.7). This technique provides an elegant reconstruction of the vermilion, and the cosmetic outcome of this procedure is usually excellent. The aesthetic result following repair of a V-type excision is often less satisfactory in the

---

BOX 12.2 **Wedge resection of the lip: technical tips**

- Up to 25% of the upper lip can be resected and repaired directly.
  - Up to 10% in younger patients without distortion
- Up to 30% of the lower lip can be resected and repaired directly.
- Careful approximation of the muscle layer ensures a functional repair.
- Micro Z-plasties at concavities preserves the gentle curves of lips.
- Consider a W resection for larger wedges in order to keep the scar above the mental crease.

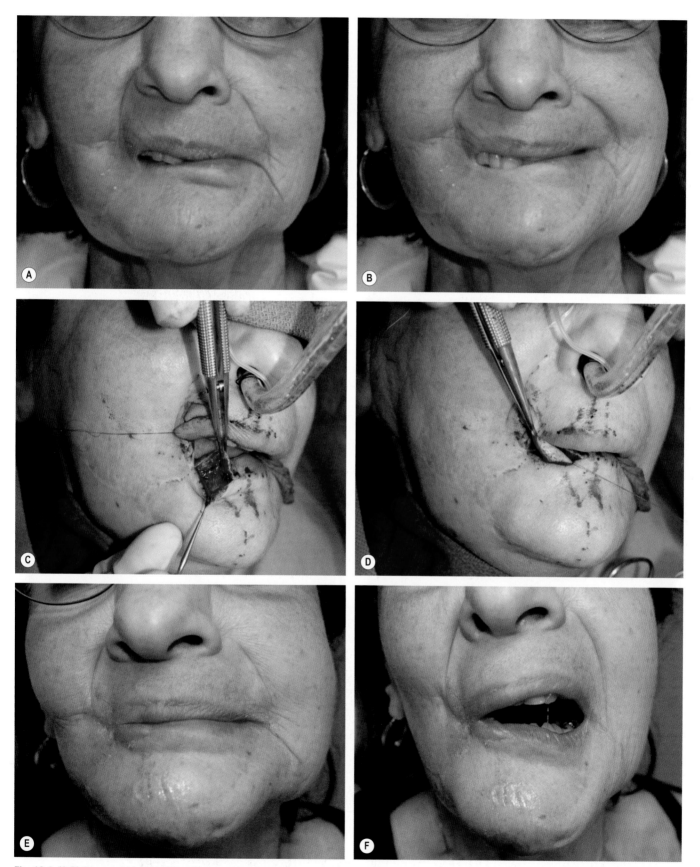

Fig. 12.4 (A,B) 74-year-old female with oral incompetence from denervated orbicularis oris muscle on right side of lower lip. She has a history of buccal mucosal cancer, osteoradionecrosis, and multiple reconstructive procedures including radial forearm free flap to right buccal mucosa and fibular osteocutaneous free flap for osteoradionecrosis. Note excess skin of right side of upper lip from previous tightening procedure of lower lip. **(C)** A modified Estlander myomucosal flap elevated with suture attached and defect created in lower lip. **(D)** Flap being transferred. **(E)** Correction of drooling and deformity in repose, although commissure is blunted. **(F)** Although drooling corrected, mild microstomia created.

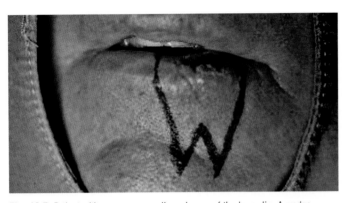

Fig. 12.5 Patient with a squamous cell carcinoma of the lower lip. A wedge excision has been planned and the patient is marked for a "W" excision in order to keep the scar above the mental crease and out of the aesthetic subunit of the chin.

upper lip, because the upper lip is able to withstand much less tissue loss before distortion of the philtral column or tightness becomes clinically apparent. The normal overhang of upper and lower lip is lost as a consequence of closure-induced tension. In addition, the anchorage of soft tissues around the pyriform aperture to the underlying bony skeleton limits compensatory movement of the remaining lip. This problem can be minimized by using a T excision, which facilitates advancement of the lateral lip elements towards the midline. The symmetry of Cupid's bow is easily lost with even minor excision in the region of the philtrum. Webster's[30] technique of crescentic perialar cheek excision is an extension of the T-excision technique that increases upper lip movement without disturbing the lateral muscle function (Fig. 12.8). Webster frequently supplements the perialar excisions with the addition of an Abbé flap lest there be too much tension[30] (Fig. 12.9). If the defect is created lateral to the philtral columns,

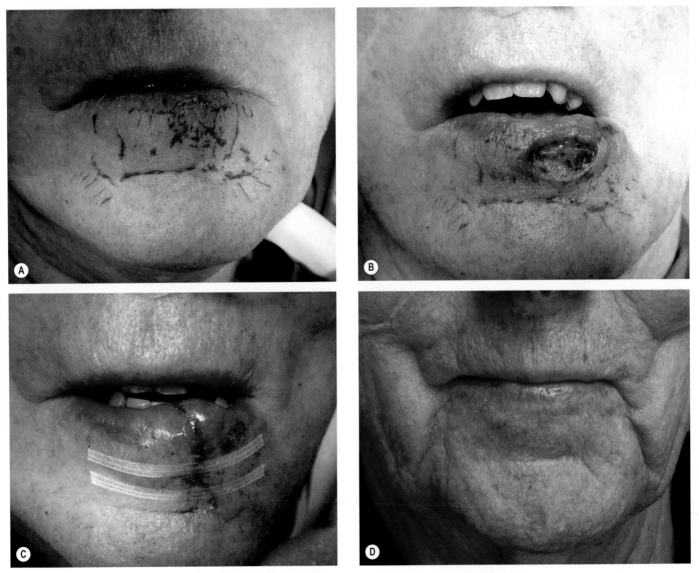

Fig. 12.6 (A) Markings for excision of basal cell carcinoma of lower lip in a 71-year-old male. Vermilion border, skin lines and rhytids marked on skin. **(B)** Defect after excision with negative margins on frozen section. **(C)** Free-style closure dictated by skin lines and rhytids, note precise alignment of vermilion and micro Z-plasty just below vermilion border. **(D)** Result 14 years postoperatively.

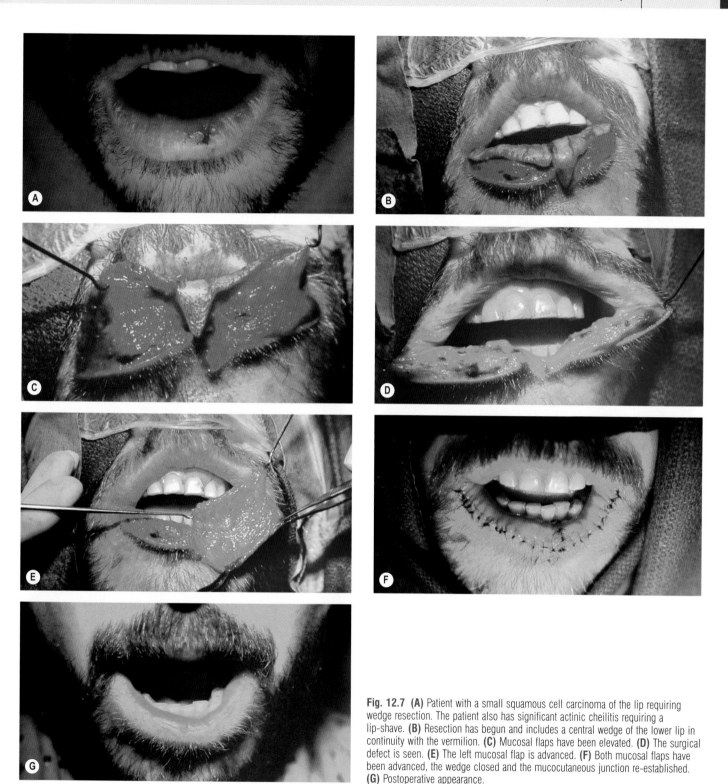

Fig. 12.7 (A) Patient with a small squamous cell carcinoma of the lip requiring wedge resection. The patient also has significant actinic cheilitis requiring a lip-shave. **(B)** Resection has begun and includes a central wedge of the lower lip in continuity with the vermilion. **(C)** Mucosal flaps have been elevated. **(D)** The surgical defect is seen. **(E)** The left mucosal flap is advanced. **(F)** Both mucosal flaps have been advanced, the wedge closed and the mucocutaneous junction re-established. **(G)** Postoperative appearance.

primary closure will frequently produce a deformity of the philtral column and lip tightness. This can be minimized by reconstructing the lateral lip subunit with a crescent-shaped lateral lip VY flap, removing the tension from the medial lip and planning all scars at the border of the aesthetic subunit or parallel to natural rhytids (Fig. 12.10). Alternatively, it is occasionally preferable to use a lip-switch flap from the lower lip, even when the defect makes up less than 25% of the lip's width. This is particularly the case with central (philtral) defects or in younger patients whose tissues are less lax and where cosmesis is often of even greater importance.

Intermediate defects

For all the reasons already described, local flaps are the best option for reconstructing larger defects involving up to

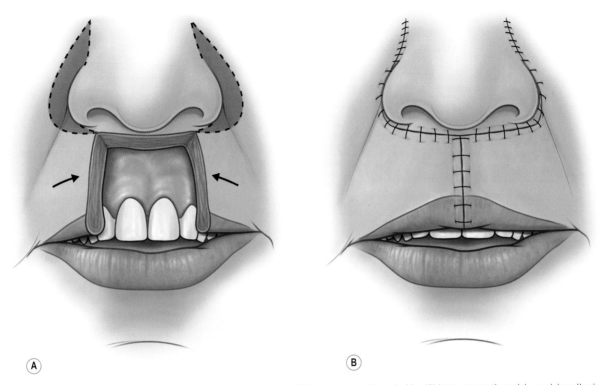

Fig. 12.8 (A) Resection of a central segment of the upper lip is shown. A "T" excision is performed with a Webster crescentic perialar excision allowing for advancement of the lip elements. **(B)** A schematic of the closure is shown.

two-thirds the width of either upper or lower lip. These flaps involve either a lip-switching maneuver, rotation of tissue from one lip to another, or recruitment and advancement of adjacent tissue, such as cheek tissue, to achieve the reconstruction. Lip-switch (cross-lip) flaps are axial flaps based on the labial arteries (Box 12.3). They replace tissue like with like,

having the capability of replacing the trilaminar defect in one lip with trilaminar tissue from the other. The classic Abbé flap can reconstruct medial or lateral lip defects with a full-thickness composite flap that reconstructs all three layers and restores continuity of the vermilion.[31] The Abbé cross-lip flap can also be used to replace any one of the trilaminar

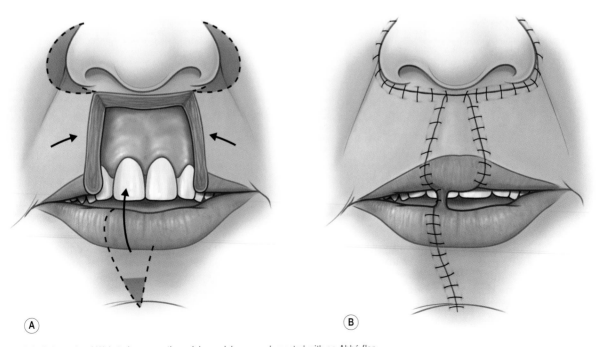

Fig. 12.9 Schematic of Webster's crescentic perialar excisions supplemented with an Abbé flap.

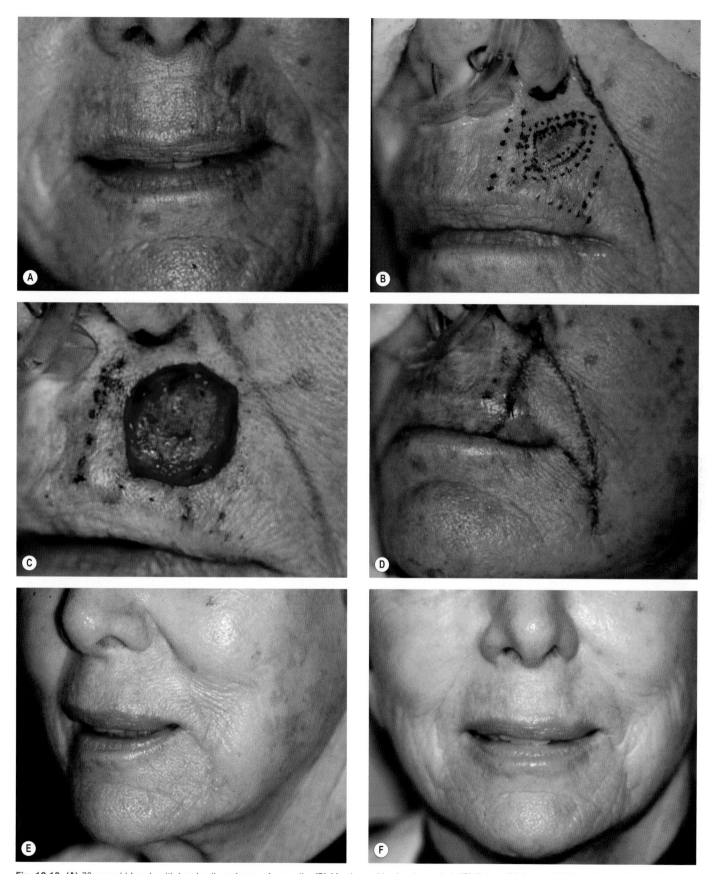

Fig. 12.10 (A) 72-year-old female with basal cell carcinoma of upper lip. **(B)** Margins and landmarks marked. **(C)** Defect. **(D)** Crescent VY flap closure with incisions along or parallel to aesthetic unit borders. **(E,F)** 5 month follow-up with no distortion of philtral column.

BOX 12.3 Lip-switch flaps: technical tips

- Subunit reconstruction demands that flap size should exactly replicate subunit size and shape.
- In non-subunit reconstruction, width of the flap should be half the width of the defect.
- Height of the flap should be the same as height of the defect.
- Pedicle of Abbé flap should be placed at the edge of defect for subunit reconstruction and at the midpoint of the defect for non-subunit reconstruction.
- Pedicle division at 14–21 days.

---

components of the lip and does not necessarily need to contain all layers throughout the flap. Ideally, the exact size of the defect should be reconstructed with an exact template of the missing aesthetic subunit. Adhering to the aesthetic subunit principle, Burget and Menick[10] suggested that defects constituting more than half of a topographic subunit of the upper lip necessitate removal of the remaining portions of the subunit so that reconstruction of the entire subunit can be performed by using an exact foil template of the defect to design the Abbé flap in the lower lip. For central defects, the lateral segments should be advanced medially so the defect remaining is the normal size of the philtrum. Reconstructing this aesthetic subunit with an exact template generally provides a more favorable aesthetic result (Fig. 12.11).

Although it is ideal to replace an exact template of what is missing, frequently the donor lip cannot "give up" all that is needed. Surgical technique is important, and there are a few technical principles that are important to follow to achieve optimal results. The first is that the width of the flap does not always need to be as big as the width of the defect. This technical trick allows for repair of the defect by taking advantage of the inherent elasticity of the lip tissues while, at the same time, reducing the amount of tissue that has to be sacrificed from the donor lip, thereby making closure of the secondary defect easier. So both lips end up a little smaller, but by taking some tissue from both lips, a better balance between the two lips is maintained. The second principle is that the height of the flap needs to match that of the defect. While one can get away with less width, less height will result in some element of notching and will produce a significantly inferior result. Finally, the position of the flap relative to the opposite lip is an important technical point to appreciate. This refers particularly to the Abbé flap and is important because the position of the flap determines the position of the pedicle. This is very important to appreciate. When the entire subunit is not being reconstructed, the pedicle should be placed roughly at the mid-position of the defect. The reason for this is that the flap will be half the width of the defect so that when the secondary defect is closed, the pedicle ends up being in precise alignment with one end of the defect. This is best explained in Fig. 12.12. Pedicle division is performed 14–21 days later as shown in Fig. 12.13.

The Estlander flap is, in reality, an Abbé flap that is brought around the commissure.[32] Once again, the width of the flap is usually one-half the width of the defect and is the same height as the defect. Using this technique, defects that involve the commissure and as much as 50% of the lower or upper lip can be adequately reconstructed with an acceptable functional

and cosmetic result. However, in this case, since the flap is rotated, no pedicle division is necessary. One disadvantage is the blunting of the commissure that is seen. However, this rarely requires any correction (Fig. 12.14). Several modifications of cross-lip flaps have also been described.

There are, however, several limitations to the cross-lip flaps. Even though the orbicularis muscle is reconstructed and continuity of the circumoral sphincter is re-established, disruption of the motor supply leads to varying degrees of abnormal lip motility. Where small flaps have been utilized, this may be barely if at all appreciable. However, where larger reconstructions have been performed, the change in motility may be more obvious. A trap-door deformity or pin-cushioning occasionally develops at the recipient site, and the cross-lip flap tends to appear thicker than the adjacent lip.[9,10,27,31,32] It also should be noted that cross-lip flaps in men will have the hair growing in the wrong direction, generally precluding one from sporting a mustache. The fan flap, initially described by Gillies and Millard[5] in 1957, is a modification of a technique described by von Bruns that utilizes quadrilateral inferiorly based nasolabial flaps.[3] This flap rotates tissue around the commissure in the same fashion as an Estlander flap, but more tissue from the nasolabial region is included.[12] A vertical releasing incision is made in the donor lip.[9] A unilateral flap can be performed to reconstruct a lip defect, but bilateral fan flaps are more frequently employed to reconstruct total or sub-total defects (Fig. 12.15).[12] Although defects involving up to 80% of the lip can be reconstructed with the Gillies fan flap, the biggest and least desirable sequel is significant microstomia as well as deficiency of the vermilion. Furthermore, denervation of the orbicularis oris can lead to oral incompetence. However, at least partial re-innervation seems to occur over a period of 12–18 months.[9,12,33] The circumoral advancement-rotation flap initially described by von Bruns in 1857 utilized full-thickness flaps that resulted in extensive denervation of the orbicularis muscle.[3] Although this technique effectively closed large composite defects of the lower lip, reconstruction was accomplished at the expense of sensation, motor function, and oral competence. These full-thickness flaps fell into disrepute until 1974, when Karapandzic[4] published a modification of von Bruns' technique. The incisional design of the Karapandzic flap, as it is now known, was identical to those advocated by von Bruns, but full-thickness flaps were not created, and the neurovascular supply to the lip was preserved via meticulous dissection (Fig. 12.16). Although most authors report its use for the closure of lip defects that involve up to two-thirds of the lip, others state that the Karapandzic flap can successfully replace 80% of the total lip length.[1,9,12,25] However, reconstructing such a large defect with this technique can result in significant microstomia. This flap may be used to reconstruct defects of the upper or lower lip in the following manner: curvilinear circumoral incisions are extended bilaterally from the base of the defect, placing the incisions within the mental crease and the nasolabial creases. The incisions are designed to maintain a uniform thickness of the flap bilaterally. Because the nasolabial crease closely approximates the commissure, the incision should be placed slightly lateral to the nasolabial crease in this region, to maintain uniform thickness of the flap. If the defect is eccentrically located, the flap should be designed so that the contralateral lower lip is the longer limb of the flap. Careful dissection of the peripheral muscle fibers and concentric

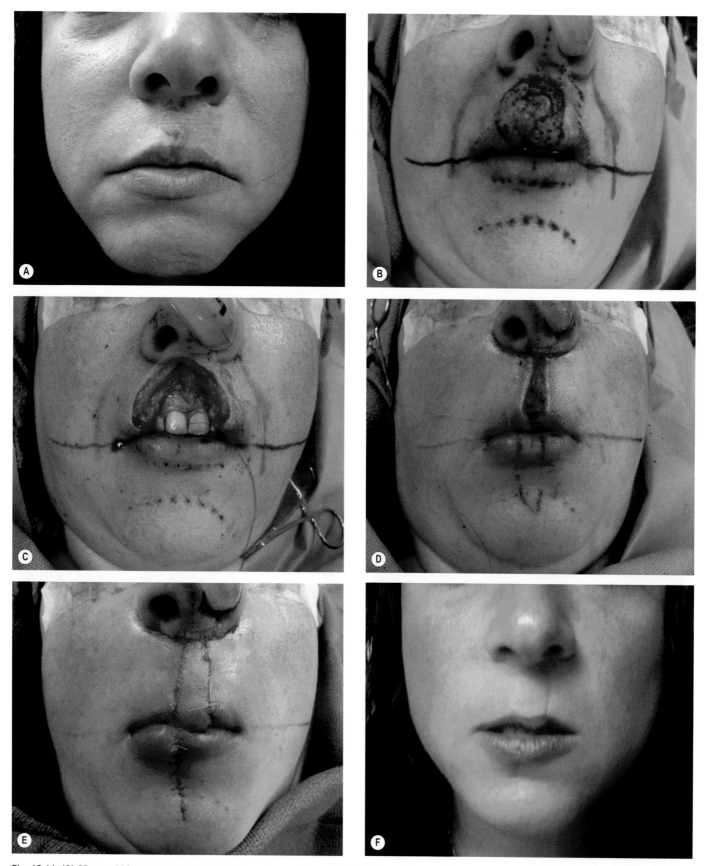

Fig. 12.11 **(A)** 35-year-old female with recurrent basal cell carcinoma of upper lip. Note skin graft from previous reconstruction. **(B)** Skin markings of tumor, scars, and landmarks with methylene blue tattoo of vermilion border. **(C)** Full-thickness excision of tumor. **(D)** Residual skin graft removed and crescentic perialar excisions performed to narrow the defect to approximate a normal philtrum. Note exact size of Abbé flap planned to fill residual defect. **(E)** Abbé flap transferred. Note micro Z-plasties of lower lip below white role and above labial mental angle. **(F)** Final result.

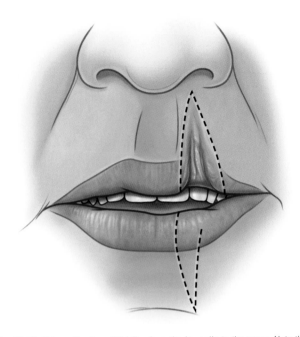

Fig. 12.12 Schematic of an Abbé flap from the lower lip to the upper. Note that the width of the Abbé flap is half the width of the defect, while the height of the flap is the same as the height of the defect. The pedicle will be planned at a point opposite the midportion of the defect and will end up at the medial end of the defect following rotation of the flap.

undermining allows advancement without any dissection of the mucosa. Preservation of the neurovascular bundles is imperative. A unilateral flap is adequate for smaller defects, whereas defects that constitute more than 50% of the lip require bilateral flaps. Function is restored because only the peripheral rim of orbicularis oris muscle is incised and the buccinator muscle is preserved. The Karapandzic flap results in blunting or rounding of both commissures, which is usually less noticeable than alteration of only one commissure. Some degree of microstomia is also inevitable, which may preclude the use of dentures. Because the combined width of the upper and lower lips is approximately 15 cm, reconstruction of a 5 cm defect results in a rounded oral aperture with a circumference that is two-thirds of the original.[9,12,21,22] However, because of the superior and predictable functional results that can be achieved with acceptable aesthetics, the Karapandzic flap is possibly the flap of choice for most larger intermediate full-thickness defects.

Frequently, a defect is too wide to close directly but is not wide enough to require a flap such as the Estlander or Abbé flap. Johanson *et al.*[34,35] proposed the stair-step advancement flap for such a defect. Though ideally suited for smaller defects, this technique is capable of reconstructing defects extending to as much as two-thirds of the lower lip (Fig. 12.17).[35] This technique involves the excision of 2–4 small rectangles arranged in a stair-step fashion that descend from medial to lateral at a 45° angle from either side of the base of

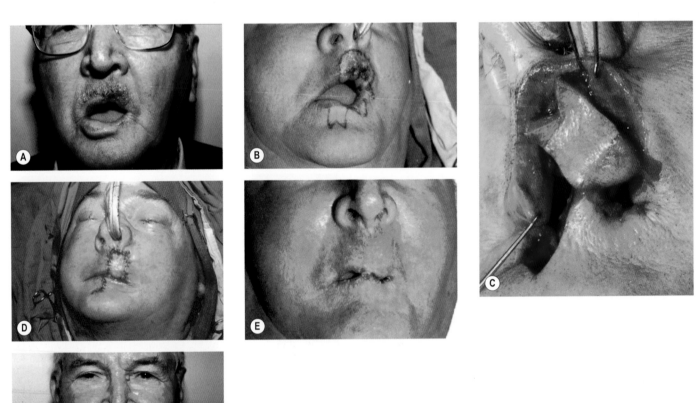

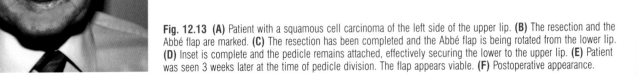

Fig. 12.13 (A) Patient with a squamous cell carcinoma of the left side of the upper lip. **(B)** The resection and the Abbé flap are marked. **(C)** The resection has been completed and the Abbé flap is being rotated from the lower lip. **(D)** Inset is complete and the pedicle remains attached, effectively securing the lower to the upper lip. **(E)** Patient was seen 3 weeks later at the time of pedicle division. The flap appears viable. **(F)** Postoperative appearance.

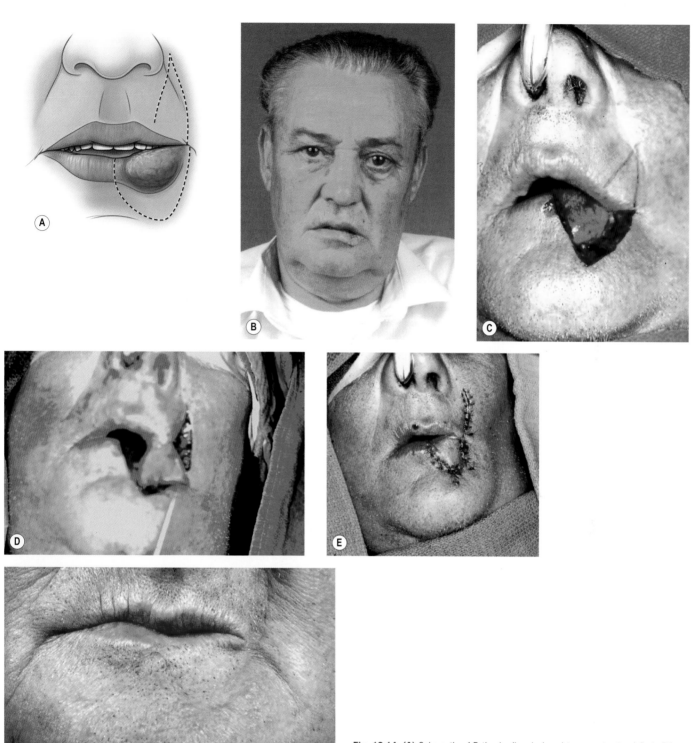

Fig. 12.14 (A) Schematic of Estlander flap designed to reconstruct a defect of the lower lip. **(B)** Patient with squamous cell carcinoma of the lower lip. **(C)** The lesion has been excised and the flap designed. Note the dimensions of the flap. The width is half that of the defect but the height is the same as the height of the defect. **(D)** The flap is being rotated into the defect. **(E)** Final inset of the flap and closure of the donor defect. **(F)** Final appearance. Note the slight blunting of the commissure.

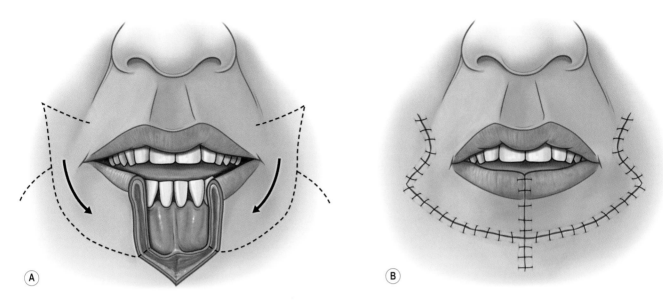

Fig. 12.15 A schematic of the Gillies fan flap is shown. Note the releasing incisions on the upper lip that allow the flap to rotate and advance.

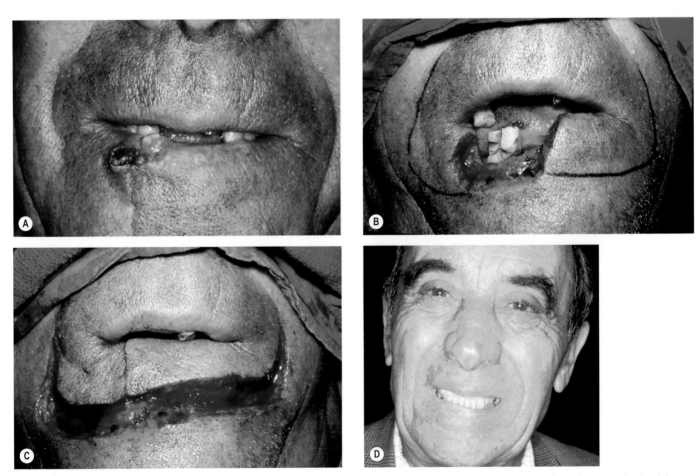

Fig. 12.16 (A) Patient with a squamous cell carcinoma of the lower lip. Note the scar from a previous wedge resection. **(B)** The resection has been completed and the markings made for a Karapandzic flap. **(C)** The flaps are rotated and advanced. Note that this is not a through-and-through dissection so that the motor and sensory nerves can be preserved. **(D)** Postoperative appearance showing good cosmesis and function.

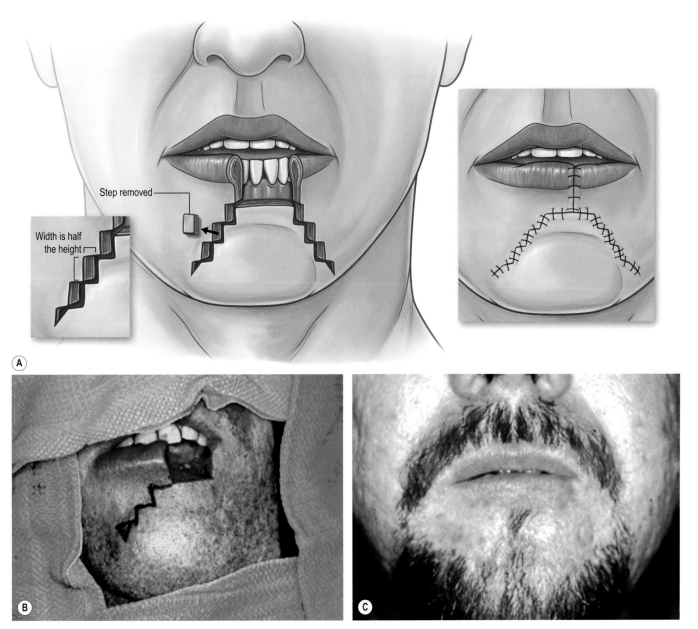

Fig. 12.17 **(A)** Schematic of a step flap reconstruction. Note that the steps are excised to allow the flaps to advance. Note also that the scar remains above the mental crease. **(B)** Patient following resection of a squamous cell carcinoma of the lower lip. Markings have been made for a unilateral step resection. **(C)** Postoperative appearance.

the defect. When the defect is located laterally, the step incision is outlined exclusively on the remaining long side of the lip.[36] If the defect is located near the midline or its horizontal length exceeds 20 mm, the staircase pattern is marked on both sides of the lower lip. The first horizontal incision is made parallel to the vermilion border and is approximately half of the width of the resected region. Usually 2–4 additional steps are necessary in the vertical direction; the width of each step is approximately one-half of its height. Finally, a triangle is excised with its apex located inferiorly. Each of the rectangles and the triangle are excised through the full thickness of the lower lip. This allows advancement of the flap in the direction of the defect with each succeeding higher step in the staircase, and the wound is closed in layers. By placing the step incisions outside of the mental crease, the aesthetic unit of the

chin can be preserved (Fig. 12.17). For this reason, the step technique is better than a wedge resection of similar size that would encroach on the chin subunit. The stair-step design allows for closure of the defect and minimizes contracture.

Large defects

Defects that involve up to 80% of the total lip length may be reconstructed with bilateral Gillies fan flaps or the Karapandzic flap, as described above.[12] Reconstruction of total or near-total defects constituting more than 80% of the lip typically leads to a poor aesthetic outcome and compromised oral competence. Because of denervation, the lip is largely adynamic. Dieffenbach (1845),[37] Bernard (1853), von Burow (1855) and von Bruns (1857)[3,12] all described techniques of

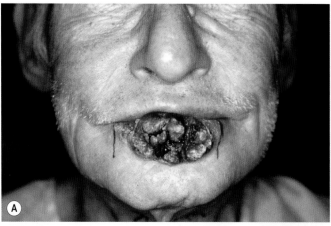

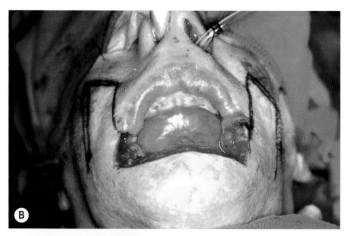

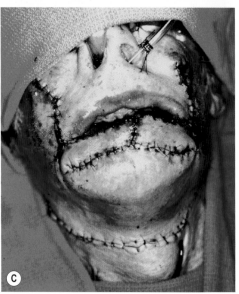

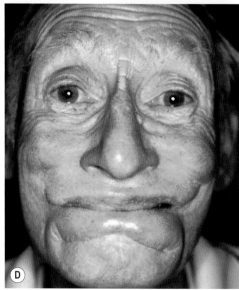

Fig. 12.18 (A) Patient with a large squamous cell carcinoma of the lower lip requiring total resection. **(B)** The resection is complete and bilateral Fujimori gate flaps have been designed. **(C)** The flaps are rotated into the defect and the secondary defects closed. **(D)** Postoperative appearance showing significant deformity of the lower face.

cheek advancement from which the current reconstructive methods that employ horizontal cheek advancement flaps have evolved. Bernard and von Burow described the transposition of full-thickness flaps to reconstruct the upper or lower lip, reconstructing the vermilion with a mucosal advancement flap.[12] Transposition of these cutaneous flaps required the excision of four triangular regions of redundant cheek skin to reconstruct the upper lip and the excision of three cutaneous triangles to reconstruct the lower lip. The reconstructive technique has become known as the "Bernard cheiloplasty" or the Bernard–Burow cheek advancement, and the triangular soft tissue excisions are referred to as "Burow's triangles".[9,30,38] Webster[27] suggested modifications of this technique that align the scars with the relaxed skin tension lines of the face. Although microstomia can be avoided with this approach, there is no functional orbicularis. Consequently, oral competence relies on the development of a tight adynamic lower lip. Prior to free tissue transfer, nasolabial flaps played a prominent role in total lip reconstruction. Dieffenbach[37] initially described the use of nasolabial flaps for upper lip reconstruction. The rectangular-shaped nasolabial flaps that von Bruns described in 1857 for lower lip defects were inferiorly-based.[3] The "gate flap" design, originally published by Fujimori[39] in 1980, rotates two nasolabial island flaps through 90°. These flaps are based on the angular artery (Fig. 12.18). Although Fujimori's technique was fashioned for

the lower lip, modifications of the gate flap have also been proposed for total upper lip reconstruction.[40] Reconstruction with any of these nasolabial flap designs is associated with suboptimal oral competence and aesthetics, and denervation of the flaps is inevitable. In an effort to address the limitations of local flaps for large lip defects, some surgeons have employed the use of multiple local flaps. Kroll[41] advocated reconstructing large lower lip defects by re-establishing the oral sphincter with an extended Karapandzic flap, followed by two sequential Abbé flaps 3 weeks apart to augment the central lower lip and a commissure plasty to widen the oral aperture. The Abbé flaps were harvested from a philtral ridge so that the scar was relatively inconspicuous and any notching of the upper vermilion from scar contraction could be disguised as a peak in the Cupid's bow. Using this technique, Kroll noted that the transfer of redundant upper lip tissue improved the appearance and volume of the lower lip, particularly near the midline. In contrast, Williams and colleagues[24,25] reconstructed these defects by simultaneously performing a modified Bernard–Burow cheek advancement flap in combination with a medially based (Abbé) cross-lip flap. In contrast to Kroll's technique, they purport that less microstomia develops, and the orientation of the modiolus is not disturbed. Kroll's technique was described for lower lip defects, whereas Williams *et al.*'s approach can be used for upper and lower defects.

As we push these concepts to larger and larger defects, one must balance the advantages of having like tissue and competent lips with the disadvantages of adding a significant amount of additional scarring to the face, distortion seen with animation and the relative microstomia produced. These concerns have moved most surgeons to consider distant or free tissue transfers for defects approaching and greater than 80% of the lip.

The radial forearm flap is the free tissue transfer technique that is most frequently employed for the reconstruction of total lower lip defects. Sakai *et al.*[8] in 1989 reported the reconstruction of a lower lip defect with a composite radial forearm–palmaris longus tendon free flap. The forearm flap is folded over the tendon sling to resurface the internal and external surfaces of the lip and cheek. A microneural anastomosis between the lateral antebrachial cutaneous nerve and the cut end of the mental nerve can be performed to achieve sensory reinnervation.[42,43] A ventral tongue flap may be used to recreate the vermilion border, although a second procedure is necessary. Following flap reconstruction, medical tattooing can also be used to create the vermilion with acceptable cosmetic results.[44,45]

Oral competence and aesthetics are optimized for lower lip reconstruction by placing the palmaris longus tendon under the appropriate degree of tension. Lip entropion can develop if the palmaris longus tendon is inset too tightly (bow-strung), and ectropion may develop if inadequate tension is placed on the tendon. Sakai *et al.*[8] sutured the palmaris tendon to the orbicularis oris muscle and dermis in the nasolabial region to suspend the reconstruction. Other surgeons have reported good outcomes by suturing the tendon to the periosteum of the malar eminence or to the orbicularis muscle of the upper lip near the philtral columns.[42,46] Our personal preference is to weave the palmaris sling through the remaining orbicularis muscle and then through itself[47] or to mobilized lateral muscle components (i.e. internal Karapandzic technique).[48] Tension can be adjusted at the time of inset to optimize lip position. If adequate tension is placed on the tendon by the facial musculature at the modioli, the muscle action from the remaining facial muscles is transferred to the neolip, resulting in a more dynamic suspension. Using this technique, the tendon assumes some degree of dynamism because the orbicularis through which it is woven retains some function (Fig. 12.19).[49] Other surgeons have similarly chosen the modiolus as the preferred site of anchorage for the tendon.[47] The design of the radial forearm free flap directly impacts the ultimate functional and aesthetic result. In our experience, optimal suspensory support for the tendon is achieved by slightly overcorrecting the tension. It is important to ensure that the pedicle is not compressed when the flap is folded over the tendon. The best functional reconstruction using free flaps suspends the reconstructed lip skin independently of orbicularis sphincter restoration. Adequate suspension of the palmaris tendon alone will not eliminate lip ptosis and ectropion. Independent suspension of the skin segment may be accomplished by de-epithelializing skin tab extensions to be tacked to the malar areas[47] or by making the width of the flap narrower than the width of the defect (approx. 75%). Because the height of the skin excision and the mucosal resection usually differ, the skin and mucosal elements of the flap must be planned accordingly. Furthermore, fibrosis following surgery and radiation therapy tends to diminish the vertical height of the lip 6–12 months after reconstruction, so the vertical height of the reconstruction should be slightly greater than the height of the defect. It is also important to note that the height of the mucosal element of the lip will usually be shorter than the

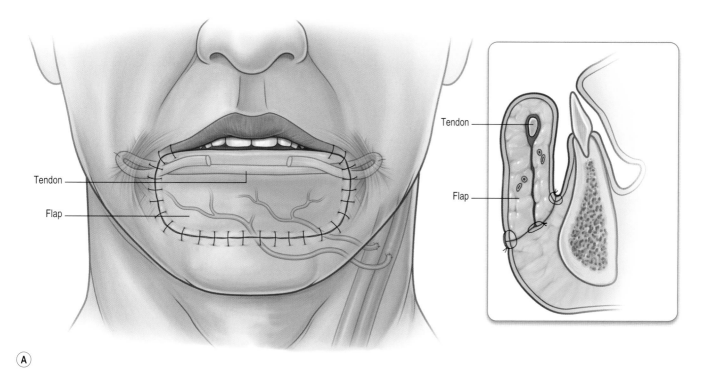

(A)

Fig. 12.19 (A) Schematic of palmaris/radial forearm flap reconstruction of the lower lip showing the Palmaris tendon woven through the remaining orbicularis muscle.

Continued

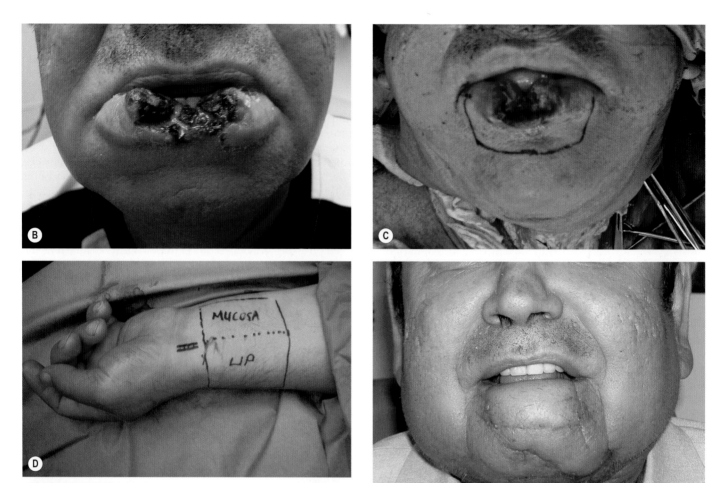

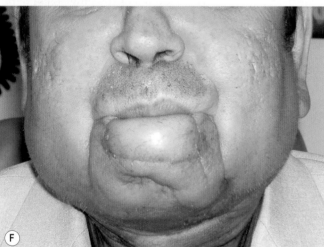

Fig. 12.19, cont'd **(B)** Patient shown with a large squamous cell carcinoma of the lower lip. **(C)** Resection of the lower lip planned. **(D)** The planned radial forearm flap. Note the different dimensions of the skin and mucosal segments of the flap. **(E)** Postoperative appearance. **(F)** Note that the patient can purse his lips and has good oral competence.

skin element. So these two elements of the defect need to be carefully measured so that the flap can be properly designed. The ultimate free flap reconstructive technique of the lip, which would also incorporate muscle between the inner and outer layers and restore the vermilion component, has not been described. Nevertheless, the composite radial forearm–palmaris longus tendon free flap has several advantages over pedicled flaps. This reconstruction allows for a single-stage procedure that results in complete skin coverage and intraoral lining. The large amount of skin that can be used with the radial forearm flap usually results in an adequate stomal size, minimizing the risk of microstomia. Although the color match between the radial forearm flap and surrounding facial tissue is frequently suboptimal, acceptable cosmetic results are attainable by respecting the borders of the aesthetic subunits during surgical resection and reconstructive planning. In Japan, temporalis, masseter, and depressor anguli oris muscle transfers have been used in place of the palmaris longus tendon to achieve a more dynamic functional result when the lower lip is reconstructed with a radial forearm flap.[50–52] Others have bridged the orbicularis muscle loss with innervated muscle flaps including a free gracilis muscle covered by a skin graft[53] or an innervated platysmal myocutaneous flap from the submental area of the neck[54]. The functional outcomes with these reconstructive approaches have not been rigorously evaluated, and a prospective assessment of oral competence and dynamic function should be conducted to compare the outcomes following the use of palmaris longus tendon and muscle transfer techniques.

Though most commonly used for the lower lip, the radial forearm flap has also been used for total upper lip reconstruction.[46] The abnormal color, texture and composition as well as the inability to recreate the fine, delicate curves and contours of the upper lip generally results in a less than acceptable aesthetic result, especially in woman and children. Reconstruction of >80% of the upper lip in men has been more successful by camouflaging the defect with hair-bearing scalp flaps.[7,48,55,56] The best results incorporate fascial spanning of orbicularis defects, a skin design that respects aesthetic units and hair growth in the correct direction.[48] These flaps tend to be thick and relatively stiff. If the patient chooses to shave the hair, multiple revisions are required to produce an acceptable aesthetic outcome.

Secondary procedures

Secondary procedures may sometimes be necessary. Simple scar revision may be necessary in situations where scarring is very prominent or where scar contracture causes a visible or functional deformity. The standard principles of scar revision apply; Z-plasty or W-plasty for tight scars, skin grafts or further local flaps to release contractures. A skin graft may be necessary, for example, to correct an entropion or ectropion of the lip that is due to scar contracture. Occasionally, a denervated lower lip will become ptotic and some sort of lip shortening procedure may be necessary. These operations, however, are not routine and which procedure to do on which patient will depend very much on the specific problem. One operation that is somewhat standardized, however, in secondary reconstruction, is the correction of microstomia. Fig. 12.20 shows a patient with post-burn microstomia corrected with

bilateral commissure plasty. This involves enlargement of the stomal opening by extending the commissure. The landmarks are the mid-pupillary lines. A vertical line dropped from the mid-pupil defines the normal position of the commissure. To correct microstomia, a through-and-through incision of the scar contracture is made from the commissure, horizontally to this line. The resulting raw areas are covered with mucosal rhomboid flaps (Fig. 12.21). Correction of microstomia caused by resection and reconstruction with, for example, Karapandzic flaps, is more challenging and surgical release as described above risks denervation and thereby limits the extent of microstomia correction possible. Initial attempts at stretching and splinting should be tried first. If surgical release is required, the continuity of the sphincteric orbicularis oris muscle should be maintained if at all possible. The boundaries of this muscle are hard to determine in these situations and it becomes a matter of judgment. In patients such as those depicted in Fig. 12.20, the microstomia is caused by scar contracture, so that when the microstomia is corrected it must be maintained by splinting.

Complications

Most of the complications encountered in lip reconstruction have already been alluded to earlier in this chapter. The standard complications that apply to any operation obviously apply in these repairs, and the patient must be counseled about the possibility of postoperative wound infection, wound dehiscence, bleeding, etc. With lip-switch procedures, and with the Abbé flap in particular, there is a risk of pedicle avulsion, and it is important to ensure that the pedicle is not too radically skeletonized. Not only can an exposed pedicle be avulsed but it can thrombose or bleed. Fortunately, this complication is rare. With free flap lip reconstruction, the standard risks of microsurgical procedures apply and include partial and total flap loss, as well as the complications associated with flap harvest. However, the complications that are most predictable are those of microstomia, denervation, oral incontinence and aesthetic deformity. All of these have been discussed earlier in this chapter.

Postoperative care

The protocol for postoperative care depends on the procedure performed. Oral hygiene is important whatever the procedure, particularly if there are sutures intra-orally. For extensive reconstructions, the patient may need to be on a liquid or soft diet for several days after the procedure. Patients often find it more comfortable to suck a liquid diet through a straw initially. This is particularly the case for patients who have had an Abbé flap. Regardless of the complexity of the reconstruction, patients are generally instructed to rinse with a mouthwash such as 0.12% chlorhexidine gluconate oral rinse after eating, for 4 or 5 days after the procedure. Patients need to be instructed about dental hygiene. Using a toothbrush in the early postoperative period may not only be uncomfortable but may disrupt suture lines. So the postoperative regimen for each patient will depend on the procedure performed and may need to be individualized. Fig. 12.22 presents an algorithmic approach to lip reconstruction.

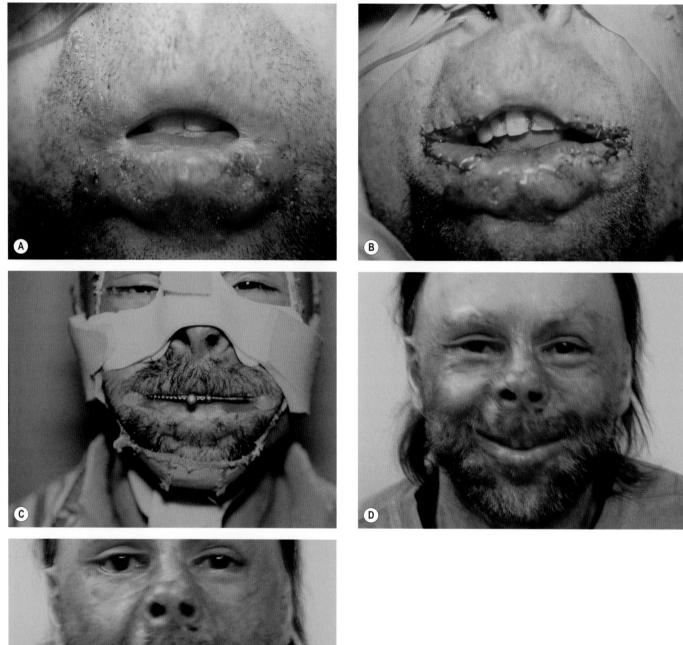

Fig. 12.20 **(A)** Patient with severe post-burn microstomia. **(B)** Patient appearance at the end of the commissure plasty. The rhomboid flaps are sutured at the mucocutaneous junction in upper and lower lips (see Fig. 12.16). **(C)** Patient seen wearing his splint postoperatively. This patient wore his splint, except to eat, for 6 months. **(D,E)** At 10 year follow-up, showing maintenance of commissure position and excellent function.

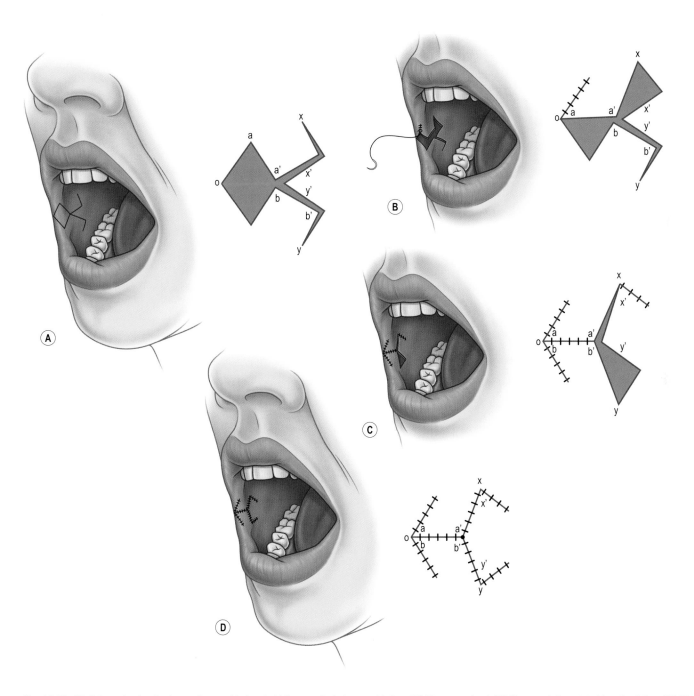

Fig. 12.21 **(A)** Schematic of split of commissure with rhomboid flaps marked above and below. **(B)** Flaps are raised. **(C)** Flaps are being rotated into the defect. **(D)** Flaps rotated into the defect; secondary defect closed by direct approximation.

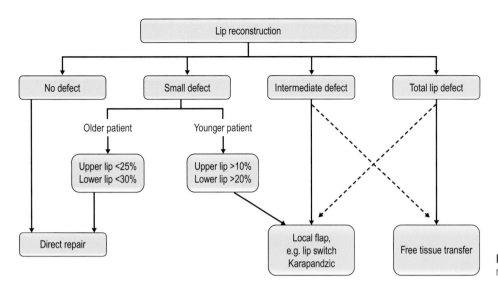

Fig. 12.22 An algorithmic approach to lip reconstruction.

🌐 Access the complete reference list online at   **http://www.expertconsult.com**

1. Neligan PC. Strategies in lip reconstruction. *Clin Plast Surg.* 2009;36:477–485. *Injury or surgical trauma can result in significant alterations of normal lip appearance and function that can profoundly impact the patient's self-image and quality of life. Neuromuscular injury can lead to asymmetry at rest and during facial animation, and distressing functional disabilities are common. Loss of labial competence may interfere with the ability to articulate, whistle, suck, kiss, and contain salivary secretions. For smaller defects, reconstruction can be very effective. Reconstructing an aesthetically pleasing and functional lip is more difficult with larger defects.*

4. Karapandzic M. Reconstruction of lip defects by local arterial flaps. *Br J Plast Surg.* 1974;27:93–97.

21. Langstein H, Robb G. Lip and perioral reconstruction. *Clin Plast Surg.* 2005;32:431–445.

23. Cordeiro PG, Santamaria E. Primary reconstruction of complex midfacial defects with combined lip-switch procedures and free flaps. *Plast Reconstr Surg.* 1999;103:1850–1856. *Free flaps are generally the preferred method for reconstructing large defects of the midface, orbit, and maxilla that include the lip and oral commissure; commissuroplasty is traditionally performed at a second stage. Functional results of the oral sphincter using this reconstructive approach are, however, limited. This article presents a new approach to the reconstruction of massive defects of the lip and midface using a free flap in combination with a lip-switch flap. This was used in 10 patients. One-third to one-half of the upper lip was excised in seven patients, one-third of the lower lip was excised in one patient, and both the upper and lower lips were excised (one-third each) in two patients. All patients had maxillectomies, with or without mandibulectomies, in addition to full-thickness resections of the cheek. A*

switch flap from the opposite lip was used for reconstruction of the oral commissure and oral sphincter, and a rectus abdominis myocutaneous flap with two or three skin islands was used for reconstruction of the through-and-through defect in the midface. Free flap survival was 100%. All patients had good-to-excellent oral competence, and they were discharged without feeding tubes.

30. Webster J. Crescentic peri-alar cheek excision for upper lip flap advancement with a short history of upper lip repair. *Plast Reconstr Surg.* 1955;16:434–464.

31. Abbe R. A new plastic operation for the relief of deformity due to double harelip. *Plast Reconstr Surg.* 1968;42:481–483.

41. Kroll SS. Staged sequential flap reconstruction for large lower lip defects. *Plast Reconstr Surg.* 1991;88:620–627.

46. Jeng SF, Kuo YR, Wei FC, et al. Total lower lip reconstruction with a composite radial forearm-palmaris longus tendon flap: a clinical series. *Plast Reconstr Surg.* 2004;113:19–23. *Large, full-thickness lip defects after head and neck surgery continue to be a challenge for reconstructive surgeons. The reconstructive aims are to restore the oral lining, the external cheek, oral competence, and function (i.e., articulation, speech, and mastication). These authors' refinement of the composite radial forearm–palmaris longus free flap technique meets these criteria and allows a functional reconstruction of extensive lip and cheek defects in one stage. A composite radial forearm flap including the palmaris longus tendon was designed. The skin flap for the reconstruction of the intraoral lining and the skin defect was folded over the palmaris longus tendon. Both ends of the vascularized tendon were laid through the bilateral modiolus and anchored with adequate tension to the intact orbicularis muscle of the upper lip. This procedure was used in 12 patients.*

13

Facial paralysis

Ronald M. Zuker, Eyal Gur, Gazi Hussain, and Ralph T. Manktelow

Access video content for this chapter online at expertconsult.com

SYNOPSIS

- Assess clinical problem: functional, psychosocial, and aesthetic.
- Understand the etiology and natural history of disease processes associated with facial paralysis.
- Knowledge of anatomy is imperative for optimizing results.
- Formulate realistic, attainable, and practical management plan.
- Surgical management is multifocal and must be individualized for each patient.

Introduction

Facial paralysis is a complex multifaceted condition with profound functional deficiencies, devastating aesthetic effects, and tragic psychological consequences. It may be congenital or acquired, affect the old and the young, and vary from mild to severe. In this chapter we will focus on the clinical problem and the surgical solutions available today.

 Access the Historical Perspective section online at
http://expertconsult.com

Anatomy

As a backdrop to the clinical management of facial paralysis, a detailed description of the anatomy of the facial nerve and the facial musculature is described below.

The facial nerve

The extratemporal portion of the seventh cranial nerve begins at the stylomastoid foramen. It is in a deep position below the earlobe but becomes more superficial before it passes between the superficial and deep portions of the parotid gland. Here it divides into two main trunks which then further divide

within the substance of the gland. In a series of anatomic dissections, Davis et al.[1] demonstrated several branching patterns of the facial nerve. Traditionally, it is taught that this results in five divisions of the facial nerve: frontotemporal, zygomatic, buccal, marginal mandibular, and cervical. In practice, however, there is no distinct separation between the zygomatic and buccal branches either in their location or in the muscles they innervate.

On leaving the parotid, the facial nerve may have eight to 15 branches making up the five divisions. Distally, there is further arborization and interconnection of these branches (Fig. 13.1). The net effect is a great deal of functional overlap between the branches. For example, a single zygomaticobuccal branch may supply innervation to the orbicularis oculi as well as to the orbicularis oris.

The temporal division consists of three or four branches[2] that run obliquely along the undersurface of the temporoparietal fascia after crossing the zygomatriarch in a location 3–5 cm from the lateral orbital margin. The lower branches run along the undersurface of the superior portion of the orbicularis oculi for 3–4 mm before entering the muscle to innervate it.[3] According to Ishikawa,[2] the upper two branches entering the frontalis muscle at the level of the supraorbital ridge are usually located up to 3 cm above the lateral canthus. The nerves usually lie approximately 1.6 cm inferior to the frontal branch of the superficial temporal artery. Because there is relatively little adipose tissue at the lateral border of the frontalis, those nerves are virtually subcutaneous and susceptible to injury.

The zygomaticobuccal division consists of five to eight branches with significant overlap of muscle innervations such that one or more branches may be divided without causing weakness. These nerves supply innervations to the lip elevators as well as to the lower orbicularis oculi, orbicularis oris, and buccinators. Functional facial nerve mapping and cross-facial nerve grafting require the precise identification and stimulation of these zygomaticobuccal branches to isolate the exact branches responsible for smiling. These nerves lie deep near the parotid-masseteric fascia in the same plane as the

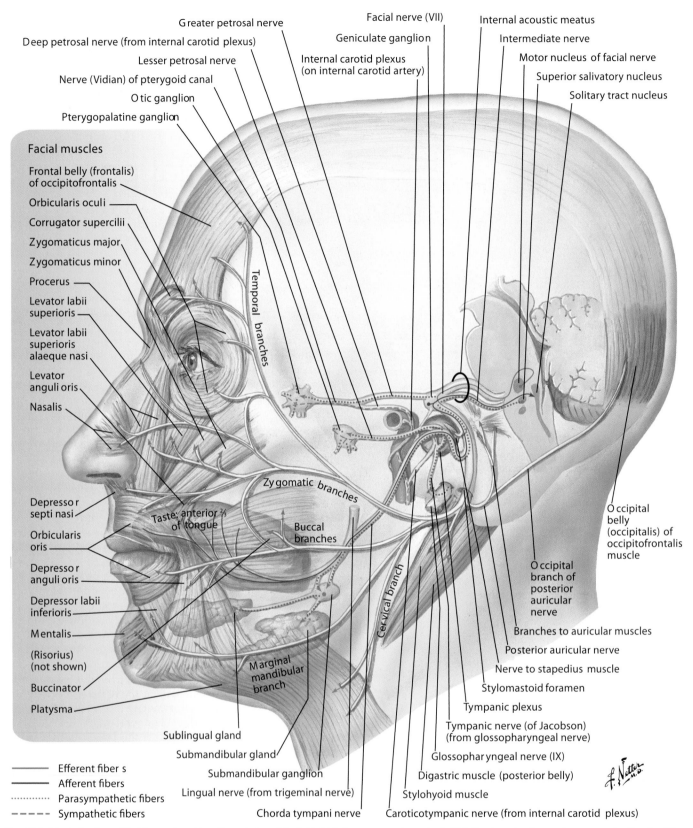

Greater petrosal nerve

Facial nerve (VII)

Internal acoustic meatus

Deep petrosal nerve (from internal carotid plexus)

Geniculate ganglion

Intermediate nerve

Lesser petrosal nerve

Internal carotid plexus
(on internal carotid artery)

Motor nucleus of facial nerve

Nerve (Vidian) of pterygoid canal

Superior salivatory nucleus

Otic ganglion

Solitary tract nucleus

Pterygopalatine ganglion

Facial muscles

Frontal belly (frontalis)
of occipitofrontalis

Orbicularis oculi

Corrugator supercilii

Zygomaticus major

Zygomaticus minor

Procerus

Levator labii
superioris

Levator labii
superioris
alaeque nasi

Levator
anguli oris

Nasalis

Temporal branches

Depressor
septi nasi

Zygomatic branches

Taste: anterior ⅔
of tongue

Buccal
branches

Occipital
belly
(occipitalis) of
occipitofrontalis
muscle

Orbicularis
oris

Depressor
anguli oris

Depressor labii
inferioris

Cervical branch

Occipital
branch of
posterior
auricular
nerve

Mentalis

(Risorius)
(not shown)

Buccinator

Platysma

Marginal
mandibular
branch

Branches to auricular muscles

Posterior auricular nerve

Nerve to stapedius muscle

Stylomastoid foramen

Tympanic plexus

Sublingual gland

Tympanic nerve (of Jacobson)
(from glossopharyngeal nerve)

Submandibular gland

Glossopharyngeal nerve (IX)

———— Efferent fibers

———— Afferent fibers

Submandibular ganglion

Digastric muscle (posterior belly)

·············· Parasympathetic fibers

Lingual nerve (from trigeminal nerve)

Stylohyoid muscle

– – – – Sympathetic fibers

Chorda tympani nerve

Caroticotympanic nerve (from internal carotid plexus)

Fig. 13.1 A typical pattern of facial nerve branching. The main branch is divided into two components, each of which then branches in a random manner to all parts of the face. The extensive distal arborization and interconnections are apparent. *(Reprinted with permission from www.netterimages.com ©Elsevier Inc. All rights reserved.)*

parotid duct. There are sometimes connections between the lower branches and the marginal mandibular division.

The marginal mandibular division consists of one to three branches[4] whose course begins up to 2 cm below the ramus of the mandible and arcs upward to cross the mandible halfway between the angle and mental protuberance. It has been well documented[2,3,5] that these branches lie on the deep surface of the platysma and cross superficial to the facial vessels approximately 3.5 cm from the parotid edge. Nelson and Gingrass[5] described separate branches to the depressor angularis, depressor labii inferioris, and mentalis, and a variable superior ramus supplying the upper platysma and lower orbicularis oris.

The cervical division consists of one branch that leaves the parotid well below the angle of the mandible and runs on the deep surface of the platysma, which it innervates by entering the muscle at the junction of its cranial and middle thirds. This point of entry is 2 or 3 cm caudal to the platysma muscle branch of the facial vessel.[6]

Facial musculature

Facial musculature consists of 17 paired muscles and one unpaired sphincter muscle, the orbicularis oris (Fig. 13.2). The subtle movements that convey facial expression require coordination between all of these muscles.

The major muscles affecting the forehead and eyelids are the frontalis, corrugator, and orbicularis oculi. There are two main groups of muscles controlling the movement of the lips. The lip retractors include the levator labii superioris, levator anguli oris, zygomaticus major and minor for the upper lip, and depressor labii inferioris and depressor anguli oris for the lower lip. The antagonist of these lip-retracting muscles is the orbicularis oris, which is responsible for oral continence and some expressive movements of the lips.

Freilinger et al.[3] have demonstrated that the mimetic muscles are arranged in four layers. The depressor anguli oris, part of the zygomaticus minor, and the orbicularis oculi are the most superficial, whereas the buccinators, mentalis, and levator anguli oris make up the deepest layer. Except for the three deep muscles, all other facial muscles receive innervation from nerves entering their deep surfaces.

The muscles that are clinically important or most often require surgical management in patients with facial paralysis are the frontalis, orbicularis oculi, zygomaticus major, levator labii superioris, orbicularis oris, and depressor labii inferioris.

The frontalis muscle is a bilateral, broad sheet-like muscle 5–6 cm in width and 1 mm thick.[4] The muscle takes origin from the galea aponeurotica at various levels near the coronal suture and inserts on to the superciliary ridge of the frontal bone and into fibers of the orbicularis oculi, procerus, and corrugators supercilii. It is firmly adherent to the skin through multiple fibrous septa but glides over the underlying periosteum. The two muscles fuse in the midline caudally; however, this is often a fibrous junction. Not only is the frontalis essential to elevate the brow, but also its tone at rest keeps the brow from descending. This tone is lost in the patient with facial paralysis, which allows the brow to fall and potentially obscure upward gaze.

The orbicularis oculi muscle acts as a sphincter to close the eyelids. Upper eyelid opening is performed by the levator palpebrae superioris muscle innervated by the third cranial

nerve and the Müller muscle, which is a smooth fiber muscle innervated by the sympathetic nervous system. The orbicularis oculi muscle is one continuous muscle but has three subdivisions: pretarsal, covering the tarsal plate; preseptal portions, overlying the orbital septum; and the orbital, forming a ring over the orbital margin. The pretarsal and preseptal portions function together when a patient blinks, whereas the orbital portion is recruited during forceful eye closure and to lower the eyebrows. According to Jelks and Jelks,[7] the preseptal portion of the orbicularis oculi is under voluntary control, whereas the pretarsal provides reflex movement.

The pretarsal orbicularis oculi overlies the tarsal plate of the upper and lower eyelids. The tarsal plates are thin, elongated plates of connective tissue that support the eyelids. The superior tarsal plate is 8–10 mm in vertical height at its center but tapers medially and laterally, whereas the inferior tarsal plate is 3.8–4.5 mm in vertical height. The skin overlying the pretarsal orbicularis is the thinnest in the body and is adherent to the muscle over the tarsal plate. The skin is more lax and mobile over the preseptal and orbital regions. The eyelid skin also becomes thicker over the orbital part of the muscle. The preseptal orbicularis provides support to the orbital septa and is more mobile except at the medial and lateral canthi, where the muscle is firmly attached to the skin. The orbital portion of the orbicularis oculi extends in a wide circular fashion around the orbit. It originates medially from the superomedial orbital margin, the maxillary process of the frontal bone, the medial canthal tendon, the frontal process of the maxilla, and the inferomedial margin of the orbit. In the upper eyelid, the fibers sweep upward into the forehead and cover the frontalis and corrugators supercilii muscles; the fibers continue laterally to be superficial to the temporalis fascia.[8,9] Because this muscle is one of the superficial group of mimetic muscles,[10] in the lower eyelid the orbital portion lies over the origins of the zygomaticus major, levator labii superioris, levator labii superioris alaeque nasi, and part of the origin of the masseter muscle. There are multiple motor nerve branches that supply the upper and lower portions of the orbicularis oculi, and these enter the muscle just medial to its lateral edge.

Freilinger et al.[3] extensively studied the three major lip elevators, zygomaticus major, levator labii superioris, and levator anguli oris, and provided data on their length, width, and thickness (Table 13.1).

The zygomaticus major takes origin from the lower lateral portion of the body of the zygoma; the orbicularis oculi and zygomaticus minor cover its upper part. Its course is along a line roughly from the helical root of the ear to the commissure

Table 13.1 Dimensions of the levators of the upper lip			
Muscle	Length (mm)	Width (mm)	Thickness (mm)
Zygomaticus major	70	8	2
Levator labii superioris	34	25	1.8
Levator anguli oris	38	14	1.7

(Reproduced from Freilinger G, Gruber, Happak W, et al. Surgical anatomy of the mimic muscle system and the facial nerve: importance for reconstructive and aesthetic surgery. *Plast Reconstr Surg*. 1987;80:686.)

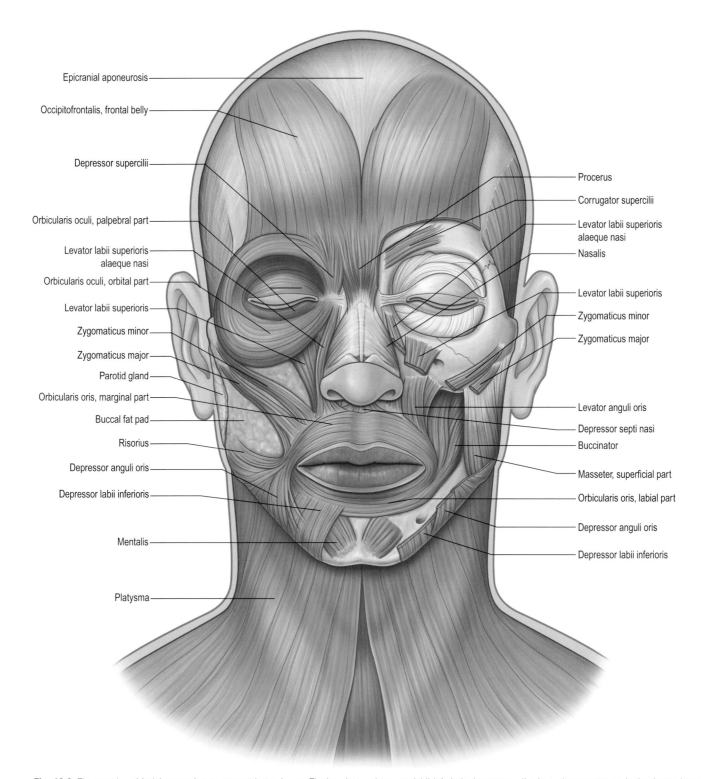

Fig. 13.2 The muscles of facial expression are present in two layers. The buccinator, depressor labii inferioris, levator anguli oris, and corrugator are in the deeper layer.

of the mouth, where it leads into the modiolus. The modiolus is the point of common attachment at which the fibers of the zygomaticus major and minor, orbicularis oris, buccinator, risorius, levator anguli oris, and depressor anguli oris come together. Deep fibers of the zygomaticus major are angled upward from the modiolus to fuse with the levator anguli oris, whereas caudal fibers continue into the depressor anguli

oris. The main nerve to the zygomaticus major enters the deep surface of the upper third of the muscle.

The levator labii superioris originates along the lower portion of the orbital margin above the infraorbital foramen. The muscle courses inferiorly, partially inserting into the nasolabial crease. The lateral fibers pass inferiorly into the orbicularis oris, and the deepest fibers form part of the

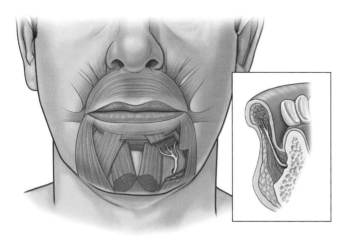

Fig. 13.3 The depressor anguli oris can be seen in the corner of the mouth. Muscle contraction pulls the corner of the mouth down as in the expression of sadness. The depressor labii inferioris goes into the orbicularis oris of the mid lateral portion of the lower lip and pulls the lip down. The muscle's function is apparent in an open-mouth smile showing the lower teeth. The mental nerve lies on the deep surface of the depressor labii inferioris.

modiolus. The nerve to this muscle reaches it by first passing underneath the zygomaticus major muscle to supply the levator labii superioris on its deep surface.

The levator anguli oris is the third lip elevator. It takes origin from the maxilla below the infraorbital foramen and inserts into the modiolus. Because this muscle belongs to the deepest layer, it is innervated on its superficial surface by the same branch that supplies innervation to the buccinator.

Three muscles along with the zygomaticus minor serve to elevate the lip. The zygomaticus muscles move the commissure at an angle of approximately 45°, the levator anguli oris elevates the commissure vertically and medially, and the levator labii superioris elevates the lip vertically and laterally to expose the upper teeth.

The orbicularis oris is a complex muscle that functions as far more than a sphincter of the mouth; it serves to pucker and purse the lips. It makes up the bulk of the lip, as skin overlies it superficially and mucous membrane is attached on its deep surface. Philtral columns are formed by the insertion of the orbicularis, and a portion of levator labii superioris, into the skin.[11] The levator labii superioris fibers reach the philtral columns by coursing above the surface of the orbicularis oris to insert into the lower philtral columns and vermilion border as far medially as the peak of Cupid's bow. Anatomically and functionally, the orbicularis oris muscle consists of two parts, superficial and deep. The deep layers of the muscle encircle the orifice of the mouth and function as a constrictor. The superficial component also brings the lips together, but its fibers can contract independently to provide expression.[12]

The lower lip depressors consist of the depressor labii inferioris, also known as the quadratus labii inferioris, and the depressor anguli oris, also known as the triangularis (Fig. 13.3). The mentalis, however, is not a lip depressor. Its indirect action on the lip is to elevate it.[8] The depressor labii inferioris arises from the lateral surface of the mandible, which is inferior and lateral to the mental foramen. It runs medially and superiorly to insert into the lower border of the orbicularis

oris and its surface. Through fibrous septa, it attaches to the vermilion and the skin of the middle third of one side of the lip.[9] Its action is to draw the lower lip downward and laterally and to evert the vermilion (e.g., as in showing the lower teeth). The depressor anguli oris arises from the mandible laterally and is superficial to the depressor labii inferioris. The medial fibers insert directly into the skin at the labiomandibular crease; the remainder blend into the modiolus.[13] It depresses the angle of the mouth (e.g., in frowning).

Diagnosis and patient presentation

Facial paralysis is a complex clinical problem with numerous consequences affecting the function, self-image, and social interactions of those afflicted and their families (Fig. 13.4). Function of the muscles vital for the protection of the eye, maintenance of the nasal airway, oral continence, and clear speech may be lost. These muscles support the face at rest and enable an individual to wink, pucker the lips, and express emotions of surprise, joy, anger, and sorrow.

Brow ptosis is more commonly a problem in the older patient. The weight of the forehead tissue may cause sagging of the eyebrow inferiorly over the superior orbital margin, which causes an asymmetric shape and obstructs the upward gaze. This may be complicated by over activity of the contralateral frontalis muscle, which increases the discrepancy between eyebrow height. At rest, the depressed eyebrow gives the impression of unhappiness or excessive seriousness. With animation, the asymmetry of the brows and wrinkling of the forehead are accentuated.

The orbicularis oculi muscle is crucial for the protection of the eye. It enables eyelid closure and provides a physical barrier against wind and foreign matter. Repetitive blinking is also important for control of the even spread of tear film in

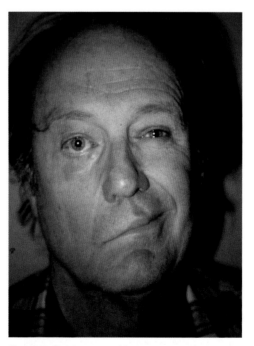

Fig. 13.4 Facial paralysis produces marked asymmetry at rest between the paralyzed side and the non-paralyzed side. The asymmetry is particularly severe in the older patient.

a lateral to medial direction to prevent drying of the cornea. The effective drainage of tears is also dependent on a functioning orbicularis oculi muscle; its action on the lacrimal sac establishes a pump-like effect that facilitates the efficient clearance of tears.

When the eyelids are open, the distance between the upper and lower eyelid is 9–11 mm at its widest point. In the neutral gaze position, the upper eyelid covers 2–3 mm of the superior corneal limbus; the lower eyelid lies at the level of the inferior corneal limbus. Thus, there is normally no sclera showing.

With eye closure, the majority of movement occurs in the upper eyelid while the lower lid remains relatively static. However, with squinting or smiling, there is up to 2 mm of upward movement in the lower eyelid. The main function of the inferior orbicularis oculi is the maintenance of lid margin contact with the globe and assistance with tear damage.

Patients with facial paralysis are troubled by significant discomfort in the eye because of corneal exposure and desiccation. This drying frequently produces a reflex tear flow. Excessive tears poorly managed by the paralyzed eyelids result in overflow. Therefore, patients with dry eyes often present with excessive tearing. This tearing problem can be distressing and is exacerbated by the downward inclination of the face (e.g., during reading).

The appearance of the paralyzed eye is also of concern to the patient. The eye has a widened palpebral aperture and is unable to convey expression. Thus, when the patient smiles, the paralyzed eyelids remain open instead of slightly closing. With the passage of time, the lower eyelid develops an ectropion, causing the inferior lacrimal punctum to pull away from the eye. An ectropion further exacerbates tearing and increases the risk of excessive corneal exposure.

The other major concern for patients with facial paralysis is the inability to control their lips. This affects the patient's ability to speak, eat, and drink properly. For example, many patients with facial paralysis have difficulty producing *b* and *p* sounds. Buccinator paralysis leads to problems in the control of food boluses. Food tends to pocket in the buccal sulcus of the paralyzed portion of the face; therefore, many patients chew only on the contralateral side. This type of paralysis also severely affects normal facial expressions. The main complaint heard from patients is their inability to smile. This should not be regarded as an aesthetic issue. It is a functional disability because it directly impairs communication. Paralysis of the orbicularis oris results in drooling and difficulty in controlling the mouth (e.g., drinking from a glass).

The emotional effects of facial paralysis cannot be overestimated. The unilaterally paralyzed face presents obvious asymmetry at rest, exacerbated by an attempt to smile (Fig. 13.5). As a result, these patients avoid situations in which they are required to smile. They become characterized as serious and unhappy, and their psychosocial functioning is frequently poor. A patient with bilateral facial paralysis has severe disability because their face cannot convey emotion.

Classification

In the formulation of a treatment plan, it is helpful to have a practical and clinically oriented classification. This will facilitate sound decision making and realistic surgical planning. Facial paralysis can take many forms. It can be classified anatomically and as congenital or acquired, and it can be

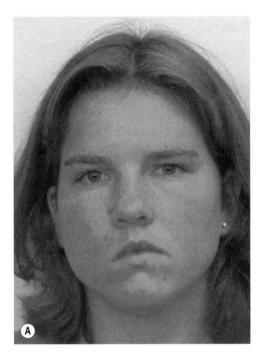

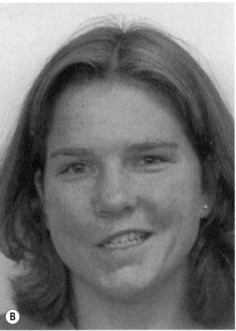

Fig. 13.5 (A) At rest, the right-sided partial facial paralysis in this young woman is minimally evident, as seen by a slight deviation of the mouth to her left and a slightly wider palpebral aperture in her right eye. **(B)** With smiling, the asymmetry becomes more apparent.

broken down further into unilateral or bilateral categories.[14] In addition, the degree of muscle involvement varies from total to partial paralysis. More than 50% of patients with facial paralysis suffer from Bell's palsy and often recover fully.

Congenital facial paralysis is present at birth. This is the most common form of facial paralysis seen in a pediatric setting. It may be isolated with the involvement of the facial nerve and its musculature only, or it may be part of a syndrome.

It is estimated that facial paralysis occurs in 2.0% of live births.[15] In the majority of patients, it is believed to be the result of intrauterine pressure on the developing fetus from the sacral prominence. The facial nerve is superficial and easily compressed. This leads to the panfacial type and buccal branch variety of congenital facial paralysis. It is believed, however, that the mandibular branch component and syndromic forms of facial paralysis may have a different etiology. In the authors' experience, the cause of unilateral facial paralysis was congenital in two-thirds of patients encountered and acquired in one-third of patients. Acquired facial paralysis resulted from intracranial tumors in 50% of patients, and acquired facial paralysis from extracranial trauma. The majority of traumas were related to surgical procedures, most commonly cystic hygroma excision. In infants, the nerve is superficial at birth and can easily be traumatized through external compression or surgical misadventure. In contrast, the cause of facial paralysis for the majority of adults is acquired, from either intracranial lesions or inflammatory processes, such as Bell's palsy.

Congenital facial paralysis may be syndromic. The most common unilateral syndromic condition associated with facial paralysis is hemifacial microsomia. All tissues of the face can be affected to a variable degree, including the facial nerve musculature. The most common bilateral congenital facial paralysis is a result of Möbius syndrome. The functional effects of congenital facial paralysis tend to worsen gradually as the influence of gravity and aging prevails.

Bilateral facial paralysis may be the result of bilateral intracranial tumors or bilateral skull base trauma, but it is usually found to be the congenital bilateral facial paralysis or Möbius syndrome. Various cranial nerves accompany the seventh nerve's involvement, specifically the sixth, ninth, 10th, and 12th. Möbius syndrome is also associated with trunk and limb anomalies in about one-third of patients, the most common being talipes equinovarus and a variety of hand anomalies, including Poland syndrome. Cranial nerve involvement is usually bilateral and severe but often incomplete. There is frequently some residual function in the lower component of the face (the cervical and mandibular branch regions). The incidence of Möbius syndrome is estimated to be about 1 in 200 000 live births.

Acquired facial paralysis may also be unilateral or bilateral through local disruption of the nerve at various locations. Damage to the nerve may be intracranial in the nucleus or the peripheral nerve, extracranial in the peripheral nerve, or the result of damage to the muscle itself. Intracranial and extracranial neoplasms, Bell's palsy, and trauma are the most common causes seen in the adult setting. Although recovery is the rule in Bell's palsy, at least 10% of patients are left with some degree of paralysis. Bilateral acquired facial paralysis is usually the result of skull base fractures, intracranial lesions, usually in the brainstem, or intracranial surgery.

Throughout all of these areas, however, facial paralysis constitutes a spectrum of involvement. It may be complete or incomplete to varying degrees, obvious in some patients, and subtle in others (Table 13.2).

Patient selection

Facial paralysis patients present with a broad spectrum of signs and symptoms. Thus, treatment varies from individual to individual. A thorough history and examination will reveal the presence of a complete or partial seventh-nerve paralysis and, if the paralysis is partial, the specific muscles affected and the extent of the paralysis. Has there been any return of function? Is this improvement continuing or has it reached a plateau? The history must include any eye symptoms, such

Table 13.2 Classification of facial paralysis
Extracranial
Traumatic
Facial lacerations Blunt forces Penetrating wounds Mandible fractures Iatrogenic injuries Newborn paralysis
Neoplastic
Parotid tumors Tumors of the external canal and middle ear Facial nerve neurinomas Metastatic lesions
Congenital absence of facial musculature
Intratemporal
Traumatic
Fractures of petrous pyramid Penetrating injuries Iatrogenic injuries
Neoplastic
Glomus tumors Cholesteatoma Facial neurinomas Squamous cell carcinomas Rhabdomyosarcoma Arachnoidal cysts Metastatic
Infectious
Herpes zoster oticus Acute otitis media Malignant otitis externa
Idiopathic
Bell palsy Melkersson–Rosenthal syndrome
Congenital: osteopetrosis
Intracranial
Iatrogenic injury
Neoplastic – benign, malignant, primary, metastatic
Congenital
Absence of motor units
Syndromic
Hemifacial microsomia (unilateral) Möbius syndrome (bilateral)

as dryness, excessive tearing, incomplete closure, discomfort when the patient is outdoors, and use of artificial tears. The patient should be questioned about the nasal airway, oral continence, speech, and level of psychosocial functioning and social interactions.

The patient's concerns and expectations must be sought. For some, attaining a symmetric appearance at rest is more important than achieving a smile. In comparison to the younger patient, the older patient is more likely to be worried about brow ptosis, ectropion, and drooping of the cheek.

The level of injury to the nerve, if it is not known, can be assessed clinically. Injury to the nerve within the bony canal may result in loss of ipsilateral taste appreciation, hyperacusis, and facial weakness because the chorda tympani and nerve to the stapedius may be injured at this level. Injury to the seventh cranial nerve near the geniculate ganglion will also result in decreased secretory function of the nose, mouth, and lacrimal gland.

Examination of the face begins with the brow. Its position at rest and with movement must be noted. The superior visual field may be diminished by the ptotic brow.

The eye must be thoroughly assessed. Visual acuity in each eye should be documented. The height of the palpebral aperture should be measured and compared with the non-paralyzed side. The degree of lagophthalmos and the presence of a Bell reflex will indicate the risk of corneal exposure. The lower eyelid position should be measured. Tone in the lower eyelid can be assessed by the use of the snap test. This is done by gently pulling the eyelid away from the globe and releasing it. The eyelid normally snaps back against the globe; however, this fails to occur in the patient with poor lid tone. The position of the inferior canalicular punctum should be assessed. Is it applied to the globe or is it rolled away and exposed? In addition, the patient should be examined for corneal irritation or ulceration.

The nasal airway is examined next. Forced inspiration may reveal a collapsed nostril due to loss of muscle tone in the dilator naris and drooping of the cheek. An intranasal examination should also be done.

Examination of the mouth and surrounding structures documents the amount of philtral deviation, the presence or absence of a nasolabial fold, the amount of commissure depression and deviation, the degree to which the upper lip droops, and the presence of vermilion inversion. With animation, the amount of bilateral commissure movement is recorded; it is also noted how much of the upper incisors show when the patient is smiling. Speech should be assessed. An intraoral examination is performed to check dental hygiene and to look for evidence of cheek biting.

The presence of synkinesis, the simultaneous contraction of two or more groups of muscles that normally do not contract together,[16] should be documented. Synkinesis is thought to occur from a misdirected sprouting of axons. The most common types of synkinesis are eye closure with smiling,[17] brow wrinkling when the mouth is moved,[18] and mouth grimacing when the eyes are closed.

An assessment of the other cranial nerves, particularly the fifth, is also performed. Cranial nerve involvement may exacerbate the morbidity of facial nerve paralysis. These nerves should also be assessed as possible donor motor nerves.

Treatment: nonsurgical and surgical

Planning, priorities, and expectations

As has been stressed previously, treatment must be individualized. However, in general, the aims of treatment are to protect the eye, to provide symmetry at rest, and then to provide movement. The ultimate goal is to restore involuntary, independent, and spontaneous facial expression. The goals of treatment for the eye are to maintain vision, to provide protection, to maintain function of the eyelids, to improve cosmesis, and to enable the eye to express emotion. The goals for the mouth are to correct asymmetry, to provide oral continence, to improve speech, and to provide a balanced symmetric smile that the patient will use in social settings. Clearly, the accomplishment of all these goals is difficult, and they cannot be achieved completely.

The patient must be counseled as to what are real and achievable expectations. It is clearly impossible to restore intricate movements to all facial muscles, and the patient who is appropriately informed is more likely to be satisfied with his or her outcome.

Nonsurgical management

Nonsurgical management of the patient with facial paralysis applies primarily to the eye and can frequently make the difference between a comfortable eye and a painful one. Nonsurgical maneuvers can protect the eye while surgery is being planned and are regularly used in concert with the surgical management of the eye. In some instances, surgery may be avoided. Nonsurgical management of the eye consists of protecting the eye and maintaining eye lubrication (Table 13.3).

Eye lubrication can be provided by a number of commercially available preparations. This includes clear watery drops containing either hydroxypropyl methylcellulose or polyvinyl alcohol along with other agents including preservatives. These drops function by absorbing into the cornea and lubricating it. Although the duration of action will vary, most are retained on the surface of the eye between 45 and 120 min.[19] Thus, to be most effective, they should be instilled frequently during the day. Thicker ointments containing petrolatum, mineral water, or lanolin alcohol are retained longer and can be used at night to protect and "seal" the eyelids during sleep. The patient who presents with excessive tearing may in fact have a dry eye and may benefit from the use of artificial tears. Corneal ulceration should be managed with prompt referral for ophthalmologic assessment.

Table 13.3 **Nonsurgical maneuvers to protect the eye**
Lid taping, particularly while sleeping
Soft contact lenses
Moisture chambers, which can be taped to the skin around the orbit
Modification of spectacles to provide a lateral shield
Forced blinking exercises in a patient with weak eye closure
Eye patches
Temporary tarsorrhaphy

Table 13.4 **Most common surgical options for each region of the face**

Brow (brow ptosis)
Direct brow lift (direct excision) Coronal brow lift with static suspension Endoscopic brow lift
Upper eyelid (lagophthalmos)
Gold weight Temporalis transfer Spring Tarsorrhaphy
Lower eyelid (ectropion)
Tendon sling Lateral canthoplasty Horizontal lid shortening Temporalis transfer Cartilage graft
Nasal airway
Static sling Alar base elevation Septoplasty
Commissure and upper lip
Nerve transfer either directly or via nerve graft to reinnervate recently paralyzed muscles Microneurovascular muscle transplantation with the use of ipsilateral seventh nerve, cross-facial nerve graft, or other cranial nerve for motor innervation Temporalis transposition with or without masseter transposition Static slings Soft-tissue balancing procedures (rhytidectomy, mucosal excision or advancement)
Lower lip
Depressor labii inferioris resection (on normal side) Muscle transfer (digastric, platysma) Wedge excision

In patients in whom there is incomplete facial nerve paralysis or recovering muscle activity after nerve injury, function may be improved with neuromuscular retraining supervised by an experienced therapist. This consists of various treatment modalities such as biofeedback, electromyography, and self-directed mirror exercises using slow, small, and symmetric movements.[20] Patients can often relearn some facial movements or strengthen movements that are weak.

Surgical management (Videos 13.1 and 13.2 ●)

Deciding on a surgical procedure can initially seem daunting. There are a number to choose from, and selecting the most appropriate reconstruction may be confusing. It is important to listen to each patient carefully to identify which aspects of the paralysis are most troublesome and to treat each region of the face separately. The age of the patient, duration of the facial paralysis, condition of the facial musculature and soft tissues, and status of the potential donor nerves and muscles will all influence treatment options. One must consider the patient's needs carefully and match the needs of the patient with the skill of the surgeon (Table 13.4).

Brow

There are at least three approaches to a brow lift: direct excision of the tissue above the brow (direct brow lift), open brow lift performed through a coronal incision, and endoscopic brow lift. Unilateral frontalis paralysis may cause a difference in brow heights of up to 12 mm. A direct brow lift is best able to correct such a large discrepancy. Direct brow lift involves excision of a segment of skin and frontalis muscle just above and parallel to the eyebrow. If the incision is placed just along the first line of hair follicles, the resulting scar is usually less noticeable. Frontalis shortening by excision and repair provides a reliable correction, which minimally relaxes over time. However, overcorrection is still required. Slight overcorrection is particularly beneficial if the person's normal side of the forehead is quite active during facial expression. Branches of the supraorbital nerve should be identified and preserved because they lie deep to the muscle (Fig. 13.6).

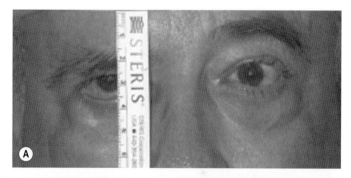

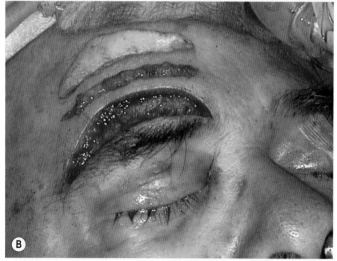

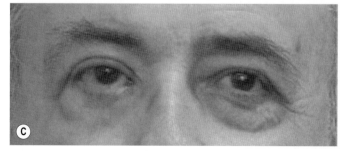

Fig. 13.6 (A) Assessment of the amount of brow depression on the paralyzed side compared with the normal eyebrow on the patient's left. **(B)** Excision of skin and a strip of frontalis muscle to correct brow ptosis. **(C)** Postoperative appearance.

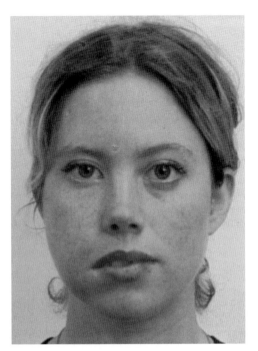

Fig. 13.7 Right facial paralysis in a young woman with total paralysis of the orbicularis oculi showing ideal eyelid configuration that allows gold weight insertion without visibility.

Brow lift may be performed through a coronal incision with or without a fascial graft to suspend the brow from the temporalis fascia or medially on the frontal bone. Whereas the scar is concealed, this is a larger operation than a direct brow lift and may not achieve as adequate a lift.

The authors have had limited experience with endoscopically assisted brow lifts for facial paralysis. The amount of lift required in the patient with facial paralysis is usually more than can be achieved from a unilateral endoscopic brow lift. It is likely that, with time, there will be gradual drooping. Therefore, the longevity of results in patients with facial paralysis has yet to be demonstrated with this procedure, especially when a large unilateral lift is required.

Weakening of the contralateral normal frontalis muscle by transaction of the frontal nerve or resection of strips of muscle is occasionally useful to control wrinkle asymmetry.

Upper eyelid

Several techniques are available for the management of lagophthalmos. These are all directed at overcoming the unopposed action of the levator palpebrae superioris. Because of its relative technical ease and reversibility, lid loading with gold prosthesis is the most popular technique. The patient's eyelid configuration is important in determining whether the bulge of the gold weight will be visible when the eye is open. If the amount of exposed eyelid skin above the lashes is more than 5 mm when the eye is open, the gold weight is likely to be noticeable to the patient. If the distance is less than 5 mm, the gold weight will roll back and be covered by the supratarsal skinfold (Fig. 13.7).

Because of its inertness, 24-carat gold is used; allergic reactions are rare, but if they occur, platinum weights are also available. Prostheses are available in weights ranging from 0.8 to 1.8 g. Adequate improvement in eye closure can be obtained with a weight of 0.8–1.2 g, giving the patient a comfortable eye without weight-related problems.[21] The appropriate weight is selected by taping trial prostheses to the upper eyelid over the tarsal plate with the patient awake. The lightest weight that will bring the upper eyelid within 2–4 mm of the lower lid and cover the cornea should be used. As long as the patient has an adequate Bell phenomenon, complete closure is not necessary. The prosthesis is fixed to the upper half of the tarsal plate by permanent sutures, which pass through the tarsal plate. Care should be taken not to interfere with the insertion of Müller muscle (Fig. 13.8). With proper placement, the prosthesis should be hidden in the upper eyelid skin crease when the eye is open. The closure produced by the gold weight is slow, and the patient must be instructed to relax the levator muscle consciously for 1–2 seconds to

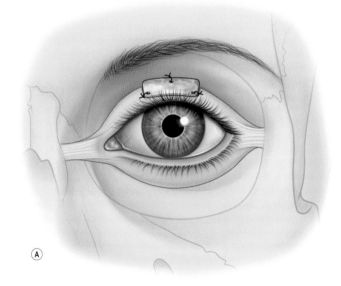

(A)

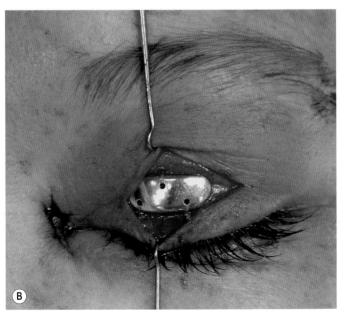

(B)

Fig. 13.8 (A) Placement of gold weight directly above the cornea on the upper half of the tarsal plate. **(B)** Gold weight sutured in place with the knots turned away from the skin.

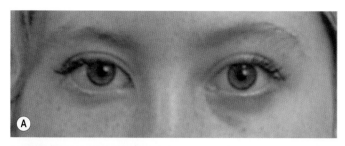

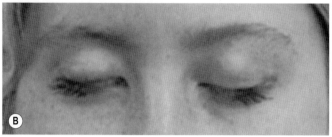

Fig. 13.9 (A) Postoperative appearance of patient shown in Fig. 13.7 after a gold weight has been fixed to the right upper eyelid. **(B)** Eye closure is shown after gold weight insertion.

allow the eyelid to descend (Fig. 13.9). Complications include extrusion, excessive capsule formation by causing a visible lump, and irritation of the eye by the weight. If these occur, the weight can easily be removed, replaced, or repositioned.

The authors have used the gold weight alone 27 times. The incidence of complications requiring removal of the weight was 2%, and 8% required revision of the weight. In 52% of patients, good symptomatic improvement was obtained. Of these patients, 64% subsequently required lower lid support with a static sling. As a result, it has become much more common to recommend both a gold weight and a lower-eyelid sling at the same operative sitting, which results in a 95% good improvement in symptoms.

An alternative procedure for the eyelid closure is the palpebral spring originally described by Morel–Fatio, which consists of a wire loop with two arms.[22] One arm is sutured along the lid margin, and the other arm is fixed to the inner aspect of the lateral orbital rim. When the eye is open, the two arms are brought close to each other; when the eyelid is relaxed, the "memory" of the wire loop moves the arms apart, causing closure of the eyelid (Fig. 13.10).

The advantage of this procedure is that it is not dependent on gravity. However, problems with malpositioning of the spring, spring breakage or weakening, pseudoptosis due to excessive spring force, and skin erosion have prevented the widespread use of this procedure. It is certainly a more involved procedure than insertion of the gold weight, and results may be dependent on the surgeon's skill level.

For short-term use, there are implantable devices. These include magnetized rods inserted into the upper and lower eyelids and silicon bands sutured to the lateral and medial canthal ligaments.

Temporalis muscle transposition has the advantage of using autogenous tissue, thereby avoiding the use of foreign materials. First described by Gillies,[23] this procedure has since been modified by several authors.[24] A 1.5-cm-wide flap of temporalis muscle based inferiorly is raised along with the overlying temporalis fascia. Because both the blood supply and motor nerve innervation enter the muscle on its inferior deep surface, the flap remains functional. The fascia overlying the temporalis muscle is then detached. It is sutured firmly to the superior edge of the temporalis muscle that is about to be transposed (Fig. 13.11). The flap is passed subcutaneously to the lateral canthus, where the fascial strips are tunneled along the upper and lower lid margins and sutured to the medial canthal ligament (Fig. 13.12). With activation of the muscle, the fascial strips are pulled tight, causing eyelid closure. This technique has the advantage of addressing both upper eyelid closure, and a static sling for the lower eyelid allows better eyelid closure. It is preferable to use a 2-mm strip of tendon; fascia appears to stretch, resulting in loss of effective eyelid movement. The disadvantages of this transfer are that, with muscle contraction, the lid aperture changes from an oval to a slit shape; there may be skin wrinkling over the lateral canthal region and an obvious muscle bulge over the lateral orbital margin. Movements of the eyelids during chewing may also be a disturbing feature for the patient. Nevertheless,

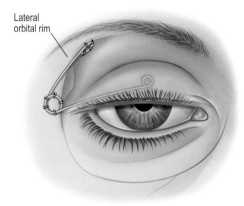

Fig. 13.10 Palpebral spring in right upper eyelid.

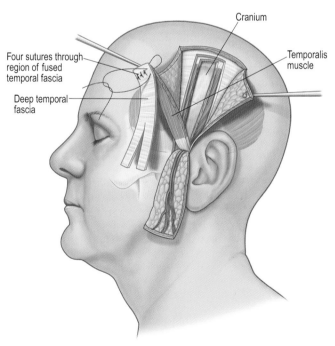

Fig. 13.11 Elevation of temporalis muscle for transfer to eye.

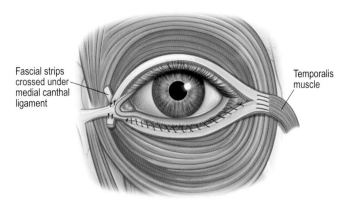

Fig. 13.12 Transplantation of temporalis muscle and fascia to upper and lower eyelids.

Fascial strips crossed under medial canthal ligament

Temporalis muscle

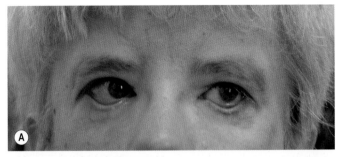

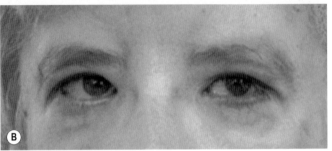

Fig. 13.13 **(A)** Marked bilateral ectropion in lower eyelids in a 52-year-old woman with Möbius syndrome. **(B)** Postoperative appearance after tendon sling insertion to lower eyelids.

this procedure usually provides an excellent static support, eye closure on command, and good lubrication of the eye through distribution of the tear film and consequent corneal protection. Microneurovascular muscle transplantation for orbicularis function is a relatively new procedure. Platysma transplantation procedures that involve revascularization with the superficial temporal artery and vein and reinnervation with a cross-facial nerve graft are tedious and complex and should be reserved for patients for whom simpler techniques have been unsuccessful. Transplantation of the platysma may also produce some undesirable thickening of the eyelids.

Historically, lateral tarsorrhaphy has been one of the mainstay treatments for paralyzed eyelids. The McLaughlin lateral tarsorrhaphy[25] may provide a reasonably acceptable cosmetic result. However, horizontal lid length is decreased, which detracts from the aesthetic appeal and obstructs lateral vision. This procedure consists of resection of a segment of lateral skin, cilia, and orbicularis from the lower lid and a matching segment of conjunctiva and tarsus from the upper lid. The two raw surfaces are sutured together, preserving the upper eyelashes. At present, the main indication for lateral tarsorrhaphy is for the patient with an anesthetic cornea, severe corneal exposure, or failure of aesthetically more acceptable techniques.

Lower eyelid

The orbicularis oculi muscle, through its attachment to the canthal ligaments, holds the lower eyelid firmly against the globe and with contraction is able to raise the lid 2–3 mm. Ordinarily, the eyelid margin rests at the level of the limbus of the eye. With paralysis of the orbicularis, tone in the muscle is lost. Gravity causes the lower eyelid to stretch and sag, resulting in scleral show. Over time, the lid and inferior canalicular punctum roll away from the globe, resulting in an ectropion (Fig. 13.13). Therefore, management is directed at resuspending the lid and reapposing the punctum to the globe.

Pronounced ectropion with lid eversion and more than 2–3 mm of scleral show is usually associated with symptoms of dryness and aesthetic concerns. This situation requires support of the entire length of the eyelid. This is best achieved with a static sling passed 1.5–2 mm inferior to the gray line of the eyelid and fixed both medially and laterally (Fig. 13.14).[26] Tendon provides longer-lasting support with less

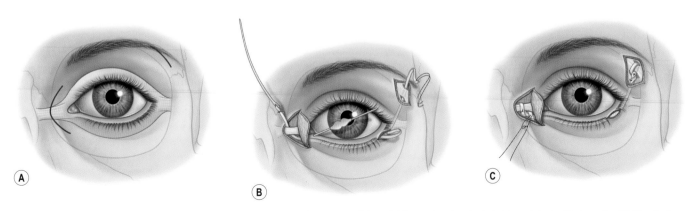

Fig. 13.14 **(A)** Incisions for insertion of static sling. **(B)** Static sling attachment to medial canthal ligament and periosteal strip on lateral orbital margin. **(C)** After fixation of sling.

stretching than the fascia lata. A 1.5-mm-wide strip of tendon (a part of either palmaris or plantaris) is sutured to the lateral orbital margin in the region above the zygomaticofrontal suture and tunneled subcutaneously along the lid anterior to the tarsal plate. Proper placement is crucial; too low a position will exacerbate the ectropion. In the elderly patient with particularly lax tissues, too superficial or high a placement may result in entropion. The sling is then passed around the anterior limb of the medial canthal ligament and sutured to itself. Subcutaneous tunneling of the tendon graft is facilitated by the use of a curved Keith needle. This procedure provides good support to the lower lid. It does not deform the eyelid, it is not apparent to an observer, and the effect appears to last well. If the sling is placed too loosely, it may be tightened at the lateral orbital margin.

Lateral examination of the eye and eyelid will determine its vector.[7] A negative vector occurs when the globe is anterior to the lid margin and the lid margin is anterior to the check prominence. In patients with a relatively proptotic eye, the lower eyelid sling will correct ectropion, but it may not decrease sclera show. In patients with a positive vector, in which the globe is posterior to the lid margin and the lid margin is posterior to the cheek prominence, the sling will be effective. However, lateral fixation of the tendon graft may need to be through a drill hole whereby the tendon is woven back to itself and sutured, 2–3 mm posterior to the lateral orbital margin, because fixation to the frontal periosteum may lift the lateral eyelid away from the globe.

The authors have used the lower lid sling on 25 occasions, and in combination with a gold weight to the upper lid, it results in 95% improvement in symptoms (Fig. 13.13B). Two patients have had complications from the lower lid sling procedure, which required the sling to be tightened. One patient required revision because the sling exacerbated the ectropion, and one required epilation of some lower eyelashes because of entropion. The lower lid tendon sling can be adjusted fairly readily if it is not in the correct position up to 1 week after placement.

Milder eyelid problems consisting of lower lid laxity and minimal scleral show may be treated with lateral canthoplasty. Jelks et al.[27] described various techniques of canthoplasty, such as the tarsal strip, dermal pennant, and inferior retinacular lateral canthoplasty. The canthal ligament must be reapproximated to the position of Whitnall tubercle, which is situated not only above the horizontal midpupillary line but also 2–3 mm posterior to the lateral orbital margin.

Horizontal lid shortening may be required to deal with redundant and stretched lower eyelid tissue. The Kuhnt–Szymanowski procedure involves the excision of a laterally placed triangular wedge of lower eyelid with its base being the lower lid margin. It can be modified not only to excise a wedge of tarsus and conjunctiva but also by resuspending the lid margin from the lateral canthus. However, this tends to distort and expose the caruncle and does not provide a lasting correction.

Cartilage grafts to prop up the tarsal plate have also been used. By augmenting the middle lamella and suturing the cartilage to the inferior orbital margin, there will be less of a tendency for the lower eyelid to migrate inferiorly. However, results may be poor because the cartilage tends to rotate into a more horizontal position rather than a vertical one, producing a visible bulge and minimal eyelid support.

In patients with isolated medial ectropion that includes punctal eversion, the lower lid can be repositioned against the globe by direct excision of a tarsoconjunctival ellipse. This causes a vertical shortening of the inner aspect of the lower lid and helps reposition the punctum against the globe. Medial canthoplasty will also support the punctum.

Nasal airway

Paralysis of the nasalis and levator alaeque nasi combined with drooping and medial deviation of the paralyzed cheek leads to support loss of the nostril, collapse of the ala, and reduction of airflow. Nasal septal deviation, which occurs in patients with congenital facial paralysis, may further accentuate any breathing difficulties. In the patient who complains of significant symptoms, correction of airway collapse is best accomplished by elevation and lateral support of the alar base with the sling of tendon and by upper lip and cheek elevation procedures. Septoplasty may be indicated to provide an improvement in airway patency.

Upper lip and cheek: smile reconstruction

The majority of patients with facial paralysis who present for reconstruction do so for either correction of an asymmetric face at rest or reconstruction of a smile. However, significant functional problems are associated with paralysis of the oral musculature, including drooling and speech difficulties. The flaccid lip and cheek can also lead to difficulties with chewing food, cheek biting, and pocketing food in the buccal sulcus due to paralysis of the buccinator. However, the main emphasis of surgery is usually centered on reconstruction of a smile.

The surgeon and patient must have clearly defined goals. Some patients only request symmetry at rest and are not concerned about animation. For these patients, static slings and soft-tissue repositioning can be most helpful. However, most patients would prefer a dynamic reconstruction.

Nerve transfers: principles and current use

Dynamic reanimation attempts to restore symmetry both at rest and while smiling. Three elements are required for the formation of a smile: neural input, a functional muscle innervated by the nerve, and proper muscle positioning. All three factor into the decision as to which would be the best for any given patient.

Reconstructive modalities for facial paralysis can be classified by two basic criteria. The first is whether reconstruction is based on the facial nerve or on a different cranial nerve,[28] and the second is whether the working muscle unit is the original facial musculature or a transferred muscle flap.[29] Reanimation based on the facial nerve can be on the ipsilateral or contralateral nerve depending on the presence of a functional and usable branch or stump. The duration of paralysis is the principal determinant for the need for muscle transfer or transplant. If duration is less than 12 months, the facial musculature is assumed to be able to be reinnervated. Muscles become irreversibly atrophic by 24 months, in which case muscle replacement is indicated. The effect of the facial musculature can be replaced by static procedures for balance or by dynamic procedures for animation. The combination of regional muscle transfer and static positioning procedure has been recently described.[30]

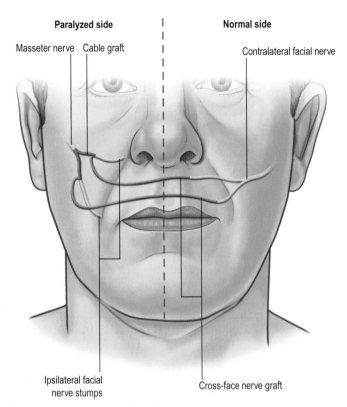

Paralyzed side   **Normal side**

Masseter nerve   Cable graft   Contralateral facial nerve

Ipsilateral facial
nerve stumps   Cross-face nerve graft

Fig. 13.15 Illustration of the "babysitter" procedure.

Primary facial nerve repair is possible in cases of recent trauma to the facial nerve.[31] A sural cable nerve graft is used to interconnect ends when there is a gap between the ipsilateral proximal stump of facial nerve to the distal stumps of zygomaticobuccal facial branches.

When the ipsilateral proximal facial nerve stump is not usable (brain tumor, head trauma and fractures, Bell's palsy, or surgery) and the facial musculature has not become irreversibly atrophic and can be reinnervated, a nerve transfer with or without nerve grafts can be very effective. This can preserve the function of the musculature on the paralyzed side and result in a more natural appearance. Recently, several innovative concepts have arisen and will be briefly outlined. This preservation of facial musculature function can be provided by another cranial nerve such as the hypoglossal nerve or portion of the trigeminal, such as the motor nerve to masseter. This is done through a nerve transfer with coaptation of the selected donor nerve to the facial nerve. The mass involvement provided by this transfer may lead to an unnatural appearing activation of the intact facial musculature, although it may provide for adequate tone. To get around this, the babysitter concept was proposed by Terzis.[32,33] The alternate motors preserve the facial musculature while awaiting appropriate, spontaneous, and synchronous innervations from a cross face nerve graft. In this procedure, a cross face sural nerve graft is used to relay facial nerve activity across the face to the paralyzed musculature. Axons from the contralateral normal facial nerve regenerate through the sheath of the graft and innervate the muscle over 4 to 8 months. Since muscle atrophy can develop while the facial nerve regenerates, an ipsilateral motor nerve (either masseter or hypoglossal) can be transposed to serve as temporary innervations or "babysitting" (Fig. 13.15). Thus, muscle tone is preserved while spontaneous smiling will in due course be restored. At the first operation, two nerve grafts are connected to the upper and lower trunks of the normal contralateral facial nerve and tunneled across the face via the upper lip. These grafts are banked on the paralyzed side. They are carefully labeled ("upper"/"lower") and placed in the temporal region to be retrieved at a second stage. Then at this first operation, a short nerve graft is used to connect the nerve to masseter or a part of the hypoglossal nerve to the distal stump of the affected facial nerve. Within 2–3 months, the paralyzed muscle will regain tone and then will begin to function in a mass pattern motion. This mass movement is then converted to softer, more spontaneous movement through the second surgery. About 6–9 months after the initial procedure,[34] the paralyzed side is re-explored. The two cross face nerve grafts are identified, split into fascicles, and coapted to the facial nerve branches distal to the prior masseter-facial nerve repair. Within 3 months, spontaneous facial nerve motion is initiated by the contralateral facial nerve (Fig. 13.16). With additional time,

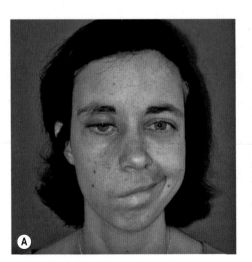
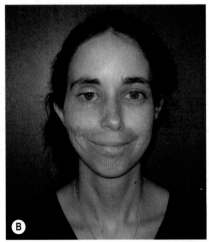
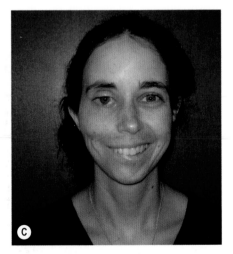

Fig. 13.16 **(A)** Preoperative photo prior to the "babysitter" procedure. **(B)** Closed-mouth smile after the "babysitter" procedure. **(C)** Open-mouth smile after the "babysitter" procedure.

these grafts will take control over the transfer. However, if the masseter nerve action is still noticeable and unwanted, the masseter nerve can be transected.

A modification of this technique proposed by Marcus utilizes the motor nerve to masseter to preserve function of the lower face and periorbital region.[35] To avoid the problem of mass action with a nerve transfer, Klebuc has suggested that the motor nerve to masseter be transferred to the buccal branch only of the facial nerve. This is done with a direct end to end coaptation.[36]

The upper face (i.e., orbicularis oculi function) can be either reconstructed with static procedures or muscle transfers as previously outlined in this chapter. Upper face function can

also be achieved in a synchronous and spontaneous fashion through cross face nerve grafting. With this technique, a sural nerve graft is connected end to side on the normal side to the upper branch of the facial nerve. It is tunneled across the upper face with the aid of small eyebrow incisions and then coapted end to end to the upper branch of the facial nerve on the paralyzed side. This is done in one single procedure along with the masseter to lower facial nerve transfer (Fig. 13.17).

A. Preoperative appearance at rest: Complete right facial paralysis.

B. Preoperative appearance with attempted smile.

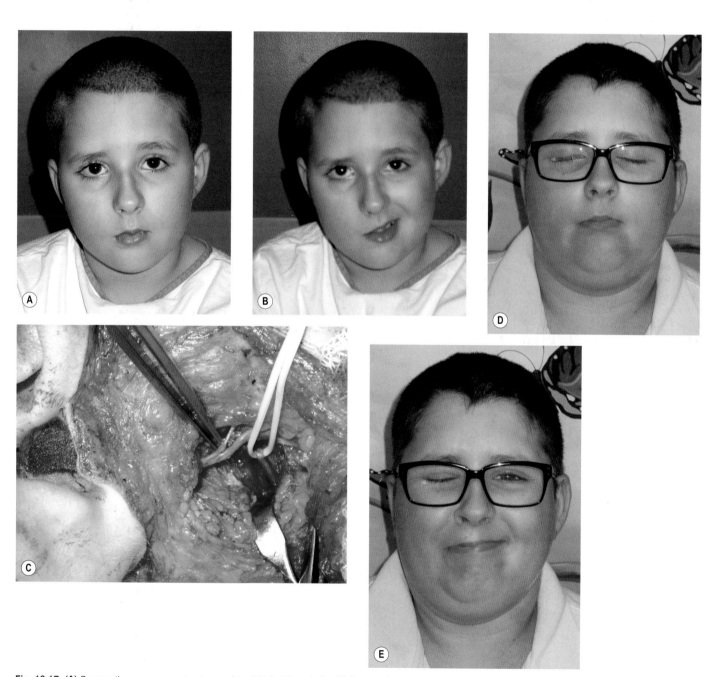

Fig. 13.17 (A) Preoperative appearance at rest: complete right facial paralysis. **(B)** Preoperative appearance with attempted smile. **(C)** Intraoperative – The motor nerve to masseter (in vessel loop) is to be transected and coapted and directly to the lower buccal branch of the facial nerve (beneath the forceps). **(D)** Two years postoperatively at rest with improvement in facial resting tone. **(E)** Two years postoperatively with smile and natural appearing nasolabial crease from the reinnervated facial musculature.

C. Intraoperative – motor nerve to masseter is transferred to lower buccal branch of facial nerve.

D. 2 years postoperatively at rest with improvement in facial resting tone.

E. 2 years postoperatively with smile and natural appearing nasolabial crease from the reinnervated facial musculature.

Microneurovascular muscle transplantation

It is not possible to restore complete symmetry of all movements because of the complexity of muscle interaction and the number of facial muscles involved. There are 18 separate muscles of facial expression, and of these, five are elevators of the upper lip and two are depressors of the lower lip. A transplanted muscle can only be expected to produce one function and movement in one direction.

If the facial nerve is used to reinnervate the transplanted muscle, the smile with laughter will be spontaneous. When other nerves are used (e.g., the fifth, 11th, or 12th), teeth clenching or other movements are required to activate the smile, at least initially. With time, the smile movement will often become less of a conscious effort and more spontaneous.

The patient's suitability for free muscle transplantation and reinnervation must be carefully assessed. This includes an assessment of the patient's ability to undergo a substantial operative procedure with general anesthesia as well as an evaluation of comorbidities that may affect the functioning of microneurovascular muscle transplantation. The patient should also be counseled with regard to the time that it could take to achieve full movement, which is usually around 18 months. It is generally recognized that reinnervation does not often occur in older individuals. However, it is difficult to determine which patient should be classified as "older" because muscle reinnervation can occur at any age. However, it is the author's practice to be reluctant to perform functioning muscle transplantations on patients who are older than 65 years.

Smile analysis

Preoperative planning is crucial. It is recognized that the unopposed smile on the normal side in unilateral facial paralysis will be an exaggerated expression of the same movement after reconstruction of the paralyzed side. Therefore, careful analysis of the patient's smile on the non-paralyzed side will instruct the surgeon in establishing a symmetric smile. As Paletz et al.[37] have shown, individuals have various types of smiles. It is important to assess the direction of movement of the commissure and upper lip. How vertical is the movement? What is the strength of the smile and where around the mouth is the force most strongly focused? What is the position of the nasolabial fold with smiling? Is there a labial mental fold? Once these features have been determined, an estimate of the muscle's size, point of origin, tension, direction of movement, and placement can be planned (Fig. 13.18).

Technique options

One-stage procedures for smile reconstruction with free muscle transplantations would seem to be the most appealing

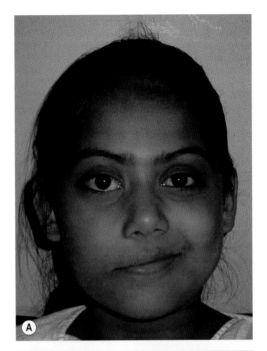

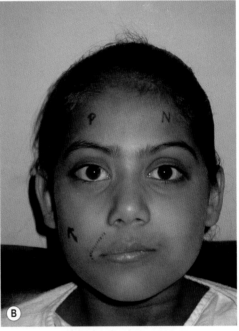

Fig. 13.18 (A) Patient shown smiling. Note direction of movement of the commissure and the mid upper lip on the normal left side, location of the fold in the nasolabial area, and shape of the upper and lower lip. **(B)** The nasolabial folds and directions of movement have been marked on the normal left side (N) and copied on the paralyzed side (P). The desired position of the muscle is outlined by two dotted lines across the cheek.

approach; however, for numerous reasons, they may not necessarily provide the best results (Table 13.4). If the ipsilateral facial nerve trunk is available, it seems to be an ideal source of reinnervation for a muscle flap. However, the exact branches to the lip elevators may be difficult to determine. If incorrect innervation is used, muscle contraction may take place only when the patient performs some facial movement

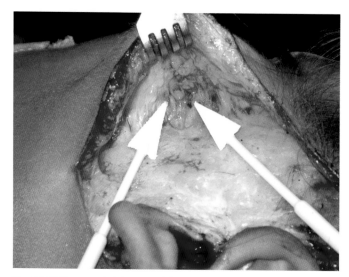

Fig. 13.19 The cross-facial nerve graft is inserted through a preauricular incision. The parotid gland can be seen immediately in front of the left ear, and branches of the facial nerve supplying the muscles of the mouth and eye are seen superficial to the background material.

Authors' preferred method: two-stage microneurovascular transplantation

Cross-facial nerve graft (Video 13.3 ▶)

The first stage of this procedure involves a dissection of the facial nerve on the unaffected side through a preauricular incision with a submandibular extension (Fig. 13.19). The zygomaticobuccal nerve branches medial to the parotid gland are meticulously identified and individually stimulated with a microbipolar electrical probe attached to a stimulator source that allows variable voltage and frequency control (Fig. 13.20). Disposable stimulators used to identify the presence of motor nerves do not provide reliable, controlled tetanic muscle contraction that will allow muscle palpation and clear visual identification of which muscle is being stimulated. Facial nerve mapping clearly identifies which nerve fibers stimulate the orbicularis oris and oculi muscles as well as the lip

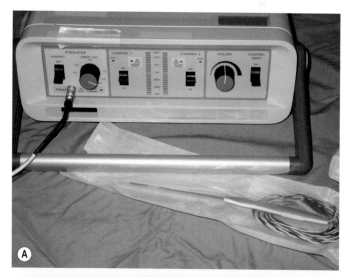

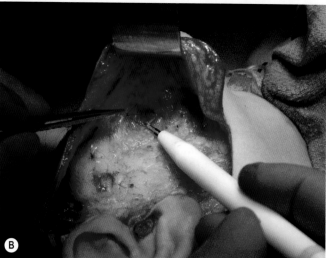

Fig. 13.20 (A) A portable electrical stimulator with variable voltage and frequency control is put in a sterile plastic bag placed close to the operating site so the surgeon can adjust the voltage as needed. **(B)** Bipolar electrical probe establishes an electrical current between the electrodes and a localized stimulus to a small area of tissue.

other than smiling, such as closing the eyes or puckering the lips.

Single-stage muscle transplants with innervation from the contralateral facial nerve have been reported. This technique requires the use of a muscle with a long nerve segment, such as the latissimus dorsi or rectus abdominis.[38] However, even the gracilis[39] has been used. The nerve is tunneled across the lip and coapted to the facial nerve branches on the opposite side of the face. The advantages here are that the patient undergoes only one operation and there is only one site of coaptation for regenerating axons to cross. There does not appear to be any significant denervation atrophy of the muscle while it awaits reinnervation. However, although the muscle may function with facial movement, it may not contract when the patient smiles. This is because the facial nerve branches used are close to the mouth and are usually found through a nasolabial incision on the unaffected side. This approach does not allow thorough facial nerve mapping to be performed; thus, the most appropriate nerve branches may not be recruited. Also, this approach does not allow an assessment of what remaining branches have been left intact.

When there is neither an ipsilateral nor a contralateral facial nerve available to act as a donor, as in Möbius syndrome or other causes of bilateral facial paralysis, another cranial nerve must be used to reinnervate the muscle transplant. It is our practice to use the nerve to the masseter muscle.[39] Zuker et al.[39] have shown that in children this provides a symmetric smile with excellent muscle excursion. These patients may never achieve involuntary movement or a truly spontaneous smile. However, in many children and 50% of adults there appears to be some cortical "rewiring" such that these people are able to activate a smile without performing a biting motion and without conscious effort.

In treatment of younger patients with unilateral facial paralysis, we prefer to perform a two-stage reconstruction consisting of facial nerve mapping and cross-facial nerve grafting, followed by a microneurovascular muscle transplantation.

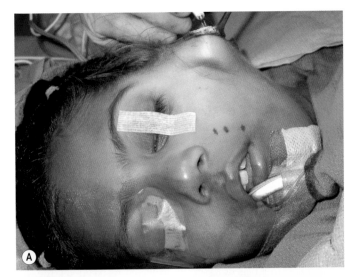

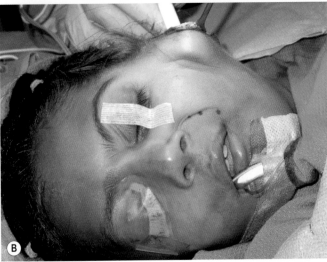

Fig. 13.21 **(A)** Patient with left facial paralysis under anesthesia. Facial nerve branches are prepared for functional nerve mapping of her right facial nerve. **(B)** Stimulation of a branch of the facial nerve to the zygomaticus major, an ideal branch for the coaptation to cross-facial nerve graft.

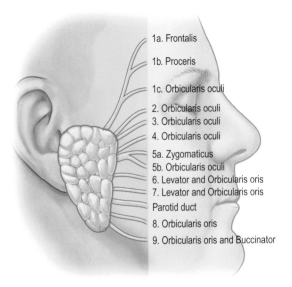

1a. Frontalis
1b. Proceris
1c. Orbicularis oculi
2. Orbicularis oculi
3. Orbicularis oculi
4. Orbicularis oculi
5a. Zygomaticus
5b. Orbicularis oculi
6. Levator and Orbicularis oris
7. Levator and Orbicularis oris
Parotid duct
8. Orbicularis oris
9. Orbicularis oris and Buccinator

Fig. 13.22 A functional nerve map is made of the branches of the facial nerve supplying the eye and mouth. The map identifies the muscles that contract when each branch is stimulated.

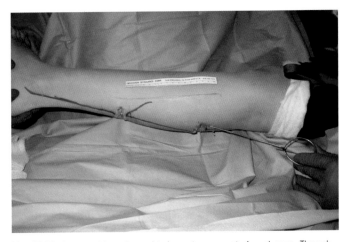

Fig. 13.23 A nerve stripper is used to harvest a segment of sural nerve. Through the posterior calf incision, the nerve is identified, dissected up to the popliteal, and cut. It is put in the stripper and the stripper passed to the midcalf. A second incision is made and the nerve is identified, cut, and withdrawn.

retractors. When stimulated, the facial nerve branches that produce a smile and no other movement are selected (Fig. 13.21). It is sometimes difficult to find "smile" branches that do not contain some orbicularis oculi function. There are usually between two and four nerve branches that do not contain some orbicularis oculi function. There are usually between two and four nerve branches that activate the zygomaticus and levator labii superioris. This allows one or two branches to be used for the nerve graft coaptation while function of the normal facial muscles is preserved (Fig. 13.22).

The sural nerve is the usual donor nerve. This is harvested with the use of a nerve stripper (Fig. 13.23). Stripping of the nerve does not appear to affect its function as a graft.[40]

The proximal ends of the donor facial nerve branches are sutured to the distal end of the nerve graft such that regenerating axons will travel in a distal to proximal direction down the graft. The current practice is to use a short nerve graft, approximately 10 cm in length, and to bank the free end in the upper buccal sulcus. This should provide a well-innervated graft. In addition, the waiting period between the first and second stages is reduced with use of a short cross-facial nerve graft from 12 months to around 6 months. Patients who have had short nerve grafts achieve stronger muscle contraction than was previously obtained with traditional long cross-facial nerve grafts (Table 13.5).

Table 13.5 Options for microneurovascular muscle transplantation	
One-stage	Muscle innervated by ipsilateral facial nerve (if available)
	Muscle with long nerve segment innervated by contralateral seventh-nerve branches
	Muscle innervated by masseter, hypoglossal, or accessory nerve
Two-stage	Cross-facial nerve graft followed by the muscle transplantation

Table 13.6 Muscles available for microneurovascular transplantation

Gracilis
Pectoralis minor
Rectus abdominis
Latissimus dorsi
Extensor carpi radialis brevis
Serratus anterior
Rectus femoris
Abductor hallucis

In addition to using a short nerve, one of the senior authors has been using the proximal end of the sural nerve as the cross-face nerve. The proximal segment from the popliteal fossa to the midcalf is thin, lacks branches, and is an excellent size match for both the selected branches of the seventh nerve and the motor nerve to gracilis.

Gracilis muscle transplantation (Video 13.4 ⊙)

Many muscles are available for functioning muscle transplantation for lower facial reconstruction (Table 13.6). The muscle should be transplantable by vascular anastomoses and have a suitable motor nerve for nerve coaptation to the face. Initially, surgeons attempted to find a muscle that was exactly the right size for the face. However, a more suitable approach is to pare down a muscle to the desired size before transplantation.[41] This concept allows the surgeon to use many different muscles and to customize the muscle to fit the functional requirements of the face. For example, a lightly structured face with only a partial paralysis will require a small piece of muscle. A large face with a strong movement of the mouth to the normal side and a total paralysis will require a large piece of muscle.

The gracilis muscle is suitable for facial paralysis reconstruction. The neurovascular pedicle is reliable and relatively easy to prepare. A segment of muscle can be cut to any desired size based on the neurovascular pedicle. This allows the surgeon to customize the muscle to the patient's facial requirements. There is no functional loss in the leg. Because the scar is in the medial aspect of the thigh, it is reasonably well hidden. However, the scar usually does spread. The thigh is far enough removed from the face that a simultaneous preparation of the muscle and the face is easily accomplished. The gracilis is the preferred muscle for transplantation because the anatomy is well known and the technique of preparing it for transplantation is well described (Figs. 13.24–13.27).[42]

The muscle is usually split longitudinally, and the anterior portion of the muscle is used. The amount of muscle that is taken varies from 30% to 70% of the cross-section of the muscle, depending on the muscle size and needs of the face. The muscle can usually be split longitudinally without concern; however, on occasion, the vascular pedicle enters in the middle of the muscle on the deep surface. In this situation, it may be necessary to remove a portion of the anterior part of the muscle as well as the posterior to pare down the width of the muscle. After facial measurements are taken, a piece of muscle with a little extra length is removed. The end of the muscle that is to be inserted into the face is oversewn with

mattress sutures, placing one more than the number of sutures inserted about the lips.

Attaching the muscle to the mouth is a critical part of the procedure (Fig. 13.27). It is usually inserted into the fibers of the paralyzed orbicularis oris above and below the commissure and along the upper lip (Fig. 13.28A,B). Preoperative smile analysis determines the points of insertion. The preoperative smile analysis is also crucial for determining the origin of the muscle, which may be attached to the zygomatic body, arch, temporal fascia, or preauricular fascia. Intraoperative traction on the obicularis oris while the movement of the mouth is observed will verify the correct placement of the sutures. The correct tension is difficult to determine because the mechanical tension within the muscle, the degree of tone that the muscle develops, and the gravitational and muscle forces within the face will influence the eventual position (Fig. 13.28C).

The vascular pedicle is usually anastomosed to the facial vessels; however, the facial vein may occasionally be absent.

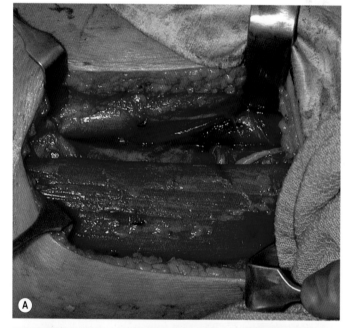

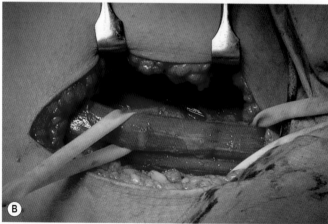

Fig. 13.24 (A) Preparation of gracilis muscle in right thigh. The motor nerve is seen in the right upper corner of the dissection adjacent to the vascular pedicle. **(B)** A longitudinal split of the anterior half of the gracilis muscle.

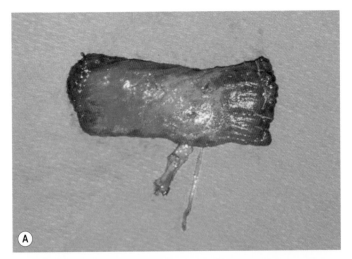

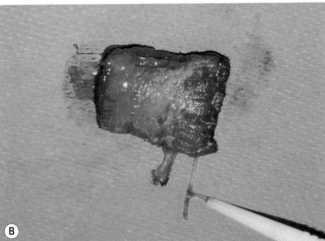

Fig. 13.25 (A) After removal of the segment of gracilis muscle, the motor nerve can be seen to the lower left and the pedicle inferiorly. The right-hand side demonstrates the distal end of the muscle, which has been oversewn with multiple mattress sutures. **(B)** Marked muscle shortening is possible in the gracilis muscle with motor stimulation.

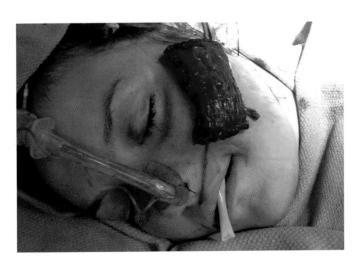

Fig. 13.26 The muscle has been removed and placed on the face to demonstrate its approximate position. The muscle's motor nerve is placed across the cheek in the position for coaptation to the cross-facial nerve graft in the upper buccal sulcus.

There is invariably a large transverse facial vein that may be used instead. The superficial temporal vessels may also be used. The gracilis is positioned so that its hilum is close to the mouth and the motor nerve can be tunneled into the upper lip. The upper buccal sulcus incision is reopened, and the free end of the nerve graft is identified and coapted to the gracilis muscle motor nerve.

Movement does not usually occur until 6 months or more have elapsed, and maximal movement is usually gained by 18 months. At this stage, an assessment is made of the resting tension in the muscle and its excursion with smiling. It is not uncommon for the patient to require a third procedure to adjust the muscle (i.e., either tightening or loosening), and this can be combined with other touch-up procedures such as debulking or an adjustment of the insertion of origin.

With this procedure, patients usually gain around 50% as much movement on the paralyzed side as on the

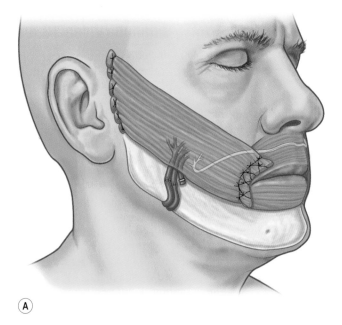

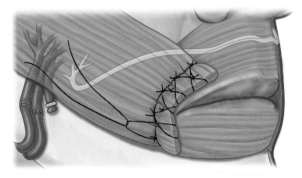

Fig. 13.27 (A) The muscle is placed in the face and revascularized by vascular anastomosis to the facial artery and the vein. Nerve coaptation to the cross-facial nerve graft is accomplished. The muscle is attached about the mouth and to the preauricular and superficial temporal fascia. **(B)** Insertion into the paralyzed orbicularis oris is accomplished with figure-of-eight sutures placed through the orbicularis oris and behind the mattress sutures at the end of the muscle. This ensures strong muscle fixation to the mouth, which should prevent dehiscence.

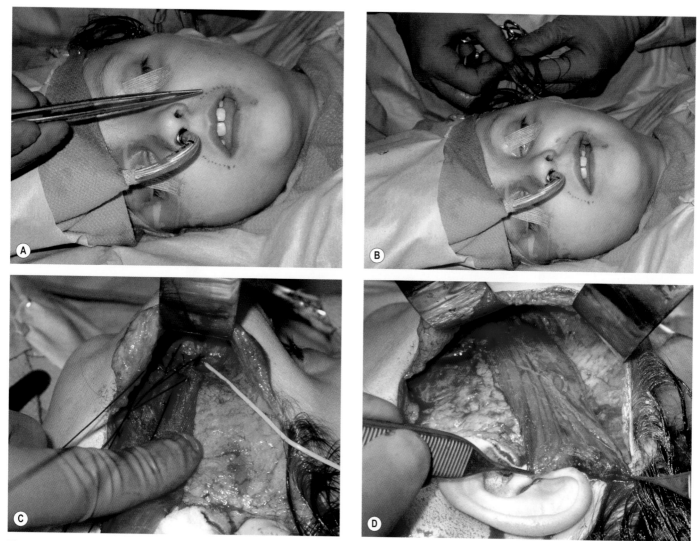

Fig. 13.28 **(A)** Anchoring sutures have been placed in the oral commissure and upper lip. The sutures can be seen at the top of the photograph. There is just enough traction to bring the commissure to an even position with the normal commissure on the right. **(B)** Traction is being placed on the anchoring sutures to the oral commissure and upper lip. A simulation of the smile that will occur can be seen. Our goal is to make this activity as close as possible to the normal side in vector and location of nasolabial crease formation. **(C)** The muscle is being inserted into the commissure and upper lip. The anchoring sutures are being placed behind the line of mattress sutures in the muscle so as to anchor the muscle securely and avoid any postsurgical drift of the insertion. **(D)** The muscle has been secured to the oral commissure and upper lip, revascularized, and reinnervated. It is now placed under the appropriate tension and secured to the fascia in the temporal and preauricular region. The muscle is pulled out to length, and just enough tension to barely move the oral commissure is affected. With this, the location of the anchoring sutures to the temporal and preauricular fascia can be determined. The muscle is then secured in position, the wound thoroughly irrigated, and the flap closed over a Penrose drain.

non-paralyzed side. This provides them with an excellent resting position and a pleasing smile that is totally spontaneous.

Muscle transplantation in the absence of seventh-nerve input

The concept of muscle transplantation in the absence of seventh-nerve input can be applied to bilateral facial paralysis and Möbius syndrome. An effective motor nerve must be used to power the muscle. The use of the 11th and 12th nerve has been described, but preference is now given to the motor nerve to the masseter. This is a branch of the trigeminal (fifth nerve) and as such is almost always normal in patients who have bilateral facial paralysis, including Möbius syndrome. The nerve courses downward and anteriorly from the

superoposterior border of the masseter in an oblique fashion. The nerve is always on the undersurface of the masseter muscle and enters this surface of the muscle belly approximately 2 cm below the zygomatic arch. The nerve courses through the muscle, giving off a variety of branches. Thus, the nerve can be traced distally, divided, and reflected proximally and superiorly to be in a position suitable for neural coaptation. The muscle transplant procedure is done much the same as described in the section on unilateral facial paralysis.

The origin and the insertion are the same, as is the revascularization process. The motor nerve to the transplanted muscle (segmented gracilis) is coapted to the motor nerve of the masseter. There is a remarkable similarity in size, and excellent reinnervation can be achieved. In fact, Bae et al.[43] have shown for patients with Möbius syndrome that the oral commissure movement accomplished by a gracilis transplant

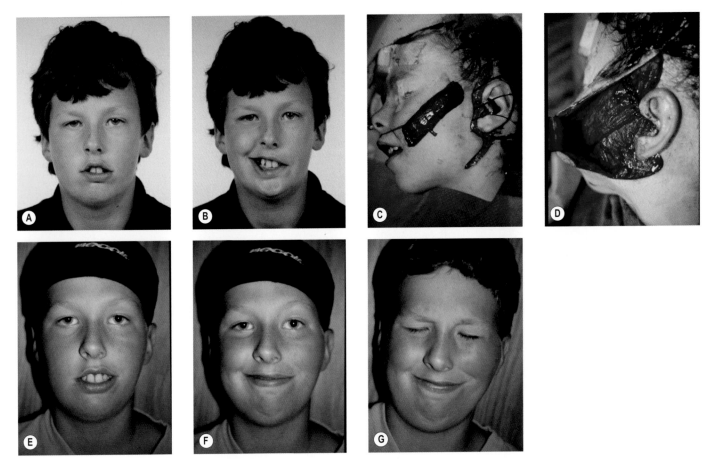

Fig. 13.29 **(A)** Preoperative view of child with congenital facial paralysis at rest. Note slight droop on affected side and shift of upper lip to normal side. **(B)** With smile. Note slight tension on affected side but no elevation. **(C)** Intraoperative view following cross-face nerve as segmental gracilis microneurovascular transport lies on check. Note vascular pedicle to be anastomosed to facial vessels and motor nerve to be coapted to cross-face nerve graft in upper buccal sulcus. **(D)** Intraoperative view. Microneurovascular transplant has been fixed at both ends, revascularized to the facial vessels, and reinnervated with previously placed cross-face nerve graft. **(E)** Postoperative view following cross-face nerve graft and microneurovascular muscle transplantation at rest. Note reasonable symmetry with no excess bulk. **(F)** With moderate smile. Note reasonable active movement with good commissure elevation and minimal bulk. **(G)** With full forced smile. Note good excursion and nice nasolabial crease formation.

innervated by the masseter motor nerve comes within 2 mm of normal movement. There is approximately 15 mm of movement normally achieved at the oral commissure. With gracilis muscle transplantation innervated by the motor nerve to masseter, commissure movement of 13.8 mm on one side and 14.6 on the other side was achieved in 32 patients. With a cross-face nerve in a similar group of patients, only 7.9 mm of commissure movement was noted. The benefit of the cross-facial nerve graft, of course, is that it provides for spontaneity of activity, whereas the motor nerve to masseter does not and initially requires conscious activity. With a muscle that is innervated with cross-facial nerve graft, the patient develops spontaneous expression because the muscle is controlled by the facial nerve on the normal side. However, when the masseter motor nerve is used, the smile movement must be learned as part of a conscious effort. Many patients are able to animate their face after some practice and biofeedback without moving their jaws and even without conscious effort. This is an area that is undergoing further study, but we feel that there is a significant role for rehabilitative services after the muscles begin to contract.

Patients with Möbius syndrome are excellent candidates for this form of surgery as usually they have limited or no seventh-nerve activity and normal fifth-nerve activity so their masseter muscles are normal. We prefer to do each side separately, spaced at least 2 months apart. The excursion of the muscle and resultant animation has been very satisfying. Innervation of the segmental gracilis muscle transplant by the motor nerve to masseter is now the preferred reconstruction for these patients. It has proved to be extremely effective in helping improve lower lip incompetence and drooling as well as speech irregularities, especially those requiring bilabial sound production. Most importantly, however, it is effective in providing the patient with an acceptable level of smile animation that is not possible with other techniques (Figs. 13.29 & 13.30).

Regional muscle transfer

Patients who are not suitable candidates for free muscle transplantation may be candidates for regional muscle transfer. These techniques, which have been in use for many

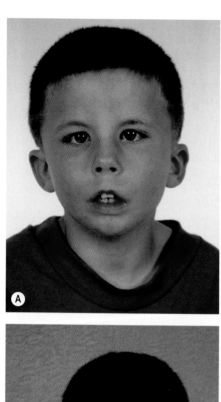

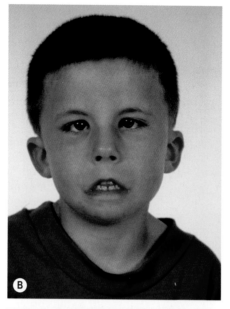

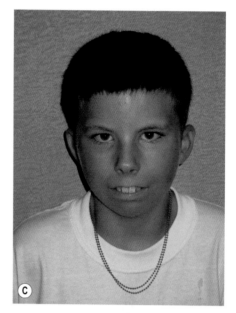

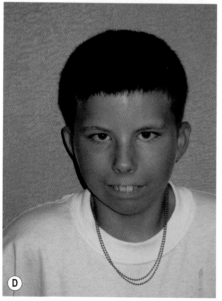

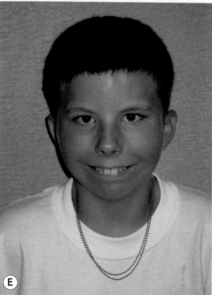

Fig. 13.30 (A) Preoperative view of child with Möbius syndrome at rest. **(B)** With attempted smile. Commissures actually turn down, giving a grimace appearance. **(C)** Postoperative view following segmental free gracilis microneurovascular muscle transplantation innervated by the motor nerve to masseter at rest. Note static support of oral commissures. **(D)** With small controlled smile. Note even elevation and tightening of oral commissures. **(E)** With full smile. Note fairly symmetrical commissure movement with nasolabial crease formation.

decades, involve the transfer of either the temporalis or masseter muscle or both. Because these muscles are innervated by the trigeminal nerve to activate a smile, patients must initially clench the teeth. With practice they can activate the muscle without moving their jaws, and some patients may achieve a degree of spontaneity.

The retrograde or turnover temporalis muscle transfer, as described by Gillies,[23] involves detaching the origin of the muscle from the temporal fossa and turning it over the zygomatic arch to extend to the oral commissure. Frequently, a fascial graft is required to achieve the necessary length to reach the mouth. This leaves a significant hollowing in the temporal region that can be filled with an implant. Baker and Conley[44] recommend leaving the anterior portion of the temporalis behind to partially camouflage the temporal hollowing. Another aesthetic disadvantage of the temporalis

transfer is the bulge of the muscle present where it passes over the arch of the zygoma. To avoid these complications, McLaughlin[25] described an antegrade temporalis transfer. Through an intraoral, scalp, or nasolabial incision, the temporalis muscle is detached from the coronoid process of mandible and brought forward. Fascial grafts are used to reach the angle of the mouth.

Labbe and Huault modified this procedure to create a true myoplasty with a mobile insertion and fixed origin and without the use of fascial grafts.[45] A further recent modification avoids undermining the anterior part of the temporalis muscle, thus simplifying the procedure and ensuring an enhanced blood supply. The coronoid is now osteotomized through the nasolabial incision, avoiding the transverse incision parallel to the zygoma arch and the osteotomy of the zygoma.[46] One of the key differences is that the temporalis

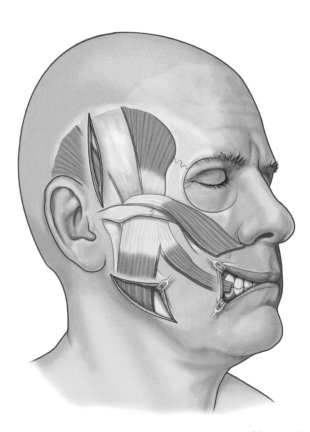

Fig. 13.31 Transplantation of both the temporalis and a portion of the masseter muscle to the periorbital region.

insertion is tunneled through the buccal fat pad, thus aiding tendon gliding and consequently commissure excursion. It may be a good alternative in the older patient or when a muscle transplant is not possible.

The masseter muscle transplantation as described by Baker and Conley[44] involves transplanting the entire muscle or the anterior portion from its insertion on the mandible and inserting it around the mouth. Rubin[47] recommends separating the most anterior half of the muscle only and transposing it to the upper and lower lip. During the splitting dissection, the surgeon must be cautious not to injure the masseteric nerve, which enters the muscle on the deep surface superior to its midpoint.

Good static control of the mouth can be achieved with the masseter transplantations; however, it lacks sufficient force and excursion to produce a full smile, and the movement produced is too horizontal for most faces. Patients frequently have a hollow over the angle of the mandible.

Rubin[47] has advocated transplanting the temporalis and masseter muscles together (Fig. 13.31). The temporalis provides motion to the upper lip and nasolabial fold; the masseter provides support to the corner of the mouth and lower lip.

Static slings

Static slings are used to achieve symmetry at rest without providing animation. They can be used alone or as an adjunct to dynamic procedures to provide immediate support. The goal is to produce a facial position equal to or slightly overcorrected from the resting position on the normal side. The slings

can be made of fascia (tensor fascia latae), tendon, or prosthetic material such as Gore-Tex®. In our experience, Gore-Tex® produces an undesirable inflammatory reaction. When fascia lata is taken from the thigh, it is preferable to repair the donor defect or an uncomfortable and unsightly muscle hernia may develop. The authors' preference, however, is to use tendon (palmaris longus, plantaris, or extensor digitorum longus) (Fig. 13.32). Tendon can easily be harvested and woven through tissues. Curved, pointed forceps are useful for inserting the tendon through the tissues of the oral commissure and upper lip and the temporalis and zygomatic fascia. Exposure can be through a nasolabial combined with a preauricular approach or a preauricular approach alone.

When tension is applied to the grafts, the force should be distributed evenly around the mouth with a little overcorrection. This is done to compensate for the difference in facial tone when the patient is awake and for postoperative stretching. The graft is then attached to the temporal fascia or to the zygoma, depending on the desired direction of pull. Multiple grafts should be inserted, usually three, to provide an even lift to the corner of the mouth and upper lip (Fig. 13.30). It is important to position the sling properly to achieve the correct elevation with regard to the upper lip and corner of the mouth (Fig. 13.33). It is possible to insert the static sling too tightly, particularly in the upper lip, which establishes a corridor through which air and liquid can escape.

Soft-tissue rebalancing

Soft-tissue procedures are useful adjuncts to both dynamic and static management. These procedures involve suspension and repositioning of the lax structures. This will include rhytidectomy with or without plication or suspension of the superficial musculoaponeurotic system; midface subperiosteal lifts may also be beneficial. Procedures on the nasolabial fold usually do not help define this important structure. Asymmetry of the upper lips may be corrected by mucosal excisions. These procedures, which may be minor, will often be of great benefit to patients.

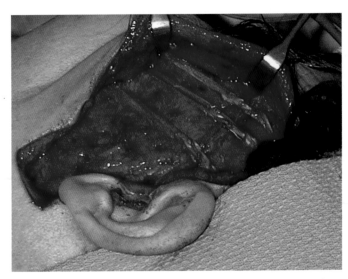

Fig. 13.32 Static slings of plantaris tendon in place to support the mouth and cheek.

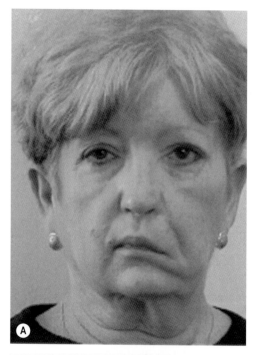

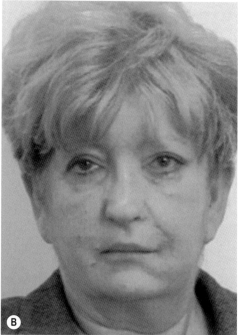

Fig. 13.33 (A) Preoperative view of an older patient at rest with marked facial asymmetry. Previous surgery elsewhere had placed a visible scar in the left nasolabial area. **(B)** Improvement in facial symmetry after insertion of static slings to the mouth.

Lower lip

The lower lip deformity caused by marginal mandibular nerve palsy may be part of a generalized facial paralysis or may occur in isolation as a congenital defect or secondary to trauma or surgery. It is a particular risk during rhytidectomy or parotid and upper neck surgery. The marginal mandibular nerve consists of one to three branches and supplies the

depressor labii inferioris, depressor anguli oris, mentalis, and portions of the lower lip orbicularis oris. The orbicularis oris also receives innervation from buccal branches and the contralateral marginal mandibular nerves. The muscle function that is missed most by the patient is that of the depressor labii inferioris. Paralysis of this muscle results in the inability to depress, lateralize, and evert the lower lip. In the normal resting position, the deformity is not usually noticeable, as the lips are closed and the depressors are relaxed. However, when the patient is talking, the paralyzed side is able to move inferiorly and away from the teeth. The deformity is most accentuated when the patient attempts a full smile, showing his or her teeth.

Problems with speech and eating may occur, but most patients are concerned primarily with the asymmetric appearance of the lower lip during speech and smiling. The inability to express rage and sorrow, which require a symmetric lower-lip depression, is also of concern.

Many techniques have been described for the correction of marginal mandibular nerve palsy, including operating on the affected side to try to animate it or operating on the unaffected side to minimize its function. Puckett et al.[48] described a technique of excising a wedge of skin and muscle but preserving orbicularis oris on the unaffected side. Glenn and Goode[49] described a full-thickness wedge resection of the paralyzed side of the lower lip. Edgerton[50] described transplantation of the anterior belly of the digastric muscle. The insertion of the digastric muscle to the mandible on the paralyzed side is divided and attached to a fascia lata graft that is then secured to the mucocutaneous border of the involved lip. Conley et al.[51] modified this technique by leaving the mandibular insertion intact but divided the tendon to the lateral aspect of the lower lip. As branches of the nerve to mylohyoid innervate the anterior belly of the digastrics, activation of the muscle requires a movement other than smiling. This is difficult to coordinate for most patients, and the result is that the digastric transplantation tends to act more as a passive restraint on the lower lip rather than as an active depressor. Terzis and Kalantarin[6] have further modified the digastric transplantation by combining it with a cross-facial nerve graft coapted to a marginal mandibular nerve branch on the unaffected side, thereby allowing the possibility of spontaneous activation with smiling.

In patients in whom the facial paralysis is less than 24 months in duration and there is evidence of remaining depressor muscle after needle electromyography, Terzis recommends mini hypoglossal nerve transplantation to the cervicofacial branch of the facial nerve. This involves division of the cervicofacial branch proximally and coaptation of the distal stump to a partially transected (20–30%) hypoglossal nerve. In patients with long-standing paralysis with a functional ipsilateral platysma muscle (i.e., an intact cervical division of the facial nerve), Terzis suggests transplantation of the platysma muscle to the lower lip.

The approach to depressor muscle paralysis has been to achieve symmetry both at rest and with expression by performing a selective myectomy of the depressor labii inferioris of the non-paralyzed side. This was first reported by Curtin et al.[52] in 1960 and later by Rubin,[47] although details of their techniques are not provided. The depressor resection can be performed as an outpatient procedure under local anesthetic and can be preceded by an injection of either long-acting local

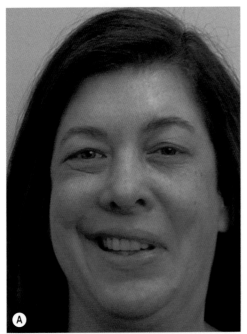

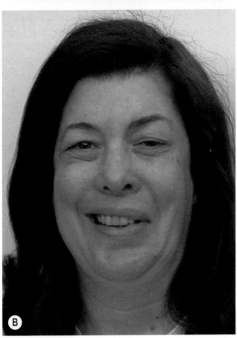

Fig. 13.34 Patient showing a "full dental" smile before depressor resection **(A)** and after depressor resection **(B)**, with marked improvement in symmetry of the lower lip.

is identified; it is partly hidden by the orbicularis oris, whose fibers must be elevated to reveal the more vertically and obliquely oriented fibers of the depressor labii inferioris, which measures approximately 1 cm in width. Care must be taken to preserve the branches of the mental nerve during the dissection (Fig. 13.3). Once the muscle has been identified, the central portion of the muscle belly is resected. Simple myotomy will not produce long-standing results, whereas results from myectomy have been permanent.

The authors have performed depressor labii inferioris resections on 27 patients, and these were reviewed with a follow-up questionnaire. Of these patients, 77% stated that their lower lip was more symmetric with smiling; half of these patients thought that their smile had changed from being significantly asymmetric to completely symmetric. Before the muscle resection, 53% of the patients were concerned about lower lip asymmetry in expressing other emotions, such as sorrow or anger. After the muscle resection, 80% of patients now thought that having a symmetric lower lip in expressing other emotions was more acceptable. Speech was unchanged in 73% of patients and improved in 27% after depressor labii inferioris resection. Some authors have suggested that depressor muscle resection will result in a deterioration of oral continence. However, in our series, 89% of patients stated that oral continence was either unchanged or improved. Three patients reported a slight increase in drooling after depressor labii inferioris resection.

Postoperative care

The postoperative care of all patients must be individualized as to their general medical health and postanesthetic management. However, some generalizations can be made relative to specific procedures. Following muscle transplantation, it is important to maintain an adequate circulating blood volume, guarded mobilization to prevent hypotension, appropriate pain control, and perioperative antibiotics. We prefer to restrict nicotine and caffeine for 6 weeks as we feel they may cause vasoconstriction and increase the risk of vessel thrombosis. In Table 13.7, a typical postoperative order set is outlined following muscle transplantation to the face.

anesthetic or botulinum toxin into the depressor labii inferioris. This injection allows the patient a chance to decide whether to proceed with the muscle resection based on the loss of function of the depressor. As a result of this operation, the shape of the smile is altered on the normal side, and the lower lip is now symmetric with the opposite side (Fig. 13.34).

The depressor labii inferioris is marked preoperatively by asking the patient to show the teeth and palpating over the lower lip. The muscle can be felt as a band passing from the lateral aspect of the lower lip inferiorly and laterally to the chin. Through an intraoral buccal sulcus incision, the muscle

Table 13.7 Postoperative regimen following muscle transplantation
Fluids to soft diet as tolerated
Bed rest day 1 then up in chair with assistance and gradual guarded ambulation
Cefazolin in appropriate age-related dosage for 3 doses
Morphine PRN for 48 h
Tylenol scheduled maximum dose for 3 days
No nicotine for 6 weeks
No caffeine for 6 weeks
No pressure on surgical site
Restrict sports or rough activities that may lead to trauma on surgical site for 6 weeks
After muscle begins to function, active exercises may be helpful with biofeedback to increase excursion, achieve symmetry, and facilitate spontaneity

Outcomes, prognosis, and complications

As in all aspects of surgical intervention, the surgeon and patient must consider the risk-to-benefit ratio. In facial paralysis reconstruction, we cannot completely replicate normality. However, we can improve the functional limitations imposed by the lack of corneal protection, the lack of oral competence with consequence leading to drooling, speech problems, and facial expression. Facial asymmetry can also lead to significant psychosocial problems. When the effects are subtle, however, one must weigh the benefits to be obtained, and this is often a function of how severe the paralysis is perceived by the patient and an assessment of this impact on the patient's general well-being. In the study by Bae et al.,[43] it was found that the average commissure movement following cross-face nerve graft and muscle transplantation was about 75% of the normal side (12 versus 15 mm). Thus, if an individual has 7–8 mm of movement, the two complex procedures would only potentially increase movement by 4–5 mm if all went well. This improvement may be worthwhile in some individuals but not in others. Each case must be assessed individually.

The potential complications are numerous but fortunately not very common. The early complications are bleeding, infection, and vascular compromise in a muscle transfer or transplant. The late complications are more common and much more difficult to deal with. They include firstly incorrect muscle positioning. This relates to the insertion at the oral commissure and upper lip which must be accurate and permanent, as previously outlined. The origin needs to be accurately placed, spread out to reduce bulk, and lead to the correct vector of the muscle being created. Secondly, great care needs to be taken to reduce bulk at the side of muscle placement. This will involve the use of only a small strip of muscle (5–15 g in a 5-year-old child and up to 15–25 g in an adult). In addition, the muscle should be spread out at its origin. The removal of the buccal fat pad and a segment of the deep fat that will overlie the newly placed muscle may also aid in lessening the likelihood of excess bulk. Thirdly, the excursion of either a transferred muscle or transplanted muscle may not meet the expectations of the surgeon or the patient and be quite disappointing. We feel that excursion is related to the power of the motor nerve utilized and to the physical placement of the muscle as it must be under the appropriate tension to maximize excursion. A poorly functioning muscle may also be related to the vascularity of the muscle or the effects of a single or double nerve repair, although it may be related to a combination of the above factors. Unfortunately, these insufficient excursion problems are not easy to correct and will be addressed in the next section.

Secondary procedures

Secondary procedures following muscle transfer or transplant are often palliative and not curative. The problems can be listed as incorrect muscle positioning, excess bulk at the side of the muscle, and poor excursion.

Muscle slippage at the insertion side is the most difficult to correct. Open reinsertion can be done but may leave the commissure too tight and the mouth distorted. This can be avoided by using a tendon graft to connect the displaced muscle to the oral commissure and upper lip. If the muscle is too tight, it can be released at its origin and slid toward the mouth. However, this may require a radical freeing of the muscle and put the neuromuscular pedicle at risk. If the vector is incorrect, it can be repositioned but only with great difficulty and again with significant risk to the pedicle. Whenever the position of the muscle is adjusted, one can expect a reduction in excursion. However, this may be a reasonable price to pay to correct the distortions imposed by poorly positioned muscle.

Excess bulk at the side of the transferred or transplanted muscle can be addressed by defatting and shaving of the outer surface of the muscle. To facilitate this, it is helpful to position the motor nerve on the deep surface of the muscle at the time of the muscle transplantation. This is particularly true when a cross-face nerve graft is used.

When the problem is poor excursion, the options are few. It may help to tighten the muscle if it has been inserted too loosely but care must be taken not to distort the mouth.

If this is not possible, then a thorough open discussion with the patient is required. Is there sufficient support or movement to alleviate the functional problems and position the mouth evenly at rest? How much movement with muscle activation is present? Is the patient content with the present situation, in view of the fact that improvement will not be easy or perhaps even possible?

If further surgery is requested after a full discussion and knowledge that improvement will be difficult, one must redo with transplantation of a second muscle. If the cause of the failure is not clear, it may be wise to use a motor nerve to power the new muscle that was not used before. This may be the motor nerve to masseter in the case of a failed cross-face nerve graft, muscle transplantation combination. The results of putting a muscle into scarred bed, and reusing the previous vessels and possibly nerve, will not be as likely for success as the primary procedure, but yet may be very helpful for selected patients.

Further considerations

Facial paralysis crosses many subspecialty lines. Limited eye closure, tear transport, and ectropion dictate the involvement of ophthalmologists as well as oculoplastic surgeons. Intranasal airflow may be limited and symptomatic, necessitating involvement of nasal surgeons often with otolaryngology background. Otolaryngologists may also be consulted for associated hearing loss, stapedial malfunction, or other components involving the middle ear. In certain patients, brainstem involvement may cause difficulty in dealing with oral secretions, aspirations, and swallowing. This may occur congenitally, such as in patients with Möbius syndrome, or it may be acquired, such as in patients with intracranial tumors. These situations may require the involvement of otolaryngologists.

There are other functional issues that may need to be addressed by subspecialists. For example, feeding may be a problem for infant or adult patients. Feeding experts from occupational therapy may be helpful in providing techniques for mechanical assistance. After surgical intervention, occupational therapy is also helpful in assisting with an exercise program to improve muscle excursion and symmetry of smile.

Speech is often affected by facial paralysis. Speech therapy can help improve articulation errors and provide appropriate lip placement.

The psychosocial aspects of facial paralysis are enormous. Surgeons tend to focus on the physical, but it is extremely important to keep the entire patient in mind. A battery of psychosocial support personnel should be available to work with the surgeon for the overall benefit of the patient. This team should include social workers, clinical psychologists, developmental psychologists, and psychologists. It is important to sort out the various needs of the patient, not just from a physical standpoint but also from a psychosocial standpoint. Only then can true success in surgical management be achieved. A majority of patients with congenital facial paralysis have unilateral and isolated involvement. It is believed to be the result of a compression of the fetal face that limits facial nerve development. Consequently, there are no genetic implications. Parents have no predisposition for additional children with facial paralysis, nor does the patient have any greater increased likelihood of having a child with facial paralysis than that of the general population. The same can be said for patients with unilateral syndrome, which occurs with hemifacial microsomia, for example. This is thought to be acquired at an early stage of fetal development because of environmental factors. Thus, again, there are no genetic implications. The same is not true, however, for all patients with Möbius syndrome. Although most are thought to be sporadic, there has been a surge of interest in the genetics of the conditions.[53] Pedigrees have been described indicating that certain forms of Möbius syndrome are inherited by an autosomal-dominant gene with variable expressivity (Fig. 13.35).

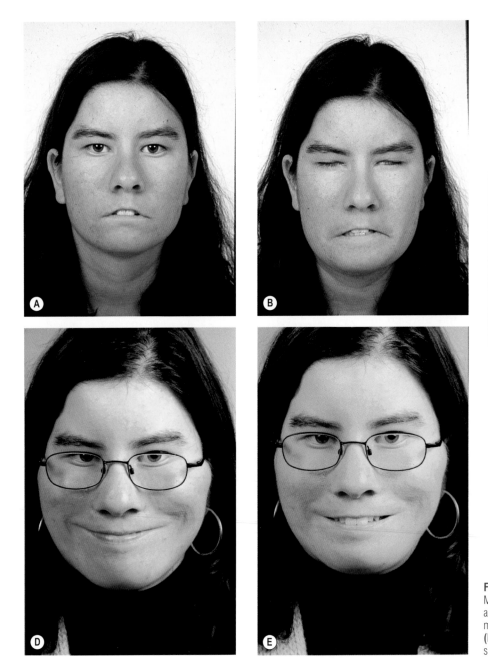
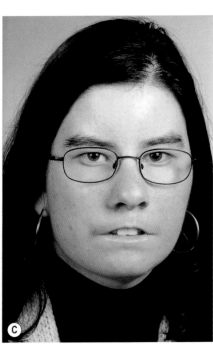

Fig. 13.35 (A,B) Preoperative views of a patient with Möbius syndrome at rest and with maximum animation. **(C)** Postoperative view of a patient after muscle transplantation to the lower face at rest. **(D)** Patient with closed-mouth smile. **(E)** Patient smiling and showing teeth.

Incomplete penetration is also thought to account for the inconsistency of involvement. Certain chromosomes have also been identified in specific patients,[54] and a reciprocal translocation between the long arm of chromosome 13 and the short arm of chromosome 1 has been described.[55] A great deal of interest has been stimulated relative to the genetic aspects of Möbius syndrome and its relationship to other behavioral conditions.[55,56] Research is under way in these areas and will undoubtedly shed light on inheritance features as well as the etiologic factors involved in Möbius syndrome.

Conclusions

Although significant progress has been made in the management of facial paralysis, much is yet to be done. Acceptable commissure movement can be achieved, but upper lip elevation is far more difficult. The short distance of the muscle involved and the challenging access have proved difficult to overcome. However, new techniques are emerging, and work in this area continues.

Across any nerve repair, there is considerable loss of axonal continuity. Improved nerve coaptation techniques with the use of neurotrophic factors will undoubtedly be instrumental in providing further improvement. From a physical standpoint, does the length of the nerve graft affect recovery? Does its vascular nature or the technique of harvest result in alteration of function? Laboratory research in these areas is ongoing and could again provide some level of improvement in recovery. The placement, anchorage, and direction of movement of the muscle transplant are critical to success. Improvements

have been made in these areas, but asymmetry continues to be a challenge. Further attention needs to be drawn to the direction of the smile and the positioning of the muscle relative to the oral commissure and nasolabial crease.

Fundamental to progress in any field is an assessment tool that is reliable, universally acceptable, and as simple as possible to use. In facial paralysis, it is necessary to measure muscle excursion, direction of movement, volume symmetries, and contour irregularities to assess the results of repair and reconstruction. For comparison of results from center to center, a common tool is needed. Also, to assess results from a psychosocial standpoint, a reliable common instrument of evaluation is needed if meaningful conclusions are to be drawn. Progress has been made on physical measurement and psychosocial profile tools,[56] and there is hope that these will be universally accepted and applied in the future.

In addition to these technical issues, concepts need to evolve with respect to new areas of development. Eye expression is an area that has not as yet been directed at commissure and upper lip elevation. Orbicularis oris function or reconstruction of the depressors has not been addressed. Finally, there is not as yet an effective method of managing synkinesis. This is an extremely disturbing phenomenon with psychosocial and functional implications. We are just beginning to see how Botox injection techniques can be effective in other areas of muscle overactivity, and perhaps some level of synkinesis control will evolve with this technique. Much is yet to be done for the patient with facial paralysis, and further research and development in this area will continue to yield improvements.

In summary, facial paralysis reconstruction continues to be an exciting evolving area of surgical development.

🌐 Access the complete references list online at **http://www.expertconsult.com**

9. Rubin L, ed. *The Paralyzed Face*. St. Louis: Mosby-Year Book; 1991. *This is a classic text on facial expressions and how to produce them surgically.*

14. Westin LM, Zuker RM. A new classification system for facial paralysis in the clinical setting. *J Craniofac Surg*. 2003;14:672–679. *This classification of facial paralysis was created as an aid to the clinician in understanding the breadth of this diverse condition.*

16. May M. Microanatomy and pathophysiology of the facial nerve. In: May M, ed. *The Facial Nerve*. New York: Thieme; 1986:63. *This classic text is a must for all students of facial paralysis.*

26. Carraway JH, Manktelow RT. Static sling reconstruction of the lower eyelid. *Operative Techniques Plast Reconstr Surg*. 1999;6:163. *Eyelid surgery must be precise and well executed to be successful.*

28. Manktelow RT, Tomat LR, Zuker RM, et al. Smile reconstruction in adults with free muscle transfer innervated by the masseter motor nerve: effectiveness and cerebral adaptation. *Plast Reconstr Surg*. 2006;118:885–899. *In this paper, evidence is presented to suggest cerebral adaptation is a real entity in the adult population.*

30. Michaelidou M, Chieh-Han J, Gerber H, et al. The combination of muscle transpositions and static procedures for reconstruction in the paralyzed face of the patient with limited life expectancy on who is not a candidate for free muscle transfer. *Plast Reconstr Surg*. 2009;123:121–129. *This is an excellent article that provides the surgeon with practical alternatives to complex microsurgical procedures.*

33. Terzis JK, Tzafetta K. The "babysitter" procedure: minihypoglossal to facial nerve transfer and cross-facial nerve grafting. *Plast Reconstr Surg*. 2009;123:865–876. *This is the first article to resurrect the nerve transfer principle for facial paralysis. Use of the entire hypoglossal had serious and permanent negative effects on speech, food manipulation, and tongue bulk.*

39. Zuker RM, Goldberg CS, Manktelow RT. Facial animation in children with Möbius syndrome after segmental gracilis muscle transplant. *Plast Reconstr Surg*. 2000;106:1. *This article describes the problems of the Möbius syndrome from a reconstructive surgeon's viewpoint and suggests a surgical procedure for function and animation.*

43. Bae Y, Zuker RM, Mantelow RM, et al. A comparison of commissure excursion following gracilis muscle transplantation for facial paralysis using a cross-face nerve graft versus the motor nerve to the masseter nerve. *Plast Reconstr Surg*. 2006;117:2407–2413. *In this paper the strong input of the masseter motor nerve is shown to translate into increased commissure excursion.*

45. Labbe D, Huault M. Lengthening temporalis myoplasty and lip reanimation. *Plast Reconstr Surg*. 2000;105:1289–1297. *This is an excellent article that provides the surgeon with practical alternatives to complex microsurgical procedures.*

14

Pharyngeal and esophageal reconstruction

Edward I. Chang and Peirong Yu

 Access video and video lecture content for this chapter online at expertconsult.com

SYNOPSIS

- Pharyngoesophageal defects are most commonly the result of a total laryngopharyngectomy for squamous cell carcinoma in the laryngeal region or hypopharynx. Other etiology includes benign strictures, pharyngocutaneous fistulas, and thyroid cancer involving the esophagus
- Radiotherapy has become the primary treatment for early stages of squamous cell carcinoma in these regions. Many pharyngoesophageal defects are the results of salvage laryngopharyngectomy following neoadjuvant radiation therapy, making reconstruction more challenging.
- Commonly used flaps for pharyngoesophageal reconstruction include the jejunal flap, radial forearm flap, and the anterolateral thigh (ALT) flap. In recent years, the ALT flap has become the most popular flap for this type of reconstruction
- Major complications following pharyngoesophageal reconstruction include anastomotic strictures and fistulas.
- The ultimate goals of reconstruction are to provide alimentary continuity, protection of important structures such as the carotid artery, and restoration of functions such as speech and swallowing
- Most patients (greater than 90%) can eat an oral diet after reconstruction without the need for tube feeding
- Speech rehabilitation is typically provided with tracheoesophageal puncture (TEP), and fluent speech can be achieved in greater than 80% of patients. Speech quality is superior with a fasciocutaneous flap than an intestinal flap
- Many patients with pharyngoesophageal defects have a frozen neck due to previous radiotherapy and surgery, making reconstruction extremely difficult with high surgical risks. Careful planning, use of transverse cervical vessels as recipient vessels, and a two-skin island ALT flap to simultaneously resurface the neck for a through-and-through defect can simplify the procedure and reduce surgical risks.

Introduction

Reconstruction of pharyngeal and esophageal defects presents unique challenges to the reconstructive surgeon.

Reconstruction is aimed at restoring continuity of the gastrointestinal tract in order to allow patients to resume a normal diet postoperatively. A number of reconstructive options are now available for reconstructing pharyngoesophageal defects; however, optimizing outcomes and postoperative functions require careful consideration of a variety of different factors. Flap selection, recipient vessel selection, neck skin resurfacing, and minimizing complications are critical to achieve maximal function following reconstruction.

Pharyngoesophageal defects can result from a variety of etiologies, most commonly tumor extirpation, but can also result from trauma or ingestion of caustic agents. In the setting of cancer, such defects are most often associated with laryngeal cancer that is often treated with radiation initially. Consequently, reconstruction often occurs in the setting of prior radiation which can have a significant impact on ultimate outcomes and postoperative function.

Reconstruction can be accomplished with local flaps or free flaps, but the modality of reconstruction depends on surgeon comfort and preference, hospital nursing and operating room staff, and hospital infrastructure. The first reported cervical esophageal "reconstruction" was documented by Mikulicz[1] in 1886 in which the proximal and distal cervical esophageal ends were connected with a rubber tube over the neck skin and the skin was later tubed to close the gap. The Wookey flap[2,3] was popular until the 1960s when Bakamjian[4] described the use of the deltopectoral flap for cervical esophageal reconstruction. However, these flaps are no longer used for pharyngoesophageal reconstruction today due to a variety of problems. The gastric pull-up procedure was introduced in the mid-1900s to reconstruct thoracic esophagectomy defects and was later used for pharyngoesophageal defects.[5–10] Subsequently, the pedicled colon and jejunum also became popular flaps for such reconstructions[11–13] but have largely been abandoned due to the need for performing a total esophagectomy to utilize these intestinal flaps which had significant comorbidity and risks for complications.

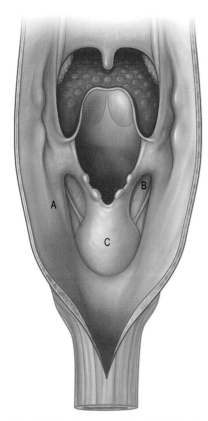

Fig. 14.1 The hypopharynx is located behind the larynx and in continuity with the oral pharynx superiorly and the cervical esophagus inferiorly. The hypopharynx is arbitrarily divided into three areas for purposes of tumor classification: the pharyngeal wall (**A**), pyriform sinuses (**B**), and postcricoid area (**C**).

The pectoralis major flap became the flap of choice for pharyngoesophageal reconstruction[14–16] in the early 1980s until free flaps became popular. Although Seidenberg *et al.*[17] reported the first clinical use of free jejunal flaps for cervical esophageal reconstruction in 1959, it did not gain popularity until the 1980s.[18–21] Although the jejunal flap has several advantages, such as rapid healing, low fistula rate, and a relatively simpler inset as the jejunum is already a tubular conduit, its abdominal morbidity and poor speech reproduction with tracheoesophageal puncture techniques make it less ideal for

pharyngoesophageal reconstruction. Since the beginning of 2000s, the anterolateral thigh flap has largely replaced both the jejunal and radial forearm flaps for pharyngoesophageal reconstruction and become the new "gold standard" in many centers due to its many advantages.[22–26]

This chapter aims to provide a brief global overview of reconstruction of pharyngeal and esophageal defects focusing on anatomy, defect classification, reconstruction, and postoperative management and complications.

Anatomy

The oropharynx is bounded by the nasopharynx superiorly, the oral cavity anteriorly, and the hypopharynx and larynx inferiorly. The superior border of the oropharynx is at the plane of the soft palate, and the inferior border is defined by the level of the hyoid bone. The main structures in the oropharynx are the base of tongue, tonsillar pillars, lateral and posterior oropharyngeal walls, and soft palate. Common oncologic defects in the oropharynx are the result of surgical resections of cancers in the base of tongue which may extend to and involve the pharyngeal wall and tonsillar pillars. Some of these defects that need not be resurfaced with a free flap can be allowed to remucosalize spontaneously. The hypopharynx extends from the level of the hyoid bone to the lower border of the cricoid cartilage and ultimately continues to become the cervical esophagus caudally (Fig. 14.1). This is a critical area that is responsible for airway protection and swallowing and speech functions. Common defects of the hypopharynx and cervical esophagus are the result of surgical resection of cancers in the hypopharynx and larynx, advanced thyroid cancers, radiation strictures, and chemical injuries. Isolated tumors in the cervical esophagus, although rare, may also require segmental esophagectomy and reconstruction (Table 14.1).

Patient evaluation

Patients anticipated to undergo surgical resection and reconstruction for malignancy should have a thorough history and physical including preoperative imaging and laboratory studies. As most laryngeal tumors are treated initially with

Table 14.1 Types of pharyngoesophageal defects requiring reconstruction		
Pathology	**Defect location**	**Type of defect**
Primary SCC	Hypopharynx and cervical esophagus	Most commonly partial
Recurrent SCC	Hypopharynx and cervical esophagus	Most commonly circumferential
Advanced or recurrent thyroid cancer	Hypopharynx and cervical esophagus	Most commonly circumferential
Isolated esophageal tumors	Cervical esophagus with an intact larynx	Most commonly partial
Pharyngoesophageal or tracheoesophageal fistulas	Cervical esophagus or hypopharynx	Most commonly partial
Anastomotic strictures	Cervical esophagus	Most commonly circumferential
Radiation-induced strictures	Hypopharynx or cervical esophagus	Partial or circumferential, depending on the degree of stricture
SCC, squamous cell carcinoma		

chemotherapy and radiation, these factors can have a significant impact when patients are scheduled to undergo surgical salvage. Discussion should also include patients' postoperative function in this setting, as a laryngectomy would have compromised function compared to an esophagectomy where the larynx can usually be preserved with relatively normal postoperative speech function. Questioning should also include pertinent prior surgeries especially if patients have had a prior resection or neck dissection which can drastically complicate salvage surgery and the availability of recipient vessels.

Other comorbidities also need to be considered in patients undergoing surgery. The overwhelming majority of patients who suffer from laryngeal and esophageal malignancy have a history of tobacco and alcohol use which may contribute to postoperative complications and impact wound healing. Further, patients with history of peripheral vascular disease in conjunction with smoking should be evaluated for donor sites as well as recipient vessels. As most patients undergoing surgery and treatment of malignancy have already had imaging studies, the studies should be reviewed to assess the availability and patency of potential recipient vessels. If patients are severely malnourished, consideration should be given to placement of a feeding tube preoperatively in order to optimize patients' nutritional status prior to surgery if possible.

The physical exam should certainly include evaluation of the donor site and local surgical sites. In the setting of prior radiation, evaluation of the pliability of the neck skin is critical. Following a visor type incision to complete the resection and subsequent reconstruction, there is a definite possibility that the skin incision cannot be closed primarily without risk of dehiscence and exposure of vital structures. The physical exam should also include a thorough vascular exam. In general the vasculature supplying the thigh and therefore the anterolateral thigh (ALT) flap are preserved since it is supplied by the profundus femoris artery. Regarding the upper extremity, an Allen's test on the upper extremity is commonly performed prior to reconstruction with a radial or ulnar artery based flap. While the utility has been questioned, it is important to assess adequate hand perfusion prior to harvesting one of the vessels for pharyngoesophageal reconstruction. Typically the non-dominant arm is utilized and, therefore, patients should be questioned regarding which side is their dominant arm. As most patients will require a tracheostomy in the immediate postoperative period or permanently in the setting of a laryngectomy, patients will only be able to communicate with writing initially and, therefore, the dominant arm should be preserved, if possible.

Flap selection

The decision for which flap is used for reconstruction is dependent on a myriad of important factors, not least of which is surgeon's preference, experience, and comfort with flap elevation. In general, a thinner, more pliable flap is recommended, and the surgical plan should always include an algorithm in the setting that the primary flap of choice is not usable. Whether a free flap or a pedicle flap is utilized is largely dependent on surgeon expertise, and both have been utilized successfully for pharyngoesophageal reconstruction.

Postoperative function can be restored with either a free or pedicle flap with most flaps being fasciocutaneous. However, one unique flap consideration is an intestinal flap either via a free jejunum or a supercharged jejunum for total esophagectomy reconstruction. The swallowing function is comparable between fasciocutaneous flaps and intestinal flaps. However, speech function is superior with fasciocutaneous flaps.[24,26] Similar consideration should be given to donor site morbidity as well. Harvesting of a fasciocutaneous flap is typically well tolerated with minimal donor site morbidity, while harvest of a segment of jejunum requires a laparotomy which may predispose patients to risk of significant fluid shift, adhesions, bowel obstruction, and an incisional hernia in the future. The advantages and disadvantages of commonly used free flaps are listed in Table 14.2.

Table 14.2 Advantages and disadvantages of commonly used free flaps

	ALT	Jejunum	Radial forearm
Flap elevation	Moderately difficult	Moderately difficult	Easy
Flap reliability	Good	Good	Good
Flap thickness	Can be too thick	Good	Good
Primary healing	Good	Best	Good
Donor site morbidity	Low	High	Moderate
Recovery time	Quick	Can be slow	Quick
Fistula rates	Low	Low	Moderate
Stricture rates	Low	High	Moderate
TEP voice	Good	Poor	Good
Swallowing	Good	Good	Good
Use for circumferential defects	Yes	Yes	Second choice
Use for partial defects	Yes	No	Yes
Contraindications	Obesity, with a very thick thigh	Severe comorbidity, prior abdominal surgery	Thin patient with a small arm, radial dominance

ALT, anterolateral thigh flap; TEP, tracheoesophageal puncture

Pedicle flaps such as the pectoralis major myocutaneous flap, deltopectoral flap, internal mammary artery perforator (IMAP) flap, and supraclavicular flap have been well-described and performed successfully for pharyngeal and esophageal reconstruction; however, at our institution, we typically reserve pedicle flaps for salvage in the setting of a leak or fistula. However, in the setting of severe carotid stenosis or the lack of recipient vessels, a local pedicle flap may be necessary in order to reconstruct the defect or resurface the radiated neck.

Pedicle flaps

The algorithm for pharyngoesophageal reconstruction should include pedicle flaps which can be used as the primary modality for reconstruction or in the setting of salvage in the case of loss of a free flap or pharyngocutaneous fistula.

Pectoralis major myocutaneous flap

The pectoralis major myocutaneous (PMMC) flap has traditionally been a workhorse flap for head and neck reconstruction.[27–29] In our institution, the PMMC flap is typically reserved for salvage situations or in situations when a free tissue transfer cannot be performed. The flap can be reliably harvested as a muscle-only flap for reinforcement of a pharyngeal closure or for closure of a fistula. An incision is made in the inframammary fold, and the muscle is identified. The muscle is released off the chest wall with the aid of a lighted retractor, and large intercostal perforators are ligated with hemoclips. The pedicle is readily identified on the deep surface of the muscle and taken as cranial as possible to the level of the clavicle. The superficial dissection is performed next preserving the fascia with the muscle that provides more robust tissue to hold sutures for the flap inset. The medial muscle is released preserving 2–3 cm of medial muscle to avoid the large internal mammary perforators that can lead to significant bleeding that can be difficult to control if injured. The lateral muscle is then released and tapered for the pedicle to islandize the muscle and minimize the bulk of the muscle proximally. A counter-incision is often made in an axillary skin fold to release the muscle from its origin at the humeral attachments. The pectoralis muscle can then be easily rotated into the neck for coverage of the pharyngeal defect with or without skin grafting for lining.

A skin paddle can also be harvested; however, the skin paddle is less reliable distally and can be prone to partial flap necrosis. Perforators arising from the pectoralis major muscle can be detected in the skin paddle using a hand-held Doppler; however, prior studies have demonstrated the utility of intraoperative indocyanine green angiography to design the skin paddle over the area of maximal perfusion. The skin paddle from a PMMC flap can be used to repair a partial pharyngectomy defect; however, circumferential defects are often difficult to reconstruct secondary to the bulk of the flap.

Supraclavicular artery perforator flap

The supraclavicular artery flap is an axial pattern flap and has been well-described based off the supraclavicular branches arising from the transverse cervical vessels. [30–33] The flap is typically thin and pliable allowing the flap to be tubed for circumferential defects or as a patch for partial defects. The flap can be islandized for inset as well. The main pedicle arises off the thyrocervical trunk and passes between the sternocleidomastoid and trapezius muscles to supply branches that will perfuse the overlying skin. The pedicle has been described to be 1.1–1.5 mm in diameter with a length up to 7 cm, but the pedicle can maintain a flap up to 35 cm in length. However, the width is limited to approximately 6 cm in greatest width to allow primary closure of the donor site (Fig. 14.2). In the setting where a radical neck dissection has been performed, or when the neck dissection includes level 5, there is a high likelihood that the transverse cervical vessels have been ligated and, therefore, a supraclavicular artery flap is contraindicated. Further, if the skin has been involved in prior radiation treatment, the use of the supraclavicular flap is also not recommended as using radiated tissue to reconstruct a pharyngeal esophageal defect would likely be at high risk for partial flap loss and subsequent fistula formation.

Internal mammary artery perforator flap

The internal mammary artery supplies a number of perforators to the overlying skin allowing design of the internal mammary artery perforator (IMAP) flap.[34–36] Multiple studies have confirmed the second internal mammary perforator is often the dominant perforator supplying the overlying skin, and a perforator dissection can provide a pedicle up nearly 10 cm for reconstruction of head and neck defect.[37,38] The size of the skin paddle is limited to the degree of laxity in the chest allowing for primary closure. The flap is typically thin and pliable and can be utilized for reconstruction of partial pharyngectomy defects or for closure of fistulae.[39] Alternatively, it can also be used for neck resurfacing or tracheal stoma reconstruction (Fig. 14.3).[34] The use of the IMAP flap for circumferential defects is limited and an alternate flap should be chosen.

Latissimus dorsi flap

The latissimus dorsi flap can also be used as a salvage flap when the initial reconstruction failed.[40] The dominant pedicle to the latissimus dorsi muscle is the thoracodorsal artery and its venae comitantes, a branch of the subscapular artery and vein. For a muscle only flap, an oblique incision is created starting in the posterior axilla and extending inferiorly for 10 to 20 cm. The subcutaneous tissue is then dissected free from the underlying latissimus dorsi fascia to the anatomical borders of the muscle. The muscle fibers of origin are divided from the posterior iliac crest and thoracolumbar fascia. The deep surface of the muscle is then elevated toward the axilla. As the flap elevation approaches the axilla, the thoracodorsal vessels are identified on the costal surface of the latissimus dorsi and protected throughout the remainder of the dissection. The majority of the tendon of the latissimus dorsi is divided while maintaining constant visualization of the underlying thoracodorsal vessels to avoid pedicle injury. A sleeve of tendon is left intact to take the tension off the vascular pedicle once the flap is transferred to the neck.

A subcutaneous tunnel is created to reach the neck. The flap is pulled through the tunnel to the neck. A skin graft is used as lining to repair the pharyngoesophageal defect. The skin graft is sewn to the remaining pharyngeal mucosa over a 14 mm Montgomery salivary bypass tube as a stent (Fig. 14.4).

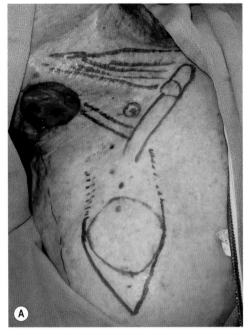

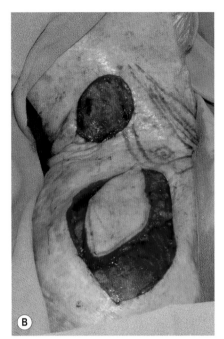

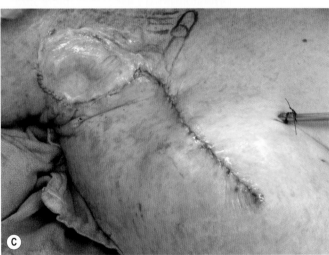

Fig. 14.2 The supraclavicular flap. **(A)** Design of the flap; **(B)** flap islandized; **(C)** primary closure of donor site.

The latissimus muscle is then used to cover the skin graft and the major vessels. In thin patients, a skin paddle can be included to repair the pharyngoesophageal defect instead of using skin grafts. The salivary bypass tube is left in place for 6 weeks.

Free flap choices

With the increasing comfort and popularity with perforator dissection and improved outcomes in free tissue transfer, the use of free flaps has become the gold standard for reconstruction of pharyngoesophageal defects. The different donor sites are virtually endless and depend predominantly on patient body habitus, donor site morbidity, and surgeon experience. An algorithm for free flap pharyngoesophageal reconstruction is outlined in Fig. 14.5. Other considerations that are critical prior to embarking on a free tissue transfer are the availability of recipient vessels, especially in the setting of prior radiation and surgery. The flap should have adequate pedicle length to reach the recipient vessels, and the potential need for vein grafts should also be entertained in the previously operated and radiated neck.

Anterolateral and anteromedial thigh flaps

The anterolateral thigh (ALT) flap has become the workhorse flap for head and neck free flap reconstruction. The flap can typically be harvested at the time of the resection to minimize operative and anesthesia time. In obese patients, the ALT flap may be too thick for pharyngeal esophageal reconstruction and alternate donor sites should be considered. The main vascular pedicle is the descending branch of the lateral circumflex femoris artery, which is a branch of the profundus femoris (Video 14.1 ▶).

Flap harvest

The patient is positioned with the axis of the leg in line and towel clips can be placed in order to prevent the legs from

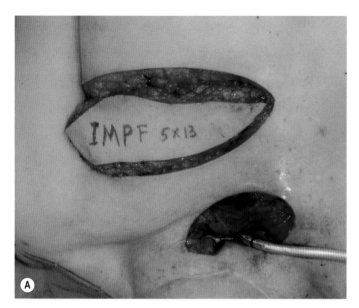
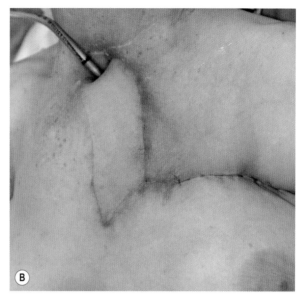

Fig. 14.3 Internal mammary artery perforator (IMAP) flap for tracheostoma reconstruction. **(A)** Flap design based on the perforator in the second intercostal space. **(B)** Healed reconstruction.

external rotation that will affect the location of the perforators and flap design. The right side is typically used for right-handed surgeons; however, either leg can be utilized and they are independent of each other.

A line is drawn connecting the anterior superior iliac spine (ASIS) to the lateral patella, the so-called A-P line.[41] The line is divided in half marking the location of the "B" perforator. The "A" and "C" perforators are located 5 cm proximally and distally, respectively (Fig. 14.6). The perforators can arise through the vastus lateralis muscle, or they can arise as sep-tocutaneous perforators between the vastus lateralis muscle laterally and the rectus femoris muscle medially. The perfora-tors typically enter the fascia approximately 1.4 cm lateral to the A-P line. In general, 93% of patients should have at least one perforator in the A-B-C location allowing for the use of the ALT flap as a potential donor site.

For circumferential defects, a 9.5 cm wide skin paddle is often needed in order to provide a diameter of approximately 3 cm (circumference equals diameter × π) to minimize the chance of stenosis of the conduit and dysphagia (Fig. 14.7A). For partial defects, the width of the remaining mucosa is subtracted from 9.5 cm to give the width of the skin paddle. The anterior skin incision is made and dissection proceeds down to the fascia (Fig. 14.7B). We typically harvest an addi-tional 1–2 cm of fascia with the flap that can be used as a second layer for closure and flap inset (Fig. 14.7C). The fascia is then elevated laterally to identify the perforators (Fig. 14.7D). The main pedicle, the descending branch of the lateral circumflex femoral vessels, is identified between the vastus lateralis and rectus femoris muscles. In general, 8–10 cm pedicle length can be obtained with the ALT flap. If a more distal perforator is present, the pedicle length can be extended. If more pedicle length is needed, the proximal branches to the rectus femoris muscles can be ligated. The size of the artery is generally 2.0–3.0 mm and vein, 2.5–3.5 mm. Once the main pedicle and the perforators have been isolated, the posterior incision is made adjusting the

size of the skin paddle to accommodate either a partial or circumferential defect.

Once the posterior incision is made, dissection proceeds down to the fascia, and again an additional 1–2 cm cuff of fascia is harvested to serve as a second layer to reinforce the closure and minimize the risk of a leak or fistula. Once the fascia is incised, the fascia is elevated off the underlying vastus lateralis muscle until the perforators are encountered. The perforators are freed from the muscle posteriorly, and the flap elevation can be completed at this time.

If two perforators are present, the skin paddle can be divided into two separate skin paddles, one used for recon-struction of the pharyngoesophageal defect, and the second dedicated to resurfacing the neck or for monitoring (Fig. 14.8). If there is only one perforator present, then a distal cuff of the vastus lateralis muscle can be harvested and utilized as either a monitoring segment or to resurface the radiated neck along with a skin graft (Fig. 14.9).

If no usable perforators can be identified in the ALT flap territory, which occurs in 4.3% of thighs, the medial skin paddle should be explored through the same incision to pos-sibly harvest the anteromedial thigh (AMT) flap (Fig. 14.10).[42–44] The main vascular pedicle for the AMT flap is the rectus femoris branch that usually originates from the descending branch 1–2 cm from its take-off (Fig. 14.11). It travels along the medial edge of the rectus femoris muscle and sends out one or two perforators to the skin (Fig. 14.10). Most perfora-tors are septocutaneous ones or pierce the medial edge of the rectus femoris muscle. The AMT flap can be harvested inde-pendently or a multi-component flap (AMT, ALT, vastus lateralis muscle, rectus femoris muscle) can be harvested depending on the needs (Fig. 14.12). Overall, AMT perforators are only present in about half of the cases. However, when there are no ALT perforators, the chances of finding a usable AMT perforator are near 100%, avoiding the need for an entirely new flap. The AMT flap may be thicker as the medial thigh tends to have thicker subcutaneous tissue than the

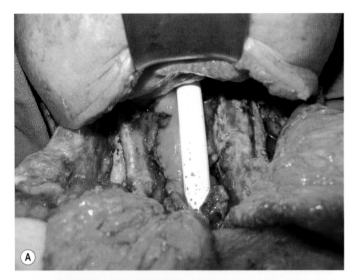

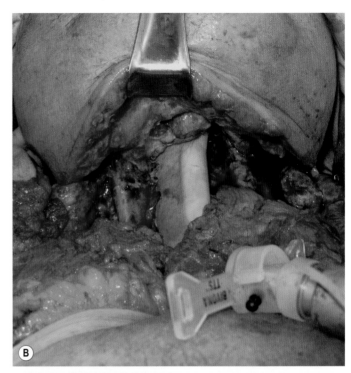

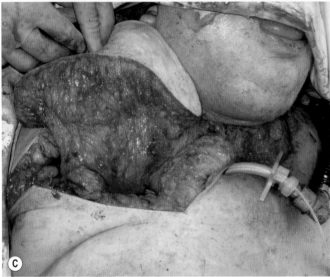

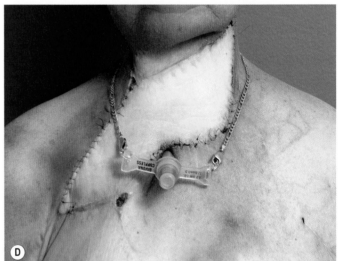

Fig. 14.4 Salvage reconstruction with a latissimus dorsi flap. **(A)** Failed primary anterolateral thigh flap reconstruction due to infection. **(B)** Skin grafting for lining and bilateral pectoralis major muscle flaps to cover exposed great vessels. **(C)** Latissimus dorsi muscle to cover the skin graft for pharyngoesophageal reconstruction and skin paddle for neck resurfacing. **(D)** Well-healed reconstruction. Patient tolerated a soft diet.

lateral thigh, and the pedicle length is often shorter than the ALT flap.

Flap inset

The flap inset is typically performed using 3-0 Vicryl sutures placing the knots inside the lumen and paying careful attention to invert the skin edge and mucosa as much as possible. For partial defects, the flap is inset around the entire defect, and once the flap has been inset, the additional cuff of fascia that was harvested with the flap can be sutured to the remaining constrictor muscles as a second layer to minimize the risk of a fistula. The flap can be thinned if necessary (Fig. 14.13). In most cases, thinning the periphery of the flap is all that is needed. When more aggressive thinning is desired, thinning should fan out from the perforator to avoid perforator injury. It is always critical to preserve a strip of mucosa, if possible,

as this will decrease the risk of developing a stricture postoperatively. For circumferential defects, the ALT flap can be tubed either in the leg or in the neck depending on the authors' preference. In general, the flap is inset, placing the seam posteriorly against the prevertebral fascia that will again hopefully contain a leak should the patient develop one. This places the perforator anteriorly and minimizes the risk of compression of the perforator (Fig. 14.14). The proximal anastomosis is usually completed first, and it is helpful to cut the proximal skin paddle in a curvilinear fashion as the proximal inset into the tongue base typically has a larger length than the distal inset into the esophageal remnant. Next, the longitudinal seam is closed suturing the skin paddle to itself in order to tube the flap. The distal inset is typically performed with a "dart" in the distal skin paddle that is inset into the cervical esophagus (Fig. 14.15). A longitudinal full-thickness

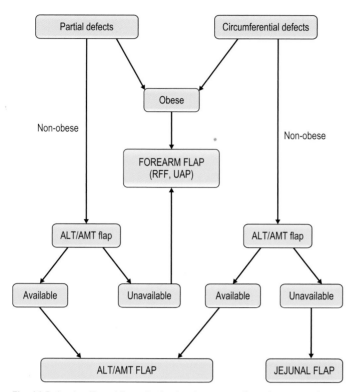

Fig. 14.5 An algorithm of flap selection for pharyngoesophageal reconstruction.

incision in made in the anterior esophagus, and the dart is inset into this spatulated esophagus to increase the diameter of the distal anastomosis and to minimize the risk of developing a stricture (Fig. 14.16). Once the flap is inset, the additional cuff of fascia is again used as a second layer to cover the distal anastomosis. For circumferential defects, a Montgomery salivary bypass tube with a diameter of 14 mm can be placed in the reconstructed esophagus through the mouth (Fig. 14.17). It is usually removed 6 weeks after surgery. We only use it in difficult cases when the distal anastomosis to the esophagus is below the tracheostoma and the tissue quality is poor and prone to leakage.

Prior to closure of the neck skin, the wound should be inspected for hemostasis and irrigated with ample amounts of normal saline. It is our preference to use antibiotic combination irrigation also prior to closure as these cases are long and contaminated. Closed suction drains are also critical to minimize the risk for a seroma that can subsequently become infected and lead to wound dehiscence and even flap thrombosis. The patient's neck should be taken out of extension, and the microvascular anastomosis should be inspected one last time prior to final closure to make certain there is no twist, kink, or compression of the pedicle or perforator. The tracheostoma is then matured to the chest skin anteriorly and to the neck skin posteriorly using 3-0 PDS sutures burying the cartilage under the skin.

If there is not ample laxity of the neck skin to achieve primary closure, as often happens in the setting of prior radiation, the second skin paddle or the vastus lateralis muscle with skin grafting can be used to resurface the neck. The skin paddle and muscle need to be oriented, making certain that the perforator and pedicle are not twisted. The second skin

paddle or skin graft is sutured to the posterior tracheal wall inferiorly and to the neck skin superiorly.

Radial forearm flap

The radial forearm free flap (RFFF) is an excellent choice for pharyngoesophageal reconstruction especially for partial defects.[45–47] Circumferential defects, however, would require harvesting of a significant portion of the forearm in order to have adequate skin to tube the flap, incurring significant donor site morbidity. Under these circumstances, an alternate flap may be necessary to avoid the donor site morbidity. For shorter defects, the flap can be oriented longitudinally so that the flap can be tubed from distal to proximal rather than from lateral to medial. Regardless, the RFFF donor site requires a skin graft to provide coverage of the underlying tendons and muscles. The pedicle for the RFFF usually is more than adequate with over 10 cm of length. The venae comitantes of the radial artery are the dominant venous outflow for the flap, but may be small in certain patients. The venae comitantes may join into a single larger vein or may converge with the cephalic vein to provide a larger caliber vein for the microvascular anastomosis. Incorporating the cephalic vein into the flap is not routinely performed in our practice unless the distal venae comitantes are less than 1 mm at the level of the wrist.

Flap harvest

The non-dominant arm is typically used as the donor arm in order to minimize the donor site morbidity. The arm should be preserved during the initial consultation to make certain that lab draws and IVs are not placed into the arm that can injure the vessels of the flap. The flap harvest can be performed with or without the use of the tourniquet based on surgeon preference. Exsanguination with an Esmarch is not necessary, and elevation prior to tourniquet inflation is adequate.

The dimensions of the flap are outlined based on the size of the defect. In most cases, the width of the flap allows the inclusion of the cephalic vein. When a smaller flap is desired, we explore the venae comitantes at the wrist crease, first by making a small incision (Fig. 14.18). If one of the veins is larger than 1 mm, as it is for most cases, the flap can be safely based on the venae comitantes. Otherwise, the flap design is shifted more laterally to include the cephalic vein as the draining vein. The radial vessels at the distal incision are dissected out, ligated, and divided. Flap dissection from the ulnar side

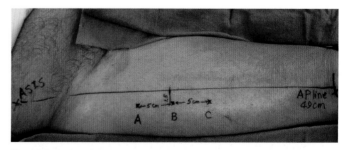

Fig. 14.6 Design of the anterolateral thigh flap. The midpoint of the line connecting the anterior superior iliac spine and the superolateral corner of the patella (A-P line) is marked. Perforator B is usually located 1.5 cm lateral to the midpoint. Perforators A and C are located 5 cm proximal and distal to perforator B, respectively.

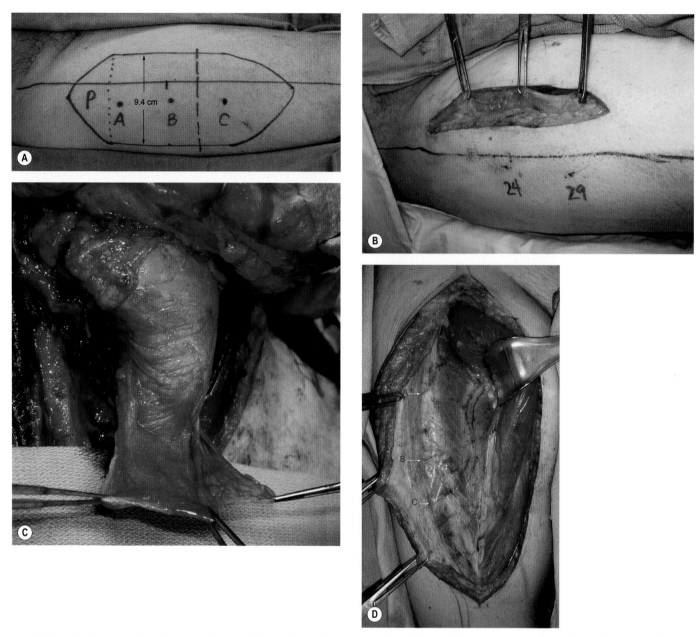

Fig. 14.7 The flap is designed to include two or three potential perforators so that a second skin paddle, usually based on perforator C, can be used for neck resurfacing or monitoring. A lip of the flap is extended proximally (P) to form an elongated oblique opening of the tube flap to accommodate the wider opening in the floor of the mouth **(A)**. A wider fascia than skin is included in the ALT flap **(B)** so that the fascia can be used to cover the suture line **(C)**. Subfascial dissection proceeds laterally until the perforators are seen **(D)**.

proceeds in a suprafascial plane until the brachioradialis tendon is reached, at which point in time, the fascia is incised to gain access to the main pedicle. The radial side dissection is also carried out in a suprafascial plane until the flexor carpi radialis tendon is found, and again the fascia is incised. The sensory branches of the radial nerve should be identified and preserved to minimize the resultant numbness over the dorsum of the thumb postoperatively. The thenar branch of the sensory nerve can only be preserved with the suprafascial technique. The flap is then elevated from a distal to proximal direction and small muscular perforators are ligated with hemoclips. Once the flap is dissected, the incision is extended toward the antebrachial fossa and the pedicle is dissected

proximally to gain length and caliber. Following release of the tourniquet, the hand should be assessed for adequate perfusion, checking capillary refill, and palpating a pulse in the ulnar artery. The inset is similar to that described for the ALT flap except often there is no additional layer of fascia that can be utilized to achieve a second layer closure.

Unlike other fasciocutaneous flaps, the donor site for the RFFF often requires a skin graft for coverage and resurfacing. A split or full thickness skin graft can be utilized and is dressed for a minimum of 5 days with either a pressure bolster or using a negative pressure dressing. A closed suction drain can be placed depending on surgeon's preference. The senior author does not use drains for forearm flap donor sites and

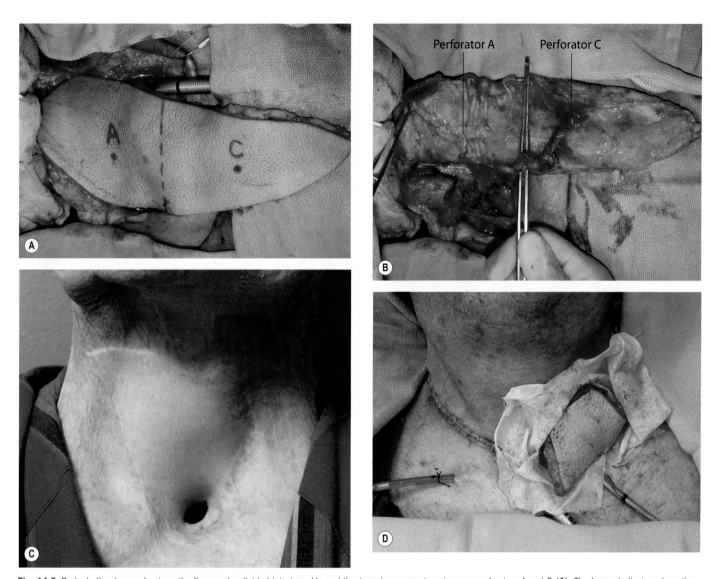

Fig. 14.8 By including two perforators, the flap can be divided into two skin paddles based on separate cutaneous perforators A and C **(A)**. The forcep indicates where the division line is **(B)**. The second skin paddle can be used for neck resurfacing **(C)** or as a monitor **(D)**.

seromas have not been seen. The majority of patients do not suffer any permanent debilitation, pain, weakness, or temperature sensitivity following flap harvest.

Ulnar artery perforator flap

The ulnar artery perforator (UAP) flap represents an excellent alternative to the radial forearm flap.[48,49] Two to three perforators can usually be found along the ulnar artery in the medial aspect of the forearm. The UAP flap is a true perforator flap that also provides thin, pliable skin that is ideal for such defects and typically provides adequate pedicle length and vessel caliber for free tissue transfer in head and neck reconstruction.[48,49] The pedicle length of the UAP flap is considerably shorter than the RFFF and on average is approximately 5–7 cm. Careful attention must be paid to avoid any injury to the ulnar nerve which lies directly adjacent to the main pedicle ulnar vessels. The UAP flap is beneficial as it often provides somewhat thicker tissue, is often not hair-baring, and tendon exposure is rare.

Flap harvest

Like the RFFF, the UAP flap should be harvested from the non-dominant arm. A line connecting the medial epicondyle to the pisiform is drawn which marks the axis for the UAP flap. Typically, the flap is harvested 5 cm proximal to the pisiform to avoid exposure of the tendons. In our experience, the location of the perforators are reliably found at approximately 7 cm, 11 cm, and 16 cm proximal to the pisiform (Fig. 14.19A), namely the A-B-C perforators.[48] The "B" perforator was the most commonly found perforator and was present in 95% of patients.

After elevation exsanguination, the radial incision is made first, and dissection begins in a suprafascial plane until past the flexor digitorum superficialis (FDS) tendons. The perforators arising from the main ulnar vessels should be visible now. The fascia is then incised exposing the ulnar neurovascular bundle, which travels between the FDS and flexor carpi ulnaris (FCU) (Fig. 14.19B). The ulnar nerve is carefully separated from the vessels and the use of electrocautery should be

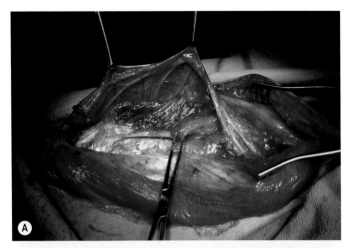

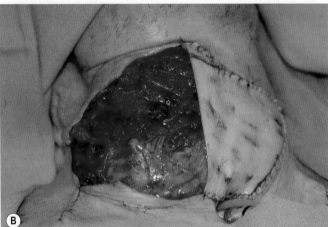

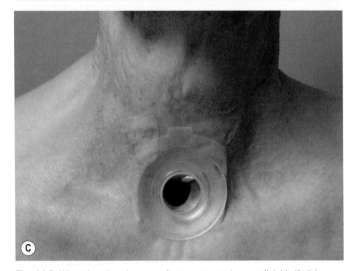

Fig. 14.9 When there is only one perforator present, the superficial half of the vastus lateralis muscle is included to support skin grafts. The descending branch travels alongside the medial edge of the vastus lateralis muscle. The superficial half of the muscle is separated from the deep half immediately below the muscular branches **(A)**. A thin and broad muscle is thus obtained to cover the neck defect with skin grafting **(B)**. Such a thin muscle produces minimal bulk so as not to obstruct the tracheostoma **(C)**.

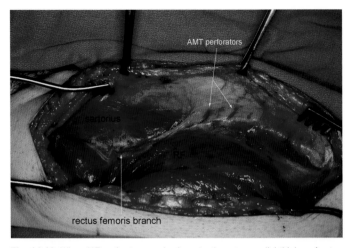

Fig. 14.10 When ALT perforators are inadequate, the anteromedial thigh perforators are explored over the rectus femoris muscle through the same incision.

avoided during the dissection to minimize any trauma to the ulnar nerve. The pedicle at the distal incision is ligated and divided. The ulnar side incision is then made, and subfascial dissection proceeds radially toward the vascular pedicle. The thin septum with the perforators is carefully dissected off the FCU, and any muscular branches are clipped and divided (Fig. 14.19C). The venae comitantes are often of adequate caliber, and the basilic vein is not routinely included. In our experience, the arterial diameter was routinely 2 mm with a vein of 2.5 mm, more than adequate for microvascular anastomoses. The vascular pedicle is dissected proximally to the bifurcation with the common interosseous vessels where the median nerve can be seen, which should be protected from traction injury (Fig. 14.19D). The inset of the flap is performed as previously described; however, careful attention is imperative as the UAP flap is a true perforator flap, and the perforators tend to be smaller than the ALT and may be prone to kinking or traction. A second skin paddle for neck resurfacing is also possible since there are usually more than one perforator (Fig. 14.19E). Prior to closure of the neck, as with all head and neck microvascular free flaps, the head is returned to a neutral position, and the pedicle and perforators should be inspected before definitive closure.

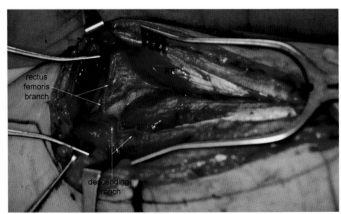

Fig. 14.11 The main vascular pedicle of the AMT flap is the rectus femoris branch that usually originates from the descending branch soon after its take-off.

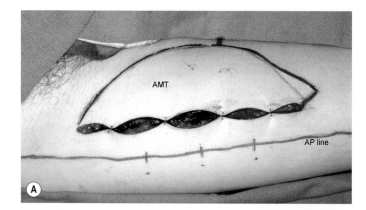

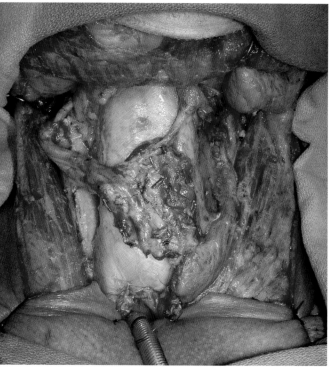

Fig. 14.14 The tubed flap is positioned with the longitudinal seam facing posteriorly against the prevertebral fascia. This will also position the perforators anteriorly to avoid compression.

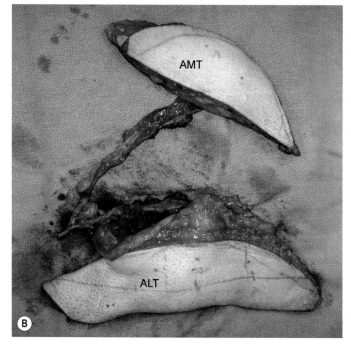

Fig. 14.12 The AMT flap can be harvested independently (A) or with the ALT flap (B) based on the common trunk proximal to the take-off of the rectus femoris branch.

The donor site for a small UAP flap can often be closed primarily given the more proximal location and redundant laxity on the ulnar aspect of the forearm. The distal tendons are not exposed as the flap is designed more proximal and, therefore, the skin graft can typically be placed directly over muscle. This minimizes the risks of complications with poor graft take over the tendons as commonly seen in the radial forearm flap donor site. The donor site is usually well-tolerated with no patients suffering from an ulnar nerve palsy or diminished grip strength in the authors' experience.

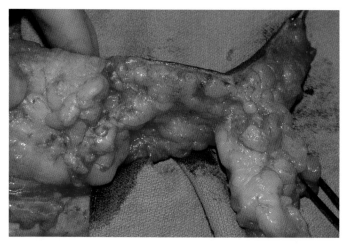

Fig. 14.13 The ALT flap can be thinned by trimming away the subcutaneous tissue. The trimming should fan out from the perforator to avoid perforator injury.

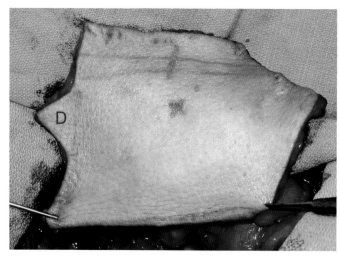

Fig. 14.15 A dart is created in the distal flap skin.

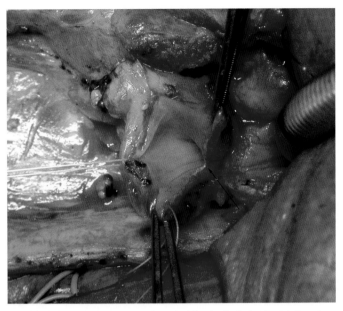

Fig. 14.16 The cervical esophagus is opened longitudinally for about 1.5 cm to spatulate the anastomosis.

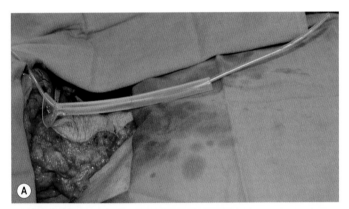

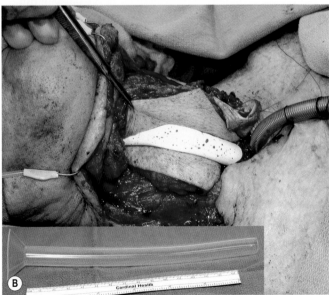

Fig. 14.17 A Montgomery salivary bypass tube with a diameter of 14 mm can be used to temporally stent the neopharynx for 2–6 weeks **(A,B)**.

Lateral arm flap

The lateral arm flap is another excellent alternative for pharyngoesophageal reconstruction in the setting that the ALT flap is too thick as occurs in obese patients, or when a forearm flap is too thin.[50–52] The lateral arm flap has a reliable pedicle that is typically 5–7 cm in length which is usually adequate to reach most recipient vessels in the neck. The radial nerve is within close proximity to the pedicle and must be carefully dissected away from the pedicle and preserved during the dissection. The lateral arm flap is more appropriate for partial pharyngoesophageal defects in order to achieve primary closure of the donor site unless the patient has lost significant weight with large amount of redundant skin available in the upper arm. The main disadvantage of this flap is the small caliber of the pedicle artery which is usually no more than 1.5 mm. The main advantage of this flap is minimal donor site morbidity.

Flap harvest

The arm is placed across the patient's torso, and the deltoid insertion and lateral epicondyle are marked. The septum is palpated between the triceps and biceps muscles and the flap designed centering on the septum (Fig. 14.20A). The posterior incision is made, and a subfascial dissection is performed from a posterior to anterior direction. The septum is approached, and the perforators are identified (Fig. 14.20B). The muscle fibers of the triceps are detached from the septum. The septum is then incised close to the periosteum, exposing the vascular pedicle. Careful attention must be paid to identifying the radial nerve which travels in close proximity to the pedicle (Fig. 14.20C). The pedicle can then be dissected as proximally as possible to obtain longer pedicle length and larger caliber

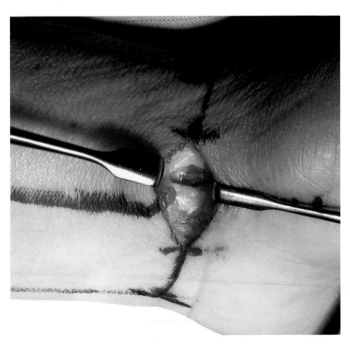

Fig. 14.18 A small exploratory incision was made first at the wrist crease to confirm the size of the venae comitantes of the radial forearm flap vascular pedicle. If both venae comitantes are less than 1 mm in diameter, the flap design is shifted more laterally to include the cephalic vein.

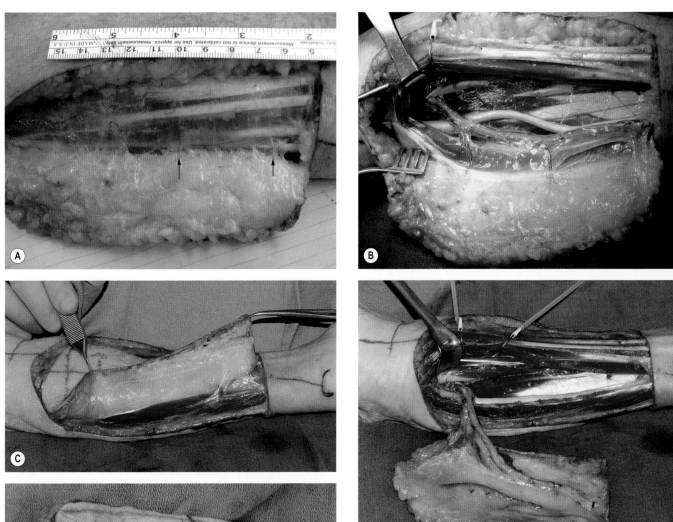

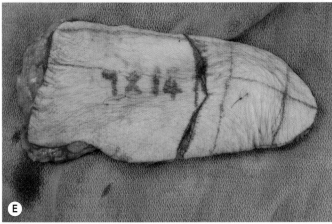

Fig. 14.19 Up to three perforators are present in the ulnar artery perforator flap at approximately 7 cm, 11 cm, and 16 cm above the pisiform, respectively. The flap designed with the distal margin 5 cm proximal to the pisiform **(A)**. The ulnar nerve travels closely with the vessels and should be carefully separated **(B)**. The septum and perforators are dissected off of the flexor carpi ulnaris (FCU) through the posterior incision **(C)**. The median nerve is near the origin of the vascular pedicle and should be protected from traction injury **(D)**. A second skin paddle can be created for neck resurfacing based on a separate perforator **(E)**.

vessels. Some of the deltoid insertion can be divided in order to gain further pedicle length if necessary. The anterior incision is made, and subfascial dissection proceeds posteriorly toward the septum. The distal pedicle is ligated, and the flap can be elevated from a distal to proximal direction.

The donor site for the lateral arm flap is closed primarily over a closed suction drain (Fig. 14.20D). Skin grafting to the upper arm is not recommended. If a larger flap is needed, a different flap is chosen.

Free jejunal flap

In circumstances when fasciocutaneous flaps are not an option for reconstruction of circumferential defects, the jejunal flap represents an excellent option.[53–55] The jejunal segment is harvested through a midline celiotomy incision but can also be harvested using a minimally invasive laparoscopic approach depending on surgeon skill and comfort. The jejunal flap provides excellent swallowing function as the normal

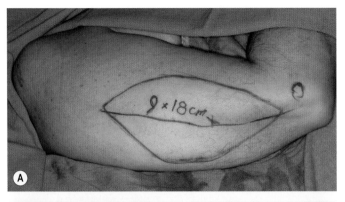

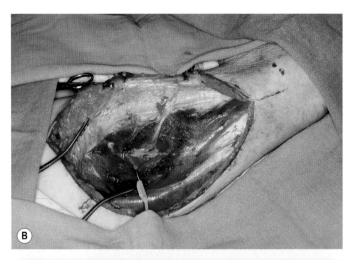

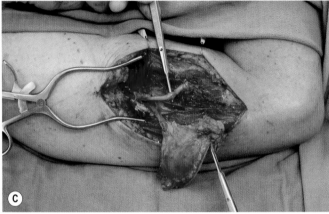

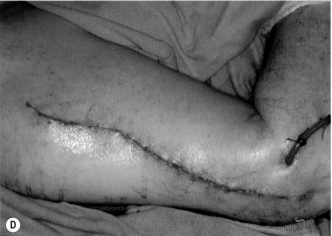

Fig. 14.20 The lateral arm flap is designed over the septum between the biceps and triceps muscles **(A)**. Dissection is carried out through the posterior incision first to identify the perforator **(B)**. The radial nerve should be carefully separated from the vascular pedicle as they travel closely together **(C)**. The donor site is closed primarily over a drain **(D)**.

mucosa provides adequate lubrication to facilitate the passage of the food bolus. It heals well with low risk for fistula formation and avoids a longitudinal suture line for circumferential reconstruction. There are, however, several serious disadvantages. Tracheoesophageal speech through tracheoesophageal puncture (TEP) is difficult and often unsuccessful. Donor site complication with bowel resection can be more serious than fasciocutaneous flaps.

Flap harvest

A midline laparotomy incision is made, and the small bowel is eviscerated in order to visualize the mesentery. Backlighting of the mesentery allows visualization of the vascular arcades supplying the jejunum (Fig. 14.21A), and typically the second arcade is selected as the pedicle for the flap. Once the arcade is identified, the pedicle is dissected to the root of the mesentery but need not proceed to the origin from the superior mesenteric trunk, and an injury to the main trunk would be catastrophic. The branches to the neighboring arcade are divided up to the serosa which isolates a segment of jejunum of 10–15 cm (Fig. 14.21B). The bowel is then divided and can be rejoined using staplers. It is important to mark the proximal end of the bowel to make certain the inset is performed in alignment with normal peristalsis.

Flap inset

The flap inset is completed in a similar fashion compared to other circumferential defects using 3-0 Vicryl sutures. The proximal anastomosis may need to be spatulated to widen the jejunum to the appropriate size to match the oropharynx. Conversely, the distal anastomosis may require spatulation of the esophagus in order to match the size of the jejunum. The anastomosis is typically performed in a single layer, although some may prefer to perform an additional layered closure in a Lembert fashion. The flap should be inset with the neck in neutral position and with some slight stretch to avoid any redundancy in the jejunum which can cause dysphagia.

A portion of the jejunum is divided creating a segment of 2–3 cm that remains attached to the terminal arcade vessels (Fig. 14.21C). This segment is externalized through the neck skin and wrapped in petroleum impregnated gauze to preserve the moisture within the monitoring segment. The segment can be used to monitor the viability of the jejunum both by color, turgor, Doppler, and peristalsis. Prior to discharge, the pedicle to the monitoring segment can be ligated with a simple suture. We prefer to place a 2-0 silk around the terminal arcade vessel outside the skin closure. When the monitoring segment is ready to be removed, one can simply tighten the silk tie and remove the bowel segment.

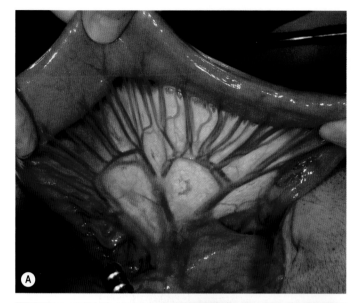

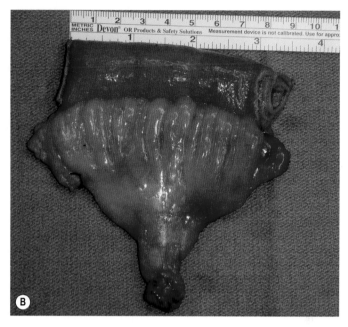

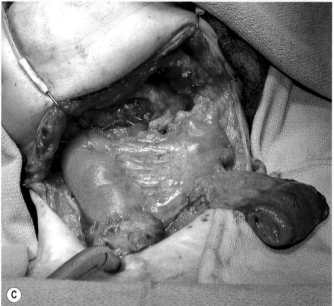

Fig. 14.21 During jejunal flap harvesting, the mesentery arcades of the jejunal flap are transilluminated with fiberoptic backlighting to facilitate vessel dissection **(A)**. A segment of jejunum 10–15 cm long is harvested for circumferential pharyngoesophageal reconstruction **(B)**. A short bowel segment is created and externalized as a monitoring segment, which is removed before the patient is discharged from the hospital **(C)**.

Donor site

The donor site should be closed meticulously as with any laparotomy incision to minimize the chance of developing an incisional hernia. If there is any concern for tension on the abdominal closure, consideration should be given to placement of mesh to reinforce the closure or performing a component separation in order to allow a tension free closure. Either a gastrostomy or jejunostomy feeding tube is placed before abdominal closure. Tube feeding is started when bowel function is returned which may take 3–5 days.

Flap monitoring

Flap monitoring is critical to optimize outcomes and minimize complications. If a microvascular thrombosis is detected, earlier intervention is the most critical factor for maximizing flap salvage. Flap monitoring is best achieved with physical exam which is the gold standard. Despite the emergence of a myriad of new technologies claiming to improve flap outcomes and provide earlier detection of microvascular complications, no current technology supplants clinical exam and experience. Therefore, nursing staff and trainees should be carefully instructed to examine the flap for signs of microvascular compromise. The flap should be inspected for color, capillary refills, turgor, temperature, and the presence of a Dopplerable arterial or venous signal should all be noted regularly. At the authors' institution, free flaps are monitored hourly for the first 3 days, and then every 2 h for the next 2 days, and then every 4 h until the patients are discharged.

For pharyngoesophageal reconstruction, however, the primary flap is buried and, therefore, not accessible for clinical examination. With the jejunal flap, a short segment of bowel based on a terminal arcade vessel can be externalized for monitoring purpose (Fig. 14.21C). Similarly, a second skin

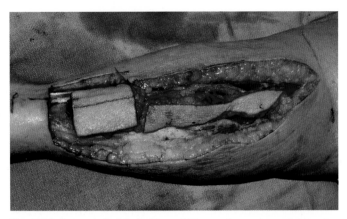

Fig. 14.22 A second skin island of the radial forearm flap can be created based on a separate proximal perforator.

paddle from a fasciocutaneous flap, being either the ALT (Fig. 14.8D), radial forearm (Fig. 14.22), or UAP flap (Fig. 14.19E), can usually be created based on a second perforator either for neck resurfacing or solely for monitoring purposes.[56] A segment of the vastus lateralis muscle can also be externalized for monitoring (Fig. 14.23). In the setting where a second paddle was not necessary or if a monitoring segment was not included with the flap harvest, alternate means of flap monitoring need to be employed. The use of the implantable Cook–Swartz Doppler has been used for monitoring buried flaps and can be placed on the artery, vein, or both. Recently, the introduction of the Flow coupler (Synovis Inc., Birmingham, AL, USA) combines an implantable venous Doppler with the coupler device used to complete the venous anastomosis (Fig. 14.24). The utility of these new technologies remains to be determined; however, in the setting when no monitoring segment or skin paddle is available, these devices represent a useful adjunct to detect microvascular thromboses.

The loss of the implantable Doppler signal should prompt immediate exploration following clinical evaluation with the potential for a high false positive rate. Nonetheless, a negative exploration for malfunction of the implantable Doppler is preferable to delaying exploration and having to manage a dead flap.

Recipient vessel selection

The recipient vessels are critical for any microvascular free tissue transfer and should be confirmed prior to committing to a free flap reconstruction. When available, the authors prefer to use branches off the external carotid such as the lingual or facial arteries which are usually an adequate size match for an ALT flap, jejunal flap, or forearm flap. The superior thyroid artery, which is anatomically the first branch off the external carotid, is often smaller at 1.5–2 mm but may serve as an excellent size match for a lateral arm flap which usually has an artery comparable in size. Recipient veins are usually a branch off the internal jugular vein such as the facial vein or its branch so that end-to-end anastomosis can be completely using a coupler. However, if there are no branches available, an end-to-side anastomosis can also be completed in a hand-sewn fashion.

In the setting of a "frozen neck", there may be a paucity of recipient vessels. The great vessels can be encased in scar, and dissection to expose these vessels can pose significant risk for carotid artery rupture. We prefer using the transverse cervical vessels as potential recipients.[57] The right side is preferred over the left side to avoid injury to the thoracic duct (Fig. 14.25A); however, both sides can be used safely with careful dissection. In most cases, the transverse cervical artery arises from the thyrocervical trunk which originates from the subclavian artery. However, there are a number of anatomical variations as the artery can arise directly from the subclavian in 21% of cases and even the internal mammary artery in 2% of cases. The transverse cervical artery crosses anterior to the

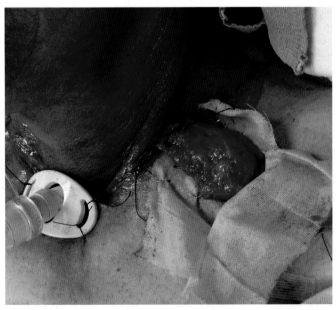

Fig. 14.23 A vastus lateralis muscle can be externalized as a monitor during anterolateral thigh flap reconstruction.

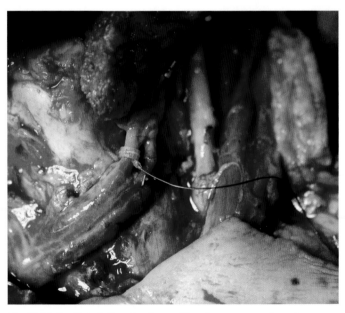

Fig. 14.24 The Synovis Flow Coupler combines the venous coupler and an internal Doppler probe that is used for simultaneous venous anastomosis and flap monitoring.

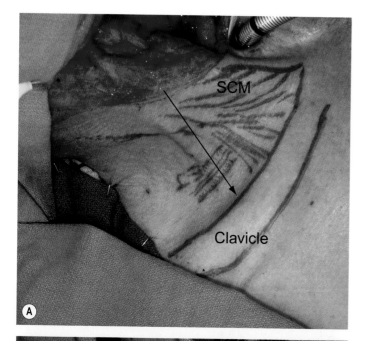

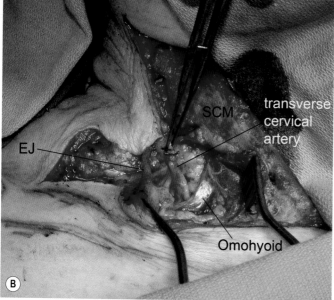

Fig. 14.25 To explore the transverse cervical vessels, an incision was made toward the mid-clavicle, lateral to the sternocleidomastoid muscle. The right side is preferred to avoid injury to the thoracic duct **(A)**. The omohyoid muscle is a good landmark to locate the transverse cervical vessels **(B)**.

recipient vein. The transverse cervical vessels are available in 92% of the cases in our experience even in the presence of a frozen neck.[57] The supraclavicular region is usually free from radiation damage and surgical scars from previous neck dissection as modern neck dissections for laryngeal cancer often spare level V.

In certain circumstances, the use of vein grafts may be necessary to reach more distant recipient vessels. The internal mammary vessels can serve as excellent recipient vessels in the setting that no other vessels are readily available.[58,59] However, vein grafts are typically necessary in order to reach the internal mammary vessels. We recommend isolating the vessels in the third intercostal space after removing the third costal cartilage. Careful attention should be paid to avoid puncturing the pleura during this dissection. Alternatively, with the help of a thoracic surgeon, the clavicular head and manubrium are resected and the internal mammary vessels dissected out all the way to their origin and turned upward to the neck to avoid vein grafting.

Reconstruction of post-laryngectomy pharyngocutaneous fistulas

Since radiotherapy became the primary treatment for early stages of laryngeal and hypopharyngeal cancers, physicians have faced a new problem in these patients: higher rates of pharyngocutaneous fistulas after salvage total laryngectomies for recurrent cancers. Although the overall incidence of post-laryngectomy pharyngocutaneous fistulas has decreased significantly in the past decade, it remains very high in previously irradiated patients.[60–62] McCombe *et al.* reported that the incidence increased from 4% to 39% when radiation was included in multi-modal therapy.[61]

Once fistulas develop, the radiation effects are compounded by salivary contamination of the neck, leading to chronic inflammation and hypoxia of the neck skin and vasculature and putting the patient at risk for loss of neck skin and the remaining pharynx, tracheostoma compromise, and even carotid artery rupture. Longstanding fistulas will inevitably promote scar formation leading to pharyngeal stricture. These more severe cases create a very difficult challenge for even the most experienced reconstructive surgeon.

The goals of surgical reconstruction should be to minimize surgical morbidity and mortality in addition to providing reliable reconstruction that achieves primary healing and a reasonable appearance and restores swallowing and speech functions. The strategies for reconstruction are the same as those for managing a frozen neck. During surgery, the fistula track and scar tissues are excised, without exposing the great vessels in the neck if they are cancer free. All patients have various degrees of pharyngeal stricture, particularly those with a longstanding fistula. The hypopharynx is opened superiorly to the base of the tongue, where the pharyngeal inlet is incised laterally and widened to approximately two to three fingers wide. This is important because primary closure of the pharynx following a total laryngectomy inevitably narrows the pharyngeal inlet. In patients with a relatively normal pharynx and cervical esophagus and no complications, a small degree of narrowing may not cause dysphagia. After pharyngoesophageal reconstruction,

brachial plexus and middle scalene muscle on its way to the lateral border of the levator scapulae muscle. The artery typically lies deep to the omohyoid which serves as a good landmark to identify the vessels (Fig. 14.25B). The supraclavicular artery which is the pedicle for the supraclavicular flap usually arises from the transverse cervical artery. The main transverse cervical artery continues laterally, and its descending branch enters to supply the trapezius muscle. The transverse artery is dissected out proximal to the take-off of the supraclavicular artery or even to the thyrocervical trunk to gain adequate caliber and flow. There is usually a transverse cervical vein that accompanies the artery. Alternatively, the external jugular vein near the clavicle can be used as a

however, food transit through the reconstructed conduit is compromised no matter what type of flap is used. Any narrowing in the pharyngeal inlet or weakness of the base of the tongue thus further compounds the problem and causes dysphagia. Once the pharyngoesophageal defect is recreated, the transverse cervical vessels are explored and a multi-island ALT flap is employed to reconstruct the defects as described earlier.

We have seen that delayed repair of post-laryngectomy fistulas often result in a severe frozen neck and a circumferential pharyngoesophageal defect. Therefore, early surgical intervention to reconstruct the neck in these patients once large fistulas develop is strongly recommended.[63] Reconstructive surgery can be performed shortly after the development of the fistula (within days) before severe fibrosis sets in. Surgical dissection in the neck is therefore much easier than in patients with a longstanding fistula. The use of various amounts of the well-vascularized vastus lateralis muscle to repair neck defects may help to achieve primary healing.

Reconstruction of isolated cervical esophageal defects with an intact larynx

The vast majority of tumors arising in the cervical esophagus are malignant, and laryngectomy is often required to achieve tumor-free margins.[58,64] For benign tumors such as schwannomas and granular cell tumors, smaller margins are acceptable, but resection of a portion of the cricopharyngeus muscle increases the risk of reflux and aspiration. Therefore, the reconstruction of isolated cervical esophageal defects can be challenging. With an intact larynx and trachea, exposure of the cervical esophagus is limited, making reconstruction technically difficult. Given the small space around the esophagus, a free tissue transfer offers the best flexibility for insetting the flap; a thin flap is required for the same reason. The radial forearm flap is, therefore, the author's flap of choice for both partial and circumferential defects. These defects are usually only a few centimeters long, so the radial forearm flap can be oriented 90° to the conventional flap design so that the width of the flap becomes the length of the neoesophagus. The longitudinal length of the flap is rolled along the vascular pedicle to form a tube. The transverse cervical vessels are preferred since they are closer to the defect.

Reconstruction of tracheostoma recurrence

Trachesostoma recurrence following a previous total laryngectomy often requires tracheal resection and sometimes a total esophagectomy. For small recurrence, the anterior tracheostoma, the manubrium, and both clavicular heads are often resected, exposing great vessels which are often radiated (Fig. 14.26A). A pectoralis major myocutaneous flap or an IMAP flap (Fig. 14.26B,C) can be used for such reconstruction.[34] The IMAP flap is based on the perforator in the second intercostal space, and the flap is designed horizontally parallel to the ribs. The distal extent of the flap

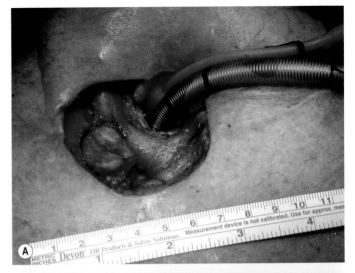

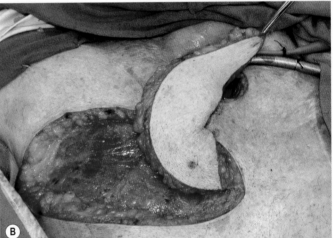

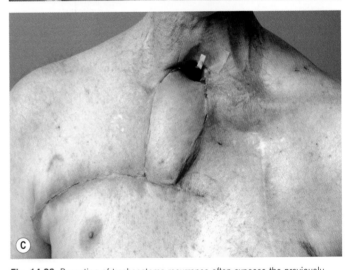

Fig. 14.26 Resection of tracheostoma recurrence often exposes the previously radiated great vessels **(A)**. An internal mammary artery perforator (IMAP) flap is a reliable and simple flap for this type of reconstruction **(B)**. The flap heals well although it may distort the nipple **(C)**.

can reach the axilla. The flap is then rotated superiorly to the defect.

When a total esophagectomy is also performed combined with tracheal resection, our preferred approach is to use the supercharged jejunal flap for total esophageal reconstruction[65] and use the ALT flap for tracheal reconstruction (Fig. 14.27).[66] Recipient vessels include the right transverse cervical vessels for the ALT flap and the left internal mammary vessels for the supercharged jejunal flap. The ALT flap is tubed and sutured to the tracheal remnant with 3-0 polydioxanone (PDS) sutures in a parachute fashion so as not to obstruct the passage of the supercharged jejunal flap. The jejunal flap is then pulled up to the neck through the substernal route and re-vascularized. The parachuting sutures of the ALT flap for tracheal reconstruction are then tied down. This sequence is important because once the jejunal flap is pulled to the neck, it is nearly impossible to suture the ALT flap to the trachea as the jejunal flap and its mesentery tend to obstruct the tracheal remnant. The superior end of the ALT flap is inset to the neck and chest skin. A Shiley tracheostomy tube is placed in the tube ALT flap to stent the lumen open. The patient should be spontaneously breathing at this time point to avoid positive ventilation

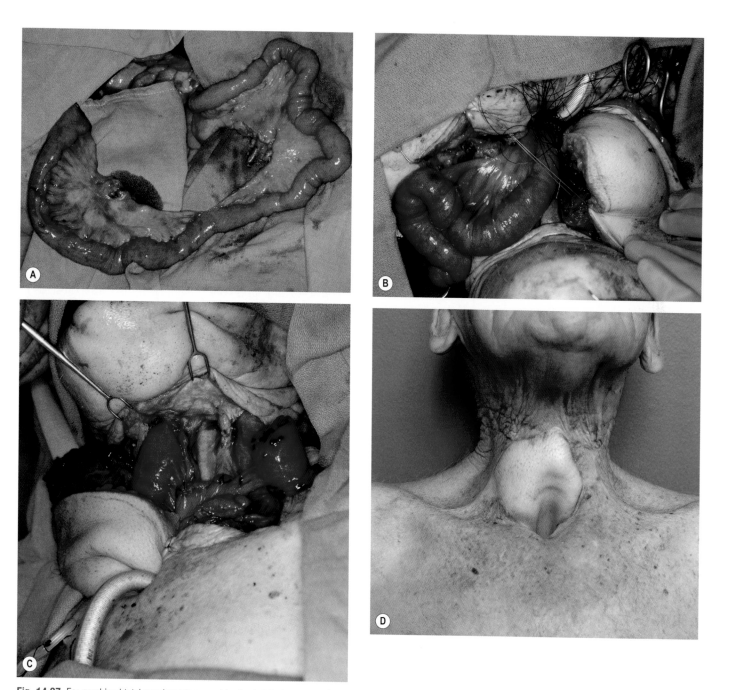

Fig. 14.27 For combined total esophagectomy and tracheal defects, a supercharged jejunal flap is used for esophageal reconstruction **(A)**. An anterolateral thigh (ALT) flap is used for tracheal reconstruction **(B)**. The ALT flap is sutured to the tracheal remnant using parachuting sutures before the jejunal flap is pulled through the mediastinum to the neck. The jejunal flap is then supercharged to the internal mammary vessels, and the ALT flap is revascularized to the transverse cervical vessels. The parachuting sutures are then tied down to the trachea **(C)**. The ALT flap provides stable tracheal reconstruction **(D)** while the patient could tolerate a soft diet.

which can cause air leakage or disruption at the ALT-trachea anastomosis. The Shiley tube is replaced with a soft Lary tube on postoperative day 3, which is managed as regular post-laryngectomy patients.

Complications

As with any complex surgery, particularly involving micro-vascular free tissue transfer, there are always the potential risks of bleeding, infection, and the most dreaded complication of loss of the free flap requiring a secondary free flap in order to reconstruct the defect. In our experience, our success rate for free flap head and neck reconstruction is greater than 97%, but 99% for pharyngoesophageal reconstruction.[67] In the setting that a flap is lost, careful analysis is necessary to identify the underlying etiology for the flap loss before embarking on another free flap.

Medical complications occur frequently since alcohol and tobacco use is prevalent in this patient population. Traditionally, these patients are kept in the intensive care unit (ICU) overnight on a ventilator after surgery. Because of the need for sedation, hypotension is common and many patients become fluid overloaded due to fluid resuscitation since vasopressors are generally considered contraindicated after free flap reconstruction. Patients with limited cardiopulmonary reserve, such as those with pre-existing cardiopulmonary conditions and elderly patients may easily develop congestive heart failure and respiratory failure. The senior author's current practice is to extubate or discontinue mechanical ventilation at the completion of surgery and allow patients to go to regular recovery and regular flap floor instead of ICU. We have shown that this practice significantly reduces the incidence of medical complications and shortens length of stay.[68] If ICU monitoring is indicated, patients are allowed to breathe spontaneously in the ICU to avoid mechanical ventilation and heavy sedation. In patients with a history of alcohol abuse and narcotic dependence, postoperative confusion and agitation are common and may cause hypertension, hematoma, anastomotic breakdowns, and avulsion of the vascular pedicle. Therefore, prompt management of these issues with the primary team, pain management, and neuropsychiatric staff is important.

Infection

Given the prior radiated and compromised tissue and long surgery time, along with the contamination from the communication with the oral cavity, there is a high risk for infection. We routinely irrigate the neck with copious amounts of antibiotic irrigation prior to closure and recommend placement of closed suction drains to minimize the risk of a fluid collection that can progress to an abscess. Patients are also maintained on intravenous antibiotics, usually Unasyn, during the entirety of their hospital stay. Hematoma can also lead to infection. Meticulous hemostasis is therefore important.

Early signs of infection, including increased swelling and erythema, can sometimes be masked by the prior radiated tissue. Occasionally, broadening the antibiotic coverage is adequate in treating a superficial cellulitis; however, any signs of a possible abscess warrant surgical exploration and

drainage. Early washout may prevent pedicle thrombosis and allow primary closure of the neck incision. Serious infections should also raise the suspicion of a fistula or a potentially even dead flap which will be described later in this chapter. In such circumstances, a staged approach is recommended with serial washouts and debridements before definitive repair.

Fistula

Pharyngocutaneous fistulas occur in 10% and 6% of patients with ALT flap reconstruction for circumferential and partial defects, respectively.[26] Proximal fistulas are rare with the ALT flap unless there is a dehiscence due to technical errors or poorly vascularized tissue. Fistulas usually develop between 1 and 4 weeks postoperatively and manifest as leakage of saliva or liquids or, in some patients, as a neck infection. Therefore, any neck infection or abscess that occurs after a pharyngoesophageal reconstruction should raise suspicion for anastomotic leakage. Risk factors for fistula formation include improper suturing techniques, poor tissue quality at the anastomosis site, previous radiotherapy, and turbulent postoperative course. At the time of surgery, any questionable tissue should be trimmed.

Once a fistula is identified, oral intake is withheld and local wound care is initiated. Small fistulas, in the absence of tumor recurrence or distal obstruction, usually heal spontaneously within 2 weeks with conservative management. Therefore, an modified barium swallow (MBS) is repeated 2 weeks later if the leakage has stopped. Larger fistulas or those with infection should be evaluated with computed tomography to rule out abscess and assess the proximity of the fistula/abscess to the carotid artery. Any dead space or abscess around the carotid artery, especially in patients who have undergone previous radiotherapy or chemoradiation, should be thoroughly but carefully debrided without jeopardizing the carotid artery. A pectoralis major muscle flap is commonly used to fill the dead space. This should be done as soon as possible to prevent rupture of the carotid artery. Attempting to repair the leak or dehiscence at this stage will not be successful and may cause more tissue damage.

Stricture

Circumferential defects and subsequent reconstruction were significantly more prone to strictures than partial defects. For these reasons, it is always critical to preserve the posterior mucosa if possible, and converting a partial pharyngectomy defect to a circumferential defect should be avoided. The proximal anastomosis is not typically prone to stricture as the base of tongue and oropharynx is usually of adequate diameter that should allow easy passage of a food bolus. The distal anastomosis is not surprisingly the source of most strictures and subsequent dysphagia. For these reasons, we recommend spatulating the distal anastomosis and insetting a dart into a longitudinal opening in the cervical esophagus. This not only widens the diameter of the distal anastomosis, but also interrupts a circumferential scar, thereby reducing the likelihood of a stricture.

If a patient develops a stricture, the assistance of a gastroenterologist is indicated to dilate the stricture. The use of a bougie with a rigid laryngoscopy to dilate the stricture is no longer recommended since there is a risk for perforation of the esophagus. At our institution, endoscopic balloon dilation is the preferred method of dilating an anastomotic stricture. Unfortunately, while dilation may provide some initial relief, the majority of patients will develop progressive dysphagia and will likely need to have the dilation repeated in the future and will eventually require surgical correction or depend on tube feeding. Surgical repair may be achieved with a radial forearm flap or by turning the external skin paddle inward for small strictures.

Postoperative function

The goal of reconstruction for pharyngoesophageal defects is to restore gastrointestinal continuity so patients will be able to tolerate an oral diet and also potentially be able to undergo a TEP for speech rehabilitation. In our experience, swallowing function is comparable between a fasciocutaneous flap and an intestinal flap, although patients will likely need to drink more fluid to help lubricate the food bolus down the reconstructed conduit. However, speech function tends to be much superior with fasciocutaneous flaps compared to intestinal flaps.[24,26]

Speech rehabilitation

Tracheoesophageal puncture (TEP) is the preferred method of voice rehabilitation and affords patients the possibility of speech after a total laryngectomy. The TEP can be performed at the time of surgery (primary TEP) or several months after surgery with use of endoscopy (secondary TEP); however, in our experience, a secondary TEP has higher success rates compared to a primary TEP and, therefore, it is our preference to perform the TEP secondarily several months following the reconstruction. The TEP is performed by puncturing the common wall between the esophagus and trachea 1.5 cm or 2 cm below the rim of the tracheostoma. In patients with a very low resection of the cervical esophagus below the tracheostoma, the puncture needs to go through the flap and the posterior tracheal wall, which is more difficult to do. Initially, a 14 Fr. red rubber catheter is inserted through the TEP and subsequently changed to voice prosthesis in 2–4 weeks once the tract has matured. The patients are followed up regularly by speech pathologists to adjust the prosthesis to obtain a tight fit so the device cannot be dislodged. Complications include widening of the puncture site with leakage around the voice prosthesis, frequent mucus plugs inside the prosthesis, and fungal infections. In our series of 349 patients, 147 patients received a TEP and 87% of them were able to achieve fluent speech.[69]

Swallowing function

For patients who have received prior radiation, an MBS is performed to assess for a leak approximately 6 weeks following a fasciocutaneous flap reconstruction and 2 weeks in patients that have not received radiation. In cases when small leaks are noted, patients are maintained on tube feeds and the MBS is repeated in 2 weeks, and most will heal spontaneously. Large leaks are usually apparent clinically and managed as previously described. If there is no evidence for a leak, patients are started on a liquid diet and then advanced to a soft or pureed diet in 3 days.

🌐 Access the complete reference list online at **www.expertconsult.com**

1. Mikulicz J. Ein Fall von Resection des Carcinomatosen Esophagus mit Plastischem Ersatz des Excidirten Stuckes. *Prag Med Wchnschr.* 1886;2:93.

2. Wookey H. The surgical treatment of carcinoma of the hypopharynx and the oesophagus. *Br J Surg.* 1948;35:249.

3. Wookey H. The surgical treatment of carcinoma of the pharynx and upper esophagus. *Surg Gynecol Obstet.* 1942;75:499.

4. Bakamjiam VY. A two-stage method for pharyngoesophageal reconstruction with a primary pectoral skin flap. *Plast Reconstr Surg.* 1965;36:173.

5. Shefts LM, Fischer A. Carcinoma of the cervical esophagus with one-stage total esophageal resection and pharyngogastrostomy. *Surgery.* 1949;25:849.

6. Leonard JR, Maran AGD. Reconstruction of the cervical esophagus via gastric anastomosis. *Laryngoscope.* 1970;80:849.

7. Harrison DFN, Thompson AE, Buchanan G. Radical resection for cancer of the hypopharynx and cervical oesophagus with repair by stomach transposition. *Br J Surg.* 1981;68:781.

8. Lam KH, Won J, Lim S, et al. Pharyngogastric anastomosis following pharyngolaryngectomy. Analysis of 157 cases. *World J Surg.* 1981;5:509.

9. Frederickson JM, Derrick JH, Wagenfeld MB, et al. Gastric pull-up vs. deltopectoral flap for reconstruction of the cervical esophagus. *Arch Otolaryngol.* 1981;107:613.

10. Spiro RH, Shah JP, Strong EW, et al. Gastric transposition in head and neck surgery: indications, complications, and expectations. *Am J Surg.* 1983;146:483–487.

15

Tumors of the facial skeleton: Fibrous dysplasia

Alberto Córdova-Aguilar and Yu-Ray Chen

 Access video and video lecture content for this chapter online at expertconsult.com

SYNOPSIS

- Tumors of the facial skeleton may arise from multiple cellular lineages. However, tumor-like lesions are more common than true bone tumors.[1] The most common craniofacial tumor-like lesion encountered by plastic surgeons is fibrous dysplasia.[2]
- Fibrous dysplasia is a benign fibro-osseous lesion in which normal bone is replaced by fibro-osseous tissue. It can present as an isolated disease or in association with other syndromes.
- Craniofacial fibrous dysplasia commonly presents as a gradual, painless, immobile mass enlargement resulting in facial asymmetry.
- Diagnosis is based on a combination of clinical, radiographic, and sometimes histological findings.
- Indications for surgical intervention include aesthetic consideration, functional impairments, relief of symptoms, and in situations where malignancy cannot be ruled out.
- The two main approaches to reach the facial skeleton are through the coronal and intraoral incisions. Surgery can be divided into conservative bone contouring or radical excision with immediate reconstruction. Planning these reconstructions usually requires a multidisciplinary team.
- Many of the principles applied in the management of fibrous dysplasia can be extended to other tumors of the facial skeleton.

Introduction

Since the skeletal framework basically determines the facial appearance, many factors come into play when treating a patient with a craniofacial tumor. Understanding the features of these tumors, the interaction of surface deformities, and their underlying anatomic counterpart is paramount to design an individualized solution for each patient. Due to the complexity of the craniofacial region and the consequences of inappropriate treatment, planning these reconstructions usually requires a multidisciplinary team.

The facial skeleton includes the frontal bone, the midface bones, and the mandible. Tumors of these bones may arise

from multiple cellular lineages; however, primary malignant tumors are rare. In contrast, tumor-like lesions are more common than true bone tumors.[1] The most common craniofacial tumor-like lesion encountered by plastic surgeons is fibrous dysplasia;[2] therefore, by using it as a model, many of the principles applied in the management of this pathology can be extended to other tumor types. As will be seen, this chapter reviews the clinical considerations, including a detailed differential diagnosis with other bone tumors and surgical approaches in patients with fibrous dysplasia. Moreover, the surgical techniques presented here give the surgeon full access to the facial skeleton, as well as various strategies for the resection and reconstruction of other craniofacial tumors.

 Access the Historical Perspective section online at
http://www.expertconsult.com

Basic science/disease process
General considerations

Tumors of the facial skeleton can be classified as either primary or secondary, but also as benign or malignant. Primary tumors may arise from osteogenic, chondrogenic, fibrogenic, vascular, hematopoietic, and other elements of the bone, as opposed to secondary tumors which originate in other organs and metastasize to the skeleton. By definition, benign osseous tumors do not metastasize and may vary in etiology (developmental, traumatic, infectious, or inflammatory). Many lesions of the facial skeleton that may mimic primary bone tumors, such as metastatic lesions and non-neoplastic processes, overwhelmingly exceed the incidence of true bone tumors.[1] Frequent craniofacial conditions simulating primary bone tumors or tumor-like lesions are giant cell reparative granuloma, Langerhans cell histiocytosis, Paget's disease, and fibrous dysplasia. The most common craniofacial tumor-like lesion encountered by plastic surgeons is fibrous dysplasia.[2]

Fibrous dysplasia (FD) is a non-inherited genetic hamartomatous disorder characterized by an intramedullary fibro-osseous lesion of affected bones. Although FD can occur in any bone, the most common locations are the craniofacial bones, proximal femur, and rib. In the craniofacial region, it frequently involves the maxillary bone, followed by mandible, frontal, sphenoidal, ethmoidal, parietal, temporal, and occipital bones.[12]

Demographics

The incidence and prevalence of FD are difficult to estimate, but it is reported to be approximately 1 : 4000–1 : 10 000 and 1 : 30 000 individuals, respectively.[13,14] FD represents 3% of all bone tumors and around 7% of benign bone tumors.[15] The disease does not appear to have any gender predilection, except in McCune–Albright syndrome, which is more commonly found in females. Lesions tend to appear unilaterally without side predominance.[16]

Etiology and pathophysiology

The precise etiology of FD is currently unknown but has been hypothesized to be associated with a genetic predisposition. The pathogenesis involves a sporadic postzygotic mutation in somatic cells located on the GNAS1 (guanine nucleotide binding protein, α-stimulating activity polypeptide 1) gene found on chromosome 20q13.2-13.3, which is responsible for the formation of the alpha subunit of stimulating G-proteins.[17] The mutation leads to sustained activation of adenylate cyclase, thus producing increased cyclic adenosine monophosphate (cAMP) activity. In skeletal tissues, overproduction of cAMP impairs the ability of bone-forming mesenchyme to transition from stem-like immature cells to mature osteogenic cells. In addition, one of the downstream effectors of cAMP is an increased secretion of interleukin-6 and expression of receptor activator of nuclear factor κ-B ligand (RANK-L), which increases the number of osteoclasts leading to bone resorption.[18] Incidentally, an overactive cAMP signaling pathway also stimulates the growth of certain tissues such as gonads, thyroid, adrenal cortex, and melanocytes, leading to endocrinopathies and skin pigmentation.[19]

Classification and associations

The classic forms of FD (Fig. 15.1) can present in a single bone or *monostotic (80–85%)*, and multiple bones or *polyostotic (15–25%)*. A variant, termed craniofacial fibrous dysplasia, involves lesions that are confined to contiguous bones of the craniofacial skeleton. Therefore, this pattern cannot be categorized as monostotic or polyostotic owing to the involvement of multiple adjacent bones of the craniofacial skeleton. Typically, bones outside of the craniofacial complex are usually not involved. Approximately 50–100% of patients with polyostotic disease will have craniofacial involvement, whereas only 10% with monostotic lesions will have involvement of these bones.[20] Skull involvement occurs in 27% of monostotic patients and up to 50% of polyostotic patients. Maxillary lesions may extend to include the zygoma, sphenoid bone, maxillary sinus, and floor of the orbit. The mandibular body is the most frequently affected region of the mandible.

The polyostotic form is a sine qua non for syndromic cases, such as Mazabraud, Jaffe–Lichtenstein, or McCune–Albright syndromes. *Mazabraud syndrome* is FD with soft tissue myxoma, usually intramuscular. *Jaffe–Lichtenstein syndrome* is FD with café-au-lait (coffee with milk) pigmentation of the skin. *McCune–Albright's syndrome* is FD lesions with café-au-lait skin pigmentation and multiple endocrinopathies. Endocrine dysfunction may produce gonadal hyperfunction leading to sexual precocity (particularly in females), hyperthyroidism, hyperparathyroidism, Cushing's disorder, acromegaly, and pituitary adenomas. In addition, the borders of the skin lesions are typically serrated or irregular usually described like the "coast of Maine", as opposed to the regular margins observed in the café-au-lait spots of patients affected with neurofibromatosis. Specific not just to FD but also observed in Paget's disease, and secondary to chronic renal failure is a clinical term "leontiasis ossea".[21] Leontiasis ossea refers to a rare condition in which facial skeleton overgrowth results in a lion's face appearance. Recognizing the aforementioned syndromic constellations of symptoms allows early diagnosis and appropriate treatment.

Natural progression and clinical behavior

FD lesions develop during skeletal growth and have a variable natural evolution (Fig. 15.2). The phenotype depends on the stage of development and timing of where the mutation occurs; the earlier during embryogenesis the mutation, the more widespread and severe the disease.[14] Genetic studies have shown that as FD lesions age, more of their mutated stem cells fail to regenerate and their previous offspring die by apoptosis, leading to normal bone cells increasing in population and allowing for more normal skeleton to be produced. This explains why lesions typically stop progressing after adolescence; however, pregnancy may stimulate their growth.[22] Even though reactivation in females may be due to the elevation in sex hormone receptors in the mutated cells, this event is also exhibited in males.[23]

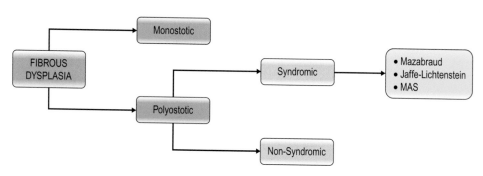

Fig. 15.1 Classification of fibrous dysplasia. MAS (McCune–Abright syndrome).

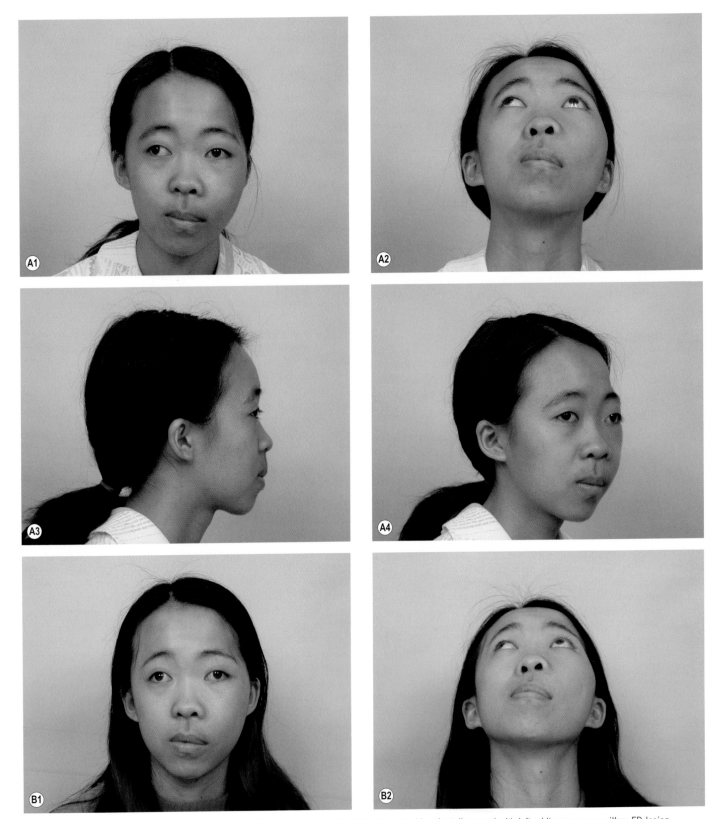

Fig. 15.2 Natural progression in a patient with craniofacial fibrous dysplasia. **(A1–A4)** A 11-year-old patient diagnosed with left orbito-zygoma-maxillary FD lesion. **(B1–B4)** Ten-year follow-up without surgical treatment.

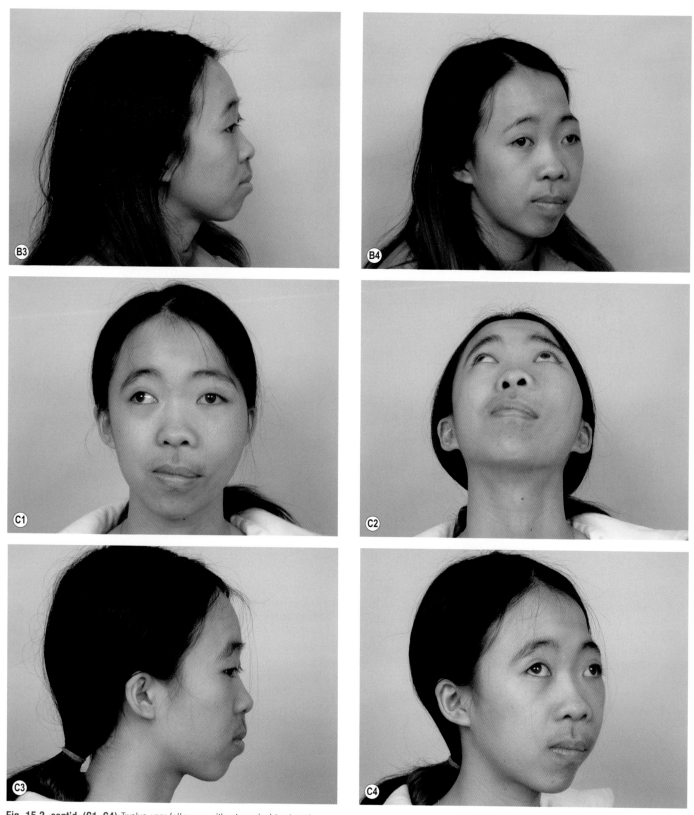

Fig. 15.2, cont'd (C1–C4) Twelve-year follow-up without surgical treatment.

Continued

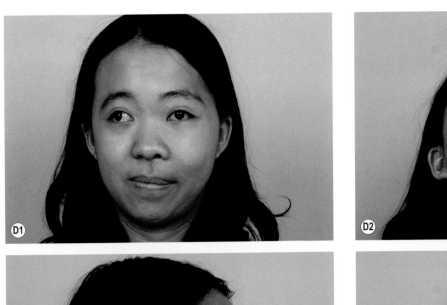

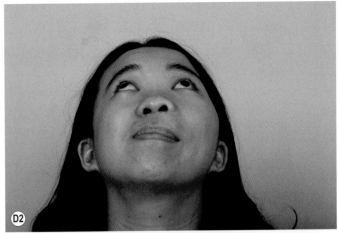

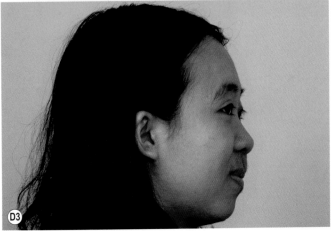

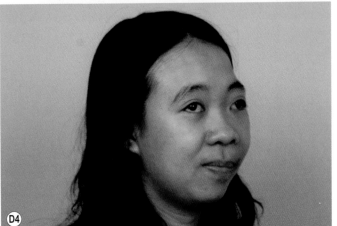

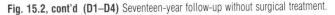

Fig. 15.2, cont'd (D1–D4) Seventeen-year follow-up without surgical treatment.

Clinical presentation may occur at any age; however, the polyostotic form usually manifests before the age of 10 and the monostotic form between 5 and 20 years old. A longitudinal study has shown that monostotic FD does not progress to any polyostotic form.[24] In McCune–Albright syndrome, while growth of the bone lesions may also diminish after puberty, the overall degree of bony enlargement and deformity is often more severe and disfiguring than in patients with monostotic or polyostotic non-syndromic FD.

Histopathology

While almost all the facial skeleton arises from intramembranous ossification, the cranial base arises from an endochondral process. This is important because FD is more common in membranous rather than endochondral bones.

FD bone lesions are characterized by woven ossified tissues, increased formation of bone matrix which does not mineralize normally with extensive marrow fibrosis. Failure of bony maturation leaves a mass of immature isolated trabeculae enmeshed in dysplastic fibrous tissue that are turning over constantly without completion of the remodeling process. This is why the macroscopic appearance of FD

may appear as white and brown rigid mass located in the medullary cavity.[25]

Microscopically, there are three main subtypes of the disease. The *Chinese writing* type is commonly found in the long bones and axial skeleton (rib, vertebrae). The bone trabeculae are thin and disconnected, with ongoing osseous resorption by osteoclasts. Frequently, resorption of the interior of bone trabeculae, so-called "dissecting resorption", similar to findings in hyperparathyroidism. The osteogenic cells are star-shaped, and numerous Sharpey fibers are present. Another pattern, described as a *sclerotic or pagetoid* type is commonly found in cases of fibrous dysplasia involving nongnathic craniofacial bones. The appearance is similar to osseous tissue found in Paget's disease, with dense and sclerotic trabecular tissue. The last one, the *hypercellular* type, is characterized by the presence of discontinuous bone trabeculae distributed in an ordered and sometimes parallel fashion. Typically, the sides of trabeculae are associated with multiple osteoblasts which are arranged in multiple layers. This type appears to occur commonly in gnathic bones. Like the *pagetoid* variant, a significant amount of bone is present in the *hypercellular* type.[26] It is notable that histology of FD does not predict the biological behavior of these lesions.[27]

Malignant potential

Malignancies can occur in any form of FD, but they are rare, ranging from 0.5% to 4%. Malignant transformation is higher in polyostotic forms and previously irradiated sites, commonly occurring in the third or fourth decade of life. The most common malignancies in descending order are osteosarcoma, fibrosarcoma, chondrosarcoma, and malignant fibrous histiocytoma.[28]

Diagnosis/patient presentation

Medical history and examination

The anamnesis and clinical evaluation guides the diagnosis of FD, but radiographic studies are necessary to determine the extent of disease and form (monostotic or polyostotic). Sometimes biopsy findings are required for a definitive diagnosis. Because radiographs cannot distinguish FD from various tumors of the facial skeleton, the information about tumor location and patient's age are sufficient to raise a suspicion of the disease. The medical history should also include the onset and types of symptoms as well as the presence of functional impairments and duration. Although signs and symptoms depend on the site, extent, and nature of the disease, FD of the facial skeleton commonly presents as a gradual, painless, immobile mass enlargement resulting in facial asymmetry.[27]

In general, the signs and symptoms correlate well with the primary bone involved and the extent of the involvement. As a consequence of the enlarging lesion, adjacent structures may be invaded or compressed, resulting in various symptoms such as orbital dystopia, proptosis, diplopia, strabismus, blindness, epiphora, anosmia, facial paralysis, tinnitus, hearing impairment, sinusitis, pain, paresthesia, tooth loss, and malocclusion. When the frontal bone is involved, the globe is usually displaced inferiorly with or without proptosis. The most feared ocular manifestation is the compressive optic neuropathy secondary to sphenoid bone disease, which may present as an acute or chronic loss of visual acuity and fields (Fig. 15.3).[29]

Specific documentation in FD cases include onset of menarche in females to rule out precocious puberty, endocrine disorders (hyperthyroidism, pituitary abnormalities, and renal phosphate wasting), growth abnormalities, skin lesions (café-au-lait spots), and history of fractures to rule out the presence of other FD lesions in the extremities. Thereby, a referral to an endocrinologist is strongly recommended to rule out McCune–Albright syndrome.[27] Moreover, if the symptoms include rapid expansion, new onset of pain, visual change or loss, hearing change or loss, evidence of airway obstruction, new onset of paresthesia, or numbness, a referral to a surgical specialist should be made imminently. In some FD patients, rapid growth is associated with other pathological lesions such as aneurysmal bone cysts or mucoceles, or rarely with malignant transformation.[30] The most common symptoms of sarcomatous change are swelling and pain, usually developing rapidly. A coexisting aneurysmal bone cyst, or cystic degeneration of FD, may clinically mimic a sarcomatous change. In addition, malignancies arising from pre-existing FD lesion are typically aggressive, thus, urgent evaluation is needed if rapid swelling and pain occur in a pre-existing FD lesion.[31]

Imaging

Since many patients are asymptomatic, the diagnosis is often made as an incidental radiologic finding. However, as a general principle, almost all patients in which FD is suspected, as well as other tumors of the facial skeleton, should undergo radiological imaging. Radiographic features of any craniofacial tumor should evaluate location, margins and zone of transition, periosteal reaction, mineralization, size and number of lesions, and involvement of a soft-tissue. While benign tumors usually grow slowly with cortical expansion, have well-defined and often sclerotic borders, and may produce a solid or smooth periosteal reaction; malignant lesions usually show poor marginal definition, along with cortical destruction, a soft tissue mass, and a spiculated or interrupted periosteal reaction.[32]

Plain films

Radiography constitutes the initial imaging tool for describing primary bone tumors and tumor-like conditions. However, owing to the overlapping of adjacent structures, plain radiographs are not recommended for diagnostic purposes for craniofacial FD lesions, although dental films, Panorex, or a conebeam computed tomography (CT) are appropriate to evaluate lesions around the dentition. A skeletal survey may be indicated if there is a suspicion of polyostotic FD, particularly in patients skeletally immature. Additional FD lesions beyond the craniofacial region require further evaluation by an orthopedic surgeon.[27]

Computed tomogram (CT)

Usually from the top of the head to the thyroid region, a CT scan without contrast and with slice thickness 3.75 mm or less is adequate to diagnose tumors of the facial skeleton.[27] Similar requirements should be used for monitoring lesions radiographically or evaluating for recurrence of disease. CT provides more detailed information about the tumor size, location, any local invasion or compression, the mineralization within the lesion, and may demonstrate periosteal reaction earlier than plain radiography.[32]

According to the bone–fibrous matrix ratio within the lesion on CT scan, three distinct patterns have been described in FD patients.[33] The *Pagetoid* pattern lesions shown a mixture of radiodense and radiolucent areas of fibrosis. *Sclerotic* pattern is the most common of craniofacial FD lesions showing a homogeneous, dense, or "ground-glass" appearance with a thin cortex devoid of distinct borders. *Radiolucent* or *cystic* pattern lesions contain one or more ovoid lucencies that are surrounded by a dense periphery. The radiolucency is because of cystic degeneration, simple bone cyst, and aneurismal bone cyst.

Even though CT findings are characteristic, variability of FD lesions may be due to the stage of development within the lesion. Polyostotic FD lesions on CT and the natural radiographic progression may vary. As these patients enter the second decade of life, the FD lesions progress to a mixed appearance, often stabilizing in adulthood but without homogeneity on appearance (Fig. 15.4). This may explain the non-pathognomonic radiographic findings such as absence of "ground-glass", "pagetoid", "lytic", and "cystic"; making it difficult to differentiate FD from other conditions such as ossifying osteoma and Paget's disease. In addition, this period of change in CT appearance coincides with case reports of increased activity of the FD lesions either through rapid growth, worsening facial asymmetry, malignant transformation, or association with other pathologic, radiolucent lesions such as an aneurismal bone cyst and accelerated expansion.[34,35] Thus, an updated CT is crucial in the context of the

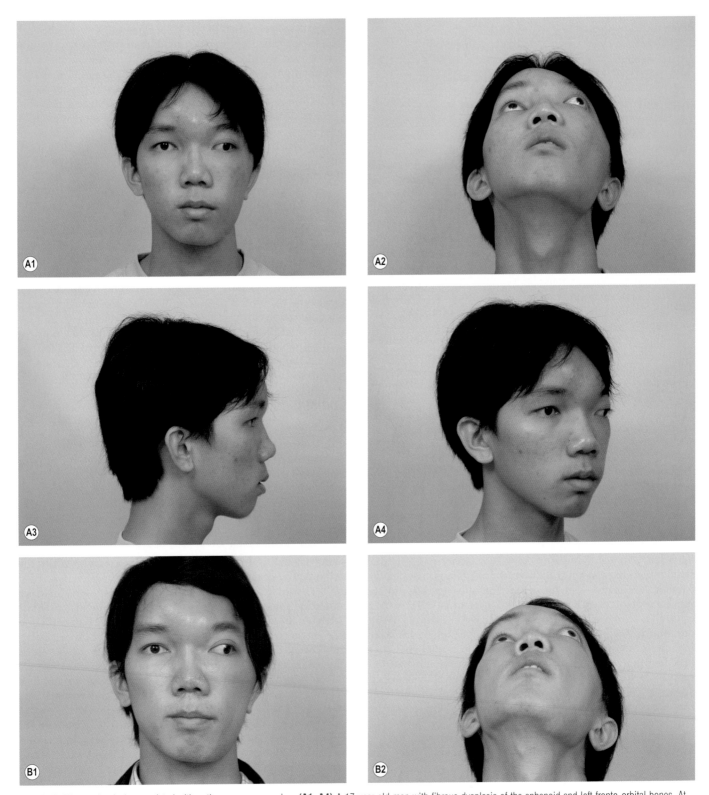

Fig. 15.3 Fibrous dysplasia associated with optic nerve compression. **(A1–A4)** A 17-year-old man with fibrous dysplasia of the sphenoid and left fronto-orbital bones. At the time of initial consultation he only has mild proptosis. **(B1–B4)** Five-year follow-up without surgical treatment.

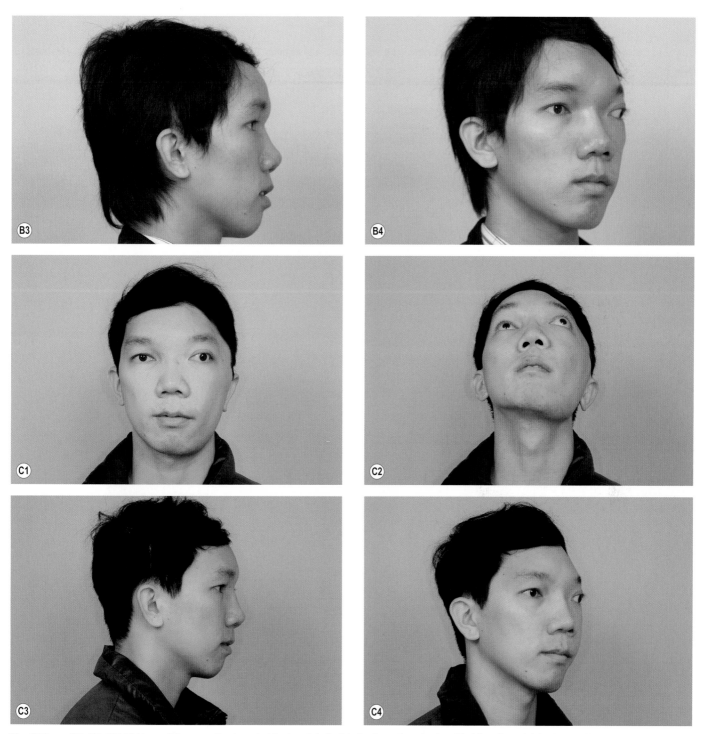

Fig. 15.3, cont'd (C1–C4) Eight-year follow-up without surgical treatment. In the interim, the patient developed insidious loss of vision in the left eye.

new onset of symptoms or rapid enlargement of the lesion at any age.

Magnetic resonance imaging (MRI)

Although MRI does not use any ionizing radiation and has been suggested by some authors as a diagnostic modality for FD, it is a complementary exam to CT.[36] MRI features of FD do not share the characteristics seen on plain radiography and CT. Moreover, MRI images of FD often resemble other tumors. This heterogeneity results from a combination of calcification, cysts, fatty areas, and septations, which shows evidence of intermediate signal intensities on T1-weighted images, high signal intensities on T2 images, and enhancement after injection of contrast material.[37] The likelihood of correctly diagnosed FD by MRI is high only when the signal intensities on

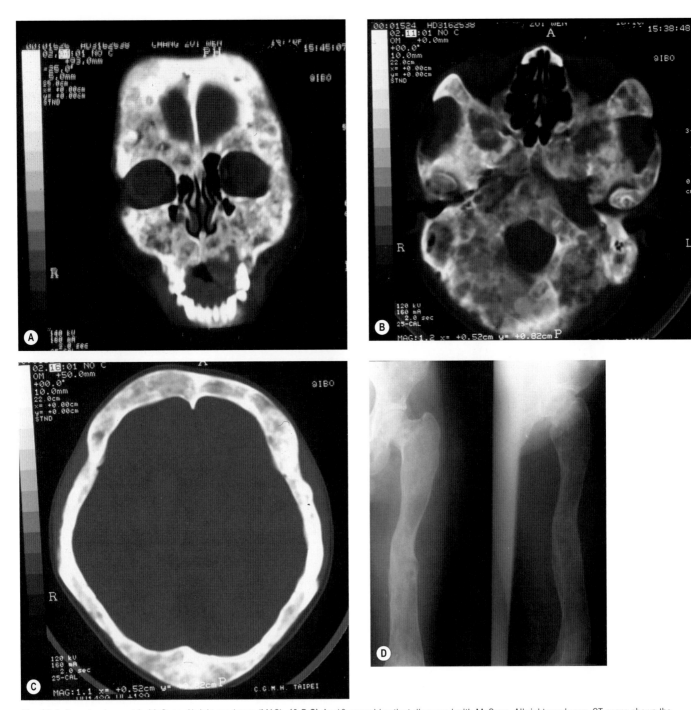

Fig. 15.4 Bone involvement in McCune–Abright syndrome (MAS). **(A,B,C)** An 18-year-old patient diagnosed with McCune–Albright syndrome. CT scans shown the severity and extension of the disease. These FD lesions showed a mixed appearance on CT such as "ground-glass", "pagetoid", "lytic", and "cystic". **(D)** Plain films also showed the bone lesions outside the craniofacial skeleton.

both T1- and T2-weighted images are low despite the injection of contrast material.[38]

Nuclear medicine

Radionuclide scan is highly sensitivity but has low specificity in diagnosing fibrous dysplasia. It may be used for assessing of the extent of skeletal involvement in polyostotic disease. In these cases, a full-body $_{99}$Tc-methylene diphosphonate bone scan is recommended to estimate the biologic

activity of the index lesion and to detect any additional lesions that may exist throughout the skeleton. The appearance of FD on a bone scintigraphy scan is the result of increased tracer uptake in the diseased bone, especially if the lesion is metabolically active, especially in the adolescent period. The detectable bony activity decreases as the lesion maturates.[39]

Another imaging modality, single-photon emission computed tomography (SPECT) has been also reported to be sensitive in the detection of lesions that are not seen on CT.[40]

The scenario and select timing for use of SPECT remains unclear.

Optical coherence tomography (OCT)

Many tumors of the facial skeleton including craniofacial FD may affect the orbit, causing partial or total loss of vision. OCT is a useful test to help diagnose optic neuropathy. It uses high resolution cross-sections of the optic nerve to determine the thickness of the retinal nerve fiber layer (RNFL). This modality may be useful for examining patients that cannot undergo a visual field exam, such as children, or may predict visual recovery after optic nerve decompression surgery. In the case where the RNFL may be thin prior to surgery, it is unlikely that surgery will improve vision while a patient with a normal RNFL may have some improvement after surgical treatment.[27]

Biopsy

Patient history and physical examination, in combination with the classic radiographic presentation, are often adequate to establish the diagnosis of various craniofacial tumors, including FD. However, in some cases, an isolated incisional bone biopsy by the appropriate surgical specialist is indicated for histologic confirmation whenever the site is accessible. As the histopathologic differential diagnosis may be difficult, the size of the biopsy should be as large as possible. Biopsy of FD does not induce growth of the lesion.[27,29] Tissue samples can be obtained at the time of surgical resection of the lesion itself. The caveat of the latter is that decision for a more radical resection cannot hinge on the result of the tissue biopsy. To avoid this scenario, it is recommended to do the biopsy as a separate procedure and wait for the result before the resection. When the histologic sample is to be obtained during the operation, and if there are any doubts intraoperatively regarding the nature of the lesion, the resection part of the operation is deferred until final histological results are available. The surgeon must biopsy with caution, as FD lesions may be quite vascular and bleed profusely. Meticulous hemostasis is imperative even with tissue biopsy. Cytological studies such as fine-needle aspiration are limited and not recommended.

Differential diagnosis

In general, the differential diagnosis of monostotic FD includes solitary unicameral cyst, aneurismal bone cyst, giant cell bone tumor, Langerhans cell histiocytosis, and plasma cell myeloma; whereas the polyostotic form includes hyperparathyroidism, Paget's disease, unilateral enchondromatosis, neurofibromatosis, and cherubism.[41] Nevertheless, the basic purpose of this chapter is to differentiate craniofacial FD from other tumors of the facial skeleton. Thus, we will focus on the most common related pathologies: ossifying fibroma, giant cell granuloma, Langerhans cell histiocytosis, and aneurysmal bone cyst.

Ossifying fibroma (OF)

OF, also known as juvenile ossifying fibroma or psammomatoid ossifying fibroma, like FD, is a hamartomatous fibro-osseous bone lesion that affects adolescents and young adults. Though less frequent than FD, it is more common in females with maxillary and mandibular predominance. Unlike FD, it grows centrifugally and is clearly demarcated from the surrounding normal bone. On CT, it presents as a well-delineated sclerosing mass with osseous trabeculae. Histopathology reveals irregular bony spicules surrounded by extensive osteoblastic activity. This feature differs from FD, in which bone deposits lack of osteoblastic activity.[29] The aim of treatment is early surgical removal.

Giant cell granuloma (GCG)

As FD, giant cell reparative granuloma, also called GCG, is a reactive, benign process within the first two decades of life that is more common in females. Radiographically, the central part of the lesion forms a well-demarcated, radiolucent, multiloculated lesion. These lesions have a hemorrhagic appearance on gross inspection and microscopically consist of groups of spindle-shaped fibroblasts that are mixed with collagen and numerous, multinucleated osteoclast-like giant cells. This means that the lesion is identical to brown tumor and only the absence of biochemical findings of hyperparathyroidism would differentiate these two pathologies.[29] The best management is aggressive surgical curettage.

Another craniofacial entity is cherubism or multilocular cystic disease of the jaws; although sometimes classified as a variant of fibrous dysplasia, cherubism is likely to be a form of giant cell reparative granuloma. Cherubism is a very rare autosomal-dominant benign fibro-osseous disorder that is characterized by symmetrical bone involvement limited to the mandible and maxilla, which typically first appear at the age of 2 to 7 years. Bone lesions are filled with soft, fibrous, giant cell-rich tissue that can expand and infiltrate the orbital floor and cause the characteristic upward tilting of the eyes causing scleral show, and hence the "cherubic" phenotype reflects jaw hypertrophy. The radiographic hallmark of cherubism is the development of symmetrical, multilocular, radiolucent, expansile lesions in the mandible and/or the maxilla. Bilateral mandibular involvement and preservation of the mandibular condyles is considered pathognomonic of cherubism.[42] In most cases, the dysplastic expansile masses begin to regress with the onset of puberty. Because cherubism is usually self-limiting, operative treatment may not be necessary.

Langerhans cell histiocytosis (LCH)

LCH or eosinophilic granuloma of bone is another rare disease with a variable clinical involvement that presents usually during the first decade with a female predominance. Despite unknown etiology, the pathogenesis involves an abnormal proliferation of antigen-presenting histiocytes (Langerhans cells) causing medullary bone resorption. Although the lesions may arise in any hematopoietically active bone, in the craniofacial skeleton they are most common in the skull and jaw. Patients may present with painful or painless bone lesions, and solitary lesions are more frequent than multiple bone involvement. Radiographic findings on plain films and CT vary widely. The early stage shows a poorly defined, lamellated periosteal reaction, and the later stage is characterized by ovoid, well-defined, and homogeneously lytic, with variable marginal sclerosis. Treatment depends on the clinical presentation and may include chemotherapy, radiotherapy, and/or surgery.[32]

Aneurysmal bone cyst (ABC)

ABC is neither a cyst nor an aneurysm, but an expansile osteolytic lesion, usually multilocular, with blood-filled spaces separated by fibrous septa.[43,44] It occurs more commonly in the second decade of life within a pre-existing or *de novo* bone lesion. Although these lesions are most often seen in long bones, they may occur at any site in any bone. Microscopy shows blood-filled cystic spaces lined not by endothelial cells but with plump, fibroblast-like cells.[29,32] The etiology still remains unclear. Radiographs and CT demonstrate an expansile, multilocular "soap bubble" (honeycomb) radiolucency, resulting in cortical thinning. Rapidly expanding lesions may have poorly defined margins and an aggressive periosteal reaction. MRI commonly shows cystic spaces with internal septa and septal contrast enhancement. On skeletal scintigraphy a "donut sign" is commonly seen due to the intense uptake at the periphery and little activity in the center of the lesion.[45] Treatment of ABC is surgical excision.

Patient selection

Surgical indications and contraindications

Since many small solitary bone lesions remain asymptomatic and static, craniofacial FD, like many other tumors of the facial skeleton, is not in itself an indication for medical or surgical intervention. Nonetheless, the four main surgical indications in any tumor include aesthetic concern, functional impairment, symptom relief, and situations in which malignancy cannot be ruled out. From these, the most common surgical indication in craniofacial FD is a progressively enlarging bony lesion that causes visible and disfiguring deformity. Common functional impairments include malocclusion. Surgical intervention is also warranted with persistent pain. As a general principle for non-malignant lesions, any surgical procedure performed must not result in aesthetic and functional impairment worse than the original deformity. The contraindications for surgical intervention of any tumor of the facial skeleton include the patient not medically fit for general anesthesia, the patient not keen for operation intervention, and if the surgical procedure is unlikely to meet the patient's expectations.

Preoperative considerations

Tumors of the facial skeleton are optimally treated through a multidisciplinary approach. Depending on the location of the lesion, referrals are made to appropriate specialists for discussion and collaboration. In general, specialists involved in a craniofacial team include craniofacial surgeons, neurosurgeons, oral and maxillofacial surgeons, otolaryngologists, neuroophthalmologists, audiologists and dentists.[27] After consultation and discussion with the patient, a treatment plan is organized. While the overall treatment is multidisciplinary in nature, usually the craniofacial surgeon must coordinate all the physicians involved and act as the principal caregiver to the patient, making sure that all goals and expectations are understood by all parties involved. To enhance the long-term partnership between the surgeon and the patient, it is important to remain somewhat flexible and acknowledge the patient's role and control in the management process. Understanding and managing patient's expectations is likely to improve patient satisfaction.

Timing of operation

A patient may present to the craniofacial surgeon at any point in time during the course of the disease, frequently during early childhood. Because FD lesion growth stops after childhood, surgery is delayed until after adolescence. This is to minimize recurrence and to intervene only after facial growth is complete. In cases of cystic degeneration, in which significant lesion expansion is associated with functional and aesthetic problems, surgery, even in childhood, is appropriate. In addition, lesions suspicious for malignant change should be investigated and treated promptly.

Variability in the growth rate of lesions combined with variation in patient age affects timing of surgery quite differently. The decision for surgical intervention must be balanced based on patient maturity, ability to cope with the disease process, and ability to balance daily responsibility (which affects school and job schedule). The degree of patient concern about the condition provides the surgeon with some leeway in the timing of the operation. This largely depends on when the patient and family feel is the right time, with the surgeon offering guidance based on their knowledge and experience of the clinical behavior of the lesions. Moreover, the degree of deformity resulting from FD is variable, as is a patient's perception of this. At some time points during the disease process, the surgeon may feel that the deformity, whether it is initial or residual, is of a minor degree such that they are not capable of achieving a level of improvement sufficient to meet the patient's expectations. In such cases, it is better to defer operation. Through serial examinations, photographic comparisons, and revisiting both surgeon's and patient's expectations, both will decide together when the optimal timing for operation or reoperation is.

Treatment/surgical technique

Although medical therapy can be used in FD associated pain and minimizing bone resorption, the mainstay of treatment is surgery. Future therapies may encompass stem cells with regenerative capacity to differentiate into bone, bringing a novel treatment strategy to genetic diseases of the skeleton. A hypothetical approach using lentivirally expressed hairpin RNA (shRNA) to silence target gene expression via RNA interference (RNAi) serves to alter an FD-causing mutation.[46] However, this has not been implemented clinically.

Nonsurgical treatment

Medical treatment has not proven to be effective in preventing the progress of the disease but plays an adjunctive role. It is focused on optimizing function and minimizing morbidity related to skeletal as well as the extraskeletal involvement. Medical therapy may vary according to the extraskeletal disease location including aromatase inhibitors, estrogen receptor modulators, growth hormone receptor antagonist, and bisphosphonates. Because the most severe deformities and symptoms occur in patients who have poorly controlled growth hormone excess, it is recommended for management of aggressively expanding lesions.[47–49] On the other hand, for

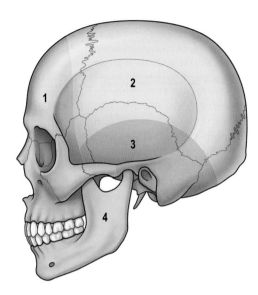

Fig. 15.5 Four zones of craniofacial fibrous dysplasia. *(Redrawn from Chen YR, Morris DE. Craniofacial tumours (fibrous dysplasia). In: Guyuron B, Eriksson E, Persing JA (eds). Plastic Surgery: Indications and Practice. Philadelphia: Saunders Elsevier; 2009:437–454.)*

skeletal involvement, bisphosphonates, human monoclonal antibodies, vitamin D and calcium supplement may be used. Radiotherapy is not advisable in the management of FD because of the possibility to induce sarcomatous change.[28,50]

Pain is a common skeletal symptom in FD yet is more frequent in the lower extremities than the craniofacial region.[51–53] Non-steroidal anti-inflammatory drugs (NSAIDS), bisphosphonates, and opiates are the most common analgesics used in FD.[52,53] Despite the possibility of bisphosphonate-related osteonecrosis of the jaws (BRONJ), bisphosphonates are still being used to reduce pain and bone turnover in FD.[52] A bisphosphonate, pamidronate (60 mg/day administered intravenously for 3 successive days given every 6 months for 18 months), has been shown to inhibit osteoclastic bone resorption by inducing apoptosis in actively resorbing osteoclasts. This mechanism increases bone density and leads to improvement in radiologic appearance and reduces bone pain associated with FD.[54] A newer drug on the market, denosumab, is a human monoclonal antibody, which binds to receptor activator of nuclear factor κ-B ligand (RANK-L) inhibiting osteoclast recruitment from precursor cells. Likewise, it may represent a potential treatment for FD bone pain.[55] Some authors recommend the use of vitamin D and calcium supplementation, as serum calcium is noted to be low in a subset of patients.[52]

Surgical treatment

The surgical approach is determined by tumor location, though many approaches to a specific skeletal region are possible. The objective of the surgery is to restore a more aesthetically pleasing and symmetrical facial appearance. Although there are some basic principles specific to craniofacial reconstruction, an artistic talent and imagination helps the surgeon reconstruct challenging deformities (Video 15.1 ⏵).

Being mindful of facial cosmesis, selection of incisions is critical in order to hide scars. The two main approaches to

reach the facial skeleton are through the coronal and intraoral incisions. Craniofacial defects resulting from resection of many tumors of the facial skeleton are reconstructed immediately using autogenous bone grafts. Traditionally, calvarium, rib, and iliac crest are the common donor sites. Calvarial bone graft is very useful, especially when the scalp has been elevated for exposure during the procedure. In addition, the resorption rate of calvarial bone graft is also noted to be low. Moreover, segments of the resected specimen have also been used as graft material to reconstruct defects.

According to Yu-Ray Chen and Samuel Noordhoff,[56] for the appropriate surgical management of FD the craniofacial skeleton can be divided into four zones (Figs. 15.5 & 15.6):

- *Zone 1* comprises the fronto-orbital, zygomatic, and upper maxillary regions. This is the most aesthetically apparent area in the whole craniofacial region; consequently, complete resection of the lesion is advisable here to minimize the possibility of recurrence. Reconstruction is performed immediately, usually with bone grafts.
- *Zone 2* represents the hair-bearing cranium. Since cosmesis is of less consequence in this area, zone 2 lesions are generally treated with a more conservative surgical approach, for example, by shaving, which tends to restore a more normal bony contour.
- *Zone 3* encompasses the central cranial base, petrous mastoid, and pterygoid bones. Given the important vascular structures and various cranial nerves, surgical intervention in this area is avoided when possible. Lesions here are observed unless they develop symptoms such as visual disturbance secondary to optic nerve compression. In such a scenario, optic canal decompression is recommended.
- *Zone 4* refers to the teeth-bearing bones, which are the maxillary alveolus and the mandible. For lesions in this zone, a more conservative approach is also preferred, at least at the initial stage. This is because resection of teeth-bearing bones will result in the patient having to require dentures, which are less functional than the original dentition.

Zone 1: Surgical technique

The eyes are protected by temporary tarsorrhaphy sutures. The head is positioned on a Mayfield head rest. The whole head is prepped to allow movement of the head during the

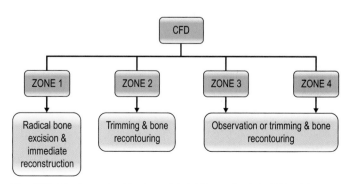

Fig. 15.6 A treatment algorithm in craniofacial fibrous dysplasia (CFD). Although this algorithm is made for CFD, it also can be extended to other benign tumors of the facial skeleton.

operation for bone graft harvest and assessment for symmetry. A bicoronal or bi-temporal approach is used to gain adequate exposure to different areas of the upper and midface, including the zygomatic arch. The planned incision is roughly 8 cm posterior to the mid-anterior hairline; from the midline, the incision is extended laterally and inferiorly to the root of the helix.

Dissection and elevation of the flap are easily performed in the subgaleal plane, however, at about 1.5 cm above the supraorbital rim, the dissection changes from subgaleal to subperiosteal plane. Dissection and soft-tissue elevation continue over the orbital roof, nasal dorsum, zygomatic arch, and anterior maxilla to obtain adequate exposure. Care should be taken to identify and preserve the lacrimal apparatus.

The planned osteotomy lines are marked. The osteotomies are designed to excise all abnormal-appearing bony lesions completely. For superficial lesions, these osteotomies are used to excise the actual bony lesions. For lesions situated deeper in the skull base, these same osteotomies may be used in the osteotomy and replacement approach. In this scenario, the osteotomized bone segment is removed to expose the deeper underlying lesion (for example, in the midline cranial base or nasal septum). After the lesion has been resected and removed, the osteotomized segment is placed back into position.

The supraorbital osteotomy is used in the resection of lesions of the superior half of the orbit (Figs. 15.7A). The neurosurgeon performs a frontal craniotomy and removes the bony plate to expose the frontal lobe. With gentle retraction of the frontal lobe and the placement of a malleable plate to protect the orbital contents, osteotomies are made through the supraorbital rim and orbital roof to remove the segment of bone containing the lesion. The osteotomies are made using a combination of burrs and saws. The orbitomaxillary osteotomy is used to resect lesions affecting the lateral orbital wall, maxilla, zygomatic body, and zygomatic arch. A frontotemporal craniotomy combined with osteotomies through the superolateral orbit and zygomatic arch are made to facilitate the removal of corresponding lesions (Fig. 15.7B).

For lesions involving the inferior aspect of zone 1, the coronal flap alone may be insufficient for adequate exposure. In this case, a combination of coronal flap and Weber–Ferguson incision or degloving face incision along the buccal sulcus is employed. Osteotomies are performed through the glabella, orbit, nasal bones, and maxilla above the level of the dental roots (Fig. 15.7C). In this situation it is particularly important to seal the extradural space from the nasopharynx, usually by using the galeal-frontalis flaps.

After the bone segment containing the lesion is removed, the defect is assessed for reconstruction. For defects involving the orbit, the goals of reconstruction are to restore symmetric skeletal form, symmetric orbital position and volume, normal anatomic compartmentalization, and to protect vital structures (i.e., globe and brain). Split calvarial grafts can be assembled into a three-dimensional construct. Alternatively, a

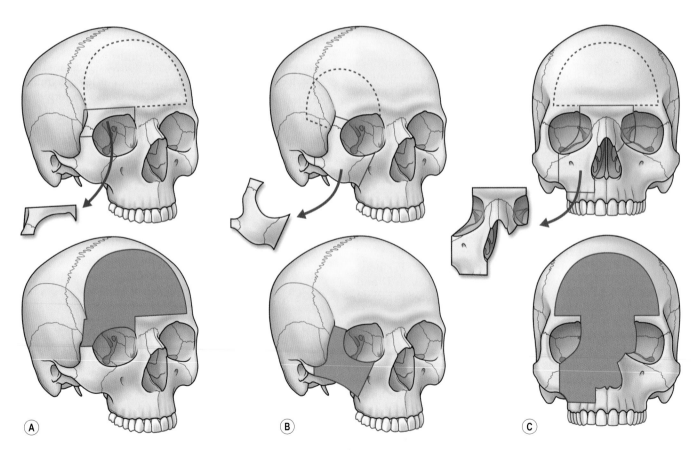

Fig. 15.7 Osteotomies used in resection of craniofacial fibrous dysplasia. **(A)** Supraorbital osteotomy. **(B)** Orbitomaxillary osteotomy. **(C)** Osteotomies through the glabella, orbit, nasal bones, and maxilla above the level of the dental roots. *(Redrawn from Chen YR, Morris DE. Craniofacial tumors (fibrous dysplasia). In: Guyuron B, Eriksson E, Persing JA (eds). Plastic Surgery: Indications and Practice. Philadelphia: Saunders Elsevier; 2009:437–454.)*

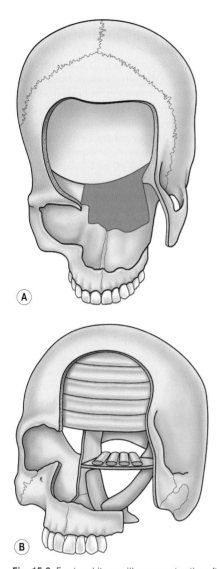

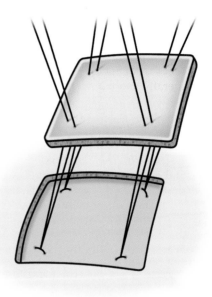

Fig. 15.9 Dural tenting sutures. Sutures are placed through the dura and tied; they are then passed through the holes drilled through the bone graft and retied.

Fig. 15.8 Fronto-orbito-maxillary reconstruction after tumor resection. **(A)** Anatomic configuration of the defect. **(B)** Configuration of the bone graft segments. Note the placement of bone grafts on the orbital floor to achieve a symmetrical height with the opposite roof.

into which the bone graft is inset (Fig. 15.11). This is to provide additional support and increase the contact area between the graft and the adjacent native bone.

Hemostasis is secured and the wound is irrigated with saline, taking care to remove all bony debris. Any dural tears should be repaired with sutures. Before the scalp is closed, fibrin glue is sparingly sprayed into the wound, and pressure is applied for a few minutes over the redraped forehead to promote adhesion and minimize potential dead space.[57] The galeal layer is closed with interrupted 3-0 Vicryl® sutures,

segment of titanium mesh can be plated to the construct to reconstruct one wall of the orbit. Bone tumors may reduce orbital volume and push the orbital floor inferiorly, thus the new orbital roof should be positioned at a height symmetrical with the opposite roof (Fig. 15.8).[58] Canthoplasty is performed using clear nylon sutures. The new canthal position is determined by comparison to the disease-free side.

Edges of the bone graft are burred to ensure a flush fit with no areas of prominence. Dural tenting sutures are placed to minimize dead space between the dura and the graft (Fig. 15.9). To avoid palpable instrumentation or even a visible prominence, we prefer to use low-profile plates and screws in an area anterior to the hairline. In some cases, the hardware is inset into a small groove burred on the graft and the adjacent native bone so that the plate and screws do not rise above the level of the graft and adjacent bone (Fig. 15.10). In placing bone grafts, a step is burred along the native bone margin,

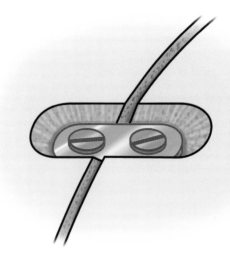

Fig. 15.10 Burying the plates. Plates are inset into the bone to create a smooth contour. A groove is burred into the graft and the adjacent native bone just larger than the plate to allow inset.

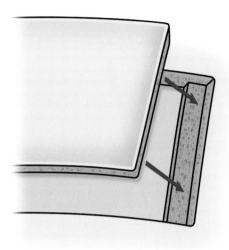

Fig. 15.11 Beveling of the bone edges. A bony step is burred along the margin of the adjacent native bone to facilitate inset and support of the graft segment. Note the inner cortex ledge medially (arrows) that allows inset of the construct, and avoidance of a step-type defect.

and the skin is closed with staples. Two suction drains are placed (one anteriorly and one posteriorly) beneath the scalp flap, each exiting through a separate stab wound in the post-auricular hair-bearing scalp. The scalp flap is closed in layers, and the tarsorrhaphy sutures are removed at the conclusion of the operation.

Zone 2: Surgical technique

Zone 2 lesions are approached through a coronal incision as described above. For lesions posterior to the hairline, bone shaving is completed using burrs. The goal here is to restore anatomic form, contour, and symmetry. In these cases, adequate bilateral exposure allows visual comparison and palpation for symmetry.

For more anterior lesions bordering on zone 1, a more aggressive approach is often taken, as this is a more visible location. A better cosmetic result can be achieved through excision, and the defect is immediately reconstructed with autogenous bone graft. Reconstruction with bone graft is much simpler in zone 2 compared to zone 1, as a single segment of bone graft is often sufficient.

Zone 3: Surgical technique

This region contains major vessels and cranial nerves; thus, tumor resection in this region is to be avoided whenever possible. The indication for surgery in this region is for those lesions that cause functional deficits, for example, visual impairment.

Optic nerve decompression

Prophylactic decompression is not advised to be performed as a primary procedure owing to the risks of failure of visual improvement after decompression or even blindness. In patients with optic canal encasement but without visual symptoms, regular observation with clinical examination and diagnostic imaging is more appropriate. Therapeutic

decompression is advocated in patients with progressive deterioration of vision. For cases with sudden visual loss, it is recommended that decompression should be performed within 1 week of the onset of the symptom to maximize the chance of visual improvement.[59] When indicated, optic nerve decompression is done with neurosurgical collaboration and may be done through a frontal craniotomy approach to the orbital roof. The neurosurgeon proceeds with decompression of the optic canal under loupe or microscopic magnification. Microburrs are used to free the optic nerve completely from any bony impingement along its entire course within the optic cone. Alternatively, a frontotemporal craniotomy or endoscopic nasal/transsphenoidal approach can be performed.

Zone 4: Surgical technique

For lesions in zone 4, the goals of surgery are to re-establish a normal symmetrical three-dimensional skeletal form and to preserve a stable dental arch support. Radical resection might cause greater deformity or functional deficit than the lesion itself; therefore, a more conservative approach such as shaving is preferred whenever possible. In some cases, shaving may not be adequate. In this situation, the lesion is excised; however, as mentioned, it is important to preserve the tooth-bearing portion of the maxilla. Successful facial bone contouring surgery in FD patients relies on first establishing the patient's goals and expectations and then identifying the anatomic basis responsible for the patient's complaints (Fig. 15.12).

For maxillary lesions, the preferred approach is through an upper gingivobuccal incision. The soft tissues are elevated from the skeleton in the subperiosteal plane to expose the lesion widely. The extent of the lesion, or the portion that is causing deformity, is marked. Care should be maintained to avoid injuries to the infraorbital nerve and dental roots. With the assistant protecting the overlying soft tissues, the lesion is shaved with burrs. The wound is irrigated with a copious amount of saline to remove bone particles and closed with absorbable sutures. If the medial and/or lateral buttresses of the maxilla are sacrificed, these structures need to be reconstructed. For immediate reconstruction, rib bone grafts are preferred. This avoids exposing and potentially contaminating the dura while harvesting the calvarial graft in the same surgery involving the oral cavity. The graft segments are placed to reconstruct the medial and lateral maxillary buttresses, vertically supporting the facial height. A step is burred along the periphery of the defect to facilitate inset of the grafts. This increases the area of contact between the graft and the adjacent native bone and enhances stability of the inset graft. Additional graft segments are placed to reconstruct the remainder of bony defects. Reference is made to the contralateral side and to disease-free landmarks (e.g., infraorbital foramina, sides of the pyriform aperture) to achieve symmetry. Bone grafts are fixed with plates and screws.

For lesions of the mandible, exposure is through a lower gingivobuccal incision. The lesions are marked and shaved. An attempt is made to preserve a symmetrical mandibular contour. With this approach, the mandibular arch remains in continuity. The level of the dental roots and mental foramina are marked to avoid injuries to these structures.

Despite a seemingly ideal reconstruction, some patients will require a subsequent orthognathic operation to correct a vertical height asymmetry or malocclusion (Fig. 15.13). This may be secondary to bone graft resorption or to progressive FD. In these cases, the operation is planned carefully with the orthodontist. The goals of such an operation are to correct malocclusion and to level a canted occlusal plane. This usually involves an asymmetric Le Fort 1 osteotomy in which the right and left sides are impacted or distracted to different degrees. Intraoperatively, we find that the facebow combined with direct measurements is helpful in assessing symmetry.[60]

For direct measurement, we expose both eyes and measure from the lower lid margin to the oral commissure, comparing both sides.

Postoperative care

Generally, the patient is extubated in the operating room. If the operation involves craniotomy and exposure of the dura then the patient is admitted to the neurosurgical intensive care unit for neurological monitoring, and a postoperative CT

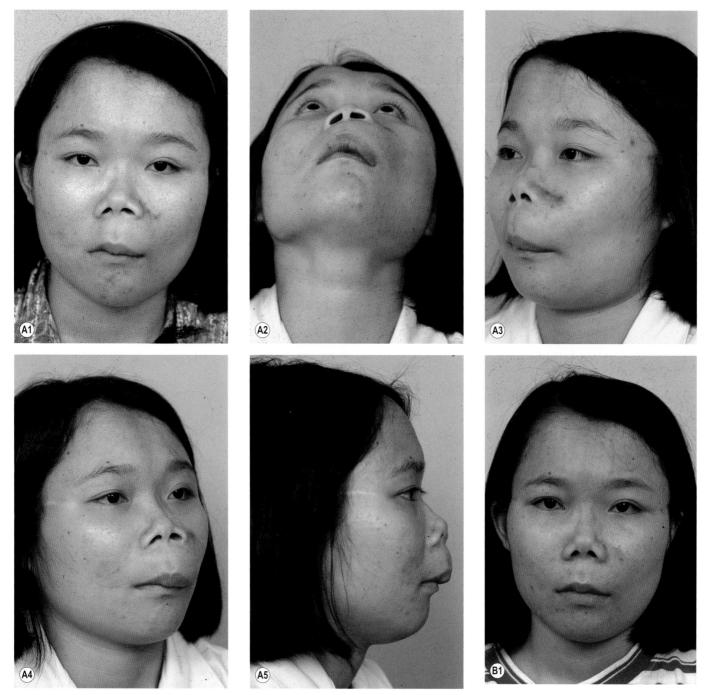

Fig. 15.12 McCune–Abright syndrome. An 18-year-old woman diagnosed with McCune–Albright syndrome who shown a FD maxillary lesion. **(A1–A5)** Preoperative photographs. **(B1–B5)** One year after shaving of FD lesion and bone contouring of the maxilla.

Continued

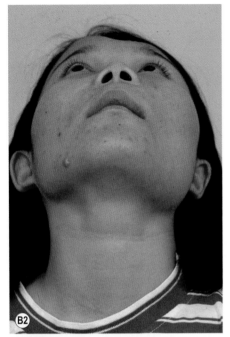

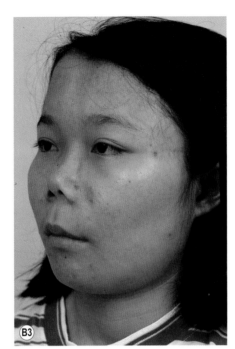

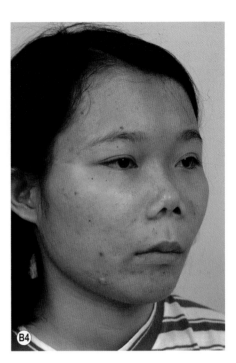

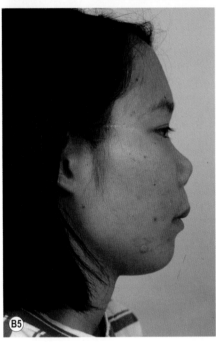

Fig. 15.12, cont'd

scan is done in the same evening or the next morning. Visual acuity is checked immediately postoperatively and serially while the patient is in the hospital. To reduce edema, the head of the bed is kept elevated to at least 30°. Cold packs are placed over the upper face beginning immediately postoperatively and continuing every hour for the next 24 h. For all patients intravenous antibiotics are continued for 2 days and changed to oral antibiotics to complete a 1-week course. If inserted, suction drains are left in place for 2–3 days, and scalp staples are removed after approximately 10 days. Patients are advised to avoid engaging in strenuous activity for 2 weeks. When transoral approaches are used, postoperative instructions include eating a soft diet and to maintain good oral hygiene.

Outcomes, prognosis, and complications

Prognosis and follow-up

Prognosis for many tumors of the facial skeleton including craniofacial FD depends on the location and severity of the pathology. Despite the lack of reliable prognostic biochemical marker for FD, some biomarkers such as serum alkaline phosphatase and urinary hydroxyproline are used occasionally to monitor disease progression and the response to the nonsurgical treatment.[34,61]

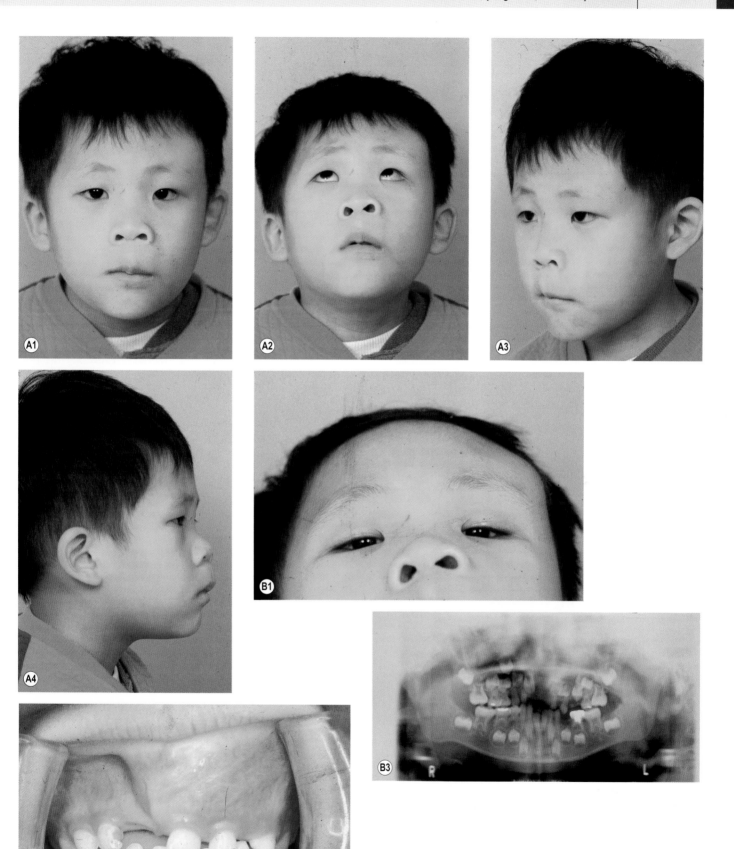

Fig. 15.13 Long-term surgical outcomes in a patient with craniofacial fibrous dysplasia. **(A1–A4)** A 6-year-old patient with fibrous dysplasia of the left fronto-orbital and maxillary bones. **(B1–B3)** Preoperative photographs. Important to notice the deciduous dentition on the Panorex, thus a more conservative technique is preferred for the maxilla. *Continued*

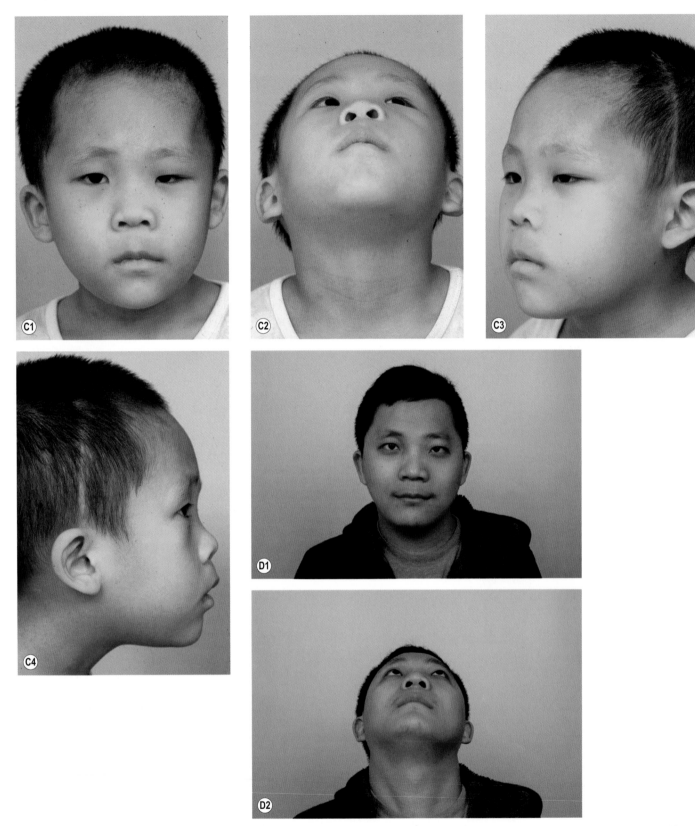

Fig. 15.13, cont'd (C1–C4) One year after subradical tumor excision (zone 1) and immediate calvarial bone graft reconstruction, and bone recontouring of the maxilla (zone 4). **(D1–D4)** Twenty-four-year follow-up after surgery.

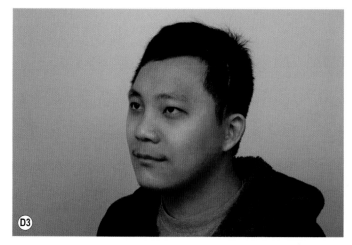
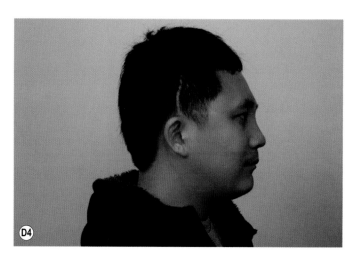

Fig. 15.13, cont'd

As part of follow-up, patients are seen at the outpatient clinic weekly for the first month after surgery and then at 3 months, 6 months, and 1 year postoperatively for potential late complications and to monitor the long-term surgical results as well as tumor recurrence. Patients with craniofacial FD should have yearly ophthalmologic and audiologist evaluations. In addition, the patient who undergoes optic nerve decompression requires repeated formal ophthalmologic assessment.

Prevention and management of potential complications

1. The superior sagittal sinus can be injured if an osteotomy is performed too close to the midline. If this occurs, it is treated in collaboration with the neurosurgeon, by using Gelfoam® packing, local pressure, and sutures.
2. Communication between the nasopharynx and the intracranial cavity can lead to epidural infection and meningitis. During reconstruction, the nasopharynx and intracranial cavity must be separated by well-vascularized tissues. The galea-frontalis flap serves well for this purpose.
3. Errors in orbital reconstruction may result in improper globe positioning. This may lead to enophthalmos, telecanthus, or dystopia. There is a tendency for the globe to assume a more inferior position. To avoid this, additional strips of bone graft may be placed along the orbital floor for reinforcement.
4. Patients may complain of a palpable or even visible prominence of the plating beneath the skin. If there is no sign of infection, the patient is reassured and the hardware removed after bony union has occurred. This problem can be avoided by several means. When possible, place instrumentation posterior to the hairline, use low-profile plating, and use the minimal quantity required to achieve stability. In addition, the groove is burred into the graft and the adjacent native bone and the plate is inset into the groove to create a smooth contour.
5. Globe injury is best avoided by gentle anteroinferior traction of the scalp flap during exposure at and below the supraorbital rim.
6. Care should be taken to level the canthi at the end of the procedure. Visual comparison and measurements should be made to place the medial and lateral canthi at the same level compared to the contralateral side. In performing the canthopexy, a non-absorbable suture is used to fix the canthal ligament to the periosteum.
7. If extensive dissection has been done to facilitate exposure of the bone, the patient may develop postoperative descent or "sagging" of the soft tissues. During reconstruction, sutures should be placed at sites of periosteal incision, to reattach and thereby resuspend the soft tissues.
8. Scalp alopecia is a complication to be avoided. Prepping and draping the entire head allow periodically lifting and slightly rotating the head during the procedure, reducing prolonged pressure at any one location. The skin closure should be tension-free, and any tension should be taken up by galeal sutures. After placing key sutures to mark the vertex, wound closure is performed in a lateral to medial direction bilaterally. This allows slight advancement of the coronal flap from its bilateral inferior aspects towards the midline, thus reducing tension in the vertex region. Should alopecia occur, this is treated as a delayed secondary procedure, at least 6 months later. A small area of alopecia can be treated through excision and a local flap; a larger area may require tissue expansion.
9. Long-term neurosensory disturbances after coronal or transoral approaches can occur and are a common source of complaints from patients. Although the majority of neurosensory changes resolve by 6 months, occasionally they may persist for up to 12 months. This possibility must be clearly communicated to the patient before surgery.
10. For resection involving the maxillary alveolus and mandible, injuries to the dental roots and inferior alveolar nerve/mental nerve can be avoided by proper surgical planning and meticulous surgical technique. Minor injury to the nerve causes temporary

hypoesthesia in the lower lip which usually will recover after few months. Severe nerve damage might lead to permanent sensory loss.

11. For resection involving the intraoral route, early complications include hematoma and intraoral wound dehiscence. These are largely preventable through mindful surgical technique. We prefer to close intraoral wounds in two layers. For the maxillary wound, several interrupted sutures are placed in the periosteal-muscular layers prior to mucosal closure. For the mandibular closure, the dissected periosteal edge is resuspended before the mucosa is closed. For cases involving an orthognathic procedure, and for cases where there has been significant exposure of the mandibular angle, bilateral closed suction drains are placed. The tip is placed at the angle, and the drain exits from the anterior aspect of the mucosal wound and is sutured around a tooth or to the orthodontics. These drains reduce edema and fluid accumulation within the dissected cavity. They are usually removed on postoperative day 1. Patients with a wound dehiscence are taken back to the operating room for irrigation and reclosure. Those with a palpable hematoma are also taken back to the operating room for evacuation and reclosure.

12. Infection of the intraoral wounds, if it occurs, usually presents subacutely from weeks to a few months after surgery. There may be a nidus such as a segment of free bone. Small, well-localized pus collections, or those that have spontaneously begun to drain intraorally, are treated in the clinic. Under local anesthetic, a portion of the wound overlying the fluctuance is opened. The wound is packed with single gauze. A more extensive collection warrants formal exploration, irrigation, and drainage in the operating room. For the patient with a recurring infection, formal exploration is recommended to remove any necrotic bone segment.

Secondary procedures

Patients may present after surgical treatment with residual or recurrent asymmetry; this possibility should be discussed with the patient preoperatively. For instance, some patients with craniofacial FD lesions may present months to years following the initial resection with an occlusal cant. This may be due to recurrent disease or graft resorption, thus CT scan is required for evaluation. Depending on the cause of the recurrent deformity, the treatment could be resection, additional bone grafting, or an orthognathic surgery. Special mention should be made of the patients with a recurrent FD of the mandible who can be treated with hemimandibulectomy and immediate reconstruction using a microvascular bone flap. The surgeon must carefully decide whether reoperation is likely to improve the degree of deformity. It is advisable to wait at least 6 months before any decision is made. This gives adequate time for edema to resolve so that a more accurate evaluation is made. In cases where reoperation is not warranted, the patient is counseled accordingly.

Conclusion

Tumors of the facial skeleton can cause significant functional and aesthetic deformities. Since these bone lesions are often located adjacent to important structures, management is best done through a multidisciplinary approach. The craniofacial surgeon coordinates input from various members in the team and decides with the patient and family the ideal timing for operation. When surgical treatment is undertaken, the goal is to resect the lesion and reconstruct an adequate skeletal framework within the same setting. It is important to be sure of the diagnosis prior to planning a treatment approach. Despite multiple surgical options, the ideal surgical technique is chosen based on the histopathology, extent of tumor growth, patient's anatomy, and surgeon's experience. While this chapter focuses on fibrous dysplasia, many of the aforementioned operative principles are also useful for treating other tumors of the facial skeleton.

 Access the complete reference list online at   **http://www.expertconsult.com**

1. Kindblom LG. Bone tumors: epidemiology, classification, pathology. In: Davies MR, Sundaram M, eds. *Imaging of Bone Tumors and Tumor-Like Lesions.* Berlin Heidelberg: Springer Press; 2009.

2. Gabbay JS, Yuan JT, Andrews BT, et al. Fibrous dysplasia of the zygomaticomaxillary region: outcomes of surgical intervention. *Plast Reconstr Surg.* 2013;131:1329–1338.

16. Wu H, Yang L, Li S, et al. Clinical characteristics of craniomaxillofacial fibrous dysplasia. *J Craniomaxillofac Surg.* 2014;42:1450–1455.

26. Riminucci M, Liu B, Corsi A, et al. The histopathology of fibrous dysplasia of bone in patients with activating mutations of the Gsα gene: site-specific patterns and recurrent histological hallmarks. *J Pathol.* 1999;187:249–258.

27. Lee JS, FitzGibbon EJ, Chen YR, et al. Clinical guidelines for the management of craniofacial fibrous dysplasia. *Orphanet J Rare Dis.* 2012;7(suppl 1–2).

31. Chen YR, Wong FH, Hsueh C, et al. Computed tomography characteristics of non-syndromic craniofacial fibrous dysplasia. *Chang Gung Med J.* 2002;25:1–8.

32. Wootton–Gorges SL. Tumors and Tumor-Like Conditions of Bone. In: Stein-Wexler R, Wootton-Gorges SL, eds. *Pediatric Orthopedic Imaging.* Berlin Heidelberg: Springer Press; 2015.

34. Chen YR, Chang CN, Tan YC. Craniofacial fibrous dysplasia: an update. *Chang Gung Med J.* 2006;29:543–548.

56. Chen YR, Noordhoff MS. Treatment of craniomaxillofacial fibrous dysplasia: how early and how extensive? *Plast Reconstr Surg.* 1990;86:835–842.

16

Overview of head and neck tumors

Andrew Foreman and Patrick J. Gullane

SYNOPSIS

■ Cancer of the oral cavity and pharynx is thought to be caused by accumulated genetic alteration initiated by toxins from tobacco and promoted in the United States by alcohol intake.

■ Tumors are staged according to the TNM system that considers anatomic subsite in the upper aerodigestive tract, size, and adjacent extension for the primary tumor (T), number, and laterality of cervical lymph nodes (N), and presence or absence of distant metastases (M).

■ Surgery or radiotherapy are both effective in early stage tumors, but surgery followed by postoperative adjuvant radiotherapy is preferable in Stage III or above tumors.

■ The primary site and the cervical metastases, or in some cases micrometastases, are treated together as a composite resection or resection of the primary and neck dissection.

■ Because of the anatomical complexity of the area, surgery and radiotherapy often interfere with the critical functions of respiration and alimentation. Resection and reconstruction should be designed to completely remove the cancer and preserve or restore as much function as possible.

■ Extensive surgery with or without previous radiotherapy may result in difficult and dangerous complications such as osteoradionecrosis, fistula, carotid exposure, and hemorrhage.

Introduction

Despite being rare, cancers of the upper aerodigestive tract (UADT) and salivary glands can have devastating consequences for patients because of the impact the disease and its treatment have on the critical functions of respiration and alimentation, in addition to the cosmetic implications of major surgery in the head and neck region. The most significant risk factors for head and neck cancers are tobacco smoking and alcohol ingestion. Consequently, this is a patient population with significant comorbid disease. Thus, tailoring treatment plans to the individual patient is essential to maximize oncologic control and minimize the associated

morbidity. Unfortunately, most patients with head and neck cancers present with late stage disease necessitating multimodality treatment, which increases the risk of subsequent complications, deformity, and dysfunction. This dysfunction has, in part, been ameliorated by the widespread application of primary reconstructive procedures, including free tissue transfer. The reconstructive surgeon needs to have a clear understanding of the underlying disease, the therapeutic approach to these cancers, and the unique challenges of reconstructing complex defects of the head and neck in order to restore form and function to the UADT.

Epidemiology

Cancers of the head and neck are relatively rare. Within the United States, they comprise 3.2% of new cancers (40 000 cases/year) but 22% of cancer deaths (12 460/year).[1] The majority (90%) of mucosal head and neck cancers are squamous cell carcinomas (SCC). Adenocarcinomas arising from minor salivary gland tissue are less common, as are sarcomas, which may be of many types. In the United States, the male:female incidence ratio is 3:1, and a racial predilection for the black population has also been reported. Patients are typically in the fifth or sixth decade, although the advent of human papilloma virus (HPV)-associated cancers has seen a reduction in age at presentation.[2]

The epidemiology of head and neck cancers is changing. Public health measures have seen a decline in tobacco use in the western world and a commensurate reduction in the incidence of smoking-related head and neck cancer.[3] However, there has been a rapid increase in the incidence of HPV-positive cancers, which predominantly affect the oropharynx. In the 20 years up to 2004, the number of oropharyngeal SCCs that were HPV-positive rose from 16.9% to 71.9% (Fig. 16.1), amounting to a 225% increase in the population incidence of this disease.[4] In 2010, the incidence of HPV-positive oropharyngeal cancers in men surpassed the incidence of HPV-positive cervical cancers (Fig. 16.2). By 2020, it is expected

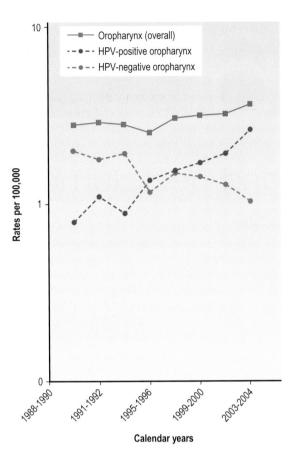

Fig. 16.1 The rising incidence of HPV positive oropharyngeal cancers saw a cross over between HPV-positive and HPV-negative tumors in the late 1990s such that HPV-positive tumors now account for >70% of all oropharyngeal malignancies in the United States. *(From Chaturvedi AK, Engels EA, Pfeiffer RM, et al. Human papillomavirus and rising oropharyngeal cancer incidence in the United States.* J Clin Oncol. *2011;29(32):4294–4301.)*

that the overall incidence of HPV-positive oropharyngeal cancer, that is both men and women, will have exceeded the incidence of cervical cancer. With the incidence of cervical cancer declining due to early cancer detection screening programs and the HPV vaccine, HPV-related oropharyngeal cancer is becoming a hugely significant public health problem. It is hoped that the introduction of vaccination against HPV infection will reverse this rapid increase, although the uptake of population-wide vaccination has varied amongst population groups and remains a significant public health challenge.[5]

Pathophysiology

Head and neck cancer represents a prototypical model of chemical carcinogenesis.[6] Multiple genetic hits enable cells to escape the normal cell cycle regulatory mechanisms.[7] Alone, smoking is the most common initiating carcinogen and increases a patient's cancer risk by eight times, whereas alcohol increases risk four fold, and these show clear dose-response associations.[8] Tobacco smoking and alcohol consumption are synergistic in their effect and using both results in a 32-fold increase in the risk of developing a head and neck cancer. The production of polycyclic aromatic hydrocarbons

is the most frequently cited carcinogenic effect of cigarette smoking, although multiple other mechanisms are known to exist.[9] While they directly contact the lining of the respiratory tract, for example the larynx, these carcinogens will also enter the blood stream from where they are secreted via saliva and can then bathe the other UADT sites such as the oral cavity and oropharynx. In the Western world, alcohol is the most common promoter in UADT cancer and is strongly associated with cancers of the hypopharynx, as this is the highest exposure site of the head and neck. In Southern Asia, betel nut chewing is common and it is also a potent cancer promoter. Betel nut chewers have a younger age of cancer onset with a reduced 5-year survival on top of the 28-fold increase in oral cavity SCC incidence.[10,11] Other pathogenic associations include Plummer–Vinson syndrome, occupational exposures (nickel, radium, mustard gas and wood dust), and viruses, in particular Epstein–Barr virus (EBV) and human papilloma virus (HPV).

Relatively recently, the role of HPV has come to the fore in SCC of the oropharynx.[12] The appreciation of HPV as a carcinogen has caused a significant paradigm shift in the management of oropharyngeal malignancies as the underlying genetic alterations as well as the clinical presentation and prognosis differ markedly from the traditional smoking and

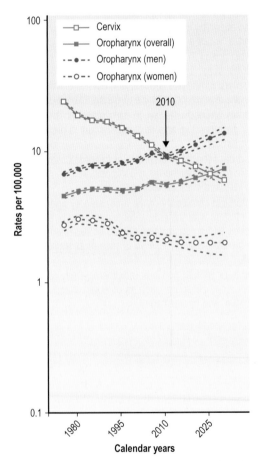

Fig. 16.2 In 2010, the incidence of HPV-associated oropharynx cancer in men exceeded that of cervical cancer in women. By 2020, the overall number of HPV-related oropharyngeal cancers will exceed the number of HPV-related cervical cancers. *(From Chaturvedi AK, Engels EA, Pfeiffer RM, et al. Human papillomavirus and rising oropharyngeal cancer incidence in the United States.* J Clin Oncol. *2011;29(32):4294–4301.)*

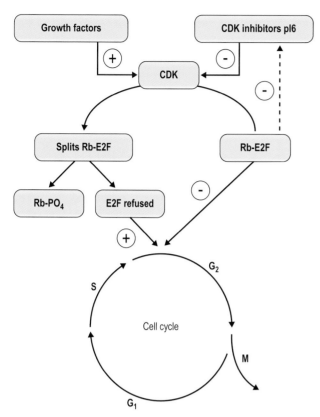

Fig. 16.3 Cell cycle implications of the interaction between the HPV E7 protein and the retinoblastoma protein. In the normal cell cycle control mechanisms, the interaction of Rb and E2F causes a transcription block and controls the cell cycle at the S-G2 transition. The phosphorylation of Rb releases E2F to drive the cell cycle forward. This is normally tightly regulated by cyclin dependent kinases. E7 prevents interaction of Rb-E2F and maintains Rb in the hyperphosphorylated state. This releases E2F to bind to DNA and drive uninhibited progression at the G2-S cell cycle checkpoint. This in turn interrupts the negative feedback loop to the cyclin dependent kinase inhibitors (including p16), thereby leading to uninhibited p16 production, which manifests as p16 overexpression on immunohistochemistry. CDK = cyclin dependent kinase

Work-up of the head and neck cancer patient

Unfortunately, more than 60% of patients with head and neck cancer present with advanced stage disease. This is due to both the non-specific nature of the early symptoms of these cancers and the fact these cancers may access lymphatic channels early in their course. 25% of oral and oropharyngeal cancers and 50% of nasopharyngeal cancers will present with neck nodal disease, thus rendering them at least Stage III disease. Dysphonia, dysphagia, odynophagia, sore throat, hemoptysis, referred otalgia, and weight loss are worrisome presenting symptoms for a UADT malignancy.

After a complete history focused on these symptoms, as well as risk factors for head and neck cancer, the physician should undertake a complete head and neck examination. Inspection and palpation of the oral cavity, oropharynx, ear, nasal cavity, and neck are mandatory. Endoscopic examination of the entire UADT with in-office flexible nasopharyngoscopy has become a routine part of the head and neck examination. Mucosal abnormalities such as red or white patches, ulcerations, or masses should be noted as suspicious. Other signs such as loose dentition, the presence of trismus, unilateral middle ear effusion, a nasal mass, or proptosis are all concerning signs the surgeon should note during the examination.

Imaging plays a crucial role in the work-up of these patients.[14] Contrast-enhanced computed tomography (CT) scanning of the head, neck, and chest has become the standard for assessing the primary tumor along with any regional and distant metastatic disease. Magnetic resonance imaging (MRI) may be helpful, in addition, to provide increased soft tissue detail. This is particularly useful in sites such as the oropharynx, base of skull and parotid gland. Positron emission tonography (PET-CT) imaging is also developing a place in the work-up of patients with head and neck cancer (Fig. 16.4).

alcohol induced cancers. HPV is a DNA virus from the papovirus family that infects basal keratinocytes and has a predilection for sites with single epithelial cell layers, such as the tonsillar crypts. There are greater than 120 subtypes that have been broadly categorized into high, intermediate, and low risk groups. HPV subtype 16 accounts for more than 90% of HPV-associated oropharyngeal SCCs. HPV exerts its oncogenic potential through the E6 and E7 proteins it produces during its life cycle. These proteins interact with p53 and the retinoblastoma (Rb) gene, respectively. E6 promotes degradation of p53, rather than mutating the protein, such that wild-type p53 is maintained albeit in greatly reduced quantities.[13] This has important implications for treatment response in HPV-associated malignancies as the normal cell cycle repair mechanisms are preserved. E7 binds Rb, maintaining it in a hyperphosphorylated state (Fig. 16.3). This releases the protein E2F from its binding site on Rb, enabling E2F to drive unregulated cell cycle progression at the G2-S transition point. As a result of the interruption of the negative feedback loop at the level of the cyclin dependent kinases (CDK), there is overexpression of the CDK inhibitor p16, an important surrogate marker for HPV infection.

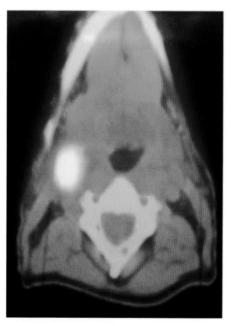

Fig. 16.4 Positron emission tomography (PET) image of a metastatic cervical node. Hypermetabolism within the cancerous node results in increased uptake of the labeled-FDG enabling functional staging. Combining PET with CT improves the anatomical localization of involved structures.

Assessment of the patient presenting with carcinoma of unknown primary, those at high risk of having distant metastatic disease, and evaluating treatment response in patients undergoing non-surgical therapy are all evolving indications for the use of PET-CT.[15]

Along with appropriate imaging that enables accurate staging of the patient a tissue diagnosis is essential. Fine needle aspirate (FNA) biopsy of enlarged neck nodes or in-office biopsy of an obvious primary site is recommended at the earliest available opportunity. Traditional work-up of the head and neck cancer patient included panendoscopy (nasopharyngoscopy, laryngoscopy, bronchoscopy, and esophagoscopy) under general anesthesia; however, this has largely been superseded by advances in imaging techniques and is reserved for patients in whom home in-office biopsy is not possible or when tumor extent is unclear from the imaging, and critical decisions with respect to management cannot be made without direct visualization under anesthesia.

Finally, assessment of nutritional status, dental hygiene, employment status, and social situation are all-important considerations when preparing a patient for potentially multi-modality, intensive treatment that is often required for these patients.

Staging

Head and neck cancers are staged using the tumor, nodal metastasis, metastasis systemic (TNM) models developed by the American Joint Committee for Cancer (AJCC) and the Union Internationale Contre le Cancer (UICC).[16] Through its iterations, it has increasingly been able to predict prognosis, provide guidance in determining treatment plans, and enable comparisons of treatment efficacy.[17] The relevant T staging systems are included throughout this chapter with the relevant primary site. Nodal metastasis staging encompasses size, number, and laterality of nodes for all head and neck sites except for nasopharynx, whereas distant metastases are recorded as present or absent (Table 16.1). The TNM classifications can then be combined to produce an overall stage designation (Table 16.1), which is often applied for determining therapeutic plans and comparing therapeutic interventions in the research setting.

Decision-making in head and neck cancer treatment

Following appropriate work-up and staging, decisions regarding head and neck cancer treatment should be made in the context of a multidisciplinary tumor board setting. In general terms, early stage disease (Stages I and II) requires single modality treatment, whereas advanced stage disease (Stages II and IV) necessitates multimodality therapy. The traditional approach to head and neck tumors was to perform surgery initially and supplement this with adjuvant radiation therapy, with or without chemotherapy, depending on stage and pathological analysis of the surgical specimens. However, in the last 30 years, there has been increasing acceptance of the significant morbidity and quality of life implications of this ablative surgery such that in some settings the use of non-surgical therapy as primary treatment has gained increasing acceptance in order to preserve critical anatomical structures, in particular the larynx. In these cases, surgery is

Stage	Description
Table 16.1 N staging, M staging, and overall UICC staging for cancers of the head and neck mucosa	
N stage	
Nx	Nodal status cannot be assessed
N0	No evidence of nodal metastasis
N1	Single ipsilateral node <3 cm
N2a	Single ipsilateral node 3–6 cm
N2b	Multiple ipsilateral nodes <6 cm
N2c	Bilateral or contralateral nodes <6 cm
N3	Any node >6 cm
M Stage	
Mx	Metastatic status cannot be assessed
M0	No distant metastasis
M1	Distant metastasis present
Overall stage	
I	T1N0M0
II	T2N0M0
III	T3N0M0, T1-3N1M0
IVa	T4aN0-1M0, T1-4aN2M0
IVb	T4bN1-2M0, T1-4bN3M0
IVc	Any M1

reserved for salvage treatment of persistent or recurrent disease. The concurrent advances in head and neck reconstructive techniques have certainly aided the success of surgery in this setting, which is often associated with an increased risk of complications.

The traditional approach to surgical management of head and neck cancer has been to resect the primary tumor with an adequate margin of normal tissue (>5 mm in the pathological specimen) and treat the regional nodal basins of the neck. While surgery remains the mainstay of treatment for many head and neck cancers, it is well established that advanced stage disease requires multi-modality therapy. Selecting patients at high-risk of locoregional recurrence after surgery forms the basis for recommending postoperative adjuvant therapy. Historically, this was largely based on anecdotal evidence and experience of the treating physicians until the results of two randomized controlled trials were published in 2004.[18,19] A comparative analysis of these two trials (RTOG #9501 and EORTC #22931) has subsequently enabled physicians to make informed choices about their patients by defining risk levels for locally advanced head and neck cancer, and this has been incorporated into the National Comprehensive Cancer Network (NCCN) guidelines.[20] Microscopically involved surgical margins and the presence of extracapsular extension are the most significant prognostic factors for poor outcome – both locoregional recurrence and survival. Patients with one or both of these risk factors have improved outcome if they receive adjuvant chemotherapy in addition to radiotherapy. A number of minor risk factors were also identified,

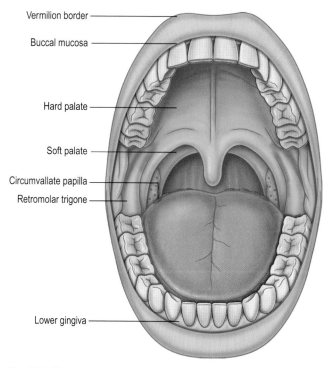

Fig. 16.5 The anatomy of the oral cavity. The oral cavity extends from the vermillion border to the hard palate and soft palate junction. Note the location of the seven subsites of the oral cavity: lip, buccal mucosa, dentoalveolar ridge, retromolar trigone, hard palate, floor of mouth, and oral tongue.

Vermilion border
Buccal mucosa
Hard palate
Soft palate
Circumvallate papilla
Retromolar trigone
Lower gingiva

Table 16.2 Oral cavity T staging as per AJCC, 7th Edition

T stage	Oral cavity	Lip
Tx	Primary tumor cannot be assessed	
T0	No evidence of primary tumor	
Tis	Carcinoma *in situ*	
T1	Tumor 2 cm or less in greatest dimension	
T2	Tumor larger than 2 cm but 4 cm or less in greatest dimension	
T3	Tumor larger than 4 cm in greatest dimension	
T4a	Tumor invades adjacent structures (e.g., through cortical bone, extrinsic tongue muscles, maxillary sinus, skin of face)	Tumor invades through cortical bone, inferior alveolar nerve, floor of mouth, skin of face (i.e., chin or nose)
T4b	Tumor invades masticator space, pterygoid plates or skull base or encases internal carotid artery	

including greater than two positive nodes, perineural invasion, vascular tumor embolisms, Stages III–IV disease or levels IV–V nodes in oral cavity, and oropharyngeal primary tumors. The presence of one of these factors is typically an indication for postoperative radiotherapy. When a number of these are present, chemoradiotherapy is again the recommended treatment in patients deemed fit enough to tolerate this.[21,22]

Oral cavity cancer

The oral cavity extends from the vermillion border of the lip to the junction of the hard and soft palate superiorly and the circumvallate papillae inferiorly and is anatomically subdivided into seven subsites: lip, buccal mucosa, dentoalveolar ridge, retromolar trigone, hard palate, floor of mouth and oral tongue (Fig. 16.5). Oral cavity cancer makes up 14% of all head and neck cancers with 55% of these patients presenting with early stage disease due to the ease of detection and surveillance of the oral cavity (Table 16.2). Treatment of oral cavity cancer can affect critical physiologic functions including speech, mastication, and swallowing. For these reasons, as well as the widespread application of free flap reconstruction, primary surgery is preferable for almost all oral cavity cancer patients barring those who are not medically fit or those who refuse surgery.

While oral cavity cancer is often grouped as a single entity, it is important to recognize that each subsite has unique characteristics that impact the management of the cancers that arise within them. The lip is the most common site of head and neck cancer, excluding cutaneous malignancies. Lip cancers are most often related to sun exposure, and they occur

more frequently on the lower lip. Pipe smoking may also predispose to lower lip cancers. The surgical management of lip cancer is of interest to the reconstructive surgeon and poses unique challenges (Fig. 16.6). By dividing the lip into thirds and determining how many thirds are removed in the resection, the head and neck surgeon can tailor the defect reconstruction using a number of well-established local techniques (Table 16.3). Only when greater than two-thirds of the lip has been resected does free tissue transfer need to be considered.

The oral tongue is the most common intraoral site for cancer to occur, and most often they present along the lateral border of the middle third of the tongue. Transoral excision is possible for most of these lesions with excellent visualization usually possible with this approach. The greatest controversy in managing these lesions is whether or not to treat the clinically node negative neck electively. It is now recognized that for early stage (T1 and T2) oral tongue SCC, depth of invasion is the most important predictor of risk of nodal metastasis.[23] Using the 20% cut-off proposed by Weiss *et al.*,[24] most studies have determined that 4 mm is the cut-off for recommending elective neck dissection in these patients. The buccal mucosa is a rare site for cancer in the western world, accounting for <10% of all oral cavity cancers. However, in South Asia, it is one of the most common sites for cancer because the habit of chewing betel nut exposes the mucosa of the buccogingival sulcus to

Table 16.3 Lip reconstruction is based on the extent of resection by dividing the lip into thirds

Lip	< ⅓	⅓ – ⅔	> ⅔
Lower	Wedge W-flap	Abbe–Estlander (lateral) Karapandzic (middle)	Gilles fan flap Bernard–Burrows Webster advancement Free flap
Upper	Wedge	Abbe +/– Estlander	Burrow–Diffenbach

Abbe = lip switch, based on sup/inf labial artery. Divide pedicle 2–3 weeks later
Estlander modification if commissure involved

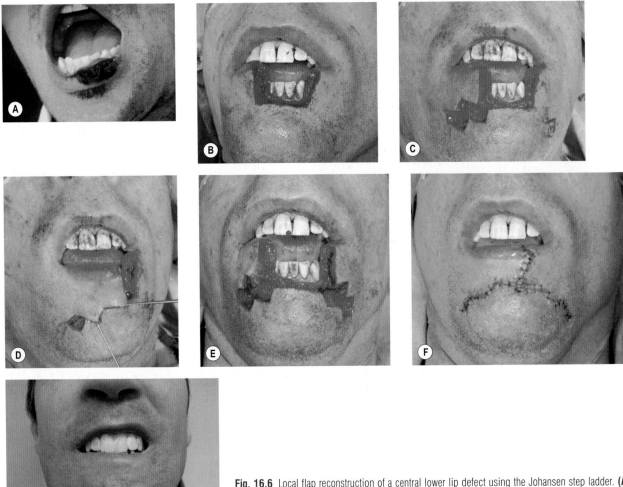

Fig. 16.6 Local flap reconstruction of a central lower lip defect using the Johansen step ladder. **(A)** Lower lip melanoma occupying ⅓ to ⅔ of the lip. **(B)** Post-tumor excision. **(C)** The step-ladder around the mental prominence is created by excision of skin wedges. **(D)** Advancement of the lip up the step ladder. **(E)** Bilateral step ladders in preparation for defect closure. **(F)** End of procedure result. **(G)** Three months postoperative image demonstrating well-healed incision and no microstomia.

carcinogens for extended periods of time. The reconstruction of such defects, typically with a fasciocutaneous free flap, is aimed to reduce the debilitating effect of the severe trismus that can result if large areas of the buccal mucosa are either closed primarily or allowed to heal by secondary intention.

The floor of mouth can be a challenging area to both assess clinically and to resect with clear margins. The proximity to the mandible often necessitates at least a marginal mandibulectomy to obtain adequate clearance of the tumor. Again, reconstruction of this site needs to maintain the mobility of this anatomic region to preserve near normal swallowing and, in particular, speech. When performed in conjunction with neck dissection, free flap reconstruction also recreates the watertight seal that separates the oral cavity from the neck, an important consideration in preventing the spread of infection to the neck. The dentoalveolar ridges, hard palate, and the retromolar trigone account for only a small percentage of oral cavity cancers (Fig. 16.7). Uniquely, however, the thin mucosal layer that covers bone in these subsites predisposes these tumors to early invasion of the mandible or maxilla. Therefore, maxillectomy and/or mandible resection, be it marginal or segmental, needs to be considered in many of these tumors.

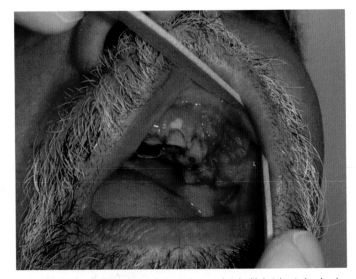

Fig. 16.7 Upper alveolus cancer. Commonly associated with betel nut chewing in Southern Asia. Although these tumors are rare, it is important to recognize tumors in this location are prone to early bone invasion.

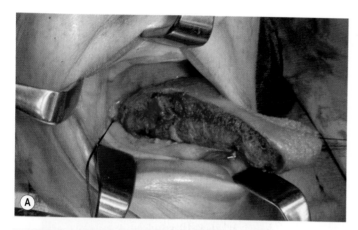

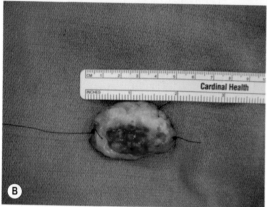

Fig. 16.8 (A) Transoral resection of a lateral tongue border squamous cell carcinoma. Note access to the posterior limit of the oral cavity. **(B)** The surgical specimen demonstrating that adequate resection margins are obtainable with this technique, which avoids the morbidity of mandibulotomy.

Surgical approaches to the oral cavity

Most oral cavity cancers not involving the mandible can be accessed transorally (Fig. 16.8). This approach results in minimal morbidity for the patient and is the preferred approach where possible. Management of the mandible is discussed below, but the approach to accessing the mandible is most commonly achieved through a lip-split approach or may be performed by raising a visor flap superiorly over the mandible. This latter approach places the mental nerves at risk, which is not desirable unless the mental foramina on both sides need to be resected for oncologic purposes. Upper alveolus cancers can often be accessed transorally as well. On occasion, the upper lip may need to be split and connected to a lateral rhinotomy incision (i.e., the Weber–Ferguson incision) to expose a greater portion of the anterior and lateral aspects of the maxilla and enable wider resection of the maxilla (Fig. 16.9). Finally, the transoral and facial approaches may be combined in the midface degloving where an extended sublabial incision is made and, as the skin flap is elevated superiorly, rhinoplasty incisions are also made to deroof the nose and enable more superior elevation of the flap (Fig. 16.10).

Management of the mandible

In managing oral cavity cancer, consideration of the adjacent bony structures, mandible and maxilla, is important from both oncologic and reconstructive perspectives. Tumors of the dentoalveolar ridges, floor of mouth, and retromolar trigone are the most likely primary sites to invade bone. Additionally, metastatic neck disease in level 1 can become fixed to the mandible, necessitating surgical management of the mandible. The optimal imaging modality for assessing the mandible is debated in the literature. CT is generally the standard investigation for staging patients with head and neck cancer.[22] It is also excellent at assessing the mandible with sensitivity for cortical bone involvement reported to be 97–100% accompanied by a specificity of 88% (Fig. 16.11).[25] MRI, on the other hand, may be better at assessing marrow space invasion; however, its specificity is only 54% reflecting a high false positive rate. SPECT scan has also been proposed as a secondary investigation to definitively exclude mandible involvement after a negative CT scan because its reported specificity is 100%.[26]

Through appropriate clinical and radiological evaluation, involvement of the mandible can be reasonably predicted prior to surgery.[27] The mandibular periosteum is thought to be a strong barrier to cancer spread, and in select cases stripping of the periosteum may be adequate therapy,

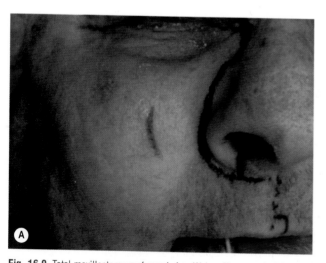

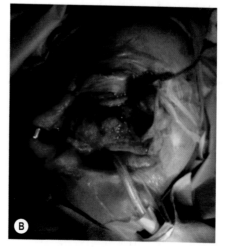

Fig. 16.9 Total maxillectomy performed via a Weber–Ferguson incision. **(A)** Preoperative marking of the Weber–Ferguson incision. **(B)** Exposure of the anterior face of the maxilla.

Continued

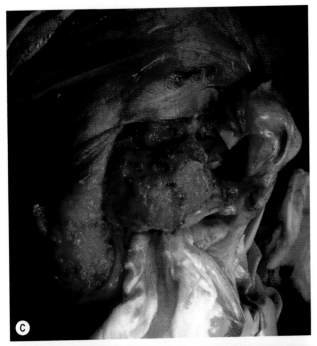

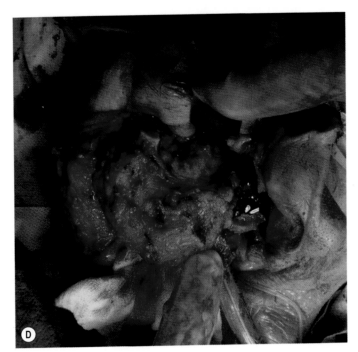

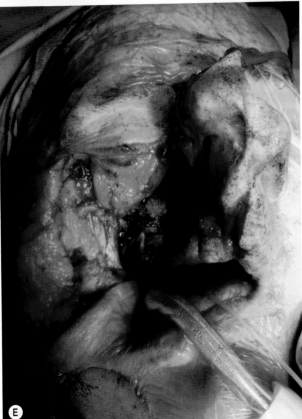

Fig. 16.9, cont'd (C) Osteotomies performed through the floor of the nose (i.e., the hard palate), medial, and lateral. **(D)** Reflecting the maxilla inferiorly to perform posterior orbital floor release. **(E)** Post-ablation defect with orbital fat on view and pterygoid plexus visible at posterior limit of dissection.

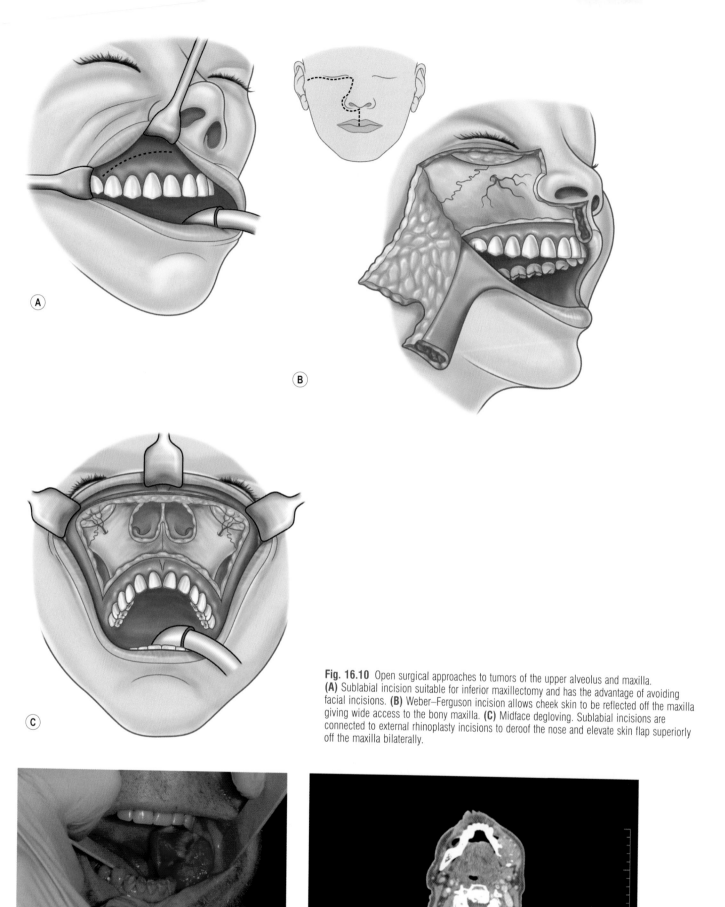

Fig. 16.10 Open surgical approaches to tumors of the upper alveolus and maxilla. **(A)** Sublabial incision suitable for inferior maxillectomy and has the advantage of avoiding facial incisions. **(B)** Weber–Ferguson incision allows cheek skin to be reflected off the maxilla giving wide access to the bony maxilla. **(C)** Midface degloving. Sublabial incisions are connected to external rhinoplasty incisions to deroof the nose and elevate skin flap superiorly off the maxilla bilaterally.

Fig. 16.11 **(A)** Large left mandibular alveolus and retromolar trigone squamous cell carcinoma. **(B)** Frank bony erosion on CT scan.

particularly if the tumor is close but not abutting the bone. Tumors that abut the mandible but do not obviously invade it, as well as tumors that only superficially invade the bony cortex, can be managed with a marginal mandibulectomy.[28] This involves resection of part of the mandibular diameter either as a rim resection or a lingual resection (Fig. 16.12). In these cases, the resected mandible provides an appropriate deep margin for the resection (Fig. 16.13). Partial resection of the mandible reduces the bone stock available to counteract the significant loads applied to the mandible. As a general rule, at least 1 cm of mandible height should be preserved in these cases to prevent pathologic fracture of the mandible. This is particularly difficult in the edentulous patient. In patients in whom this cannot be achieved, segmental resection and appropriate reconstruction provide a more predictable and durable functional result for the patient.

Significant invasion of the mandibular cortex, involvement of the marrow space, or paresthesia of the mental nerve suggesting inferior alveolar nerve involvement are all indications to perform a segmental mandibulectomy (Fig. 16.14). Preoperative imaging is useful in planning

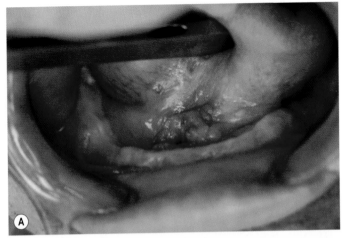

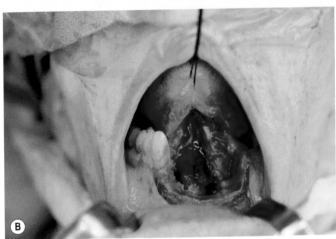

Fig. 16.13 (A) Floor of mouth tumor abutting the mandible. **(B)** Marginal mandibulectomy in this site provides a bony margin, as well as providing excellent access to the deep margin of these tumors, allowing adequate visualization to appropriately resect the deep muscular margin.

osteotomy sites such that a sufficient margin can be obtained around the tumor.

Oropharynx cancer

The oropharynx extends from the level of the hard palate superiorly down to the tip of the epiglottis inferiorly (Fig. 16.15). It is continuous with the nasopharynx superiorly and hypopharynx inferiorly as well as the oral cavity anteriorly. The anterior tonsillar pillars and circumvallate papillae mark the transition from oral cavity to oropharynx. The subsites of the oropharynx are the palatine tonsils, base of tongue, soft palate, and posterior pharyngeal wall (Fig. 16.16). The tonsil is the most common site of tumor origin (60%), followed by base of tongue (25%), soft palate (10%), and pharyngeal wall (5%). A paradigm shift has occurred in oropharyngeal cancer with the recognition of HPV as a strong and independent risk factor for oropharyngeal SCC. HPV-associated oropharynx cancer is different to the traditional smoking and alcohol related cancers.[2] HPV-associated cancers are seen in younger patients who often do not smoke or drink alcohol, and an even greater proportion of these are males. The gene expression profile is different (see pathophysiology of head and neck

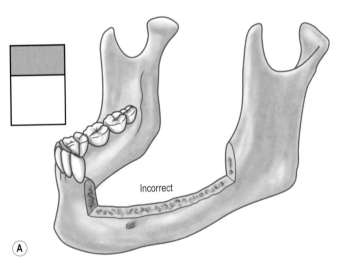

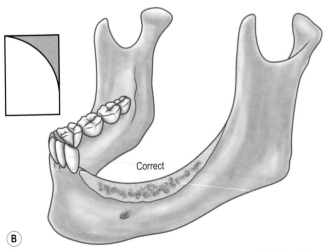

Fig. 16.12 Marginal mandibulectomy. **(A)** Incorrect technique with right angle osteotomies. This increases risk of subsequent fracture during to loading these segments. **(B)** Curved marginal mandibulectomy reduces the chance of creating weak points in the bone and more evenly distributes load across the mandible.

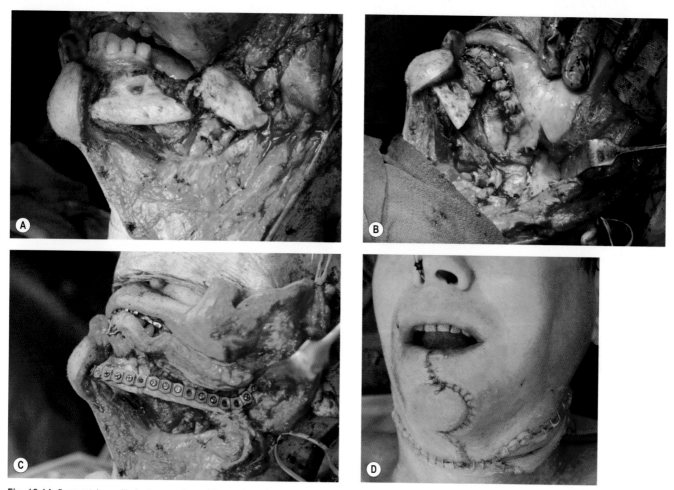

Fig. 16.14 Segmental mandibulectomy performed in a patient with osteoradionecrosis after primary chemoradiotherapy for a left tonsil squamous cell carcinoma. **(A)** A pathological fracture of the left mandible is demonstrated. **(B)** Following segmental mandibulectomy. **(C)** Fibula free flap reconstruction inset with mandibular plating system. **(D)** End of procedure photo demonstrating the circumental lip split incision.

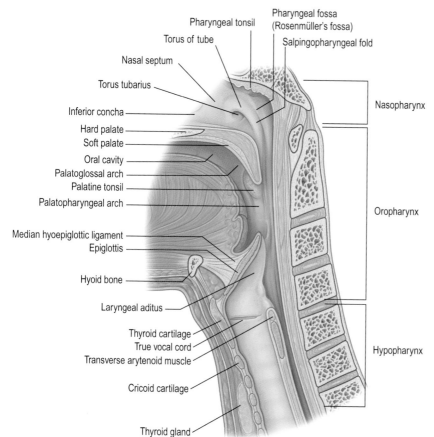

Fig. 16.15 Anatomy of the oropharynx. The oropharynx is continuous with nasopharynx above and the hypopharynx below. The subsites are visualized in this image also: tonsil, base of tongue, soft palate, and posterior pharyngeal wall.

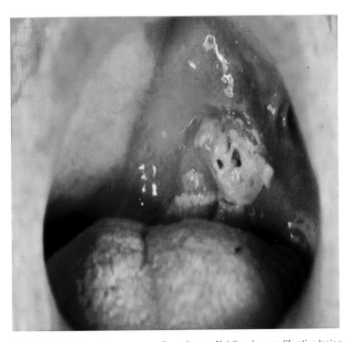

Fig. 16.16 A left tonsil squamous cell carcinoma. Not the ulceroproliferative lesion arising in the left tonsil fossa, extending onto the soft palate.

Table 16.4 Oropharynx T staging as per AJCC, 7th Edition	
T stage	**Oropharynx**
Tx	Primary tumor cannot be assessed
T0	No evidence of primary tumor
Tis	Carcinoma *in situ*
T1	Tumor 2 cm or less in greatest dimension
T2	Tumor larger than 2 cm but 4 cm or less in greatest dimension
T3	Tumor larger than 4 cm in greatest dimension or involves lingual surface of epiglottis
T4a	Tumor invades larynx, deep/extrinsic muscle of tongue, medial pterygoid, hard palate, mandible
T4b	Tumor invades lateral pterygoid, pterygoid plates, lateral nasopharynx, skull base, or carotid artery

cancer above) and the histology more commonly poorly differentiated and basaloid in morphology due to the predilection for HPV to infect basal keratinocytes. Finally, the clinical behavior is significantly different. The 3-year overall survival for HPV positive patients who do not smoke is 93%, compared with 46.8% for the typical non-HPV, tobacco-related oropharynx cancer (Fig. 16.17).[29] Thus, HPV-associated oropharyngeal cancer is recognized as a unique clinical entity, a fact that may be reflected in future iterations of the AJCC staging of this primary site and already is driving change in treatment selection for such patients (Table 16.4).

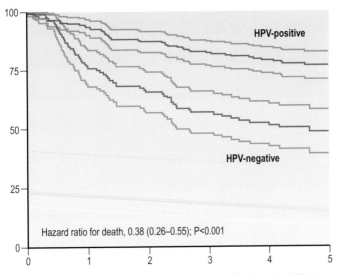

Hazard ratio for death, 0.38 (0.26–0.55); P<0.001

Fig. 16.17 Overall survival from oropharyngeal SCC stratified based on HPV status and smoking history. HPV positive cancers in non-smoking patients has a 3-year overall survival in excess of 90% compared with less than 50% for non-HPV positive tumors in patients with a smoking history. *(From Ang KK, Harris J, Wheeler R, et al. Human papillomavirus and survival of patients with oropharyngeal cancer. N Engl J Med. 2010;363(1):24–35.)*

Surgical approaches to the oropharynx

The traditional approach to the oropharynx (Fig. 16.18) has been through a mandibulotomy or alternatively via a transcervical approach (pharyngotomy or lingual release). All of these open surgical procedures are associated with significant morbidity due to the interruption to the suprahyoid musculature that is critical for swallowing function (Fig. 16.19). In addition, mandibulotomy is associated with potential complications such as non-union, malocclusion, and chronic infection of mandibular hardware. With advances in head and neck irradiation techniques, in particular intensity modulated radiation therapy (IMRT), and extrapolation of organ-preservation strategies from the larynx, non-surgical treatment of oropharyngeal malignancies became increasingly common. However, it is also recognized that this treatment is not benign either, and the early and late effects of radiation can significantly impair a patient's quality of life. Thus, there has been renewed interest in transoral approaches to the oropharynx.[30] Initially, this was with transoral laser microsurgery (TLM), but the advent of the surgical robot systems has sparked interest in transoral robotic surgery (TORS), which is now FDA approved for early stage oropharyngeal cancers.[31–34] The advantage of a transoral surgical approach is primarily the avoidance of a mandibulotomy and its inherent morbidity. Patients return to a normal diet more quickly, are less likely to require free flap reconstruction, and have a shorter hospital stay.[35] TORS also offers the benefit of distal chip telescopes that can be angled to visualize around corners, the use of multiple instruments in the mouth at one time to facilitate dissection and articulated arms for increased maneuverability. Evaluation of the oncologic and functional outcomes of transoral surgery is currently underway in earnest. It appears that TORS is associated with similar oncologic outcomes to primary radiotherapy for p16 positive oropharyngeal SCC, however, a difference in adverse event profile does exist between the two modalities.[36] Furthermore, this can be achieved in a cost-effective manner.[37] TORS is currently undergoing evaluation through multi-center randomized controlled trials in the management of oropharynx SCC.

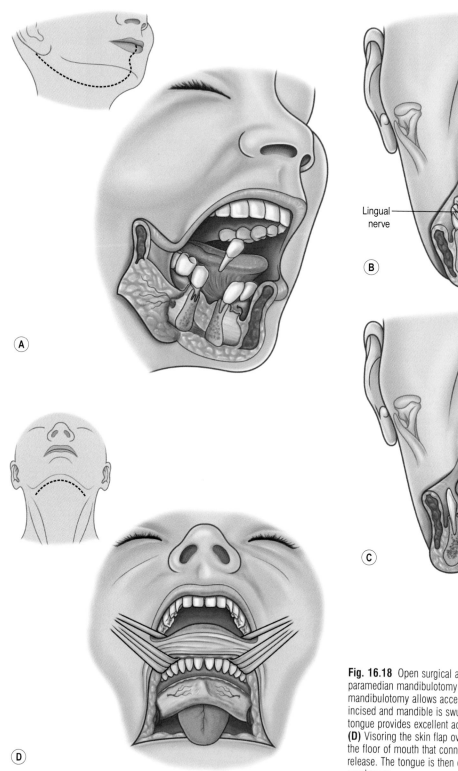

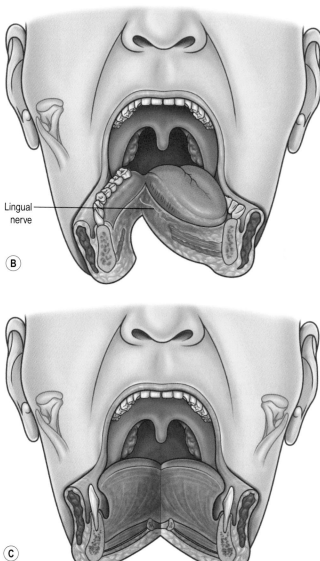

Lingual nerve

Fig. 16.18 Open surgical approaches to the oropharynx. **(A)** Preparation for paramedian mandibulotomy with lip split incision and tooth removal. **(B)** Paramedian mandibulotomy allows access to the oropharynx when the floor of mouth mucosa is incised and mandible is swung away from the midline. **(C)** The midline split of the tongue provides excellent access to the posterior pharyngeal wall and cervical spine. **(D)** Visoring the skin flap over the mandible and then making mucosal incisions in the floor of mouth that connect to the neck dissection perform comprises a lingual release. The tongue is then delivered into the neck, allowing visualization of the oropharynx.

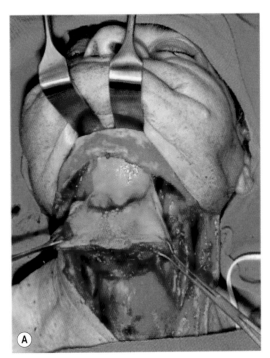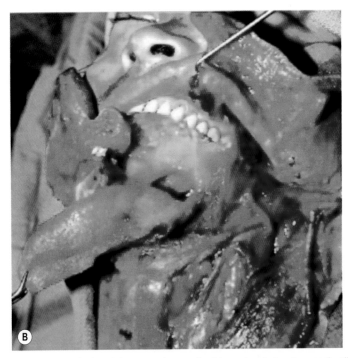

Fig. 16.19 Surgical approaches to the oropharynx. **(A)** Lingual release enables visualization of the tongue base, soft palate, and posterior pharyngeal wall. **(B)** Paramedian mandibulotomy and mandibular swing also allows excellent visualization of the oropharynx.

Larynx and hypopharynx cancer

The larynx occupies a unique place in the anatomical and functional make-up of the head and neck. The primary functions of the larynx are respiration, airway protection, and voice production; thus disease or surgery of the larynx can inhibit critical functions that contribute to both the patient's medical health and psychosocial well-being. The hypopharynx wraps around the posterior larynx and provides a portal of entry for food to the esophagus, meaning that cancers that arise here can significantly alter swallowing and thus nutritional intake. The larynx extends from the tip of the epiglottis to the inferior border of the cricoid cartilage and is subdivided into the supraglottis, glottis, and subglottis (Fig. 16.20). Of particular relevance to cancer treatment, the glottis is an area of lymphatic watershed, meaning that only advanced glottis cancers will attain lymphatic access for cancer dissemination

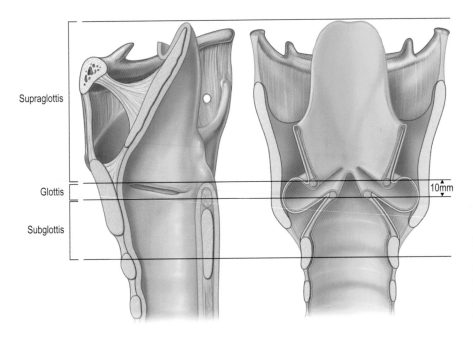

Supraglottis

Glottis

Subglottis

10mm

Fig. 16.20 Anatomy of the larynx. The subsites of the larynx, supraglottis, glottis, and subglottis can be appreciated. The glottis is a watershed area for lymphatic drainage; hence cancers at the glottis level metastasize relatively late. The supraglottis has abundant lymphatic drainage to the neck bilaterally and typically presents with early regional metastatic disease.

Table 16.5 Larynx T staging as per AJCC, 7th Edition

Note the different staging systems for the different subsites of the larynx: supraglottis, glottis, subglottis

T stage	Supraglottis	Glottis	Subglottis
Tx	Primary tumor cannot be assessed		
T0	No evidence of primary tumor		
Tis	Carcinoma *in situ*		
T1	Tumor limited to one subsite* of supraglottis with normal vocal cord mobility	Tumor limited to vocal cord(s) (may involve anterior or posterior commissure) with normal mobility. T1a: tumor limited to one vocal cord, T1b: tumor involves both vocal cords	Tumor limited to the subglottis
T2	Tumor invades mocusa of more than one adjacent subsite of supraglottis or glottis or region outside supraglottis (e.g., mucosa of base of tongue, vallecula, medial wall of piriform sinus (without fixation of the larynx)	Tumor extends to supraglottis and/or subglottis, and/or with impaired vocal cord mobility	Tumor extends to vocal cord(s) with normal or impaired mobility
T3	Tumor limited to larynx with vocal cord fixation and/or invades any of the following: postcricoid area, pre-epiglottic space, or paraglottic space	Tumor limited to the larynx with vocal cord fixation and/or invasion of paraglottic space and/or inner cortex of thyroid cartilage	Tumor limited to larynx with vocal cord fixation
T4a	Tumor invades through the thyroid cartilage, and/or extends into soft tissues of the neck, thyroid, and/or esophagus	Tumor invades through outer cortex of thyroid cartilage and/or to other tissues beyond the larynx (e.g., trachea, soft tissues of neck including deep extrinsic tongue muscles, strap muscles, thyroid, esophagus)	Tumor invades through cricoid or thyroid cartilage and/or extends to other tissues beyond the larynx (e.g., trachea, soft tissues of neck, thyroid, esophagus)
T4b	Tumor invades prevertebral space, encases carotid artery or invades mediastinal structures		

*subsites include the following: ventricular bands (false cords), arytenoids, suprahyoid epiglottis, infrahyoid epiglottis, aryepiglottic folds (laryngeal aspect)

to the regional lymph nodes. The supraglottis, on the other hand, has rich lymphatic supply, and cancers arising here present with clinically evident neck metastasis early in their disease course (Table 16.5).

The hypopharynx extends from the tip of the epiglottis (level of the hyoid) to the cricopharyngeus muscle at the entry to the upper esophagus (lower border of the cricoid) and contains three subsites – piriform fossa, posterior pharyngeal wall, and post-cricoid region (Fig. 16.21). Cancer of the hypopharynx is the least common of the upper aerodigestive tract malignancies accounting for less than 5% of all head and neck cancers. In addition, they have a dismal prognosis that is in part due to their advanced stage at presentation due to their concealed primary location, their unique propensity to spread submucosally, making resection with clear margins difficult as well as their ready access to abundant lymphatic channels. 80% of hypopharynx cancers will have neck nodal disease and 25% have distant metastatic disease at the time of presentation (Table 16.6).

Evidence for treatment of larynx and hypopharynx cancer

The management of laryngeal and hypopharyngeal cancer has changed significantly over the last 30 years with the emergence of new surgical tools and data from large clinical

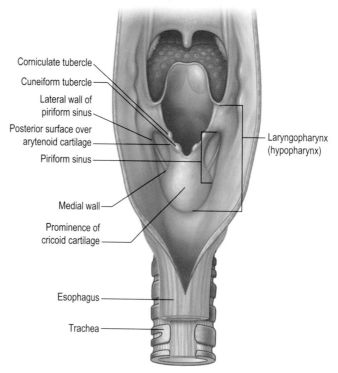

Fig. 16.21 Anatomy of the hypopharynx. The hypopharynx wraps around the posterior aspect of the larynx and can be subdivided into the piriform fossa, post-cricoid region, and posterior pharyngeal wall.

Table 16.6 Hypopharynx T staging as per AJCC, 7th Edition

T stage	Hypopharynx
Tx	Primary tumor cannot be assessed
T0	No evidence of primary tumor
Tis	Carcinoma *in situ*
T1	Tumor limited to one subsite of hypopharynx <2 cm
T2	Tumor invades more than one subsite of hypopharynx or an adjacent subsite or 2–4 cm in greatest diameter without fixation of hemilarynx
T3	>4 cm in greatest dimension or with fixation of hemilarynx
T4a	Tumor invades thyroid/cricoid cartilage, hyoid bone, thyroid gland, esophagus, or central compartment soft tissue
T4b	Tumor invades prevertebral space, encases carotid artery, or invades mediastinal structures

trials presenting patients and their physicians multiple treatment options.[38] As with other head and neck sites, early larynx and hypopharynx cancer is treated with single modality therapy. The options for treatment of early laryngeal cancers are open partial laryngeal surgery (e.g., vertical partial laryngectomy, horizontal supraglottic laryngectomy), TLM, or radiation therapy. All of these approaches have similar oncologic control rates, which exceed 85% 5-year locoregional control and overall survival.[39–41] The morbidity profile of each is different, and decision-making involves a detailed discussion between the treating physician and the patient. TLM offers the advantage of a single treatment episode and avoids the side effects of radiation treatment. In general, TLM and radiation therapy are the primary treatment options with open partial laryngeal surgery reserved for patients who refuse radiotherapy and have poor endoscopic access precluding TLM. Early voice outcomes after treatment are better for radiation when compared to laser; however, the long-term results do not demonstrate significant difference.[42–44] Transoral approaches, such as TLM or TORS for early hypopharyngeal lesions, located away from the post-cricoid region and medial wall of the piriform fossa may be appropriate; however, these cases represent a small subset of patients with most patients presenting with more advanced disease.[45] The neck should always be treated electively in supraglottic tumors and hypopharynx cancers, by way of the modality used to treat the primary site.

While the historical standard treatment for advanced laryngeal cancer has been surgery with total laryngectomy, followed by postoperative radiation therapy, this paradigm changed significantly in the late 1980s and became more broadly accepted following the publication of the VA study in 1991.[46] This study of 332 patients compared induction chemotherapy followed by radiotherapy in patients who had a partial or complete response (non-responders proceeded to surgery) with a control arm that underwent the standard therapy of surgery (total laryngectomy plus neck dissections) and postoperative radiation. At 2 years, the survival was 68% for both groups with 64% of the study group having the added benefit of keeping their larynx. A subsequent study of 547 patients (RTOG #91-11) attempted to further define the contribution of radiotherapy and chemotherapy by comparing three groups – radiotherapy alone, concurrent chemoradiotherapy, and induction chemotherapy followed by radiotherapy.[47] While overall survival did not differ between groups, the concurrent chemoradiotherapy group had the highest rate of larynx preservation and locoregional control. Thus, it has become the standard non-surgical therapy for advanced laryngeal cancer. Involvement of the laryngeal cartilages and pre-treatment laryngeal dysfunction remain indications for primary surgery; however, in the absence of these features concurrent chemoradiation has become the favored treatment approach with the hope of preserving laryngeal function. It is important to acknowledge the long-term morbidity associated with non-surgical treatment of larynx cancer. In a review of 230 patients from three RTOG trials (91-11, 97-03 and 99-14), 43% had a severe late toxicity (severe laryngopharyngeal dysfunction, feeding tube dependence beyond two years or death related to effects of treatment).[48] Organ preservation does not always equate with function-preservation, and the effects of radiation therapy progress well beyond the follow-up time points referenced in many clinical trials.

The VA study design has also been applied in a study of 194 patients with hypopharynx SCC.[49] The 10-year survival was not different between the induction chemotherapy and radiation group (13.1%) and the surgical group (13.8%); however, more than half (8.2%) of the survivors in the non-surgical group kept their larynx at the 10-year follow-up point. With the same caveats of advanced laryngeal cancer, primary non-surgical therapy is typically recommended to these patients with surgery being reserved for salvage of persistent or recurrent disease.

Surgical approaches to the larynx and hypopharynx

The surgical approaches to early larynx cancer have already been discussed. The gold standard surgical management of advanced laryngeal cancer is total laryngectomy. This involves removal of the airway from above the hyoid to the upper tracheal rings and creation of a permanent tracheostome to the anterior neck skin. The pharynx is closed primarily to allow near-normal swallowing. Voice rehabilitation following total laryngectomy is preferentially achieved through use of a trachea-esophageal valve speaking prosthesis. Esophageal speech and electrolarynx devices are less desirable methods of restoring the voice. The anatomical location of these tumors dictates that primary surgery in these cases is complicated by the almost universal need for laryngectomy in addition to pharyngectomy (partial or total) in all but the earliest of hypopharyngeal cancers.

Management of the neck

The neck is the most common site of metastasis for head and neck malignancy. In addition, it is the most important determinant of prognosis with it being well established that the presence of neck disease reduces survival by approximately 50%. Thus, rational decisions about treating the neck are paramount in head and neck cancer decision-making. Treatment of the neck may be either therapeutic or elective depending on whether or not there is clinically detectable nodal disease at the time of presentation. In the setting of clinically evident neck disease, a therapeutic neck dissection is warranted with adjuvant therapy decided based on the pathologic features. In the patient without clinical evidence of neck disease, the decision to treat or not to treat the neck is based on the probability of occult neck disease being present, as treating this disease while it is microscopic confers an improved prognosis for the patient compared with attempting salvage surgery after recurrence becomes clinically evident.[50] In a landmark study, Weiss *et al.* determined that above an occult metastasis risk of 20%, the benefits of elective neck treatment outweighed the risks.[24] In the head and neck, this encompasses all subsites except for T1 lip and glottis cancers as well as thin early stage tumors of the oral cavity.[51,52] The choice of treatment modality for the neck is dictated by the treatment of the primary site – surgery or radiation therapy.

Surgical approaches to the neck: neck dissection

First described by George W. Crile in 1906, the neck dissection is an *en bloc* resection of the nodal drainage stations of the UADT. In its original form, the radical neck dissection was a systematic removal of the lymph nodes from the mandible to the clavicle and from the midline to the trapezius in addition to the sternomastoid muscle, internal jugular vein, and accessory nerve (Fig. 16.22). This package of nodal tissue is now divided into a number of levels, which allow accurate description of the procedure and indicate most common sites of metastatic spread from different subsites of the head and neck (Fig. 16.23). The radical neck dissection is undoubtedly a morbid procedure, in particular the sacrifice of the accessory

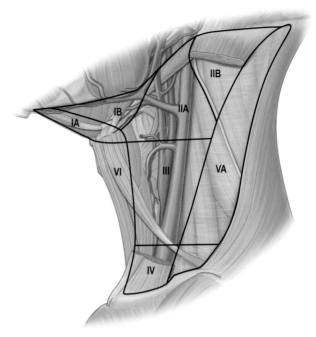

Fig. 16.23 The levels of the neck that enable description of the neck dissection. IA is the submental triangle between the anterior bellies of digastric and the mandible. IB is the submandibular triangle. Levels II, III, and IV are the jugular chain of lymph nodes divided by the hyoid bone and the cricoid cartilage. Level II is further subdivided to IIA and IIB by the accessory nerve. Level V is the posterior triangle, divided into VA and VB by the omohyoid muscle. *(From Robbins KT, Clayman G, Levine PA, et al. Neck dissection classification update: revisions proposed by the American Head and Neck Society and the American Academy of Otolaryngology–Head and Neck Surgery. Arch Otolaryngol Head Neck Surg. 2002:751–758.)*

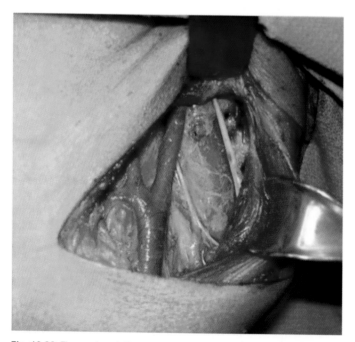

Fig. 16.22 The non-lymphatic structures that can be preserved in a modified radical neck dissection: internal jugular vein, accessory nerve, and sternomastoid muscle.

nerve leads to the debilitating shoulder syndrome that was encountered almost universally amongst patients undergoing radical neck dissection. With improved recognition of the drainage patterns of the UADT mucosal sites, more conservative procedures are now advocated.[51,53] Preservation of at least the accessory nerve can improve function considerably for these patients (Fig. 16.24). The move towards conservatism in neck surgery is particularly relevant for the clinically negative neck whereby only the "most likely" nodal levels are dissected in order to pathologically stage the neck and provide guidance for adjuvant therapy and prognosis. For the clinically positive neck, a comprehensive neck dissection remains the recommended procedure, although even in the setting of early stage nodal disease, a selective neck dissection may still be adequate therapy.

Just as the neck dissection has evolved as a surgical technique, so too the classification of this procedure has also changed. Currently, neck dissections are classified as per the system agreed on by the American Head and Neck Society and the American Academy of Otolaryngology-Head and Neck Surgery (Box 16.1).[54] This classification fundamentally reports the number of levels dissected and the preservation or resection of non-lymphatic structures, including the sternomastoid muscle, accessory nerve, internal jugular vein, overlying skin, hypoglossal nerve, carotid artery, and vagus nerve, amongst others. The most commonly performed neck dissection is a selective I–IV neck dissection, and the steps of this procedure are listed in Box 16.2. It is important to

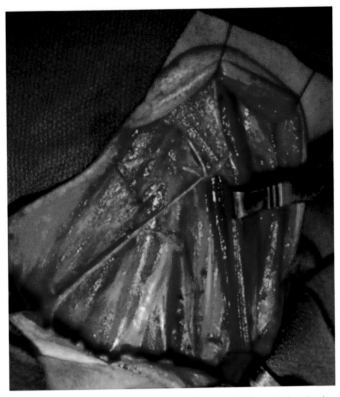

Fig. 16.24 Accessory nerve dissected through its course in the posterior triangle. Preservation of this nerve can reduce the dysfunction that characterizes radical neck dissection.

BOX 16.1 **The current classification of neck dissection. Broadly, neck dissections are comprehensive (all five levels) or selective (less than five). The updated classification described here removes the descriptive names (e.g., supraomohyoid) from selective neck dissections and rather uses description by the levels dissected**

1. Radical neck dissection
2. Modified radical neck dissection
3. Selective neck dissection: each variation is depicted by "SND" and the use of parentheses to denote the levels or sublevels removed
4. Extended neck dissection

(From Robbins KT, Clayman G, Levine PA, et al. Neck dissection classification update: revisions proposed by the American Head and Neck Society and the American Academy of Otolaryngology-Head and Neck Surgery. *Arch Otolaryngol Head Neck Surg* 2002:751–758.).

recognize the density of anatomical structures within the neck and thus the list of potential complications from this operation is extensive (Table 16.7).

Salivary gland neoplasms

Salivary gland neoplasms represent a diverse group of neoplasms, both benign and malignant, that are potentially challenging to the head and neck surgeon with respect to their accurate preoperative diagnosis and surgical management given their proximity to the facial nerve within the parotid gland. The salivary gland system consists of paired parotid, submandibular, and sublingual glands along with hundreds of minor salivary glands throughout the oral cavity and pharynx.

BOX 16.2 **Steps of the selective I–IV neck dissection**

1. Patient is positioned supine with an inflatable shoulder roll
2. Cervical incision marked and infiltrated with vasoconstrictor
3. Skin incised and subplatysmal flaps raised to the level of the mandible and clavicle
4. Start by raising fascia off the anterior border of the sternomastoid muscle, ligating and dividing the perforating vessels
5. Identify accessory nerve 1 cm above the most superior perforator and deep to the sternomastoid tendon
6. Dissect the accessory nerve superomedially to identify posterior belly of digastric muscle and superior end of internal jugular vein
7. Dissect level IIB at this time (if required) and release nodal package underneath accessory nerve to join with remaining dissection
8. Continue to raise fascia from sternomastoid muscle to identify the roots of the cervical plexus, representing the floor of dissection
9. Divide omohyoid muscle or release fascia from omohyoid to enable access to level IV
10. Dissect lower limit of the neck dissection with identification of the transverse cervical vessels and phrenic nerve
11. Control the thoracic duct and/or its feeding lymphatic channels
12. Dissect nodal package forward off the cervical plexus and prevertebral fascia
13. Fascia is then rolled over the internal jugular vein to release the carotid sheath
14. Posterior belly of digastric muscle followed anteriorly to tendinous insertion to hyoid bone
15. Identify and preserve hypoglossal nerve
16. Turn attention to level I dissection by incising the submandibular fascia and raising this off the submandibular gland. This maneuver protects the marginal mandibular branch of the facial nerve
17. Ligate the facial artery and vein superiorly
18. Release the contents of level IA off the midline and anterior belly of digastric
19. Continue level one dissection by releasing submandibular fascia and skeletonizing the mylohyoid muscle
20. Retract the mylohyoid muscle anteriorly to expose the submandibular triangle
21. Ligate ganglionic branch from lingual nerve, submandibular duct and associated veins, preserving hypoglossal nerve
22. Dissect gland down to posterior belly of digastric to meet up with II–IV dissection
23. Ligate facial artery again and deliver specimen
24. Check hemostasis with particular attention to chyle leak in low level IV
25. Place suction drain
26. Close platysmal with 3-0 Vicryl and skin with running subcuticular 4-0 Biosyn or skin staples

Table 16.7 Complications of neck dissection	
General	**Specific**
Hematoma	Neural injury- CN XI, CN XII, marginal mandibular branch of CN VII, lingual nerve, brachial plexus, phrenic nerve, vagus nerve
Infection	Vascular injury: carotid artery, internal jugular vein
Wound dehiscence	Chyle leak
Seroma	Air embolism
Atelectasis, PE, UTI, DVT	

Epidemiology

The incidence of salivary gland tumors in the US is in the range of 1–3 per 100 000 population.[55] The distribution of frequency and malignancy amongst the salivary glands is of particular note (Table 16.8). In terms of frequency, the proportion of tumors found in the parotid gland compared to the submandibular gland and sublingual gland is 100:10:1.[56] Interestingly, however, 80% of parotid tumors are benign, in contrast to 60% of submandibular, 40% of sublingual gland, and 20% of minor salivary gland tumors, making the risk of malignancy inversely proportional to the size of the gland (Table 16.8).

Work-up of a salivary gland neoplasm

The first consideration in assessment of an enlarged salivary gland is to differentiate neoplastic and non-neoplastic causes. Sialadenosis, sialadenitis (viral, bacterial), and sialolithiasis along with autoimmune conditions (Sjögren's syndrome, sarcoidosis) are all non-neoplastic causes that need to be excluded. Once a neoplastic cause is considered most likely, the history is important in aiding differentiation of benign from malignant tumors. Features such as pain, rapid growth, and cranial nerve neuropathies are all warning signs for malignancy. On examination, the presence of fixation to skin or the deeper structures such as muscle and bone, as well as cervical lymphadenopathy, should also alert the clinician to the potential for malignancy.

While ultrasound is a rapid, non-invasive, and relatively cheap test, cross-sectional imaging is preferred for preoperative planning. The size and location of the mass as well as its relationship to surrounding structures, in particular any

Table 16.8 Tumors of the salivary glands		
Gland	**Benign (%)**	**Malignant (%)**
Parotid	80	20
Submandibular	60	40
Sublingual	40	60
Minor salivary glands	20	80
Note the inverse relationship between size of salivary gland and risk of malignancy		

extension to the parapharyngeal space or invasion of skin, subcutaneous tissues, or underlying muscle should all be specifically examined for (Fig. 16.25). The availability and cost of CT scanning has made it the modality of choice in many centers. MRI does have a number of inherent benefits when assessing salivary gland neoplasms. The superior soft tissue definition enables improved delineation of the margins of a lesion, and the signal intensities may aid diagnosis. High-grade malignancies tend to have low to intermediate signal intensities on all imaging sequences, whereas low-grade malignancies and benign tumors typically have low T1 signal and high T2 signal.[57] Gadolinium enhanced sequences are critical in assessing perineural invasion and cervical lymph node metastasis.

Fine needle aspiration (FNA) plays a key role in the preoperative work-up of a patient with a salivary gland tumor. While the decision to operate does not solely depend on the findings of a needle biopsy, it does have a number of benefits. Firstly, it may identify inflammatory causes as well as lymphoma, which do not require surgery. Secondly, the preoperative identification of a high-grade malignancy enables the surgeon to determine surgical urgency and to counsel the patient with respect to the need for neck dissection, possible sacrifice of the facial nerve, and the need for postoperative adjuvant therapy. It is critical for the clinician to also understand the potential pitfalls in its use.[58] FNA cytology is highly dependent on the experience of the reporting pathologist and yields a non-diagnostic sample more frequently than FNA of other head and neck masses. Finally, and most importantly, the sensitivity and specificity of this test even for differentiating benign from malignant pathology is not 100%. A meta-analysis of the diagnostic accuracy of FNA cytology for parotid lesions examined 64 studies, including 6169 cases, and concluded the sensitivity of this test was 79% and its specificity 97% when attempting to differentiate malignant from

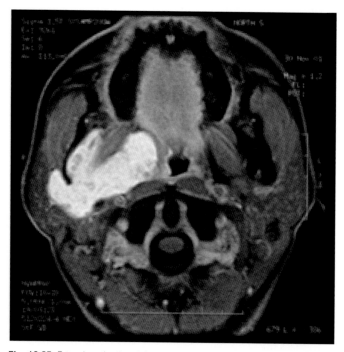

Fig. 16.25 Extension of a deep lobe parotid tumor to the parapharyngeal space.

benign tumors.[59] A study by the same authors examining ultrasound-guided core biopsy found the sensitivity to be 92% and specificity 100% when analyzing the data from 277 cases reported in five studies.[60] Interestingly, a two-step procedure of FNA followed by core biopsy, if the FNA was non-diagnostic, yielded a sensitivity of 99% and a specificity of 96%. Thus, in a clinical sense, the addition of core biopsy to FNA can reduce the false negative rate from 21% to just 1%.

In the event of a malignant diagnosis, the combination of clinical examination and radiologic imaging enables accurate staging using current AJCC TNM staging for major salivary gland cancer (Table 16.9), which assists in guiding treatment decisions. Minor salivary gland cancers are staged according to their anatomic site of origin.

Pathology of salivary gland neoplasms

Salivary gland neoplasms are a particularly diverse group of tumors. Their clinical behavior reflects this diversity and is often driven by histologic grade. Thus, a detailed understanding of salivary gland pathology is essential in order to guide appropriate treatment for patients (Box 16.3).

Pleomorphic adenoma is the most common benign salivary gland neoplasm, and it demonstrates some unique clinical and pathological features (Fig. 16.26). Despite being an encapsulated tumor, it does often contain pseudopodia that project from its surface.[61] It is thought that these can contribute to post-surgical recurrence and hence why parotidectomy in

some form, rather than enucleation, is recommended for these lesions.[62] This reduces the recurrence rate from 4% to less than 1% (Fig. 16.27).[63] It also has a known risk of malignant transformation.[64,65] One large study highlighted the importance of disease duration in assessing malignant

Table 16.9 AJCC TNM staging for major salivary gland cancer

Note N stage and M stage are as for the upper aerodigestive mucosal sites

T stage	Salivary gland
Tx	Primary tumor cannot be assessed
T0	No evidence of primary tumor
Tis	Carcinoma *in situ*
T1	Tumor 2 cm or less in greatest dimension without extraparenchymal extension
T2	Tumor larger than 2 cm but 4 cm or less in greatest dimension without extraparenchymal extension
T3	Tumor larger than 4 cm in greatest dimension and/or has extraparenchymal extension
T4a	Tumor invades skin, mandible, ear canal, and/or facial nerve
T4b	Tumor invades pterygoid plates or skull base or encases internal carotid artery

---

BOX 16.3 World Health Organization (WHO) classification of parotid neoplasms

Malignant epithelial tumors

Squamous cell carcinoma 8070/3

    Verrucous carcinoma 8051/3

    Papillary squamous cell carcinoma 8052/3

    Basaloid squamous cell carcinoma 8083/3

    Spindle cell carcinoma 8074/3

    Adenosquamous carcinoma 8560/3

    Acantholytic squamous cell carcinoma 8075/3

Lymphoepithelial carcinoma 8082/3

Sinonasal undifferentiated carcinoma 8020/3

Adenocarcinoma

    Intestinal-type adenocarcinoma 8144/3

    Non-intestinal-type adenocarcinoma 8140/3

Salivary gland-type carcinomas

    Adenoid cystic carcinoma 8200/3

    Acinic cell carcinoma 8550/3

    Mucoepidermoid carcinoma 8430/3

    Epithelial-myoepithelial carcinoma 8562/3

    Clear cell carcinoma N.O.S. 8310/3

    Myoepithelial carcinoma 8982/3

    Carcinoma ex pleomorphic adenoma 8941/3

Polymorphous low-grade adenocarcinoma 8525/3

Neuroendocrine tumors

    Typical carcinoid 8240/3

    Atypical carcinoid 8249/3

    Small cell carcinoma, neuroendocrine type 8041/3

Benign epithelial tumors

Sinonasal papillomas

    Inverted papilloma

    (Schneiderian papilloma, inverted type) 8121/1

    Oncocytic papilloma

    (Schneiderian papilloma, oncocytic type) 8121/1

    Exophytic papilloma

    (Schneiderian papilloma, exophytic type) 8121/0

Salivary gland-type adenomas

    Pleomorphic adenoma 8940/0

    Myoepithelioma 8982/0

    Oncocytoma 8290/0

Soft tissue tumors

Malignant tumors

    Fibrosarcoma 8810/3

    Malignant fibrous histiocytoma 8830/3

BOX 16.3 World Health Organization (WHO) classification of parotid neoplasms—cont'd

Leiomyosarcoma 8890/3

Rhabdomyosarcoma 8900/3

Angiosarcoma 9120/3

Malignant peripheral nerve sheath tumor 9540/3

Borderline and low malignant potential tumors

Desmoid-type fibromatosis 8821/1

Inflammatory myofibroblastic tumor 8825/1

Glomangiopericytoma

(Sinonasal-type hemangiopericytoma) 9150/1

Extrapleural solitary fibrous tumor 8815/1

Benign tumors

Myxoma 8840/0

Leiomyoma 8890/0

Hemangioma 9120/0

Schwannoma 9560/0

Neurofibroma 9540/0

Meningioma 9530/0

Tumors of bone and cartilage

Malignant tumors

Chondrosarcoma 9220/3

Mesenchymal chondrosarcoma 9240/3

Osteosarcoma 9180/3

Chordoma 9370/3

Benign tumors

Giant cell lesion

Giant cell tumor 9250/1

Chondroma 9220/0

Osteoma 9180/0

Chondroblastoma 9230/0

Chondromyxoid fibroma 9241/0

Osteochondroma (exostosis) 9210/0

Osteoid osteoma 9191/0

Osteoblastoma 9200/0

Ameloblastoma 9310/0

Nasal chondromesenchymal hamartoma

Hematolymphoid tumors

Extranodal NK/T cell lymphoma 9719/3

Diffuse large B-cell lymphoma 9680/3

Extramedullary plasmacytoma 9734/3

Extramedullary myeloid sarcoma 9930/3

Histiocytic sarcoma 9755/3

Langerhans cell histiocytosis 9751/1

Neuroectodermal

Ewing sarcoma 9260/3

Primitive neuroectodermal tumor 9364/3

Olfactory neuroblastoma 9522/3

Melanotic neuroectodermal tumor of infancy 9363/0

Mucosal malignant melanoma 8720/3

Germ cell tumors

Immature teratoma 9080/3

Teratoma with malignant transformation 9084/3

Sinonasal yolk sac tumor (endodermal sinus tumor) 9071/3

Sinonasal teratocarcinosarcoma

Mature teratoma 9080/0

Dermoid cyst 9084/0

Secondary tumors

1 Morphology code of the International Classification of Diseases for Oncology (ICD-O) {821} and the Systematized Nomenclature of Medicine (http://snomed.org).
Behavior is coded /0 for benign tumors, /3 for malignant tumors, and /1 for borderline or uncertain behavior.
(From Barnes L, World Health Organization, International Agency for Research on Cancer. *Pathology and Genetics of Head and Neck Tumors.* Lyon: IARC; 2005:1.)

---

risk when their review found the risk to be 1.5% at 5 years, increasing to 10% at 15 years.[66] Carcinoma ex pleomorphic adenoma is an aggressive malignancy that is histologically high-grade and demonstrates an overtly infiltrative growth pattern. Avoidance of this entity is a good reason to recommend surgery for pleomorphic adenoma despite its otherwise benign nature.

Warthin's tumor is the second most common benign salivary gland tumor and is found almost exclusively in the parotid gland. In contrast to pleomorphic adenoma, it demonstrates no risk of malignant transformation and may potentially be observed. It is pathologically represented by its former name – papillary cystadenoma lymphomatosum. Bilayer epithelium grows in papillary fronds projecting into cystic spaces, surrounded by lymphoid follicles with germinal

centers. Its unique clinical features include its predilection for older males, an association with smoking, and its unique ability to concentrate Technetium-99.[67,68] It is bilateral in 10% of cases and multicentric within the ipsilateral gland in a further 10%.[69]

The diagnosis of salivary gland malignancies has evolved considerably in recent years with the World Health Organization (WHO) now recognizing 24 distinct pathological entities (Box 16.3).[70] These tumors demonstrate a broad range of morphological diversity and, coupled with the relative rarity of many of these, can make accurate diagnosis difficult. Pathologists continue to rely on microscopic appearance as the immunocytochemical profiles are rarely useful in aiding diagnosis.[71,72] Clinically, it is most useful to consider these malignancies as either low-grade or high-grade.[73] High-grade

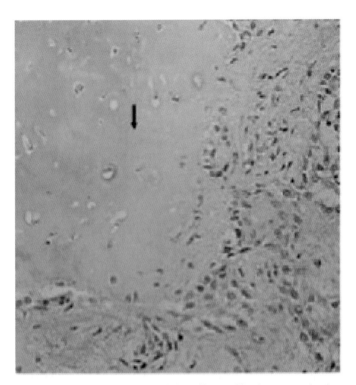

Fig. 16.26 Pleomorphic adenoma pathology. Pleomorphic adenoma contains three components histologically: epithelial, myoepithelial, and stromal components. The stroma may be myxoid, chondroid, osteoid, fibroid, or vascular.

malignancies include high-grade mucoepidermoid carcinoma, adenocarcinoma, squamous cell carcinoma, salivary ductal carcinoma, and carcinoma ex pleomorphic adenoma. Low-grade malignancies include low-grade mucoepidermoid carcinoma, acinic cell carcinoma, basal cell adenocarcinoma, and low-grade polymorphous adenocarcinoma. Adenoid cystic carcinoma (ACC) is an intermediate grade malignancy that can span either end of the histologic grading spectrum. In any case, however, it is a high-risk tumor in terms of disease recurrence.[73] This differentiation helps to guide treatment (see below).

Mucoepidermoid carcinoma is the most common salivary gland malignancy with the majority occurring in the major salivary glands although oral cavity minor salivary glands are not infrequently involved.[74] Various histologic grading systems have been developed, but in essence high-grade lesions are those with increased epidermoid cells, whereas low-grade lesions tend to have a greater mucinous component with less cytologic atypia and a lower mitotic rate (Fig. 16.28). Grading correlates strongly with clinical behavior of these tumors. ACC is a salivary gland malignancy that demonstrates unique clinical features. Pathologically, it demonstrates three distinct growth patterns that may overlap within the same tumor – tubular, cribriform, and solid (Fig. 16.29). The solid lesions are more aggressive with a higher tendency to nodal metastasis, whereas the cribriform pattern is the most common and most easily recognized with its "Swiss cheese" appearance histologically. ACC is a relentless disease with a propensity for perineural spread and late recurrences. While 5-year survival approaches 80%, 10-year survival is 10–30% and 15-year

survival is 1–10% with many of these late failures being lung metastases.

Squamous cell carcinoma warrants special discussion in parotid surgery. While primary SCC of the parotid gland is rare, metastatic cutaneous SCC is the most common malignant parotid gland tumor, particularly in countries with high sunlight exposure such as Australia.[75] The parotid gland contains approximately 15–20 lymph nodes within the parotid gland, mostly within the superficial lobe, and these are the first echelon nodes for an extensive area of the face and scalp anterior to a vertical line through the external auditory meatus.[76] These tumors are aggressive, with a propensity for extracapsular extension, neck nodal metastasis, and perineural spread of disease.[77] Hence, they most often require multi-modality treatment with surgery targeted to extent of disease (Fig. 16.30) and adjuvant therapy based on disease extent and the features of the surgical pathology report (Fig. 16.31).[76,78,79]

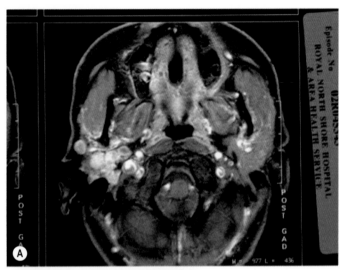

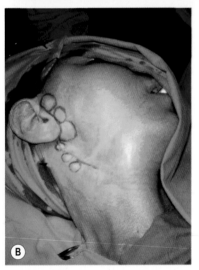

Fig. 16.27 (A) MRI of recurrent pleomorphic adenoma demonstrating multifocal disease through the superficial and deep lobes. **(B)** Extensive multifocal disease. Recurrent pleomorphic adenoma represents a difficult management problem for the head and neck surgeon. Pleomorphic adenoma recurrence is often multifocal as demonstrated in these images. Operation in a previously operated field places the facial nerve at significant risk during these procedures.

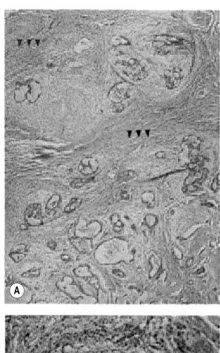

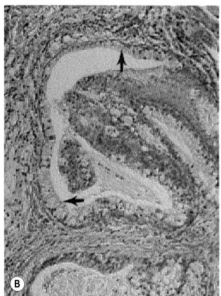

Fig. 16.28 Mucoepidermoid carcinoma. **(A)** High grade. **(B)** Low grade

Decision-making in salivary gland neoplasms

The management of salivary gland neoplasms is predominantly surgical. The decision to operate rather than observe most salivary gland neoplasms is based on four considerations. Firstly, the lack of certainty in differentiating benign from malignant pathology using preoperative FNA behests the surgeon to seek diagnostic certainty via surgical removal. Secondly, pleomorphic adenomas have a potential for malignant transformation that has already been discussed. Thirdly, the surgical procedure may become more difficult as the tumor increases in size, potentially increasing the risk to the facial nerve in parotid surgery. Finally, many patients have cosmetic concern with a salivary gland neoplasm that can only be reconciled with surgical excision.

Effective management of salivary gland malignancies requires an understanding of the pathologic considerations discussed above. Application of these principles enables clinicians to target appropriate therapy to individual patients based on tumor histology, grade, and stage. Division to high-grade and low-grade malignancy enables the surgeon to tailor their surgical intervention. Parotidectomy alone is adequate therapy for low-grade malignancies. With a preoperative diagnosis of a high-grade salivary gland malignancy, consideration should be given to elective neck dissection because of an increased risk of occult regional metastatic disease.[80] Obviously, the presence of clinical or radiological evidence of neck nodal disease necessitates therapeutic neck dissection.

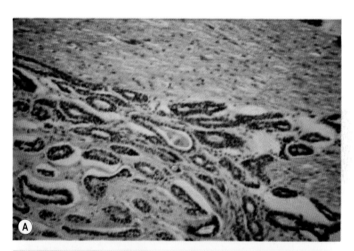

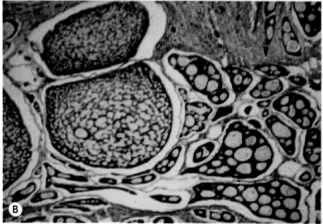

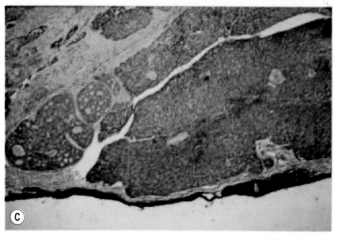

Fig. 16.29 Adenoid cystic carcinoma. **(A)** Tubular; **(B)** cribriform; **(C)** solid.

		NECK	
		Positive	**Negative**
PAROTID	**Positive**	Parotid + CND **PORT**: parotid + neck	Parotid + Staging Neck: • Ant 1°- I-III SND • Post 1°- II-V SND • Unknown 1°- CND **PORT**: parotid + neck (if SND +ve, otherwise don't include neck)
	Negative	CND **PORT**: parotid + neck	No evidence for SND ?? SNB ***Watch + wait***

Fig. 16.30 Management of the parotid and neck in metastatic squamous cell carcinoma. *(From D'Souza J, Clark J. Management of the neck in metastatic cutaneous squamous cell carcinoma of the head and neck.* Curr Opin Otolaryngol Head Neck Surg. *2011;19(2):99–105.)*

Furthermore, high-grade malignancies, advanced stage tumors, or those with local invasion as well as low-grade malignancies with positive surgical margins should be considered for postoperative radiation therapy.[81]

Surgical management of salivary gland neoplasms

Multiple surgical procedures have been described for managing tumors of the parotid gland. The classical approach to benign tumors has been a superficial parotidectomy, which extirpates the entire parotid gland superficial to the plane of the facial nerve (Fig. 16.32). With improved understanding of the biology of salivary gland disease, partial parotidectomy is more commonly performed currently. This involves identification of the facial nerve trunk and dissection tailored to enable removal of the tumor with a cuff of normal tissue. This often does not equate to a full superficial parotidectomy, reducing dissection of distal facial nerve branches and minimizing cosmetic deformity. For malignant tumors, a total conservative parotidectomy is recommended in which all parotid tissue is removed while sparing the facial nerve. The deep lobe is removed in piecemeal fashion between nerve branches. Finally, parotid tumors presenting with preoperative facial nerve palsy should undergo radical parotidectomy in which the entire parotid tissue is removed *en bloc* with facial nerve sacrifice. In these cases, preoperative Gadolinium-enhanced MRI is essential to determine the proximal extent of facial nerve involvement, which may be within the parotid gland or may extend through the stylomastoid foramen and up the fallopian canal of the temporal bone. In the latter case temporal bone surgery, mostly commonly lateral temporal bone resection, is indicated.

Management of submandibular gland neoplasms should take into consideration the greater risk of malignancy. Tumors either suspected or proven to be malignant should be removed along with the overlying fascia, as opposed to subfascial dissection that characterizes a submandibular gland excision for inflammatory disease or sialolithiasis. Furthermore, the same principles that guide elective neck dissection in parotid

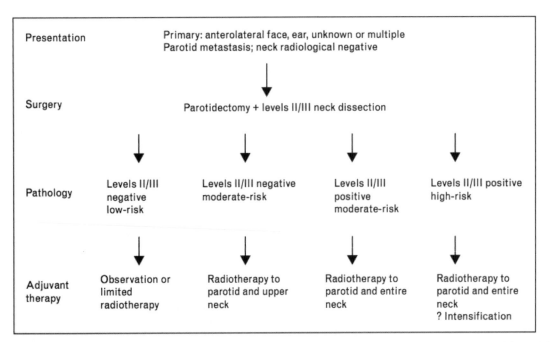

Fig. 16.31 Management algorithm for postoperative adjuvant therapy in metastatic SCC to the parotid gland. *(Adapted from D'Souza J, Clark J. Management of the neck in metastatic cutaneous squamous cell carcinoma of the head and neck.* Curr Opin Otolaryngol Head Neck Surg. *2011;19(2):99–105.)*

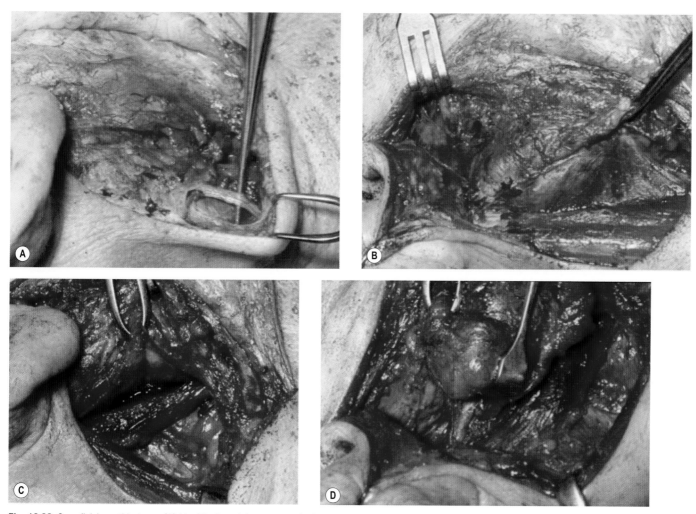

Fig. 16.32 Superficial parotidectomy. **(A)** Identification of the greater auricular nerve and preservation where possible. **(B)** Raising the parotid fascia off the sternomastoid muscle. **(C)** Identification of posterior belly of digastric, a useful landmark for the depth of the facial nerve. **(D)** Dissecting tumor off the main trunk of the facial nerve.

surgery hold true for the submandibular gland also. Sublingual and minor salivary gland tumors are removed transorally as a wide local excision.

Postoperative adjuvant treatment

The addition of radiotherapy in the postoperative period after resection of salivary gland malignancy is thought to improve locoregional disease control.[81] As already discussed, postoperative radiotherapy is indicated in patients with high grade histologic types, advanced stage disease, positive surgical margins, or local invasion including perineural spread or bone involvement. Primary radiotherapy may be considered for patients not fit for surgery. The role of chemotherapy has been limited. In contrast to mucosal sites of the head and neck, platinum-based chemotherapy has not been employed in combination with radiotherapy. However, a recent trial from the Trans-Tasman Radiation Oncology group (TROG) has completed recruitment to compare radiation alone with concurrent chemoradiotherapy for high-risk metastatic cutaneous SCC (TROG 05.01). The results of this trial have not yet been analyzed.

There is some enthusiasm for targeted therapies for selected salivary gland malignancies. Case reports have reported success in the use of Trastuzumab in the adjuvant setting for management of salivary ductal carcinoma, a cancer with an otherwise dismal outcome.[82,83] Similarly, targeted therapy for adenoid cystic carcinoma has also been reported with c-KIT tyrosine kinase inhibitors.[84,85] None of these would be considered standard practice at this time, however.

Conclusions

Head and neck tumors represent a diverse group of diseases that require the treating physician to have an in depth understanding of in order to provide evidence-based care plans. The treatment of these cancers has evolved significantly in recent years with technological advances and large-scale clinical trials. Ablative treatment of head and neck cancer has significant functional and cosmetic consequences for the patient and the post-treatment defects represent some of the most challenging scenarios that the reconstructive surgeon will encounter.

⊕ Access the complete reference list online at   **http://www.expertconsult.com**

2. Gillison ML. Human papillomavirus-associated head and neck cancer is a distinct epidemiologic, clinical, and molecular entity. *Semin Oncol.* 2004;31(6):744–754.

18. Bernier J, Domenge C, Ozsahin M, et al. Postoperative irradiation with or without concomitant chemotherapy for locally advanced head and neck cancer. *N Engl J Med.* 2004;350(19):1945–1952.

19. Cooper JS, Pajak TF, Forastiere AA, et al. Postoperative concurrent radiotherapy and chemotherapy for high-risk squamous-cell carcinoma of the head and neck. *N Engl J Med.* 2004;350(19): 1937–1944.

21. Blanchard P, Baujat B, Holostenco V, et al. Meta-analysis of chemotherapy in head and neck cancer (MACH-NC): a comprehensive analysis by tumour site. *Radiother Oncol.* 2011;100(1): 33–40.

24. Weiss MH, Harrison LB, Isaacs RS. Use of decision analysis in planning a management strategy for the stage N0 neck. *Arch Otolaryngol Head Neck Surg.* 1994;120(7):699–702.

29. Ang KK, Harris J, Wheeler R, et al. Human papillomavirus and survival of patients with oropharyngeal cancer. *N Engl J Med.* 2010;363(1):24–35.

46. Induction chemotherapy plus radiation compared with surgery plus radiation in patients with advanced laryngeal cancer. The Department of Veterans Affairs Laryngeal Cancer Study Group. *N Engl J Med.* 1991;324(24):1685–1690.

47. Forastiere AA, Goepfert H, Maor M, et al. Concurrent chemotherapy and radiotherapy for organ preservation in advanced laryngeal cancer. *N Engl J Med.* 2003;349(22):2091–2098.

53. Shah JP. Patterns of cervical lymph node metastasis from squamous carcinomas of the upper aerodigestive tract. *Am J Surg.* 1990;160(4): 405–409.

81. Armstrong JG, Harrison LB, Spiro RH, et al. Malignant tumors of major salivary gland origin. A matched-pair analysis of the role of combined surgery and postoperative radiotherapy. *Arch Otolaryngol Head Neck Surg.* 1990;116(3):290–293.

17

Local flaps for facial coverage

David W. Mathes

Access video and video lecture content for this chapter online at expertconsult.com

SYNOPSIS

- After careful and complete evaluation of the defect, the surgeon should formulate a reconstructive plan that is tailored to the patient's needs
- Always assess the availability and laxity of local tissue
- Keep the reconstruction as simple as possible
- Always consider the next flap that might need to be performed (do not burn bridges)
- Local tissue is far superior to free flap reconstruction of the face as it provides like tissue and should be the first thought when reconstructing facial defects
- Choose a flap that will both restore function and achieve a good cosmetic result

Introduction

The face is the most common location for neoplasms of skin, and the incidence of these tumors is increasing due the aging of our population and increasing exposure to ultraviolet light. These patients often present to the plastic surgeon for reconstruction more than once for treatment. The face is a very cosmetically sensitive location on the body, and the reconstruction can be challenging for the surgeon as we seek to preserve form and function. The reconstruction must begin with careful evaluation of the defect. The surgeon must consider the location, regional skin laxity, size, shape, and depth of the defect.

The principles of reconstruction are the same as in other areas of the body. After careful and complete evaluation of the defect, the surgeon should formulate a reconstructive plan that is tailored to the patient's needs. This planning should, if possible, include several reconstructive options. A simple reconstructive plan can often yield superior results to the more complex options. The viable options for coverage are dictated primarily by the vascular supply in the area. The excision of a malignant lesion must be based on current

guidelines and should not be designed to fit in with the chosen method of reconstruction. In situations where there is concern as to the pathology, a temporary dressing is applied until a definitive diagnosis becomes available. The best reconstructive plans include consideration of secondary procedures and the future needs of the patient.

The design of flaps on the face is based on the fundamental concepts in plastic surgery of advancement, transposition, and rotation. However, the reconstructive design should not be limited by these basic concepts. Often it is necessary to modify the flap into an island flap. When this technique is combined with appropriate pedicle dissection, it yields a mobile flap that is relatively free of tension and reduces the incidence of congestion of the flap. In those cases where the defect is beyond your reconstructive abilities, the use of a full-thickness skin graft is acceptable provided the skin color and texture match. Once healing is complete, a more satisfactory resection and a well-designed local flap reconstruction can be performed. The other technique that can be employed at the time of skin graft placement is the use of tissue expansion. This technique can provide the ideal skin cover and allow for the transfer of like tissue to close large defects. Alternatively, the surgeon can take advantage of the fact that the skin will undergo stress relaxation (skin elongates over time) when a closure is tight or a flap appears smaller than the defect. There is a limit to the utilization of stress relaxation in facial reconstruction dictated by the tissue's blood supply.

The success of flap reconstruction of the face is dependent on making the correct defect analysis. Understanding what is missing allows for the surgeon to design a reconstruction that addresses all of the layers. After selection of the flap, the next step is to tailor the design to hide the incisions in the borders of well-known aesthetic units. Local tissue is far superior to free flap reconstruction of the face as it provides like tissue and should be the first thought when reconstructing facial defects. Only when the defect is too large or complex should the surgeon turn to more distant flap for reconstruction.

Forehead and scalp

The scalp often requires flap closure, except for very small lesions, due to its relative inelasticity. Most often, single or paired large rotation flaps are reliable local workhorses. Numerous variations exist, such as Juri flaps and Orticochea flaps, but the principles of scalp rotation flaps are the same. These flaps are best elevated in the subgaleal plane to preserve vascularity.[1-3] Care must be taken if subcutaneous undermining is performed to avoid damaging the blood supply and causing alopecia by traumatizing hair follicles. The importance of designing large (often in a 9:1 ratio) flaps cannot be overemphasized. Unlike other body areas, the scalp is inelastic. For this reason, small flaps have limited success for anything other than a small defect. Galeal scoring expands scalp flaps, but should be performed in no smaller than 1-cm intervals, to avoid disrupting the blood supply.

The forehead generally offers a limited amount of spare skin. In addition, asymmetrical movement on one side of the forehead can raise the position of the patient's brow, giving them a quizzical appearance. In reconstructing the central forehead, the options are limited. The best local flaps move skin on the horizontal access and thereby avoid raising the brow.

Bilateral horizontal advancement flaps can be designed to take advantage of the naturally occurring rhytids (Fig. 17.1). The flaps should be designed equal to size of the defect. Small Burrow's triangles can be added to allow reduce the occurrence of dog-ears.

Hatchet flap reconstruction can also be designed for reconstruction of the forehead. It generally requires the use of two flaps.[4] One flap should be based superiorly and one inferiorly (Fig. 17.2). These flaps are then elevated and transposed into the defect, again, avoiding the superior elevation of the brow.

The use of patterned flaps should be avoided in the forehead; one exception is the use of a rhomboid flap to reconstruct defects in the temple (Fig. 17.3). Provided that the flap does not shift the hairline significantly, this can provide an excellent result with the scars hidden in the rhytids of the temporal area.

The optimal treatment of large forehead defects is through the application of tissue expansion (Fig. 17.4). Once the forehead skin is expanded the reconstruction can be achieved with the use of a simple advancement of the skin. The critical part of this surgery is the planning of the type of tissue expander used and the need for overexpansion to ensure tension-free closure.

Eyebrow reconstruction

The eyebrow is complex and reconstruction is difficult; this is because hair grows in a fixed pattern that is not uniform and is difficult to reproduce exactly. A scalp island flap based on the temporal blood supply can be used, but the hair must be trimmed. The hair is often too dense and does not grow in the correct manner. An alternative technique is micro-hair transplants with frequent trimming. These, unfortunately, rarely produce the unique anatomy and the density of the eyebrow hair. Eyebrow flaps must be designed with care to maintain the correct anatomic relationship. Unfortunately, there may be a shortage of material available, and it may not be possible to

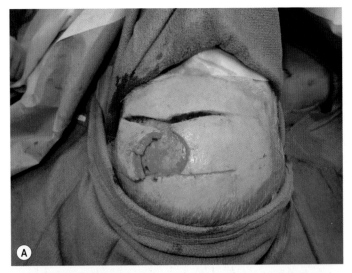

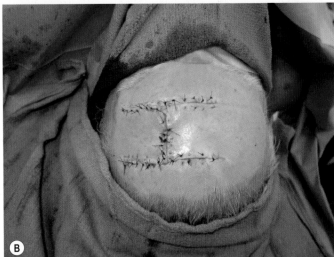

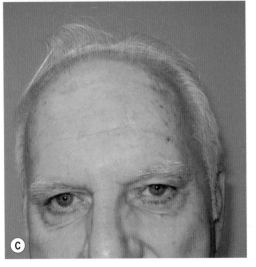

Fig. 17.1 (A–C) Bilateral horizontal advancement flaps can be designed to take advantage of the naturally occurring rhytids.

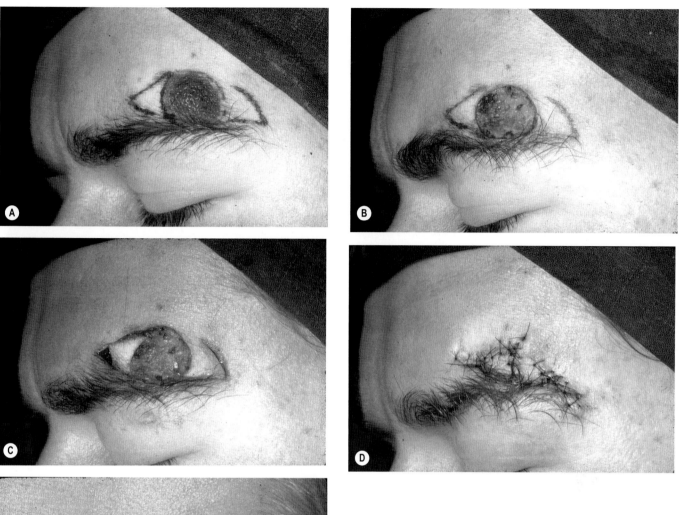

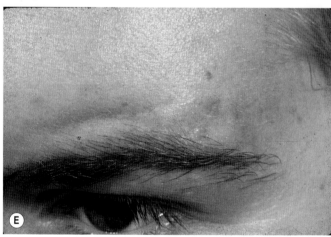

Fig. 17.2 Nevus of left supraorbital area involving eyebrow – hatchet flap reconstruction. **(A)** The planned excision has been drawn out together with bilateral hatchet flaps. **(B)** Nevus has been excised. It can be seen that the flap pedicles are superior for the lateral flap and inferior for the medial flap. **(C)** The flaps are elevated. **(D)** The flaps are transposed, and the secondary defect is closed. **(E)** Satisfactory end result with the eyebrow in a good position.

have the eyebrow in the exact desired anatomical position or size.

Eyelids

Partial upper lid defects

The reconstruction of the upper lid is critical as it is vital for the protection of the eye. Failure to adequately reconstruct the upper lid, especially in the vertical component, may cause conjunctivitis and/or impaired vision. Without an adequate upper lid, the eye will be at risk for exposure, scarring, and loss of vision. Often, some of the same techniques used in reconstruction of the lower eyelid are used in upper eyelid surgery.

An advancement flap can be designed with an incision made horizontally from the lateral canthus (Fig. 17.5). This is followed by the division of the superior limb of the lateral canthal ligament and an incision in the conjunctiva of the superior fornix. The addition of a Z-plasty can be performed

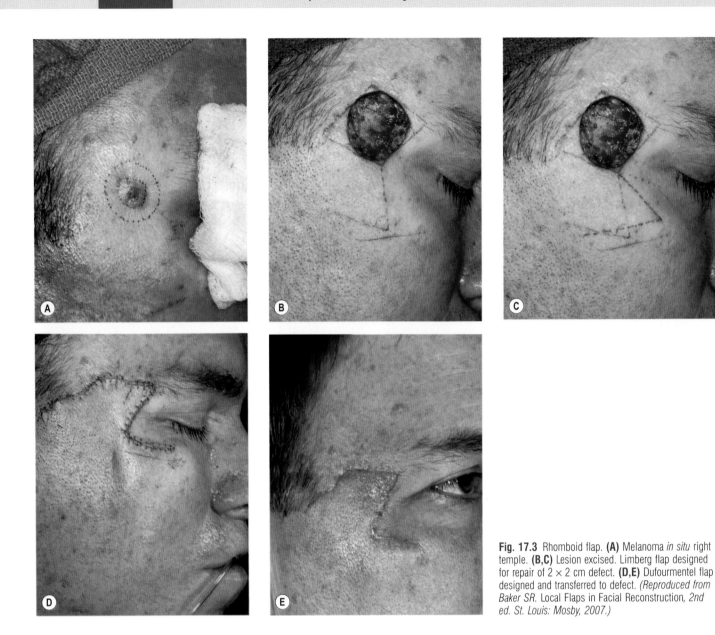

Fig. 17.3 Rhomboid flap. **(A)** Melanoma *in situ* right temple. **(B,C)** Lesion excised. Limberg flap designed for repair of 2 × 2 cm defect. **(D,E)** Dufourmentel flap designed and transferred to defect. *(Reproduced from Baker SR.* Local Flaps in Facial Reconstruction, *2nd ed. St. Louis: Mosby, 2007.)*

to deal with the dog-ear. Best results depend on accurate suturing and repositioning of the gray line, the lash line, and the rim conjunctival junction.

Defect of the upper lid can also be addressed by using a lid-switch flap (Abbé flap) (Fig. 17.6). In much the same way one would use an Abbé flap to reconstruct the lip, this can be applied to the upper eyelid with the flap based on the marginal vessels in the lid, and a full-thickness V flap (the defect of which should close easily) can be taken from the lower lid, swung up, and sutured into the upper lid in layers.

The lower lid defect closure requires the edges to come together directly without tension. If this does not occur, a small lateral canthal incision is made, and the inferior limb of the lateral canthal tendon is divided. If this is not sufficient, a long transverse incision from the canthus out to the temporal skin (incorporating a Z-plasty if necessary) will suffice to obtain tensionless closure. It is important that a preoperative examination of the mobility of the lower lid is carefully assessed. If necessary (e.g., in children), the conjunctiva is

anesthetized with drops or, rarely, general anesthesia. In adults, infraorbital nerve blocks can be used

Large and total upper lid defects

For larger defects, the lower lid is used and the significant lower lid defect is reconstructed. A large full-thickness portion of lower lid is moved up on its marginal vascular pedicle. A partial lower lid reconstruction is necessary. As the portion of lower lid is turned up, the full-thickness of the cheek is advanced medially and grafted with nasal septum on its inner surface, as required (Fig. 17.7).

To reconstruct the upper lid, the whole lower lid can be turned up. The lower lid reconstruction is based on an advancement cheek flap lined with nasal septum, cartilage, and mucosa as above. These pedicled lid reconstructions are left attached for 2–3 weeks, depending on the vascularity of the upturned flaps. Once the upper lid reconstruction is in position, small adjustments are often necessary. Rearrangements

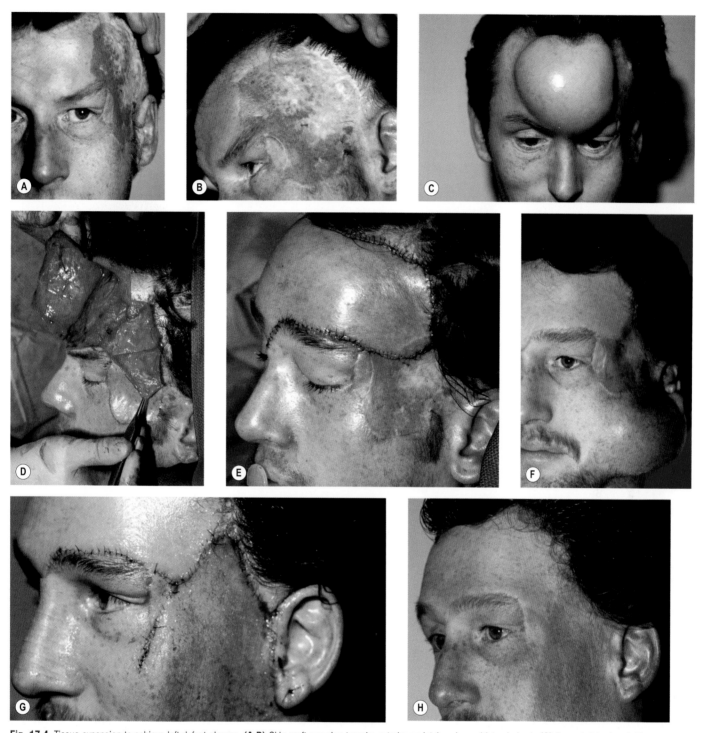

Fig. 17.4 Tissue expansion to achieve left defect closure. **(A,B)** Skin graft covering temple, anterior parietal scalp, and lateral cheek. **(C)** Expanded forehead skin. **(D)** Following tissue expansion, expanded forehead skin used to cover defect created by partial resection of skin graft. **(E)** Expansion provided sufficient skin to cover temple. **(F)** Tissue expander beneath lateral cheek skin. **(G)** Six days following removal of skin graft from cheek and reconstruction with expanded cheek advancement flap. **(H)** Six months postoperative. *(Reproduced from Baker SR. Local Flaps in Facial Reconstruction 2nd ed. St. Louis: Mosby, 2007.)*

are usually required for the lateral canthus and occasionally to the edge of the lower lid or to provide adjustment of lower lid height. With meticulous technique, a good cosmetic and functional result can be obtained.

When a healthy eye is present, a lid can be prefabricated on the forehead. A pocket the size of the lid is designed and a mucosal graft is inserted. When this reconstruction is complete, it is brought down on a vascular pedicle to replace the lid. The pedicle is divided at 3 weeks. This protects the eye, but movement is minimal, unless there is some remaining orbicularis which can be used immediately or at a later date (Fig. 17.8).

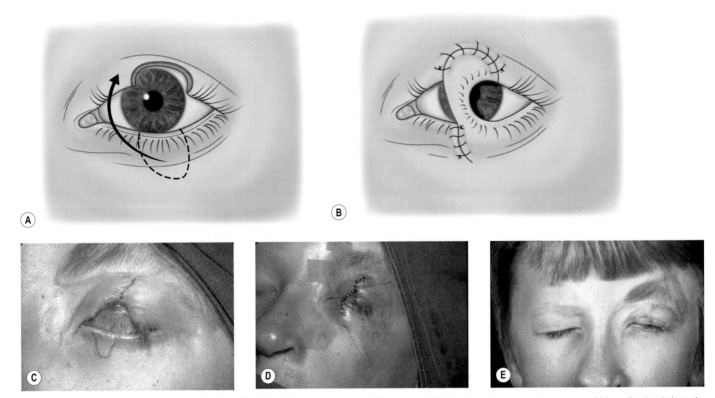

Fig. 17.5 Coloboma of the upper eyelid – Abbé flap. **(A–C)** The defect can be seen, and the planned Abbé flap from the lower to the upper eyelid is outlined and shown in diagrammatic form. **(D)** The flap is in position. **(E)** The patient can close his eyelid satisfactorily.

Partial lower lid defects

Lesions are frequently resected in a V fashion and the resulting defect can be carefully closed in layers. If this is not possible, the lower portion of the lateral canthal ligament is divided through a small lateral canthal incision. This allows the lid to move medially, and closure can be obtained without tension. If there is too much tension, the incision and dissection are taken further laterally on the cheek. Closure is then obtained without difficulty. The lateral incision is closed with a Z-plasty in order to reduce any skin tension.

An extensive defect requires that a portion of nasal septum, with mucosa attached on one side, be inserted with the mucosa toward the globe in order to form an internal lamella. A portion of ear cartilage, with perichondrium in place of the mucosa, can also be used for support. Mucosalization of the inner surface occurs fairly rapidly. A cheek rotation flap of the required size then provides external cover. If the cheek skin is insufficient, prior expansion of the lateral cheek skin should be performed, or a narrow midline forehead flap can be used. The latter has the advantage of being a little more rigid. This, however, requires accurate sizing in all dimensions; also there will be a forehead scar.

Total lower lid defects

These result from tumor resection, from trauma, or when the lower lid is used to reconstruct the upper lid (Fig. 17.7). Reconstruction of the total lower lid is primarily performed

for cosmesis. The lower lid can be reconstructed with a cheek rotation flap which is lined with oral mucosa or more satisfactorily using nasal septal cartilage with its perichondrium intact as shown in Fig. 17.7. In other instances, a forehead flap may be necessary. This has the disadvantage of bulk, which can result in poor aesthetics. With time, however, the latter can be improved upon by debulking. With experience, there is no longer so much concern about ischemia resulting in skin or lid loss.

Lid-switch flap (Abbé flap)

By using the same principles as the Abbé flap on the lip, a similar reconstruction can be used for defects of the upper lid (Fig. 17.7A–D) There are marginal vessels in the lid, and a full-thickness V flap (the defect of which should close easily) can be taken from the lower lid, swung up, and sutured into the upper lid in layers. The lower lid defect closure requires the edges to come together directly without tension. If this does not occur, a small lateral canthal incision is made, and the inferior limb of the lateral canthal tendon is divided. If this is not sufficient, a long transverse incision from the canthus out to the temporal skin (incorporating a Z-plasty if necessary) will suffice to obtain tensionless closure. It is important that a preoperative examination of the mobility of the lower lid is carefully assessed. If necessary (e.g., in children), the conjunctiva is anesthetized with drops or, rarely, general anesthesia. In adults, infraorbital nerve blocks can be used.

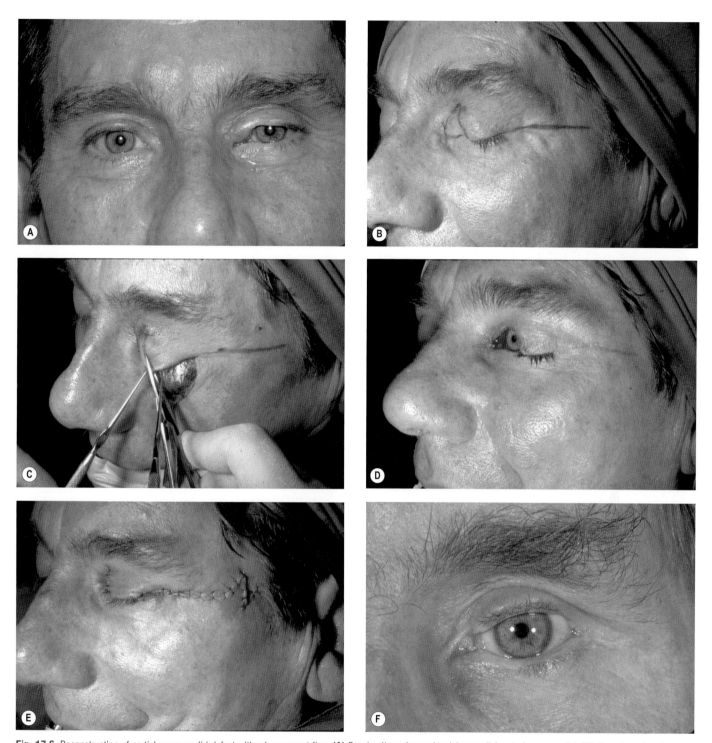

Fig. 17.6 Reconstruction of partial upper eyelid defect with advancement flap. **(A)** Basal cell carcinoma involving medial end of upper eyelid. **(B)** Operative plan of excision and rotation and advancement of the upper lid. **(C)** Excision of upper lid basal cell carcinoma. Note spoon to protect eye and the use of sharp pointed scissors to resect the lid. **(D)** Defect after excision of medial portion of the upper eyelid. **(E)** Lateral canthotomy performed superiorly. The lid is advanced with lateral Z-plasty in the temporal region. **(F)** End result.

Medial canthal defects

Generally, forehead flaps provide a reliable and reasonably good method of reconstruction. These flaps must be lined with mucosa; however, additional support is not required because of the inherent flap rigidity. It is very important to place a flap of sufficient size into the medial canthal area. Failure to do this results in troublesome epiphora.

Nasal reconstruction

The nose is a complex structure comprised of three critical layers (skin, bone, and cartilage) and lined by mucoperichondrium. The outer layer of skin has different properties depending on location. The skin of the dorsum and the sidewalls are thin and smooth while the skin of the tip and ala is thick and stiff and contains sebaceous glands. The nasal bones and cartilage provide the structural integrity and projection of the nose. Finally, the lining of the nose consists of specialized tissue that is thin and well vascularized with dry, hair-bearing skin at the vestibule and moist mucosa in the nasal vault. The surgeon must identify and define the defect in terms of size, depth, orientation, and location on the nose. The

reconstruction is based on the analysis of what is missing and the plan to provide suitable replacement of these tissues to restore the nose to its premorbid condition.

The outer skin of the nose has been divided into aesthetic subunits based on adjacent areas of characteristic skin quality, contour, and border outline. These subunits are the dorsum, tip, columella, and paired sidewalls, alae, and soft triangles.[5]

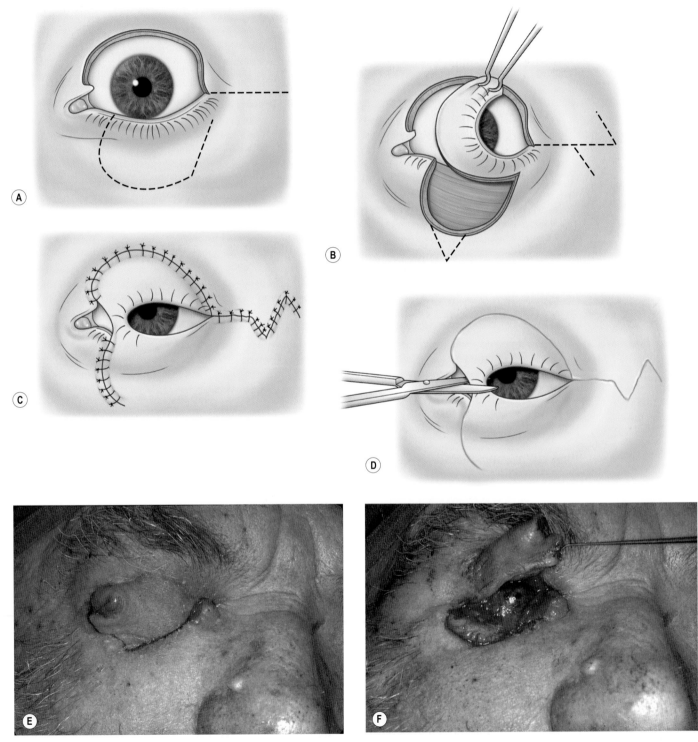

Fig. 17.7 (A–D) Reconstruction of total upper eyelid defect with lower lid transposition. **(E)** Preoperative markings indicate the upper eyelid area to be resected. **(F)** The total upper eyelid is resected; the lower eyelid will be rotated up to reconstruct the upper eyelid with use of a medial pedicle.

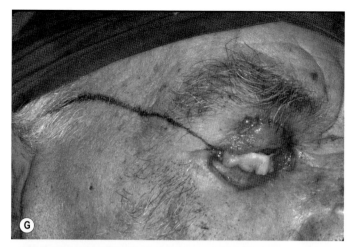

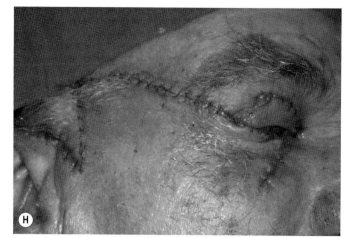

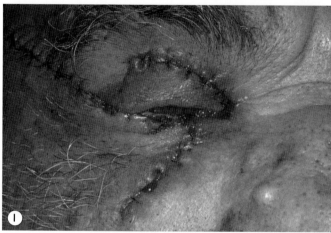

Fig. 17.7, cont'd (G) The medial pedicle is divided, and the medial end of the lower lid is inset into the defect of the medial side of the upper lid. **(H)** A nasal septal chondromucosal graft is placed in position, and the cartilage is scored to make it bend as favorably as possible. A lateral cheek rotation flap is performed. Note the lateral Z-plasty to give as much medial movement as possible. This will give a good end result. **(I)** A nasal septal chondromucosal graft is placed in position, and the cartilage is scored to make it bend as favorably as possible.

According to the subunit principle, if greater than 50% of a subunit is involved, excision of the entire subunit before reconstruction is recommended. However, this is not universally applicable, as enlarging small defects may result in increased use of the forehead flap for defects where smaller local flaps may suffice. The subunit principle is a tool, not a rigid rule, and should be modified to fit the individual needs of the patient.[6,7]

Flap section in nasal reconstruction is based on defect location and orientation (Table 17.1), with the nose divided transversely into three zones (proximal third, middle third, and distal third). Many of these reconstructions can be performed under local anesthesia in an outpatient setting. However, once defects exceed the 2 cm in size, it can become difficult to rotate local tissue.

Proximal third

Defects most often encountered in the proximal third of the nose can be centrally located on the dorsum or radix area or laterally on the upper sidewalls. These defects often have exposed periosteum or bone but rarely require bone reconstruction.

Defects in the upper third are often reconstructed with a glabella flap (Fig. 17.9) transposed from the midforehead or glabella region.[8] If the lesion is centrally located, it can often be reconstructed with a dorsal nasal advancement flap (Fig.

17.9). Lateral defects that are horizontally orientated can be reconstructed with the glabellar flap, whereas those defects that are vertically orientated can be treated with a V–Y flap from the dorsum of the nose (Fig. 17.10). Larger combined defects are best treated with a forehead flap but can be amenable to an extended glabella flap or modified glabella-bilobed flap (Fig. 17.11).[9]

Medial third

The middle third of the nose is divided into central and lateral zones, and includes the nasal bones and upper lateral cartilages. The medial third is an excellent place to apply the dorsal nasal flap. The lateral defects encountered in the medial third can be closed with a V–Y flap, nasolabial flap, bilobed flap, or a dorsal nasal flap. A very useful flap is a V–Y flap based on perforators from the facial artery (Fig. 17.12).[10,11] Larger defects will most often require a forehead flap.

Distal third

The distal third zone of the nose is the most common location for nasal defects after cancer excision. Alar defects can be reconstructed with a staged nasolabial flap (Fig. 17.13). However, for alar defects sparing the rim, a V–Y advancement flap may used.[12] Any remaining alar rim will need a cartilage graft for support to prevent collapse of the rim. Small alar rim

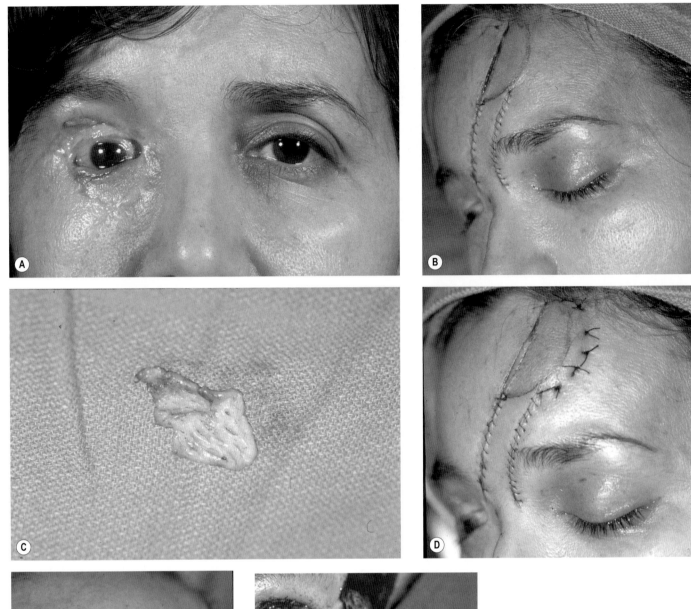

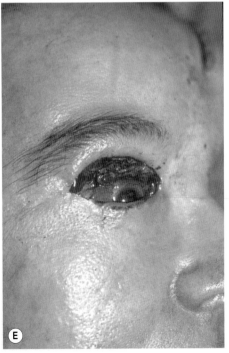

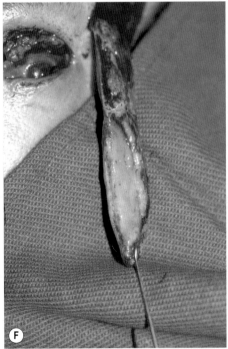

Fig. 17.8 Total reconstruction of upper eyelid by a prefabricated composite forehead flap. **(A)** The preoperative appearance with no upper eyelid whatsoever. The lower eyelid is intact. **(B)** An upper eyelid is delayed vertically on the forehead with a bucket being designed under the forehead skin and subcutaneous tissue. **(C)** A mucosal graft is harvested, and holes are made in it to stretch it. **(D)** The mucosal graft is placed, mucosal side down, into the pocket in the center of the forehead with a small pack. Sutures are holding the mucosa in position. **(E)** Upper eyelid is released as much as possible. **(F)** Upper eyelid reconstruction being brought down to reconstruct the upper lid. Note the mucosa on the undersurface of the flap.

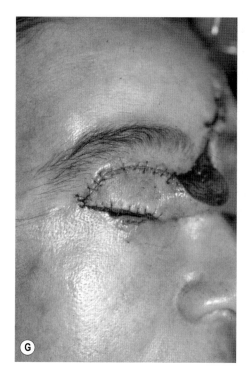

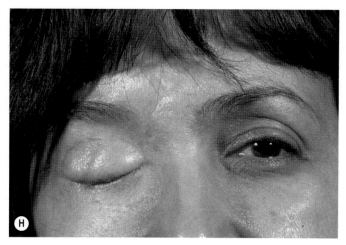

Fig. 17.8, cont'd (G) The lid is inset. **(H)** The lid reconstruction is complete and ready for levator muscle repositioning.

Table 17.1 Flap selection for nasal reconstruction with local and regional flaps based on location	
Proximal third of the nose	
Central	Horizontal defect: dorsal nasal flap Round defect: glabella flap Vertical defect: V-Y flap
Lateral	
	Horizontal defect: glabella flap, first choice; dorsal nasal flap, second choice Vertical defect: V-Y flap Combined defect: gorehead flap
Middle third of the nose	
Central	Horizontal and round defect: dorsal nasal flap Vertical defect: V-Y flap
Lateral	Horizontal defect: dorsal nasal flap Vertical defect: V-Y flap, first choice; nasolabial flap second choice Combined defect: forehead flap
Distal third of the nose	
	Alar defect: nasolabial flap, first choice; V-Y flap, second choice Domal-alar groove defect — nasolabial flap, first choice; V-Y flap, second choice Dome defect: bilobed flap Central tip defect — bilobed flap Columella defect: composite graft, skin graft, ascending helical free flap Nasal sill defect: nasolabial flap Combined defect forehead flap, first choice; nasolabial or extended V-Y flap, second choice

defects (up to 8 mm) can be reconstructed with a composite graft of skin and cartilage from the root of the ear helix. If the defect is full-thickness, then lining can be provided by turnover flaps or skin graft, cartilage from the nasal septum or ear concha (placed along the alar edge), and skin from nasolabial flap or forehead flap.

Defects located in the domal-alar groove can be reconstructed with a nasolabial flap but, more recently, these defects are often reconstructed with the V–Y flap advanced laterally to cover the defect in a single stage. Those defects confined to the dome of the nose are usually best reconstructed with a forehead flap. Alternative options include the use of the dorsal nasal flap or the use of a bilobed flap.[13,14] Cartilage tip grafts may need to be placed if there is deficient or weakened cartilage. Lining can be reconstructed with a mucoperichondrial flap or full-thickness skin graft (FTSG).

If the defect involves only the columella and is small then a composite graft from the antihelix of the ear can be used. If no cartilage is deficient and there is intact periosteum, an FTSG may be placed. If the columella defect is large or encompasses the entire columella, a multi-staged nasolabial flap may be required.[15] When a more complex reconstruction is required (e.g., bilateral alar rims and columella), the total central forehead flap should be used (Fig. 17.14). The best approach to the more complex lower third defect is to use the three-stage technique described by Menick (Fig. 17.15).[16]

The key to complete survival of the flap is the position of its base; this should be at the medial canthal level or below. In this way, the vascular anastomosis on the side of the nose between the cheek and forehead vessels can provide a satisfactory flap to close the defect. With the base correctly positioned, the midline flap will comfortably reconstruct the nasal tip and the columella without tension. The forehead is closed

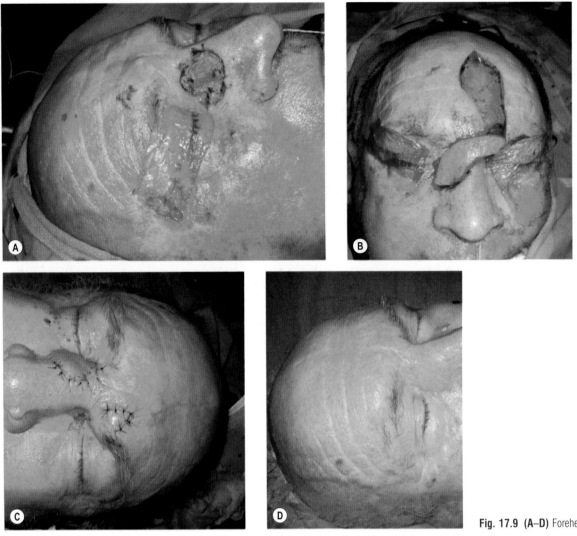

Fig. 17.9 (A–D) Forehead flap for Medial canthus.

directly, but if there is tension in the area just anterior to the hairline, it should be left to close spontaneously. The scar resulting from this rarely, if ever, requires any reconstruction The pedicle is divided at 3 weeks, depending on the inset, and the nasal tip is fashioned. Apart from thinning, it is unusual

to require further adjustments. If there is any concern about vascularity, the flap base is delayed.

If a total nasal reconstruction is required, a larger amount of forehead skin is harvested in the transverse dimension, but again, the base should be positioned at or below the medial

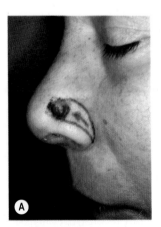
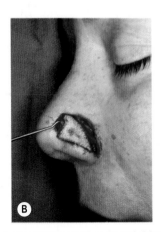
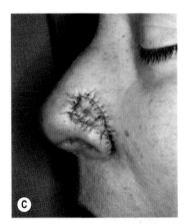
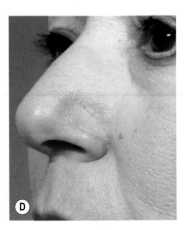

Fig. 17.10 (A–D) This defect is closed with a V-Y flap based on the underlying Nasalis.

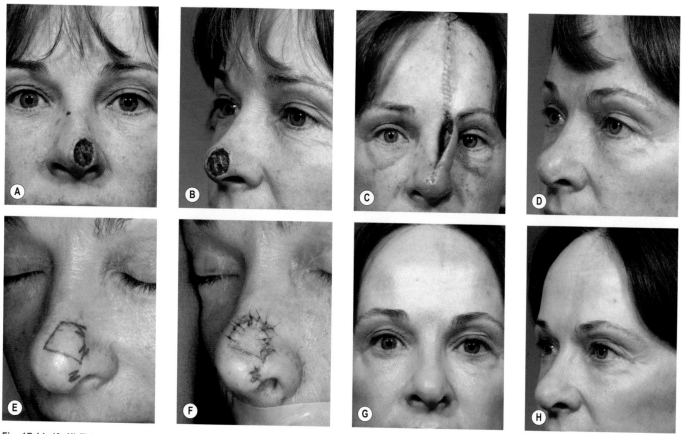

Fig. 17.11 (A–H) This lesion on the nasal dorsum is reconstructed with a forehead flap.

canthal ligament. The septal mucosa is used for lining. For closure of the midline forehead defect, the skin can frequently be mobilized extensively and advanced. If there is concern, a tissue expander can be inserted to expand the whole forehead.

This gives a large amount of skin with a good blood supply. If nasal support is needed, a cranial bone graft from the outer table of the skull is taken from an area where the curvature is similar to that required for the defect reconstruction, and the shape can be chosen to some extent. This may be done at the same time as secure screw stabilization of the bone graft in

the forehead/nose junction. It may be safer to delay grafting to the time of flap division or to a third procedure. Noses may be prefabricated elsewhere (e.g., on the forearm using a radial flap) and subsequently transferred by microvascular techniques.

Cheek

The cheek is the largest aesthetic subunit of the face. The cheek is broad and has a smooth convex contour that makes

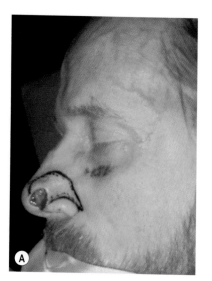

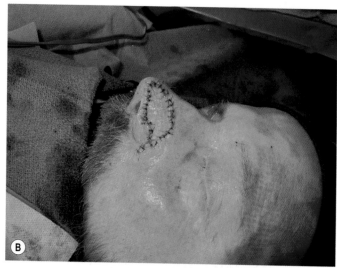

Fig. 17.12 (A,B) V–Y flap from the dorsum of the nose.

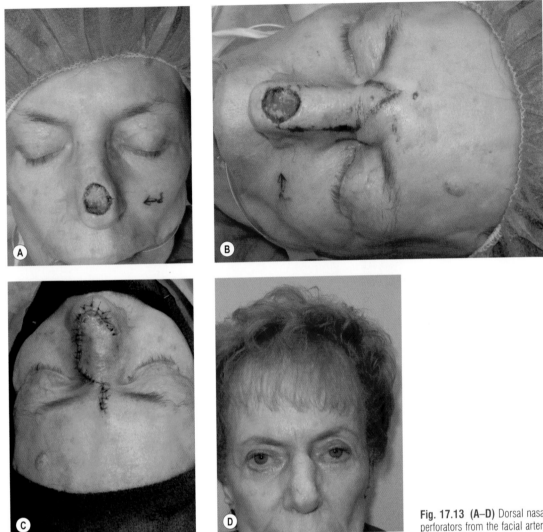

Fig. 17.13 (A–D) Dorsal nasal flap. This is a V-Y flap based on perforators from the facial artery system.

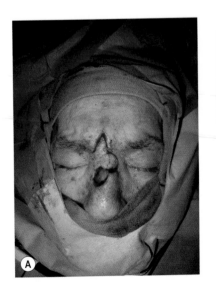
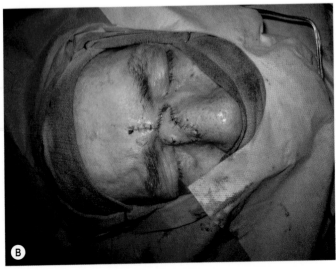

Fig. 17.14 (A,B) Modified glabellar-bilobed flap.

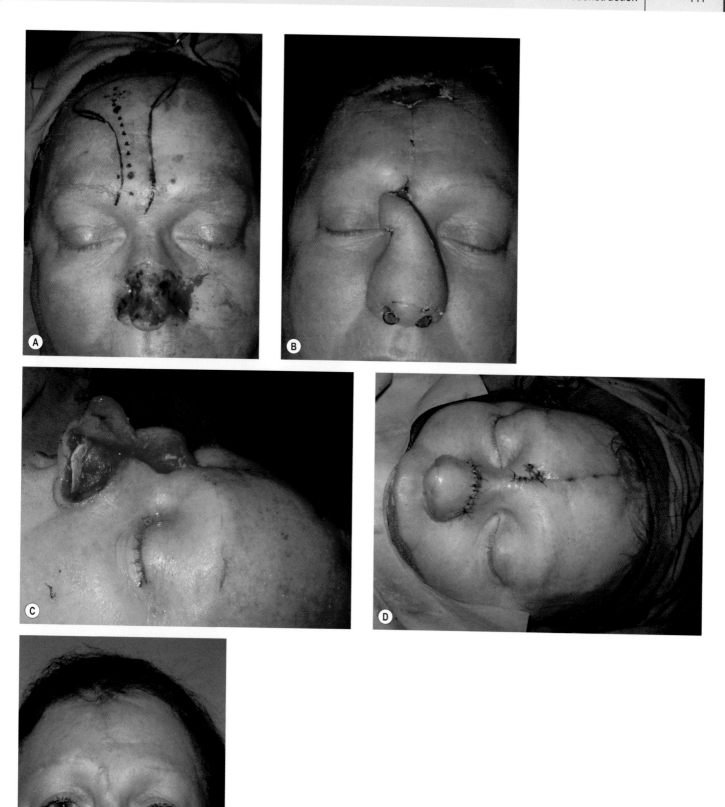

Fig. 17.15 (A–E) Three stage technique described by Menick.

it difficult to hide incisions in this region. For this reason, it is important to limit the use of geometric flaps such as bilobed or rhomboid flaps on the cheek. However, when reconstructing the cheek, the surgeon must consider the effect on the adjacent structures such as the lower eyelid, nasal ala, and the lip. The boundaries of the cheek include the infraorbital rim and zygomatic arch, superiorly, the nasofacial junction, nasolabial fold, and labiomandibular crease, medially, the border of the mandible, inferiorly, and the preauricular crease, laterally. Whenever possible, the incisions of the flap used should be placed in these boundaries to minimize the visibility of the scars.[17] There are four main subdivisions of the lateral cheek. These include the medial, zygomatic, buccal, and lateral units. Each of these areas has unique characteristics that the surgeon must account for while planning the reconstruction. The whole range of flaps can be used (Table 17.2) – rotation, advancement, transposition, and island type – with many variations required and usually available for each type of reconstruction.[18]

Rotation and advancement flaps for cheek closure

The cheek area is large and, therefore, rotation flaps can be designed to close the skin defect (Fig. 17.16). The design of rotation can be calculated by placing one end of a thread on the angle apex and the other at the edge of the defect. By rotating the outer end of the flap on the skin, the required circumference can be marked. Often, flap closure of the cheek is best achieved with a combination of rotation and advancement. This is especially true in the medial cheek subunit. The incisions for these flaps should be placed in the borders of the aesthetic subunits (Video 17.2 ▶).

The defects that are encountered in the medial subunit can be closed with a large anteriorly based cheek flap. The incisions of this flap extend laterally along the zygomatic arch, up into the temple and then inferiorly in the preauricular skin fold and can be extended into the neck when more skin is needed. The soft tissues are raised in the subcutaneous plane and rotated anteriorly to close the defect.

Another option for a large defect in the medial subunit includes a posteriorly based cheek flap. The incision is carried along the nasolabial fold and then down into the cervical skin (if necessary). The skin is then rotated superiorly to fill the defect and the standing cone deformity is created over the zygomatic arch is excised (Fig. 17.17). If the defect is located laterally then a flap can be designed that recruits skin from anterior and inferior to the defect. The tissue is rotated superiorly and an anterior standing cone deformity is then excised.

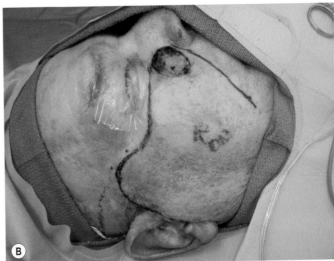

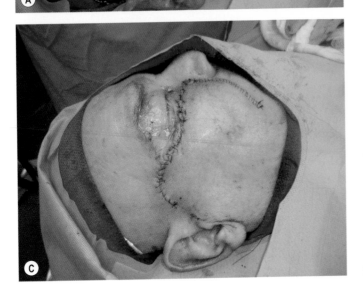

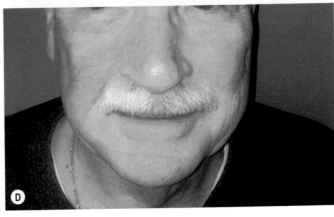

Fig. 17.16 (A–D) Cheek rotation flap.

Table 17.2 Flap considerations based on size and location of cheek defect

Location	Size of defect	Reconstructive choice
Lateral		
	Small	Primary closure
	Medium	Cheek advancement
	Large	Cervicofacial rotation flap
Zygomatic		
	Small	Primary closure
	Medium	Transposition flap
	Large	Cervicofacial rotation flap/large bilobed flap
Medial		
	Small	Primary Closure/V–Y island advancement flap
	Medium	V–Y island advancement flap/cheek advancement flap
	Large	Cervicofacial rotation flap (anterior/posterior based)
Buccal	Small	Primary closure
	Medium	Primary closure/transposition flap
	Large	Cervicofacial rotation flap/large bi-lobe flap

These flaps should be suspended to the underlying periosteum with suture support of 4-0 or 3-0 polyglycolic suture at multiple sites along the flap. This is especially true in those medial defects and this technique will minimize the chance of ectropion of the lower lid or distortion of the nose or lip.

V–Y island advancement flap

The V–Y island advancement flap can be used in cheek reconstruction.[19] The best places to design this flap are the nasolabial and perialar area. The V–Y flap can be modified with a curvilinear incision and this provides some element of rotation when the flap is advanced into place (Fig. 17.18). The donor site is then closed, primarily creating base of the Y. The V–Y island advancement flap requires preservation of at least one third of the subcutaneous tissue beneath the skin. However, depending on the vascular anatomy, this can also be harvested as a perforator flap. The closure of the Y limb pushes the flap into the defect. There is a higher incidence of pin cushioning of the flap in the early postoperative period that resolves over time.

Transposition

A transposition flap is elevated from a nearby area with excess laxity and moved to close a defect while the base of the flap remains intact. These flaps may be used for defects in the buccal and lateral subunits; however, the patterns of these flaps can create challenges during reconstruction of cheek defects. These flaps are based on geometric patterns such as the rhomboid flap. The lesion is resected in a rhomboid design and then the location of the excess skin is determined with a pinch test. The flap can then be taken from the area with the most available skin. The flap is rhomboid and should fit perfectly into the defect. As the flap is fitted into the defect, the donor site becomes significantly reduced. Because the design has corners, pin cushioning rarely, if ever, occurs. The donor site can be closed directly. Any excess skin is resected. These flaps maybe used for small- to medium-sized defects in the mid portion of the cheek although in the authors' practice, rhombic flaps are used primarily in the temple area. Bilobed flaps may be used to close small preauricular defects and small- to medium-sized defects located in the central cheek. A large bilobed cheek flap can be created, recruiting tissue from the preauricular area for the first flap and the postauricular skin for the second flap.[20] The cervical skin is then advanced for closure of the second flap donor site.

Large cheek defects

When large areas of the cheek require resection, it is possible to elevate the inferior skin of the cheek and neck. This large amount of skin can be moved upward and medially, a combination of advancement and rotation. Such a flap will allow significant defects to be closed with the correct skin match and, more importantly, it is tension-free. The scar can be hidden in the pre-auricular and pre-hairline area. The results from this technique can be excellent. It may be necessary to remove a lateral triangle of excess skin that results from the rotation. Care must also be taken when reconstructing defects in the male face. If possible, hair-bearing skin should not be placed in the non-hair-bearing areas of the face.

Lips

The upper and lower lips are each made up of a red portion and a white portion with the vermilion border serving as the demarcation between the two. The upper lip consists of a medial and two lateral subunits, demarcated by the philtral ridges and the nasolabial folds. The philtral ridges are the elevated ridges of white lip extending vertically from the highest point of the vermilion on either side to the base of the columella. The common lip reconstruction paradigm is based on the amount of horizontal lip involved in the defect. The upper lip and lower lip must be considered individually because the methods used for reconstruction are not always applicable to both locations.

Upper lip

The Cupid's bow, the central mucosal excess, the position of the base of the nose, and the oral commissure are the areas to be considered in upper lip reconstruction. Any method that compromises the symmetry of these areas is not satisfactory. Unfortunately, when the defect is large, an optimal result may not be obtainable.

Direct closure

Direct closure is used whenever possible, but care should be taken to realign the mucocutaneous margin and the white roll. In some instances, to prevent a notch on the free margin, a mucosal Z-plasty may be employed. This must be done with care. Dry (external) mucosa should be extraoral, and

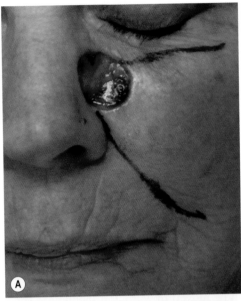

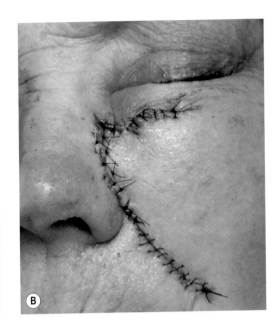

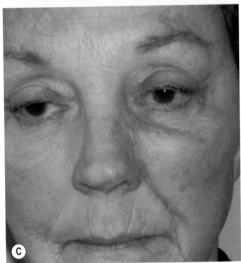

Fig. 17.17 (A–C) Posteriorly based cheek flap.

wet (internal) mucosa should be intraoral. If wet mucosa is exposed, it will be obvious because it is red and shiny and tends to crust when dry. The Cupid's bow is an important aesthetic area and should always be managed with great care. Its symmetry should not be compromised unless this is unavoidable. In full-thickness defects, accurate muscle reconstruction is critical to ensure symmetrical upper lip function.

Lateral and central defects can be closed directly, but judgment must be used. Any degree of asymmetry should be minimal. The muscle must be dissected out from the mucosa and the skin and reconstructed with accuracy. Magnification helps greatly and should always be used. In lip repair, there should be equal emphasis on aesthetics and function.

Larger defects

In the lateral and central areas of the upper lip, the perialar crescentic flap can be used. To allow the lip to advance without tension, a crescent of skin and deep subcutaneous tissue is

removed from around the lateral area of the alar base by careful layered closure. It is important to construct the lower part of the crescent end at the alar base. This maintains the correct vertical height of the lip. In addition, the mucosa is incised transversely in the upper buccal sulcus. A fringe of mucosa should be left on the alveolus for accurate closure. This allows the whole lip segment to move medially, and large closure can be performed without tension. When there are large midline defects, these can sometimes be closed with bilateral perialar crescentic advancement flaps. The problem with this reconstruction is that it may result in a tight lip. In addition, the Cupid's bow may more than likely be compromised, but this is unavoidable and further surgery may be required, as indicated.

Abbé flap

Traditionally, the Abbé flap was a full-thickness V-shaped portion of the lower lip, which was taken up to expand the

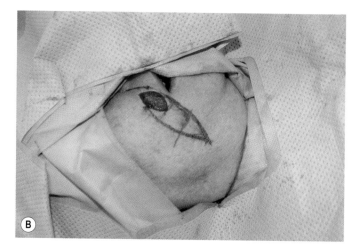

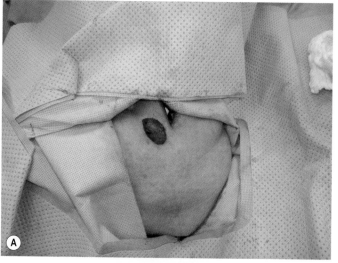

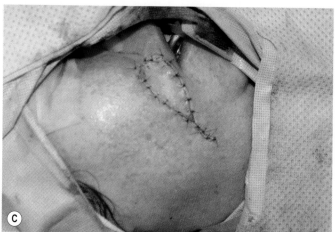

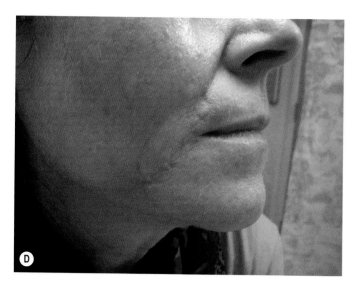

Fig. 17.18 (A–D) V–Y island advancement flap.

upper lip transversely.[21] The labial vessels provide the blood supply. The upper lip is released by a vertical incision and the V-shaped defect of the upper lip is reconstructed using the Abbé flap. The lower lip vessel is then divided at 2–3 weeks. Although this gives nice release of the upper lip and provides bulk, there is a tendency to have a convexity bilaterally on either side of the flap and there tends also to be more movement in the lateral segments of the upper lip, with little or no movement of the flap.

In order to prevent these problems and to create a mobile upper lip that would give a more satisfactory result aesthetically and functionally, Jackson changed the design of the Abbé flap.[22] He advocated that the flap be incised anteriorly on the lower lip skin and posteriorly on the mucosa. On one side of the flap, the incision is taken from the buccal sulcus over the lip mucosa and on to the skin. The lower lip muscles are dissected out, leaving the mucosa and skin free of attachments. At this point, the muscles of the lower lip are intact and the mucosa and skin are sutured. In the upper lip, an incision is made and the orbicularis muscles are dissected out so that they can be freed and joined in the midline. This

muscle dissection is extensive so that the muscles can be interdigitated in the midline. Care is taken not to disturb any nerves. This having been done, the lip dimensions are now satisfactory in terms of lip height and muscle bulk. The lower lip segment is now swung up into the upper lip defect and is sutured in position. Because of the very narrow pedicle, it is possible to have the flap placed in exactly the required position. This is almost like a full-thickness graft of the skin and mucosa and, therefore, the division of the supplying vessel can be carried out in 2–5 days, although five is most frequent.

At the second-stage procedure, it is necessary to rearrange the mucocutaneous junction with additional trimming of the flap. If the flap described above can be used, the lower lip muscle is left intact and the upper lip muscle is reconstructed. This results in good function of both lips in most cases.

Fan flaps

Fan flaps can be used for hemi-lip or total upper lip defects. These defects may be skin only or a full-thickness lip defect.

Fan flaps can be standard or full-thickness and are based on the perioral vasculature. The commissures are maintained and the flaps are rotated around them; thus, the anatomy of the mouth is maintained. However, fan flaps yield a much better result on the lower lip. This type of reconstruction has largely been overtaken by the perialar crescentic advancement flap.

Lower lip

In the lower lip, skin defects can be reconstructed with nasolabial flaps. These can be transferred as a two-stage procedure or in one stage, as island flaps. Pin cushioning is a problem regardless of whether the flaps are round or square.

Full-thickness defects

In the lower lip, as opposed to the upper lip, larger defects can be closed directly because of the greater lip laxity. The closure should be performed in a careful, layered fashion in the following order: mucosa, muscle, and skin.

Karapandzic technique

By use of the Karapandzic technique, three-quarters of the lower lip can be reconstructed without difficulty (Fig. 17.19).[23] It has some resemblance to the perialar crescentic advancement flap, but it is a superior method. The reconstruction should replace the full-thickness and depth of the lip. The skin is incised in a transverse direction to just beyond the nasolabial fold. Laterally, the vessels and nerves are dissected out and carefully preserved. The orbicularis muscle fibers are spread apart as far laterally as necessary. After this, it should be possible to move the leading edge to the midline or beyond, if necessary. It is best to use bilateral flaps and to perform a layered closure where they meet. In this way, a loose and symmetric lip is obtained, and the blood and nerve supply are maintained. Also, a properly functioning lip with a virtually normal anatomy is formed. The scars settle well and are acceptable from a cosmetic viewpoint.

Gillies fan flap

Until the Karapandzic procedure was published, the Gillies fan flap was considered to be the method of choice. Full-thickness nasolabial flaps based on the labial vessels are swung around the commissure into the lower lip defect. These flaps can be unilateral or bilateral.

Comparison between Karapandzic and Gillies techniques

In the Karapandzic technique, the commissures are maintained and the width of the commissure is satisfactory.[23] There is no need to supply lower lip mucosa. The flaps are neurotized and results in good lower lid function and sensation. In the Gillies reconstruction, the mouth is narrowed, and there is no mucosal cover of the flaps at the lip margin. Mucosal cover is supplied by advancing intraoral mucosa. Unfortunately, mucosa from this area is always red and shiny, and frequently has a tendency to crust when exposed to the air. The nerves are not kept intact, thus lip function and sensation are compromised. In spite of this, the function may be better than expected, especially in hemi-lip reconstruction.

Tongue flaps

Tongue flaps can be used to replace the lip red margin in reconstructions that do not supply the required amount of mucosa.[24] Tongue flaps are also used in patients with advanced and extensive leukoplakial involvement of the lip mucosa. The traditional method is to use the dorsum of the tongue, but its color and surface irregularity make it aesthetically unsuitable as a lip mucosal substitute. The undersurface of the tongue mucosa is smooth, may have good color, and can easily be transferred in a staged procedure. The flap is based anteriorly. It should be of a sufficient length and width. It is sutured into the lip defect. In 10 days, under local anesthesia, the flap is divided and inset. The tongue defect is closed directly. The mucosa tends to be a deeper shade of red and shinier than normal tongue mucosa. Crusting may occur and may require frequent application of petroleum jelly. Sensation is reduced as with any free transplant on the lip.

Total lower lip reconstruction

The Karapandzic technique can be used for total lower lip reconstruction, but the reconstructed lip is frequently too tight. The method of choice is bilateral fan flaps with resurfacing of the red lip with a flap from the undersurface of the tongue.[25] The Webster advancement technique, in which bilateral full-thickness horizontal advancement cheek flaps can be brought into place by excision of bilateral upper and lower vertical triangles at their bases, is another possibility. The mucosa is again supplied from the undersurface of the tongue. The scars in the nasolabial lines and around the chin heal well. The main problem is that the reconstructed lip is flat and tight and tends to trap-door. On occasion, two Abbé flaps from either side of the prolabial segment of the lip can be turned down to increase lip volume, but the end result is not particularly satisfactory from a cosmetic point of view. Function (e.g., drooling) may be improved to a variable degree. Not infrequently, free tissue transfer will be required to reconstruct a total lip defect.

Commissure reconstruction

The commissure mucosa occasionally requires reconstruction. When analyzed, this can be divided into two rhomboids, one for each lip. Rhomboid flaps from the intraoral cheek area can resurface the defects without difficulty, and the donor sites can be closed directly. However, this is wet mucosa and is redder than the normal lip. Another method for larger defects (e.g., electrical burns) is to develop a large triangular mucosal island flap, advance its base to the commissure, and then use the considerable amount of tissue obtained as required. The donor site is closed directly. Later rearrangement of the mucosa is always required but, fortunately, a sufficient supply is available after the procedure. Finally, in some instances, lateral tongue flaps can be used to cover the upper and lower lip region at the commissure. These are divided after 10 days. These flaps are not widely used because anteriorly-based mucosal flaps have proved to be more satisfactory in terms of position and patient comfort.

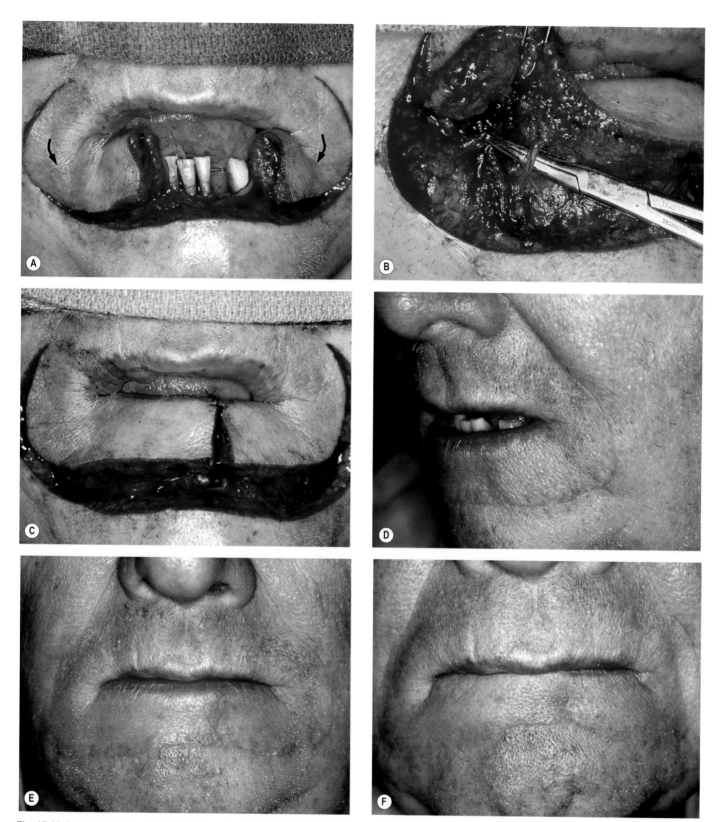

Fig. 17.19 Reconstruction of partial defect of lower lip with Karapandzic rotation-advancement flaps. **(A)** Full-thickness defect of the lower lip. Bilateral Karapandzic flaps incised. **(B)** Demonstration of vessels preserved with "Karapandzic" technique of dissection. Compared to central lip, identification of peripheral margin of orbicularis muscle in the vicinity of commissures is more difficult. Releasing facial muscular attachments to orbicularis muscle may be performed lateral to actual peripheral margin of orbicularis muscle near commissures to insure consistency of thickness of muscular layer of flaps. **(C)** Flaps approximated. **(D,E)** Six months postoperative. For proper lip height, flaps are designed with uniform width throughout length of flaps. For this reason, it is necessary to design flaps lateral to melolabial crease near commissure. **(F)** One year postoperative. Reconstructed lip has tightened, resulting from scar contraction. Such long-term changes are common. *(From Renner G. Reconstruction of the lip. In: Baker SR, Swanson NA (eds). Local flaps in facial reconstruction. St. Louis: Mosby, 1995:368, with permission.)*

Ear

The areas of the ear most often requiring excision and reconstruction are the rim and the conchal area.

Rim defects

It is frequently possible to excise a rim lesion and advance the rim by incising full-thickness down to the lobule. There is no residual defect with this method (Fig. 17.20).[26] If there is concern about the viability of the tip of this flap or if the defect is larger, the posterior skin is dissected up and may be included into the rim. A larger flap with a large base has a better blood supply and is more likely to survive. It does not result in any ear deformity. In some instances, superior and inferior rim flaps will be used in conjunction with one another. Even larger defects are better reconstructed by postauricular flaps (Fig. 17.21). The flap is elevated and sutured to the anterior edge of the defect. After 3 weeks, a large flap is incised in the postauricular area, dissected up to provide laxity, and brought to the ear rim to provide more tissue. It is trimmed as necessary and sutured in place. Deep sutures can help in forming the shape as required. Further adjustments will most likely be necessary following on healing.

Anterior concha

If a lesion of significant size occurs in the anterior concha, resurfacing will be required.[27] To achieve this, the lesion is resected together with the underlying conchal cartilage. The ear is then distracted forward, and a flap is designed with a central vertical pedicle based on the ear mastoid groove. The skin anterior and posterior to the groove is elevated, and with some division of the subcutaneous hinge superiorly and inferiorly, it can be rotated into the ear defect. The posterior edge of the postauricular island is sutured to the posterior edge of the defect, and the anterior edge of the island is sutured to the anterior edge of the defect. The posterior defect is closed directly. This will give an excellent result both on the anterior aspect of the concha and in the postauricular groove (Fig. 17.22).[28] In a large degloving of the ear, a temporal fascial flap is used to cover the defect. The flap is then covered with a

full-thickness skin graft. This is a rare injury, but this technique can also be used in reconstruction of the congenitally absent ear. The end result is suboptimal because of the poor color of the skin graft. It may also have a shiny surface, especially if a split-thickness graft is used.

Perforator flaps in the face

Facial artery perforator flap (Video 17.1 ⊙)

The facial artery flap is a relatively new addition to the flap options in facial reconstruction.[29] It can be designed with an aesthetic donor site and due to the reliability of the presence of perforators these flaps can have a large arc of rotation. They are commonly used as a V–Y flap or as a propeller flap (Fig. 17.18).[30,31] For clinical application, the identification of the facial artery and its perforators can be identified with the use of a hand-held Doppler. The facial artery travels from the midpoint of the mandibular edge towards the nasal alar margin medial to the labial crease. There are generally four to five cutaneous perforators of greater than 0.5 mm that arise along the course of the artery.

Submental flap

The submental flap is very useful perforator flap for reconstruction of the lower face. It can be used both intraorally as well as for cutaneous reconstruction.[32,33] It is based on the submental artery (a well-defined branch of the facial artery). This vessel arises deep to the submandibular gland and passing forward and medially across the mylohyoid muscle and can be either superficial or deep to the digastric muscle and terminates behind the mandibular symphysis on the anterior belly of digastric. It gives off several cutaneous branches that pierce the platysma and this allows a large flap to be raised, from mandibular angle to mandibular angle, with width determined by the flaccidity of the neck skin allowing direct closure (up to 18 × 7 cm). This flap has a pedicle length of 8 cm and an arc that allows it to reach the lower two-thirds of the face.[34] It provides excellent donor tissue with a well-hidden donor site (Fig. 17.23).

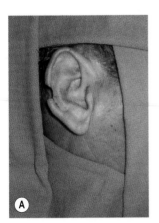 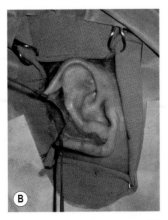 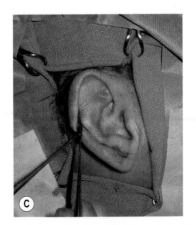 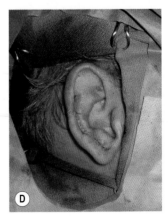

Fig. 17.20 (A) Helical defect following resection of a basal cell carcinoma. **(B)** Helical flaps are raised based on the posterior skin. **(C)** Flaps are dissected until advancement and closure without tension is possible. **(D)** Final appearance following closure. *(Courtesy of Dr. David Mathes.)*

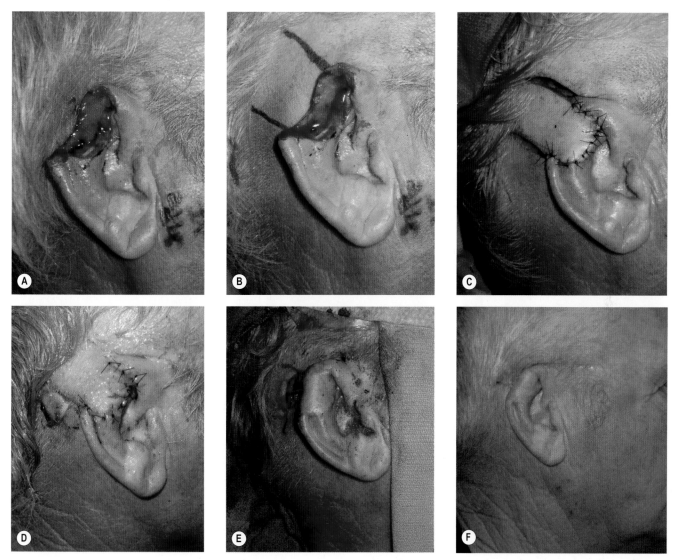

Fig. 17.21 **(A)** Defect of upper ear after resection of squamous cell carcinoma. **(B)** Post-auricular flap is designed, **(C)** raised and inset into defect. **(D)** Appearance prior to pedicle division and **(E)** following pedicle division. The intervening defect is skin grafted most easily with a post-auricular graft harvested more inferiorly than the defect and closed directly. **(F)** Late appearance. *(Courtesy of Dr. David Mathes.)*

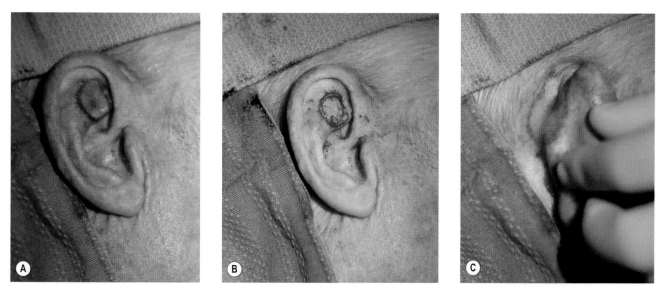

Fig. 17.22 **(A)** A 72-year-old man with a basal cell in the upper ear, marked for excision. **(B)** Defect includes anterior skin and underlying cartilage. **(C)** Postauricular, superiorly based flap outlined.

Continued

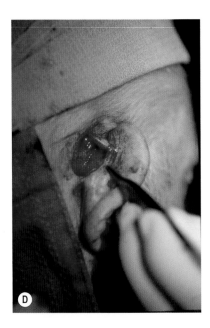

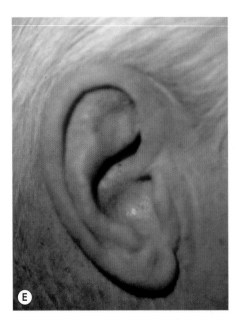

Fig. 17.22, cont'd (D) Flap raised and tunneled into anterior defect. Small segment of flap is de-epithelialized and secondary defect is closed directly. **(E)** Final appearance of healed flap. *(Courtesy of Dr. Peter Neligan.)*

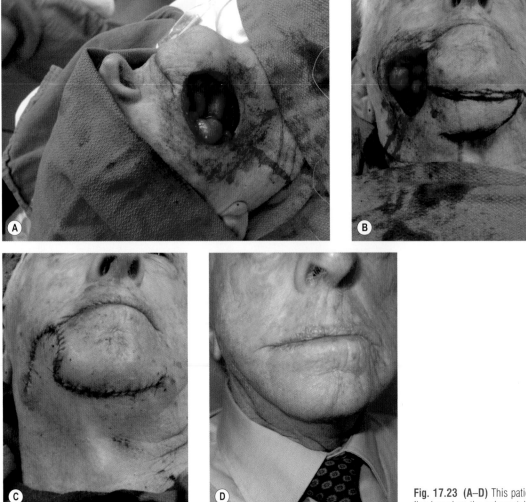

Fig. 17.23 (A–D) This patient is reconstructed with a submental flap based on the submental branch of the facial artery.

References

1. Juri J, Juri C, Arufe HN. Use of rotation scalp flaps for treatment of occipital baldness. *Plast Reconstr Surg.* 1978;61(1):23–26.

2. Orticochea M. Four flap scalp reconstruction technique. *Br J Plast Surg.* 1967;20(2):159–171.

3. Orticochea M. New three-flap reconstruction technique. *Br J Plast Surg.* 1971;24(2):184–188.

4. Zilinsky I, Farber N, Haik J, et al. The hatchet and bilobed flaps revisited: shedding new light on traditional concepts. *J Drugs Dermatol.* 2012;11(1):99–102.

5. Burget GC, Menick FJ. The subunit principle in nasal reconstruction. *Plast Reconstr Surg.* 1985;76(2):239–247.

6. Parrett BM, Pribaz JJ. An algorithm for treatment of nasal defects. *Clin Plast Surg.* 2009;36(3):407–420.

7. Rohrich RJ, Griffin JR, Ansari M, Beran SJ, Potter JK. Nasal reconstruction–beyond aesthetic subunits: a 15-year review of 1334 cases. *Plast Reconstr Surg.* 2004;114(6):1405–1416, discussion 1417–1409.

8. Koch CA, Archibald DJ, Friedman O. Glabellar flaps in nasal reconstruction. *Facial Plast Surg Clin North Am.* 2011;19(1):113–122.

9. Panizzo N, Colavitti G, Papa G, et al. Reconstruction after wide excision in medial canthal region: the extended bilobed glabellar-palpebral flap. *J Plast Reconstr Aesthet Surg.* 2015;68(1):131–132.

10. Staahl TE. Nasalis myocutaneous flap for nasal reconstruction. *Arch Otolaryngol Head Neck Surg.* 1986;112(3):302–305.

11. Wee SS, Hruza GJ, Mustoe TA. Refinements of nasalis myocutaneous flap. *Ann Plast Surg.* 1990;25(4):271–278.

12. Constantine VS. Nasalis myocutaneous sliding flap: repair of nasal supratip defects. *J Dermatol Surg Oncol.* 1991;17(5):439–444.

13. Zitelli JA. Design aspect of the bilobed flap. *Arch Facial Plast Surg.* 2008;10(3):186.

14. Zimany A. The bi-lobed flap. *Plast Reconstr Surg (1946).* 1953;11(6):424–434.

15. Menick FJ. Aesthetic refinements in use of forehead for nasal reconstruction: the paramedian forehead flap. *Clin Plast Surg.* 1990;17(4):607–622.

16. Menick FJ. A 10-year experience in nasal reconstruction with the three-stage forehead flap. *Plast Reconstr Surg.* 2002;109(6):1839–1855, discussion 1856–1861.

17. Jowett N, Mlynarek AM. Reconstruction of cheek defects: a review of current techniques. *Curr Opin Otolaryngol Head Neck Surg.* 2010;18(4):244–254.

18. Garrett WS Jr, Giblin TR, Hoffman GW. Closure of skin defects of the face and neck by rotation and advancement of cervicopectoral flaps. *Plast Reconstr Surg.* 1966;38(4):342–346.

19. Pribaz JJ, Chester CH, Barrall DT. The extended V–Y flap. *Plast Reconstr Surg.* 1992;90(2):275–280.

20. McGregor JC, Soutar DS. A critical assessment of the bilobed flap. *Br J Plast Surg.* 1981;34(2):197–205.

21. Abbé R. A new plastic operation for the relief of deformity due to double harelip. *Plast Reconstr Surg.* 1968;42(5):481–483.

22. Jackson IT, Soutar DS. The sandwich Abbé flap in sceondary cleft lip deformity. *Plast Reconstr Surg.* 1980;66(1):38–45.

23. Karapandzic M. Reconstruction of lip defects by local arterial flaps. *Br J Plast Surg.* 1974;27(1):93–97.

24. Rees TD, Tabbal N, Aston SJ. Tongue-flap reconstruction of the lip vermilion in hemifacial atrophy. *Plast Reconstr Surg.* 1983;72(5):643–647.

25. Jackson IT. Use of tongue flaps to resurface lip defects and close palatal fistulae in children. *Plast Reconstr Surg.* 1972;49(5):537–541.

26. Antia NH, Buch VI. Chondrocutaneous advancement flap for the marginal defect of the ear. *Plast Reconstr Surg.* 1967;39(5):472–477.

27. Brent B. The acquired auricular deformity. A systematic approach to its analysis and reconstruction. *Plast Reconstr Surg.* 1977;59(4):475–485.

28. Masson JK. A simple island flap for reconstruction of concha-helix defects. *Br J Plast Surg.* 1972;25(4):399–403.

29. Hofer SO, Posch NA, Smit X. The facial artery perforator flap for reconstruction of perioral defects. *Plast Reconstr Surg.* 2005;115(4):996–1003, discussion 1004–1005.

30. Kannan RY, Mathur BS. Perforator flaps of the facial artery angiosome. *J Plast Reconstr Aesthet Surg.* 2013;66(4):483–488.

31. Camuzard O, Foissac R, Georgiou C, et al. Facial artery perforator flap for reconstruction of perinasal defects: An anatomical study and clinical application. *J Craniomaxillofac Surg.* 2015;43(10):2057–2065.

32. Ishihara T, Igata T, Masuguchi S, et al. Submental perforator flap: location and number of submental perforating vessels. *Scand J Plast Reconstr Surg Hand Surg.* 2008;42(3):127–131.

33. Curran AJ, Neligan P, Gullane PJ. Submental artery island flap. *Laryngoscope.* 1997;107(11 Pt 1):1545–1549.

34. Faltaous AA, Yetman RJ. The submental artery flap: an anatomic study. *Plast Reconstr Surg.* 1996;97(1):56–60, discussion 61–52.

18

Secondary facial reconstruction

Julian J. Pribaz and Rodney K. Chan

SYNOPSIS

- Secondary revision is an inevitable and indispensable part of facial reconstruction.
- An accurate diagnosis of the missing parts is as important in secondary reconstructions as during the primary reconstruction.
- A comprehensive reconstructive plan is needed from the start, including bailout strategies.

Introduction

The goal of any reconstruction is to restore to normal – or close to normal – form and function. This could only be completely achieved by replantation or, in the future, transplantation. All of our current reconstructive methods will always fall short of the ideal due to specific tissue characteristics. Hence the need for secondary, tertiary, or in fact multiple revisional procedures to achieve the best possible functional and aesthetic result. Indeed, the meaning of the word *plastic*, which is derived from the Greek *plastikos*, means to make or mold.

This chapter will address the principles and techniques utilized to enhance the final result of the initial primary reconstructive procedure. The sequence of reconstruction and timing in the application of these different techniques should be guided by basic principles. A well-thought-out reconstructive path is needed from the start so as not to "burn any bridges". Secondary facial reconstructions can be broadly separated into (1) those that were part of the initial reconstructive plan and (2) those that were unplanned and which may present to a different surgeon as a challenging case.

Access the Historical Perspective section online at
http://www.expertconsult.com

Basic science/disease process

Secondary facial reconstruction assumes a previous operative procedure, the cause of which in the head and neck may have a wide range of etiologies, from congenital malformations to various types of trauma, including burns, ballistic injuries, motor vehicle accidents, and animal bites. Tumors involving both bone and soft tissues and infections may also have been the culprit. Each one of these etiologies has its own unique consequences.

Tissues may have been lost, displaced, or distorted. Both bone and soft tissues may have been involved. A common feature of all these etiologies is that, along the way, wounds were created and treated. These may have been simple and superficial but, more likely, deep and complex. Healing may have been facilitated by primary or secondary closure, or involved a prior operative procedure utilizing tissue locally or afar. It should be remembered that there is renewed swelling and scarring at each interface, and that this occurs with each operative procedure, which in turn makes the outcome after each procedure somewhat unpredictable. It is usual and safe practice to allow the patient and the involved tissue to heal, the swelling to subside, and the scarring to mature before embarking on secondary and tertiary operative procedures.

Diagnosis/patient presentation

An accurate diagnosis of the deformity and an appraisal of the missing parts are essential. The deformity is compared with what is considered to be the "perceived normal". If the deficit is unilateral, the best guide is a comparison with the opposite side. With more extensive defects where both sides are involved, a consideration of baseline appearance as seen on an old photograph may serve as a guide to reconstruction. However, realistic goals must be set from the start as to what might be achievable with reconstruction.

An evaluation for secondary facial reconstruction begins with a thorough investigation into the history of the patient, in particular the operations and flaps that were previously utilized, paying close attention to the remaining donor vessels in the head and neck.[2] Next, an accurate diagnosis of the missing parts has to be made. While it is generally obvious what the missing parts are for a primary reconstruction that immediately follows extirpation, it is less obvious in secondary reconstructions where tissues have been pulled closed or healed secondarily. It takes an astute plastic surgeon to visualize what constitutes adequate contracture release and the resulting defect. This attention to making the correct comprehensive diagnosis is especially important when evaluating a patient whose primary reconstruction was performed elsewhere. Subsequent revisions are individualized and dictated by the area and underlying cause that required reconstruction. Therefore, a surgeon who specializes in secondary facial reconstructions needs to be well versed in all rungs of the reconstructive ladder, especially when many first-line options have already been utilized.

Patient selection

Facial defects and deformities should be evaluated in a systematic manner, starting from:

1. Overall magnitude and extent of the deformity and its anatomical location.
2. Displacement of major facial subunits; for example, the eyebrows, eyelids, nose, ears, and lips.
3. The extent of contour distortion.
4. Location and quality of the scarring that is present.
5. The color, texture, and quality of the skin.
6. The presence, absence, and distortion of specialized cutaneous features; for example, the hairline, sideburn, and beard area.
7. The quality of the subcutaneous tissues, volume, and distribution.
8. The function or lack thereof of the underlying musculature.
9. The integrity or deformity of the underlying bony or cartilaginous support structures.
10. The status and quality of tissues lining the oral and nasal cavity.
11. The loss of other specialized components such as the lacrimal apparatus, teeth, and an adequate and mobile tongue.

The status of all these elements should first be appraised and a decision made regarding the best method of restoration.

In consideration of secondary reconstruction it is understood that a primary procedure has already been performed. The effectiveness of the first reconstruction has to be evaluated and sometimes it is necessary to advise the complete removal of an inadequate first reconstructive effort, to recreate the defect, and start again from scratch. For complex reconstruction, it is ideal to have an expert evaluate the initial presenting problem and develop an appropriate and often-staged treatment plan. No complex facial defect or deformity can be expected to be adequately repaired in a single stage and thus if a staged repair is required, it is necessary to plan a correct sequence of procedures so to avoid "burning future bridges".

Treatment and surgical technique

Meticulous technique and planning should be emphasized at every step of a multistage facial reconstruction, as this makes subsequent operations more predictable. Planning and initial flap tailoring are critical first steps. Radiographs are useful to visualize the missing bony elements. We recommend the liberal use of preoperative and intraoperative models to simulate the missing soft tissues and/or bone in developing the plan.[3] This maneuver at the commencement of an operative procedure allows for tailored flaps to be designed at the most ideal donor site.

In general, the principles that are observed in secondary facial reconstructions are:

1. Restore uninjured or partially injured anatomical features to their normal location.
2. Repair scar contracture and, if possible, place the scars along the natural crease lines.
3. Restore the contour, which may involve debulking or augmenting soft facial parts with dermis fat grafts or autogenous fat grafting.[4,5]
4. Restoration of contour is more important than the presence of scars.
5. Replace "like with like", thus, soft tissues should be replaced with soft tissues, and bony tissues with bone or bone substitutes.
6. Use local flap options with better color and texture match as advancement or transposition flaps to provide better cutaneous coverage of de-epithelialized, previously placed distant free flaps that may have been used.
7. Local specialized flaps, for example, hair-bearing flaps, to reconstruct specific subunits previously covered by large distant flaps are also used to help break up the scars and create an illusion of a more normal appearance.
8. If local flaps are not available to improve the color mismatch of distant flaps, consider the use of thin split-thickness skin grafts harvested from the scalp as overgrafts to resurface these areas after de-epithelialization of the existing flap.[6]
9. Carry out functional restoration of absent muscles of facial expression, especially for restitution of a smile and adequate closure of the eyelids and mouth. The options of free muscle transfer, with and without nerve grafts or local or regional muscle transfers of functioning muscle, can all be considered.
10. Restore adequate bony platform to repair bony contour deformities, or allow for dental rehabilitation with osseointegrated implants.
11. Carry out supplemental prosthetic reconstruction of non-reconstructible parts, for example, orbital and ear prostheses.

A few recurrent themes encountered in complex facial reconstructions are worthy of mention: (1) reconstruction of deficient intraoral and intranasal lining; (2) reconstruction of hair-bearing regions; as well as the use of (3) prefabrication and (4) prelamination as adjunctive techniques.

Intraoral and intranasal lining

Deficiency in intraoral and intranasal lining must be suspected in cases of internal or external perioral contractures, or when the lining is known to have been excised or irradiated. Deficiency in intraoral lining can manifest as dry mouth, lack of facial movement, or lack of oral competence. Therefore, prior to commencement of any perioral reconstruction, intraoral scars must be fully released and the lining reconstructed. Otherwise, any attempts at external skin replacement will be suboptimal. Replacements of intraoral lining include skin grafts, regional flaps, and distant flaps. While skin graft might appear to be most appealing because of its availability and simplicity, we have not found it to be durable, especially in scarred or irradiated beds. Distant flaps such as anterolateral thigh flaps and radial forearm free flaps are certainly reliable methods of replacing lining. However, in cases of multiple prior operations, those flaps may have already been utilized or may be needed elsewhere. Furthermore, donor vessels are usually scarce. The facial artery musculomucosal (FAMM) flap, a composite flap with mucosa and muscle taken from the lateral cheek, should be considered as an option. This is best done at the first operation when wide exposure and easy access to supple mucosa are available. When harvested with the overlying buccinator muscle, this is a robust flap that can cover widths of 2–2.5 cm. It can be based either superiorly (retrograde flow) or inferiorly (antegrade flow) to cover a variety of oronasal mucosal defects, including defects of the palate, alveolus, nasal septum, antrum, upper and lower lips, floor of the mouth, and soft palate (Fig. 18.1).[7]

With larger mucosal defects involving the floor of the mouth, the submental flap based on the submental branch of the facial artery is another useful regional option. Our experience indicates that this flap is generally very reliable with minimal donor site morbidity but should be used with caution if there was prior irradiation. Further, it can be easily combined with the need for a neck dissection, though it is imperative to raise the flap and preserve its blood supply prior to commencement of the extirpative procedure.[8]

While vermilion is not strictly intraoral lining, it is a specialized type of tissue that is impossible to reproduce. When vermilion is missing and cannot be borrowed from its neighboring areas, its appearance is much better matched with the use of non-keratinized mucosa than the use of keratinized skin. In the early days of vermilion reconstruction, jejunal and gastric mucosa were attempted but were fraught with problems. The use of gastric mucosa in particular can be hypersecretory and its acidic contents ulcerogenic. FAMM flap, based superiorly for the upper lip and inferiorly for the lower lip, can give a good match for this specialized tissue.[9] Alternatively, the use of lingual mucosa or tattooing of keratinized skin can also be acceptable.

Hair-bearing flaps

Successful facial reconstructions, especially in males, need to recognize the pattern of hair growth particularly in the

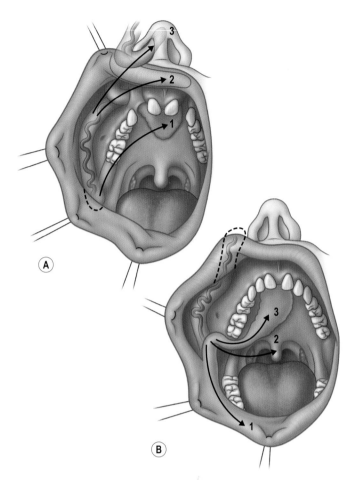

Fig. 18.1 (A) Superiorly based facial artery musculomucosal (FAMM) flap may be used for defects of the anterior palate, alveolus, maxillary antrum, nose, upper lip, and orbit. **(B)** Inferiorly based FAMM flap may be used for defects of the posterior palate, tonsillar fossa, alveolus, floor of mouth, and lower lip.[7]

sideburn and beard areas in order to maintain symmetry. However, few sites are available as hair-bearing donors. The temporal scalp, frontal scalp, and the submental region can all give satisfactory results.[10] The frontal scalp can be transferred using the supratrochlear artery and the submental region can be transferred on the submental branch of the facial artery, though these areas may not be available. Temporal scalp skin contains an abundance of hair follicles and needs implantation of a heterotopic vessel as a first-stage reconstruction (see prefabrication, below).

Prefabrication

Prefabrication refers to the pretransfer implantation of a nonnative vascular pedicle into the tissue desired for reconstruction. It is used when the tissue desired for reconstruction cannot be practically transferred by alternate means. To optimize aesthetics in facial reconstruction, prefabrication is typically used to hand-pick thin tissues with cutaneous qualities most similar to the pre-disfigured part. The donor vessel can be any good length of vessel, including its surrounding fatty tissue.[11,12] The radial forearm fascial flap, the temporal parietal fascial flap, and the descending branch of the lateral femoral circumflex pedicles are all reliable donor vessels of good caliber. This is placed under the desired area of transfer and, if needed, can be placed over a tissue expander. This is an especially useful adjunct in cases of secondary facial reconstructions as first-line donor options are exhausted and new donor options need to be explored. This technique essentially creates a limitless number of donor sites.

Prelamination

Flap prelamination is a term first coined by Pribaz and Fine in 1994, referring to the pretransfer implantation of anything other than a vascular pedicle in the territory of an existing axial vascular bed.[13,14] In aesthetic facial reconstruction, prelamination is often used to assemble composite flaps that can be transferred as a unit that more closely approximates the pre-disfigured part.[11] Prelamination is a useful adjunct in both primary and secondary facial reconstructions of complex multifaceted defects.

Each of the selected cases of secondary facial reconstructions below demonstrates many of the basic dictums previously described. While secondary reconstructions can be broadly separated into two categories: (1) those that were part of the initial reconstructive plan and (2) those that were unplanned and usually followed multiple other unsatisfactory reconstructions done elsewhere, it is on the second category that we want to focus. In the cases of secondary reconstructions that follow, we will first demonstrate our diagnosis of the missing elements and then the principles used to arrive at the reconstructive plan.

Case example 1

This patient is a 16-year-old girl with severe facial burns from a hot-oil spill as a baby. She underwent initial reconstruction with staged tube pedicle flap from her groin for nose and chin reconstruction which unfortunately was totally inadequate (Fig. 18.2).

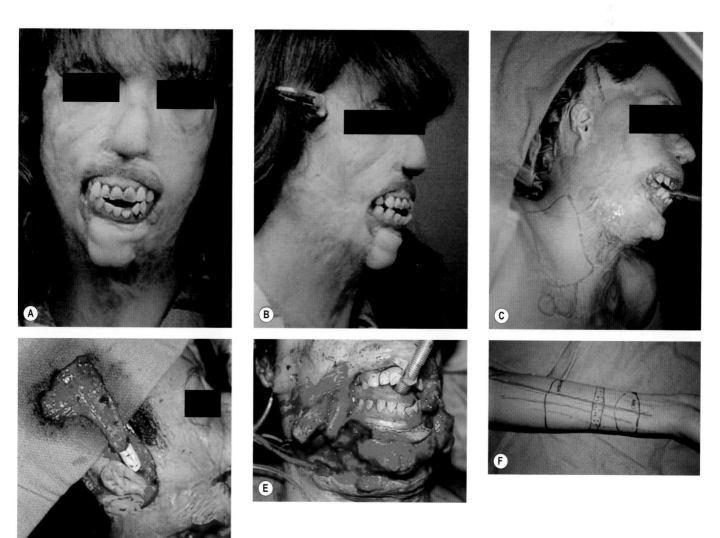

Fig. 18.2 A 16-year-old girl with severe facial burns from a hot-oil spill as a baby. **(A,B)** Her initial reconstruction with staged tube pedicle flap from her groin for nose and chin reconstruction was unfortunately inadequate to give her oral competence and facial expression. **(C,D)** At the first stage, right neck skin is prefabricated using pedicled temporal parietal fascia flap over a tissue expander for upper lip reconstruction. **(E,F)** Lower lip and chin were reconstructed with free folded radial forearm flap and bilateral facial artery musculomucosal flaps.

Continued

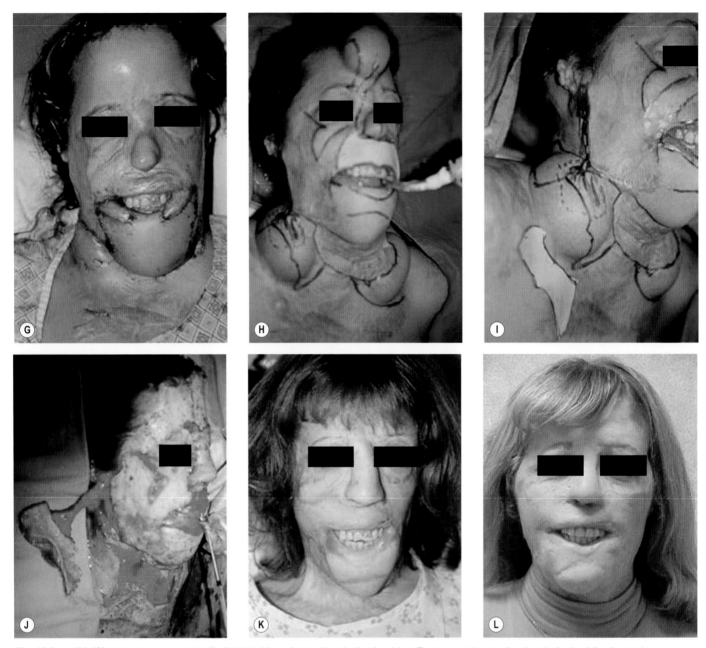

Fig. 18.2, cont'd (G) Her interim appearance with diminished lower incisor show is already evident. Tissue expander was placed under forehead flap for nasal reconstruction. At the second stage, her upper lip was reconstructed with the prefabricated expanded pedicle neck flap. **(H,I)** Template of the upper lip defect is seen and the course of the transposed pedicle outlined. **(J)** Her nose was reconstructed with the expanded forehead flap over lining flaps and cartilage grafts. **(K)** She was seen 3 months postoperatively with lower lip sagging. Dynamic temporalis muscle slings were designed to support her lower face and lips (not shown). **(L)** A satisfactory outcome is achieved 2 years following initial presentation. She has achieved oral competence and improved nasal aesthetics.[2]

Diagnosis

1. Full-thickness upper and lower lip loss and consequent lack of oral competence manifested as frequent oral caries and lack of facial expressions.
2. Nasal deformity with lack of tip projection and ill-defined facial-alar groove.

Reconstructive plan

Additional oral lining and external skin are needed to correct her upper and lower lip deficiencies. No local options are available. A radial forearm free flap is planned for lower lip reconstruction and a prefabricated neck flap is planned for upper lip reconstruction. Forehead flap and cartilage grafts will increase nasal projection and nasal skin quality. At the first stage, right neck skin was prefabricated using a pedicled temporal parietal fascia flap over a tissue expander for upper lip reconstruction. A tissue expander was also placed under forehead flap for nasal reconstruction. The lower lip and chin were reconstructed with free folded radial forearm flap. A three-dimensional template of the defect was made following contracture release which was then converted into a two-dimensional pattern before transposing on to the radial forearm.

She was seen immediately following lower lip free folded radial forearm flap and bilateral FAMM flap for vermilion reconstruction. At the second stage, her upper lip was reconstructed with the prefabricated expanded pedicle neck flap. Template of the upper lip defect is seen and the course of the transposed pedicle outlined. Her nose was reconstructed with a forehead flap over lining flaps and cartilage grafts. Sculpting of the supramental crease was also done at this time.

She was seen 3 months postoperatively with lower lip sagging. Bilateral dynamic temporalis muscle slings were designed to support her lower face and lips. She is seen immediately after her lower lip revision as well as sculpting of her nose. The mouth closes when the patient bites down. A satisfactory outcome is achieved 2 years following initial presentation. She has achieved oral competence and improved nasal aesthetics.[2]

This case illustrates multiple principles of secondary facial reconstruction:

1. Comprehensive diagnosis from the outset.
2. Use of templates for planning.
3. Prefabrication to bring in additional tissue, saving her from an additional free tissue transfer.
4. Use of FAMM flap for vermilion reconstruction.
5. Delayed use of forehead flap for resurfacing after previous distant flap.
6. Restoration of contour following free tissue transfer through debulking and placement of scars along natural creases.
7. Functional reconstruction of the lower lip with bilateral temporalis muscle flaps.

Case example 2

This patient is a 23-year-old female with a history of extensive burns and multiple facial skin grafts and releases who now desires better texture and uniformity (Fig. 18.3).

Diagnosis

The skin is irregular and noncompliant with no subcutaneous fat throughout her face and neck. She suffers from loss of normal nasal and facial contours from contractures of the face and nose.

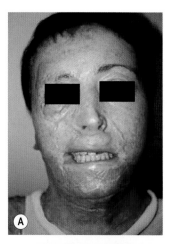
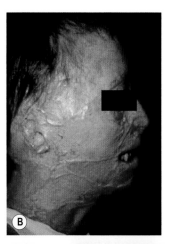
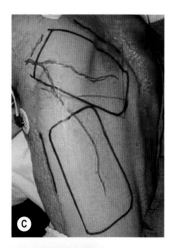
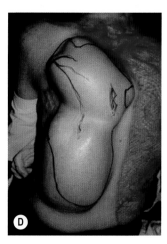

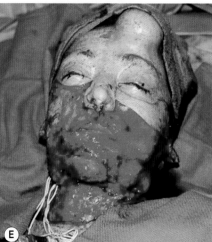
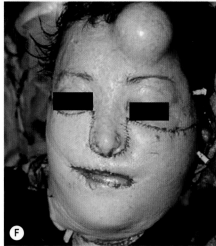
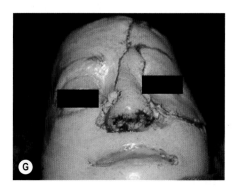

Fig. 18.3 A 23-year-old female with a history of extensive burns and multiple facial skin grafts and releases who now desires better texture and uniformity. **(A,B)** She suffers from loss of normal nasal and facial contours from contractures of the face and nose. **(C,D)** Facial resurfacing using an expanded free scapular/parascapular free flap was designed and outlined. **(E)** Following expansion, hypertrophic burn scar was excised from her face and neck. **(F)** She is seen immediately following free tissue transfer. **(G)** Expanded forehead flap was used for nasal resurfacing.

Continued

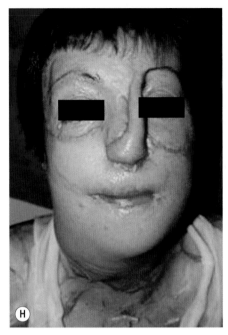 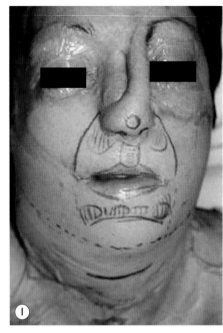 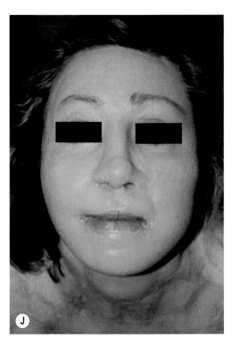

Fig. 18.3, cont'd **(H)** She is seen following healing of her free flap which still lacks normal facial and nasal contours. **(I)** Facial aesthetic units were recreated through debulking and placement of scars in lines of natural creases to recreate lines of the cheek, the philtrum, the upper lip, and chin. **(J)** Resurfacing of unstable skin has achieved a more uniform appearance of her face and neck.

Reconstructive plan

The intention was to carry out facial resurfacing using an expanded free scapular/parascapular free flap. She has few unburned donor sites large enough to resurface this area. Following expansion, hypertrophic burn scar was excised from her face and neck. Templating over the back was performed. She is seen immediately following free tissue transfer. Expanded forehead flap was used for nasal resurfacing. She is seen following healing of her free flap, which still lacks normal facial and nasal contours. Facial aesthetic subunits were recreated through debulking and placement of scars in lines of natural creases to recreate separation between the cheeks, the philtrum, the upper lip, and chin. Resurfacing of unstable skin has achieved a more uniform appearance of her face and neck. Attempts at further improving facial skin tone with laser resurfacing were partially successful, and the patient is satisfied with her appearance with use of additional makeup.

This case illustrates multiple principles of secondary facial reconstruction:

1. Comprehensive diagnosis from the outset.
2. Use of templates for planning.
3. Delayed use of forehead flap for resurfacing.
4. Uniform resurfacing of the face and neck with expanded free flap.
5. Restoration of contour following free tissue transfer through debulking and placement of scars along natural creases.

Case example 3

The patient is a 17-year-old male (see preinjury in Fig. 18.4B) following self-inflicted gunshot wound to the central one-third of his face with loss of bony support and left mandible. Reconstruction was first done elsewhere including open reduction, internal fixation of multiple bony fractures, rib grafts, and radial forearm free flap to separate the oro- and nasopharynx. Cantilever bone graft and forehead flap were performed for nasal reconstruction and subsequent Abbé flap for upper lip deficiency. The patient presented for secondary facial reconstruction 24 months after initial injury.

Diagnosis

1. Midface retrusion with lack of bony support.
2. Lack of nasal projection and ill-defined facial alar groove, deficient left alar.
3. Asymmetric lip with upper lip contracture and intraoral contracture.

Reconstructive plan

The intention was to carry out release of all intraoral contracture and reconstruct bony platform using free fibula flap. The contralateral facial artery is outlined in anticipation of extensive lining deficits. Midfibula osteotomy was performed to give support to both the maxilla and the mandible as a single free osteocutaneous flap. A large lining deficit is indeed seen following release. Both the fibular skin paddle as well as a superiorly based right FAMM flap can be seen during inset.

At a second stage, deficient left alar is reconstructed with free auricular flap of ascending helix and root of helix. Sixty-three months postinjury, after healing and edema subsided, a second forehead flap was done for nasal resurfacing. He is seen 8 years after the initial injury with symmetric lips lacking any external or internal oral contractures, improved midface, nasal projection, and nasal appearance.

This case illustrates multiple principles of secondary facial reconstruction:

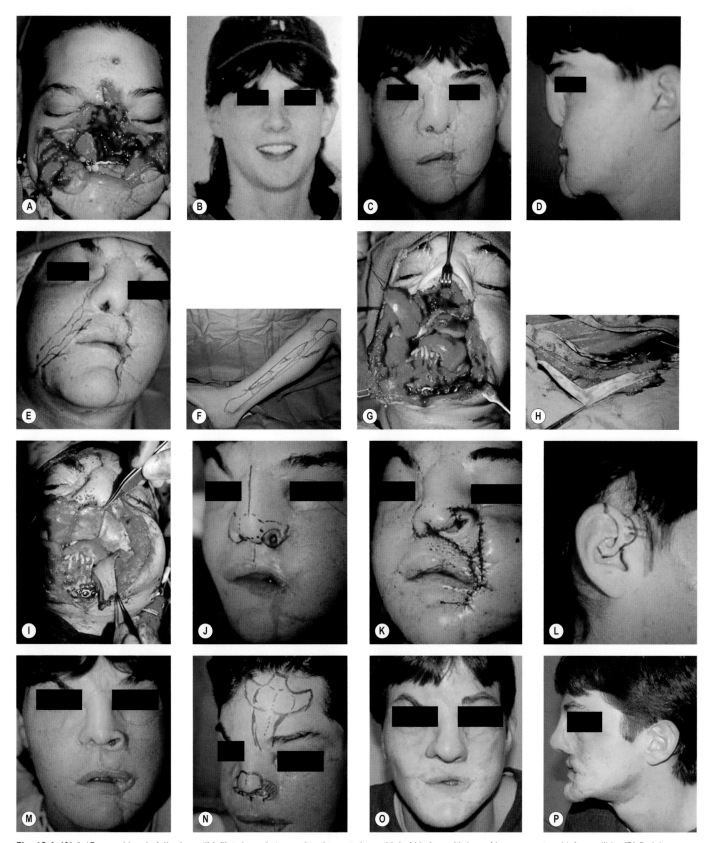

Fig. 18.4 **(A)** A 17-year-old male following self-inflicted gunshot wound to the central one-third of his face with loss of bony support and left mandible. **(B)** Preinjury appearance from an old photograph used as reference. Reconstruction first performed elsewhere included open reduction, internal fixation of multiple bony fractures, rib grafts, and radial forearm free flap to separate the oro- and nasopharynx. Cantilever bone graft and forehead flap were performed for nasal reconstruction and subsequent Abbé flap for upper lip deficiency. **(C,D)** The patient presented for secondary facial reconstruction 24 months after initial injury, lacking mid facial bony support, nasal projection, and asymmetric lip with upper lip and intraoral contractures. **(E)** The contralateral facial artery is outlined in anticipation of extensive lining deficits. **(F)** Reconstructive plan included release of all intraoral contracture and reconstruction of bony platform using free fibula flap. **(G)** A large lining deficit is indeed seen following release. **(H)** Midfibula osteotomy was performed to give support to both the maxilla and the mandible. **(I)** Both the fibular skin paddle, as well as a superiorly based right facial artery musculomucosal flap, are used for coverage. **(J–L)** At a second stage, deficient left alar is reconstructed with free auricular flap of ascending helix and root of helix. **(M,N)** Sixty-three months postinjury, after healing and edema subsided, a second forehead flap was done for nasal resurfacing. **(O,P)** He is seen 8 years after the initial injury with symmetric lips lacking any external or internal oral contractures, improved midface, nasal projection, and nasal appearance.

1. Comprehensive diagnosis from the outset, starting reconstruction from "scratch".
2. Adequate release of intraoral contracture a must, using FAMM flap and cutaneous portion of the free flap.
3. Reconstruction of stable bony platform.
4. Delayed use of second forehead flap for resurfacing.

Case example 4

A 39-year-old male presents with extensive left facial arteriovenous malformation (Fig. 18.5).

Diagnosis

He has a large deficit involving his cheek, upper and lower lip, intraoral lining, muscles of facial expression, and bony maxillary platform.

Reconstructive plan

This is a case of a planned multiple-stage reconstruction. He was primarily reconstructed using a tailored radial forearm folded flap, customized to defect with an alginate model. The folded portion was used for intraoral lining. Palmaris longus slings were used to suspend the lip and a contralateral FAMM flap was used for vermilion reconstruction. A planned delayed

reconstruction of the maxillary platform was performed using a free fibula flap with osseointegrated implant for future dental rehabilitation. This was complicated by dehiscence of the radial forearm flap from the lateral alar with exposed plate. An extended forehead flap including a hair-bearing segment which was initially planned for mustache reconstruction was also able to cover the cheek defect. He was seen at 6 months postoperatively with excellent cheek projection and a symmetric mustache. At the time, he was still lacking all the facial mimetic muscles and thus had an asymmetric smile. A functional platysma-submental flap based on the submental branch of the facial artery and the cervical branch of the facial nerve was used for cheek reconstruction. One week later, muscle function was evident; 2 years later, he achieved a symmetric smile and symmetric hair growth.

This case illustrates many principles of secondary facial reconstruction:

1. Comprehensive diagnosis from the outset.
2. Planning for a multiple-stage reconstruction from the start.
3. Use of alginate to model a three-dimensional volume loss and then converted to a two-dimensional defect on the donor site that can later be folded.
4. Use of FAMM flap for vermilion reconstruction.

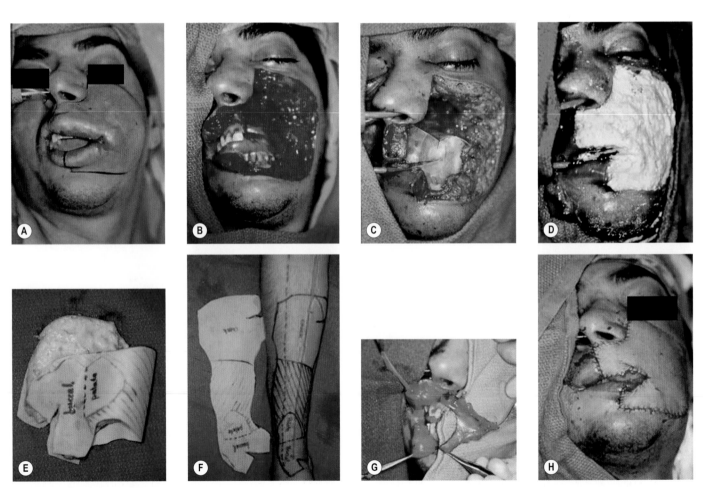

Fig. 18.5 (A) A 39-year-old male presents with extensive left facial arteriovenous malformation. **(B)** He has a large deficit involving his cheek, upper and lower lip, intraoral lining, muscles of facial expression, and bony maxillary platform. **(C,D)** He was primarily reconstructed using a tailored radial forearm folded flap, customized to the size, shape, and volume of the defect with an alginate model. **(E,F)** The folded portion was used for intraoral lining. **(G,H)** Palmaris longus slings were used to suspend the lip and a contralateral facial artery musculomucosal flap was used for vermilion reconstruction.

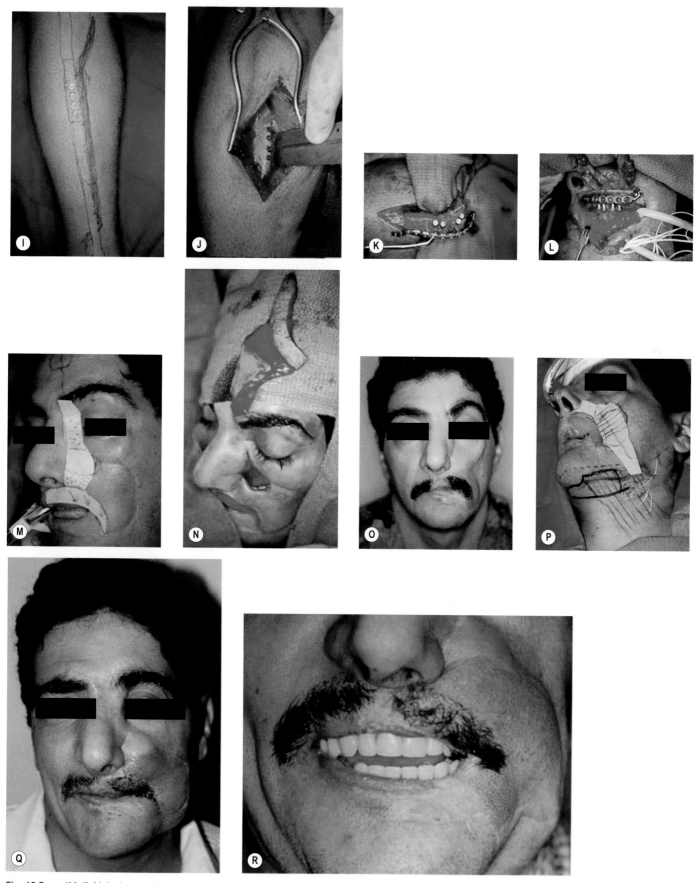

Fig. 18.5, cont'd (I–L) A planned delayed reconstruction of his maxillary platform was performed using a free fibula flap with osseointegrated implant for future dental rehabilitation. This was complicated by dehiscence of the radial forearm flap from the lateral alar with exposed plate. **(M,N)** An extended forehead flap, including a hair-bearing segment which was initially planned for mustache reconstruction, was also used to cover the cheek defect. **(O)** He was seen at 6 months postoperatively with excellent cheek project and symmetric mustache, though he still was missing all the facial mimetic muscles and had an asymmetric smile. **(P)** A functional platysma flap based on the submental branch of the facial artery and the cervical branch of the facial nerve was planned for cheek reconstruction. **(Q)** One week later, muscle twitching was evident. **(R)** Two years later, he achieved a symmetric smile and symmetric hair growth.

5. Reconstruction of stable bony platform with dental implants in place.

6. Delayed use of forehead flap for resurfacing both the cheek and mustache reconstruction.

7. Use of local flaps secondarily to provide better color match and hair-bearing segments.

As evident from the patients presented, each case of secondary reconstruction is unique. While thinking "outside the box" is no doubt necessary at times, adherence to the basic principles demonstrated above will help guide the reconstruction.

Postoperative care

Postoperative care for each patient is unique and depends on the specific procedure performed. In the early postoperative period, this uniformly involves flap monitoring, perioperative antibiotics, and appropriate scar management. It is usual and safe practice to allow the patient and the involved tissue to heal, the swelling to subside, and the scar to mature before embarking on another tertiary procedure.

Outcomes, prognosis, and complications

Multiple operations are often required to achieve a finally acceptable outcome. This is discussed in detail with the patient from the start and the plan modified on an "as needed" basis. Realistic goals need to be communicated. Depending on the complexity of reconstruction, the number of secondary revisions necessary ranges from 2–3 for relatively simple defects to exceeding 20–30 for more complex defects. Once composite tissue allotransplantation becomes more widely available, patients with certain defects, especially those involving the central triangle of the face, should be pursued as transplant candidates. As such, local and regional flap options might actually become "lifeboats".

On assessing our own outcomes, it is of foremost importance as reconstructive surgeons to listen to our patients as they serve as our best teachers. Persistent complaints following reconstruction can be a hint as to what we can do better. To that end, we must strive to reintegrate the patient back to normalcy through our reconstructive means.

Complications are, unfortunately, a part of performing any complex reconstruction. Especially in areas of previous irradiation and severe scarring, blood supply is suboptimal and donor vessels are lacking. As Millard preached in his writings, each reconstructive plan must have a lifeboat, preferably even a lifesaver in a lifeboat.[15] For this reason, when first approaching a problem, the surgeon should go through the mental exercise of considering all the different options before deciding on the best one. The other options, hence, will serve as lifeboats when they become needed.

🌐 Access the complete reference list online at   **http://www.expertconsult.com**

3. Pribaz JJ, Morris DJ, Mulliken JB. Three-dimensional folded free-flap reconstruction of complex facial defects using intraoperative modeling. *Plast Reconstr Surg.* 1994;93:285–293. *Multifaceted free flaps are often needed in the reconstruction of complex facial defects. The article describes a simple technique to determine both the volume of tissue required and the localization of the various epithelial surfaces, thereby simplifying these complex reconstructions using an intraoperative alginate moulage.*

7. Pribaz J, Stephens W, Crespo L, et al. A new intraoral flap: facial artery musculomucosal (FAMM) flap. *Plast Reconstr Surg.* 1992;90:421–429. *First description of the FAMM flap by Pribaz et al. combining the principles of nasolabial and buccal mucosal flaps. The flap has proven to be reliable based either superiorly (retrograde flow) or inferiorly (antegrade flow) to reconstruct a wide variety of difficult oronasal mucosal defects, including defects of the palate, alveolus, nasal septum, antrum, upper and lower lips, floor of the mouth, and soft palate.*

8. Taghinia AH, Movassaghi K, Wang AX, et al. Reconstruction of the upper aerodigestive tract with the submental artery flap. *Plast Reconstr Surg.* 2009;123:562–570. *The article demonstrates the versatility of FAMM flaps specifically in lip and vermilion reconstruction. While lip and vermilion are specialized tissues that cannot be easily reproduced,*

FAMM flap has features similar to those of lip tissue that makes it an option when such losses are encountered. In this article, the anatomy, dissection, and clinical applications for the use of the FAMM flap in lip and vermilion reconstruction are discussed.

11. Mathy JA, Pribaz JJ. Prefabrication and prelamination applications in current aesthetic facial reconstruction. *Clin Plast Surg.* 2009;36:493–505. *A review of prefabrication and prelamination techniques in facial reconstruction. Some of their unique abilities are presented, and their advantages, limitations, and technical pointers are provided. Relevant features and interdependencies among these procedures as they relate to aesthetic facial reconstruction are discussed.*

13. Pribaz JJ, Fine NA. Prelamination: defining the prefabricated flap – a case report and review. *Microsurgery.* 1994;15:618–623. *First paper to coin the term "prelamination" as modification of flaps prior to local or distant transfer were gaining wide acceptance. This article also clarifies the use of the term "prefabrication" which, until then, was used to describe all possible modifications. In this article, the term "prelamination" is used to refer to the implantation of tissue or other devices into a flap prior to transfer and suggests that prefabrication be restricted to the implantation of vascular pedicles.*

19

Facial transplant

Michael Sosin and Eduardo D. Rodriguez

Access video lecture content for this chapter online at expertconsult.com

SYNOPSIS

- Feasibility of face transplantation is well-established, and an extensive vetting process for candidate selection using a multidisciplinary team is recommended and likely to optimize patient outcomes.
- Most facial defects will not warrant face transplantation, but those patients considered for face transplantation should meet the established indications and avoid contraindications and relative contraindications described from the current experience.
- Face transplantation requires meticulous technical planning and practice using cadaveric and translational models. Computer aided techniques increase the precision of technical outcomes.
- Each facial defect and facial allograft is different; a combination of craniofacial, microsurgical, and aesthetic principles of plastic surgery should guide allograft design.
- Face transplantation improves patient's quality of life, but is not considered lifesaving.
- Allograft acute rejection is a phenomenon that must be recognized clinically and initiation of treatment should not be delayed.
- Standard maintenance immunosuppression includes orally administered tacrolimus, mycophenolate mofetil, and corticosteroids. Patients may deviate from the regimen based on co-morbidities and the side-effect profiles of immunosuppressive agents.
- Sensory and motor functions have a predictable pattern of restoration ranging from days to months, and months to years, respectively.

Introduction

Clinical face transplantation has entered its 12th year in existence and, as of June 2017 there have reportedly been 38 face transplants performed worldwide.[1] This constantly evolving surgical discipline is categorized as a specialty within a broader field known as vascularized composite tissue allotransplantation (VCA), defined as the transplantation of multiple tissue types including bones, cartilage, tendons, ligaments, muscles, nerves, blood vessels, and skin. Facial transplantation is reserved for a specific group of patients that have

suffered devastating facial deformity which is unable to be adequately reconstructed using traditional reconstructive techniques. Advances have been predicated on prior advances including techniques and experience gained in reconstructive microsurgery, innovation in new pharmacological agents in solid organ transplantation, and pioneering surgical approaches dedicated to improving their patients' quality of life, autonomy, and ability to socially integrate back into society. Although the burgeoning field continues to expand at a rapid pace, the broader application of face transplantation for patients in need has yet to occur. Understanding the fundamental principles of facial transplantation is crucial to interpreting outcomes and propelling future breakthroughs in the field. This chapter specifically focuses on providing the reader with a historical overview of facial VCA, ethical dilemmas, the process by which patients are evaluated for facial VCA candidacy, allograft design within anatomical and technological contexts, an overview of outcomes, immunology of face transplantation, and the future of the specialty.

Access the Historical Perspective section online at
http://www.expertconsult.com

Selection of patients

To consider a patient for face transplantation, a multidisciplinary team of specialists must evaluate multiple patient factors. Commonly, patients have sustained severely deforming facial injury and may have undergone multiple reconstructive procedures. The results of prior surgery often fail to meet patient and surgeon expectations. Consequently, patients will have lived with a facial deformity for years, often relegating them to psychological, social, and daily challenges. Aside from patients understanding the technical obstacles of performing such complex surgery, other purposes of the evaluation is to determine whether the patient fully understands the risks and benefits of face transplantation. The transplantation team must also assess the patient's ability to adhere to life-long medication and to cope with the changes of self-identity.

Once patients are identified to have facial disfigurement that is not amenable to microsurgical reconstruction, they are evaluated as potential candidates for face transplantation. Identification of absent facial subunits, specific components missing (such as bone, muscle, mucosa, etc.), and investigation of vascular integrity and anatomy are crucial in the initial evaluation. The patient will also undergo rigorous psychosocial evaluation including but not limited to:

a. Assessment of understanding and expectations of procedure and alternatives
b. Patient quality of life, behavioral trends
c. Cognitive ability
d. Coping skills
e. Body image
f. Medical compliance
g. Social support network
h. History or risk of substance abuse.

Involvement of the transplant surgical service, infectious disease specialty, radiologists, speech pathologists, social services, and a nutritionist provide an all-encompassing evaluation to optimize the patient selection process. Establishing a patient–provider relationship early in the evaluation process allows for the development of a sound relationship among team members and a long-term relationship between the patient and provider. A multidisciplinary approach cannot be overemphasized.

Indications

Early in face transplantation, specifically defined indications for performing the procedure were not defined, leaving most discretion to the surgeon and patient. Nevertheless, as more patients have undergone facial transplantation, a set a multiple conditions and patterns of facial defects have formed tangible indications for face transplantation. Moreover, enough time has elapsed since transplantation that complications associated with the care of face transplant patients have helped guide various centers in developing indications and contraindications. There are minor differences among the indications of various institutions that perform facial transplantation, but there is a broad consensus for most of the indications, which are presented in this chapter.

The Brigham and Women's Hospital institutional review board has openly described their protocol in selecting face transplant candidates. Indications for facial transplantation involved the most difficult or impossible defects to reconstruct, defects had to comprise greater than 25% of the facial area or involve the central face such as the eyelids, nose, or lips, and, lastly, patients had to have alternative reconstructive methods considered and deemed unfavorable or unsatisfactory.[16] Other groups have deviated from the 25% facial defect as necessary for transplantation. Rather, a closer examination by all groups has focused on the etiology of the facial deformity, which may vary considerably. Patients have undergone face transplants secondary to animal attacks (bear, dog, non-human primate), tumor (malignant and benign), burn

(thermal and electrical), ballistic and blunt trauma (Table 19.1).[1] Each select group of patients harbors inherent challenges. Preformed antibodies to multiple transfusions and skin grafts can make burn patients and trauma patients more difficult to find an ideal donor. Patients with malignancies are at an increased risk for developing recurrence of their malignancy, especially in the setting of chronic immunosuppression. As the field expands, the indications and set of injuries are likely to converge onto a specific subset of patients. Once outcomes become more predictable, surgeons may be more cavalier to expand the indications to incorporate a broader group of patients.

Absolute and relative contraindications

Indications for facial transplantation are largely balanced by the patient's benefit from the procedure outweighing the risks of surgery and life with allograft. However, contraindications vary amongst the various groups performing such procedures. Chronic conditions such as HIV and malignancy within a 5-year period remain absolute contraindications, and blindness is considered a controversial comorbidity to be transplanted.[1,15] In the setting of immunosuppression, the infectious complications and susceptibility to tumor growth and spread is considered extremely high for patients with HIV and malignancy.[16] Many of this data has been gleaned from the solid organ transplant literature, but also has been drawn from the some of the early face transplants performed. The Spanish group had transplanted an HIV-positive patient, which was initially considered a success.[17] Unfortunately, the patient developed recurrence of the initial malignancy, which led to his death.[18] Other chronic conditions are also considered when selecting patients for transplantation.

Blindness is considered a controversial topic among various groups in their willingness to transplant such patients. The condition in which a patient sustains facial deformity with blindness poses significant challenges such as inability to visualize biofeedback physiotherapy and the dangerous inability to recognize early signs of acute rejection. On the contrary, others[19,20] describe the principle of justice mandating that surgeons be obligated to provide facial reconstruction to blind patients, ultimately leading to a blind patient receiving a face transplant.[19] The challenges to the blind patient must be mitigated with extensive family support, which may limit the reintegration into society. Furthermore, the cost of failing to detect acute rejection or delayed presentation of acute rejection will result in decreased allograft longevity and is likely to result in chronic rejection, as seen in upper extremity/hand transplantation. This remains an ongoing controversy.

There are concerns of performing simultaneous upper extremity and face transplantation. Two patients, one from the French group[21] and another from the Brigham group[22], have undergone simultaneous bilateral hand transplantation and face transplantation. Both patients developed an early postoperative *Pseudomonas* infection, ultimately resulting in sepsis and death in one patient and sepsis leading to bilateral hand amputations and facial allograft survival in the other patient.[22] The issues related to simultaneous hand and face transplantation within a single stage surgery include a large antigenic burden, prolonged anesthesia time, large-volume

Text continued on p. 469

Table 19.1 Face transplants performed worldwide

	Team leader(s)	Date	Location	Recipient (age, sex)	Indication	Extent of defect	Functional deficit	Facial allograft	Death (cause, time from transplant)	Acute rejection (episodes)	Chronic rejection
1	Devauchelle and Dubernard	November, 2005	Amiens, France	38 years, Female	Dog bite	Cheek, nose, lips, chin	Labial competence, speech	Partial	Death	Yes (2)	Yes
2	Guo	April, 2006	Xi'an, China	30 years, Male	Bear bite	Cheek, nose, upper lip, maxilla, orbital wall, zygoma	-	Partial	Death (noncompliance, -)	Yes (3)	No
3	Lantieri	January, 2007	Paris, France	29 years, Male	Neurofibromatosis	Forehead, brows, eyelids, nose, lips, cheeks	Labial competence, speech	Partial	Alive	Yes (2)	No
4	Siemionow	December, 2008	Cleveland, OH, USA	45 years, Female	Ballistic trauma	Lower eyelids, nose, upper lip, orbital floor, zygoma, maxilla	Speech, eating	Partial	Alive	Yes (3)	No
5	Lantieri	March, 2009	Paris, France	27 years, Male	Ballistic trauma	Nose, lips, maxilla, mandible	Labial competence, speech	Partial	Alive	Yes (1)	No
6	Lantieri	April, 2009	Paris, France	37 years, Male	Third degree burn	Forehead, nose, eyelids, ears, cheek	Blink	Partial	Death (sepsis, 2 mo.)	No†	No
7	Pomahac	April, 2009	Boston, MA, USA	59 years, Male	Electrical burn	Lower eyelid, cheek, nose, lips, maxilla, zygoma	Labial competence, speech	Partial	Alive	Yes (3)	No
8	Lantieri	August, 2009	Paris, France	33 years, Male	Ballistic trauma	Cheek, nose, lips, maxilla, mandible	Labial competence, speech	Partial	Alive	Yes (1)	No
9	Cavadas	August, 2009	Valencia, Spain	42 years, Male	Cancer/radiation therapy	Lower lip, tongue, floor of mouth, mandible	Labial competence, speech	Partial	Death (cancer, -)	Yes (2)	No

Continued

Table 19.1 Face transplants performed worldwide—cont'd

	Team leader(s)	Date	Location	Recipient (age, sex)	Indication	Extent of defect	Functional deficit	Facial allograft	Death (cause, time from transplant)	Acute rejection (episodes)	Chronic rejection
10	Devauchelle and Dubernard	November, 2009	Amiens, France	27 years, Male	Ballistic trauma	Nose, lips, mandible	Labial competence, speech, eating	Partial	Alive	Yes (8)	Yes
11	Gomez-Cia	January, 2010	Seville, Spain	35 years, Male	Neurofibromatosis	Cheek, lips, chin, mandible	Labial competence, speech	Partial	Alive	Yes (1)	No
12	Barret	March, 2010	Barcelona, Spain	30 years, Male	Ballistic trauma	Eyelids, nose, lips, lacrimal apparatus, zygoma, maxilla, mandible	Labial competence, speech	Full	Alive	Yes (3)	No
13	Lantieri	June, 2010	Paris, France	35 years, Male	Neurofibromatosis	Eyelids, ears, nose, lips, oral mucosa	Blink, speech	Full	Alive	Yes (1)	No
14	Pomahac	March, 2011	Boston, MA, USA	25 years, Male	Electrical burn	Forehead, eyelids, left eye, nose, cheek, lips	Blink, speech	Full	Alive	Yes (3)	No
15	Lantieri	April, 2011	Paris, France	45 years, Male	Ballistic trauma	Nose, mandible, maxilla	Labial competence, speech	Partial	–	–	No
16	Lantieri	April, 2011	Paris, France	41 years, Male	Ballistic trauma	Nose, mandible, maxilla	Labial competence, speech	Partial	Death (suicide, 36 mo.)	–	No
17	Pomahac	April, 2011	Boston, MA, USA	30 years, Male	Electrical burn	Forehead, eyelids, nose, cheek, lips	Labial competence, speech	Full	Alive	Yes (5)	No
18	Pomahac	May, 2011	Boston, MA, USA	57 years, Female	Animal attack	Forehead, eyelids, eyes, nose, lips, maxilla, mandible	Blink, speech	Full	Alive	Yes (4)	No

Table 19.1 Face transplants performed worldwide—cont'd

	Team leader(s)	Date	Location	Recipient (age, sex)	Indication	Extent of defect	Functional deficit	Facial allograft	Death (cause, time from transplant)	Acute rejection (episodes)	Chronic rejection
19	Blondeel	December, 2011	Ghent, Belgium	54 years, Male	Ballistic trauma	Eyes, eyelid, cheek, nose, maxillae, mandible, lip	Speech, eating	Partial	Alive	Yes (1)	No
20	Ozkan	January, 2012	Antalya, Turkey	19 years, Male	Burn	Forehead, nose, cheeks, lips	-	Full	Alive	Yes (7)	No
21	Nasir	February, 2012	Ankara, Turkey	25 years, Male	Burn	-	-	Full	Alive	-	No
22	Ozmen	March, 2012	Ankara, Turkey	20 years, Female	Ballistic trauma	Nose, upper lip, maxilla, mandible	-	Partial	Alive	-	No
23	Rodriguez	March, 2012	Baltimore, MD, USA	37 years, Male	Ballistic trauma	Forehead, eyelids, nose, cheek, lips, zygoma, maxilla mandible	Speech, blink	Full	Alive	Yes (3)	No
24	Ozkan	May, 2012	Antalya, Turkey	34 years, Male	Thermal burn	Forehead, eyelids, nose, cheeks, lips	-	Full	Alive	Yes (-)	No
25	Devauchelle and Dubernard	September, 2012	Amiens, France	-, Female	Vascular tumor	Lower eyelid, maxilla, tongue	Eating	Partial	Alive	Yes (-)	No
26	Pomahac	February, 2013	Boston, MA, USA	44 years, Female	Chemical burn	Nose, lips, eyelids, forehead, cheek, ears, eyes, neck	Speech, blink, labial competence	Full	Alive	Yes (4)§	No
27	Maciejewski	May, 2013	Gliwice, Poland	32 years, Male	Blunt trauma	Nose, lips, eyelid, cheek, maxilla	Speech	Partial	Alive	Yes (1)	No
28	Ozkan	July, 2013	Antalya, Turkey	27 years, Male	Ballistic trauma	Forehead, eyelids, left eye, nose, cheek, mandible	-	Full	Alive	Yes (-)	No

Continued

Table 19.1 Face transplants performed worldwide—cont'd

	Team leader(s)	Date	Location	Recipient (age, sex)	Indication	Extent of defect	Functional deficit	Facial allograft	Death (cause, time from transplant)	Acute rejection (episodes)	Chronic rejection
29	Ozkan	August, 2013	Antalya, Turkey	54 years, Male	Ballistic trauma	Scalp, forehead, eyelids, nose, left eye, maxilla, mandible, tongue	-	Full	Death (lymphoma and respiratory failure, 12 mo.)	Yes (2)‡	No
30	Maciejewski	December, 2013	Gliwice, Poland	26 years, Female	Neurofibromatosis	Forehead, eyelids, nose, maxilla, lips, mandible	Speech, eating	Full	Alive	Yes (-)	No
31	Ozkan	December, 2013	Antalya, Turkey	22 years, Male	Ballistic trauma	Forehead, lips, nose, maxilla, mandible	-	Partial	Alive	Yes (-)	No
32	Pomahac	March, 2014	Boston, MA, USA	-, Male	Ballistic trauma	Forehead, nose, lips, lower face	Speech, eating	Full	Alive	Yes (5)	No
33	Papay	September, 2014	Cleveland, OH, USA	-, Male	Blunt trauma	Scalp, forehead, eyelids, nose, eye, maxilla, cheeks	Speech	Partial	Alive	Yes (1)	No
34	Pomahac	October, 2014	Boston, MA, USA	31 years, Male	Ballistic trauma	-	-	Full	Alive	Yes (2)	No
35	Barret	February, 2015	Barcelona, Spain	45 years, Male	Arteriovenous malformation	Lower face, neck, lips, tongue, pharynx	Speech	Full	Alive	-	No
36	-	May, 2015	St. Petersburg, Russia	-, Male	Electrical burn	Forehead, nose, lips		Partial	Alive	-	-
37	Rodriguez	August, 2015	New York, NY, USA	41 years, Male	Thermal burn	Scalp, forehead, eyelids, nose, cheeks, lower face, ears, lips, neck	Labial competence, blink	Full	Alive	No	No
38	Mardini	June, 2016	Rochester, MN, USA	32 years, Male	Ballistic trauma	Nose, cheeks, maxilla, lips, mandible, teeth	-	Partial	Alive	-	No

Reprinted with permission from Sosin M, Rodriguez ED. The face transplantation update: 2016. *Plast Reconstr Surg.* 2016;137:1841–1850.
†Discrepancy between reports. The patient was described as having skin biopsy findings of grade I rejection with ongoing graft ischemia and another report stating no clinical rejection was evident.
‡Underwent removal of allograft and had an anterolateral thigh flap for coverage of the facial wound.
§Antibody-mediated rejection was observed in this patient.

resuscitation, and impaired cortical adaptation.[23,24] However, these issues are not supported by well conducted studies and remain anecdotal explanations for such poor outcomes. Interestingly, the other VCA experiences and animal models offer refutable data to each of the aforementioned concerns. The amount of transplanted tissue has shown to have a positive impact in animal models[25] and clinical solid organ transplants[26–28]. Extensive face transplants with successful outcomes[29,30] continue to contradict the theory of antigenic burden and the concerns of extended anesthesia time and requirement of blood products during allograft procurement.[31] Both the France and Boston groups propose a more cautious approach to patients requiring combined hand and face transplants by performing staged transplantations.[22]

Other relative contraindications with a larger ethical dilemma may surface. These issues include a recent history of substance abuse or severe depression, which pose many challenges to the patient. A major psychological burden of face transplantation on self-identity, impact on mental and physical health, and need for adherence to strict lifelong medication may act as stressors that may cause substance abuse and depression to resurface. Careful psychiatric evaluation must elucidate whether depression is secondary to the facial deformity or if the patient's depression has an organic etiology preceding the facial deformity. Despite the transformative potential of face transplantation, prior depression and suicidal attempts should limit the application of face transplantation. This has been recognized firsthand by Lantieri et al. reporting one of their patients (from a series of seven patients) eventually committing suicide after a prior attempt pre-transplant.[32] However, the overwhelming positive outlook from patients that undergo facial VCA is well-established. Following face transplantation, patients have a decreased prevalence of depression and verbal abuse, improved body image, quality of life, sense of self, are able to reintegrate socially, and some return to work.[12,32–39]

Once the patient has passed the screening process for facial transplantation and is selected as a candidate recipient for facial VCA, immunological testing is pursued. Once a potential donor is identified, HLA-testing, donor-recipient crossmatch, and donor specific antibody (DSA) titers are obtained. Historically, partial HLA-compatibility with a negative crossmatch and low DSA reactivity was considered a universal practice in VCA, but the last several years have challenged these principles. Similar to kidney transplantation, a donor-recipient crossmatch is completed with peripheral blood using flow cytometry.[40,41] However, peripheral blood crossmatching may potentially have increased false negative results, especially in patients exposed to multiple transfusions.[42] This has led to most VCA centers adopting the use of donor lymph nodes in the majority of transplantation procedures.[40] Achieving an immunologically compatible donor amongst a small donor pool is even further narrowed by skin tone, hair color, cephalometrics, and age.

In addition to antigenic compatibility, the consequences of Epstein–Barr virus (EBV) and cytomegalovirus (CMV) mismatches have elucidated themselves as important factors in the immunosuppressed patient. It is postulated that the propensity of the skin endothelium to retain a greater viral load relative to endothelial cells of the kidney, liver, or heart allografts contributes to an increased risk of rejection.[43] Hand and kidney transplantation demonstrates a high incidence of CMV infection.[44] This been implicated as the nidus of an immune response within the allograft and associated with decreased graft survival.[45–47] Cytomegalovirus mismatches have been reported in at least nine face transplant patients[47] leading to ganciclovir-resistant and valganciclovir-resistant infection in two patients.[35] Additionally, CMV seropositivity is problematic because the treatment of CMV viremia involves decreasing immunosuppression, which may itself predispose the patient to rejection.[47,48]

The risk of *de novo* malignancy is increased in immunosuppressed solid organ transplant recipients approximately two to four times compared with that of age-matched controls.[49] Moreover, EBV naïve recipients receiving EBV-positive allografts may carry an increased risk of developing a future malignancy.[47] The clinical VCA experience has largely focused on technical aspects of surgery and viral status has poorly been reported. Of two known recipients who were mismatched for EBV,[1,37] one patient (Amiens, France) developed a monoclonal B-cell lymphoma at several months post-transplant, requiring Rituximab and reduction of immunosuppression.[50,51] Although EBV status was not reported, Ozkan reported one patient that developed post-transplant lymphoproliferative disorder (PTLD) (a known consequence of immunosuppression and EBV infection), which was followed by graft failure requiring an ALT flap for coverage of the patient's facial wound and ultimately resulting in the patient's death.[1] With the limited experience of viral mismatching and poor outcomes, it is recommended that CMV and EBV mismatching be avoided, particularly as patients require lifelong immunosuppression.

Technical approach

Defect assessment

Evaluation of a potential face transplant recipient involves conducting a thorough assessment of the craniomaxillofacial injury. Commonly, patients with composite tissue loss will have a deficit of bone and skin with variable involvement of essential functional anatomy inevitably impacting deglutition, respiration, oral competence, and blinking. Previously, a classification system designed for oncologic midface defects was proposed as a system to stratify patients being evaluated for face transplantation. Although this system was popularized for selection of free tissue transfer for midface defects, there were shortcomings in its application for face transplantation. Specifically, the defects of candidates being evaluated for face transplantation seem to vary drastically as compared with those defects created surgically from oncologic resections.

A more encompassing classification system was described by Mohan et al.[52] with a goal of predicting the optimal transplant design. This system was developed from the experience of actual face transplants performed worldwide. Although this algorithmic approach is broad, it serves as a primer to the surgeon in considering pattern of injury, principles of aesthetic subunit(s) design, and incorporates an already familiar Le Fort-based classification scheme. The diagram in Fig. 19.1 details this classification system and illustrates the extent of hard tissue and soft tissue defects.

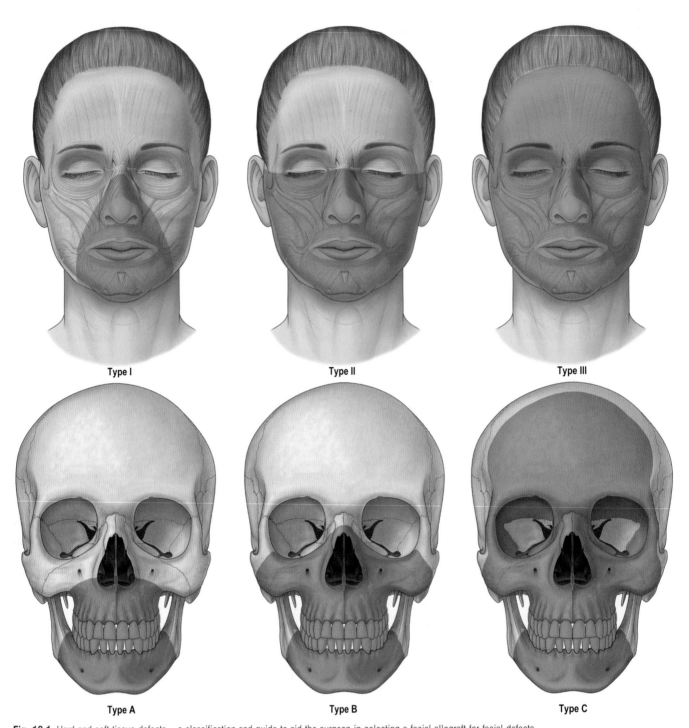

Type I   Type II   Type III

Type A   Type B   Type C

Fig. 19.1 Hard and soft tissue defects – a classification and guide to aid the surgeon in selecting a facial allograft for facial defects.

Imaging and operative planning

Preparation for facial allograft design and the completion of a successful procedure involves the use of cutting edge technology, cadaveric surgical simulations, and anatomical perfusion studies. In order to achieve optimal functional and aesthetic outcomes, a planning process is essential. The principles of craniofacial surgery, aesthetic surgery, and microsurgery help guide the allograft design process. Rigid fixation of the facial buttress is the basis for soft tissue reconstruction.

Special attention should be made to preserve ligamentous and canthal attachments to mitigate the degree of ptosis and maintain muscular insertions to best sustain facial animation, and, ultimately, allograft survival is dependent upon healthy perfusion of the allograft.

Preparation for transplantation should incorporate multiple radiologic and technological adjuncts. This includes a three-dimensional craniomaxillofacial computerized tomographic scan, a triple phase angiogram to evaluate arterial and venous anatomy, and CAD/CAM technologies are strongly

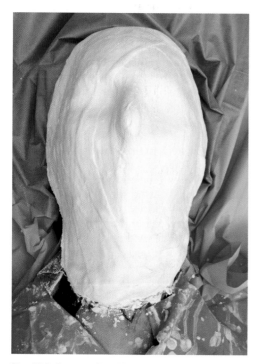

Fig. 19.2 Donor mask mold reservoir creation.

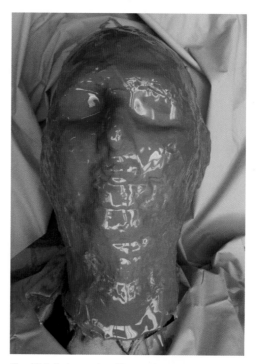

Fig. 19.3 Donor mask mold reservoir creation continued.

recommended to precisely design osteotomy site location, print cutting guides, and allow for re-evaluation of mock transplantation for attaining optimal outcomes. With multiple technical strategies of allograft preparation, recipient preparation, and allograft inset exist, the tenets of craniofacial, microsurgical, and aesthetic surgery are reviewed below in describing surgical principles of face transplantation.

Synchronization of teams

The ideal donor is able to provide multiple organs for life saving procedures, in addition to providing a life-altering facial allograft. Due to the nature of face transplantation being the most novice specialty, the onus of establishing an organized team approach for all transplant teams relies on the reconstructive surgeon. It is well-established that simultaneous allograft preparation of the face, chest organs, and abdominal organs is feasible and has technically been successful. However, optimization of timing can minimize cold ischemia time and it is recommended for the facial allograft to be harvested prior to cross-clamping of the aorta, with immediate division of the allograft pedicles prior to aortic cross-clamping.

Mask

Formulation of a silicone-based prosthetic mask is typically fashioned prior to any allograft procurement (Fig. 19.2–19.5). This allows for coverage of the donor defect upon completion of the procedure, and it also provides a dignified means of transportation from the operating room facilitating a dignified return of the remains for the family of the deceased.

Surgical planning

Pre-operative computed tomography scans are obtained of the donor and recipient to develop a virtual surgical plan. This provides optimal design of Le Fort III osteotomies, bilateral mandibular sagittal split osteotomies, or uniquely designed osteotomies specific to the patient's specific bony deficit (Figs. 19.6 & 19.7). Additionally, stereolithographic models of the recipient can be manufactured for intraoperative use to ascertain the precision of the allograft. Specific cutting-guides

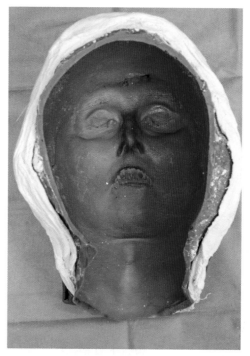

Fig. 19.4 Donor mask mold reservoir created. *(Printed with permission from and copyrights retained by Eduardo D. Rodriguez, M.D., D.D.S.)*

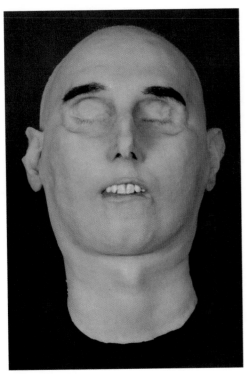

Fig. 19.5 Donor mask. *(Printed with permission from and copyrights retained by Eduardo D. Rodriguez, M.D., D.D.S.)*

are processed and manufactured for all recipient and donor osteotomy sites to decrease operative time and foster more precise apposition (Fig. 19.8).

Donor allograft recovery

The description of allograft preparation will vary based upon patient defect. The description below provides an overview of a total face allograft harvest with variation in anatomic components included and excluded.

Neck and lower face

Markings are made on the donor to incorporate the neck and total face, which should avoid inclusion of the tracheostomy site. Skin markings are crucial to hide or camouflage, to better foster an aesthetically pleasing result with inconspicuous scars. Neck incisions are placed over the sternal notch extending bilaterally just above the clavicles, ascending along the posterolateral portions of the neck to the pre-auricular region. Markings are completed below the occipital groove of the posterior hairline and sagittally in the midline, or in a coronal fashion within the frontal hair bearing region depending on whether the scalp is or is not included within the allograft, respectively. An incision is made along the right neck and a subplatysmal flap is elevated. The external vein is dissected and ligated. If the greater auricular nerve is encountered, it is dissected, divided, and saved for the inset of donor tissue as a potential nerve allograft. The sternocleidomastoid muscle is retracted laterally to identify the carotid sheath and its contents. The internal jugular vein is identified and dissected cranially to identify the thyrolingual facial trunk (Fig. 19.9). All branch points of the external carotid artery are also dissected cephalad to preserve the facial, occipital (if scalp is included), and lingual arteries (if the tongue is incorporated within the allograft). The sternocleidomastoid muscle may then be sharply divided as the caudal dissection proceeds to identify branches of the external carotid artery (Fig. 19.10). As mentioned earlier, division of the superior thyroid, ascending pharyngeal and associated arteries allow for mobilization of the allograft. If the lingual artery is preserved, it should be dissected to the tongue base throughout its trajectory within the mylohyoid muscle. Sacrificing the posterior auricular artery should only occur once the occipital artery has been identified. Encountering the anterior and posterior bellies of the digastrics muscle and hypoglossal nerve is expected, and division is necessary to expose the tortuous course of the facial artery (Fig. 19.11). Division of the digastric muscle laterally facilitates exposure of the submandibular gland, duct and

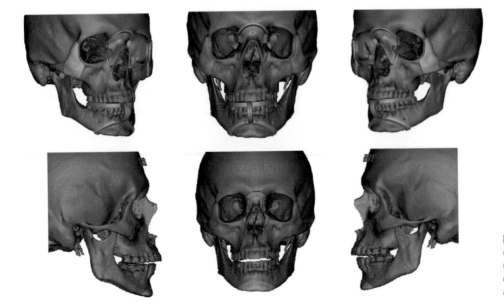

Fig. 19.6 Recipient osteotomy preparation using computerized surgical planning to design cutting guides. *(Printed with permission from and copyrights retained by Eduardo D. Rodriguez, M.D., D.D.S.)*

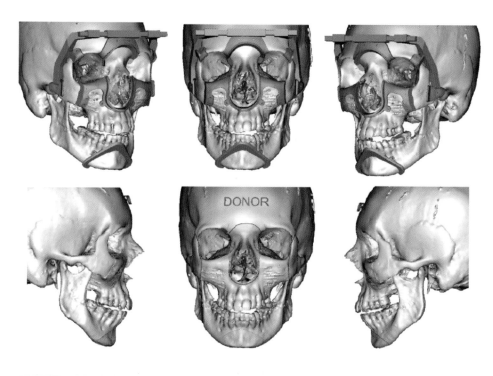

Fig. 19.7 Donor osteotomy preparation using computerized surgical planning to design cutting guides. *(Printed with permission from and copyrights retained by Eduardo D. Rodriguez, M.D., D.D.S.)*

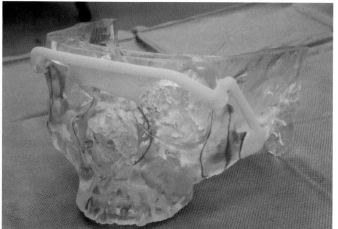

Fig. 19.8 Stereolithic 3D template of the donor for development of ideal cutting guides.

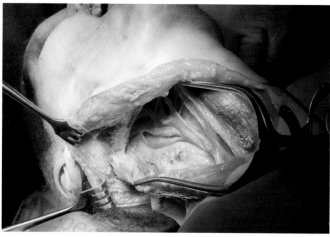

Fig. 19.10 Donor dissection of the arterial anatomy showing the external carotid artery and its branches.

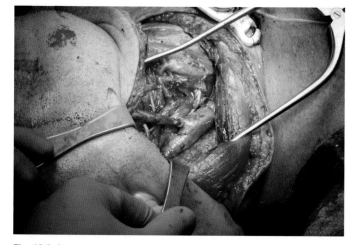

Fig. 19.9 Donor dissection of the venous anatomy showing the internal jugular vein and thyrolingual facial trunk.

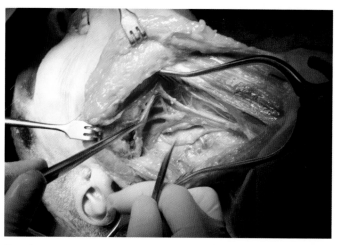

Fig. 19.11 Encountering the digastric muscle during the donor dissection; this is divided to expose the distal arterial branches.

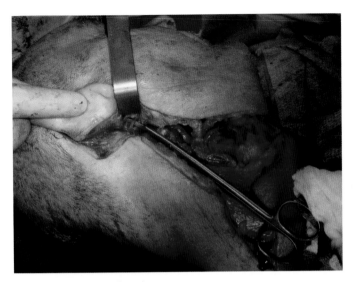

Fig. 19.12 Facial nerve dissection.

vessels, which are ligated and divided excluding the submandibular gland from the allograft. The hypoglossal nerve should be preserved as a potential nerve allograft during inset. The posterior branch of the facial vein is dissected cranially where the mandibular division of the facial nerve is identified and protected.

The neck incision is extended to a pre-auricular incision or around the neck laterally if the ears and scalp are incorporated within the allograft. If the pre-auricular dissection is pursued, it is carried down to the sub-superficial musculoaponeurotic system plane to identify the parotidomasseteric fascia. Meticulous dissection allows for visualization of Stensen's duct, which is ligated and divided, excluding the parotid duct from the allograft. All facial nerve branches are identified and dissected free individually (Fig. 19.12). If the ears and scalp are included, the dissection continues cranially along the occipital artery to identify its deeper course in the occipital groove posterolateral to the mastoid process (Fig. 19.13). Extensive retraction of a thick musculocutaneous flap is required laterally to expose the occipital vessels. The facial nerve, superficial temporal artery, and internal maxillary artery are therefore identified later in the dissection. For allografts incorporating a bilateral sagittal split osteotomy of the mandible, the pterygomasseteric sling is incised and stripped from the mandible. The internal maxillary artery is ligated and divided at this point to minimize blood loss during future Le Fort III osteotomies. Each dissection must be completed bilaterally prior to moving forward with allograft preparation.

If the tongue is included, an incision is made to the floor of the mouth along the lingual mucosa bilaterally to the tongue base. Dissection proceeds to identify the lingual nerves and divide them, while avoiding any injury to the lingual arteries. Lateral dissection allows for the alveolar ridge to be exposed and a connecting incision of the soft palate cranially allows for the pterygoids to be exposed. This perioral dissection is saved for a later point if the ears and scalp are included. Following elevation of the ears and scalp, attention is then drawn to the hair bearing scalp.

Scalp

Gentle elevation and flexion at the neck allows for the posterior midline scalp to be incised down to the subperiosteal layer. The scalp is elevated bilaterally (Fig. 19.14) and continues until the sub-superficial temporal fascia is reached. Care is taken to not violate this plane as the superficial temporal artery and vein are protected and maintained within the allograft, while excluding the temporalis muscle from the allograft. Subperiosteal elevation continues to the supraorbital rim, and a portion of the zygomaticofrontal process, zygomatic arch, and lateral orbital rim are exposed. The supraorbital and supratrochlear neurovascular contents are ligated and divided. Attention should then return to the posterior periosteal scalp elevation which continues laterally to elevate the occipital artery from the occipital groove and the ears bilaterally if attachments still remain.

Periorbital region

The eyelid structures are dissected through a transconjunctival incision. Dissection of the lower eyelid continues in a

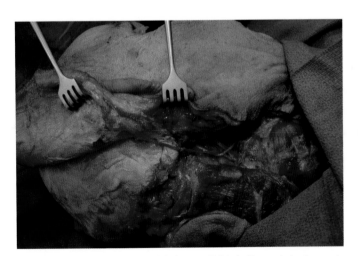

Fig. 19.13 Identification of the occipital artery. *(Printed with permission from and copyright retained by Eduardo D. Rodriguez, M.D., D.D.S.)*

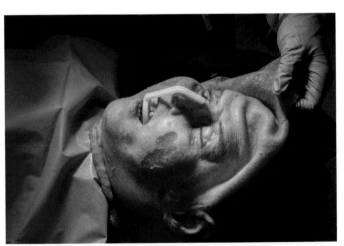

Fig. 19.14 Scalp elevation is completed bilaterally with an incision made down the middle from the vertex caudad to reach the neck allowing for adequate elevation of the allograft.

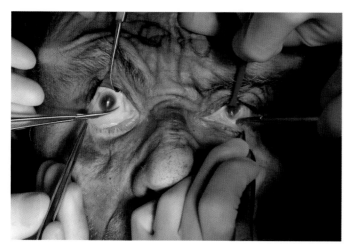

Fig. 19.15 Eyelid dissection – transconjuctival dissection.

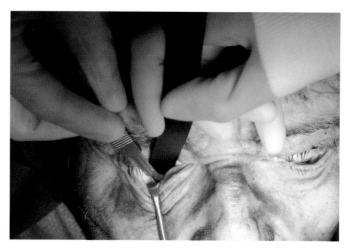

Fig. 19.17 Eyelid dissection – dissection proceeds to maintain the superior and inferior tarsal plates along with underlying orbicularis oculi muscle.

subseptal plane down to the inferior orbital rim. The upper eyelid dissection preserves the tarsus, levator palpebrae superioris, septum, and orbicularis oculi and meets the superior orbital rim. The similar lower eyelid dissection is completed to preserve the tarsal plate and orbicularis oculi meeting the inferior orbital rim (Fig. 19.15–19.17).

A coronal incision is then made in the hair-bearing region to connect the pre-auricular incisions bilaterally, if the ears and scalp are excluded from the allograft. The soft tissue of the forehead is caudally elevated in the subperiosteal plane to expose the nasofrontal segment. Care is taken not to disrupt the medial canthal attachments. The coronal incisions and the eyelid incisions are connected and the inferolateral orbital rim is stripped of soft tissue attachments. Additionally, the lateral canthal tendons are tagged and cut. Le Fort III cutting-guides are then placed over the nasofrontal and bilateral orbitozygomatic segments (Fig. 19.18).

If the ears and scalp are incorporated, the facial nerve, superficial temporal artery, and internal maxillary artery are identified via lateral access directed medially from the elevated ears. Medial retraction of the allograft facilitates a deeper dissection in the sub-superficial musculoaponeurotic system

plane of the superior pole of the parotid gland, without violating the parotid-masseteric fascia. The parotid duct and vascular branches are ligated and divided, and the facial nerve trunk is tagged and divided to preserve maximum length. The superficial temporal artery is also identified to avoid inadvertent injury. Typically, the internal maxillary artery is able to be identified and divided during initial external carotid artery branch dissection, but if it was unable to be identified, the internal maxillary artery can be identified, ligated, and divided at this point. At this juncture, prefabricated cutting-guides must be approximated for appropriate fit, which can only be ensured through adequate soft tissue exposure. Once proper hardware engagement is achieved, screw fixation of the cutting-guides is reserved for after the intraoral and eyelid dissections are completed.

Intraoral

A circumferential intraoral incision is made along the gingivobuccal mucosal junction to preserve as much mucosa as possible while avoiding the parotid papillae, bilaterally.

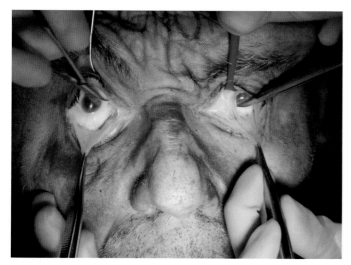

Fig. 19.16 Eyelid dissection – continued.

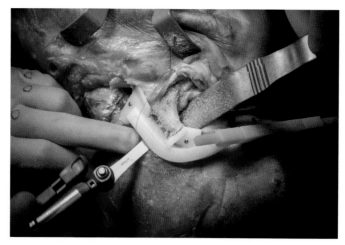

Fig. 19.18 Eyelid dissection – lateral canthii are identified with polypropylene suture and divided allowing for completion of osteotomies.

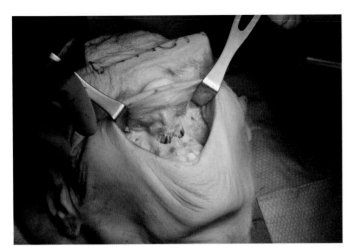

Fig. 19.19 An intraoral incision with elevation of a subperiosteal dissection of the maxilla exposes the infraorbital neurovascular contents.

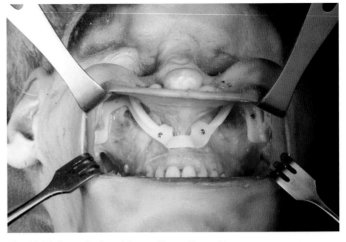

Fig. 19.21 Screw fixation of the maxillary cutting guide.

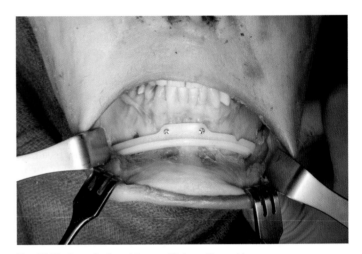

Fig. 19.22 Screw fixation of the mandibular cutting guide.

The maxilla is exposed through elevation of an osteomucosal flap to expose potential sites for osteotomies and/or cutting guide placement. Exposure of the orbitozygomatic region and anterior surface of the maxilla to expose the infraorbital foramen content is then completed (Fig. 19.19). If exposure is inadequate, snap-fit cutting guides may not be positioned properly. Further exposure is achieved through flap elevation to allow for engagement of hardware. Throughout the inferior mucosal incision, the dissection continues to the submucosa down to the mandibular symphysis for enough subperiosteal elevation to accommodate a genial segment cutting-guide (Fig. 19.20). Preservation of the mentalis muscle insertion is attempted but not always possible depending on the size of the cutting guides. The submucosal dissection must be completed laterally to divide all remaining circumferential attachments of the buccinator to complete the intraoral mucosal dissection.

Contour engagement of prefabricated cutting-guides confirms proper anatomic alignment, which is followed by screw fixation and osteotomies of the orbitozygomatic, zygomaticomaxillary, transverse maxillary, nasofrontal, and genial regions (Fig. 19.21–19.25). Infrahyoid strap muscles are then divided inferiorly liberating the allograft from all soft tissue attachments besides the bilateral vascular pedicles. Bilateral ligation and division of the internal jugular veins and external carotid arteries completes final allograft liberation.

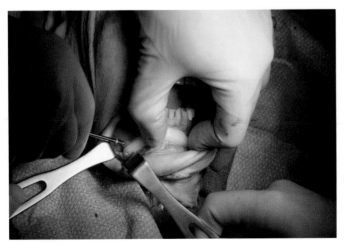

Fig. 19.20 Exposure of the mandibular symphysis and screw fixation of the cutting guide allows for a precise chin osteotomy.

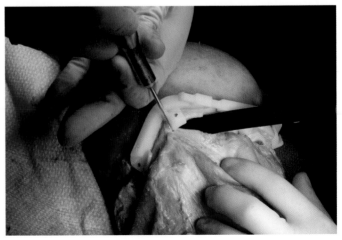

Fig. 19.23 Screw fixation of the orbitozygomatic and nasofrontal cutting guide.

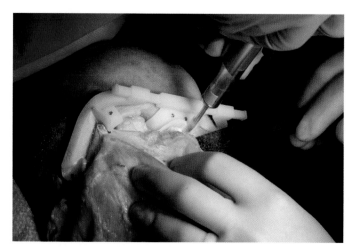

Fig. 19.24 Nasofrontal osteotomy completion with the soft tissue of the allograft protected.

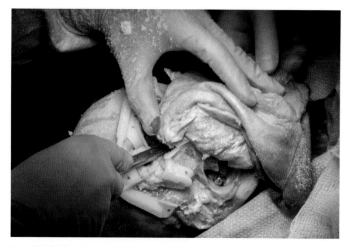

Fig. 19.26 Trimming of the allograft along the nasal septum.

Osteotomies

Allografts encompassing bilateral sagittal split osteotomies are completed through an intra- and extraoral approach. The inferior alveolar nerve is identified and divided as proximally as possible. As described earlier, Le Fort III cutting-guides can be snap-fit into place or anatomic position can be checked using an intraoperative navigation system to confirm precise placement of osteotomies. Bone cuts are made anterior to the zygomatic arches and posterior to the orbital rims. The nasofrontal osteotomy is created posterior to the medial canthus and the canalicular drainage system if possible. Completion of the Le Fort III osteotomy involves the pterygomaxillary junctions, which are cut to mobilize the bony segment of maxillomandibular complex. This freely separates, although the nasal septum may require trimming (Fig. 19.26). Any soft tissue attachments must be divided (Fig. 19.27) to leave only the vascular pedicles in continuity. At this juncture, the external carotid arteries and the internal jugular veins are ligated and divided bilaterally, ultimately liberating the allograft (Fig. 19.28–19.31). It is placed on the back table in an ice-water bath of preservation solution and immediately irrigated with tissue preservation solution (Figs. 19.32 & 19.33).

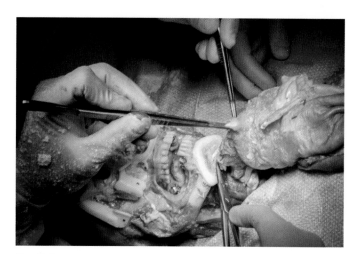

Fig. 19.27 Strap muscles and submandibular soft tissue remain intact.

Recipient preparation

The recipient preparation begins at the same time as the donor operation, but there are several distinct differences that are highlighted. Maximal preservation of neurovascular structures are typically preserved within the recipient defect. Stensen's

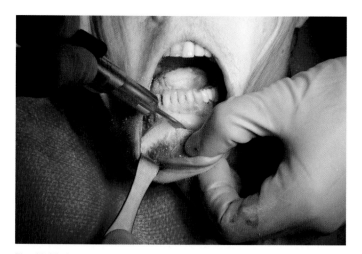

Fig. 19.25 Completion of the mandibular osteotomy.

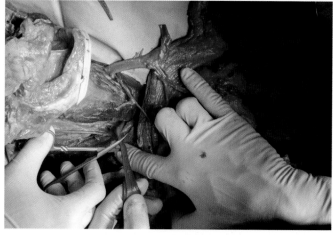

Fig. 19.28 Prior to division of the allograft pedicles.

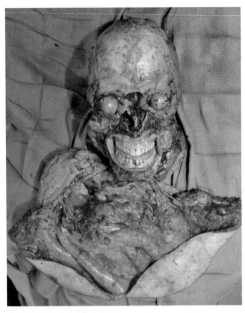

Fig. 19.29 Elevation of the allograft with bilateral pedicles intact. *(Printed with permission from and copyright retained by Eduardo D. Rodriguez, M.D., D.D.S.)*

duct is also preserved when possible. The coronal incision is carried to a more superficial plane to preserve the frontalis and orbicularis oculi. If a coronal incision is not utilized, then the defect is usually larger and accommodates the scalp and ears. All skin of the donor is typically de-epithelialized and scar tissue excised. All nerve branches are divided as distally as possible including the zygomatic, buccal, and mandibular branches of the facial nerve, as well as the sensory nerves, including the infraorbital, supraorbital nerves, and supra-trochlear nerves. Osteotomies will incorporate normal bone

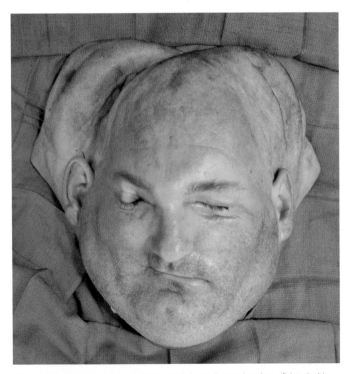

Fig. 19.30 Allograft resting on the donor defect prior to elevation. *(Printed with permission and copyrights retained by Eduardo D. Rodriguez, M.D., D.D.S.)*

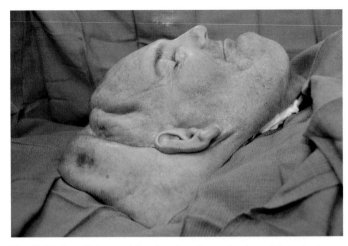

Fig. 19.31 A profile image of the allograft resting on the donor defect prior to elevation. *(Printed with permission from and copyrights retained by Eduardo D. Rodriguez, M.D., D.D.S.)*

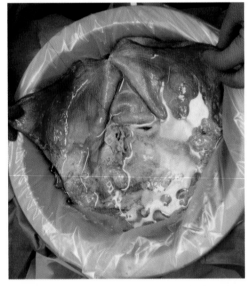

Fig. 19.32 The allograft placed onto back table in an ice-water bath of preservation solution.

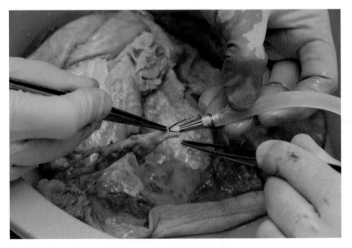

Fig. 19.33 Preservation solution is infused into the allograft.

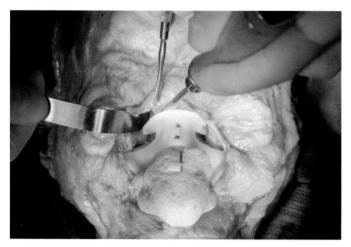

Fig. 19.34 Recipient defect preparation includes de-epithelialization and scar excision, and fixation of cutting guides.

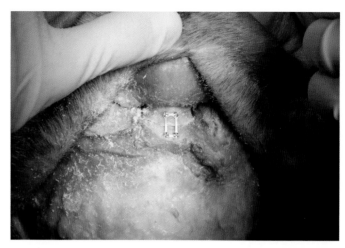

Fig. 19.36 Allograft inset – nasofrontal allograft fixation.

along defect edges at the cost of achieving better anatomic approximation with healthy wound edges (Figs. 19.34 & 19.35).

Allograft inset

Once both teams have completed their respective operative portions, the allograft is transferred to the recipient operating room where the allograft inset begins. Rigid fixations of bony elements are completed, including the nasofrontal complex (Fig. 19.36), the orbitozygomatic regions, and the mandibles (if included). Next, nerve coaptations are completed. Nerves

repaired will vary depending on the recipient functional deficits. Laying sensory nerves of the infraborbital and supraorbital nerves over their respective foramena may be required if a nerve coaptation is not feasible. Following this, the vascular anastomoses are completed with the arterial and venous pedicles anastomosed on one side, then the other. The soft tissue of the face is then re-draped and retaining sutures are placed within areas of excess tissue laxity or mobility. The lateral canthal tendons are fixed at the zygomaticofrontal sutures approximately 1 mm above the medial canthal tendon. The rest of the eyelid structures are gently re-draped and the skin is sutured in place (Figs. 19.37 & 19.38).

Immunosuppression and rejection

The concepts of transplant immunology are beyond the scope of this chapter, but an understanding of the breadth of medications and their timely use is crucial. Immunosuppression

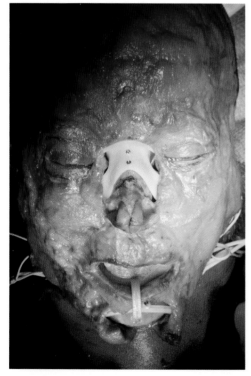

Fig. 19.35 Recipient preparation after nasal and mandibular osteotomies have been completed. *(Printed with permission from and copyright retained by Eduardo D. Rodriguez, M.D., D.D.S.)*

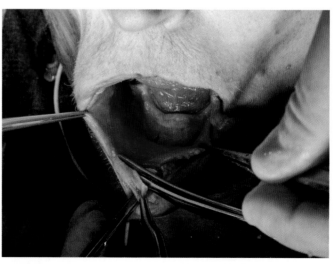

Fig. 19.37 Allograft inset – intraoral trimming of the allograft to conceal the incisional scar. *(Printed with permission from and copyright retained by Eduardo D. Rodriguez, M.D., D.D.S.)*

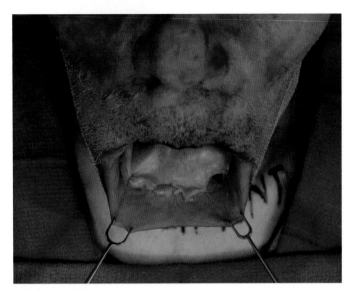

Fig. 19.38 Allograft inset – intraoral apposition of mucosa. *(Printed with permission from and copyright retained by Eduardo D. Rodriguez, M.D., D.D.S.)*

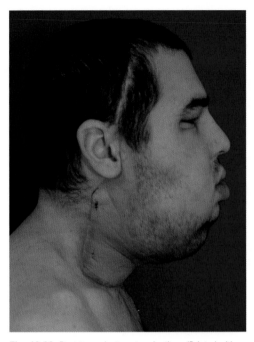

Fig. 19.39 Post-transplant acute rejection. *(Printed with permission from and copyrights retained by Eduardo D. Rodriguez, M.D., D.D.S.)*

medications can be divided into three categories: induction therapy, maintenance therapy, and rejection therapy. Typically, prior to transplantation, patients will receive an induction immunosuppressive regimen just prior to the transplantation in an attempt to blunt a lymphocytic response immediately post transplantation. Induction medications include antithymocyte globulin, or an anti-IL-2R α chain antibodies (daclizumab or basiliximab), or anti-CD52 (alemtuzumab), with or without varying combinations of mycophenolate mofetil (MMF) and FK506 (tacrolimus) and corticosteroids. Recently, anti-CD20 has been incorporated in the induction therapy protocol.[30]

Following induction therapy and completion of the transplant, patients will begin maintenance therapy consisting of tri-therapy combining mycophenolate mofetil (MMF) and FK506 (tacrolimus) and steroids. The degree of tapering and minimization of medications is tempered by the concern for patients developing an episode of acute rejection. Additionally, the metabolic side effect profile of these medications has led to acute and chronic kidney injury, diabetes mellitus, and infection.[53,54] This has prompted groups to utilize different strategies to avoid corticosteroids, and deviate from incorporating FK506 and implementing less nephrotoxic agents such as sirolimus or everolimus.[53] Despite attempts of maintenance therapy, nearly all face transplants have manifested a process known as acute rejection.

The skin has long been considered the most antigenic tissue relative to other tissues of the human body.[55] It has become well-established that the skin of the allograft is the main target of early acute rejection.[56–59] Acute rejection is recognized clinically via physical examination as erythematous macules, diffuse redness, or asymptomatic papules over the transplanted skin.[56,59,60] Early in the recovery process, residual inflammation and edema may persist and confound the physical exam (Figs. 19.39 & 19.40). Routine skin biopsies can guide the surgical team regarding suspicion for acute rejection. Early evidence of rejection is seen with perivascular lymphocytic infiltrates in the dermis. The predominant cells

are CD3+/CD4+ T-cells with occasional CD8+ cytotoxic T-cells, FoxP3+ T-regulatory cells, and CD68+ histiomonocytic cells of recipient origin. Rejection from the dermis will progress to the epidermis and then to the hypodermis if left untreated.[47] As the severity of rejection increases, epidermal findings will include keratinocyte apoptosis, necrosis, and vacuolization. Microscopically, nonspecific changes involve mainly dermis and epidermis, and gradations of involvement

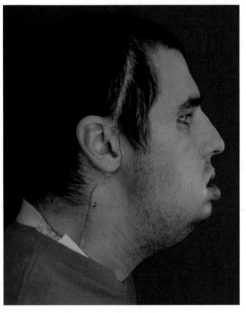

Fig. 19.40 Quiescence of allograft edema and erythema following acute rejection treatment. *(Printed with permission from and copyrights retained by Eduardo D. Rodriguez, M.D., D.D.S.)*

can complicate pathologic interpretation.[61] Based on histologic findings, a consensus scoring system known as the Banff classification[56] has been established to assess the severity of acute rejection, but there are limitations to relying on this system for treating acute rejection in the context of facial VCA. Some groups have investigated the utility of mucosal biopsies[61,62] and sentinel skin graft.[63] Both approaches have not replaced the gold standard of the allograft skin biopsy.

Once recognized, the treatment of acute rejection involves pulse intravenous steroids, and will typically require an increase in the dosing of a maintenance immunosuppression regimen. Adjunct FK506 topical based therapy has also been utilized for directed therapy to the skin. Most rejection within the face transplant literature focuses on acute rejection, its frequency, and implication of severity. However, as time has progressed, newer entities of rejection have declared themselves including: antibody-mediated rejection and chronic rejection. These entities remain enigmatic and challenging to treat.[64,65]

Pediatric facial VCA

The expansion of facial VCA to pediatric facial transplantation has been proposed by several groups and remains controversial. The largest hesitation of performing facial VCA in children pertains to the lifelong requirement of immunosuppressive medication and the long-term adverse risks of developing hypertension, dyslipidemia, cardiovascular disease, malignancy, osteoporosis, renal failure, and other systemic effects. It is well-established that children burdened with craniofacial deformity involving facial burns, capillary vascular malformations, hemifacial microsomia, and neurofibromatosis have impaired quality of life early in life and into adulthood.[66] Although allotransplantation of non-vital organs is a controversial issue in part due to synchronized skeletal growth of the patient and the allograft and development impairment associated with transplantation,[67] the principle drawback of pediatric face transplantation is noncompliance. The need for independence, known rebellious phase, and state of invulnerability is typical of adolescence and early adulthood, predisposing patients to a very high noncompliance rate. Non-adherence is reportedly as high as 22%, the major cause being graft loss or rejection in adolescent transplant recipients.[65,66] Currently, pediatric face transplantation is regarded as extremely controversial and, at present, there are no centers that have performed a pediatric face transplant. However, the future is evolving and recent arguments in support of pediatric face transplantation have been made,[65] especially in light of a recent bilateral hand transplant performed at the University of Pennsylvania with a remarkable result.[66]

Future directions

Apart from drugs, research protocols are directed towards tolerance induction. This has been studied largely in animal models to develop chimerism or even microchimerism, but this has yet to be successfully demonstrated in humans. Development of new drugs and donor specific tolerance through various protocols is only one barrier to the expansion of facial VCA. Choice selection of future candidates is just as important to optimize outcomes. Although tissue regenerative medicine has long been touted as the next great reconstructive technology, there have not been many advances to help patients with devastating facial injury. To support expansion of future transplantation, the worldwide experience must continue to report their outcomes so the reconstructive transplant community learns with each experience.[68] Just as solid organ transplantation evolved over the last 50 years, facial VCA is on a fast path to mimic a similar trajectory.

Case

A 41-year-old male retired firefighter underwent a successful total face, eyelids, ears, scalp, and skeletal subunit transplant. The recipient endured full-thickness disfiguring thermal facial injury (Figs. 19.41–19.43) while in the line of duty in 2001. The extent of injury involved cartilaginous destruction of the bilateral ears and nose. The perioral soft tissue was contracted resulting in labial incompetence and sialorrhea. Periorbital involvement led to impairment of the blink mechanism and ultimately visual deterioration. The scalp sustained full thickness burns and the neck developed contractures. The extent of soft tissue facial and scalp tissue involved in transplantation constitutes the most extensive face transplant performed to date. Early follow-up has demonstrated encouraging results both functionally and aesthetically (Figs. 19.44–19.46). Reflexive and volitional blink remains intact, the patient is able to speak, retains oral competence, has regained his sense of smell, and has improved neck range of motion. The patient satisfaction with his outcome and his dramatic improvement in quality of life has been remarkable.[30]

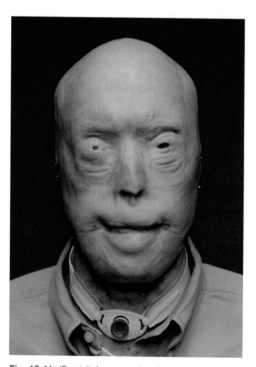

Fig. 19.41 (Frontal) A preoperative photo of a patient with thermal injury including total face and scalp burns that underwent face transplantation. *(Printed with permission from and copyright retained by Eduardo D. Rodriguez, M.D., D.D.S.)*

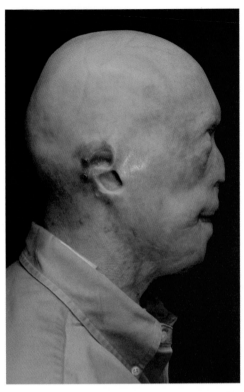

Fig. 19.42 (Profile) A preoperative photo of a patient with thermal injury including total face and scalp burns. *(Printed with permission from and copyright retained by Eduardo D. Rodriguez, M.D., D.D.S.)*

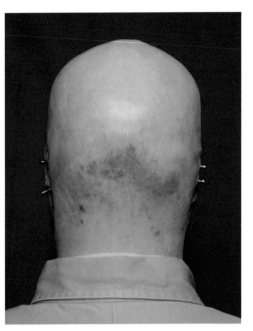

Fig. 19.43 (Posterior) A preoperative photo of a patient with thermal injury including total face and scalp burns. *(Printed with permission from and copyright retained by Eduardo D. Rodriguez, M.D., D.D.S.)*

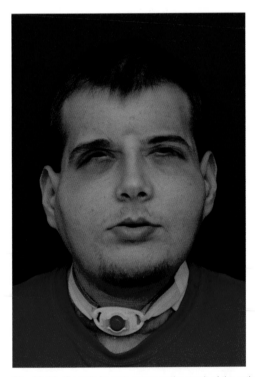

Fig. 19.44 (Frontal) An early postoperative result of the patient following face transplantation. *(Printed with permission from and copyright retained by Eduardo D. Rodriguez, M.D., D.D.S.)*

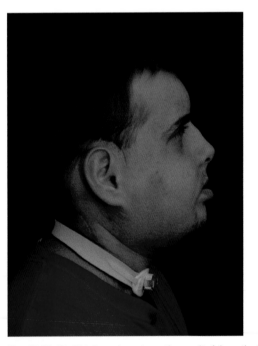

Fig. 19.45 (Profile) An early postoperative result of the patient following face transplantation. *(Printed with permission from and copyright retained by Eduardo D. Rodriguez, M.D., D.D.S.)*

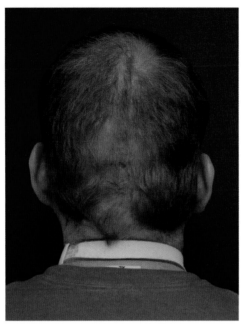

Fig. 19.46 (Posterior) An early postoperative result of the patient following face transplantation. *(Printed with permission from and copyright retained by Eduardo D. Rodriguez, M.D., D.D.S.)*

🌐 Access the complete reference list online at **http://www.expertconsult.com**

1. Sosin M, Rodriguez ED. The Face Transplantation Update: 2016. *Plast Reconstr Surg*. 2016;137:1841–1850.

12. Devauchelle B, Badet L, Lengele B, et al. First human face allograft: early report. *Lancet*. 2006;368:203–209.

15. Pomahac B, Diaz–Siso JR, Bueno EM. Evolution of indications for facial transplantation. *J Plast Reconstr Aesthet Surg*. 2011;64:1410–1416.

19. Pomahac B, Pribaz J, Eriksson E, et al. Three patients with full facial transplantation. *N Engl J Med*. 2012;366:715–722.

26. Starzl TE, Demetris AJ, Murase N, et al. Cell migration, chimerism, and graft acceptance. *Lancet*. 1992;339:1579–1582.

29. Dorafshar AH, Bojovic B, Christy MR, et al. Total face, double jaw, and tongue transplantation: an evolutionary concept. *Plast Reconstr Surg*. 2013;131:241–251.

30. Sosin M, Ceradini DJ, Levine JP, et al. Total face, eyelids, ears, scalp, and skeletal subunit transplant: a reconstructive solution for the full face and total scalp burn. *Plast Reconstr Surg*. 2016;138:205–219.

32. Lantieri L, Grimbert P, Ortonne N, et al. Face transplant: long-term follow-up and results of a prospective open study. *Lancet*. 2016;S0140–6736(16)31138–2.

35. Lantieri L, Hivelin M, Audard V, et al. Feasibility, reproducibility, risks and benefits of face transplantation: a prospective study of outcomes. *Am J Transplant*. 2011;11:367–378.

39. Coffman KL, Gordon C, Siemionow M. Psychological outcomes with face transplantation: overview and case report. *Curr Opin Organ Transplant*. 2010;15:236–240.

PART 2

Pediatrics

20

Embryology of the craniofacial complex

Jingtao Li and Jill A. Helms

SYNOPSIS

- Analysis of human craniofacial development opens the door to understanding the basis for craniofacial dysmorphologies.
- Establishment of the craniocaudal and mediolateral axes is essential for proper craniofacial development.
- Neural crest cells are a multipotent, migratory mesenchymal population of cells that give rise to the majority of the facial skeleton.
- Facial clefting is a multifactorial disorder. Single mutations in multiple signaling pathways can result in facial clefting.
- Neurocranium is comprised of a cartilaginous and a membranous portion. Cartilaginous neurocranium is derived from embryonic mesoderm, while the membranous neurocranium is derived from cranial neural crest.
- Cranial sutures remain patent during infancy through an intricate balance between maintenance of undifferentiated cells and cells that have differentiated into osteoblasts.
- Derivatives of the five pharyngeal arches form parts of the human face and the neck.
- Three well known teratogens, retinoic acid, alcohol, and cyclopamine, affect craniofacial development.

Introduction

We come into this world primed to connect with the faces around us; it is literally hardwired into our neural circuitry. There is a specialized region in our brain located in the temporal lobe in the fusiform gyrus that is filled with neurons that preferentially fire when the individual is looking at a face.[1] Within minutes of birth, babies are using this facial recognition domain; studies demonstrate that even very young infants show a strong preference for looking at faces over all other objects.[2] So in a brain that is ultimately responsible for coordinating every single activity that will maintain all body functions and ensure survival, there is allocated some terribly precious real estate whose only apparent purpose is to respond to faces. Not an object, not a tree or a rock or a banana or anything else, just a face. This is not a hominid specialization, either; other mammals including sheep have similar facial recognition sites.[3]

Our ability to "read a face" is essential for human survival. The face is the means by which we communicate with the world and each other. "The welfare of mankind depends on the expression and recognition of emotion", wrote Charles Darwin in *The Expression of the Emotions in Man and Animals*.[4] Support for Darwin's statement can be found when observing any adult with an infant: of all the motor skills that infants must master, none is as important as mimicking the facial gestures of people around them. Even at a very early age, humans devote a great deal of attention and energy to teaching infants the movements required for facial expression. In fact, we know that children who are incapable or uninterested in learning this task are often later diagnosed with conditions such as autism. This focus on the face ultimately translates into our faces becoming central to our sense of identity. This chapter is devoted to an explanation of how this remarkable part of our anatomy comes about. We begin at the beginning, just after fertilization of the egg by the sperm, when the head is first distinguished from the tail; we continue throughout the embryonic, and then into the fetal periods. The explosion of genetic research provides a framework for understanding how mutations create asymmetries and imbalances in the proportions of the human face. This wealth of new data represents an important step towards understanding the molecular, cellular, and environmental causes of craniofacial birth defects; our next challenge is to figure out how to use this information to reduce, ameliorate, or possibly even prevent these birth defects from happening.

The craniofacial complex

Ralph Waldo Emerson wrote, "A man finds room in the few square inches of the face for the traits of all his ancestors; for the expression of all his history, and his wants"[5] and in doing so he succinctly summarized the significance of the craniofacial complex. This region of our anatomy is how others distinguish us, and it is how we see ourselves and, therefore, has been the study of intense investigation for hundreds of years.

The craniofacial complex is primarily derived from cranial neural crest cells and mesodermal cells that interact though elaborately choreographed movements to form composite tissues including the skeleton, the musculature, the connective tissues, and the epithelial specializations unique to the head region. Both passive cell displacement and active cell migration are involved in gastrulation and neurulation, which establish the head region and the stage for craniofacial development. As one might suspect, disruptions that affect the timing, rate, or extent of cell migration often result in craniofacial defects; these will be discussed in detail later in the chapter.

The craniofacial complex also houses the organs responsible for sight, taste, smell, and sound and, therefore, must integrate these sensory inputs into the architecture of the head.

Like other tissues, the craniofacial complex develops through a synchronized series of reciprocal tissue–tissue interactions. In the head, however, these interactions occur between neural and non-neural ectoderm; between ectoderm and endoderm; and between ectoderm, endoderm, and mesoderm. The molecular signals mediating these interactions have, in large part, been identified and, accordingly, there is a growing understanding of how perturbations in a particular signaling pathway manifest as a given craniofacial malformation. Clearly, decades of research have provided us with an understanding of the etiologies of many craniofacial deformations, which has surely the stage set for developing therapeutic interventions to treat – or perhaps prevent – such anomalies in the future.

Distinguishing head from tail

Lewis Wolpert famously described not birth, marriage, or death, but gastrulation as the most important phase of one's life[6] and it is during this period that the "head" and "tail" orientation of an embryo is firmly established. Prior to gastrulation, a newly formed zygote must generate sufficient numbers of cells to eventually form an entire embryo. To that end, the zygote divides repeatedly to generate a solid, mulberry-like cell mass known as a morula. It is at this stage that the morula traverses the fallopian tube and enters the uterus. With further cell division, the morula becomes a blastocyst, which itself has two components. The first component is the trophoblast, which contributes to the formation of placental structures that support and nourish the developing embryo; the second component is the embryoblast that differentiates into the embryo itself.

Gastrulation begins in the third week of human life and it is an event that is restricted to the embryoblast, and it begins when an invagination that spans the length of the pancake-like human embryo is visible. This invagination is called the primitive streak and cells from the ectoderm stream into this invagination in a head (cranial) to tail (caudal) gradient. As they migrate past the most caudal extent of the primitive streak, the cells pass by an anatomical landmark called Hensen's node. It is in this moment that cells are exposed to chemical morphogens that will influence their ultimate behavior.

Patterning the craniofacial complex

Whereas gastrulation creates the three germ layers – ectoderm, mesoderm, and endoderm – it is neurulation that creates the fourth germ layer, the neural crest. During neurulation the flat neural plate is transformed into a neural tube (Fig. 20.1). This transformation has an important impact of facial development, because the *medial* domain of the neural plate becomes the *ventral* surface of the neural tube, and *lateral* domains of the neural plate constitute the *dorsal* surface of the neural tube (Fig. 20.1). Some of the most important signaling pathways that control craniofacial development are actually involved in specifying the medial and lateral domains of the neural plate. For example, the medial domain of the anterior neural plate is patterned by signals in the Hedgehog (HH) family of secreted proteins. Sonic Hedgehog (SHH) is expressed in this midline domain around the time of neurulation and there its primary function is to repress activity of the transcription factor PAX6 (Fig. 20.1). PAX6 is a master transcriptional regulator of eye development.[7] SHH normally represses PAX6 function in this medial domain where the expression domains of the two molecules overlap; as a consequence, a single PAX6-expressing eye domain separated into two, bilaterally symmetrical PAX6-positive eye fields.[8] When SHH signaling is lost or blocked, such as happens in congenital cases of holoprosencephaly (HPE), PAX6 expression persists in the medial domain. Consequently, the single, PAX6-positive eye field is not sub-divided and the affected fetus exhibits cyclopia[9,10] (Fig. 20.1). Other midline structures are also affected in HPE:[11] the nose may be completely absent or fetuses may have in place of the nose a tubular-shaped structure called a proboscis. In less severe cases of HPE, the affected fetus' eyes can be set very closely. In milder forms of HPE, the affected individual can exhibit hypotelorism[12]; in a microform of HPE, patients may only exhibit a single central incisor. All of these anomalies share a common feature: they represent a collapse in the mediolateral growth of the craniofacial complex, which can be attributable to disruptions in midline Hedgehog signaling.[13]

SHH is involved in specifying the medial domain of the neural plate; the lateral domains of the neural plate are specified by signals in the bone morphogenetic protein (BMP) family. Like HH proteins, BMPs are secreted growth factors, and a gradient of BMP signaling is instrumental in defining which region of the neural plate will give rise to neuroectoderm (and thus form the brain) and which region will give rise to non-neural ectoderm (and thus form epidermis). Just as loss of SHH can lead to HPE, so too can elevated BMP signaling; BMP signals are normally restrained to the lateral borders of the neural plate, but in cases where their domains are expanded they can interrupt medial SHH function. Embryos affected in this manner exhibit narrowing of the midfacial region and microform versions of HPE (Fig. 20.1).[14] BMPs are also critically important dorsal signals that specify the roof plate of the developing forebrain.[15]

Genesis of the cranial neural crest

During neurulation, a new population of neural crest cells form the dorsal region of the folding neural tube, specifically

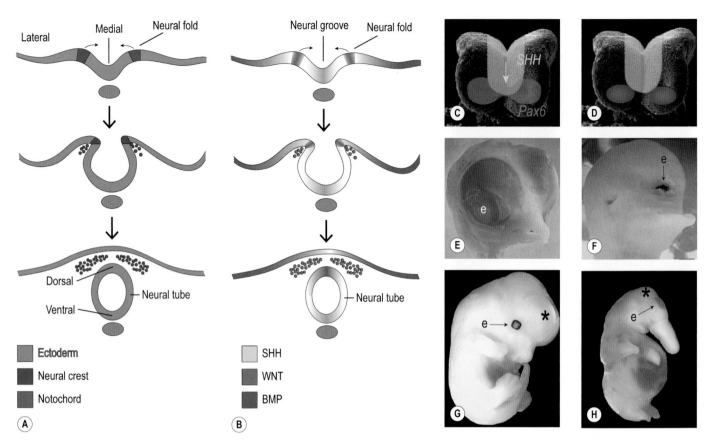

Fig. 20.1 (A,B) Expression pattern of Sonic hedgehog (SHH, yellow), WNT (red) and BMP (green) signaling during the process of neurulation. **(C)** SHH expression (yellow) in the medial neural plate with Pax-6 expression (orange) in the dumbbell-shaped area which corresponds to the feature eye field. **(D)** Subdivision of Pax6 expression into two bilateral domains through expression of SHH. **(E)** Wild-type chick embryo. **(F)** Chick embryo exhibiting cyclopia. **(G)** Wild-type mouse embryo at embryonic day 15.5. **(H)** Mouse embryo exhibiting cyclopia with proboscis as a result of loss of SHH in the neural plate which has led to persistence of a single Pax6 anterior midline. e=eye.

from a region called the neural folds; this neural fold defines the boundary between neural and non-neural ectoderm (Fig. 20.1). Neural crest cells are generated at this boundary region when columnar ectodermal cells detach and transform into elongated mesenchymal cells (Fig. 20.2). This process is referred to as an epithelial-to-mesenchymal transition (EMT) and is a unique feature of normal neural crest cells; it is also a feature shared by metastatic cells.[16] Neural crest and metastatic cells share other features, for example, both being highly invasive.[17] As a consequence of this similarity, considerable effort has gone into understanding the molecular regulation of neural crest cell migration.[18] For example, neural crest cell migration is specified in part by the action of the transcription factor Slug and after migration is complete, Slug expression is typically shut off.[19] Highly invasive cancer cells, however, continue to express high levels of Slug and what is more, cancer cells derived from Slug-expressing neural crest cells are much more invasive than cancer cells derived from mesodermal cells.[20] When Slug is inactivated, even in neural crest-derived cancer, cells become non-metastatic.[21] These studies demonstrate important parallels between the molecular programs governing neural crest behavior and cancer cell behavior, and underscore how understanding the development of the craniofacial complex can have direct implications for understanding processes such as cancer metastasis.

The generation of neural crest cells is also intimately dependent upon the Wnt pathway of secreted proteins. Wnt proteins are first expressed in the neural folds; if Wnt signaling is experimentally blocked at this stage then neural crest cells fail to be generated.[22] Wnt signals in turn drive expression of a number of transcription factors including Slug (mentioned previously) as well as Sox9 and FoxD3.[23] Disruptions to these neural crest transcription factors result in a range of severe congenital defects. For example, Sox9 is expressed in neural crest cells,[24] and mutations in this transcription factor are associated with campomelic dysplasia,[25] a condition where the appendicular skeleton exhibits bowing and angulation defects; in addition, affected infants exhibit macrocephaly, hydrocephalus, hypertelorism, a small or flat nasal bridge, micrognathia, and cleft palate.[26]

Mutations in the neural crest inducer Sox10[27] cause peripheral demyelinating neuropathy, central dysmyelination, Waardenburg syndrome, and Hirshsprung disease (PCWH[28]). Clinical features of this condition include neurosensory deafness and extensive peripheral neuropathies. Given the important role of neural crest cells in the generation of glia,[29] a basis for this complex congenital syndrome can readily be appreciated.

Exodus of the neural crest

Once specified, cranial neural crest cells must begin an extensive migration from the dorsal neural tube into the ventrally

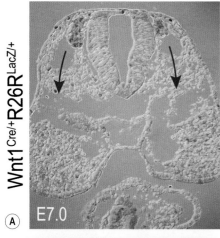

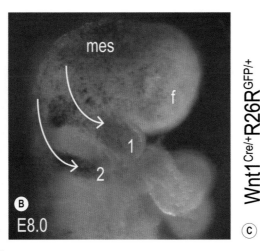

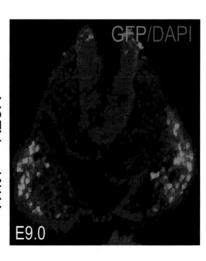

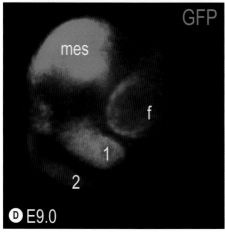

Fig. 20.2 Neural crest migration in mouse embryo. **(A)** Specification of neural crest cells at embryonic day 7. **(B)** Neural crest cells begin to migrate at embryonic day 8. **(C)** Coronal section and **(D)** wholemount sample showing the migrated neural crest cells at embryonic day 9. mes=mesencephalon; f=frontal prominence; 1=first pharyngeal arch; 2=second pharyngeal arch.

positioned pharyngeal arches (Fig. 20.2). A disruption in this migratory process underlies the classification of malformations known as neurocristopathies.

CHARGE syndrome is a well-recognized example of a neurocristopathy, which manifests as ocular coloboma, heart defects, choanal atresia, and ear abnormalities. Mutations in the gene CHD7 are responsible for 70–90% of CHARGE syndrome cases.[30] Loss of CHD7 leads to activation of p53, a tumor suppressor gene,[31] and an increase in the expression of the p53 protein inhibits genes related to neural crest migration, including SNAIL2 and ETS1. As a consequence of disrupted neural crest migration, craniofacial morphogenesis and heart development are perturbed.[32]

Clearly, the control of neural crest migration is important but how do neural crest cells know which pathway to take, and their ultimate destination? New data now demonstrate that migrating neural crest cells contain receptors on their cell surfaces that specifically recognize guidance cues found on adjacent epithelial cells. Relative to neural crest, the epithelial (i.e., endodermal and ectodermal) cells are stationary and therefore can provide directions to the neural crest as they make their way to the pharyngeal arches.[33] Guidance cues can function as positive (attractive) and negative (repulsive) signals, and chief among them are the Ephrins.[34] These same guidance cues also direct axons to their correct targets.[35]

Efficient neural crest migration is governed in part by chemotaxis, i.e., the movement of a cell towards a directive substance. Neural crest cells make use of a surface organelle called the primary cilium to sense these "directive substances". These primary cilia are required for the transduction of HH signals,[36] and their importance in regulating neural crest cell behavior has been demonstrated through loss-of-function analyses. For example, loss of component of the intraflagellar transport system, which moves proteins up and down the primary cilia, leads to perturbations in HH signaling and craniofacial defects including frontonasal dysplasias.[13,37] Several other factors essential for neural crest migration, including SDF-1, PDGF-AA, and VEGFA, have their receptors positioned on the primary cilia. For an excellent review of the subject, see Chang et al.[38]

Differentiation of the cranial neural crest

Once their migration into the pharyngeal arches is complete, neural crest cells must expand, through the process of proliferation, and then differentiate. Neural crest cells have been referred to as stem cells because of the enormous diversity of cell types into which they differentiate.[39] In the head region, neural crest cells give rise to neural, odontogenic, and skeletogenic tissues, as well as melanocytes, some intrinsic eye muscles, pericytes that encase blood vessels in the head, and

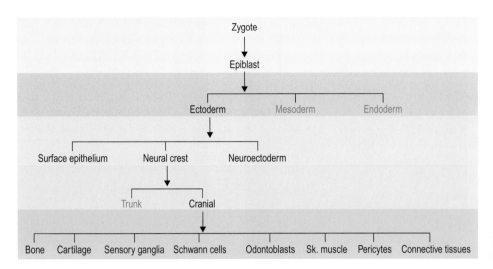

Fig. 20.3 Differentiation of the cranial neural crest.

adipocytes (Fig. 20.3). In the trunk region, neural crest cells give rise to sensory neurons and glia of the peripheral nervous system, including the enteric nervous system.[40]

The factors controlling this range of cellular phenotypes have been the focus of considerable investigation. What is clear from new studies is that epigenetics plays an important role in the process (reviewed in Hu *et al.*[41]). For example, craniofacial cartilage, bone, and muscle are all derived from a single population of neural crest cells; but, until recently, it was not clear how a set of cells that share the same genetic information could differentiate into such a variety of cell types. Joanna Wysocka and colleagues have now demonstrated that regulatory elements in the DNA called enhancers are responsible for the activity of transcription factors, which in turn regulate the transcriptome in a given population of

neural crest cells.[42] Epigenomic mapping of neural crest cells has been used to identify the enhancer "signatures" in human neural crest cells predicting which genes will be turned on and off as cranial neural crest cells differentiate,[43] and even which enhancer signatures are thought to be responsible for creating the features of a human (versus primate) face.[44,45] These studies have provided some of the first clues into how craniofacial variation in primates is established.[46]

Organization of the pharyngeal arches

The neural crest pharyngeal arches are the starting material from which the face develops (Fig. 20.4). The pharyngeal arches are separated by pharyngeal clefts, each of which gives

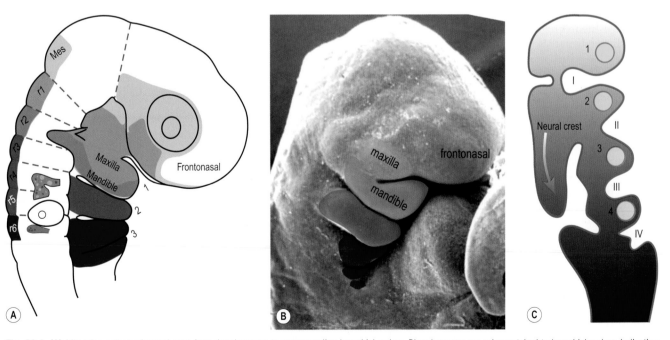

Fig. 20.4 (A) Migration pattern of neural crest from rhombomeres to corresponding branchial arches. Rhombomeres are color-matched to branchial arches, indicating which rhombomere the neural crest cells in a particular arch or facial prominence comes from. **(B)** Scanning electron image of pharyngeal arches. The arches are indicated by different colors. **(C)** The outgrowth of the pharyngeal clefts and pouches (Roman numerals). The arches (1,2,3,4) are composed of a core of neural crest (purple) and mesoderm (orange) surrounded by both surface ectoderm (blue) and pharyngeal endoderm (green).

rise to a variety of structures. Pharyngeal cleft 1 gives rise to the auditory tube and middle ear, and part of the tympanic membrane. Cleft 2 contributes to part of the middle ear and the palatine tonsil, and cleft 3 gives rise to the inferior parathyroid glands and cells in the thymus. The fourth cleft contributes to the superior parathyroid glands and to the thymus, and along with cleft 6 contributes to the musculature and cartilage of the larynx (Fig. 20.4). The pharyngeal arches form in an anterior-to-posterior gradient: the first arch appears on day 22; the second and third arches appear sequentially on day 24; and the fourth through sixth arches appear sequentially on day 29. A summary of the derivatives of each arch and cleft is available in Table 20.1.

The face is predominantly derived from the first pharyngeal arch. As neural crest cells within the arch proliferate, the arch expands in an anterior (cranial) to posterior (caudal) fashion. The cranial swelling gives rise to the maxillary prominence, which will form the upper jaw and the caudal swelling gives rise to the mandibular prominence, which will form the lower jaw. As the upper and lower jaws develop, the second pharyngeal arch (also known as the hyoid arch) serves as a bracing element to support them. The third pharyngeal arch forms the lower rim of the hyoid bone as well as the root of the tongue, epiglottis, and thyroid and inferior parathyroid. The fourth and sixth arches together give rise to the larynx.

Disorders of arch development

Underdevelopment of the first and second pharyngeal arches lie at the foundation of one of the most common groups of facial malformations, which are collectively referred to as craniofacial microsomia. Clinical manifestations of craniofacial microsomia include asymmetries due to hypoplasia of the external and middle ear, the mandible, zygoma, maxilla, temporal bone, facial muscles, muscles of mastication, palatal muscles, tongue, and parotid gland.[47] The severity of the craniofacial macrosomia sequence can range from subtle facial asymmetries with small preauricular skin tags to severe,

bilateral malformations that include microtia, microphthalmia, and mandibular hypoplasia that can compromise the airway. In the vast majority of cases, the etiology of craniofacial microsomia is unknown, but there are several risk factors including maternal use of vasoactive drugs, diabetes mellitus, and second trimester bleeding. The molecular basis for this malformation sequence is still under debate but some data suggest that it is due to insufficient cranial neural crest proliferation, leading to smaller than normal arches. The root cause of the inadequate proliferation may arise from ischemia, secondary to a defect in the stapedial artery that provides the initial blood supply to this region.[47]

Another class of malformations that are attributable to abnormal development of the first and second pharyngeal arches is a spectrum of etiologically heterogeneous craniofacial anomalies referred to as mandibulofacial dysostoses. Mandibulofacial dysostosis are similar to craniofacial microsomia in that both are characterized by malar and mandibular hypoplasia; the distinguishing feature, however, is that in mandibulofacial dysostosis the manifestations of the syndrome are symmetrical.[26] One well-studied mandibulofacial dysostosis is Treacher–Collins syndrome, an autosomal dominant genetic disorder characterized by bilateral deficiencies in pharyngeal arch-derived structures that includes mandibular and malar hypoplasia, microtia, and macrostomia. The genetic basis for Treacher–Collins syndrome is due to perturbations in the expression of nucleolar phosphoprotein, Treacle.[48] Autosomal dominant mutations in the TCOF1 gene that encodes Treacle interrupt neural crest cell formation and proliferation, leading to hypoplastic features of Treacher–Collins patients.[48]

Another example of mandibulofacial dysostosis is 22q11.2 deletion syndrome, also known as DiGeorge syndrome, which is characterized by cleft palate, cardiovascular anomalies, and agenesis or hypogenesis of the derivatives of the third and fourth pharyngeal clefts (i.e., the thymus and parathyroid glands). The 22q11.2 deletion syndrome is caused by haploinsufficiency of the TBX1 gene.[49] TBX1 encodes a transcription factor that regulates the expression of as-yet-unknown genes

Table 20.1 Derivatives of the pharyngeal arches

Arch	Skeletal element	Musculature	Nerve	Artery
1st (mandibular and maxillary)	Incus, malleus, zygomatic, squamous. Part of the temporal, mandible and maxilla	Muscles of mastication	Trigeminal	Maxillary artery
2nd (hyoid)	Stapes, styloid process of temporal bone, stylohyoid ligament. Lesser horn and body of hyoid bone	Muscles of facial expression	Facial	Stapedial artery
3rd	Greater horns and lower body of hyoid	Muscles of the stylopharyngeus (throat)	Glossopharyngeal	Common carotid/internal carotid
4th and 6th	Cartilages of the larynx	Muscles of pharynx constriction, muscles of phonation, palatoglossus (tongue), muscles of upper esophagus	Vagus	Arch of aorta, right subclavian artery, original sprouts of pulmonary artery, ductus arteriosus, roots of pulmonary arteries

Modified from Moody SA (ed). *Principles of Developmental Genetics.* Burlington, MA: Academic Press; 2007, Ch. 30, Table 1).

that are involved in controlling neural crest migration.[50] TBX1 is not required in neural crest cells *per se*; rather, using a mouse model of DiGeorge syndrome,[51] scientists demonstrated that aberrant neural crest cell migration was caused because of a lack of guidance cues provided by pharyngeal pouch endoderm.[52] These analyses clearly demonstrate that neural crest migration is intimately dependent on cues from the surrounding ectoderm and endoderm,[53] and that deficiencies in neural crest cells – caused by disrupted migration, inadequate proliferation, or excessive cell death – underlie many of the craniofacial syndromes characterized by underdeveloped structures.[54]

Building the face

The basic morphology of the face is established between the fourth and 10th weeks of human development, and between embryonic days 10–15 of murine development (Fig. 20.5). In both mammals, the face is formed as a result of fusion of the midline frontonasal prominence, and three paired prominences, the maxillary, lateral nasal, and mandibular prominences. Each of these prominences is filled with cranial neural crest cells. Each of the prominences, and the structures that arise from them, are discussed below. Despite their obvious phenotypic differences, the faces of human and mouse embryos share a very similar blueprint at the phylotypic stage of development (Fig. 20.5). Through selective cell proliferation, where one facial prominence expands relative to another in a species-specific manner,[55–57] the final phenotype of each face is established.

As expected based on its moniker, the unpaired, midline frontonasal (median nasal) prominence develops in the midline of the embryo, and is characterized by a deep furrow called the infranasal depression (Fig. 20.5). Structures derived from the frontonasal prominence include the forehead, the middle of the nose, the philtrum, septum, middle portion of the upper lip, and primary palate (Fig. 20.5). Together, the frontonasal-derived primary palate and nasal septum fuse with the bilateral palatal shelves (derived from the maxillary prominences, see below) to create the anterior portion of the roof of the mouth.

During early craniofacial development, the lateral nasal prominences are nearly equal in size to the frontonasal prominence in both humans and mice (Fig. 20.5) but with time, cell proliferation in the lateral nasal prominences is significantly reduced compared to that in the frontonasal prominence; as a consequence, the resulting structures to which they give rise (i.e., the alae of the nose) are considerably smaller (Fig. 20.5).

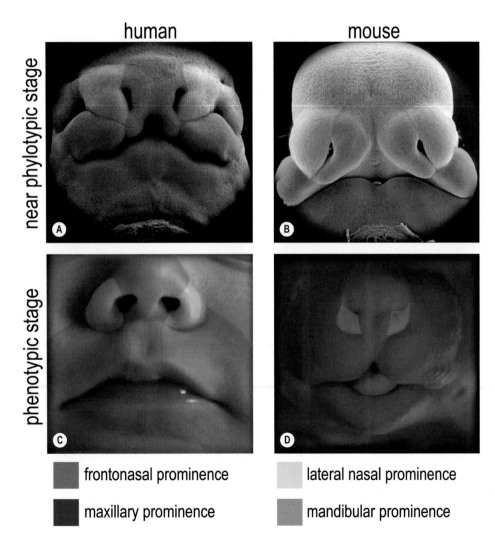

human   mouse

near phylotypic stage

phenotypic stage

A   B   C   D

frontonasal prominence

maxillary prominence

lateral nasal prominence

mandibular prominence

Fig. 20.5 Prominences of the vertebrate face (**A–D**). Frontonasal prominence (purple) contributes to the forehead, middle of the nose, philtrum, and primary palate; maxillary prominence (blue) contributes to the sides of the face and lip and the secondary palate; lateral nasal prominence (yellow) forms the sides of the nose; and the mandibular prominence (red) produces the lower jaw.

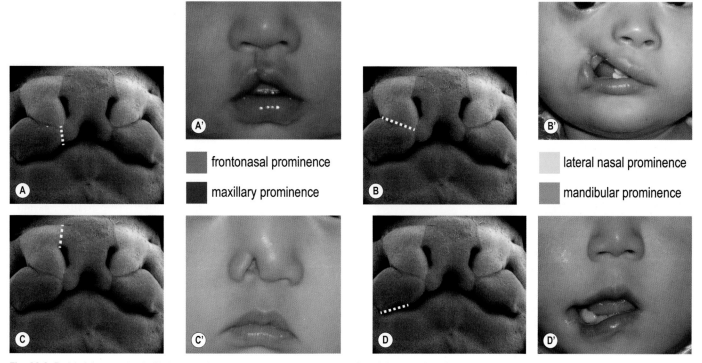

Fig. 20.6 Facial clefts associated with interrupted fusion between facial prominences. **(A, A')** Cleft lip; **(B, B')** oblique facial cleft; **(C, C')** alar cleft; **(D, D')** transverse facial cleft.

The maxillary prominences are initially equal in size to the lateral nasal prominences (Fig. 20.5) but exuberant neural crest proliferation ultimately results in the maxillary prominences contributing to the upper cheek, the lateral upper lip, maxilla, and the secondary palate (Fig. 20.5). The mandibular prominence grows as a single unit from the first pharyngeal arch with a separating notch in the center (Fig. 20.5). The notch between bilateral mandibular prominences is obliterated through mesenchyme proliferation and ectoderm migration, and the prominences eventually merge, rather than fuse, with each other. Ultimately, the mandibular prominence forms the lower cheek, the lower lip, the lower jaw including the floor of the mouth and the submental area, as well as part of the middle ear, and the anterior two-thirds of the tongue (Fig. 20.5). Thus, in mammals, the blueprint of the face is conserved, and selective neural crest cell proliferation leads to species–specific variations in facial form.

Facial fusions and clefting defects

Cell proliferation results in growth of the facial prominences and brings them into proximity to one another; the next critical step is to create a seamless unification of the prominences. This process is achieved in two integrated steps: adhesion and fusion. As they touch, the ectoderm enveloping each prominence must "get out of the way" in order to create a unified facial structure. One mechanism by which ectodermal cells appear to be removed is through regional programmed cell death that results in superficial layers of the ectoderm/epithelium "peeling off" and leaving only a basal epithelial layer intact.[58] When the facial prominences fuse, cell connections are reinforced and stabilized by the formation of adhesion junctions, such as desmosomes.[58] Mutations in the

interferon regulatory factor IRF6 result in inappropriate adhesions between the palatal shelves and the tongue, resulting in palatal clefting phenotypes in mice and humans.[59] Therefore, disruptions in extent of growth of each facial prominence or the process of fusion can result in facial clefting.

Clefts can be categorized in a number of ways; here we present an embryologic point of view of the etiology of facial clefting. When the frontonasal and maxillary prominences fail to fuse, the result is cleft lip (Fig. 20.6). When the lateral nasal and maxillary prominences fail to fuse, the result is an oblique facial cleft (Fig. 20.6). When the frontonasal and lateral nasal prominences fail to fuse the result is an alar cleft (Fig. 20.6). The maxillary and mandibular prominences must fuse and, in the absence of this event, the result is a transverse facial cleft (Fig. 20.6). Other facial clefts can arise (e.g., median upper lip cleft, median lower lip cleft) but these are rarer events.

Palatogenesis

The secondary palate separates the nasal passage from the mouth. In a stepwise manner, the palatal shelves extend vertically on either side of the tongue then subsequently rotate to a horizontal plane dorsal to the tongue, and fuse (Fig. 20.7). Initially, the palatal shelves are lined by an epithelium (the medial edge epithelium, MEE); as the shelves grow towards the midline, the MEE of each shelf approximates and forms the midline epithelial seam (MES). The MES is then removed through the process of mesenchymal to epithelial transition (MET, the opposite of EMT), which leads to a confluence between the mesenchyme of the palatal shelves. Perturbations caused by genetic, mechanical, or teratogenic factors can occur at any of these steps, and frequently result in a cleft of

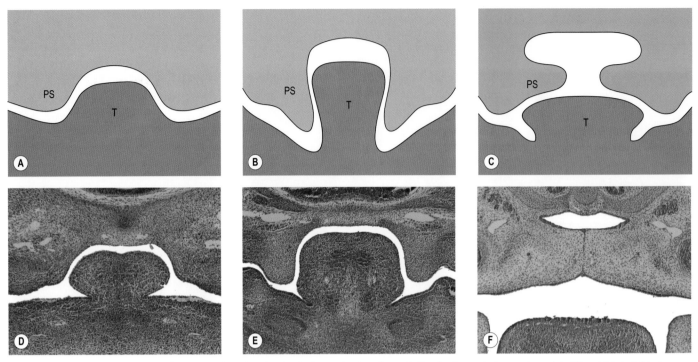

Fig. 20.7 (A–F) Schematic diagram and coronal sections through a developing murine face demonstrating development of secondary palate. PS=palatal shelf (blue); T=tongue (red).

secondary palate. Another type of secondary palatal clefting is palatal insufficiency, which is often caused by inadequate outgrowth of the maxillary prominences.

The neurocranial base

The neurocranium comprises the bones that protect the brain. The ventral portion of the neurocranium is called the basicranium and includes the sphenoid and ethmoid bones, the mastoid and petrous portions of the temporal bone, and the base of the occipital bone. Using experimental manipulations[60] and genetic fate-mapping approaches in mice[61] the embryonic origins of the bones of the basicranium have been established as arising from mesodermal cells that originate as part of the occipital somites and somitomeres. Skeletal elements that comprise the basicranium form through endochondral ossification, where a cartilaginous template or anlage is first established and then is gradually replaced with a bony matrix through the process of vascular invasion.

Cranial vault and sutures

The cranial vault is comprised of seven neural crest-derived[60] bones: the paired frontal, squamosal, and parietal bones, and the occipital bone. The majority of the cranial vault forms through the process of intramembranous ossification, where mesenchymal cells condense and directly differentiate into osteoblasts without forming a cartilaginous intermediate. The occipital bone is a composite structure where the inferior portion forms via endochondral ossification and the superior portion forms via intramembranous ossification.

The bones of the cranial vault are separated by fibrous tissue called sutures, which include the frontal sutures lying between the frontal bones; the sagittal suture interposed between the parietal bones; the coronal suture that separates the frontal and parietal bones; and the lambdoid suture that is positioned between the parietal and occipital bones (Fig. 20.8).

Sutures remain patent (open) into postnatal life. The expansion of the brain, which continues well into young adulthood, stimulates the continued growth of the cranial vault bones. The bones expand in size by adding new bone at their edges; while this osteogenic differentiation is taking place, a subset of cells between the cranial vault bone edges must be maintained in a fibrous state in order to keep the sutures patent. This leads to an interesting situation: cells in the middle of the suture complex must remain undifferentiated while adjacent cells differentiate into osteoblasts and add to the growing calvarial bones. How these states of proliferation and differentiation are so precisely synchronized is still unknown, but it is clear that

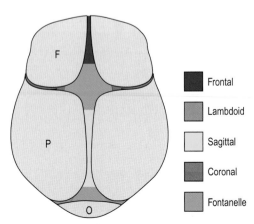

	Frontal
	Lambdoid
	Sagittal
	Coronal
	Fontanelle

Fig. 20.8 Cranial sutures.

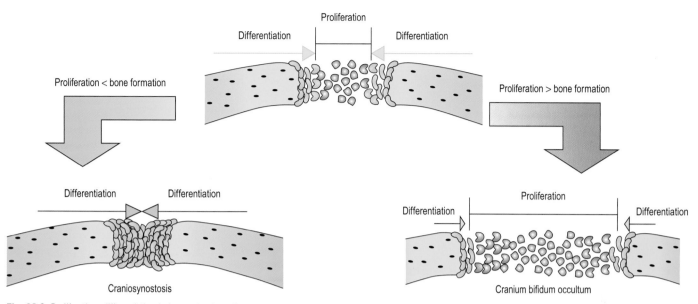

Fig. 20.9 Proliferation–differentiation balance at suture sites.

destabilization of this balance is the basis for both craniosynostoses and cranium bifidum occultum (Fig. 20.9).

In pathological conditions such as cleidocranial dysplasia[62] or frontonasal dysplasias[13] the skull bones fail to grow adequately. In these situations, the result is fibrous tissue covering the cerebral hemispheres without the benefit of ossification, clinically referred to as cranium bifidum occultum (Fig. 20.9). Craniosynostoses, on the other hand, arise when cells in the suture region prematurely differentiate into osteoblasts and inadvertently fuse the cranial bones to one another. Craniosynostoses can be either inherited or isolated.[63] Isolated, non-syndromic craniosynostoses have a frustratingly obscure etiology, but more is known about the molecular basis for the craniosynostotic phenotypes that arise as a result of an inherited mutation.

Patients with Saethre–Chotzen syndrome have mutations in the transcription factor *Twist*.[64] A mouse model of the Saethre–Chotzen syndrome has been generated; and, based on analyses of this animal, the premature suture fusion is a result of inappropriate intermixing of neural crest-derived cells in the frontal bone with mesoderm-derived cells in the parietal bone.[65] Humans with the same mutations exhibit nearly identical skeletal defects,[66] which suggests that interventions to prevent this suture fusion phenotype may be tested on an appropriate animal model.

Mutations in the Wnt target gene, Axin2, are also associated with a craniosynostotic phenotype[67] and, in this case, *in vitro* data indicate that cells in which Wnt signaling is amplified have a tendency to differentiate prematurely into osteoblasts.[67] Axin2 mutant mice have shorter snouts and premature fusion of the metopic suture, data that argue for a tight balance on the level of Wnt signaling for proper growth of the calvarial bones.

Conclusions

In 1657, the physician William Harvey wrote, "Nature is nowhere accustomed more openly to display her secret mysteries than in cases where she shows tracings of her workings apart from the beaten paths; nor is there any better way to advance the proper practice of medicine than to give our minds to the discovery of the usual law of nature, by careful investigation of cases of rarer forms of disease". Over hundreds of years, physicians have followed this guidance and carefully cataloged craniofacial anomalies in their patients. Other than careful scrutiny of the phenotypes, however, there was little additional help that physicians and scientists could provide to affected patients and their families.

The World Wars brought about horrific injuries, which forced surgeons to make dramatic improvements in surgery and patient care. These techniques and tools resulted in new ways to save lives, which also had a profound influence on the care of patients with craniofacial deformities. Some of these techniques (i.e., free flaps, distraction osteogenesis, tissue expansion) found direct application in the surgical repair of congenital defects.

In 1966, another leap forward came with the work of Victor McKusick, an internist and medical geneticist who published that year the first catalog of all known genes and genetic disorders. This critically important knowledgebase, *Mendelian Inheritance in Man* (MIM), was made available online in 1987 as *Online Mendelian Inheritance in Man* (OMIM) and is still updated daily. It remains the world's largest repository for genetic information on craniofacial disorders, and as our understanding of the role of genetics in many craniofacial anomalies improves, so too has the ability to detect and discriminate among apparently similar patient phenotypes. The last few decades have led to a deep understanding of the molecular and cellular basis for craniofacial conditions and, with it, a burgeoning concept that some of these anomalies may be treatable by genetic or cellular interventions. Coupling this information with continued surgical innovation will undoubtedly lay the groundwork for better management of the defects created by nature.

Access the complete reference list online at   http://www.expertconsult.com

9. Chiang C, Litingtung Y, Lee E, et al. Cyclopia and defective axial patterning in mice lacking Sonic hedgehog gene function. *Nature*. 1996;383:407–413. *Using targeted gene disruption model, this study verified the critical role of Sonic hedgehog signaling in the patterning of midline structures.*

13. Brugmann SA, Allen NC, James AW, et al. A primary cilia-dependent etiology for midline facial disorders. *Hum Mol Genet*. 2010;19:1577–1592. *This study demonstrated direct correlation between Hedgehog signaling and the medial-lateral patterning and development, especially in the craniofacial region. Over- and under-expression of Sonic hedgehog signaling would respectively lead to hypertelorism and hypotelorism.*

17. Yang J, Weinberg RA. Epithelial-mesenchymal transition: at the crossroads of development and tumor metastasis. *Dev Cell*. 2008;14:818–829. *The epithelial-mesenchymal transition is a highly conserved cellular program that allows polarized, immotile epithelial cells to convert to motile mesenchymal cells. This review summarized major signaling pathways that regulate the epithelial-mesenchymal transitions during both development and tumor metastasis, which furthered our molecular understanding of cell migration and morphogenesis.*

22. Garcia–Castro MI, Marcelle C, Bronner–Fraser M. Ectodermal wnt function as a neural crest inducer. *Science*. 2002;13: 13. *Neural crest cells, which generate peripheral nervous system and facial skeleton, arise at the neural plate/ectodermal border via an inductive interaction between these tissues. Along with recognized role of Wnts and BMPs in neural crest induction in amphibians and zebrafish, this study showed that Wnt molecules are necessary and sufficient to induce neural crest cells in avian embryos.*

37. Brugmann SA, Cordero DR, Helms JA. Craniofacial ciliopathies: A new classification for craniofacial disorders. *Am J Med Genet A*. 2010;152A:2995–3006. *This study examined a group of craniofacial disorders that are the result of defects in primary cilia. Based on the frequent appearance of craniofacial phenotypes in diseases born from defective primary cilia, it proposed a new class of craniofacial disorders referred to as craniofacial ciliopathies.*

40. Couly GF, Coltey PM, Le Douarin NM. The triple origin of skull in higher vertebrates: a study in quail-chick chimeras. *Development*.

1993;117:409–429. *This study used the quail-chick chimera technique to study the origin of the bones of the skull in the avian embryo. The data obtained allow us to assign a precise embryonic origin from either the mesectoderm, the paraxial cephalic mesoderm or the five first somites, to all the bones forming the avian skull.*

45. Prescott SL, Srinivasan R, Marchetto MC, et al. Enhancer divergence and cis-regulatory evolution in the human and chimp neural crest. *Cell*. 2015;163(1):68–83. *This study used epigenomic profiling from human and chimpanzee cranial neural crest cells to systematically and quantitatively annotate divergence of craniofacial cis-regulatory landscapes.*

53. Barriga EH, Mayor R. Embryonic cell–cell adhesion: a key player in collective neural crest migration. *Curr Top Dev Biol*. 2015;112:301–323. *This review summarized the molecular mechanisms underlying cadherin turnover, showing how the modulation and dynamics of cell-cell adhesions are crucial in order to maintain tissue integrity and collective migration in vivo, and concludes that cell-cell adhesion during embryo development cannot be considered as simple passive resistance to force, but rather participates in signaling events that determine important cell behaviors required for cell migration.*

55. Helms JA, Brugmann SA. The origins of species-specific facial morphology: the proof is in the pigeon. *Integr Comp Biol*. 2007;47:338–342. *This review approached how diversity was created by using the domesticated pigeon as a model organism, and focused on exploiting the unique properties of domesticated pigeons to gain critical insights into the molecular and cellular basis for craniofacial variation.*

61. Jiang X, Iseki S, Maxson RE, Sucov HM, Morriss–Kay GM. Tissue origins and interactions in the mammalian skull vault. *Dev Biol*. 2002;241:106–116. *Using a transgenic mouse with a permanent neural crest cell lineage marker, this study showed that cranial sutures are formed at a neural crest-mesoderm interface, and intramembranous ossification of mesodermal bones required interaction with neural crest-derived meninges, whereas ossification of the neural crest-derived frontal bone is autonomous. These observations provided new perspectives on skull evolution and on human genetic abnormalities of skull growth and ossification.*

21.1

Overview of the unilateral cleft lip and nose deformity

Michael R. Bykowski and Joseph E. Losee

SYNOPSIS

- A multidisciplinary team approach, including the craniofacial surgeon, orthodontist, speech pathologist, otolaryngologist, social worker, and psychologist.
- Essential that this team builds a focused collaboration around the patient from infancy to adulthood to achieve self-confidence, social integration, and optimal functionality.
- Cleft care can begin prior to the child being born when the cleft is diagnosed prenatally.
- Further treatment of the cleft can start before any surgical intervention with different types of pre-surgical interventions.
- The patient will undergo several stages of treatment through adolescence to achieve excellent facial aesthetics, normal dental occlusion, and normal speech.
- These are the goals that are introduced in this chapter and are expanded upon in the subsequent chapters by cleft surgeons who seek to join the others who have previously pushed cleft care to its modern limits.

Introduction

The repair of a bilateral cleft lip has been described as the "most important day in the child's life",[1] which is a sentiment that extends to a unilateral cleft lip repair. The repair is a gift to the infant, their family, and the surgeon. While the ancient ignorance based on religion and superstition regarding the etiology of this congenital deformity no longer exists, the social stigma does. It has been the life work of many cleft surgeons to identify deficiencies in treatment and, further, to push the leading edges of new cleft lip treatment. Indeed, it is the responsibility of current and future cleft surgeons to persist and persevere to achieve excellent facial aesthetics, normal dental occlusion, and normal speech. These are the goals that are introduced in this chapter and are expanded upon in the subsequent chapters by cleft surgeons who seek

to join the others who have previously pushed cleft care to its modern limits.

 Access the Historical Perspective section online at
http://www.expertconsult.com

Embryology

While the details of facial development are dynamic and extremely complex, a general understanding is critical to the craniofacial surgeon. In the first week following fertilization of the ovum, the zygote divides repeatedly into a mulberry-like cell mass known as the "morula". While the morula migrates through the fallopian tube and enters into the uterus it continues to divide into a blastocyst – which is composed of an inner and outer layer. The outer layer is the trophoblast, which contributes to the placental structures. The inner layer is the embryoblast, which develops into the embryo. During the second week of development the blastocyst implants into the uterine endometrium.

In the third week of human development, the embryoblast divides into three layers through a process called "gastrulation", which leads to the three primary germ layers: ectoderm, mesoderm, and endoderm. Due to its major role in development, some refer to the neural crest as the "fourth germ layer". The neural crest is especially important in craniofacial development and gives rise to the much of the neural, odontogenic, and skeletogenic tissues of the craniofacial region.

The orofacial region can be identified in the fourth week post-conception. At this point, an area of the trilaminar germ disk (typically consisting of the ecto-, meso-, and endoderm) lacks mesoderm, forming a bilaminar oropharyngeal membrane. The cavity adjacent to the oropharyngeal membrane marks the stomodeum (the primitive mouth), around which five facial prominences swell during the fourth week of embryogenesis. The stomodeum is bordered rostrally by the

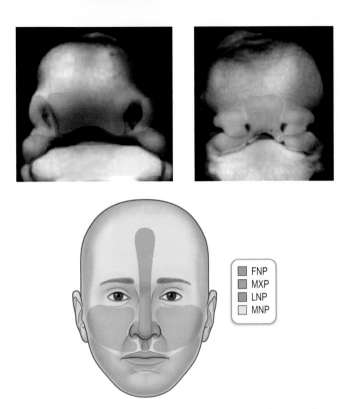

Fig. 21.1.1 Prominences of the face. Frontonasal prominence (FNP), maxillary prominence (MXP), lateral nasal prominence (LNP), mandibular prominence (MNP).

median frontonasal prominence, laterally by the paired maxillary prominences, and caudally by the paired mandibular prominences (Fig. 21.1.1).

During the 4th through 10th weeks post-conception, the basic morphology of the face is developed, which is formed due to fusion of the frontonasal prominence and the maxillary, lateral nasal, and mandibular prominences (Fig. 21.1.1).

The frontonasal prominence – as its name indicates – forms the forehead, midline of the nose, the central lip (philtrum), and the primary palate. Disruptions of the frontonasal development can lead to a bilateral cleft lip with a "fly-away" primary palate. On the inferior and lateral aspects of this prominence form the bilateral nasal placodes, which then submerge to form the nasal pits. Each nasal pit communicates posteriorly with the stomodeum.

The medial nasal process of both sides gives rise to the middle portion of the nose, the middle portion of the upper lip, and anterior portion of the maxilla, as well as the primary palate. The maxillary process grows medially and approaches the lateral and medial nasal processes. As a result, the maxillary process pushes the medial nasal process towards the midline, which it then merges with its anatomic counterpart from the opposite side (Fig. 21.1.1). The merging of the two medial nasal processes results in the formation of that part of the maxilla which carries the incisor teeth, and the primary palate and the central upper lip. The upper lip is therefore formed from the fusion of the maxillary process of each side and the medial nasal process. Thus, clefting of the lip is a result of failed fusion of the maxillary process and medial nasal process. The lateral nasal prominences give rise to the alae of the nose (Fig. 21.1.1). The maxillary prominences give

rise to the upper jaw and the sides of the face, the sides of the upper lip, and the secondary palate.

Formation of the secondary palate commences around 7–8 weeks and completes around the third month of gestation. Three outgrowths appear in the oral cavity. The nasal septum grows downward from the frontonasal process along the midline. Two palatine shelves, one from each side, extend from the maxillary processes toward the midline. At first, the shelves are directed downward along each side of the tongue. After the seventh week, the head of the embryo tilts back and the tongue is withdrawn from between the shelves. The shelves then elevate and fuse with each other above the tongue and anteriorly with the primary palate. The septum and the two shelves converge, fuse along the midline, and hence separate the primary oro-nasal cavity into the nasal *and* oral cavities.

The closure of the secondary palate proceeds gradually from the primary palate in a posterior direction. The extent of clefting found in a child reflects the time when closure of the secondary palate was affected. Full clefting results from interference at the start of closure and partial clefting later as the process proceeds posteriorly.

As discussed above, clefts of the lip and the anterior maxilla are a result of defective development of the embryonic primary palate. Often when such clefts occur, the distortion of the facial development prevents the palatine shelves from making contact when they swing into the horizontal position. Thus, clefts of the primary palate are often accompanied by clefts of the secondary palate, both hard and soft.

Epidemiology

The genetics of cleft lip with or without a cleft palate, or an isolated cleft palate, are complicated and do not follow a Mendelian inheritance pattern. The etiology of cleft lip and palate is thought to be multifactorial involving genetic and environmental factors. This consensus is supported by the concordance rate of 30–60% among monozygotic twins compared to 1–5% among dizygotic twins. Families with "cleft lip with or without palate" and "cleft palate only" are at a higher risk of having another child with the deformity when compared to the general population. Table 21.1.1 lists the increased risk for having the next child having the deformities based on current family members.[6,7] A recent cohort study from Denmark evaluating more than 54 000 relatives of cleft lip and palate probands reports recurrence risks for first, second, and third degree relatives, respectively: 3.5%, 0.8 %, and 0.6%.[8] Individuals affected by the most severe oral cleft had a significantly higher recurrence risk among both offspring and

Table 21.1.1 **Risk of cleft lip and/or cleft palate**		
Family members	**CL and CL/P**	**CP only**
One child with a deformity	4%	2%
One parent with a deformity	4%	6%
One parent and one child with deformities	17%	15%
Two children with deformities	9%	

siblings – e.g., the recurrence risk for siblings of a proband with isolated bilateral cleft lip with cleft palate was 4.6% (3.2 to 6.1) versus 2.5% (1.8 to 3.2) for a proband born with a unilateral defect.

Anatomy

An in-depth understanding of the anatomic deformity of the cleft lip and nose is critical to achieving successful surgical correction. While the soft tissues of the upper lip and nose are most visually affected and appreciated by peers, this deformity is a composite tissue deformity involving skin, muscle, cartilage, and bone. Early in the child's life, the attention of cleft surgeons is focused on all of these structures. The normal upper lip is characterized by complex positioning of the mucosa and vermillion, white roll, central tubercle, philtral dimple, philtral columns, and columellar–labial junction.

The adult nose is made up of nine convex and concave surfaces: the nasal subunits.[9] However, because cartilaginous and bony growth is not complete at the time of primary cleft lip and nose repair, it is useful to appreciate that there are differences in the nasal anatomy of the adult and a newborn.

The orbicularis oris is the main intrinsic muscle that encircles the mouth, which consists of two functional components – the superficial (pars superficialis) and the deep (pars marginalis) components. The pars superficialis is located under the skin of the lip and functions with nearby facial muscles of expression primarily to retract the upper lip. Furthermore, the pars superficialis consists of an upper and lower muscle bundle. The lower bundle originates from the depressor anguli muscle on each side, decussates in the midline attaching its fibers into the skin, thus forming the philtral columns on the contralateral side. The pars marginalis – which runs under the vermillion across from one modiolus to the other – provides the sphincteric action of the mouth.

Obviously, the cleft interrupts the continuous encirclement of the mouth by the orbicularis oris. The abnormal muscular attachments of the orbicularis oris contribute to the lip and nasal deformity. On the cleft side, the orbicularis oris attaches to the ipsilateral alar base, displacing the lower lateral cartilage inferiorly, posteriorly, and laterally, which produces the collapsed, concave deformity. On the non-cleft or medial side, the orbicularis oris attaches to the caudal septum and displaces it ipsilaterally.

As discussed above, the pars superficialis decussates in the midline to form the philtral columns. However, on the cleft side, the pars superficialis runs from the modiolus towards the midline but redirects superiorly to abnormally attach to the nasal ala and periosteum of the piriform rim. These attachments are responsible for the lateral displacement of the nostril, a lateral bulge when the muscle contracts, and the underlying bony piriform rim's inferior and lateral displacement. On the non-cleft side, the pars superficialis continues from the modiolus into the cleft edge perpendicularly. The pars marginalis is interrupted by the cleft but largely does not appear to cause further deformation.

The bony deformity is most pronounced by the alveolar cleft, which usually extends from the incisive surface of the alveolus, creating a greater and lesser cleft maxillary segments. The bony deformity extends cephalad to the piriform rim, nasal septum, and nasal alar region. The maxillary dentition is usually affected, often with a missing permanent lateral incisor as well as frequent supernumerary teeth, which may extrude into the cleft.

Presurgical infant orthopedics

Cleft lip deformities not only distort the soft tissues of the lip but are associated with significant alveolar (bony tissues) and nasal (cartilaginous tissues) deformities. While there are several preoperative treatment modalities for cleft lip/nose, the overall goals are similar: to more closely approximate the cartilaginous, bony, and soft tissues to convert a complete cleft lip/nose into an "incomplete" cleft lip/nose phenotype. Historically, a head bonnet with an elastic strip had been used to ventroflex the protruding premaxilla, in bilateral clefting, to accomplish these goals. Currently, the most common options for pre-surgical infant orthopedics (PSIO) include simple lip taping, cleft lip-nose adhesion, the application of a Latham appliance and naso-alveolar molding (NAM). Each has its advantages, disadvantages, and different levels of success.

Taping

The use of adhesive strips has the potential to apply a force that slowly narrows the cleft gap. The DynaCleft® device consists of an adhesive tape connected by an elastomeric strip that bridges the cleft segments. It can be used for both unilateral and bilateral clefts. The elastic core applies a constant controlled force to better approximate the lip and alveolus. Over time and serial applications of the device, the bony and soft tissues are guided toward approximation, allowing for a possibly easier primary repair of the lip. Placement of the device occurs shortly after birth.

Lip–nose adhesion

Lip–nose adhesion (typically performed prior to 2–3 months of age) involves creation of rectangular "book flaps" from the medial and lateral cleft margins within the nostril sill and upper lip. When the flaps along the medial edges of the cleft lip and nostril sill are sewn together, an incomplete cleft phenotype is created. The goals are to ultimately mold the maxillary dental arch towards a more normal position, to reposition the ala of the nose, and finally to release tension of the lip in preparation of the definitive lip repair.[10] This procedure, however, is felt to be associated with additional scarring and abnormal tethering of the lip and nasal elements.

Latham device

Although primarily used for *bilateral* clefts, the Latham device is worth noting. The device is a form of active PSIO used to align cleft tissues. The Latham device requires an additional surgery for placement and is secured with surgical pins. This device requires the child's guardian to turn the screw daily as well as weekly visits to the orthodontist. While effective, the Latham device may have lost some popularity due to the advent of naso-alveolar molding (NAM). Such active PSIO has opponents who claim retraction of the premaxilla results in adverse facial growth and occlusal outcomes.[11,12]

Naso-alveolar molding

Naso-alveolar molding (NAM) is a passive form of PSIO, accomplishing a change to the alveolus and lip as well as changes to the nose. NAM is most indicated in wide unilateral clefts and for all complete bilateral clefts. The goal of NAM is to narrow the cleft gap by aligning the maxillary arch; and, this subsequently brings the edges of the clefted lips together. As well, NAM addresses the cleft lip nasal deformity, particularly with the bilateral cleft where it extends the columella through tissue expansion, improves sagittal projection, as well as the size, shape, and symmetry of the nasal apertures.

Surgical techniques

While differences between surgical techniques can be significant and have evolved over years, the overall goal is similar – to create a functional and aesthetically pleasing lip and nose. Unilateral cleft lip and nose repair can be conceptualized as "philtral subunit reconstruction" – with the goal of creating a symmetric and normally shaped philtrum with a balanced Cupid's bow – placing the incision along the philtral column. Basically, this can be accomplished with straight or curved incisions, with or without the use of triangular flaps. In the next three chapters, three common and unique techniques for unilateral cleft lip and nose repair will be described. Four techniques are briefly described here.

The Randall–Tennison repair

Charles Tennison initially described this triangular flap repair in 1952,[13] which was later modified by Peter Randall.[14] Tennison used a sterilized paper clip that he sculpted to determine the position of a nearly equilateral triangular flap on the lateral lip element superior to the vermillion. This lateral lip based triangular flap is inset into the medial lip element above the white roll, thereby lengthening the medial flap and balancing Cupid's bow.

The rotation-advancement repair

The rotation-advancement technique was described by D. Ralph Millard and has subsequently undergone many revisions. In this technique, a curved rotation incision is created on the medial lip element that allows for inferior rotation of the central lip element, balancing Cupid's bow. The lateral lip is then advanced into the defect created by the rotation and sewn in place. In its original conception, three flaps were described: A, the medial rotation flap; B, the lateral advancement flap carrying the alar base on the cleft side; and C, the triangular flap attached to the columella that is advanced across the nasal floor. The rotation-advancement repair is further described by Dr. Philip Chen in Chapter 1.1.

Extended Mohler repair

Lester Mohler's technique theoretically positions the scar to simulate the "mirror image" of the unaffected philtral column.[15] This technique is compared to Millard's repair where the incision (and subsequent scar) approaches the midline of the philtrum as it advances superiorly near the columella–lip junction. In Mohler's repair, the marking for the medial lip segment was modified in the superior portion, and extends onto the columella, using columellar base tissue to achieve adequate height to balance Cupid's bow. The extended Mohler repair is further described by Dr. Roberto Flores in Chapter 1.2.

Fisher anatomic subunit repair

Similar to the Mohler repair, David Fisher described a technique that leaves the cleft side incision symmetric to the unaffected philtral column.[16] Moreover, borrowing from Burget's subunit principles in nasal reconstruction,[9] Fisher uses the concept of anatomic subunits of the lip. His technique borrows from the Tennison–Randal technique where frequently a small triangular flap is inside above the white roll when needed to balance Cupid's bow. The anatomic subunit repair is described by Dr. David Fisher in Chapter 1.3.

Postoperative considerations

While postoperative management protocols for unilateral cleft lip and nose repair vary between surgeons, there is a short list of issues that must be considered, and these include airway protection, analgesia, arm restraints, antibiotic use, lip scar management and taping, and nasal stenting.

Early postoperative monitoring of the airway is required, as blood and secretions, coupled with changes in the airway from endotracheal intubation and alterations in the lip and nose, put the infant at risk. As with any surgery, pain control is an important aspect of postoperative care; nerve blocks often decrease the need for analgesic medication.

The use of arm restraints has been a controversial subject. However, one research group conducted a review of primary cleft surgeries with different protocols for postoperative restraints – one surgeon routinely used restraints whereas the other did not.[17] There was no difference in early complications (i.e., infection, fistula, dehiscence) in patients who were required to wear arm restraints versus those who were not.

As with most procedures in plastic surgery, there is no consensus regarding the use of antibiotics in cleft surgery. Given the nature of the lip and nose surgery, most surgeons likely administer at least a preoperative dose of antibiotics. Some surgeons performing more invasive nasal surgery prefer to administer a postoperative course as well.[18]

There is no consensus regarding use of external skin sutures on the cleft lip and nose repair. If external sutures are used, their removal or dissolution protocol is unique to each surgeon. If absorbable sutures are utilized, many surgeons choose fast-absorbing sutures to minimize scarring. Absorption can be expedited by gently wiping the suture line with normal saline or dilute hydrogen peroxide starting early postoperatively. Due to an infant's inability to cooperate, they have been brought to the operating room for permanent suture removal in the past. Others have removed permanent sutures in the clinic during the initial postoperative visit. One protocol instructs the caregiver to bring the child to clinic *nil per os* (NPO) and hungry. The child is then placed supine with the head in the surgeon's lap. Giving the hungry child a bottle allows for the sutures to be removed in a much more calm and controlled fashion.

Once the initial wound healing has commenced, many surgeons employ various protocols for lip scar management that include scar massage and scar taping. Some recommend extended courses of lip scar taping with micropore tape and/or silicone-impregnated tape. The authors recommend that their patients receive 3 months of silicone-impregnated lip scar taping. For hypertrophic scars that do not respond to massage and taping, steroid impregnated tape and/or steroid injections have been employed.

Some surgeons recommend a postoperative course of nasal stents use (Fig. 21.1.2). Postoperative nasal stenting is utilized to maintain the reconstructed nasal shape and prevent deleterious changes that result from wound scarring, cartilage memory, and nasal scar contracture. Silicone nostril conformers are placed at the time of primary rhinoplasty to maintain the form and position of the reconstructed nasal deformity and are used for weeks to months.

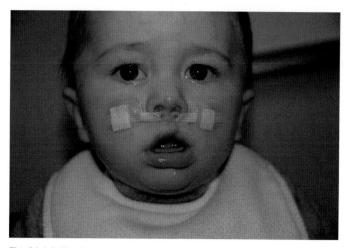

Fig. 21.1.2 Nasal stent.

Complications

The above-mentioned postoperative considerations are instituted to prevent complications. Unfortunately, each surgery is joined with a set of potential complications. These complications can be classified as early or late. Early complications are those that occur within the hospital stay and may prolong the hospital stay. A recent retrospective review demonstrates a wide array of potential complications,[19,20] which include: airway obstruction, hematoma, infection, anesthesia-related problems, and dehiscence. Longer-term potential complications include: stitch granuloma, hypertrophic scarring, nostril floor breakdown with use of nasal stents, oronasal fistula, and notching. Complications specific to nasal stenting include infections, pressure necrosis, or soft tissue loss.[18]

 Access the complete reference list online at **http://www.expertconsult.com**

9. Burget GC, Menick FJ. The subunit principle in nasal reconstruction. *Plast Reconstr Surg.* 1985;76:239.

13. Tennison CW. The repair of the unilateral cleft lip by the stencil method. *Plast Reconstr Surg.* 1952;9:115–120.

14. Randall P. A triangular flap operation for the primary repair of unilateral clefts of the lip. *Plast Reconstr Surg.* 1959;23:249–259.

15. Mohler LR. Unilateral cleft lip repair. *Plast Reconstr Surg.* 1987;80(4):511–517.

16. Fisher DM. Unilateral cleft lip repair: an anatomical subunit approximation technique. *Plast Reconstr Surg.* 2005;116(1): 61–71.

17. Michelotti B, Long RE, Leber D, Samson T, Mackay D. Should surgeons use arm restraints after cleft surgery? *Ann Plast Surg.* 2012;69(4):387–388.

18. Alef M, Irwin C, Smith D, et al. Nasal tip complications of primary cleft lip nasoplasty. *J Craniofac Surg.* 2009;20(5):1327–1333.

19. Zhang Z, Fang S, Zhang Q, et al. Analysis of complications in primary cleft lips and palates surgery. *J Craniofac Surg.* 2014; 25(3):968–971.

20. Schönmeyr B, Wendby L, Campbell A. Early Surgical Complications after Primary Cleft Lip Repair: A Report of 3108 Consecutive Cases. *Cleft Palate Craniofac J.* 2015;52(6):706–710.

21.2

Rotation advancement cheiloplasty

Philip Kuo–Ting Chen, Jeremiah Un Chang See, and M. Samuel Noordhoff

 Access video content for this chapter online at expertconsult.com

SYNOPSIS

Pre-surgical nasoalveolar molding/nasal molding
Key steps in surgery
- Determine the landmarks.
- Determine the incision line for rotation: Mohler's incision versus traditional rotation incision.
- Determine the incision lines for advancement including a white skin roll flap, orbicularis marginalis flap, L-flap, and turbinate flap (if necessary). Eliminate the perialar incision.
- Adequate release of muscle in both the rotation and advancement flaps. Adequate mobilization of the alar base on the cleft side.
- Nasal floor reconstruction using mucosal flaps without leaving raw surface. Overcorrection of the nostril width on the cleft side.
- Anchoring of the advancement flap to nasal septum to centralize the Cupid's bow.
- Approximate the orbicularis muscle in overlapping fashion for philtral reconstruction.
- Reconstruct the white skin roll according to subunit principle.
- Correct central vermilion deficiency with triangular vermilion flap from lateral lip.
- Semi-open rhinoplasty with reverse U incision on the cleft side and rim incision on the non-cleft side.
- Atraumatic dissection to release the fibrofatty tissue from lower lateral cartilages.
- Advancement and fixation of the cleft side lower lateral cartilage to the non-cleft side lower lateral cartilage and skin in an over-corrected position.
- Define the ala–facial groove with alar transfixion sutures.
Postoperative maintenance of over-correction with silicone nasal conformer.

Introduction

The techniques presented here are based on the experiences at Chang Gung Craniofacial Center over a period of 30 years in a Taiwanese population. They have also been tested in other racially diverse centers. The improved outcomes result from an integrated approach with pre-surgical management, surgical refinements, and post-surgical maintenance.

Preoperative plan

Multidisciplinary care

A multidisciplinary approach is essential to the satisfactory treatment of cleft patients. This includes surgeons, orthodontists, speech pathologists, pedodontists, prosthodontists, otolaryngologists, social workers, psychologists, as well as a photographer.[1] In addition, the Center's coordinator serves to coordinate all these specialties for the benefit of the patients as well as gathering and recording vital information. These contribute to the comprehensive care of cleft patients from infancy to adulthood.

First visit

At Chang Gung Craniofacial Center, the initial visit is made as soon as possible after birth. An orthodontist and plastic surgeon carefully examine the infant to record tissue deficiencies and distortion. The coordinator and social worker provide psychological support to the patient's family and essential information regarding the subsequent care. The baby is also evaluated by a pediatrician for other systemic abnormalities.

Nasoalveolar molding/nasal molding

Pre-surgical nasoalveolar molding (NAM, for complete cleft lips) or nasal molding (for incomplete cleft lips) is started soon after the first visit. Usually it takes 3–4 months for the completion of the molding process.

During the past 28 years, several techniques have been used for pre-surgical management. They vary from simple to very sophisticated techniques. These include sleeping in prone position,[2] lip taping,[3] pre-surgical orthopedics with an acrylic plate[4] with lip taping and three different NAM techniques. Among these three techniques, modified Grayson's and Liou's (modified Figueroa's) are commonly used. Both molding techniques require outpatient adjustments every 1–2 weeks.

Modified Grayson's technique

A passive orthopedic appliance is used together with taping of the lip. The alveolar molding is started first to narrow the alveolar gaps while molding the premaxilla into a proper position. Upon achieving a certain alveolar narrowing and arch alignment, a nasal mold is added to the orthopedic appliance. The nasal mold will lengthen the columella and reshape the alar dome. Taping across the upper lip also acts as a lip adhesion that decreases the nasal width (Fig. 21.2.1A,B ⊕).[5]

Fig. 21.2.1 appears online only.

Liou's technique (Modified Figueroa technique)

This device is composed of a dental plate, nasal molding components, and adhesive tape (Micropore™). The dental plate is held to the palate with dental adhesive. Micropore™ tape is placed across the clefts to minimize the alveolar cleft, retract the pre-maxilla, and keep both alar bases medial. The nasal components project forward in a sagittal direction from the dental plate. Columella lengthening is achieved by the combined forces of backward movement of the premaxilla and forward movement of the nasal tip. Both the alveolar and nasal molding processes are performed simultaneously (Fig. 21.2.2A,B).[6]

A prospective randomized controlled trial showed there were no differences between these two NAM techniques in terms of frequency of clinical visit, total cost, nostril height, and nostril area ratio. The modified Grayson technique reduced nostril width more efficiently but caused more alveolar ulceration. However, there was no difference in nostril width following surgery. Overall, these two NAM techniques produced similar nasal aesthetic outcomes.[7]

Nasoalveolar molding with a spring device

To decrease the burden of care for the parents, a new molding device using the spring mechanism was developed from the modification of Liou's technique. The molding prongs are made from 0.032-inch β-titanium wire with a helix. It only needs four clinic visits before lip repair, thus significantly decreasing the number of follow up visits. This can be very important for patients with limited resources, as it saves cost and travel time (Fig. 21.2.3A,B ⊕).

Fig. 21.2.3 appears online only.

Nasal molding with silicone nasal conformer

For incomplete cleft lips, nasal molding can be achieved by using silicone nasal conformers.[8] Nasal conformers with different heights can gradually increase nasal dome height by stretching the columella as well as molding the shape of deformed lower lateral cartilage (LLC). Parents are instructed to change to a larger size conformer every 2–3 weeks (Fig. 21.2.4A–D ⊕).

Fig. 21.2.4 appears online only.

Operative techniques

Treatment plan for lip repair in Chang Gung Craniofacial Center

There are several different treatment plans leading to the surgical correction of the deformity. With effective pre-surgical nasoalveolar molding, definitive cheiloplasty with anterior palate repair is done at the age of 3–5 months. Whenever pre-surgical orthopedics is not available or if the child is older than 3 months at presentation, cleft width determines the protocol. If the cleft width is less than 12–15 mm, the child proceeds to surgery. If there is a wide cleft (>12–15 mm) or significant tissue deficiency, nasolabial adhesion cheiloplasty is done at 3 months, followed by a definitive cheiloplasty at about 9 months old.[9]

Rotation advancement cheiloplasty for complete clefts (Videos 21.2.1 and 21.2.2 ▶)

Markings

Cupid's bow, vermilion, commissure, columellar base, and alar base

The points of the Cupid's bow (CPHR, LS, CPHL) are marked on the epidermis–vermilion junction line along with the white skin roll (WSR) as described by Millard. Usually, point CPHR is easy to identify. Gentle upward lift on the nasal tip with a finger helps to define point LS (Fig. 21.2.5A,B). This is essential because it is easier to level the Cupid's bow if LS is marked toward CPHR, making Cupid's bow somewhat narrower. However, the shape of the Cupid's bow can be partially deformed. If one places point LS toward the cleft margin, point CPHL will be moved higher, and it will be more difficult to level the Cupid's bow. The distance between LS and CPHL is determined by the measurement between CPHR and LS. The vermilion–mucosa junction line, the red line,[10,11] is also marked. This clearly defines the intervening vermilion below the heights of the Cupid's bow. It also identifies the vermilion deficiency beneath the height of Cupid's bow near the cleft margin. Next, one marks out the midpoint of columella base (SN), highest points of the philtral columns (CPHSR, CPHSL), bilateral base of the ala (SBAR, SBAL) and commissure (CHR, CHL). Lastly, the width of the WSR at point CPHR is marked out. The width of the WSR is usually around 2 mm at the age of 3–6 months old (Fig. 21.2.6A).

Base of philtral column on the cleft side

The base of the philtral column on the cleft side (CPHL') is a definite anatomic point but somehow difficult to identify. The red line always converges and meets the WSR medially. Frequently, there is a distinct point where the WSR changes directions and makes a slight curve 3–4 mm before meeting the red line. Point CHPL' is where the WSR changes direction and the vermilion first becomes widest which is usually 3–4 mm lateral to the converging point of red line and WSR.[12] This is an important anatomic point for the cleft-side philtral column and seldom requires adjustment unless there is a severe discrepancy in the horizontal or vertical length (Fig. 21.2.6B). As mentioned earlier, the width of the WSR flap

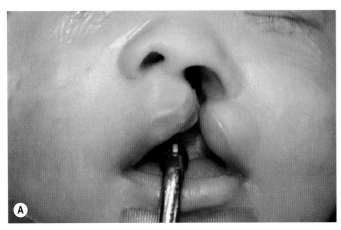
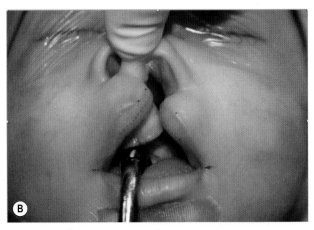

Fig. 21.2.5 (A,B) The different shape of Cupid's bow when pushing the nasal tip upward with a finger. This maneuver helps to define the point LS.

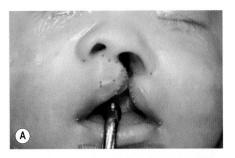
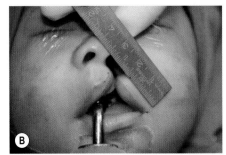
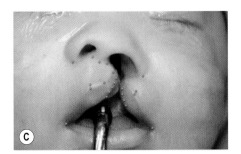
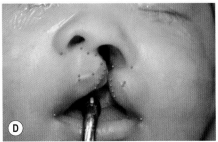

Fig. 21.2.6 (A) The points: CPHR, LS, CPHL, SN, CPHSR, CPHSL, SBAR, SBAL, CHR, CHL and the red lines. (B) The point CPHL'. Although the horizontal lip length is shorter on the cleft side, this point is still chosen at its anatomical position. (C) Besides the points in (D) shows the split point of nasolabial groove.

corresponds to the measurement on the non-cleft side (Fig. 21.2.6C). The split point of the nasolabial groove (the point where the skin-mucosal junction changes its direction at the deepest point of the nasal vestibulum on the cleft side) is also marked (Fig. 21.2.6D).

Proposed point of medial nasal sill

Gentle inward pressure on the cleft side ala base helps to define the position and direction of the cleft side nasal sill. The proposed point of the medial nasal sill, which is usually the highest point of the philtral column on the cleft side (CPHSL'), is the point where the nasal sill ends medially and meets the base of columella during skin closure (Fig. 21.2.7). This point is marked approximately 8 mm from a tangential line on the ala–facial groove in a 3–6-month-old baby. This distance helps to achieve an over-corrected nostril width on the cleft side.

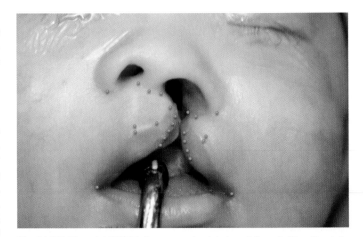

Fig. 21.2.7 The point CPHSL', the proposed point of medial nasal sill on the cleft side.

Measurements

Various measurements are made, based on the anthropometric points marked (Fig. 21.2.8). Important measurements for the

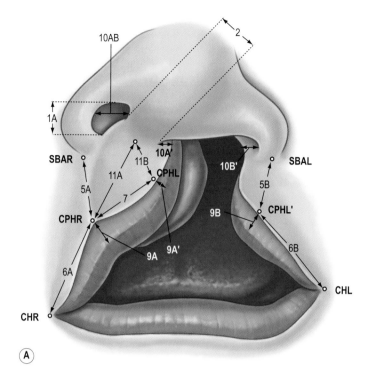

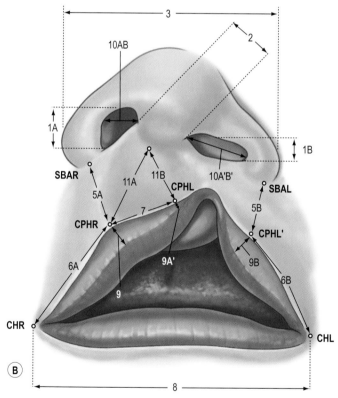

Fig. 21.2.8 **(A)** Unilateral complete cleft with anthropometric markings for measurements. **(B)** Similar markings for unilateral incomplete cleft lip. *(From Noordhooff MS, Chen YR, Chen KT, Hong KF, Lo LJ. The surgical technique for the complete unilateral cleft lip-nasal deformity. Opera Tech in Plast Reconstr Surg. 1995;2(3):167–174.)*

surgeon to evaluate include the vertical length (5A, 5B) and the horizontal width (6A, 6B) of the lip.

Peaking of Cupid's bow

The discrepancy between the heights from the central columella base (SN) to the two peaks of the Cupid's bow (CPHR and CPHL) is critical for leveling the Cupid's bow. The authors favor Mohler's incision for rotation if the discrepancy is over 2 mm. A shorter rotation incision from CPHL to CPSHL is carried out if the discrepancy is less than 2 mm (Fig. 21.2.9A,B).

Lateral lip height and length

The short horizontal length on cleft side (HL) can be lengthened by adjusting point CPHL' medially; however, this would shorten the vertical length (VL) (Fig. 21.2.10A). Vertical length is more important aesthetically compared with the horizontal length. Therefore, vertical length is seldom sacrificed for horizontal length. The short vertical length can be increased by adjusting point CPHL' laterally, but this would result in an even shorter horizontal length which is pre-existing (Fig. 21.2.10B). The traditional method of extending the upper rotation-advancement incision around the ala can also increase the short vertical length. However, this results in an unacceptable perialar scar and should be avoided. Point CPHL' is as

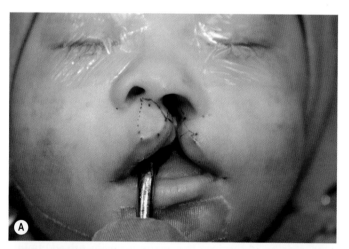

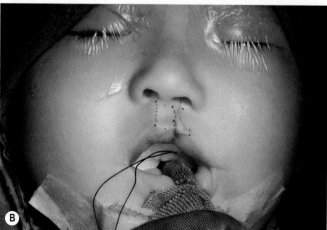

Fig. 21.2.9 **(A)** Markings for the Mohler incision if the height discrepancy is more than 2 mm. **(B)** Marking for the simple rotation incision if the height discrepancy is less than 2 mm.

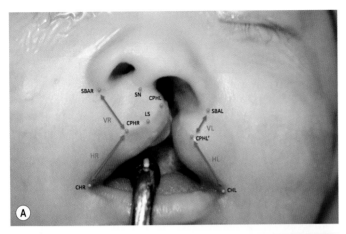

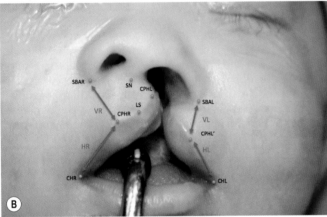

Fig. 21.2.10 (A) Moving point CPHL' medially will increase the horizontal lip length but shorten the vertical lip height. **(B)** Moving the point CPHL' laterally will have the opposite effect.

important as other anatomic points and should not be adjusted until all incisions, muscle dissection, and approximation are completed. This is because an increase in vertical length – up to 4 mm – can be achieved by adequate muscle dissection and redraping of the skin over the muscle, thus eliminating the need of perialar incisions or adjusting the point CPHL'. This lengthening effect should be taken into consideration rather than strictly observing the mathematically fixed points marked during lip repair. The preoperative measurements between points will differ after muscle release, muscle approximation, and skin redraping; therefore, they must be re-checked after muscle approximation.

Incomplete clefts often appear to have a vertically long lateral lip. However, the measurement of the cleft side vertical height is usually similar to the non-cleft side because the cleft side lateral lip and the alar base are inferiorly displaced (Fig. 21.2.11A). Therefore, the vertically long lateral lip, seen in incomplete clefts, is just an illusion. Adequate mobilization of the cleft side alar base and lateral lip, prior to advancing the entire lateral complex superiorly and medially, always levels Cupid's bow without vertically shortening the lateral lip (Fig. 21.2.11B).

White skin roll

The width of the WSR is usually widest above point CPHR. The WSR remains quite prominent between points CPHR and

LS but becomes narrower toward point CPHL. The authors routinely measure the width of WSR at point CPHR and transfer this measurement to the cleft side. The measured WSR at point CPHR is always wider (e.g., 2 mm wide at the age of 3–6 months old) than the observed WSR at point CPHL'. A triangular WSR flap is designed above point CPHL'. This 2 mm WSR flap helps to level Cupid's bow and corrects the WSR deficiency at point CPHL. In addition, it helps reconstruct the upper lip contour line in accordance to the subunit concept as advocated by Onizuka (Fig. 21.2.12A–D).[13]

Vermilion width

The vermilion width beneath point CPHL is always deficient compared with the counterpart vermilion at point CPHR or CPHL'. Inadequate reconstruction of this vermilion deficiency will result in free border deformities like exposed mucosa, color mismatching, and dry crusting as seen in a straight-line vermilion closure (Fig. 21.2.13). Therefore, the vermilion medial to point CPHL' should be used to correct the vermilion deficiency beneath the Cupid's bow.[10]

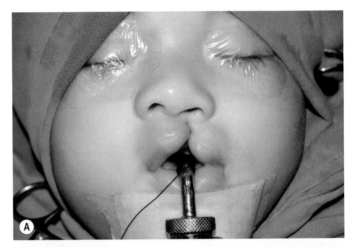

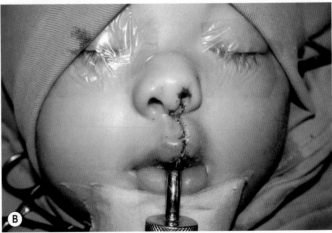

Fig. 21.2.11 (A) Although the vertical lip height seems longer on the cleft side, the height measurement between the two sides shows a similar result. The long lip is a false impression due to the downward displaced alar base. **(B)** Moving the whole lateral lip/alar base upward can achieve a symmetrical lip without shortening of the skin and muscle.

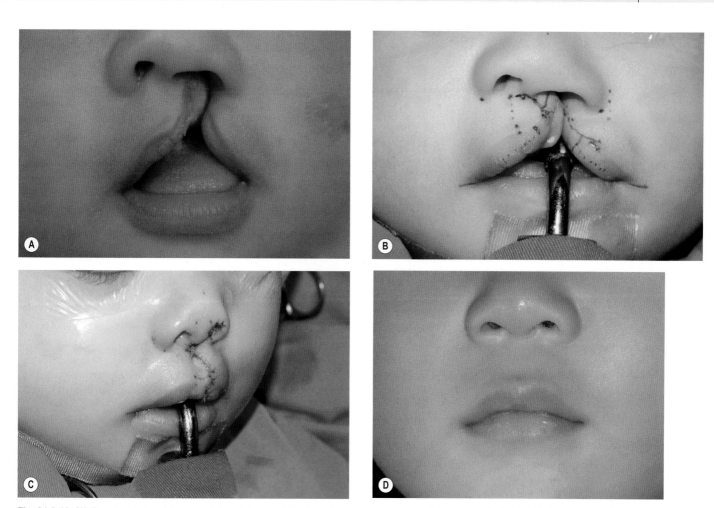

Fig. 21.2.12 **(A)** The width of the white skin roll is widest at point CPHR and becomes narrower toward the point CPHL. **(B)** A WSR flap is designed above the point CPHL' according to the width of WSR above CPHR. **(C)** The WSR flap helps to level the Cupid's bow, correct the WSR deficiency at the point CPHL while reconstructing the upper lip contour line. **(D)** The upper lip contour line. There is a horizontal groove at the upper margin of the WSR.

Incision lines

Incisions on the non-cleft side

Mohler incision

A Mohler incision[14] is designed for rotation if the discrepancy is over 2 mm. The incision is marked as a curvilinear line from

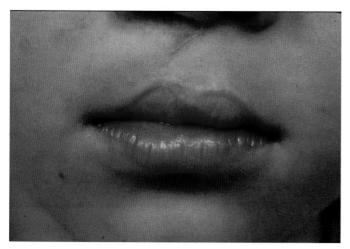

Fig. 21.2.13 Vermilion deficiency at the central free border after a straight line closure in this area.

CPHL extending upward into the base of columella then back-cut to the nasolabial junction of the non-cleft side philtral column (Fig. 21.2.13). The height of this rotation incision should match the height of the non-cleft side philtral column. The angle of the back-cut depends on the width of columella, ideally should be around 90° (Fig. 21.2.14A). If the columella is narrow, e.g., in the presence of median facial dysplasia,[15] a Mohler rotation incision would result in a very narrow columella base and should be avoided.

The incision across the free border of the lip at CPHL should be at a right angle to the axis of the white skin roll, facilitating subsequent lip closure. The lip is stabilized with a hook and finger while the incision is made with a #67 blade (Fig. 21.2.14B). The end point of the back-cut is at the point CPHSR. The incision should never extend across point CPHSR as this will lengthen the lip on the non-cleft side.

Simple rotation incision

A shorter rotation incision from CPHL to CPSHL is used if the discrepancy is less than 2 mm (Fig. 21.2.9B). This will avoid the scar across the nasolabial junction which is usually more obvious than the vertical scar on the lip. If the amount of rotation is inadequate, the incision line can be easily converted into a Mohler incision with extension into the columellar base.

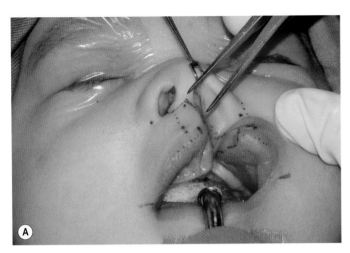

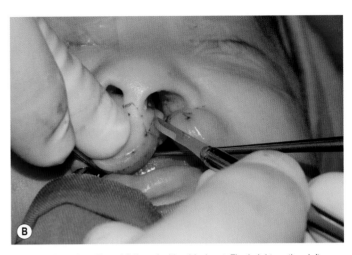

Fig. 21.2.14 (A) Markings for the Mohler technique are designed with the incision extending into the columella and followed with a black cut. The height on the cleft margin is similar to the height of philtral column on the non-cleft side. The angle of the back cut is around 90°. (B) The lip is stabilized with hook and finger while incised with #67 blade to ensure an accurate cut.

Mohler[14] and Onizuka[13] analyzed the shape of philtrum and concluded that the majority have philtral columns in an outward curvilinear configuration. Therefore, the authors strongly feel the curvilinear incision of Mohler gives a better philtral morphology compared to a straight line incision.

Adequate rotation

Adequate muscle dissection should reach the nasal floor of the non-cleft side as this releases the abnormal muscle insertion to the columellar base (Fig. 21.2.15A). Downward traction on the free border of the lip will determine if the rotation is

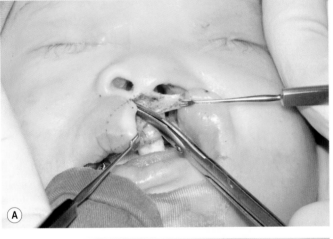

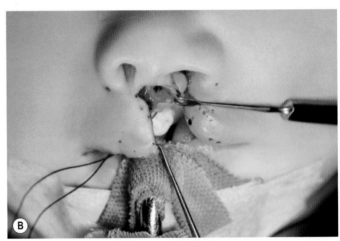

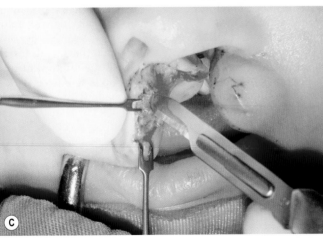

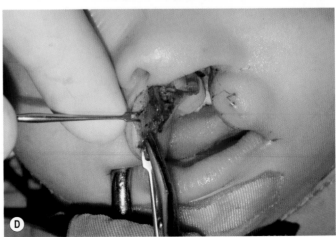

Fig. 21.2.15 (A) Adequate muscle dissection should reach the nasal floor of the non-cleft side as this releases the abnormal muscle insertion to the columellar base. (B) Downward traction on the free border of the lip will determine if the rotation is adequate, that is, both points CPHR and CPHL are at the same level. (C) Muscle layer is dissected along the skin edge initially with blade. (D) The muscle dissection is then continued with a pair of tenotomy scissors. The abnormal muscle insertion beneath the columellar base and nasal floor is released, followed by muscle attachment to the skin in the subdermal plane for a distance of 2–3 mm. The dissection plane is deeper, initially leaving a cuff of muscle on the incision edge and gradually to the subdermal level for better philtral ridge morphology.

adequate, that is, both points CPHR and CPHL are at the same level (Fig. 21.2.15B). If the rotation is inadequate, extending the back cut beyond the non-cleft side philtral column should never be attempted. This will result in a vertically long lip. At this point, if the Cupid's bow is not leveled, no further action is to be taken until the muscle dissection and repositioning has been completed. The back cut down the non-cleft side philtral column, advocated by Millard, leaves a wider and lower defect at the apex of the rotation, compared to the Mohler incision. This defect is then filled with a square-shaped advancement flap, always closed with much tension. This results in a conspicuous oblique scar across the upper philtrum. Therefore, this back cut on the non-cleft side philtrum should be avoided.

As mentioned, the authors routinely insert a WSR flap for lip subunit repair. This WSR flap provides an additional 1–2 mm of lip length, lowering and balancing Cupid's bow. This decreases the necessity of a back-cut.

Muscle dissection on the rotation flap

The muscle layer is dissected along the skin edge initially with a blade, then continued with a pair of tenotomy scissors. The abnormal muscle insertion beneath the columellar base and nasal floor is released. Following this, the muscle attachment to the skin, in the subdermal plane, is released for a distance of 2–3 mm. Initially, along the free edge of the lip, the dissection plane is deeper, leaving a small cuff of muscle on the incision edge. The dissection then moves gradually to the subdermal level. This provides for better philtral ridge morphology (Fig. 21.2.15C,D).

C-flap and footplate of medial crura

The C-flap incision is made on the line extending from point CPHL along the skin and mucosa junction to the deepest point of the skin on the premaxilla. At this point, the incision turns superiorly, for 5 mm or more, along the columellar skin and septal mucosa junction. The intercrural space beneath the columella is separated by tenotomy scissors (Fig. 21.2.16A,B). This allows mobilization of the C-flap and for repositioning the downward displaced medial crural foot plate on the cleft side LLC. The medial tip of the C-flap (at point CPHL) will be used to fill in the defect at the columellar base created by the Mohler incision. For patients with a simple rotation incision, it will be trimmed accordingly.

Septal dissection

The authors favor anterior palate repair during primary lip repair. The septal incision behind the C-flap is extended downward behind the premaxilla along the junction of the vomer and hard palate (Fig. 21.2.17A). Instead of a caudal septal dislocation, advocated by other surgeons, a septal mucosal flap is raised subperichondrially in continuity with the vomer flap used for the anterior palate repair (Fig. 21.2.17B,C).

Incisions on the cleft side lateral lip element

White skin roll flap and L-flap

A triangular WSR flap above point CPHL' is marked according to the width of the WSR at point CPHR (Figs. 21.2.9A,B & 21.2.12B). Usually the width and length are around 2 mm in a 3–6-month-old baby. An L-flap is marked based on the

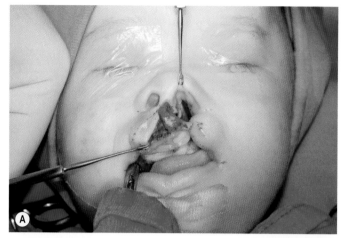

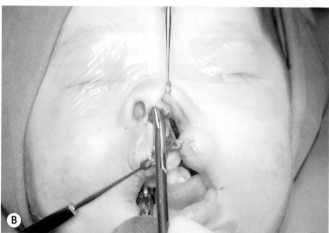

Fig. 21.2.16 (A) The C-flap extends from point CPHL along the skin and mucosa junction to the deepest point of the skin overlying the premaxilla. At the premaxilla, the incision turns superiorly for 5 mm or even longer along the columellar skin and septal mucosa junction. The CM flap is separated from the C-flap. **(B)** Use a tenotomy scissors to separate the foot plate of the medial crura in the C-flap.

alveolar margin, extending along the free border of the lip to the point where the red line and WSR converge. The width of the L-flap is around 5 mm. The upper margin of the L-flap corresponds to the skin incision from the WSR flap distally to point CPHSL'. The upper L-flap incision line is extended inwardly to the "split point" of nasolabial groove, or the skin-mucosal junction on the piriform rim. This incision meets the inferior edge of the turbinate (Fig. 21.2.18A,B).

Inferior turbinate (T) flap

An inferior turbinate (T) flap, pedicled anteriorly, is created by making incisions on the lower and upper edges of the turbinate for 1.5 cm. A transverse incision is made posteriorly, connecting the upper and lower incisions and pedicling the flap anteriorly. This flap is helpful to fill the mucosal defect created by releasing the alar base from the retro-positioned lesser maxillary segment (Fig. 21.2.18A).

Incision and dissection

The lateral lip is stabilized with a hook and finger. The WSR flap incision is made with #11 blade, followed by #67 blade for the vermilion and skin incision along the cleft margin. The

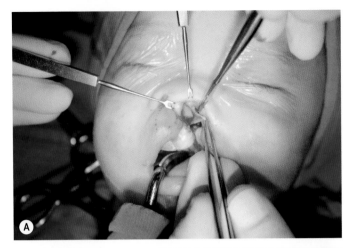

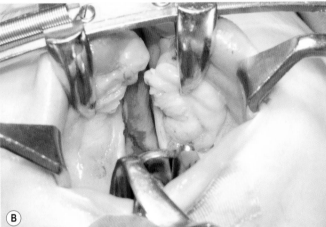

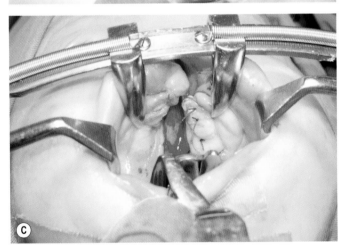

Fig. 21.2.17 **(A)** The septal flap is extended backward connecting the vomer flap if the anterior palate is repaired together with lip repair. **(B)** Intraoral view shows the design of the vomer flap. Its anterior part is connecting with the septal flap. **(C)** Repairing the anterior palate with vomer flap. The vomer flap is imbricated under the mucoperiosteum of the lesser segment.

the LLC and the lateral lip. The lateral lip is released from maxilla in a pre-periosteal plane (Fig. 21.2.18C). The extent of maxillary dissection is usually close to the infraorbital foramen. Even in wide clefts, adequate mobilization of the lip and alar base can be accomplished with a more extensive dissection over the maxilla.

The lateral lip mucosa is incised and dissected 2 mm from the muscle edge. Excessive mucosal dissection will result in thick scarring and should be avoided. The orbicularis peripheralis muscle is bunched up as a disorganized mass of fibers with numerous dermal insertions. Using a tenotomy scissors, the orbicularis peripheralis muscle is dissected along the edge of the dermis to a line extending from the base of the ala (SBAL) to the base of the philtral column (CPHL'). The dissection is continued in a subdermal plane superiorly around the alar base. This releases the abnormal insertions of the paranasal muscles, including the transverse portion of the nasalis muscle, depressor septi, and levator muscles of the upper lip and ala. The extent of muscle dissection should be lateral to the angular artery; ensuring most of the abnormal muscle insertions to the alar base are completely released (Fig. 21.2.18D–G). Adequate muscle release allows the tethered and bunched-up muscle to be stretched out, thus lengthening the lateral lip effectively to gain a substantial increment of vertical height and horizontal length. Similar to the non-cleft side, the dissection plane is deeper initially and gradually becomes subdermal, thus leaving a cuff of muscle on the edge of the incision, for better philtral ridge morphology.

Removal of fat pad under the vestibulum

Upon adequate muscle dissection beneath the alar base, a cuff of fat pad will usually bulge out from the nasal vestibule. Removal of this bulging fat pad will decrease some tissue thickness at the alar base, thus improving the vestibular webbing which is a common deformity seen after primary lip repair (Fig. 21.2.18H).

Mulliken uses a lenticular excision at primary repair to effectively eliminate the vestibular web.[16,17] However, this results in a linear scar on the lateral nasal vestibule, which might tether the LLC from medial advancement in secondary rhinoplasty.

Creation of the orbicularis marginalis flap

The orbicularis marginalis (OM) flap is incised along the free border of the lip and includes the orbicularis marginalis muscle, the vermilion medial to point CPHL', and the corresponding mucosa posteriorly.[9] The incision line of the OM flap is perpendicular to the skin. The muscle volume at CPHL' is preserved similar to the volume at point CPHR on the non-cleft side (Fig. 21.2.18I). Gentle downward traction of the OM flap can determine the tissue adequacy along the free margin, and the lip contour should be in a smooth line (Fig. 21.2.18J).

Nasal floor reconstruction and alar base repositioning

When the anterior palate repair is done simultaneously with primary lip repair, the vomer flap is imbricated beneath the mucoperiosteal edge of the lesser segment. The nasal floor is reconstructed by the septal and L-flaps. The septal flap is sutured to the lower margin of the L-flap, while the

L-flap is raised with a tenotomy scissor, and including a thin layer of muscle to ensure adequate blood supply. The T-flap is elevated in a retrograde fashion, and is pedicled on the lateral nasal vestibular skin (Fig. 21.2.18A, inset). After elevation of the L- and T-flaps, the attachments of the LLC to the maxilla and ULC are released, allowing easy mobilization of

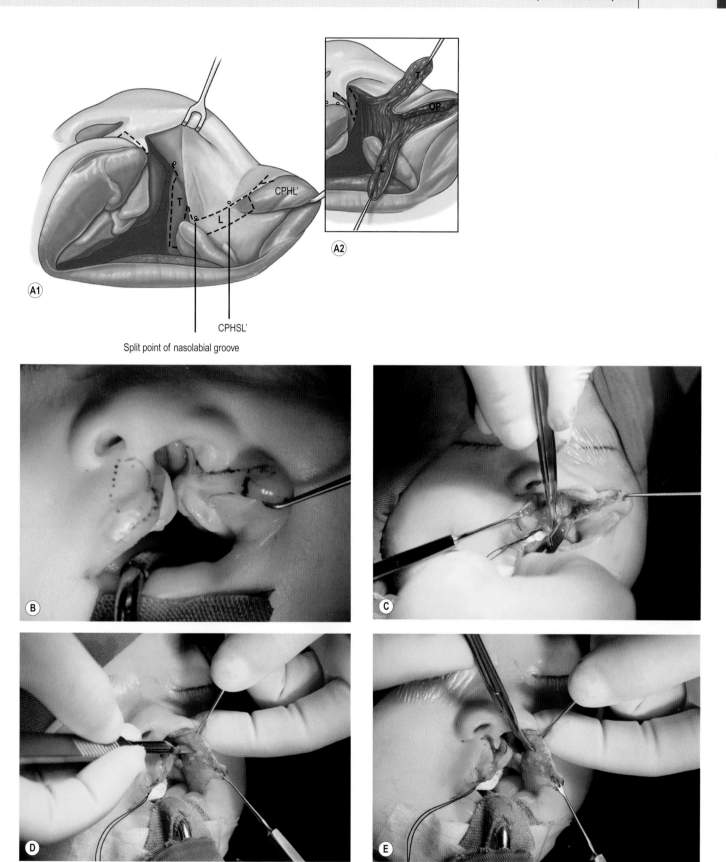

Fig. 21.2.18 **(A)** An inferior turbinate flap is designed to provide enough soft tissue coverage on the lateral nasal wall if there is lip repair alone without anterior palate repair. The L-flap will be brought across the nasal floor suturing to the septal incision. **(B)** The design of the L-flap. The width is around 5 mm and the length is depending on the width of the cleft. Its upper margin incision goes from the WSR flap above the CPHL' through CPHSL' to the split point of nasolabial junction, then turns 90° along the skin-mucosal junction on the piriform area. **(C)** The lateral lip is released from maxilla above the periosteum plane. The extent of the maxillary dissection is usually close to the infraorbital foramen. **(D)** The orbicularis peripheralis muscle is released from skin. The dissection is started with a blade. **(E)** Dissection is then continued with tenotomy scissors, which is initially deep and then becomes more superficial leaving a cuff of muscle on the wounds edge.

Continued

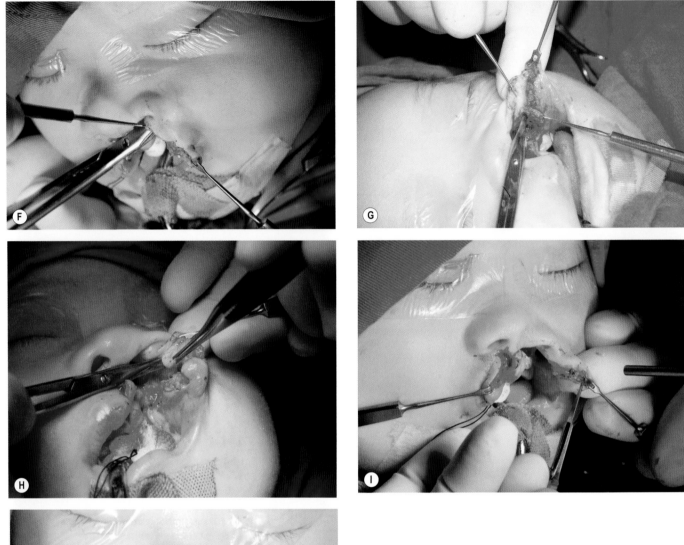

Fig. 21.2.18, cont'd **(F)** The abnormal muscle insertions around the alar base are adequately released. The bulging lateral to the alar base created by the tip of scissors showing the extent of the dissection. **(G)** The angular artery is used as a landmark for muscle dissection. **(H)** Removal of this bulging fat pad under the nasal vestibulum will decrease some tissue thickness at the alar base, thus improving the vestibular webbing which is a common deformity seen after primary lip repair. **(I)** The incision line of the OM flap is perpendicular to the skin. Similar muscle volume is preserved at CPHL' and point CPHR on the non-cleft side. **(J)** Gentle downward traction of the OM flap can determine the tissue adequacy along the free margin and the lip contour should be in a smooth line.

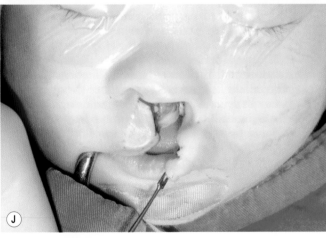

upper margin of the L-flap is sutured to the lower margin of the piriform incision (Fig. 21.2.19A,B). As the anterior part of the vomer flap is in continuity with the septal flap, a complete nasal floor closure is obtained. The vestibular skin with attached ala is advanced medially and superiorly. The upper margin of the piriform incision is sutured to the septal/L-flaps, while the split point of nasolabial groove is sutured to the uppermost point of the septal incision (Fig. 21.2.19C). This provides a two-layer closure of the nasal

floor. The alar base is advanced medially to achieve a 2 mm over-correction on nostril width.[6] The vertical position of the alar base should be at the same level as the non-cleft side. Final positioning of the alar base can be adjusted after nasal reconstruction.

When the lip repair is separated from anterior palate repair, the T-flap, based on vestibular skin, is rotated 90° to fill in the defect on piriform rim. Its superior edge is sutured to the inferior edge of the piriform incision. The T-flap corrects the

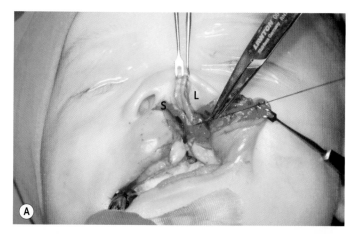

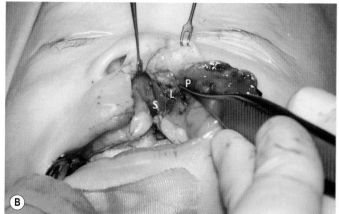

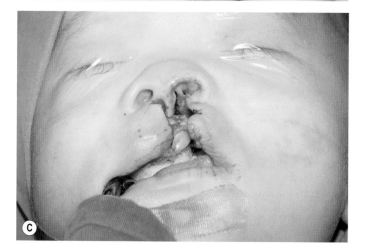

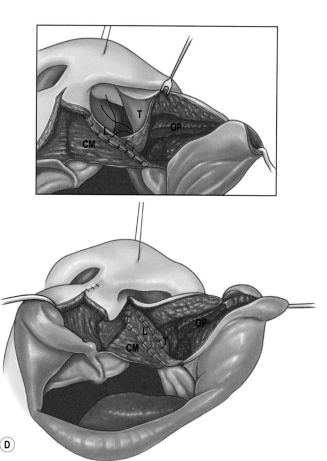

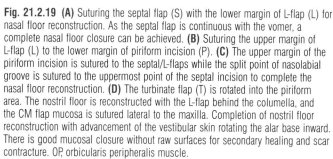

Fig. 21.2.19 **(A)** Suturing the septal flap (S) with the lower margin of L-flap (L) for nasal floor reconstruction. As the septal flap is continuous with the vomer, a complete nasal floor closure can be achieved. **(B)** Suturing the upper margin of L-flap (L) to the lower margin of piriform incision (P). **(C)** The upper margin of the piriform incision is sutured to the septal/L-flaps while the split point of nasolabial groove is sutured to the uppermost point of the septal incision to complete the nasal floor reconstruction. **(D)** The turbinate flap (T) is rotated into the piriform area. The nostril floor is reconstructed with the L-flap behind the columella, and the CM flap mucosa is sutured lateral to the maxilla. Completion of nostril floor reconstruction with advancement of the vestibular skin rotating the alar base inward. There is good mucosal closure without raw surfaces for secondary healing and scar contracture. OP, orbicularis peripheralis muscle.

mucosal deficiency and allows repositioning of the LLC and ala base without restriction. The L-flap is brought medially behind the columella and sutured to the mucoperichondrial flap of the posterior septal incision. The inferior edge of the T-flap is sutured to the superior edge of the L-flap. The C-flap mucosa is turned laterally and placed anterior to the L-flap. Its tip is sutured to the base of L-flap and its upper margin is sutured to the inferior edge of the L-flap. This gives good mucosal coverage of the nostril floor and lateral nostril wall without exposing any raw surface or tension. The vestibular skin with attached ala is advanced as described previously (Fig. 21.2.19D).

Muscle reconstruction

The muscle is approximated with 5–0 polydioxanone. A key suture is placed in the muscle approximating points CPHL to CPHL′. Downward traction is placed on this suture to level the Cupid's bow, and assures correct placement of subsequent muscle sutures (Fig. 21.2.20A). The superior-most stitch is placed through the tip of the advancement flap muscle (which was released from the superolateral attachment to the alar base) and is anchored to the caudal edge of the nasal septum, in a vertical mattress fashion (Fig. 21.2.20B). This anchoring suture helps to pull the lateral lip medially, centralizing Cupid's bow and correcting the possible lateral deviation of

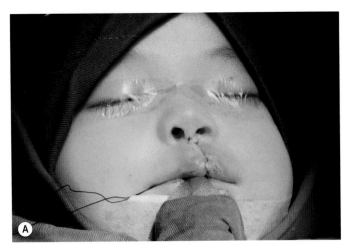

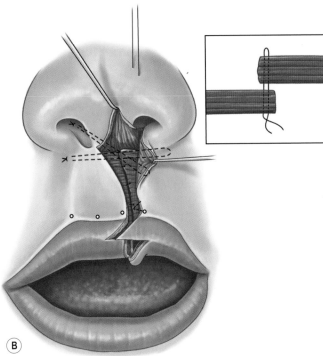

Fig. 21.2.20 (A) A key suture is placed in the center of the muscle apposing of points CPHL to CPHL'. This is to align the lip position by downward traction to level the Cupid's bow, making sure correct placement of each subsequent muscle suture. **(B)** Orbicularis peripheralis muscle closure (with septal anchoring suture). Inset: Overlapping the lateral muscle on the medial muscle for philtral column reconstruction.

the cleft side lip due to tissue deficiency. The muscle sutures are placed in such a way that the lateral muscle overlaps above the medial muscle, increasing muscle thickness and simulating a philtral column (Fig. 21.2.20B, inset).[18] To help restore the philtral dimple, the subdermal layer at the midline of philtrum is captured during muscle approximation. The muscle in OM flap is carefully sutured to avoid any depression in the vermilion post operatively.

Philtral column reconstruction

For a better aesthetic result of the philtral column, several key steps are necessary. (1) *Skin incision*: The authors favor the Mohler incision, which is more vertical and laterally placed, compared to the traditional rotation-advancement. Its curvature is more natural looking compared to the straight line technique. The final position of a Mohler incision mimics the natural curve of the non-cleft philtral column, and this holds to the subunit concept. (2) *Muscle reconstruction*: The overlapping muscle approximation, with vertical mattress sutures, increases the muscle thickness and simulates the philtral column. (3) *Subdermal suture placement*: Catching the subdermal layer at the midline of the philtrum, during muscle approximation, helps to restore the philtral dimple. (4) *Soft tissue laxity*: In addition to the increased muscle thickness created by overlapping muscle approximation, the muscle repair is made tighter than the overlying skin. This will produce slightly excess skin during closure and is necessary to reconstruct a bulging philtral column. The "excessive" skin after muscle reconstruction should be preserved, as it provides sufficient soft tissue laxity for a better philtral column appearance.

Insertion of the WSR flap

Point CPHL and CPHL' are approximated with 5–0 polydioxanone subcuticular suture followed by 7–0 polyglactin suture for skin. Following the WSR contour, the width of the WSR is measured and marked at the point CPHL. An incision, according to the length of WSR flap, is carefully designed to place the WSR flap tip at the horizontal groove of the lip contour line, as advocated by Onizuka.[13] The natural contour line is at the upper margin of the WSR. This helps to restore the continuity and fullness of the WSR, in addition to leveling the Cupid's bow (Fig. 21.2.21A–D).

Incisions for the triangular vermilion flap

The vermilion flap, based on the lateral lip element, is marked and incised on the OM flap. While the OM flap is held under tension, a #11 blade is used to ensure an accurate cut. After muscle approximation, the vermilion flap is inserted into the medial lip incision, made along or above the red line beneath the Cupid's bow CPHL point. The main purpose of this vermilion flap is to correct the vermilion deficiency beneath the Cupid's bow, and not for increasing the tissue bulk on the central free border. The tip of the vermilion flap should not cross the natural lip tubercle that is always present in a unilateral cleft. This natural tubercle should never be violated by the vermilion flap (Fig. 21.2.22A,B).

Closure of the free border of the lip

The excess mucosa below the vermilion flap is trimmed accordingly to approximate the free border of the lip edges without excessive tissue. Careful attention during excision of the excessive mucosa and muscle is important. The most common error is to leave too much muscle or mucosa on the free border. Incisions on the vermilion are closed with continuous 7–0 polyglactin suture. The lateral lip buccal mucosa is trimmed and closed with interrupted 5–0 polyglactin sutures. The upper edge of the buccal mucosa is sutured to the lower edge of C-flap mucosa that bridges the alveolar gap. This gives a complete mucosal closure without tension.

Incisions on nasal floor

The medial tip of the C-flap is used to fill the defect on columella base after a Mohler incision; or, it is trimmed when

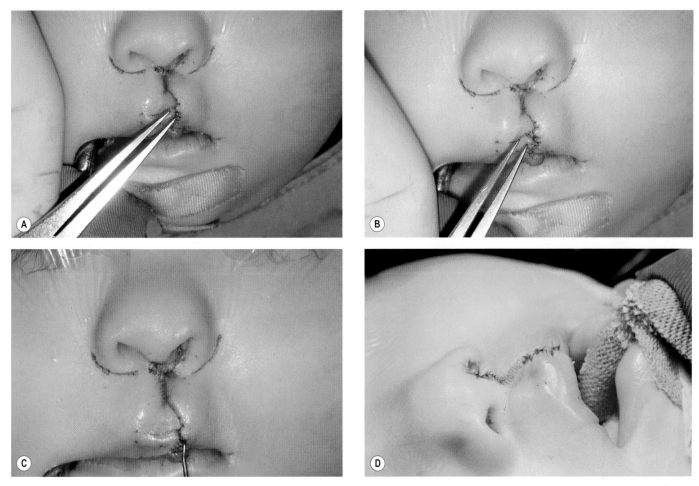

Fig. 21.2.21 **(A)** The width of the WSR is measured and marked at the point CPHL following the WSR contour. **(B)** An incision line according to the length of WSR flap is carefully designed to place the WSR flap tip at the horizontal groove of the lip contour line. **(C)** Careful insertion of the WSR flap to restore the natural lip contour line. **(D)** The appearance of the lip contour line after wound closure.

using a simple rotation incision. The lateral edge of the C-flap is brought laterally inside the nasal sill.

In an attempt to limit or eliminate incisions around the alar base, no horizontal incisions on the lateral advancement flap are made initially. At this point, the surgeon can better visualize how to proceed. Incisions around the ala base leave conspicuous scars, an unnatural ala–facial groove, and should be avoided. If the alar base on the cleft side lateral lip element is high, an incision is made inside the cleft side nasal sill (Fig. 21.2.23A). This incision can vertically lengthen the lip and level the alar base and Cupid's bow. If the alar base is already leveled after muscle reconstruction, a vertical nasal floor incision is made, as shown in Fig. 21.2.23B. Every attempt is made to preserve the natural nasal sill. The nasal sill is unique tissue, very difficult to reconstruct in secondary deformities, and should be carefully preserved in primary repairs. During the primary repair, the nostril width on the cleft side is slightly over-corrected (2 mm narrower than the non-cleft side) as the authors' experience shows the cleft side nostril will widen with time after the primary operation.[6]

Final skin closure on lip

The point CPHSL' is sutured to CPHSL and the rotation flap creates a suture line that mimics the philtral ridge. Excess skin

on the nostril floor is excised accordingly; however, careful preservation of the nasal sill is maintained. The nasal floor is closed with 5–0 polyglactin sutures and lip skin is closed with 7–0 polyglactin sutures (Fig. 21.2.24).

Adjustments during the final stage

The preoperative markings and measurements will differ after adequate muscle dissection and approximation. Therefore, these should be continuously checked while deciding the necessary adjustments to achieve a satisfactory result. Every cleft surgery is different; and, minor adjustments are necessary in most patients – herein lies the enjoyment, yet challenge, of each case.

Long vertical length of cleft side lip

A vertically long lateral lip is seldom encountered. It can be avoided by the septal anchoring suture used to suspend the lateral lip upward and trimming the excessive tissue from the nasal floor.

Short vertical length of cleft side lip

This is a common problem in most complete clefts. Adequate release and approximation of the orbicularis muscle will

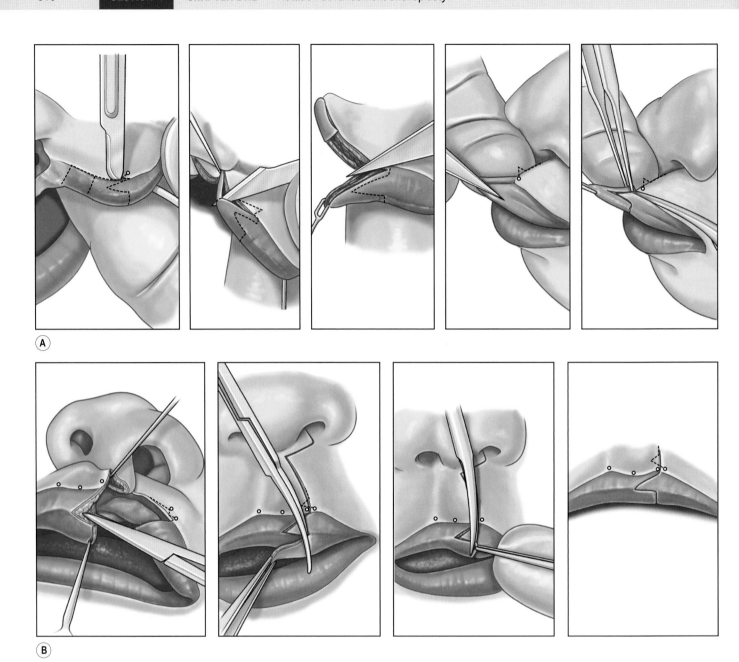

Fig. 21.2.22 **(A)** The vermilion flap is marked and incised on the OM flap while the OM flap is held under tension. The width of the vermilion flap should correct the vermilion deficiency under the Cupid's bow. The tip of the vermilion flap should not cross the natural lip tubercle. **(B)** Medially, the lip is incised on the red line beneath the Cupid's bow for insertion of the vermilion flap. The excessive tissues on both medial and lateral lips are carefully trimmed.

increase the vertical length by 3–4 mm, while an additional 2 mm is provided by the WSR flap designed on the lateral lip. If the lip is still short, point CPHL' can be shifted 1 mm laterally without sacrificing much on the horizontal lip length. This can also increase the length of the WSR flap, thus achieving further downward rotation. Lastly, a perialar incision can be made, lengthening the vertical lip height with cheek tissue; however, this should be avoided if possible.

Long horizontal length of cleft side lip

This is a relatively simple problem. Point CPHL' can be moved as lateral as necessary to shorten the horizontal length.

Short horizontal length of cleft side lip

This problem is almost impossible to solve. After adequate muscle dissection and approximation, the horizontal lip length on the cleft side will usually increase by several millimeters. A horizontally short lip is aesthetically acceptable compared to a vertically short lip with peaking of the Cupid's bow.

Long vertical height of non-cleft side lip

Any vertical length exceeding 12 mm on the non-cleft side lip (in a 3-month-old baby) is excessively long and difficult to manage. Shortening this length could be performed by excising a portion of a full-thickness lip segment (at the junction of the lip and nasal floor) and is seldom performed.

Free border of the lateral lip

If the lateral lip is too thin or deficient, the mucosa can be released further (by extending the buccal sulcus incision) but this seldom corrects the problem. A poorly placed septal anchoring suture will pull the lateral lip too high and thus worsen the problem. Lateral lip deficiency can be corrected with lip augmentation using a temporoparietal fascia graft as a secondary procedure.[19] On the other hand, one often finds a bulging free border in incomplete clefts. The most accurate way of correcting this excessive tissue is to incise along the

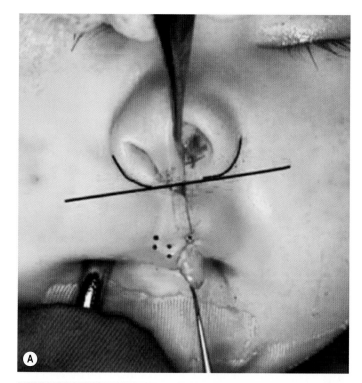
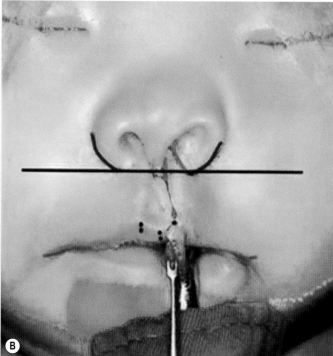

Fig. 21.2.23 (A) If the alar base and the peak of the Cupid's bow on the cleft side are still high, incision as the direction shown is made inside the cleft side nasal floor. This incision can vertically lengthen the lip and level the alar base and Cupid's bow. **(B)** If the alar base is already leveled after muscle reconstruction, incision is made as the direction shown to keep the alar base position.

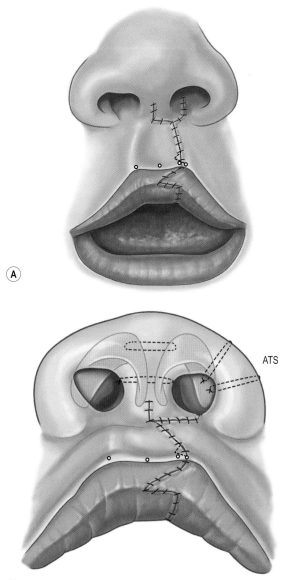

Fig. 21.2.24 (A) Complete wound closure with columella elongation achieved by the Mohler's rotation incision; note the laterally positioned philtral column. **(B)** Alar transfixion sutures (ATS) using 5–0 absorbable monofilament are placed with traction on the LLC. One suture is placed in the vestibular skin. The remaining sutures catch the leading edge of the LLC, pass through the alar-facial groove and back near the rim of the ala, and are tied on the inner side. Notching of the skin disappears within 1–2 weeks.

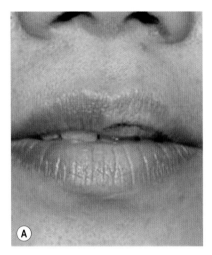 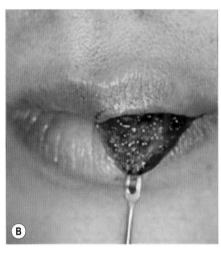 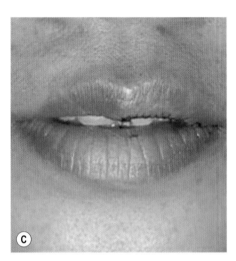

Fig. 21.2.25 The most accurate way to correct the excess mucosa is to make incision along the extension of the red line from medial lip **(A)**, raising an inferiorly based mucosal flap with a thin layer of marginalis muscle **(B)**, re-draping the flap and trimming the excess tissue **(C)**.

red line, raise an inferiorly based mucosal flap with a thin layer of marginalis muscle, and redrape the flap while trimming the excessive tissue (Fig. 21.2.25).

Semi-open rhinoplasty

Many techniques have been reported for primary nasal reconstruction in unilateral clefts.[16,20–28] Several reports on the long-term results in primary nasal correction have not shown any adverse effect on nasal growth.[29–34] For the past 30 years, several techniques have been used in the Chang Gung Craniofacial Center for nasal reconstruction in unilateral clefts.[9,12,23,35] In the authors' experience, a semi-open rhinoplasty can achieve a precise and less traumatic dissection of the cartilaginous framework, providing better visualization and repositioning of the displaced cartilages. It can also preserve and elongate the cleft side columella.

Incision

A rim incision on the non-cleft nostril and a reverse U incision on the cleft nostril is marked. The reverse U incision is made 2 mm higher than the alar rim to achieve an over-correction on the cleft nostril.

Release of fibrofatty tissue from LLCs

The nasal rim incisions (an inverted U Tajima incision on the cleft side and an alar rim incision on the non-cleft side) are made with #67 blade followed by dissection above the LLCs with tenotomy scissors. The caudal edges of both LLCs can be easily visualized through these incisions, thus avoiding any risk of iatrogenic injury to the cartilaginous framework. The fibrofatty tissue of the nasal tip is released from both LLCs. This dissection pocket should be connected to the earlier created pocket created by the intercrural space dissection. The cleft side nostril dissection should extend lateral to the groove of the LLC caudal edge.

Repositioning of LLCs

The LLCs are approximated with a medial rotation of the cleft side LLC cartilage, and united with 5–0 polydioxanone mattress sutures. The stitches are placed 5 mm more laterally on the cleft side cartilage for over-correction. A second

through-and-through suture is placed on the medial crura, lower than the first stitch, for further crural support.

Trimming the excessive skin

After repositioning of the LLCs, the columella on the cleft side will be lengthened by recruitment of tissue along the medial limb of the reverse U incision. There is always excess skin on the upper part of the cleft side columella; and, this is responsible for the soft triangle webbing found in secondary cleft nasal deformities. This excessive skin is trimmed with sharp scissors, and the wound is closed with 5–0 polyglactin sutures.

Alar base position

The most important factor in achieving alar base symmetry is adequate release of the abnormally attached paranasal muscles. The alar–facial groove is further accentuated by the approximation of the lip musculature.

Creation of the alar–facial groove

Dissection between the skin and LLC releases the fibrous attachments and leaves behind a significant dead space. Furthermore, mobilization of the cleft side alar base will accentuate the vestibular webbing within the nostril. Removal of the fat pad (beneath the alar base) and two alar transfixion sutures (correcting the intra-vestibular mucosal webbing) help solve these problems while defining the alar–facial groove. The lower suture obliterates the dead space and tacks down the vestibular webbing. The upper suture catches the leading edge of the LLC and provides support the LLC. Skin dimpling from these sutures usually disappears 2 weeks after surgery (Fig. 21.2.26).

Patient examples are shown as Figs. 21.2.27 and 21.2.28.

Rotation advancement cheiloplasty for incomplete clefts

Surprisingly, incomplete cleft lips are sometimes as difficult or more challenging to reconstruct.[36] Moreover, the expectations for an excellent result are higher, and surgeons tend

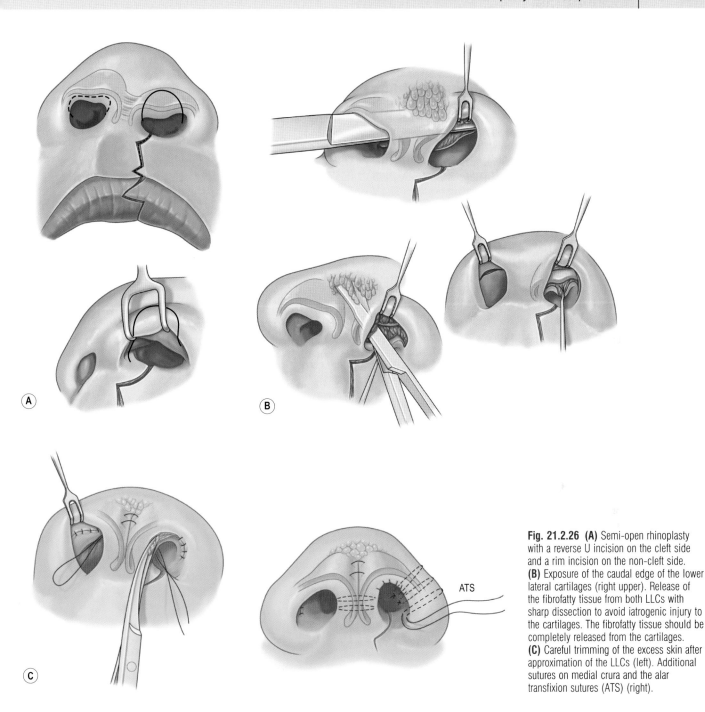

Fig. 21.2.26 (A) Semi-open rhinoplasty with a reverse U incision on the cleft side and a rim incision on the non-cleft side. **(B)** Exposure of the caudal edge of the lower lateral cartilages (right upper). Release of the fibrofatty tissue from both LLCs with sharp dissection to avoid iatrogenic injury to the cartilages. The fibrofatty tissue should be completely released from the cartilages. **(C)** Careful trimming of the excess skin after approximation of the LLCs (left). Additional sutures on medial crura and the alar transfixion sutures (ATS) (right).

to underestimate the pathology and do less of a procedure during reconstruction. It is a common mistake to think that a vertically long lateral lip exists and then try to shorten the lip during the operation without proper repositioning of the alar base. In fact, intraoperative measurements usually show both vertical heights are equal. The appearance of a vertically long lateral lip results from the downward displacement of the cleft side alar base. Therefore, it is important to mobilize completely the alar base and reposition it cephalically instead of vertically shortening the lateral lip.

Markings and incisions

The rotation incision and muscle dissection are performed similar to complete clefts, using either the Mohler technique or a simple rotation-advancement, together with the C-flap design. The incision on the advancement flap is made along the cleft edge after designing the WSR flap (Fig. 21.2.29A).

Nasal floor incision

A transverse incision is made inside the nasal floor at the junction of the skin and mucosa, leaving ample tissue on the piriform area and premaxilla (Fig. 21.2.29B). A subperiosteal dissection is performed from the nasal septum and along the nasal floor towards the piriform rim, raising a mucoperiosteal flap that will be used for correction of the nasal floor deficiency. The authors have been using a technique of minimal skin flap paring since the mid-1990s, as advocated by Koh;[37] however, we feel that the nasal floor transverse incision is essential for adequate alar base mobilization and restoring nasal floor symmetry.

Dissection of muscle and elevation of OM flap

The technique and extent of muscle dissection is similar to that performed in complete clefts. Less muscle dissection tends to leave the abnormal muscle insertions to the alar base, and results in a lateral and downward displacement of the alar base, often seen in secondary deformities. The OM flap is raised as in complete clefts.

Nasal floor reconstruction

The raised mucoperichondrial flap from the nasal septum and the mucoperiosteal flap of piriform area is folded over and sutured to each other, matching the height of the nasal floor on non-cleft side nostril (Fig. 21.2.29C). The alar base is turned inward, and its leading edge, at the vestibular incision, is sutured to the mucosa on the nasal floor as in complete clefts. Theoretically, placing Surgicel under the periosteum of the cleft side nasal floor could stimulate new bone formation, thus correcting the bony

deficiency in this area. However, in a study performed by the authors, no benefit was achieved in the overall aesthetic outcome.[38]

Muscle reconstruction

Muscle reconstruction is performed as in complete clefts, using an anchoring suture to the septum for centralizing the Cupid's bow. Overlapping mattress muscle sutures are used to reconstruct the philtral column ridge.

Nasal correction

Nasal correction is performed as in complete clefts with a rim incision on non-cleft side nostril and reversed U incision on cleft side. The cartilage dissection, cartilage repositioning, and alar transfixion sutures are performed as mentioned above. The cleft side nostril needs to be over-corrected (a higher and narrower nostril).

Excessive free border

Although the "long lateral lip" is usually an illusion in incomplete clefts, it is not uncommon to have some excessive tissue

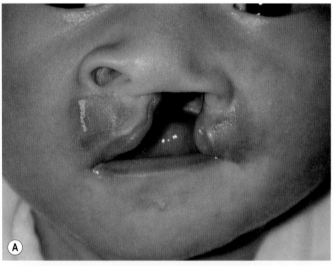
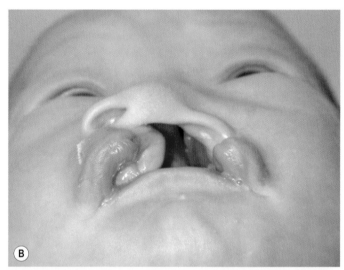
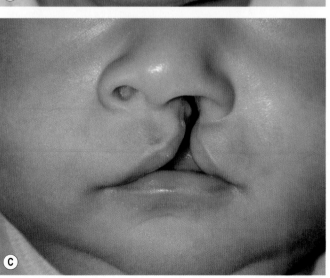
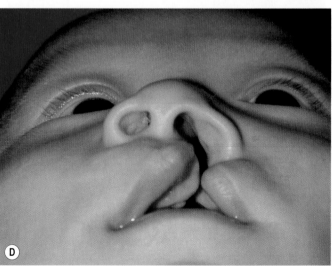

Fig. 21.2.27 (A,B) A 2-week-old boy with left complete cleft of primary and secondary palate. **(C,D)** 3 months after nasoalveolar molding, before lip repair.

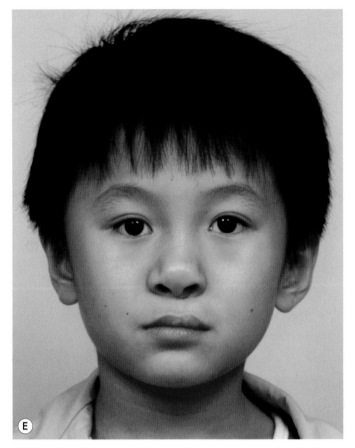

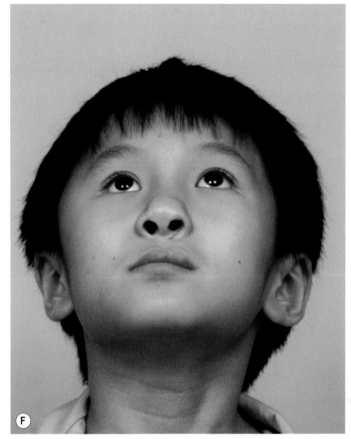

Fig. 21.2.27, cont'd (E,F) Postoperative views at the age of 7 years.

(vermilion, orbicularis marginalis, and mucosa) along the free border of the cleft side lateral lip after leveling the Cupid's bow. If it is too obvious, the excessive free border tissue can be trimmed using the technique shown in Fig. 21.2.25.

A patient example is shown in Fig. 21.2.30.

Complete cleft of primary palate

Patients who present with complete clefts of primary palate (complete cleft lip and alveolus anterior to the incisive foramen, UCLA) are notorious for having inferior results, when compared to their peers with unilateral complete

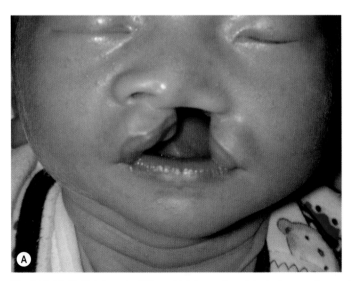

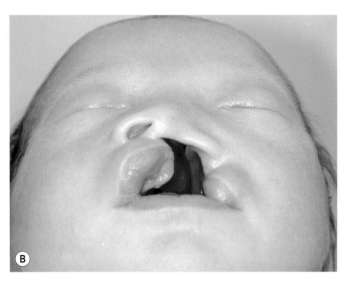

Fig. 21.2.28 (A,B) A 2-week-old boy with left complete cleft of primary and secondary palate.

Continued

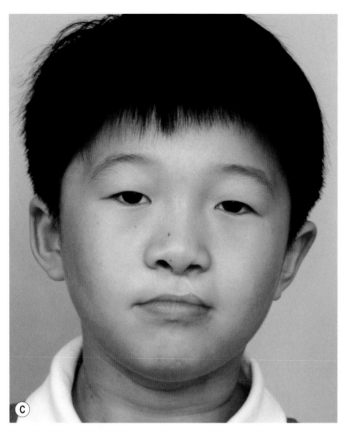

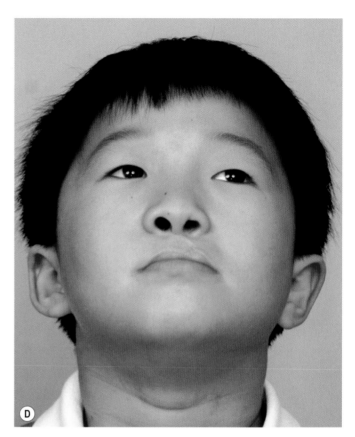

Fig. 21.2.28, cont'd (C,D) Postoperative views at the age of 7 years.

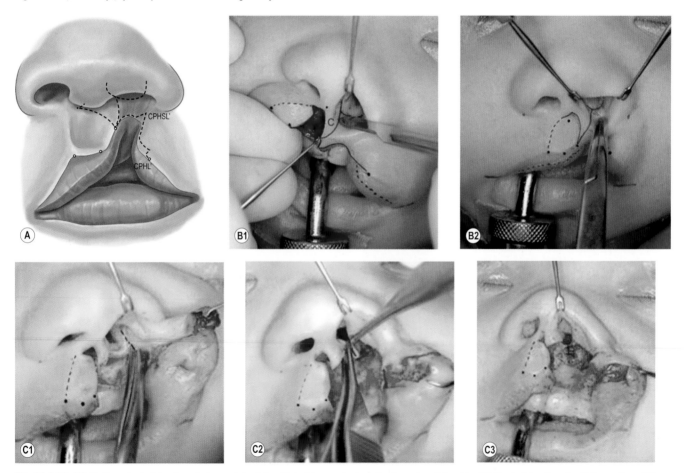

Fig. 21.2.29 (A) Markings for incision lines in incomplete clefts with incision made along the free edge of the skin. **(B)** The incision lines for C-flap and nasal floor: a transverse incision is made inside the nasal floor at the junction of skin and mucosa leaving ample tissue on piriform area and premaxilla. **(C)** The local tissue on nasal septum and piriform area (C1) is turned over (C2) and sutured with each other to match the height of the nasal floor on non-cleft side nostril (C3).

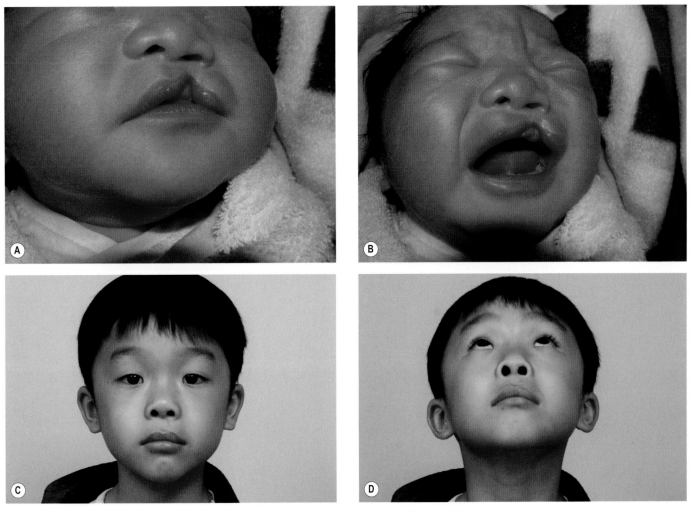

Fig. 21.2.30 **(A,B)** A 3-week-old boy with left side incomplete cleft lip. **(C,D)** Postoperative views at the age of 7 years.

clefts of both the primary and secondary palate (UCLP). These inferior results are because the protruding premaxilla is resistant to movement during pre-surgical NAM. As well, there often exists a short vertical lip height on the cleft side (Fig. 21.2.31A–D). Quite often, a persistent downward displacement of the nasal sill and alar base remains after surgery.

The surgical modifications for patients with isolated complete clefts of primary palate are:

- Mainly using the vertical lip height to determine the point CPHL′, i.e., by moving CPHL′ more laterally (Fig. 21.2.31E). As aforementioned, a short horizontal lip does not look as obvious as compared with a short vertical lip with peaking of the Cupid's bow or downward displacement of the alar base.
- Using the septal flap, nasal floor tissue, and the L-flap for nasal floor reconstruction. The nasal floor tissue and L-flap are undermined subperiosteally (Fig. 21.2.31F,G).

A patient example is shown in Fig. 21.2.31H–K.

Microform cleft lip

Surgical correction of the microform cleft lip has received less attention in the literature, likely because of its minor

deformity. Efforts have been made to eliminate the external scar that results from traditional rotation-advancement or straight-line closures. Cho[39] advocated orbicularis muscle interdigitation through an intraoral incision. Mulliken[40] has suggested the double uni-limb Z-plasties, muscle approximation, and philtral ridge augmentation with a retro-auricular graft. The authors' preference remains a modified rotation-advancement cheiloplasty as discussed in incomplete cleft lips. This is because with this technique the surgeon has the ability to (1) release the misaligned muscle completely while mobilizing the displaced alar base, (2) reconstruct the philtral column in both height and direction, and (3) over-correct the cleft side nostril. In addition, it allows for the excision of the cleft groove or striae which is not parallel to the non-cleft side philtral column. The repair also requires a WSR flap above the non-cleft side Cupid's bow to correct the high peaking of the Cupid's bow. Although scarring is the major concern, scars are usually inconspicuous if surgery is performed early (i.e., at 3 months) and parents are compliant to the postoperative scar care (Fig. 21.2.32 ⊕). A recent prospective randomized controlled trial showed that intraoperative injection of Botulinum toxin A along the suture line helps to improve the scar in primary lip repair.[41]

Fig. 21.2.32 appears online only.

Postoperative care

Postoperative monitoring and care begins immediately in the recovery room. The caregiver is allowed to enter the recovery room to hold the baby and be briefed on the essentials of maintaining a patent airway. Postoperative management is continued by a specialized cleft nurse, giving further instructions about the airway and subsequent care upon returning to the ward. These instructions include removal of oral and

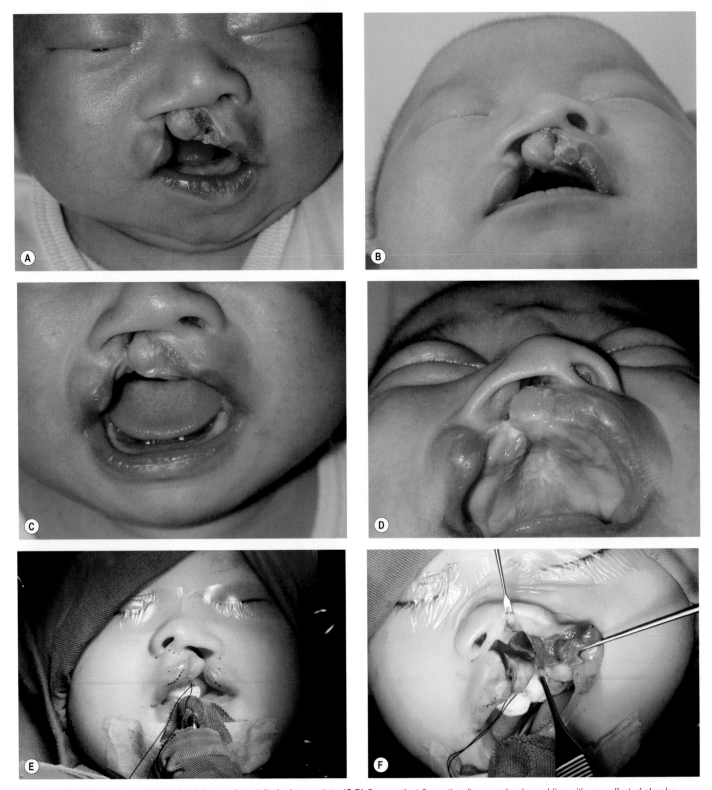

Fig. 21.2.31 (A,B) A 2-week-old girl with right complete cleft of primary palate. **(C,D)** Same patient 3 months after nasoalveolar molding with poor effect of alveolar molding. **(E)** Markings for the lip landmarks. The vertical height on the cleft side is more important in determining the point CPHL'. **(F)** Using septal flap, L-flap and local nasal floor/piriform periosteal flaps for nasal floor reconstruction.

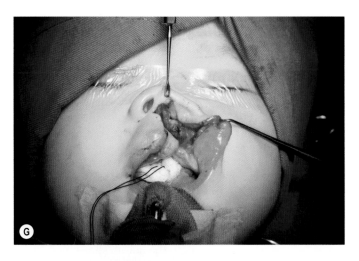

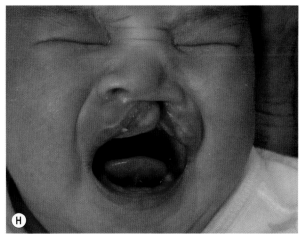

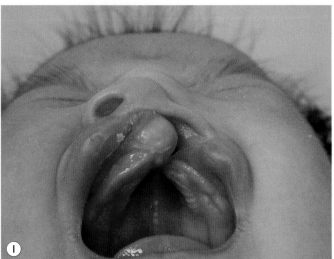

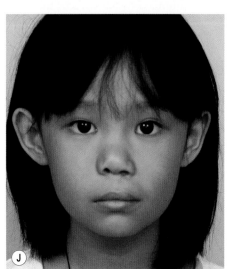

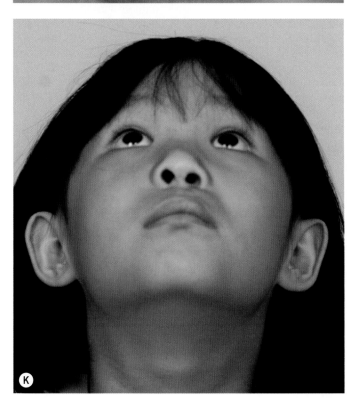

Fig. 21.2.31, cont'd (G) The result of nasal floor reconstruction using the aforementioned tissue. The height of the nasal floor is similar to the height in non-cleft side. **(H,I)** A 2-week-old girl with left complete cleft of primary palate. **(J,K)** Postoperative views at the age of 8 years.

upper airway secretions, wound dressings of normal saline, and bottle feeding with a "good flow" soft nipple. Feeding can be started as soon as the baby desires. No arm restraints are used.

Any blood clots or mucus on the wound is cleaned with normal saline-soaked swabs every 2–6 h, and then antibiotic ointment is applied to the suture line. It is important to keep the incision from drying out or crusting. Normal saline dressings also reduce pain and swelling. The baby and mother are discharged home the day following surgery and return to the outpatient department in 5 days. At that time, skin sutures are removed under oral chloral hydrate sedation. Postoperative scar care begins immediately with Micropore™ tape and silicone sheet compression. The patient is usually seen monthly for the first 3 months and then periodically. This is to ensure that parents are compliant with postoperative scar care. Lip scar massage is usually encouraged to hasten scar maturity and correct any elevation of the Cupid's bow secondary to scar contracture.

Postoperative maintenance of nasal shape

Post-surgical nasal molding was first introduced in 1969 by Osada[42] and Skoog.[43] Friede[44] used an acrylic conformer and demonstrated improvement in nasal contour. Matsuo[8] first reported pre-surgical molding in the unilateral incomplete cleft with a silicone conformer which was continuously used for 3 months and then only at night for up to 12 months of age postoperatively. It is believed that the deformed nasal cartilage can be easily molded and manipulated while it is still malleable.

Subsequently, silicone nasal conformers have been used in many centers to support the LLC during the healing phase and prevent nasal contracture and stenosis. Silicone nasal conformers have been used at the Chang Gung Craniofacial Center since the late 1980s.[45] At present, a modified set of nasal conformers are used. This set contains five conformers with increasing height (1 mm increments). Parents are instructed to change to the next larger size conformer every 2–3 weeks until achieving the largest size of 4 mm on the cleft side. The conformer is used at all times for 6 months to 1 year postoperatively if possible. Success in nasal conformer application depends much upon the cooperation and perseverance of the parents (Fig. 21.2.33 ⬤).

Fig. 21.2.33 appears online only.

Outcomes, prognosis, and complications

Long-term results of lip morphology

Lip symmetry is the main goal for cleft lip repair. A study was performed at the Chang Gung Craniofacial Center evaluating the long-term (at least 4 years follow-up) lip morphology in 19 complete unilateral cleft lip patients, who were operated on in 2002. The surgical technique was similar to the technique herein described, except no septal anchoring muscle suture was placed. The results (with at least 4 years follow-up) revealed that Cupid's bow was deviated to the cleft side (Fig. 21.2.34 ⬤).[46] Therefore, the authors routinely place a septal

anchoring suture to affix the cleft side lateral lip medially, thus centralizing the Cupid's bow.

Fig. 21.2.34 appears online only.

Long-term result of nasal morphology

It is also important to document the long-term nasal morphology following the integrated approach with pre-surgical nasoalveolar molding, surgical refinement, and post-surgical maintenance. Several studies conducted at Chang Gung Craniofacial Center evaluating the long-term nasal morphology outcomes. The initial study evaluated 25 patients operated on between 1997 and 1999. All these patients underwent Liou's technique of pre-surgical nasoalveolar molding. The surgical technique for nasal reconstruction was performed as described above, except no cartilage dissection or repositioning was performed. Although the nasal shape was quite symmetrical immediately following surgery, at 3 years follow-up, there were significant differences among measurements of nostril height, columellar length and nostril width. The cleft side nostril and columellar height were significantly shorter than the non-cleft side, while the cleft side nostril was significantly wider (Fig. 21.2.35 ⬤).[6] The next study included a group of patients who received the modified Grayson technique of nasoalveolar molding. The surgical technique included repositioning of the LLCs through bilateral rim incisions. This study demonstrated better results when compared with the previous study; nonetheless, there was a similar trend in terms of nasal relapse.[47] Based on these observations, the authors' current practice includes performing a reverse U incision on the cleft side and over-correction of the cleft side columellar height, nostril height, and width. Postoperatively, the cleft nostril needs to be maintained in the over-corrected position using the modified silicone conformer. The third study compared the outcome of primary nasal reconstruction among four different techniques, namely, closed rhinoplasty alone, NAM alone, NAM plus semi-open rhinoplasty and NAM plus semi-open rhinoplasty with over-correction in a group of 76 patients during 11 years. The final technique had the best overall result including nostril height ratio, one-fourth medial part of nostril height ratio, nasal sill height ratio, nostril area ratio, nostril height to width ratio and panel assessment.[48]

Fig. 21.2.35 appears online only.

Satisfaction of patients

Patient and parent satisfaction are largely dependent upon psychosocial adaptation. A study performed in early 2000 at the Chang Gung Craniofacial Center evaluated the results in 77 patients who underwent cleft lip repair in 1996.[9] A total of 24% of patients required no further revision of the nose or lip; 36% required nasal correction, while 10% lip correction; 28% required both nasal and lip revision. Approximately 60% of the patients requested lip or nose revision before school age. With our integrated approach and improvement in outcomes in recent years, only a few patients request revision before school age. Therefore, secondary nasal deformity correction can usually be delayed until completion of facial growth and the completion of psychological development. A large number of our patients were satisfied with the outcome of primary nasal reconstruction and did not request any secondary rhinoplasty procedure.

Complications

A total of 112 patients underwent unilateral cheiloplasty at the Chang Gung Craniofacial Center from January 2008 to November 2009, and were evaluated for postoperative complications. No instances of wound dehiscence were encountered. There was one minor separation of the nasal floor and two minor separations of the nasolabial junction which healed uneventfully. There were no significant wound infections reported except for five cases of stitch abscess (4.5%) and no instances of postoperative bleeding. Hypertrophic scarring was noted in only 3% of the patients.

Summary

The integrated approach to treating the cleft lip and nose presented here is based on the vast experience at the Chang Gung Craniofacial Center. It represents a 30-year ongoing evolution, with periodic evaluation of our operative results and refinements in treatment protocols. The pre-surgical management has evolved from simple lip taping and prone sleep position to very sophisticated nasoalveolar molding. The surgical refinements include modifications of our own technique and those adopted from other surgeons. Postoperative care also has changed with time, aiming to achieve the best result. Although our approach is based on the Taiwanese population, these techniques have also been tested in other racially diverse centers. In some locales without the facilities and personnel for pre-surgical management and postoperative maintenance, the surgical refinements, as discussed above, can still produce consistently improved results.

 Bonus images for this chapter can be found online at **http://www.expertconsult.com**

Fig. 21.2.1 (A) Modified Grayson molding device. **(B)** The device held in proper position by elastics and tapes. Lip taping helps to approximate the alveolus.

Fig. 21.2.2 (A) Liou's (modified Figueroa) molding device. **(B)** The device held in proper position by dental adhesives. Lip taping is also used.

Fig. 21.2.3 (A) Liou's molding device with spring mechanism. **(B)** The device held in place with dental adhesives. Lip taping is also used.

Fig. 21.2.4 (A) Nasal molding with silicone nasal conformer. **(B)** A set of nasal conformers with different heights for cleft side. **(C)** A 10-day-old baby with right incomplete cleft lip. Nasal shape before the nasal molding. **(D)** Same baby at the age of 3 months before lip repair. The nasal shape after nasal molding.

Fig. 21.2.32 (A,B) A 2-week-old boy with left side occult cleft lip. **(C,D)** Postoperative views at the age of 5 years.

Fig. 21.2.33 Postoperative care with Micropore™ tapes across the lip and silicone nasal conformer. The nasal conformer held in nostril with tape.

Fig. 21.2.34 Serial photographs of a boy with right complete cleft of primary and secondary palate. **(A)** 2 weeks old; **(B)** immediately after operation; **(C)** 1-year-old before palate repair; and **(D)** at the age of 5 years. The Cupid's bow, though leveled, is deviated to the cleft side.

Fig. 21.2.35 Serial photographs of a girl with left complete cleft of primary and secondary palate. **(A)** 2 weeks old; **(B)** during nasoalveolar molding with Liou's method; **(C)** immediately after operation (without cartilage dissection and repositioning); **(D)** 1-year-old before palate repair; **(E)** at the age of 1.5 years; and **(F)** at the age of 3 years.

 Access the complete reference list online at **http://www.expertconsult.com**

6. Liou EJ, Subramanian M, Chen PKT, et al. The progressive changes of nasal symmetry and growth after nasoalveolar molding: a three-year follow-up study. *Plast Reconstr Surg.* 2004;114(4):858–864.

7. Chang CS, Wallace CG, Pai BCJ, et al. Comparison of two nasoalveolar molding techniques in unilateral complete cleft lip patients: a randomized, prospective, single-blind trial to compare nasal outcomes. *Plast Reconstr Surg.* 2014;134(2):275–282.

9. Chen PKT, Noordhoff MS, Kane A. Repair of unilateral cleft lip. In: Neligan P, ed. *Plastic Surgery.* 3rd ed. London: Elsevier-Saunders; 2012:517–549 [Chapter 23]. vol. 3.

13. Onizuka T, Ichinose M, Hosaka Y, Usui Y, Jinnai T. The contour lines of the upper lip and a revised method of cleft lip repair. *Ann Plast Surg.* 1991;27(3):238–252.

14. Mohler L. Unilateral cleft lip repair. *Plast Reconstr Surg.* 1987;80(4):511–516.

16. Mulliken JB, Martinez–Perez D. The principle of rotation advancement for repair of unilateral complete cleft lip and nasal deformity: technical variations and analysis of results. *Plast Reconstr Surg.* 1999;104(5):1247–1260.

26. Cutting CB, Dayan JH. Lip height and lip width after extended Mohler unilateral lip repair. *Plast Reconstr Surg.* 2003;111(1):17–23.

28. Stal S, Brown RH, Higuera S, et al. Fifty years of the Millard rotation-advancement: looking back and moving forward. *Plast Reconstr Surg.* 2009;123(4):1364–1377.

31. Salyer KE, Genecov ER, Genecov DG. Unilateral cleft lip-nose repair: a 33-year experience. *J Craniofac Surg.* 2003;14(4):549–558.

48. Chang CS, Por YF, Liou EJW, et al. Long-term comparison of four techniques for obtaining nasal symmetry in unilateral complete cleft lip patients: a single surgeon's experience. *Plast Reconstr Surg.* 2010;126:1276–1284.

21.3

Extended Mohler repair

Roberto L. Flores

SYNOPSIS

- Treatment philosophy
  - Nasoalveolar molding
  - Gingivoperiosteoplasty
  - Tension-free reconstruction
  - No lip adhesion
  - Primary nasal reconstruction
  - Closure of the nasal floor
- Evolution of technique
- Markings
- Downward rotation of Cupid's bow
- Preparation of the medial lip element
- L-flap dissection
- Lateral lip element dissection
- Intranasal mucosa reconstruction
- Oral mucosa reconstruction
- Primary rhinoplasty Part I
- Alar base repositioning
- Orbicularis oris repair
- Upper lip skin and vermillion repair
- Primary rhinoplasty Part II
- Postoperative care
- Results

Summary box

Primary cleft lip and nasal repair seeks to achieve lasting symmetry to the lip and nose while camouflaging scars within the contours of the face. This surgery is often the first step in the larger treatment plan for cleft care, therefore the quality of the repair sets the direction of the function and appearance for the patient. As the surgeon should strive to effect the most change with the least amount of surgery, nasoalveolar molding should be pursued whenever possible. Primary nasal repair has been demonstrated to be safe and should be performed with slight overcorrection to the alar base and nostril rim position. The nasal floor should be closed to better prepare the patient for future alveolar bone graft. Gingivoperiosteoplasty may be considered in experienced centers. The Mohler Cutting repair, described herein, has the advantage of placing the final scars perfectly along the subunit borders. The technique can be applied to all patients with a unilateral cleft, despite the width of the cleft, or the use of pre-surgical orthopedics. The technique also has the advantage of offering a medial approach to primary cleft rhinoplasty.

Introduction

Aesthetic reconstruction of the upper lip is enhanced by adherence to the subunit principles advocated by Burget and Menick.[1] Scar placement along the subunit borders are more easily hidden and emphasize the geometric patterns recognized by the eyes as structurally normal components of the face. The Mohler cleft lip repair locates the final scars perfectly along the subunit borders of the skin-bearing upper lip, without the use of triangular flaps or curvilinear scars which disrupt the harmony of upper lip aesthetics.

The extended Mohler repair, recently popularized by Cutting, addresses some of the limitations of Mohler's original design and, in its current form, can be applied to any unilateral cleft lip deformity regardless of severity of the defect or use of pre-surgical orthopedics. Cutting's popularization of the Mohler repair, in addition to his technical modifications, justify the appropriate description of the technique as the Mohler Cutting repair. These modifications have led to the widespread acceptance of the repair and have maintained its popularity as one of the most common techniques used to repair the unilateral cleft lip deformity.

Treatment philosophy

Nasoalveolar molding

Primary cleft lip and nasal reconstruction has been made more predictable by the development of nasoalveolar molding (NAM).[2] Although the Mohler Cutting repair can be applied to any complete unilateral cleft lip deformity, regardless of severity, NAM leads to greater nasal symmetry,[3–5] facilitates gingivoperiosteoplasty,[6] and decreases the need for secondary surgery. Through weekly to biweekly modifications of the alveolar plate and nasal stent, NAM anatomically aligns the alveolar segments, lengthens the columella, increases nasal tip projection, folds the lower lateral cartilages towards its native form, transposes the lower lip and alar base towards the midline, and expands the intranasal lining. Therapy is usually completed within 8–10 weeks in patients with a unilateral cleft deformity. The summative effect of NAM is altering the severity of the cleft towards a mild phenotype. Therefore, the benefit of NAM lies in the ability for good surgeons to achieve excellent results and for experienced surgeons to more consistently obtain the near perfect result. In the author's practice pattern, NAM is used whenever feasible by the family.

As popularity has increased, a growing number of cleft centers have reported the benefit of NAM or similar technical variation.[7–13] Currently, there is an ongoing debate between the proponents and skeptics of NAM[14,15] which will require large population, multicenter analysis to resolve. Prospective multicenter analysis of the surgical and quality of life outcomes of NAM are currently ongoing, which will provide a comprehensive analysis of the benefits and limitations of this technique.

Gingivoperiosteoplasty

The "boneless" bone graft has variable numbers of supporters and remained a topic of active debate. During primary cleft lip repair or cleft palate reconstruction, the mucosal edges of the alveolus may be connected to promote bony union between the free alveolar segments. Gingivoperiosteoplasty (GPP) was originally described by Skoog[16] and later popularized by Millard[17] who used a Latham device to actively mold the alveolus prior to GPP.

Proponents state that the procedure will avoid, in most cases, the need for secondary alveolar bone graft. Indeed, successful GPP is demonstrated in 60% of patients with a unilateral cleft,[18–20] circumventing the morbidity and financial burden of an additional surgery.[21] Anterior growth appears to be unaffected through the age of mixed dentition.[22] However, other reports have suggested some impairment of midface growth after GPP.[23] Furthermore, the procedure is very technique dependent. Even a moderate dissection force can fracture the thin alveolar bone and destroy underlying tooth buds. Mucoperiosteal flap dissection must be limited to the mesial and distal faces of the alveolus with no dissection of the lingual or buccal faces. This requires perfect alignment of the alveolar segments and a gap of 1 mm. Pre-surgical orthopedics, therefore, is a necessary adjunct to gingivoperiosteoplasty.

Opponents state that gingivoperiosteoplasty has a limited success rate and will damage anterior facial growth as well as the developing teeth.[24] Indeed, GPP has a variable success rate across institutions,[6,24] implicating the technical challenges of the procedure. The majority of the clinical reports of gingivoperiosteoplasty are single institution experiences limiting a large volume analysis. More importantly, there are no published studies to date reporting on the effects of GPP on anterior facial growth in the facially mature patient with a cleft. Gingivoperiosteoplasty experienced resurgence after the development of nasoalveolar molding and the initial NAM and GPP patients of this resurgence have only recently achieved the age of facial maturity. The eventual report of complete facial growth after GPP will undoubtedly spark another active debate on the indications and benefits of this procedure.

Tension-free reconstruction

The purpose of the suture is to join together vascularized tissue so that normal healing can occur. Normal healing does not occur when sutures a placed under tension. When considering the delicate reconstruction of the three dimensional form of the lip and nose, this principle is taken a step further: even mild amounts of tension will result in relapse of the cleft deformity, cause widened scars, and predispose the patient to further surgery to the lip and nose resulting in additional scars in these areas. Tension on closure, even mild tension, should not be addressed with sutures; this is a therapy, which does not last. Tissues should be adequately freed until tension is completely eliminated in the critical aesthetic areas of the nose and upper lip skin. In cases where pre-surgical orthopedics is not used, extensive dissection may be required.

No lip adhesion

Lip adhesion is commonly advocated in cases where NAM or a similar form of pre-surgical orthopedics cannot be employed. This author's experience is that lip adhesions are unnecessary, even in the cases of very wide cleft lips, and can compromise surgical outcomes. Three points deserve mention in this regard:

1. L-flap reconstruction: The use of a lip adhesion precludes the use of an L-flap, whether based on the alveolus as described by Millard[25] or pedicled on the lateral nasal wall, as advocated by Cutting.[26] Although a lip adhesion can bring the lip and alveolar segments in greater apposition, the alar base and nose are mildly affected by this procedure. The lip adhesion, therefore, may benefit lip reconstruction at the cost of nasal reconstruction. Without an L-flap, a pyriform aperture incision defect cannot be closed with mucosal tissue. Therefore, the intranasal incision is not made at the time of nasal repair or the incision is made but not reconstructed. Both of these will compromise the quality of nasal repair in the very patients who require the full armamentarium of reconstructive techniques: patients with wide cleft lip deformities.

2. Scar: In addition to eliminating certain flap options, a lip adhesion produces a scar in the center stage of the planned repair. Lip adhesion will therefore compromise the quality of the lip tissue and this is appreciable at the time of lip repair.

3. Complete cheek and nasal dissection: One of the great challenges of wide cleft lip repair is medial

transposition of the lateral lip and alar base to achieve a tension-free closure. Although a lip adhesion can be useful in achieving this end, one can simply perform thorough cheek and lip dissection at the time of primary repair and achieve the same surgical ends of lip and alar base transposition, but without the cost of flap sacrifice and scar. This dissection requires a generous pyriform aperture incision and wide dissection across the face of the maxilla as far superior as the infraorbital rim and as far later as the medial canthus. A supraperiosteal dissection plane is maintained to limit blood loss. This dissection, by definition, will sacrifice the infraorbital nerve; however, lip sensibility does return to the level of the unaffected lip by the process of adjacent neurotization.[27]

Primary nasal repair

Previous studies have demonstrated the aesthetic benefit to primary cleft rhinoplasty[28,29] as well as the safety of infant rhinoplasty to subsequent nasal growth. Although primary cleft rhinoplasty is advocated by most surgeons, not all rhinoplasties are created equal. The great enemy of the refined soft tissue repair is scarring; therefore primary cleft rhinoplasty should execute the best and most lasting change with the least amount of dissection. Any surgeon can perform a three layer nasal dissection at the time of infancy, then "touch up" the nose with an open rhinoplasty and cartilage grafts prior to elementary school, then refine the nose again (with an open rhinoplasty, of course) at the age of adolescence. However, one would predict that by the time facial maturity is reached, the density of scar surrounding the lower lateral cartilages and embedded in the nasal tip skin would preclude any aesthetic or functional result in the patient beyond the mediocre. Costal cartilage is advocated by many surgeons who perform adult cleft rhinoplasty; however, even these rigid grafts can be deformed by the steady, persistent force of cicatrix.

Primary cleft rhinoplasty, therefore, should be directed and limited in dissection. Although removal of fibrofat in the nasal tip can certainly result in greater tip refinement at the time of repair, will that same procedure be perceived as a benefit when attempting to refine the scarred tip at the age of 22? The benefit and detriment of different types of primary rhinoplasty is an area that lacks scientific assessment. Active cleft surgeons are familiar with the scarred nasal tip resulting from excessive operations that resists the most acrobatic surgical repair. The under-operated nose can be predictably improved, although perfection is elusive. The over-operated, scarred nose can produce unfortunate, complex, and insurmountable hurdles to an already challenging operation which, in many cases, can be avoided with proper planning and appreciation for the larger picture.

There are several principles of care which are advocated to produce the most change with the least potential harm:

1. Nasoalveolar molding: pre-surgical manipulation of the nose and alveolus results in a more predictable primary cleft rhinoplasty which requires less nasal (and facial) dissection compared to patients who have not undergone nasoalveolar molding. The requirement of secondary "touch up" surgery is decreased while increasing overall nasal symmetry.[3]

2. Limited dissection: in the growing face, surgical planning should take into account the immediate and long-term effects of surgery. As adult cleft rhinoplasty remains one of the formidable challenges in plastic surgery, logic would suggest that limiting the amount of scar present in the nose at the time of facial maturity would be a wise investment for the patient. Therefore, the art of primary cleft rhinoplasty should include effecting the most change with the least surgery. This philosophy falls somewhat counter to the culture of plastic surgery, which tends to advocate more complex and a greater number of procedures to reach the holy grail of the perfect result.

3. Indications for secondary rhinoplasty: The ideal treatment plan for patients with a cleft would be an effective primary cleft rhinoplasty at the time of cleft lip repair followed by a second rhinoplasty at the time of facial maturity. This goal can be achieved in many patients; however, several others may require a "touch up" surgery prior to reaching facial maturity. It is the opinion of the author that these patients are the ones most at risk for the formation of excessive scars within the nose. Secondary rhinoplasty on the growing face should be considered if there is direct and clear request by the patient or caregiver, not because the surgeon is trying to improve their result. When performing immature cleft rhinoplasty, consideration should be given to the consequences of the procedure. Aggressive cartilage dissection, resection of nasal tip fibrofat, and cartilage implants can all look favorable for a time after surgery; however, subsequent nasal reconstruction may be compromised by overzealous application of these techniques.

Nasal floor closure

A principle of cleft surgery, which lacks emphasis, is closure of the nasal floor at the time of lip repair. The procedure requires extra work and has no bearing on the aesthetic result of the primary reconstruction. However, reconstruction of the nasal mucosa over the area of the alveolar cleft will have implications on future alveolar bone graft surgery. Nasal floor closure is commonly the most challenging part of alveolar bone graft surgery, and soiling of bone graft with nasal flora is a known source of bone graft failure. Unfortunately, exposure of the nasal floor defect during alveolar bone graft surgery can be challenging due to obstruction by the alveolar segments. At the time of primary lip repair, the nasal floor is well exposed. The vomer and lateral nasal wall are available for primary nasal floor reconstruction at the time of lip repair. This added effort at the time of infancy will be a wise investment which will be appreciated during alveolar bone graft surgery.

Evolution of technique

The Mohler Cutting repair evolved from an appreciation of the limits of the Millard rotation advancement repair and a need for a more aesthetic upper lip repair. In his signature repair, Millard placed an incision along the philtral line on the cleft side, which curves towards the philtral column on the non-cleft side at the superior aspect of the medial lip element.[25,30] This curvilinear incision produced a back cut on the upper lip, facilitating downward rotation of the medial lip element as a near total philtral unit. Cupid's bow, which is preserved in the unilateral cleft deformity, rotates downward with the medial lip element producing an anatomic reconstruction of this aesthetic structure. Cupid's bow, the philtral dimple, and most of the philtral column was preserved and orthotopically repositioned through this procedure. Downward rotation of the medial lip composite resulted in elongation of the philtrum on the cleft side and the resulting upper lip defect was filled by medial advancement of the lateral lip element.

The major limitation of the Millard repair is in its violation of the subunit borders at the superior third of the upper lip. The incision line veers away from the philtral line on the cleft side and curves towards the contralateral philtrum. This violation becomes more apparent in children with wide clefts who typically require a significant downward rotation of the medial lip element and therefore, a larger back cut. A compounding limitation is the use of the lateral lip element to fill the defect created by downward rotation of Cupid's bow. In the cases of wide cleft lips, the lateral lip element may require aggressive medialization to close the defect created by the larger back cut. As a result, the attached alar base can be excessively medialized, creating a micronostril, a deformity that lacks a definitive means of correction. Some surgeons have relied on perialar incisions in order to prevent the creation of a micronostril; however, scars in this area heal poorly and are difficult to correct.

Mohler's variation of the classic rotation-advancement repair relocates the back cut, used for downward rotation of Cupid's bow, from the medial lip to the columella. The result of this seemingly minor modification has powerful effects on upper lip aesthetics and nasolabial form. As the back cut is transposed from the lip to the nose, the defect created by the downward rotation of the medial lip element is also relocated to the columella. The inferior columellar skin, now part of the medial lip element flap, is transposed inferiorly with the medial lip to become the superior aspect of the philtrum, completely restoring the aesthetic subunit of the philtrum. The defect in the columella created by inferior rotation of the medial lip element is filled by superior rotation of the C-flap. The summation of these transpositions resembles an asymmetric Z-plasty repair rather than a rotation advancement repair. Superior rotation of the C-flap has the secondary benefit of superior transposition of the depressed medial crura and lengthening of the columella. As the lateral lip element is not used to fill the defect created by the downward rotation of Cupid's bow, less medial advancement of the lateral lip element is generally required, decreasing the risk of creating a micronostril. Moreover, there is a limited differential degree of advancement that is required between the lateral lip element (to fill the downward rotation of the Cupid's bow) and the alar base (to create an aesthetic and balanced nostril). Therefore, there is little need to separate the lateral lip from the alar with an unaesthetic perialar incision. A short, near horizontal incision at the alar base is all that is needed.

In Mohler's original design, the base of the back cut ended at the superior border of the philtral dimple, limiting the downward rotation of Cupid's bow. Millard criticized Mohler's original description of his columellar back cut as being inadequate for use in complete clefts and likely useful only in incomplete clefts.[31] In Cutting's variation, the apex of the Mohler incision was extended to just beyond the midline of the columella. The back cut was then brought down to the opposite philtral column, but no further (Fig. 21.3.1). This modification will achieve full downward rotation of the Cupid's bow in any unilateral cleft lip patient, regardless of severity.

Markings

Surgical markings for the Mohler Cutting repair start with standard tattooing of the white roll. The depth of Cupid's bow is marked on the white roll followed by the height of Cupid's bow on the non-cleft side. In patients with an indistinct philtral line, care should be taken to avoid marking the philtrum too wide. A wide philtrum will require a larger back cut for complete rotation. The ethnic background of the patient should also be considered as Caucasian people tend to have more narrow philtrums compared to Asian, African, and Hispanic people who tend toward wider philtrums. The distance between these two points is used to mark the height of the Cupid's bow on the cleft side. The white roll usually becomes indistinct at this area. The cleft sided height of the Cupid's bow is marked just medial to the desired point as the incision will pass lateral to this white roll point.

The white roll point on the lateral lip element is determined by the vertical height of the lip on the non-cleft side. This mark has been classically determined by measuring the distance from the commissure to the height of Cupid's bow on the non-cleft side and transposing this distance to the cleft side.[25] This method of marking, advocated by Millard, will restore a symmetric horizontal width of the upper lip at the sacrifice of vertical lip height at the philtral line. Even small discrepancies of vertical lip height (1–2 mm) are visible at conversation distance while discrepancies in horizontal width are less easily noticed and correct over time.[32,33] Another commonly advocated approach locates the lateral lip point to the white roll over widest width of the vermillion, Noordhoff's point.[34] In the incomplete and some complete cleft lip deformities, this mark accurately restores vertical height of the lip. However, in the cleft lip with a vertically short lateral lip, Noordhoff's point will produce a vertically short reconstruction. Therefore the vertical height of the lip on the non-cleft side is used to determine the lateral lip point on the white roll. This distance is about 10 mm in the 3-month-old child.

The back cut of the Mohler Cutting repair is angled, not curved as drawn in the rotation advancement repair. Therefore, the Mohler Cutting back cut is defined by only two points: the apex of the back cut located on the columella and the base of the back cut located at the junction of the columella with the upper lip. Minor adjustments of these two points affect the degree of achievable downward rotation, the proportion of the surrounding tissue, and location of the final scars. The apex of the back cut should be at least 1.5–2 mm superior to the base of the columella, approximately $\frac{1}{7}$ across the columellar width, towards the non-cleft side. If the apex is drawn too low then inadequate downward rotation will be the result. If the point is too far towards the cleft side, the C-flap will be narrow and inadequate to fill the defect created by the downward rotation of Cupid's bow. This may be the cause of the narrow columella that some surgeons associated

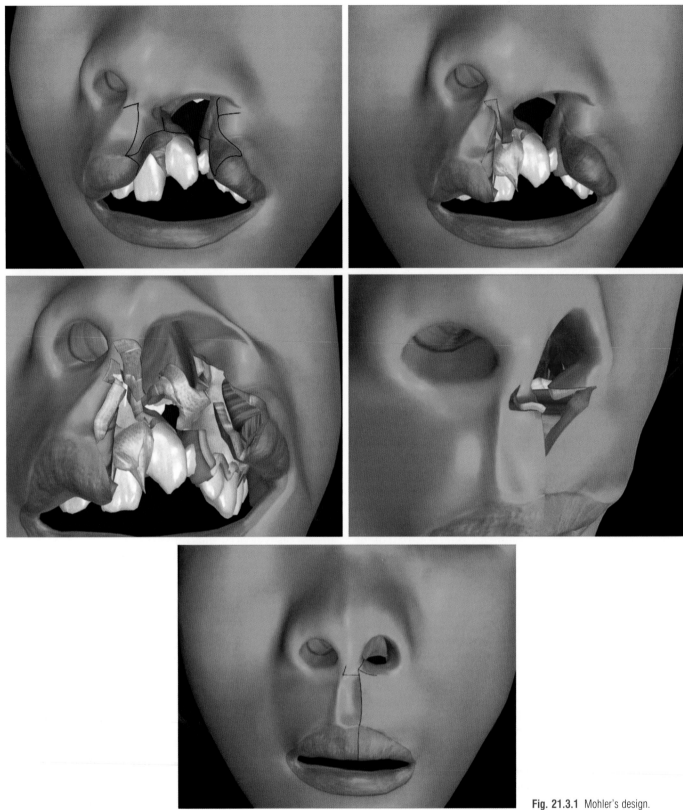

Fig. 21.3.1 Mohler's design.

with this technique. If the apex is placed too far towards the non-cleft side then the philtrum will be narrow and unaesthetic at its superior aspect. If the base of the back cut is placed lateral to the philtrum, then the upper lip will be lengthened. If the point is placed on the philtrum but inferior to the junction of the columella and upper lip then the final scars will violate the subunits of the upper lip. The learning curve of the Mohler Cutting repair is associated with appreciating the effects of subtle changes of these two points on the total repair.

A line is drawn connecting the apex of the back cut with the height of Cupid's bow on the cleft side. This line should have a subtle convexity at the lower third of the lip to create an aesthetic shield shape to the philtrum. At the base of the philtrum, the line should pass just lateral to the point marking the height of Cupid's bow on the cleft side. If the line goes through the white roll point then the tattoo point will be incised and not visible during reconstruction. The apex and base of the back cut are connected as a straight line and the C-flap and M-flap are drawn in the standard manner. The anterior border of the M-flap should be drawn perpendicular to the white roll. It is important to include the maximum amount of skin when marking the C-flap without incorporating mucosa. In cases in which pre-surgical orthopedics are not used, the greater area of the C-flap will be used to fill the defect in the columella. If mucosa is included in the C-flap then this tissue may be transposed to the nose and upper lip. An oblique line is drawn 1 mm inferior to the white roll at the anterior border of the M-flap to the red line. This line should be approximately 5 mm in length and is the receiving incision for the Noordhoff triangular flap.

Attention is now drawn to the lateral lip element. A line is drawn along the alar base crease at the border of the upper lip skin within the nostril floor skin. This line should start medially at the mucosal border and extend laterally to the medial border of the nostril rim. In the wide cleft lip with a short vertical height of the lateral lip element, the upper lip skin can be pulled into the nostril floor by aberrant attachments of the pars superficialis to the periosteum of the piriform aperture. Therefore, the medial border of the alar base crease may be pulled slightly (1 mm) within the nose. It is important not to over extend the medial border of the alar crease line into the substance of the nostril floor as this will cause a micronostril which is difficult to correct. The lateral border of the alar crease line ends at the medial border of the nostril rim. No perialar incision is used. The medial border of the lateral lip element is drawn from inferior to superior, starting 1 mm inferior to the white roll, on the vermillion. The line then crosses the white roll, in a perpendicular fashion, just medial to the white roll mark to a point 1 mm superior to the white roll. Transecting the white roll at a right angle will prevent notching of this anatomic structure. The line then quickly and gracefully curves to meet the medial border of the alar crease line at the base of the nose. This curved incision increases the vertical height of the lateral lip at the cost of horizontal lip length. Long term studies have demonstrated that discrepancies in horizontal lip length can correct over time.[32,33]

A Noordhoff triangular flap[34] is drawn on the vermillion to restore fullness to the vermillion at the area of the tubercle, prevent a whistling deformity and anatomically reconstruct the red line of the upper lip. This last benefit is of particular importance in Asian and African-American patients who commonly have a distinct border between the mucosa and vermilion. This flap capitalizes on the excess vermillion usually present in the lateral lip and transposes this tissue to the deficient medial lip element. As vermillion is delicate tissue, care is taken to incorporate a generous amount of red lip in the flap for easier handling. Excess vermillion and mucosa can be later trimmed from the triangular flap or the medial lip element. The inferior border of the L-flap is drawn to meet the medial edge of the gingivobuccal sulcus on the lesser segment.

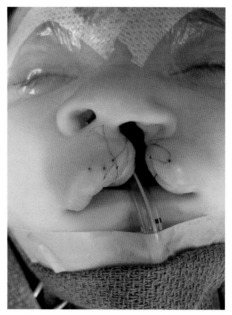

Fig. 21.3.2 Complete Mohler Cutting markings for the unilateral cleft lip repair. Note the back cut is placed on the columella rather than on the upper lip. The back cut markings are extended as a dotted line onto the upper lip. Extension of the incision onto the upper lip will lengthen the lip length on the non-cleft side. Therefore, the back cut should be limited to the columella. Note the generous Noordhoff triangular flap which incorporates the maximum amount of dry lip.

Final appearance of the cleft lip markings can be appreciated in Fig. 21.3.2.

Technical aspects of surgery

Downward rotation of Cupid's bow

The M-flap and C-flap are first mobilized with care to preserve the underlying orbicularis oris. The Mohler back cut is then incised through dermis only. A horizontal incision is then made at the base of the columella (base of the Mohler back cut) across the orbicularis oris (Fig. 21.3.3). If this incision is made at the apex of the Mohler back cut then the medial crura will be transected. The full thickness of upper lip muscle is transected with preservation of the oral mucosa. Dissection then proceeds deep to the orbicularis oris on the medial lip element, freeing a cuff of muscle from the underlying oral mucosa. This dissection plane should continue to the base of the Mohler back cut. If further downward rotation is required, a mucosal incision is made parallel to the frenulum then across its base in a hockey stick fashion. This incision will result in further downward rotation of the Cupid's bow. The frenulum defect is closed with the M-flap.

Preparation of the medial lip element

The skin of the medial element is sharply dissected from the underlying orbicularis oris muscle as far as the philtral dimple but no further. This small skin flap creates space for sutures during orbicularis oris reconstruction and frees the medial edge of the upper lip skin for further downward rotation of Cupid's bow.

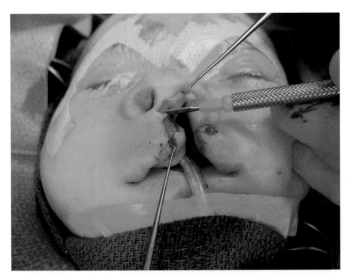

Fig. 21.3.3 Transection of the orbicularis oris is performed in a transverse manner at the junction of the columella with the upper lip. Performing this incision at the apex of the back cut will result in transection of the medial crura. A full-thickness incision of the upper lip muscle is required to fully rotate the Cupid's bow inferiorly.

L-flap dissection

The L-flap is sharply dissected from the orbicularis oris with care to preserve the muscle underlying the Noordhoff triangular flap. Without the underlying muscle, the Noordhoff flap will be flimsy and difficult to handle. As the base of the L-flap is approached, near the gingivobuccal sulcus, the level of dissection changes from a submucosal to a subperiosteal plane. Using a small periosteal elevator, a pocket is made at the inferior/lateral rim of the pyriform aperture, directly on the bone. This dissection pocket is widened to include the inferior aspect of the lateral nasal wall. A vertical, intranasal incision is made in the lateral aspect of the cleft-sided nostril at the junction of the squamous epithelium and nasal mucosa (Fig. 21.3.4). This incision is made from superior to inferior to meet the superior/posterior border of the L-flap incision. This

vertical incision should continue down to the bony edge of the pyriform aperture. A horizontal, intranasal incision is then made from posterior to anterior at the inferior border of the lateral nasal wall, joining the inferior border of the L-flap incision. Completing these two incisions will pedicle the L-flap on the lateral nasal wall (Fig. 21.3.5). This modification prevents oronasal fistula formation and aids in gingivoperiosteoplasty as well future alveolar bone grafting. A vomer flap is raised at this time for eventual closure of the anterior nasal floor. A gingivoperiosteoplasty can be performed at the discretion of the surgeon.

Lateral lip element dissection

The L-flap is tucked within the cleft-sided nostril and gingivobuccal sulcus incision is made. This incision is connected with the pyriform aperture incision by a supraperiosteal dissection across the face of the maxilla (Fig. 21.3.6). In patients with incomplete clefts or patients who have undergone NAM, there will be limited need for the gingivobuccal sulcus incision and supraperiosteal dissection. In patients with wide cleft lips who have not undergone pre-surgical orthopedics, dissection across the face of the maxilla can be extensive, extending as far superior as the supraorbital rim and as far lateral as the lateral canthus. Dissection along the medial buttress of the nose is also important to free the cartilaginous attachments from the pyriform rim. Dissection proceeds until a tension free, orthotropic transposition of the ala can be achieved. Even a small amount of tension at the time of closure will result in relapse of the deformity, despite appearances at the end of the procedure.

Intranasal mucosa reconstruction

All mucosal defects in the cleft sided nostril are closed with mucosal flaps. The pyriform aperture incision is reconstructed with the L-flap to prevent closure of this defect by secondary intention which will result in relapse of the alar deformity (Fig. 21.3.7). All excess L-flap should be meticulously trimmed as redundancy in this reconstruction will result in excess

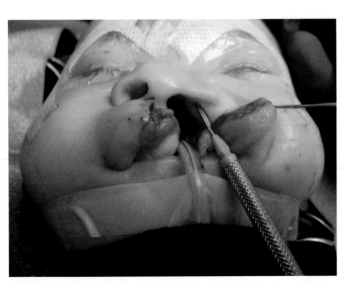

Fig. 21.3.4 A vertical pyriform aperture incision is made at the junction of the nasal mucosa with the squamous epithelium of the nostril.

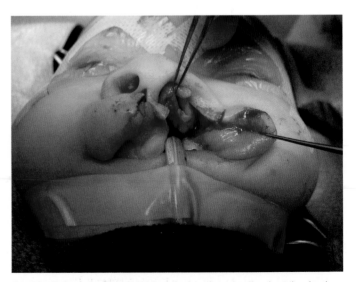

Fig. 21.3.5 The L-flap is pedicled from the lateral nasal wall and not the alveolus. This modification will prevent a persistent oronasal fistula and assist in reconstruction of the nasal floor.

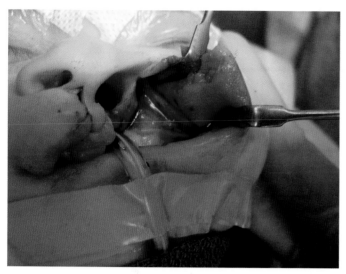

Fig. 21.3.6 The oral sulcus incision will merge with the pyriform aperture incision. Supraperiosteal dissection across the face of the maxilla will free the alar base. In cases where NAM is not used, this dissection may extend widely across the maxilla. The goal is to sufficiently release the displaced tissue as to eliminate all tension during alar base repositioning.

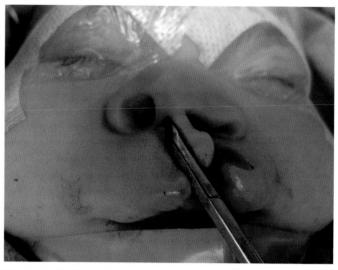

Fig. 21.3.8 The Mohler Cutting incision facilitates a medial approach rhinoplasty. At the apex of the back cut, blunt scissor dissection is used to separate the medial crura and gain access to the nasal tip.

mucosa bulging into the nose. The anterior floor of the nose is reconstructed to facilitate bony reconstruction of the alveolus. If a gingivoperiosteoplasty is performed at the time of primary cleft lip repair then nasal floor closure will be required. If a secondary bone graft is planned then closure of the nasolabial fistula will result in an easier reconstruction and in increased graft take. The vomer flap is sutured to the inferior/medial edge of the L-flap. Horizontal mattress sutures are placed from posterior to anterior to achieve a water-tight seal to the floor of the nose.

Oral mucosa reconstruction

In patients with an incomplete cleft or well-opposed alveolar segment, oral mucosa reconstruction is rarely a problem. In patients with wide unilateral cleft lips, care must be taken to

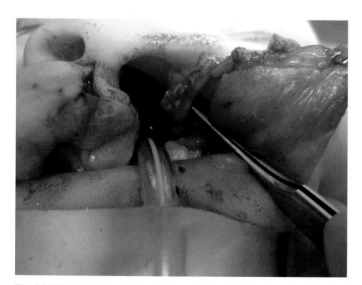

Fig. 21.3.7 The forceps point to the trimmed L-flap which has been inset into the pyriform aperture incision.

prevent tension at the midline mucosa repair as this could lead to dehiscence of the wound. At the lateral aspect of the sulcus incision, aggressive medial transposition of the oral mucosa can be achieved without risk to vascularization of the flap. Oblique sutures are placed with decreasing tension from lateral to medial. The goal is to achieve a tension-free closure at the midline, which will result in healthy healing of the intraoral lining.

Primary rhinoplasty Part I

An underappreciated benefit of the Mohler Cutting repair is the position of advantage it offers to medial approach primary cleft rhinoplasty. Access to the medial crura, nasal tip, and lower lateral cartilages is facilitated by the apex of the back cut, located on the columella. Converse scissors are inserted between the medial crura at the apex of the Mohler back cut and gentle spreading is used to separate these paired structures (Fig. 21.3.8). A hemi-membranous incision is made from the septal angle to the floor of the nose on the cleft side (Fig. 21.3.9). The hemi-membranous incision is connected to the dissection pocket created between the medial crura with care not to damage the lower lateral cartilages. The Converse scissors are then inserted underneath the nasal tip skin, over the lateral crura and lateral crus. Gentle spreading will release the skin over the upper and lower lateral cartilages on the cleft and non-cleft side (Fig. 21.3.10). Dissection between the lower lateral cartilage and nasal mucosal is unnecessary and will only create additional scar. Fibrofat is not removed from the nasal tip. The depressed lower lateral cartilage on the cleft side is elevated to a super-corrected position with a Ragnell retractor. The medial crura are affixed to each other using a long-lasting absorbable suture (Fig. 21.3.11). These sutures serve the secondary purpose of shaping the columella. Several transfixion sutures are then used to close the hemi-membranous septum incision. The columellar length on the cleft side should equal that of the non-cleft side at the end of this portion of this procedure. In patients with a wide cleft and no pre-surgical orthopedics, a nostril rim incision is added

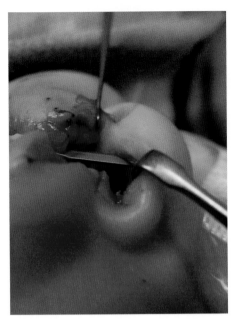

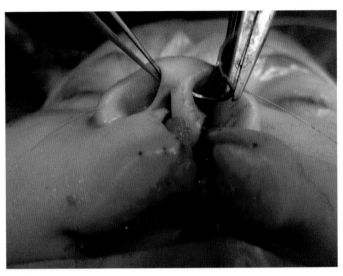

Fig. 21.3.11 The depressed lower lateral cartilage is elevated to a super-corrected position using a Ragnell retractor. Long-lasting absorbable sutures are used to affix the medial crura in its new position and to shape the columella.

Fig. 21.3.9 A hemi-membranous incision is used to free the depressed medial crura on the cleft side. This lower lateral cartilage will be elevated to a super-corrected position.

on the cleft side. The lower lateral cartilage is dissected from the overlying skin and a suspension suture is placed between the upper lateral and lower lateral cartilage. An intradomal suture is also placed at this time. Excess nostril rim skin is carefully trimmed and the nostril rim is closed.

Alar base repositioning

A flap of dermis and muscle is sharply dissected from the nasal floor skin of the cleft sided alar base. This dermomuscular pennant is sutured to the crura footplate on the unaffected side using two long-lasting absorbable sutures (Fig. 21.3.12). The caudal septum may be incorporated into the suture to straighten the anterior septum.

Orbicularis oris repair

The skin of the lateral lip element is sharply separated from the orbicularis oris as far laterally as the alar base. Excess orbicularis oris is sharply trimmed towards the level of the skin incision. The orbicularis oris is reconstructed using buried sutures. If the muscle has been properly trimmed, the upper lip skin edges will "kiss" once the orbicularis oris has been reconstructed. This will eliminate all tension from the upper lip skin repair.

Upper lip skin and vermillion repair

The upper lip skin and Noordhoff triangular flap are inset. Excess mucosa on the medial lip element is trimmed to prevent excess fullness in the area of the tubercle. The C-flap is trimmed and used to fill the entire columellar defect created by the downward rotation of the Cupid's bow (Fig. 21.3.13).

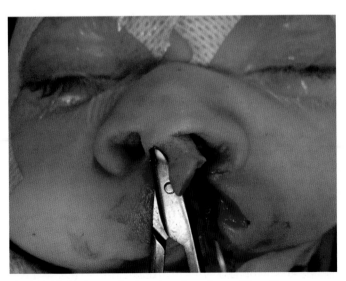

Fig. 21.3.10 Gentle spreading is performed over the nasal tip cartilages.

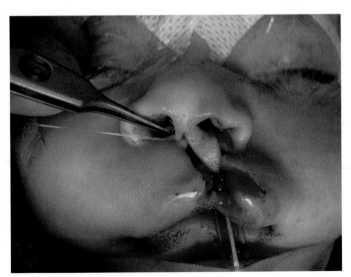

Fig. 21.3.12 The alar base is affixed to the caudal septum and medial crura on the non-cleft side.

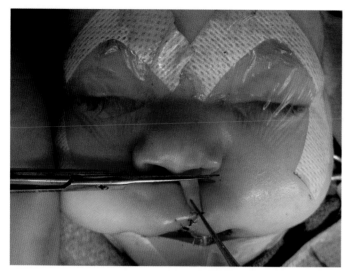

Fig. 21.3.13 The C-flap is trimmed to fill the entire defect created by the downward rotation of Cupid's bow. Note this defect is located entirely within the columella. The lateral lip element skin is not used to fill this defect.

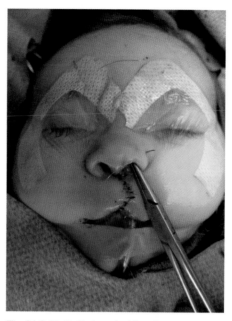

Fig. 21.3.14 Vestibular web obliterating sutures are placed intranasally behind the web and through the alar–facial groove. The suture is returned through the same percutaneous puncture and then intranasally in front of the web. Tying this suture will obliterate the vestibular web and accentuate the deficient alar–facial groove.

A straight line scar should extend along the entire length of the philtrum on the cleft side. The lateral aspect of the C-flap is united with the alar base skin to close the nostril floor. The nostril floor should be closed in a stair-step fashion in relation to the upper lip incision. This will avoid the convergence of four skin corners at the base of the nose which can produce a depressed scar. Proper skin dissection of both the C-flap and the nasal floor flap on the lateral lip element will prevent the formation of a micronostril even in cases where the C-flap is deficient.

Primary rhinoplasty Part II

Lower lateral cartilage repositioning and vestibular web obliteration is performed using internal retention sutures. An oblique horizontal mattress is placed from the cleft sided nostril to the non-cleft nostril and back again to elevate the depressed lateral crura and address nostril apex overhang. The point of maximum overhang on the nostril rim is sighted and a suture is placed through the lower lateral cartilage, into the dissection pocket underneath the nasal tip skin. The trajectory of the suture is posterior and lateral. The suture then passes through the lower lateral cartilage on the non-cleft side and into the non-cleft nasal airway. The suture is then returned to the cleft sided nostril, following a parallel trajectory, 2 mm behind the first pass. Tying this oblique, nostril to nostril, horizontal mattress suture will elevate the depressed lower lateral cartilage and medialize the lateral crus. It is critical to overcorrect the vertical height of the lower lateral cartilage in anticipation for descent of this structure over time.[5]

The vestibular web is addressed without the use of external bolsters or nasal packing. A long-lasting suture is placed behind the vestibular web, and through the alar-facial groove externally (Fig. 21.3.14). The same percutaneous hole is used return the suture into the nose but anterior to the vestibular web. Tying this suture will obliterate the vestibular web and accentuate the alar-facial groove. Two or three sutures may be required to achieve the full effect of this internal retention suture (Fig. 21.3.15).

Postoperative care

Unilateral cleft lip repair is commonly performed as an outpatient surgery. Parents are instructed to clean the upper lip twice daily with soap and water as well as dilute hydrogen peroxide. Arm braces which prevent bending at the elbows are used for 3 weeks to protect the reconstructed site. These braces are generally well tolerated. No pacifier is used during this 3-week period and a special feeding bottle is used during

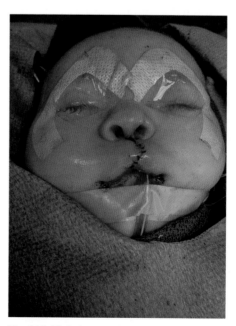

Fig. 21.3.15 At the conclusion of primary rhinoplasty, the lower lateral cartilage should be anatomically repositioned and the vestibular web obliterated.

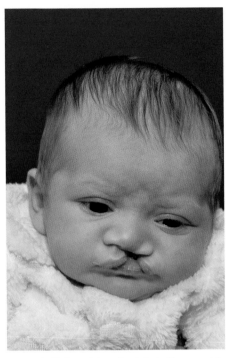

Fig. 21.3.16 Frontal view of an infant with a complete unilateral cleft lip deformity

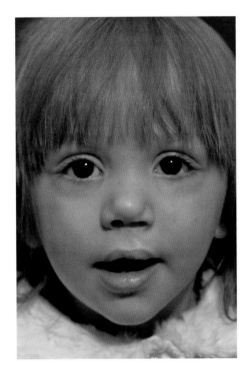

Fig. 21.3.18 Postoperative view of the same infant depicted in Fig. 21.3.16. No NAM was used in this patient. Note the placement of the final scars along the subunit borders of the lip.

this time. The patient may breastfeed normally. All permanent sutures are removed 5–7 days postoperatively. Tape is then applied to the upper lip to prevent micro-shearing at the incision line. This tape will remain in place for 2 weeks.

Results

Long-term clinical outcomes of patients undergoing the Mohler Cutting repair demonstrates restoration of the upper lip height on the affected side.[32] Surgeons and parents should appreciate that the upper lip height will initially shorten on

the affected side. This concerning appearance will peak about 6–8 weeks postoperatively when the scar is at its most prominent and firm state. As the scar eventually softens and remodels, over the course of one year, the upper lip will elongate. Scar massage is initiated 6 weeks postoperatively. Symmetrical upper lip and nasal form can be achieved with aesthetic placement of the upper lip scars along subunit borders (Figs. 21.3.16–19).

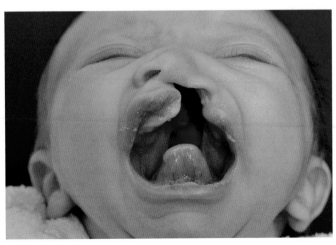

Fig. 21.3.17 Basal view the same infant in Fig. 21.3.16. Note the significant cleft nasal deformity

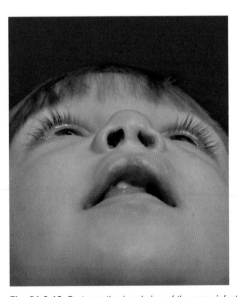

Fig. 21.3.19 Postoperative basal view of the same infant depicted in Fig. 21.3.16. Note the significant improvement in nasal symmetry. A single procedure was performed in this patient.

🌐 Access the complete reference list online at **http://www.expertconsult.com**

2. Grayson BH, Cutting C, Wood R. Preoperative columella lengthening in bilateral cleft lip and palate. *Plast Reconstr Surg.* 1993;92(7):1422–1423. *The first report of nasoalveolar molding. In this early report, the technique is applied to a patient with bilateral cleft lip and palate.*

15. Grayson BH, Garfinkle JS. Early cleft management: the case for nasoalveolar molding. *Am J Orthod Dentofacial Orthop.* 2014;145(2):134–142. *Dr. Grayson in his classic articulate fashion describes the benefit of NasoAlveolar molding to the patient with a cleft and reviews the supportive and non-supportive evidence to this therapy.*

25. Millard DR Jr. *Cleft Craft: The Evolution of its Surgery. Volume 1 - The Unilateral Deformity.* Vol. 1. Boston: Little, Brown, and Company; 1976. *The technique of the rotation advancement repair, its development and evolution is beautifully described in Millard's tome of cleft care.*

28. McComb H. Primary correction of unilateral cleft lip nasal deformity: a 10-year review. *Plast Reconstr Surg.* 1985;75(6):791–799. *Harold McComb's report demonstrates the safety and efficacy of primary cleft rhinoplasty. It is this report which demonstrated that nasal manipulation at the time of infancy is not harmful to nasal growth.*

29. Salyer KE. Primary correction of the unilateral cleft lip nose: a 15-year experience. *Plast Reconstr Surg.* 1986;77(4):558–568.

30. Millard DR Jr. *Transactions of the 1st International Congress of Plastic Surgery, Stockholm.* Baltimore: Williams and Wilkins; 1957. *Ralph Millard's critique of the original design for the Mohler repair in which he correctly points out that its ultility would be limited to patients with incomplete unilateral clefts.*

32. Cutting CB, Dayan JH. Lip height and lip width after extended Mohler unilateral cleft lip repair. *Plast Reconstr Surg.* 2003;111(1):17–23, discussion 24–16. *Long-term outcomes of the Mohler Cutting repair demonstrated a benefit to labial form and correction of horizontal shortening of the upper lip.*

33. Mulliken JB, LaBrie RA. Fourth-dimensional changes in nasolabial dimensions following rotation-advancement repair of unilateral cleft lip. *Plast Reconstr Surg.* 2012;129(2):491–498. *Long-term outcomes of the rotation advancement repair. Mulliken demonstrates that the alar base lateralizes over time and that horizontal shortening of the upper lip corrects over time.*

34. Noordhoff MS. *The Surgical Technique for the Unilateral Cleft Lip-Nasal Deformity.* Taipei: Noordhoff Craniofacial Foundation; 1997. *The Noordhoff (Chang Gung) unilateral cleft lip repair is described including the vermillion triangular (Noordhoff) flap which prevents the whistling deformity of cleft lip repair.*

21.4

Unilateral cleft lip repair, anatomic subunit approximation technique

David M. Fisher

SYNOPSIS

- The non-cleft side bow peak is marked on the vermilion-cutaneous junction where the straight part of the half bow meets the upper convexity of the lateral lip element. The cleft side bow peak is then placed an equal distance from the midline.

- A natural undulation of the cutaneous roll can only be achieved if the upwards convexity of the lateral lip element lateral to Noordhoff's point is preserved.

- The transverse length of the cleft side lateral lip element need not and should not be compromised to achieve vertical height.

- Leveling of the Cupid's bow is the result of a Rose–Thompson lengthening effect in all cases. In most cases, a small triangle is also placed above the roll.

- Orientation of the lateral lip element incisions must vary depending on the vertical height of the lateral lip element.

- Vermilion deficiency below the cleft side half of Cupid's bow should be augmented with vermilion from the lateral lip element.

- Medial incisions should be performed first. Lateral lip markings can be adjusted if necessary.

- Approximation of lip elements is along the seams of anatomic subunits.

Preoperative assessment

It is essential to ensure that the infant is optimized prior to surgery; the input of various pediatric specialists will be required for patients with syndromes and co-morbidities. Early liaison with the anesthesia team is recommended. Failure to thrive is seen in approximately 40% of children with a palatal cleft and 9% of those with an isolated cleft lip; thus all cleft patients must be closely monitored preoperatively for appropriate weight gains.[1] Close communication between the family and the cleft team (via the clinical nurse specialist, dietician, feeding specialist, and social worker) is essential at this stage.

Cleft lip repair is deferred until the age of 3–6 months to allow for the optimization of underlying medical issues, minimization of the risks of anesthesia, and the completion of pre-surgical orthopedic treatment, if indicated.

A typical treatment pathway, from antenatal diagnosis to adulthood, for a child with a complete unilateral cleft lip and palate (cUCLP), as practiced at The Hospital for Sick Children in Toronto, Canada, is outlined in Table 21.4.1. While a child with an isolated incomplete cleft lip (iCL) may require just the single operation, the burden of care in the case of a complete cleft of the lip and palate is far more substantial.

Pre-surgical orthopedics

Pre-surgical infant orthopedics is indicated for all complete clefts. It is not used for complete cases with a Simonart Band or in incomplete cleft lip. Nasoalveolar molding (NAM) as described by Grayson et al.[2] is our preferred method. The primary goal is improved alignment of the alveolar arches. Once the alveolar cleft segments are aligned the nasal component is added. The goal is anteromedial repositioning of the cleft side dome. It is important that this is done gradually and gently so as to avoid expansion of the cleft side nostril circumference.

While it is our preference to employ pre-surgical orthopedics, the anatomic subunit approximation technique does not require it. The greatest perceived benefit of pre-surgical orthopedics is an improvement of the asymmetry of the nasal base in the anteroposterior dimension and less relapse of the nasal deformity. In bilateral cases where there is protrusion of the premaxilla the benefits may be even greater.

Surgical plan: anatomical subunit approximation technique

The anatomical subunit approximation technique[3] borrows the concept of anatomical subunits first described by Burget

Table 21.4.1 Typical surgical treatment pathway for a child with a unilateral complete cleft lip and palate at the Hospital for Sick Children, Toronto.

Age	Treatment
Prenatal diagnosis	Parental consultation with cleft surgeon
2 weeks up to lip repair	Pre-surgical orthopaedics (if indicated)
3–6 months	Cleft lip repair and primary nasal correction
10–14 months	Palate repair ± myringotomy and tubes
≥ 3 years	Lip revision (if indicated)
≥ 4 years	Surgical correction of VPI (if indicated)
≥ 7 years	Lobule rhinoplasty (if indicated)
8–10 years (mixed dentition)	Alveolar bone graft
≥ 12 years	Definitive septorhinoplasty (if indicated)
≥ 16–18 years (skeletal maturity)	Orthognathic surgery (if indicated)

and Menick for nasal reconstruction.[4] The lip and nose complex are viewed in terms of their anatomical subunits and the repair aims to produce a cutaneous scar along the "ideal line of repair" – along the seams of adjacent subunits. Incisions cross the cutaneous rolls of the lip elements perpendicular to the rolls. The incision on the medial cleft side then ascends from a point above the cutaneous roll such that it mirrors the ridge of the non-cleft philtral column. It then curves superolaterally just below and, thus, preserves the lip-columellar crease to the medial point of closure in the nostril sill. Lip length is achieved by two mechanisms: firstly, a Rose–Thompson[5,6] effect as angled lines straighten upon approximation (which accounts for approximately 1 mm of lengthening) and, secondly if required, a small inferior triangle from the lateral lip element, which is positioned just superior to the cutaneous roll (a modification of the Tennison–Randall repair).[6,7] The lengthening achieved by the Rose–Thompson principle significantly reduces the size of the inferior triangle that would otherwise be required had a traditional inferior triangle repair been performed. The technique also utilizes Noordhoff's lateral vermilion triangle flap[8] to augment the deficient vermilion height of the medial lip element on the cleft side.

This technique has a number of advantages over the inferior triangle and rotation-advancement repairs. In variance with the rotation-advancement techniques.[9–11] there is minimal scarring at the base of the nose. The cutaneous scar is positioned along the seams of anatomical subunits with the exception of, when required, a small triangle above the cutaneous roll. Tension is ideally positioned above the roll accentuating the pout of the lip. Continuity of the cutaneous roll is achieved by side-to-side approximation of the roll elements. In common with the inferior triangle repair, lateral lip transverse length need not be compromised to achieve

vertical height, a commonly practiced compromise when performing a rotation-advancement type repair.[9–11] Note that the lateral lip element is almost always short in its transverse dimension when compared to the non-cleft side. As commonly seen in complete clefts, the vertical height of the lateral lip is also short.[12,13] The practice of moving the base of the incision laterally to achieve vertical height is a compromise that is not required by the anatomical subunit approximation technique.

Readers are encouraged to refer to the initial description[3] for a detailed description of the repair. Refer also to the legends accompanying Figs. 21.4.1–21.4.6. The Cupid's bow and philtral column heights are marked with the cleft side bow peak and philtral column heights being equidistant relative to the midline as the corresponding non-cleft side markings. Note that the non-cleft side Cupid's bow peak is not marked at the highest point of the curve of the lip, but rather where the straight portion of the non-cleft side half bow meets the convexity of the lateral lip element (Fig. 21.4.1). No such convexity exists on the cleft side of the medial lip element. The corresponding convexity on the cleft side will come from the lateral lip element lateral to "Noordhoff's point".

Points are marked above each bow peak just above the cutaneous roll at points above the lines perpendicular to the vermilion-cutaneous junction. The medial lip cleft side philtral column incision (equivalent to the "greater lip height") (Fig. 21.4.2) will ascend from the point above the roll to the height of the lip just below the lip-columellar crease. The incision line

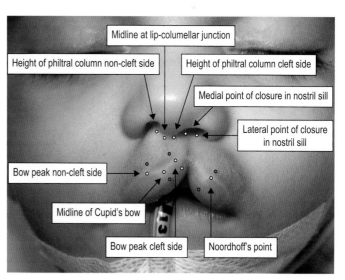

Fig. 21.4.1 The *non-cleft side Cupid's bow peak* is not marked at the highest point of the curve of the lip. It is marked where the straight portion of the non-cleft side half bow meets the convexity of the lateral lip element. Note that there is no such convexity on the cleft side of the medial lip element. This curve of the bow on the cleft side will come from the lateral lip element lateral to Noordhoff's point. The *cleft side peak of Cupid's bow* is positioned on the vermilion-cutaneous junction on the cleft side of the medial lip element equidistant from the *midline of the bow*. "Noordhoff's point" is identified on the vermilion–cutaneous junction where the cutaneous roll and the vermilion–mucosal junction lines start to converge medially. It is not necessarily the tallest portion of the red lip. At this point there is adequate vermilion height (usually matching the height of vermilion below the non-cleft side peak of Cupid's bow) and good quality cutaneous roll. Both of these features, vermilion height and quality of the cutaneous roll, diminish if this point is moved medially. The upward convexity of the lateral lip element is lateral to "Noordhoff's point".

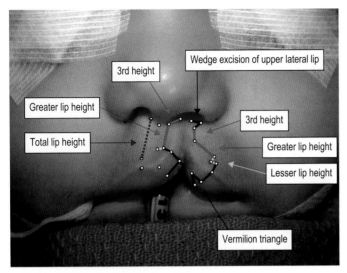

Fig. 21.4.2 Pre-surgical markings. For a complete description, the reader is encouraged to refer to DM Fisher. Unilateral cleft lip repair: An anatomical sub-unit approximation technique.[3] In minor clefts with minimal rotation of Cupid's bow, an opening incision and inferior triangle may not be necessary. When the lateral lip element is long, a wedge excision of upper lateral lip skin is required. It is placed below the lateral point of closure in the nostril sill and medial to subalare.

The point of origin of the opening incision for the medial lip back cut (if indicated) is initiated just above the cutaneous roll. The opening incision is drawn perpendicular to the greater height incision.

The medial and lateral points of closure within the nostril sill are not distinct anatomical points and are arguably the hardest points to define in this repair. The medial point of closure in the nostril sill is positioned lateral to the curve of the lip-columellar crease. It will be positioned more medial in complete cases and more lateral in incomplete cases. This will allow the operator to adjust the length of the "third height" and therefore take up less lateral lip height in a complete case (where there is vertical height deficiency), or use up height of the lateral lip height in an incomplete case (where there is vertical height excess). The lateral point of closure in the nostril sill is then chosen on the lateral lip element, relative to the medial point of closure in the nostril sill, such that when these two points are approximated, two goals are accomplished: 1) the nares are of equal circumference and 2) symmetry of the alar bases, from the anterior view, is achieved. Gentle manipulation of the medial and lateral lip elements should confirm acceptable positioning of these points. In complete clefts where the lateral lip is tethered such that the medial and lateral lip elements cannot be brought together, it is advisable to release the lateral lip element before marking the lip.

Calipers are used to measure the "total lip height" and the "greater lip height". The "total lip height" is measured with the lip at rest and is defined as the height of the non-cleft side philtral column from a point above the roll to a point just

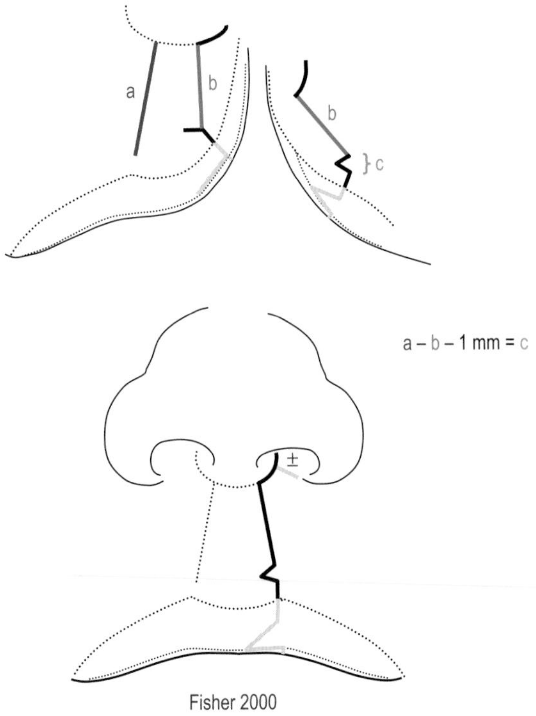

then traverses superolaterally to the medial point of closure in the nostril sill (equivalent to the "third height"). From the point above the roll, the incision line continues caudally perpendicular to the roll through the bow peak and vermilion and across the free border of the lip into the mucosa.

$$a - b - 1\ mm = c$$

Fisher 2000

Fig. 21.4.3 Pre-surgical markings and measurements. The *total lip height* and the *greater lip height* are each measured from points above the roll to the base of the columella. The *lesser lip height* (base width of the *small inferior triangle*) is equal to the *total lip height* minus the *greater lip height* less 1 mm. The 1 mm accounts for the Rose–Thompson lengthening that occurs as the angled incision lines approximate in the vertical.

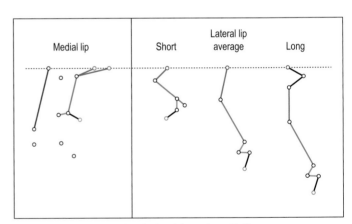

○ Medial point of closure in nostril sill
○ Cupid's bow peak cleft side
○ Lateral point of closure in nostril sill
○ Noordhoff's point

Fig. 21.4.4 Lateral lip markings will vary depending on the vertical height of the lateral lip element. In many complete clefts the vertical height of the lateral lip element will be short. In such cases, the *greater lip height* incision will be more horizontal and its lateral extreme may need to be coincident with the upper incision of the *inferior triangle* which will require an upward pointing orientation. In contrast, with many incomplete clefts, the vertical height of the lateral lip element may be excessive. In this case, it is helpful to position both the *medial* and *lateral points of closure in the nostril sill* more laterally. This essentially lengthens the *third height*. If the lateral lip remains too long despite this maneuver, a medially based wedge excision of upper lip can be performed below *lateral point of closure in the nostril sill*. The position of the lateral point of closure in the nostril sill and of "Noordhoff's point" should not be compromised.

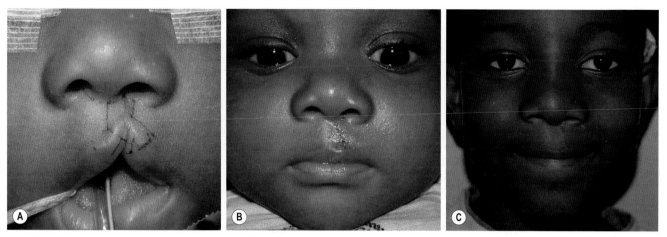

Fig. 21.4.5 An example of the *anatomic subunit approximation technique* in a patient with an incomplete unilateral cleft. **(A)** preoperative appearance and markings at age 5 months; **(B)** appearance at one week postoperatively; **(C)** age 6 years.

below the lip-columellar crease. The "greater lip height" is measured with gentle downward traction on the lip to unfurl the medial lip. It is defined as the height of the cleft side philtral column incision from a point above the roll to a point just below the lip-columellar crease and it is positioned along a line which mirrors the non-cleft side philtral column. The "lesser lip height" (equivalent to the base width of the small inferior triangle) is equal to the "total lip height" minus the "greater lip height" and less 1 mm (Fig. 21.4.3). The 1 mm accounts for the approximate length achieved by the Rose–Thompson principle. If an inferior triangle is required, the back cut for the opening incision is drawn perpendicular to the "greater lip height" incision, and of a length equal to the "lesser lip height" (the inferior triangle being equilateral). Rotation of the bow is achieved by the combination of the back cut and the Rose–Thompson effect (as the angled lines straighten). The "lesser lip height" is usually between 1 and 1.5 mm and never exceeds 2 mm. For minor form incomplete clefts, an inferior triangle is often not necessary. Note that the back cut is made perpendicular to the greater height incision and not parallel to the cutaneous roll. The latter would

produce a flattening of the Cupid's bow when the back cut is opened. The perpendicular back cut preserves tissue above the roll and thus better conserves the curve of Cupid's bow.

The base of the cutaneous incision on the lateral lip element is marked according to the recommendations of Noordhoff. "Noordhoff's point" is marked along the vermilion-cutaneous junction at the point where the cutaneous roll and red line begin to converge medially (Fig. 21.4.2). The natural upward convexity of the cutaneous roll lateral to Noordhoff's point is ideally suited for reconstruction of the cleft side curve of the bow. A point is marked just above the cutaneous roll at a point above "Noordhoff's point" along a line perpendicular to the vermilion-cutaneous junction. Between the lateral point of closure in the nostril sill and the point above the roll three lengths must be accommodated: the "greater lip height", the "lesser lip height", and the "third height" (corresponding in length to the line connecting the height of the cleft side philtral column and the medial point of closure in the nostril sill). This is readily achieved by placing the "greater lip height" caliper on the lateral lip element such that its lower tip lies the "lesser lip height" distance away from the point above the roll, and

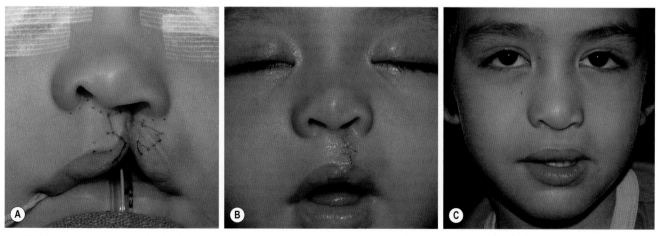

Fig. 21.4.6 An example of the *anatomic subunit approximation technique* in a patient with a complete unilateral cleft lip and palate. **(A)** Preoperative appearance and markings, age 6 months; **(B)** 1 week postoperative; **(C)** age 3 years.

its upper tip lies the "third height" distance away from lateral point of closure in the nostril sill.

In complete clefts where there is a short vertical height to the lateral lip element, the angle of the "greater lip height" incision on the lateral lip will be more horizontal and, in extreme cases, may be confluent with the upper limb incision of the inferior triangle (Fig. 21.4.4). Alternatively, in an incomplete cleft that presents a relative excess of vertical height, the "third height" may be lengthened by lateralizing the medial and lateral points of closure within the nostril. If vertical height excess persists in spite of this maneuver, it may be necessary to perform a medially based wedge excision of the upper lip below the lateral point of closure in the nostril sill. The lateral apex of this wedge excision should never extend laterally beyond subalare; this is unnecessary and leaves an unsightly scar. Care should be taken not to alter the vertical height of the lateral point of closure in the nostril sill as this will compromise the final vertical position of the alar insertion.

Any vermilion deficiency below the cleft side half of the Cupid's bow requires augmentation. An opening incision is created along the vermilion–mucosal junction below the cleft side half of the Cupid's bow. This back cut will receive a laterally based vermilion triangular flap from the lateral lip element as described by Noordhoff (Fig. 21.4.2).

In incomplete clefts, a wedge excision of the nostril sill above the medial and lateral points of nostril sill closure is performed. The excision should be sufficient to balance the circumference of the nares, with great care taken not to over-resect, as the resultant nostril stenosis presents a difficult reconstructive challenge. The mucosa of the cleft margins is removed by wedge excision; a short lateral upper buccal sulcus advancement incision may be helpful on occasions.

In complete clefts, the mucosal incisions on the medial and lateral lip elements extend cranially to the points of attachment of each lip element to the greater and lesser alveolar segments, respectively. An upper buccal sulcus incision extending laterally from the point of attachment of the lateral lip element is made. From the medial point of closure in the nostril sill, the incision continues intranasally along the caudal margin of the septum for a distance of up to 12 mm to facilitate access for septal repositioning. The lateral free edge of the septal flap will receive the medial free edge of the lateral vestibular flap. The lateral vestibular flap is fashioned by incising from the lateral point of closure in the nostril sill to the attachment point of the lateral lip element to the alveolus, and then along the piriform margin. This allows for supraperiosteal mobilization of the alar base. An anteriorly based inferior turbinate flap may be incorporated to cover the vestibular lining defect in clefts with a significant anteroposterior distance between the greater and lesser maxillary segments.

Primary nasal correction

The anatomic subunit approximation technique describes a technique for cleft lip repair. It can be accompanied by most previously describes techniques of primary rhinoplasty.

Because the cleft nasal deformity is the result of an underlying skeletal deformity,[14] it stands to reason that the skeletal deformity needs to be corrected before any correction can be fully realized in the nose. Because pre-surgical orthopedics can only partially improve the deformity (by correcting maxillary segment misalignment while not addressing maxillary hypoplasia); and, because primary bone grafting is not performed, it is unrealistic to completely correct the nasal deformity at the primary operation. A plea must be made for patience. The potential risks of a primary rhinoplasty include iatrogenic deformity to the skin envelope and cartilages and the introduction of scar that may complicate subsequent interventions. There will be future opportunities to augment the skeletal base deficiencies at the time of alveolar bone grafting and orthognathic surgery if indicated. This will set the stage for definitive septorhinoplasty. At this time, deformities such as a broad deviated nasal dorsum, which are only obvious after maturity, may be addressed. Definitive secondary septorhinoplasty will be successful only if the cartilages are intact and robust, and the skin envelope is complete and free of scar.

The authors preferred primary rhinoplasty is relatively aggressive at the nasal base and relatively conservative in the lobule. Primary rhinoplasty is performed with the following goals in mind:

1. Balanced alar bases (from the anterior view)
2. Columellar base mobilization to the midline
3. Caudal septal release and repositioning
4. Alar base release and repositioning
5. Release of the nasal attachments to the piriform margin
6. Anteromedial advancement of the cleft side dome and lateral crus
7. Creation of the scroll – internal nasal valve plication suture(s)
8. Lateralization of the cleft side lateral vestibular lining – alar transfixion suture(s)
9. No external skin incisions
10. No excision(s) of skin envelope

A nasal stent is placed and secured with a trans-septal suture. It is removed with the sutures at one week. The currently available stents do little to effect nasal tip position but are perceived to be helpful to smooth out the nostril sill closure.

Operative technique

Local anesthesia is limited to bilateral infraorbital nerve blocks and for submucoperiosteal hydrodissection of the caudal septum. In order to prevent errors in measurement and in the perception of the balance of the repair, the lip elements are not infiltrated.

It is important that the repair be performed in the proper sequence to allow the operator to assess progress and make modifications, if necessary. The medial lip incisions (without the back cut) should be made first. The *1ˢᵗ Checkpoint* is the assessment of the length achieved by the Rose–Thompson effect alone. The 1 mm of calculated lengthening is an estimate. It will be greater when the slope of the bow is steeper; the more rotated the bow, the more acute will be the angle formed by the incision across the roll and the greater height incision and, thus, the more lengthening will be achieved as this angle opens to become 180°. Conversely, the more level the bow the more obtuse will be the angle, and less lengthening will be achieved by the Rose–Thompson effect.

If the bow has been leveled by the Rose–Thompson effect, an opening incision and inferior triangle will not be necessary. If deemed appropriate, the opening incision is then made. It is made of sufficient length to level the bow. The *2nd Checkpoint* is ensuring that the triangle that has been drawn on the lateral lip element is of the exact size to fill the defect created by the opening incision in the medial lip element once the bow has been leveled. The size of the triangle can be adjusted at this point provided the lateral lip incisions have not already been performed. Finally, once the medial and lateral lip elements have been fully mobilized from their skeletal attachments, the *3rd Checkpoint* is the approximation the medial point of closure in the nostril sill with the lateral point of closure in the nostril sill. Before committing to the lateral point of closure, the surgeon will want to check that the nares are of equal circumference and the cleft side alar base has been sufficiently rotated to achieve symmetry with the non-cleft side alar base.

On the medial lip element, dissection between skin and muscle is limited to 1 mm from the incised margin so to preserve any philtral dimple. Dissection between skin and muscle on the lateral lip element is more extensive; skin is freed from the underlying muscle sufficient to advance the muscle relative to the skin and release the lateral bulge of the lip. Muscle approximation is made in a simple end to end fashion.

Absorbable monofilament sutures are used for the mucosa and muscular approximations. Skin is approximated with non-absorbable sutures. Vermilion is approximated with braided absorbable sutures. The cutaneous and vermilion sutures are removed in the operating room one week postoperatively.

Postoperative care

Elbow splints are to be worn for 2 weeks postoperatively. Children may resume oral feeding immediately in the recovery room following surgery. Patients are discharged on the following day if they are clinically well and oral intake is sufficient. Suture removal is undertaken on the seventh postoperative day under general anesthesia. The incision line is moistened with antibiotic ointment. Parents are instructed to keep the suture line clean and moist with Vaseline®. A return visit is scheduled at 3–4 weeks postoperatively, at which point parents are given instructions regarding scar massage.

🌐 Access the complete reference list online at **http://www.expertconsult.com**

1. Pandya AN, Boorman JG. Failure to thrive in babies with cleft lip and palate. *Br J Plast Surg.* 2001;54:471–475.

2. Grayson BH, Santiago PE, Brecht LE, Cutting CB. Pre-surgical nasoalveolar molding in infants with cleft lip and palate. *Cleft Palate Craniofac J.* 1999;36:486–498.

3. Fisher DM. Unilateral cleft lip repair: an anatomical subunit approximation technique. *Plast Reconstr Surg.* 2005;116:61–71. *This article describes the author's technique for unilateral cleft lip repair. Individual markings are described in detail.*

4. Burget GC, Menick FJ. The subunit principle in nasal reconstruction. *Plast Reconstr Surg.* 1985;76:239–247.

5. Tennison CW. The repair of the unilateral cleft lip by the stencil method. *Plast Reconstr Surg.* 1952;9:115–120.

6. Randall P. A triangular flap operation for the primary repair of unilateral clefts of the lip. *Plast Reconstr Surg Transplant Bull.* 1959;23:331–347.

8. Noordhoff MS. *The surgical technique for the unilateral cleft lip-nasal deformity.* Taipei, Taiwan: Noordhoff Craniofacial Foundation; 1997.

Noordhoff's repair is a modification of Millard's Rotation Advancement repair. It avoids the circumalar incision. The repair incorporates a small triangle above the cutaneous roll when required to level the Cupid's bow and a vermilion flap from the lateral lip element to augment central vermilion deficiency.

13. Boorer CJ, Cho DC, Vijayasekaran VS, Fisher DM. Pre-surgical unilateral cleft lip anthropometrics: implications for the choice of repair technique. *Plast Reconstr Surg.* 2011;127:774–780. *Pre-surgical anthropometric measurements were taken in fifty consecutive patients with unilateral cleft lip to determine the incidence of lateral lip element hypoplasia. Combined vertical height and transverse length deficiency of the cleft side lateral lip element was present in 62% of patients.*

14. Fisher DM, Mann RJ. A model for the cleft lip nasal deformity. *Plast Reconstr Surg.* 1998;101:1448–1456. *The features of the primary cleft lip nasal deformity are detailed. A model to describe the mechanisms of the deformations is presented. The model supports an external deformation theory rather than intrinsic hypoplasia.*

22

Repair of bilateral cleft lip

John B. Mulliken

SYNOPSIS

- A child born with bilateral cleft lip should not have to suffer because of an ill-conceived and poorly executed primary repair. The operative principles for synchronous nasolabial repair are established:
  - Maintain symmetry
  - Secure primary muscular continuity
  - Design proper philtral size and shape
  - Construct median tubercle from lateral labial elements
  - Position/secure lower lateral cartilages and sculpt nasal tip and columella.
- The techniques based on these principles are within the repertoire of a well-trained surgeon whose practice is focused on children with cleft lip. Formation of philtral columns and dimple are just beyond the surgeon's craft.
- Preoperative dentofacial orthopedic manipulation of the premaxilla is necessary to permit synchronous closure of the primary palate. The surgeon must repair the bilateral cleft lip and correct the nasal deformity in three dimensions based on knowledge of anticipated changes in the fourth dimension. Modifications of the techniques used in repair of the most common complete form are needed for the less common bilateral variants, such as binderoid, complete with intact secondary palate, symmetrical incomplete, and asymmetrical complete/incomplete.
- Outcomes can be assessed using preoperative and serial photography and documentation of revision rates. Direct anthropometry is the "gold standard" for quantification of the changing nasolabial features; however, it requires training and experience. Intraoperative anthropometry is used to record baseline dimensions and is repeated as the child grows. Two-dimensional photogrammetry is applicable for certain linear and angular measurements if properly scaled. Computerized three-dimensional photogrammetry is a new methodology for quantifying nasolabial appearance. It is both accurate and reliable, and can be employed in intra- and inter-institutional comparative studies.

Access the Historical Perspective section online at
http://www.expertconsult.com

Introduction

James Barrett Brown and his colleagues wrote that a bilateral cleft lip is twice as difficult to repair as a unilateral cleft and the results are only half as good.[1] Now, over half a century later, many surgeons still seem resigned that the appearance of their patients after bilateral cleft lip repair cannot match those with repaired unilateral cleft lip. Too many infants born with bilateral cleft lip undergo old-fashioned, often multi-staged procedures and later have to endure sundry revisions throughout childhood and adolescence. Despite the surgeon's efforts, the stigmata of the repaired bilateral cleft lip and nose remain painfully obvious – even at a distance.

To the contrary, I have written that the appearance of a child with repaired bilateral cleft lip should be comparable to, and in many instances surpass, that of a repaired unilateral complete cleft lip.[2] This optimistic statement is based on two major advances in the management of bilateral cleft lip over the past quarter century. First is the recognition of the need for preoperative manipulation of the protuberant premaxilla. Second is the acceptance of the principles and techniques of bilateral labial repair and especially the importance of synchronous correction of the nasal deformity.

Principles

Surgical principles, once established, usually endure, whereas surgical techniques continue to evolve. The following principles for repair of bilateral cleft lip were induced based on study of the literature and observations of residual deformities[3]:

1. *Maintain nasolabial symmetry.* Even the slightest differences between the two sides of the lip and nose will become more obvious with growth. Symmetry is the one advantage a bilateral cleft lip has over its unilateral counterpart.

2. *Secure muscular continuity.* Construction of a complete oral ring permits normal labial function, eliminates

lateral bulges, and minimizes philtral distortion and interalar widening.

3. *Design the philtral flap of proper size and shape.* The philtrum rapidly elongates and widens, particularly at the columellar–labial junction.

4. *Construct the median tubercle using lateral vermilion–mucosal elements.* There is no white roll in the prolabium. Retained vermilion lacks normal coloration and fails to grow to full height.

5. *Position the slumped/splayed lower lateral cartilages and sculpt excess soft tissue in nasal tip and columella.* These maneuvers are necessary to establish normal nasal projection and columellar length/width.

Principles 1–4 needed definition, interpretation, and confirmation. Principle 5, primary correction of the nasal deformity, was a fundamental change in surgical strategy. The so-called "absent columella" is an illusion; nearby labial tissue need not be recruited to build it. "The columella is in the nose" became this author's shibboleth. The columella can be exposed by anatomic positioning and fixation of the lower lateral cartilages and sculpting expanded skin in the soft triangles and upper columella.[4]

Third and fourth dimensions

Analogous to a sculptor working in marble, the surgeon must construct three-dimensional nasolabial features in flesh. Unlike sculpture in stone, the repaired bilateral lip and nasal deformity change with time – there will be normal growth, as well as abnormal alterations of these features. The nasolabial stigmata are attributable to the three-dimensional primary repair and the subsequent fourth-dimensional distortions.

Farkas and colleagues used direct anthropometry to document the normal patterns of nasolabial growth in Caucasians from age 1–18 years.[5] Fast-growing nasolabial features attain more than 75% of adult dimensions by age 5 years. For example, nasal height and width develop early, reaching a mean of 77% and 87% of adult size, respectively, by age 5 years. All labial landmarks grow rapidly, reaching approximately 90% of adult proportions by age 5 years. In contrast, tip protrusion and columellar length are slow-growing features; they reach a mean of only two-thirds of adult size by 5 years of age. These differences in nasolabial growth explain the well-recognized nasal stigmata and labial misproportions of a repaired bilateral cleft lip. The fast-growing features become overly long or too wide, i.e., interalar distance and philtral length and width. In an early study of a small number of patients, it was determined that from time of initial closure to age 5 years, the philtrum widened by a factor of 2.5 at the top and expanded two-fold between the peaks of Cupid's bow.[3] In contrast, nasal tip protrusion and columellar length remain abnormally short following conventional bilateral labial repair.

Applying *a posteriori* reasoning, the nasolabial features programmed for rapid growth in early childhood must be crafted on a small scale, whereas slow-growing features should be made slightly larger than the normal dimensions for an infant. Construction of the median tubercle is the exception to these guidelines. This normally fast-growing feature reaches 87% of adult height by age 5 years, but after bilateral cleft lip repair, the tubercle lags behind. Therefore, it must be fashioned to be as full as possible, anticipating insufficient growth.[2,6,7] There is also the unpredictable fourth-dimensional factor of central incisal show. Despite the surgeon's effort to craft a full median tubercle, augmentation may be necessary after eruption of the permanent central incisors and after the maxilla is in normal sagittal position.

Presentation

Bilateral cleft lip presents in three major anatomic forms: bilateral symmetrical complete (50%); bilateral symmetrical incomplete (25%); and bilateral asymmetrical (complete/incomplete) (25%).[45] The extent of the palatal cleft usually corresponds to the severity of the labial clefts. Bilateral complete cleft of the primary palate (lip and alveolus) is almost always associated with a bilateral complete cleft of the secondary palate. Bilateral symmetrical incomplete cleft lip is usually seen with minor or absent notching of the alveolar ridge with an intact secondary palate. There is more variation in palatal clefting in the asymmetrical bilateral forms: the palate can be either bilateral complete or unilateral complete on the major side.

Terminology for the contralateral bilateral asymmetric cleft lip requires further refinement. In general, the term "incomplete" cleft lip usually denotes that there is cutaneous continuity between the medial (nasomedial process) and the lateral (maxillary process). Incomplete cleft lip presents in a spectrum. At the severe end, there is a thin cutaneous band that some would argue constitutes a "complete" cleft lip. At the other end of the spectrum are the lesser-forms of incomplete cleft lip. Yuzuriha and Mulliken classified and defined these lesser-forms as *minor-form*, *microform*, and *mini-microform* as determined by the degree of disruption at the vermilion–cutaneous junction.[46]

Minor-form cleft lip extends 3–5 mm above the normal Cupid's bow peak, i.e., 50% or less of the normal cutaneous labial height. Other features are: deficient vermilion on medial side of the cleft; cutaneous groove and muscular depression; hypoplastic median tubercle; and minor nasal deformity.

Microform cleft lip is characterized by a notched vermilion–cutaneous junction with an elevated Cupid's bow peak less than 3 mm above normal. The other features are the same as in a minor-form, but they are less obvious. Nasal deformities include small depression of the sill, slightly slumped alar genu, and 1–2 mm lateral displacement (and often under-rotation) of the alar base.

Mini-microform cleft lip is distinguished by a disruption of the white roll (vermilion–cutaneous junction) without elevation of the Cupid's bow peak. Usually there is a notch at the free mucosal margin. Muscular depression (particularly noticeable below the nostril sill) is variable as is the cleft nasal deformity.

This detailed subcategorization of the contralateral side in an asymmetrical bilateral cleft lip is important because the extent of vermilion–cutaneous disjunction determines the operative strategy. Synchronous bilateral nasolabial repair is indicated for a contralateral incomplete cleft lip, including a minor-form. Correction of a contralateral microform or mini-microform is usually deferred until closure on the greater side. The type of contralateral (lesser-form) cleft lip not only

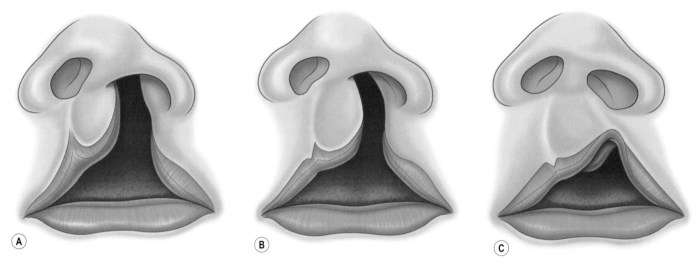

Fig. 22.1 Examples of asymmetrical bilateral cleft lip with a contralateral lesser-form. **(A)** Left complete and right minor-form; **(B)** left complete and right microform; **(C)** left incomplete and right mini-microform.

guides the primary repair, it also foretells what revisions are likely to be necessary (Fig. 22.1).[45]

Preoperative dentofacial orthopedics

Alignment of the three maxillary elements sets the skeletal stage for synchronous bilateral nasolabial repair. After retrusion and centralization of the premaxilla, the philtral flap can be designed in proper proportions, the nasal tip cartilages can be anatomically positioned, and the alveolar clefts can be closed, which stabilizes the maxillary arch and usually eliminates oronasal fistulas. Furthermore, premaxillary repositioning minimizes the nasolabial distortions that occur during the rapid growth of early childhood.

There are two dentofacial orthopedic strategies: passive and active. A passive molding plate is retained by undercuts and maintains the transverse width of the maxillary segments. An external force is needed to retract the premaxilla, such as adhesive tape from cheek to cheek or an elastic band attached to a headcap. Bilateral labial adhesions have been tried since the mid-19th century; however, they often dehisce because of tension and the absence of prolabial muscle. Cutting and Grayson have popularized a more sophisticated version of a passive plate and taping called "nasoalveolar molding" (NAM).[44,47,48] Their plate produces differential pressure on the maxillary segments by selective reduction on the inner surfaces and addition of soft acrylic on the outer surfaces. After the alveolar gap is reduced to 5 mm, nasal molding begins. The nostrils are pushed upward by a bilobed acrylic nubbin on stainless steel prongs that are attached to the palatal plate. A soft denture material is added across the nasolabial junction and a vertical tape is placed from prolabium to appliance, to give a downward counterforce to the upward force applied to the nasal tips that stretch the columella. The premaxilla is gradually retracted by serial application of tape across the outrigger to the cheeks or to the labia. These tapes are changed daily by the parents. The apparatus must be adjusted weekly to modify the alveolar molding plate so as to narrow the maxillary segments. Although usually effective, NAM is labor-intensive and slow. There is no expansion of the maxillary elements with NAM; it is difficult to retract the premaxilla into alignment with the lesser segments. Unless there is adequate space in the arch, the premaxilla will abut the labial surface of the segments.

Complications with NAM include inflammation of the oral and nasal mucosa, blistering of the cheeks, trouble in feeding the infant, and difficulty in centralizing a badly torqued premaxilla. The skin of the columellar–labial junction can ulcerate if the horizontal prolabial band is too tight. There is also a potential risk that the molding plate could become dislodged and obstruct the airway; infants are obligatory nasal breathers until about age 3 months. A 5 mm diameter hole is placed in the center of the molding plate to minimize the possibility of this complication.[49]

The active-type dentofacial orthopedic device in current use is based on the prototypic design by Georgiade and associates,[50] later refined and popularized by Millard and Latham.[51] The Latham appliance is constructed from a plaster cast of the upper jaw taken in the office. In the past, the appliance was fabricated in London, ON, Canada. A local, skilled prosthetist can also fabricate the custom device. The appliance is pinned to the maxillary shelves with the infant under general anesthesia. An elastic chain on each side is connected to a transvomerine wire that is looped under a roller in the posterior–superior section of the appliance and attached to cleats at the anterior edges of the maxillary plate. The parents turn the ratcheted screw daily to expand the anterior palatal segments. Visits are necessary at 1, 3, and 5 weeks to assure appropriate fit and to adjust the bilateral elastic chains that retrocline the premaxilla. The process normally takes 6–8 weeks. The Latham appliance is effective in correcting premaxillary position in the sagittal plane; however, the movement is more retroclination than retroposition. The appliance can also rectify premaxillary rotation through differential traction, although there is little effect on vertical position (Fig. 22.2).

The merits of passive versus active dentofacial orthopedics continue to be debated by proponents of each approach. Critics of active premaxillary orthopedics argue it causes

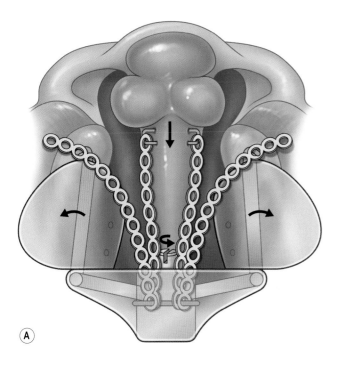

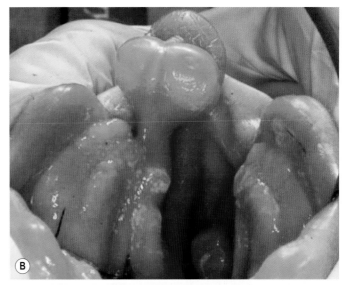

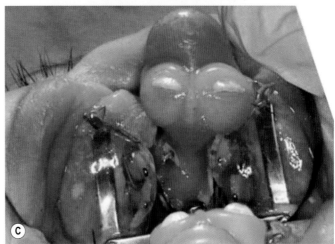

Fig. 22.2 (A) Latham appliance; **(B)** prior to insertion of device; **(C)** 6 weeks following dentofacial orthopedic manipulation.

midfacial retrusion.[52,53] Others have failed to document such an effect beyond that expected inhibition of vertical and forward maxillary growth in children with repaired bilateral cleft lip/palate followed through the age of the mixed dentition.[54] There is also recent controversy about a possible deleterious effect of alveolar gingivoperiosteoplasty.

Traditional treatment protocols place undue emphasis on efforts to minimize inhibition of midfacial growth. Some degree of maxillary retrusion is an unavoidable consequence of closure of the cleft lip and cleft palate or both. The first priorities should be nasolabial appearance and speech. Midfacial retrusion is predictably corrected by maxillary advancement with the additional aesthetic benefits to nasal, labial, and malar projection.

Operative techniques

The day of repair of a bilateral cleft lip and correction of the nasal deformity is the most important day in the child's life. It should be the first case in the morning, and probably the only operation for that day. The surgeon must work slowly and deliberately, taking as much time as necessary, without

distractions such as scheduled meetings, patients waiting in the office, and other obligations.

The technical details for repair of a bilateral complete cleft lip and nasal deformity are given below, followed by modifications used for the major anatomic variants of bilateral cleft lip. The reader will note that descriptions of the procedures do not follow the usual sequence of marking, dissection, and closure. Instead, the operative steps are portrayed as they proceed, which often requires turning attention from the lip to the nose, then back to the lip again, and ending with the final touches to the nose. Some leeway in the sequence of the operation is possible, but in general this is not advisable until considerable experience is gained in these procedures.

Bilateral cleft, complete cleft lip, and palate

Markings

A sharpened tooth pick is used for drawing and the ink is brilliant green dye (tincture) rather than methylene blue dye (aqueous). The anatomic points are designated using the standard anthropometric initialisms (see Fig. 22.3).[6] With the nostrils held upward with a double-ball retractor, the philtral

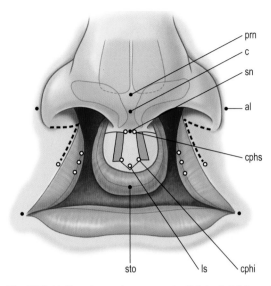

Fig. 22.3 Markings for synchronous repair of bilateral cleft lip and nasal deformity. Open circles denote tattooed dots. Anthropometric points: pronasale (prn); highest point of columella nasi (c); subnasale (sn); ala nasi (al); crista philtri superior (cphs); crista philtri inferior (cphi); labiale superius (ls); stomion (sto).

flap is drawn first. Its dimensions are determined by the child's age at repair (usually 5–6 months), and less so by ethnicity. The length of the philtral flap (sn–ls) is set at 6–7 mm (normal male 11.4±1.3 mm at 6–12 months); usually it is the same as the height of the cutaneous prolabium. If the prolabial element is overly long, the philtral flap can be shortened appropriately. The width of the philtral flap is set at 2 mm at the columellar–labial junction (cphs–cphs) and 3.5–4 mm between the proposed Cupid's bow peaks (cphi–cphi) (normal male 6.7±1.0 mm at 6–12 months). The sides of the philtral flap should be drawn slightly concave in anticipation of slight bowing with growth. Flanking flaps are drawn; these will be de-epithelialized and will come to lie beneath the lateral labial flaps in an effort to simulate philtral columns. These flanking flaps also add width and increase the vascularity of the phil- tral flap.

The proposed Cupid's bow peaks are carefully noted on the lateral labial elements and marked just atop the white roll above the vermilion–cutaneous junction. These points are situ- ated so that there is medial extension of white roll to form the handle of the Cupid's bow and sufficient vermilion height to construct the median tubercle and raphe. Curvilinear lines are drawn at the juncture of the alar bases and lateral labial elements. Anthropometric dimensions are measured and recorded before proceeding. Lidocaine with epinephrine is injected into the nose and labial segments, and after the con- ventional 5–7 min waiting time, the critical points, including the vermilion–mucosal junctions, are tattooed with tincture of brilliant green dye (Fig. 22.3).

Labial dissection

First, all labial lines are lightly scored. The philtral flanking flaps are de-epithelialized, the extra prolabial skin is discarded, and the philtral flap is elevated (including subcutaneous tissue) close to the anterior nasal spine. Leave fibrous attach- ments to maintain the columellar-labial angle. The lateral

labial elements are disjoined from the alar bases, and the basilar flaps are freed from the piriform attachments by inci- sion along the lower section of the vestibular cutaneo-mucosal junction.

The mucosal incisions are extended distal along the gingi- volabial sulcus to the premolar region. With a double hook on the muscular layer, the lateral labial elements are widely dis- sected off the maxillae in the supraperiosteal plane. The non-dominant ring finger is held on the infraorbital rim (to protect the globe) as the dissection is further extended over the malar eminence (Fig. 22.4). Extensive release of the lateral labial segments is a critical maneuver so as to minimize tension at the muscular and cutaneous closure. The orbicularis oris bundles are dissected in the subdermal and submucosal plane for 1 cm, or a little further if necessary (Fig. 22.5).

Alveolar closure

The lateral nasal mucosal flaps are released from beneath the inferior turbinates, the medial nasal mucosal flaps are elevated from the premaxilla, and the nasal floors are closed. The premaxillary mucosal incisions are continued on each side and vertical incisions are made in the facing gingiva of the lesser segments. Often digital pressure on the premaxilla is necessary to permit the alveolar gingivoperiosteal closure.

The alar base flaps are advanced medially and the inner edge is sutured to the anterior edge of the constructed nasal floor. The thin strip of vermilion is trimmed off the premaxil- lary mucosa and the remaining mucosal flange is secured high to the premaxillary periosteum to construct the posterior side of the central gingivolabial sulcus (Fig. 22.6).

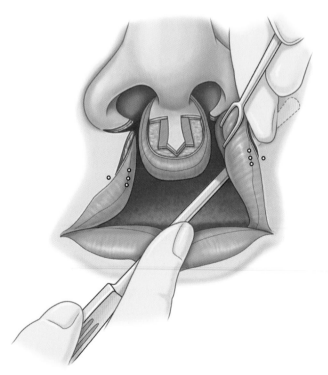

Fig. 22.4 Lateral labial elements dissected off maxilla in supraperiosteal plane, extending over the malar eminences.

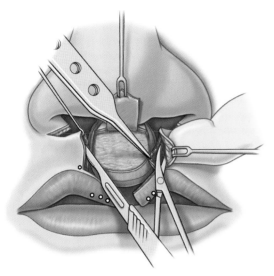

Fig. 22.5 Dissection of orbicularis oris muscle bundles in subdermal and submucosal planes.

suture is inserted through each upper lateral cartilage and then through the ipsilateral lateral crus. Often it is possible to place a second intercartilaginous suture. Holding an intranasal cotton-tipped applicator beneath the genu and tenting the nostril roof facilitates the insertion and tying of these sutures (Fig. 22.9).

The C-flap on each side of the columellar base is trimmed to 3–5 mm in length (Fig. 22.10A). The alar bases are advanced medially, rotated endonasally, and sutured side-to-end to the C-flaps. Next, the tips of the alar base flaps are trimmed and closure of the sills is completed. A "cinch suture" of polypropylene is placed through the dermis of each alar base, passing under the philtral flap, and tied to narrow the interalar dimension (al–al) to less than 25 mm (normal male 26±1.4 mm at 6–12 months). The premaxillary sutures placed earlier are brought above the muscular layer, inserted through the alar bases (near the "cinch suture") and tied. These sutures simulate the depressor alae nasi and also: (1) form the cymal shape of the sills; (2) prevent alar elevation with smiling; (3) minimize postoperative nasal widening (Fig. 22.10B).

Labial closure

It is critical to emphasize advancement of the lateral labial elements during closure of the sulci. A back-cut is made at the distal end of the sulcal incision, and each sulcus is closed while the labial flap is being pulled mesially with a double hook. The advanced lateral labial mucosa forms the anterior wall of the central gingivolabial sulcus.

The orbicular bundles are apposed (end-to-end), inferiorly to superiorly, using simple polydioxanone sutures. Prior to completion of the muscular closure, a polydioxanone suture is placed on each side of the premaxilla and left untied. A polypropylene suture suspends the uppermost muscular elements to the periosteum of the anterior nasal spine (Fig. 22.7A).

Construction of the median tubercle begins with placement of a fine chromic suture, about 3 mm medial to the tattooed lateral Cupid's bow peak-point, joining the white-roll–vermilion–mucosal flaps in the midline (Fig. 22.7B). The excess vermilion–mucosa is successively trimmed on each side, and the flaps are accurately aligned to form the median raphe. There is a natural inclination to save too much of the vermilion–mucosal flaps, resulting in a furrowed raphe. Attention is next focused on nasal repair before insetting the philtral flap.

Nasal dissection and positioning the lower lateral cartilages

The slumped/splayed lower lateral cartilages are exposed through bilateral rim incisions ("semi-open" approach). Fibrofatty tissue is dissected off the anterior surface of and between the cartilages; this is aided by elevation with a cotton-tipped applicator on the mucosal underside. Dissection is continued across the dorsal septum to expose the upper lateral cartilages (Fig. 22.8).

With direct visualization, a horizontal mattress suture of 5-0 polydioxanone (P2 reverse cutting needle, Ethicon) is placed between the genua and left untied. Another mattress

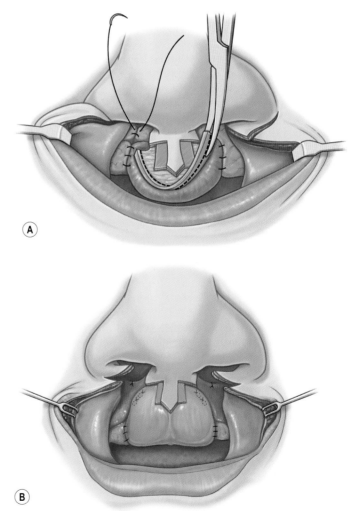

Fig. 22.6 **(A)** After completion of gingivoperiosteoplasty, redundant premaxillary vermilion is trimmed. **(B)** Remaining premaxillary mucosal flange sutured to periosteum forming posterior wall of anterior gingivolabial sulcus.

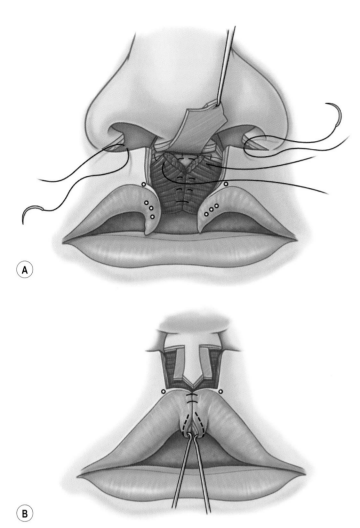

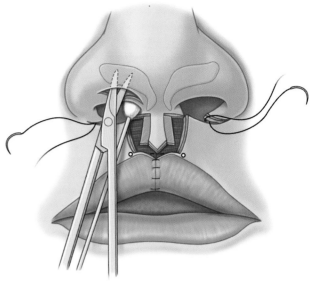

Fig. 22.8 Lower lateral cartilages exposed through rim incisions. Cotton-tipped applicator elevates nostril and helps display genua.

Fig. 22.7 (A) Apposition of orbicularis oris from inferior to superior; uppermost suture placed through periosteum of anterior nasal spine. **(B)** Lateral white-roll–vermilion–mucosal flaps trimmed to construct median tubercle and Cupid's bow.

Final touches

Fashioning a philtral dimple seems just beyond the surgeon's skill; nevertheless, it is worth trying. One way to simulate this depression is to suture the dermis in the lower one-third of the philtral flap to the orbicularis layer. The tip of the philtral flap is inset into the handle of Cupid's bow. The leading edge of the lateral labial flaps need not be trimmed before apposition to the philtral flap. A little extra lateral labial tissue helps to simulate the columns. There should be no tension at the philtral closure, which is done with fine, interrupted dermal and percutaneous sutures. The cephalic margin of the labial flaps must be trimmed, corresponding to the position and cymal configuration of the sills (Fig. 22.11). Closure of the labial flaps to the sills proceeds laterally to medially.

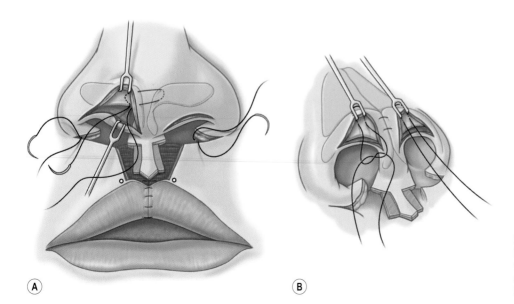

Fig. 22.9 Positioning dislocated and splayed lower lateral cartilages: **(A)** Apposition of genua with interdomal mattress suture; **(B)** suspension over ipsilateral upper lateral cartilage with intercartilaginous mattress sutures.

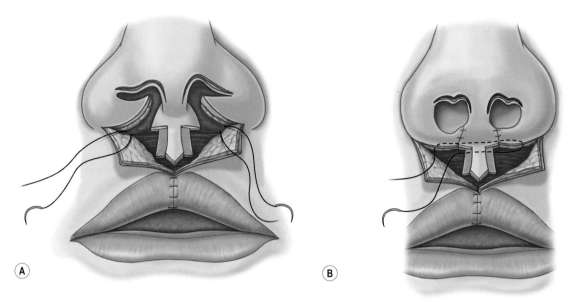

Fig. 22.10 (A) Columellar flaps shortened and alar bases trimmed. Note bilateral sutures in premaxillary periosteum below alar bases – these were inserted prior to completion of muscular closure. **(B)** Alar base flaps rotated endonasally and secured (side-to-end) to C-flaps. Interalar distance narrowed with cinch suture. Right premaxillary suture to alar base has been tied – note cymal configuration (depression) of lateral sill.

After anatomic positioning of the lower lateral cartilages, it is obvious that there is redundant domal skin in the soft triangles and in the upper columella. This extra skin is excised in a crescentic fashion from the leading edge of the rim incisions and extending inferiorly along each side of the columella (see Fig. 22.11). This resection narrows the nasal tip, defines and tapers the mid-columella, and elongates the nostrils. Apposition of the genua also accentuates the extra lining (oblique webbing) in the lateral vestibules. Lenticular excision on the cutaneous side of the intercartilaginous junction flattens this lateral vestibular ridge (see Fig. 22.11, inset).

Immediately postoperative nasolabial anthropometry is documented and placed in the child's record (Fig. 22.12).[6] The constructed columella (sn–c) is usually 5–6 mm, (normal male 4.7±0.8 mm at 5 months). After the measurements, a strip of ¼-inch Xeroform gauze is wrapped around a 19-gauge silicone tubing and a 1 cm segment is inserted into each nostril. These vented "stents" are removed after 48 h. Prolonged nostril splinting is difficult to maintain, likely to damage the sills, and probably unnecessary.

Postoperative care

A Logan bow is taped to the cheeks: (1) to protect the labial repair and (2) to hold an iced-saline sponge over the wound for 24 h postoperatively. The infant is discharged from

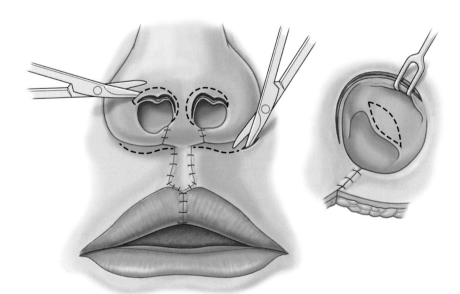

Fig. 22.11 Crescentic excision of expanded domal skin and lining extended into upper columella. Cyma-shaped resection of superior margin of lateral labial elements to fit curve of the alar base and sill. Lenticular excision of lateral vestibular web (inset).

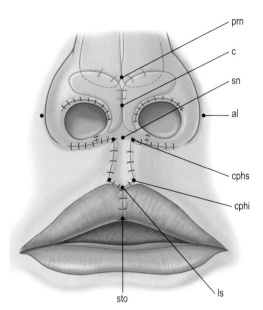

Fig. 22.12 Completed bilateral complete cleft lip/nasal repair. Pronasale (prn); highest point of columella nasi (c); subnasale (sn); ala nasi (al); crista philtri superior (cphs); crista philtri inferior (cphi); labiale superius (ls); stomion (sto).

the hospital on the second postoperative day. The parents are instructed in suture-line care and how to keep the nostrils clean. Percutaneous sutures are removed 6 days postoperatively under general anesthesia using mask induction and insufflation. A ½-inch transverse Steri-Strip (3M Health Care, St. Paul, MN) is trimmed and placed over the labial scars; the tape is changed as needed for 6 weeks. Thereafter, the parents are instructed to perform digital massage (with Pedi-Mederma, Merz North America, Raleigh, NC) for several months and counseled about the importance of application of sunblock ointment (Fig. 22.13).

Technical modifications for bilateral variations

Late presentation of bilateral complete cleft lip/palate

Dentofacial orthopedics may not be available or practical in developing countries. Even in developed nations, a child with bilateral complete cleft lip/palate can present in late infancy, and by that age the premaxilla is rigid and preoperative manipulation is not possible. Rather than attempt labial closure over a protrusive premaxilla, consider ostectomy and set-back. There are two alternatives: (1) premaxillary set-back and nasolabial repair or (2) premaxillary set-back and palatoplasty. With careful attention to mucosal blood supply, premaxillary retropositioning can be safely done along with bilateral nasolabial closure. Another uncommon indication for the first alternative is partially successful dentofacial orthopedic preparation. *Caution*: Only a bilateral narrow isthmus of septal mucosa nourishes the premaxilla after the mucosal incisions and elevation necessary for alveolar gingivoperiosteoplasties and for resection of the premaxillary neck and inferior septal cartilage. The second alternative, premaxil-

lary set-back, gingivoperiosteoplasties, and palatoplasty, is the safer procedure. It is recommended if the child is nearing age 1 year or older when speech is the first priority. Bilateral nasolabial repair on a solid maxillary foundation is scheduled later.

Primary premaxillary retropositioning is likely to accentuate midfacial retrusion; however, nasolabial appearance and speech take precedence. The majority of children with bilateral complete cleft lip/palate will need maxillary advancement.

Binderoid bilateral complete cleft lip/palate

Nasal features in this rare bilateral variant include: orbital hypotelorism, hypoplastic bony/cartilaginous elements (including short septum and absent anterior nasal spine), and conical columella. Labial features are: hypoplastic prolabium/premaxilla (with a single incisor) and thin vermilion in the lateral labial segments.[55] The floppy premaxilla usually precludes an attempt at dentofacial orthopedic manipulation; furthermore, it is often unnecessary because the premaxilla is not procumbent.

Synchronous nasolabial repair is accomplished as described above, but there are some slight differences. Sometimes the premaxilla is so small that alveolar gingivoperiosteoplasties cannot be accomplished during labial closure. If necessary, a passive palatal plate can be used to maintain anterior maxillary width following nasolabial closure. The philtral flap need not be drawn overly small in either height or width; it will expand very little with growth. The interalar dimension should be narrowed to slightly below age-matched normal because it will widen. Although the lower lateral cartilages are hypoplastic, usually they can be dissected, positioned, and secured. The thin and tapered columella can be augmented when the child is older (Fig. 22.14).

Secondary procedures are likely in a patient with the binderoid variant. These include dermal grafts to augment the median tubercle and to widen the narrow columellar base; cartilage grafts to the nasal tip, and a costochondral graft to build-up the nasal dorsum and project the tip; and maxillary advancement along with augmentation of the *fossae praenasale*.[55]

Bilateral complete cleft lip and intact secondary palate

Bilateral complete cleft lip/alveolus with intact secondary palate is another very rare form. The premaxilla is solid, thus obviating dentofacial orthopedics. If the premaxilla is not severely protrusive, it may be possible to accomplish synchronous nasolabial repair and closure of the posterior premaxillary cleft. If this strategy is chosen, alveolar gingivoperiosteoplasties should be delayed in order to preserve premaxillary blood supply. But, if the premaxilla is procumbent, consider a first-stage premaxillary ostectomy and set-back, along with closure of the alveolar clefts, and closure of the defect at the anterior edge of the hard palate. Bilateral nasolabial repair can be done safely at the second stage later in infancy. The alternative plan is premaxillary set-back, bilateral nasolabial repair, and closure of the posterior premaxillary–palatal defect, leaving the facing edges of the alveolar clefts intact (to maintain blood supply to the premaxilla). The third strategy is premaxillary set-back, gingivoperiosteoplasties,

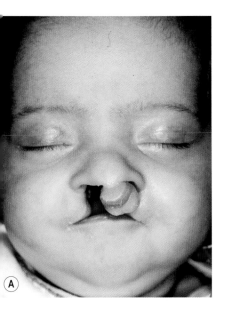

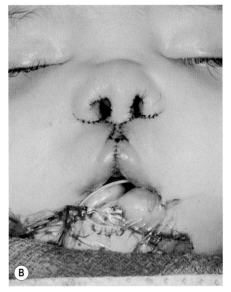

Immediate postoperative anthropometry documents undercorrected fast-growing features and overcorrected slow-growing features compared with normal values		
Intraoperative	Patient (7 months)	Normal (6–12 months)
n–sn	20.0[a]	26.9±1.6
al–al	24.5	25.4±1.5
sn–prn	10.5	9.7±0.8
sn–c	6.0[a]	4.7±0.8
cphs–cphs	1.5	NA
cphi–cphi	4.5[a]	6.5±1.1
sn–ls	5.5[a]	10.7±1.1
sn–sto	11.2[a]	16.0±0.8
ls–sto	6.2	5.3±1.4

Normal values expressed as norm±SD.
[a]Values outside SD.
SD, standard deviation; NA, not available.

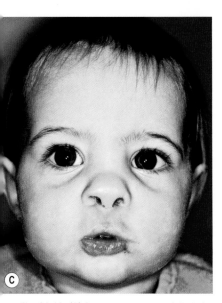

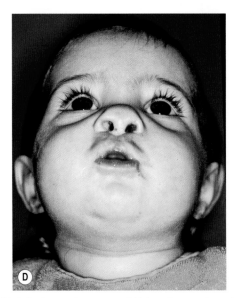

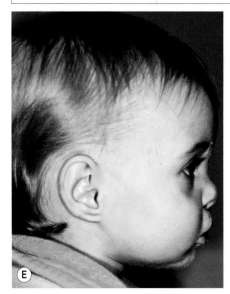

Fig. 22.13 (A) Bilateral complete cleft lip/palate. **(B)** Following synchronous nasolabial repair at age 6 months. **(C,D,E)** At 4 months postoperative. Note columella/tip projection, hint of a philtral dimple, and normal columellar–labial angle.

nasolabial repair, and delayed closure of the premaxillary–palatal cleft (the latter is technically difficult). Midfacial retrusion is very unlikely following primary premaxillary set-back because the secondary palate is intact (Fig. 22.15).

Bilateral incomplete cleft lip

One-quarter of all double labial clefts are incomplete and most are symmetrical.[45] Of all the bilateral variants, this is the most easily repaired. The design and execution are the same as for the bilateral complete form, including adjustments based on expected nasolabial changes with growth. There are two technical considerations that need to be underscored. The first relates to construction of the median tubercle. Usually, the tubercle should be formed using the lateral white-roll–vermilion–mucosal flaps. However, in the rare instance of a bilateral lesser-form (<50% of cutaneous labial height) and a

prominent central white roll, the prolabial vermilion–mucosa may be utilized as the central segment. The next consideration is columellar length: measure sn–c. If columellar length is normal for the infant's age and the lower lateral cartilages are in nearly normal position, it may be unnecessary to position the cartilages and sculpt the tip. Nevertheless, interalar narrowing is always needed as this dimension is overly wide and will increase with growth. If the columella is short and the alar domes are splayed, the lower laterals should be apposed through the semi-open approach (Fig. 22.16).

Asymmetrical bilateral (complete/incomplete) cleft lip

Symmetry, the first principle of bilateral labial repair, should be foremost in mind when planning and executing closure of

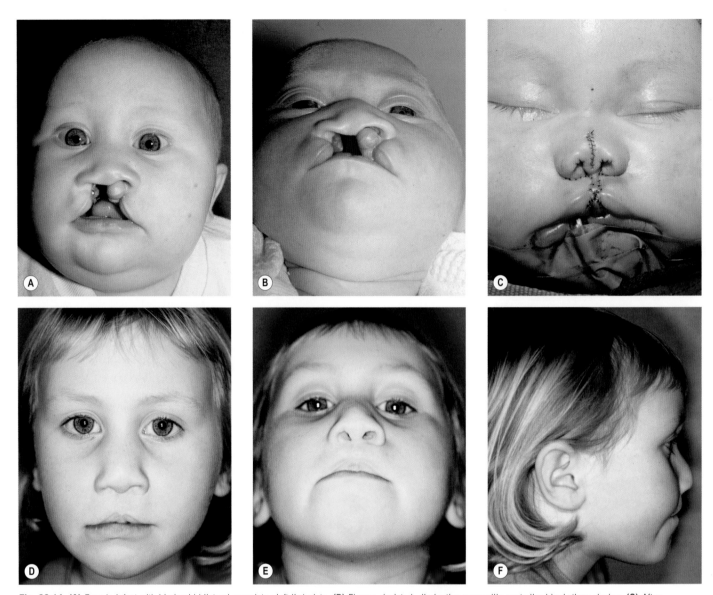

Fig. 22.14 **(A)** Female infant with binderoid bilateral complete cleft lip/palate. **(B)** Floppy, deviated, diminutive premaxilla centralized by Latham device. **(C)** After synchronous repair. Note thin vermilion in lateral labial elements. Midline tip incision is no longer used. **(D–F)** Appearance at age 5 years.

an asymmetrical variant. An algorithm for timing and techniques for repair of asymmetrical bilateral cleft lip is shown in Fig. 22.17. If both greater and lesser side clefts are incomplete or the lesser side is a minor-form, synchronous bilateral repair is indicated. However, if the greater side is incomplete and the contralateral side is microform or mini-microform, the incomplete side should be repaired first.

If the greater side is a complete cleft, it is initially managed by unilateral dentofacial orthopedics, followed by nasolabial adhesion and alveolar gingivoperiosteoplasty. Thus, the greater side is converted from a complete to an incomplete cleft. This levels the surgical field, and the options for the next stage become clear. If the contralateral (lesser side) cleft lip is a minor-form or a more severe incomplete, the second stage is simultaneous bilateral nasolabial repair. Keeping symmetry in mind, technical maneuvers on the complete side must be exaggerated because the distortions and tensions are greater than on the incomplete side. Even if the lower lateral cartilage

is in near-normal position on the incomplete side, use bilateral rim incisions and overcorrect the cartilage on the complete side. There may be inequality of vermilion height at the junction forming the median raphe. This can be adjusted by a vermilion unilimb Z-plasty, usually with the triangular flap designed on the lesser side vermilion (Fig. 22.18).

If the contralateral side is a microform cleft, it is best first to narrow the complete side by preoperative dentofacial orthopedics and repair it either in one stage or two (after preliminary nasolabial adhesion) with alveolar gingivoperiosteoplasty. In so doing, observe the contralateral microform when designing the arc and position of the medial incision for rotation-advancement repair. Try to limit the incision at the columellar base and advancement of the lateral labial element so that the philtral suture line will match the configuration of the contralateral microform. After the scar has remodeled, the contralateral microform is corrected using the double unilimb Z-plastic technique, including muscular apposition and

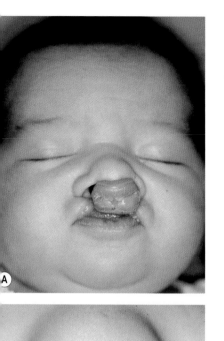

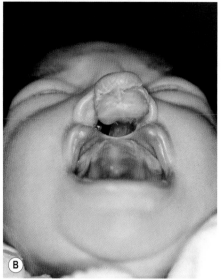

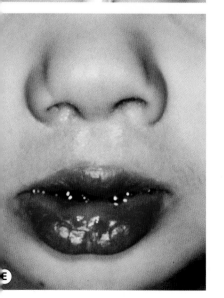

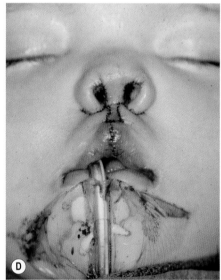

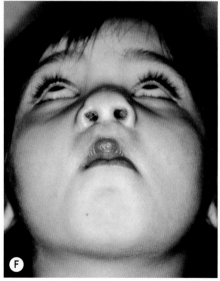

Intraoperative anthropometry: slow-growing nasal protrusion and columella were crafted larger than normal but just within 1 SD		
Intraoperative	Patient (6 months)	Normal (6–12 months)
n–sn	21.0[a]	26.9±1.6
al–al	24.5	25.4±1.5
sn–prn	10.5	9.7±0.8
sn–c	5.0	4.7±0.8
cphs–cphs	2.1	NA
cphi–cphi	4.5[a]	6.5±1.1
sn–ls	5.5[a]	10.7±1.1
sn–sto	13.0[a]	16.0±0.8
ls–sto	7.0[a]	5.3±1.4

Normal values expressed as norm±SD.
[a]Values outside SD.
SD, standard deviation; NA, not available.

Fig. 22.15 (A) Female infant with bilateral complete cleft lip/alveolus (van der Woude syndrome). **(B)** Intact secondary palate. **(C)** Markings for synchronous repair at age 6 months. **(D)** Following premaxillary set-back, alveolar gingivoperiosteoplasties and nasolabial repair. Palato-premaxillary defect closed and lower labial sinuses excised in second stage. **(E,F)** Appearance at age 2 years.

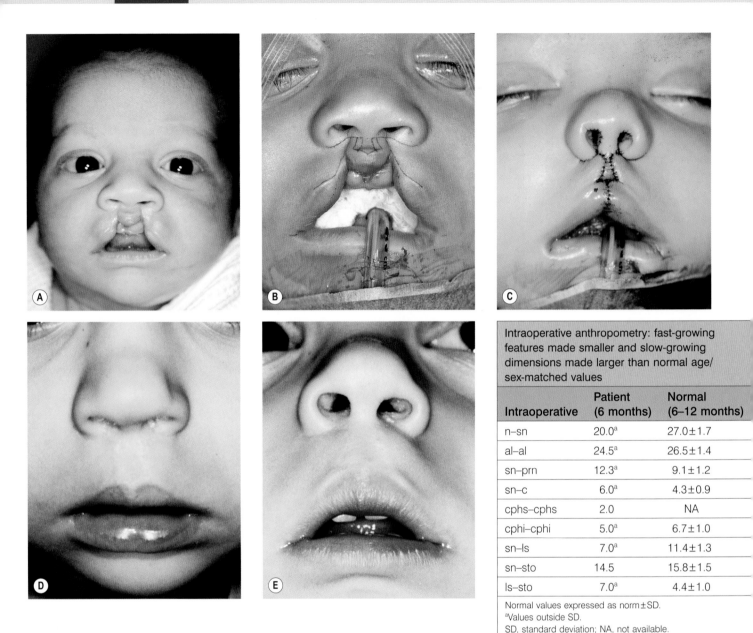

	Patient	Normal
Intraoperative	**(6 months)**	**(6–12 months)**
n–sn	20.0[a]	27.0±1.7
al–al	24.5[a]	26.5±1.4
sn–prn	12.3[a]	9.1±1.2
sn–c	6.0[a]	4.3±0.9
cphs–cphs	2.0	NA
cphi–cphi	5.0[a]	6.7±1.0
sn–ls	7.0[a]	11.4±1.3
sn–sto	14.5	15.8±1.5
ls–sto	7.0[a]	4.4±1.0

Intraoperative anthropometry: fast-growing features made smaller and slow-growing dimensions made larger than normal age/sex-matched values

Normal values expressed as norm±SD.
[a]Values outside SD.
SD, standard deviation; NA, not available.

Fig. 22.16 **(A)** Bilateral symmetrical incomplete cleft lip. **(B)** Markings for synchronous closure at age 6 months. **(C)** Following nasolabial repair. **(D,E)** Appearance at age 1.5 years.

dermal graft to augment the philtral ridge, and nasal correction.[56] If the position of the contralateral microform cannot be matched by rotation-advancement on the greater side, synchronous bilateral repair is the best strategy. Mirror-image symmetry is the goal with attention to philtral shape, Cupid's bow position, alar base placement, and nostril axis.

If the lesser side cleft is mini-microform, often this can be corrected by vertical lenticular excision at the same time as repair on the greater side, although nothing is lost by waiting. Nasolabial asymmetries between the greater and lesser sides can best be judged when the child is older. Augmentation of the median tubercle is almost always necessary. If the Cupid's bow peak is too high on the repaired greater side, it is best to lower it (by unilimb Z-plasty) rather than adjust the

mini-microform. Sometimes, a minor correction is needed to correct asymmetry of the nasal tip. Often a contralateral mini-microform does not need attention.[45]

Outcomes

The surgeon's responsibility does not end with completion of nasolabial repair. There is an obligation to periodically assess the outcome of the procedure and, if possible, to continue to do so until skeletal growth is complete. Only by so doing can the surgeon come to understand changes in the fourth dimension, learn from these observations, and apply this knowledge to succeeding infants with bilateral cleft lip.

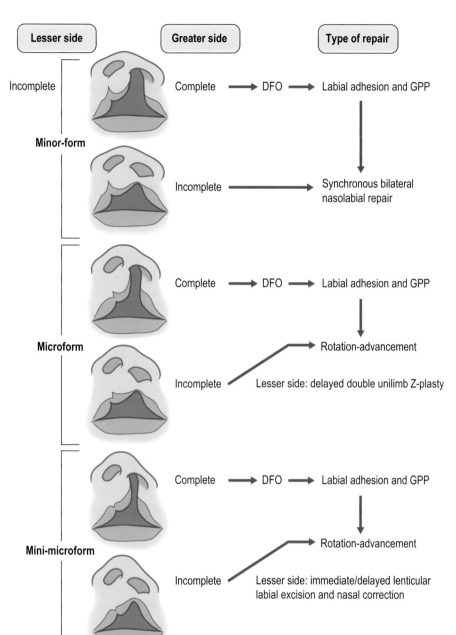

| Lesser side | Greater side | Type of repair |

Incomplete

Minor-form

Complete → DFO → Labial adhesion and GPP

Incomplete → Synchronous bilateral nasolabial repair

Microform

Complete → DFO → Labial adhesion and GPP

Incomplete → Rotation-advancement
Lesser side: delayed double unilimb Z-plasty

Mini-microform

Complete → DFO → Labial adhesion and GPP

Incomplete → Rotation-advancement
Lesser side: immediate/delayed lenticular labial excision and nasal correction

Fig. 22.17 Algorithm for correction of asymmetrical bilateral cleft lip (complete/incomplete) and contralateral incomplete or lesser-form cleft. DFO, dentofacial orthopedics; GPP, gingivoperiosteoplasty. *(Modified from Yuzuriha S, Oh AK, Mulliken JB. Asymmetrical bilateral cleft lip: complete or incomplete and contralateral lesser defect (minor-form, microform, or mini-microform). Plast Reconstr Surg. 2008;122:1494–1504.)*

Photography

Preoperative photographs are the basic minimum for documentation. Images are unacceptable if taken when the child is on the operating table with the endotracheal tube in place. The surgeon must find the time and have the patience to take preoperative frontal, submental, and lateral views of the infant. Intraoperative photographs taken after cutaneous markings and immediately after the repair are also useful. The standard angle for the submental view should align the nasal tip on a line sighted half-way between the medial canthi and eyebrows. The submental photograph is essential for assessment of nasal configuration and symmetry. Photographs must be taken periodically during childhood, as well as before and after adolescent growth.

Standardized photographs can be used for panel-assessment of repaired bilateral cleft lip.[57] Although visual-perceptive analysis using a predetermined rating scale can be reliable, it is clumsy, time-consuming, and still subjective.

Revision rate

Most surgeons keep a mental tally of the kinds of revisions that are necessary after cleft lip repairs. Documenting the types of secondary corrections guides the surgeon to make technical alterations during subsequent primary procedures. The surgeon's goal is to minimize the number of revisions. For a repaired bilateral deformity, the cutaneous lip should never need to be reopened. The nasal cartilages may require repositioning, the mucosal free margin often

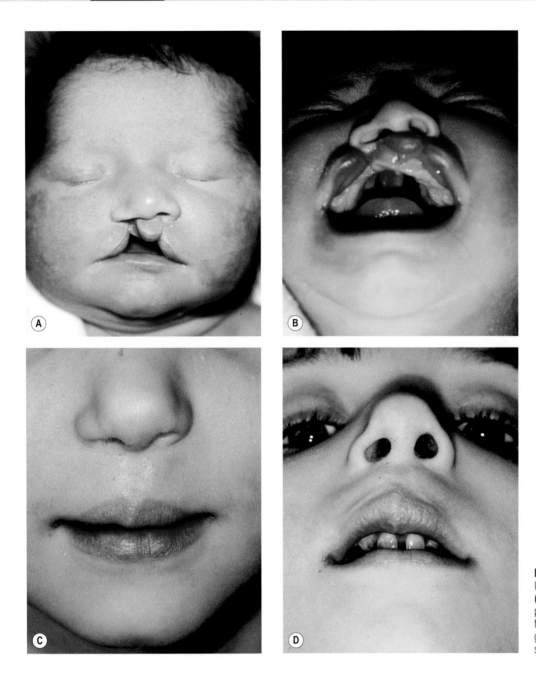

Fig. 22.18 (A) Asymmetrical bilateral cleft lip: right complete and left incomplete. **(B)** Bilateral complete cleft of secondary palate, submental view. **(C,D)** Age 6 years following first-stage right labial adhesion/ gingivoperiosteoplasty and second-stage synchronous nasolabial repair.

must be adjusted, and, sometimes, nasal width has to be narrowed.

Symmetry is the one major advantage of a bilateral complete cleft lip as compared to a unilateral complete cleft lip. Any nasolabial asymmetry following closure and further distortions with growth will become increasingly obvious before the child attends school. These asymmetries remain relatively unchanged during childhood, but they often become magnified during adolescence. The age for kindergarten is a good time to assess the child for revision.

In a study of 50 consecutive non-syndromic children (median age 5.4 years), the revision rate was 33% for those with bilateral complete cleft lip/palate as compared to 12% for those with bilateral complete cleft lip/alveolus and intact secondary palate.[58] The most common labial revision was resuspension of prolapsed anterior gingivolabial mucosa. This problem has since been minimized by trimming prolabial

vermilion and securing the remaining mucosa to the premaxillary periosteum. Augmentation of a weak median tubercle with a dermal–fat graft is also common; this was usually done at the time of alveolar bone grafting (age 9–11 years). Using the posterior iliac donor site, a thick dermal–fat graft is easily taken along with harvest of cancellous bone.[59]

The most frequent nasal distortion in this series was disproportionate widening of the interalar dimension; however, this rarely required correction during childhood. None of the children in this study required a secondary "columellar lengthening" or revision for an abnormally wide or long philtrum.

Given preoperative asymmetry, the revision rate for asymmetrical bilateral cleft lip would be expected to differ slightly from that for the more common symmetrical complete forms. Indeed, our study showed the rate of nasolabial revision correlated with the degree of preoperative asymmetry between the greater and lesser sides.[45] The lowest frequency of nasolabial revision was in the contralateral minor-form subgroup because symmetry is more likely achieved by synchronous bilateral correction. In contrast, the highest frequency of both nasal and labial revision (usually on the greater side) was in the contralateral mini-microform subgroup. This was predictable because the nearly normal configuration of a mini-microform makes it more difficult to attain primary symmetry. Conceptually, the complete/mini-microform type of bilateral cleft lip approaches the unilateral complete cleft lip deformity. In all of the contralateral lesser-forms, the most common labial deformity was a thin median tubercle, accentuated by a full mucosal free margin on the greater side. This deficiency of the tubercle can be explained by insufficient mesodermal contribution from the lesser side.

Reassessment of the frequency and types of nasolabial revisions must be undertaken after skeletal maturity. We analyzed the frequency of Le Fort I osteotomy and maxillary advancement in the major forms of bilateral cleft lip: 50% for bilateral incomplete or bilateral asymmetrical complete/incomplete and 75% for bilateral complete cleft lip/palate.[60] The high rate of maxillary advancement in our unit reflects our preference for operative correction for all patients with midfacial retrusion whatever the occlusal relationship. Le Fort I advancement is often combined with alloplastic onlay to the malar eminences to give a normal convex facial profile. Attempts to compensate for a small degree of maxillary retrusion at the dental level results in a relatively flat facial profile.

The need for secondary nasolabial correction is based on subjective criteria, determined by the surgeon's opinion and often made in agreement with the family and the older patient. Cephalometry has long been used by dental specialists to document skeletal growth in children with repaired cleft lip/palate. Similar quantitative methodology is needed to permit assessment of nasolabial appearance during childhood and adolescence.

Direct anthropometry

Farkas was the first to apply medical anthropometry to children with repaired bilateral cleft lip.[61] His reference book is invaluable.[62] It contains normative values for 28 nasal and 18 labial linear/angular measurements in a North American Caucasian population from birth (0–5 months and 6–12 months) and each year up to age 18. Direct anthropometry requires training, practice, and patience. The tools are a sliding Vernier caliper and a Castroviejo caliper. Locating the soft-tissue landmarks and measuring nasolabial dimensions are usually easily accomplished in a child older than 5 years, but difficult to impossible in a younger child. Intraoperative anthropometry is used to assess severity of the deformity prior to the procedure and immediately after repair as a record of baseline nasolabial dimensions.[6] In an analysis of 46 consecutive repairs of bilateral complete cleft lip, intraoperative anthropometry confirmed the strategy of design in three dimensions in anticipation of the fourth dimension. All fast-growing nasolabial features were set smaller than age and sex-matched normal infants. The only exception was central vermilion–mucosal height (median tubercle) that purposely was made overly full (on average 155% of normal). The slow-growing features, nasal protrusion, and columellar height, were also constructed longer than normal, 130% and 167%, respectively.

Direct anthropometry can be repeated as the child grows and compared to normal values based on sex and age. This was shown in a retrospective longitudinal analysis of 12 children with bilateral complete cleft lip who underwent repair with the same procedure as described herein.[4] Through age 4 years, nasal height and protrusion, as well as columellar length and width, were within 1 standard deviation of normal values. The interalar dimension was overly wide, about 1 standard deviation above normal. Nevertheless, the nose often did not appear wide because children with bilateral cleft lip tend to have minor orbital hypertelorbitism. The cutaneous lip was intentionally set short because this is less eye-catching than the typical long lip appearance in these patients. Thus, total lip height was 1–2 standard deviations below normal, whereas, height of the median tubercle was 1 standard deviation above normal at 4 years. Fullness of the central red lip usually falls below normal in older children. Depending on the show of the permanent incisors, the median tubercle either is augmented or excess mucosa is trimmed. An example of an 8-year-old boy with repaired bilateral complete cleft lip/palate is shown in Fig. 22.19 with intraoperative and postoperative anthropometry.

Serial direct anthropometry in 32/48 patients with repaired bilateral incomplete cleft lip was compared to Farkas's normative values.[63] Females, African-Americans, and Asians were excluded because of their small numbers, leaving 22 Caucasian males in the long-term study. Nasal measurements demonstrated: interalar dimension (al–al) widened in early childhood and followed line of normal growth thereafter; nasal tip protrusion (sn–prn) grew in parallel above the normal line; columellar height (sn–c) crossed the normal line in early childhood and remained slightly below into adulthood. Labial measurements showed: Cupid's bow width (cphi–cphi) was normal into late adolescence; upper philtral width (cphs–cphs) remained below the normal line; philtral height (sn–ls) stayed below the normal line; median tubercle (ls–sto) grew slowly, sometimes dropping below the normal line during adolescence; total labial height (sn–sto) closely approximated Farkas's normal line throughout childhood and adolescence.

Normative anthropometric measures are needed for the major ethnic groups. Farkas' book, in addition to Caucasian norms, includes data from Singapore for three age groups: 6 and 12 years (taken in school children) and 18 years (taken in army recruits and university students).[62] Indian anthropometry from infancy to adulthood is also available.[64] Kim and colleagues measured six nasolabial features in normal Korean children age 5 years and younger, and compared the mean values to 30 children who had a modified "Mulliken repair" for three variants of bilateral cleft lip.[65] They found all nasolabial features were within 2 standard deviations of normal. Nasal tip protrusion and columellar length were below, whereas nasal width was slightly above, in normal age-matched Korean noses.

Indirect anthropometry

Photogrammetry

Photogrammetry is the original type of indirect anthropometry. It eliminates any inaccuracies introduced in trying to measure the lip and nose in a frightened or fidgety child.

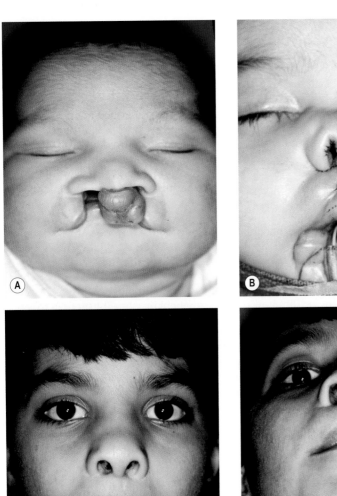

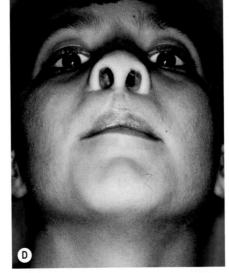

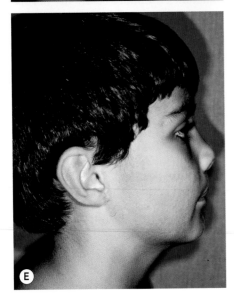

Intraoperative anthropometry: note overcorrected nasal protrusion and columellar length; nasal width is narrower than normal				
	Intraoperative		Postoperative	
	Patient (6 months)	Normal (6–12 months)	Patient (8 years)	Normal (8 years)
n–sn	22.0[a]	27.0±1.7	44.0	42.1±2.4
al–al	26.0	26.5±1.4	36.0[a]	29.8±1.5
sn–prn	15.0[a]	9.1±1.2	17.7[a]	15.9±1.3
sn–c	7.0[a]	4.3±0.9	10.5[a]	8.0±1.1
cphs–cphs	2.0	NA	7.7	NA
cphi–cphi	4.0[a]	6.7±1.0	10.4[a]	8.8±1.1
sn–ls	7.5[a]	11.4±1.3	9.0[a]	14.0±2.2
sn–sto	16.5	15.8±1.5	16.0[a]	19.7±1.8
ls–sto	7.0[a]	4.4±1.0	7.8	8.0±1.2
Normal values expressed as norm±SD. [a]Values outside SD. SD, standard deviation; NA, not available.				

Fig. 22.19 **(A)** Bilateral complete cleft lip/palate. **(B)** Submental view following closure. **(C–E)** Appearance at age 8 years. Note nasal protrusion and columellar length are longer than normal; however, nasal width and Cupid's bow width are above normal.

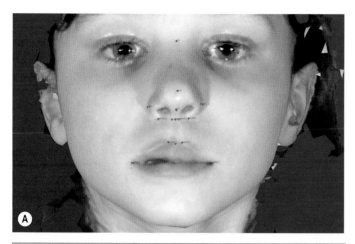

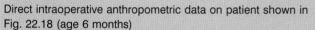

Direct intraoperative anthropometric data on patient shown in Fig. 22.18 (age 6 months)		
Intraoperative	Patient (6 months)	Normal (6–12 months)
n–sn	23.0[a]	26.9±1.6
al–al	24.0[a]	25.4±1.5
sn–prn	12.3[a]	9.7±0.8
sn–c	6.0[a]	4.7±0.8
cphs–cphs	2.0	NA
cphi–cphi	4.0[a]	6.5±1.1
sn–ls	6.8[a]	10.7±1.1
sn–sto	13.4[a]	16.0±0.8
ls–sto	6.5	5.3±1.4
Normal values expressed as norm±SD. [a]Values outside SD. SD, standard deviation; NA, not available.		

Indirect anthropometry (3D photogrammetry) at age 6 years (same patient as shown in Fig. 22.18). Note changes in fast- and slow-growing features		
Postoperative	Patient (6 years)	Normal (6 years)
n–sn	37.6	39.3±2.7
al–al	26.5	27.5±1.3
sn–prn	15.8[a]	14.5±1.2
sn–c	L, 7.0; R, 6.4	7.5±1.0
cphs–cphs	3.2	NA
cphi–cphi	6.7[a]	8.4±1.3
sn–ls	11.5[a]	12.6±1.3
sn–sto	20.3[a]	18.7±1.7
ls–sto	9.7	8.0±1.1
Normal values expressed as norm±SD. [a]Values outside SD. SD, standard deviation; NA, not available.		

Fig. 22.20 (A,B) Three-dimensional photogrammetry (Vectra 3D imaging system): anthropometric points located on frontal and submental images. (Same patient as in Fig. 24.18.)

However, measurements on two-dimensional photographs likely introduce errors due to magnification, variation in lightening, angulation, head position, and subject-to-camera distance. The magnification factor can be eliminated by including a standard metric in the photograph. Photogrammetry can only be used for linear measurements of certain nasolabial features, as well as for proportions and angles.[66] Examples of photogrammetric assessment in 15 patients with bilateral complete cleft lip repaired by the operative techniques described herein are found in a study by Kohout and colleagues.[67] The ratio of columellar length (sn–c) to nasal tip protrusion (sn–prn), the two slow-growing dimensions, was 0.47±0.08, i.e., very close to the normal of 0.53±0.02 at a mean age of 2 years. Changes in the columellar–labial angle were analyzed in a small cohort of children. This angle was obtuse in early childhood (128.5±6.5°) (normal 102.5±5.2°), but began narrowing after age 7 years and normalized by adolescence. Possible explanations for this change include either growth of the anterior-caudal septum, increasing obliquity of the lip, or increasing maxillary retrusion.

Liou and colleagues employed basilar photogrammetry to assess 22 young children with repaired bilateral complete cleft lip using the NAM protocol.[68] They determined that columellar length decreased in the first and second years postoperatively, then started to increase in the third year, but still lagged behind the normal length by 1.9 mm, whereas all other nasal dimensions increased significantly. Lee and co-workers also used photogrammetry to assess children who had undergone the NAM protocol and primary "retrograde" nasal correction.[69] They noted that columellar length was slightly less, but not statistically different, from a control group of children at an average age of 3 years.

Morovic and Cutting adapted some elements of primary nasal correction described herein and used photogrammetry with intermedial canthal distance as the scaling standard.[70] In 25 children, they calculated near-normal columellar length and tip projection, but nasal width, columellar width, and nasolabial angles were significantly greater than the control values.

Stereophotogrammetry

Three-dimensional stereophotogrammetry is the most advanced way to quantitatively assess nasolabial appearance.

Several systems are currently available: 3dMDface (3dMD, Atlanta, GA) and Vectra (Canfield Imaging Systems, Fairfield, NJ). The validity and reliability of these systems have been documented.[71,72] Synchronized high-resolution digital cameras capture images in milliseconds. Software algorithms merge the different overlapping images into a single three-dimensional image that can be viewed, turned in any direction, and analyzed on a computer. Standard anthropometric points are easily located after the image is appropriately maneuvered and the nasolabial dimensions are recorded (Fig. 22.20). Furthermore, the digital images can be manipulated to calculate soft-tissue projection and produce a numeric value for mirror-image symmetry of the nose or lip.

Conclusion

Every year, a cleft lip/palate team will treat only a few children born with a bilateral deformity or a variant. Every infant with this defect deserves a surgeon who has the requisite patience, precision, and passion to undertake the first operation. Indeed, the primary procedures are the major determinants of the child's appearance and ability to communicate. The surgeon also has the obligation to care for and assess these children well into adulthood – this requires singular commitment.

⊕ Access the complete reference list online at   **http://www.expertconsult.com**

6. Mulliken JB, Burvin R, Farkas LG. Repair of bilateral complete cleft lip: intraoperative nasolabial anthropometry. *Plast Reconstr Surg.* 2001;107:307–314.

13. Millard DR Jr. *Cleft Craft: The Evolution of Its Surgery.* Vol. II. Boston, MA: Little, Brown; 1977. *One definition of a "classic" is a great book that is often cited, but seldom read. In his conversational style of writing, Millard recounts the history of bilateral cleft lip repair as if he was an observer. The novice may find the organization of the book a little difficult to follow. Nevertheless, reading Millard's text is analogous to watching a master surgeon in the operating room. The more experienced the visitor, the more gained by the experience.*

44. Cutting CB, Grayson BH, Brecht L, et al. Presurgical columellar elongation and primary retrograde nasal reconstruction in one-stage bilateral cleft lip and nose repair. *Plast Reconstr Surg.* 1998;101:630–639. *The article describes the prototype of a nasoalveolar molding appliance in preparation for synchronous nasolabial repair by Cutting's technique. The authors underscore that expansion of nasal lining is as important as stretching columellar skin. The principle of primary positioning the lower lateral cartilages is applied as described in this chapter; however, the technique differs.*

45. Yuzuriha S, Oh AK, Mulliken JB. Asymmetrical bilateral cleft lip: complete or incomplete and contralateral lesser defect (minor-form, microform, or mini-microform). *Plast Reconstr Surg.* 2008;122:1494–1504. *This paper focuses on a subgroup of asymmetrical bilateral clefts that present with a lesser-form variant that is contralateral to a complete or incomplete cleft lip. The lesser-forms are defined based on extent of disruption at the vermilion–cutaneous junction: minor-form; microform, and mini-microform. These designations determine the methods of repair and correlate with frequency and types of revisions that are usually necessary.*

55. Mulliken JB, Burvin R, Padwa BL. Binderoid complete cleft lip/palate. *Plast Reconstr Surg.* 2003;111:1000–1010. *The authors define a rare subset of patients who have complete cleft lip/palate, nasolabiomaxillary underdevelopment, and orbital hypertelorism. One-half of the patients have a bilateral complete deformity, characterized by a diminutive single-toothed premaxilla. Necessary modifications in primary repair and in secondary correction of the hypoplastic soft tissue and skeletal elements are described.*

57. Lo L-J, Wong F-H, Mardini S, et al. Assessment of bilateral cleft lip nose deformity: a comparison of results as judged by cleft surgeons and laypersons. *Plast Reconstr Surg.* 2002;110:733–741.

58. Mulliken JB, Wu JK, Padwa BL. Repair of bilateral cleft lip: review, revisions, and reflections. *J Craniofac Surg.* 2003;14:609–620.

62. Farkas LG, ed. *Anthropometry of the Head and Face.* 2nd ed. New York, NY: Raven Press; 1994.

69. Lee CT, Garfinkle JS, Warren SM, et al. Nasoalveolar molding improves appearance of children with bilateral cleft lip–cleft palate. *Plast Reconstr Surg.* 2008;122:1131–1137. *This study provides further proof of the principle of primary nasal correction. Photogrammetry was used to document columellar length in patients with bilateral cleft lip/palate who had nasal repair by the two-stage forked flap method versus primary nasal correction after nasoalveolar molding; both groups were compared to age-matched controls. Measurements to age 3 years showed nearly normal columellar length in the primary repair group without need for further nasal procedures, whereas secondary operations were recommended for all children who had forked flap columellar lengthening.*

72. Wong JY, Oh AK, Ohta E, et al. Validity and reliability of craniofacial anthropometric measurements of 3D digital photogrammetric images. *Cleft Palate Craniofac J.* 2008;45:232–239.

23

Cleft palate

Jason H. Pomerantz and William Y. Hoffman

SYNOPSIS

- Normal speech is the primary goal of cleft palate repair; minimizing effects of maxillary growth is also important but ultimately secondary.
- Cleft palate repair prior to 1 year of age (ideally 9–10 months) results in better speech outcomes than later repairs.
- The levator veli palatini muscle is longitudinally oriented in the cleft palate patient. Realignment of the muscle to a transverse and posterior position in the soft palate is the key to a successful functional result.
- Eustachian tube function is abnormal in cleft patients due to abnormal position of the tensor veli palatini muscle; this must be addressed in every cleft palate patient, usually with ventilating tubes.

 Access the Historical Perspective section online at
http://www.expertconsult.com

Basic science

Embryology

The embryology of maxillary and palatal development is reviewed in detail in Chapter 20. In broad terms, the failure of fusion of the frontonasal and maxillary processes gives rise to the cleft of the primary palate, which includes the lip, alveolar process, and the hard palate anterior to the incisive foramen. This results in a cleft in the typical location between the premaxilla and the lateral maxilla, on either one or both sides. The lateral palatal shelves fuse later than the primary palate, around 7–8 weeks' gestation, as they rotate from vertical to horizontal orientation. This fusion proceeds from anterior to posterior, which helps us to understand the spectrum of clefts of the secondary palate.

The levator palatini and other pharyngeal muscles are derived from the fourth branchial arch and are innervated by the pharyngeal plexus, primarily cranial nerve X (vagus). The sole exception to this is the tensor palatini muscle, which arises from the first branchial arch and is innervated by cranial nerve V (trigeminal).

Anatomy of the velar muscles

Careful anatomic evaluation of each patient is of paramount importance in considering palatoplasty. Anatomic variability within the broad diagnosis of cleft palate will influence the timing and sequence of surgical repair as well as the type of repair. Optimal functional results depend directly on accurate analysis of the available structures and understanding of their long-term significance to function and facial growth (Fig. 23.1).

It is critical to understand the anatomy of the levator palatini muscle and the derangement of this anatomy that occurs in all clefts of the palate, including submucous cleft palate. Normally the levator muscle forms a transverse sling across the posterior half of the soft palate, and contraction causes the soft palate to move superiorly and posteriorly, contacting the posterior pharyngeal wall for velar closure, usually at the level of the adenoid pad. This action forms the characteristic "genu" seen on lateral views of the palate in motion.

In addition to being discontinuous across the cleft, the levator muscle runs more or less longitudinally along the cleft margin before it inserts aberrantly into the posterior border of the hard palate.[11–13] This results in ineffective contraction and inability to close the palate against the posterior pharyngeal wall. Air escape through the nose during speech produces a characteristic hypernasal quality. In addition, aberrant levator positioning, as well as an abnormal fusion with the tendon of the tensor veli palatini muscle, is thought to impair the function of the tensor muscle in assistance with Eustachian tube function, and is thought to be contributory to cleft otopathology.[14] A review of cleft otopathology is presented in the next section.

Ear pathology

Alt was the first physician to note a correlation between ear disease and cleft palate in 1878.[15] Numerous studies have

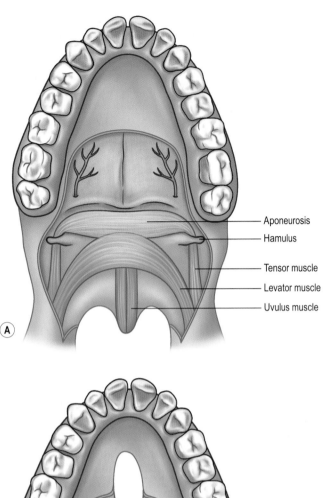

(A)

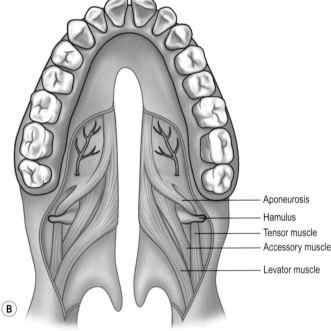

(B)

— Aponeurosis
— Hamulus
— Tensor muscle
— Levator muscle
— Uvulus muscle

— Aponeurosis
— Hamulus
— Tensor muscle
— Accessory muscle
— Levator muscle

Fig. 23.1 (A) Normal anatomy: The levator veli palatini muscle can be seen forming a sling across the soft palate; the tensor veli palatini is shown coming around the hamulus to fuse with the levator. **(B)** Cleft palate: The muscles are seen running more or less parallel with the cleft margin.

linked the presence of a cleft palate to abnormalities in Eustachian tube function. In multicenter studies, incidence of otitis media effusion has been found to be 96–100% in cleft palate patients, measured by both middle ear effusions on otoscopy and impedance testing and middle ear aspiration.[16,17] In the cleft palate, impairment of tubal dilation is thought to occur from complex misalignment of the paratubal musculature.[18,19]

Both radiologic and manometric testing techniques have demonstrated abnormalities in active dilation of the Eustachian tube.[20] In addition, intrinsic abnormalities of tubal cartilage framework rendering a Eustachian tube more collapsible have been noted. Although anatomic studies show that the levator veli palatini muscle does not directly actively open the Eustachian tube orifice, it is likely to have a secondary effect by influence on the tensor veli palatini and also with passive position of the orifice. The levator and tensor do share a common tendinous insertion near the hamulus and pulley position around the hamulus. In the cleft patient, the levator is connected solidly against the rigid posterior hard palate; the pulley effect around the hamulus cannot be activated and this impairs opening of the tube. In addition, some theorize that constant bathing of the tube orifice with oropharyngeal refluxed material leads to inflammation and obstruction of drainage. Other studies have demonstrated adenoidal tissue at the level of the tubal dilator that could potentially contribute to mechanical obstruction.[21] Anatomic paratubal abnormalities and risk for serous otitis media and chronic audiologic sequelae are present, regardless of cleft type, although Pierre Robin sequence has been postulated to be associated with even higher risk for hearing loss because of potential for concomitant ossicular malformation.[22]

Chronic obstruction of drainage leads to serous otitis media, and long-standing effusion can result in hearing loss. Estimates are 20–30% incidence of pure tone hearing loss in cleft patients by audiography[23]; decreased hearing has been found in as many as half of cleft palate patients by other authors.[24] Untreated children with clefts and severe effusions may have total deafness. Whereas hearing loss is significant in any child, it may be even more so in a cleft patient in whom speech development may be abnormal.

It has long been suggested that closure of the palate reduces risk of permanent hearing loss. In retrospective studies, children who had undergone palatoplasty had significantly lower incidence of permanent hearing loss than did children with unrepaired cleft palates.[24] Although still controversial, palatoplasty is thought by most surgeons to reduce risk of chronic serous otitis media and hearing loss. Nevertheless, serous otitis persists in most cleft patients for several years after palate repair. Although not currently recommended for every cleft palate patient (e.g., absence of effusion during examination under anesthesia), myringotomy with placement of ventilating tubes remains the mainstay of treatment for this difficult problem.[25]

Patient presentation

Cleft palate with cleft lip and alveolus

Although the primary palate and the secondary palate form at different stages of embryonic development, cleft palate is most commonly seen in combination with cleft lip. The alveolar portion of the cleft lies between the maxillary lateral incisor and canine tooth roots. This results in malposition of the maxillary lateral incisor and cuspid in both the deciduous and permanent dentition.[26,27] The maxillary lateral incisor on the cleft side is absent in 80–90% of cleft patients; when present, it may be smaller than the contralateral tooth or significantly dysmorphic[27–29] Absence of other teeth is not uncommon,[30] but it may be related to the surgery itself because adults who have not been operated on do not show the same patterns of hypodontia.[31] Asymmetry is common, resulting in alterations in first maxillary molar position.[32–34] In comparison to non-cleft individuals, patients with unilateral cleft lip and palate have overall reduction in crown size[35] and delay of eruption of permanent dentition.[36] These findings support the theory of global dental growth potential disturbance associated with clefting. Interestingly, eruption of deciduous dentition is not significantly delayed.[37]

Unilateral complete cleft palate is characterized by direct communication between the entire length of the nasal passage and oropharynx (see Fig. 23.3D). Absence of a portion of the inferior piriform aperture, along with hypoplasia of the lateral nasal bony platform at the maxillary wall, contribute to the cleft nasal deformity; the nasal base is depressed, the ala collapses, and the floor widens. The superior and posterior nasal septum is deviated and buckled toward the cleft side, and when viewed intraorally from inferiorly, the vomer and caudal septum slants towards the non-cleft side. The soft palate muscles are discontinuous in the midline and insert along the cleft margins in an abnormal manner. The unilateral complete cleft is thus a full-thickness palatal defect of nasal mucosa, bony palate, velar musculature, and oral mucosa; all of these deficiencies must be addressed during the cleft palate repair or later at the time of alveolar cleft bone grafting.

In the bilateral complete cleft lip and palate, the premaxillary segment, containing the central and lateral incisor tooth roots, is discontinuous from the alveolar arch. The lateral segments often collapse inward and lingually, resulting in "locking out" of the premaxilla. Preoperative management with presurgical infant orthopedics (PSIO) may help prevent or treat lateral segment collapse and correct the anterior position of the premaxilla. If untreated, the anterior location of the premaxilla in this situation may result in anterior fistulas, which may in turn cause significant speech problems and nasal regurgitation of fluid. Later orthodontic treatment of the maxillary arch can expand the lateral segments before bone grafting; however, repositioning of the premaxilla at this age is usually not possible.

Kernahan and Veau proposed standardized reporting schemes, each of which is commonly used to distinguish the variable presentations of clefts of the palate, shown in (Fig. 23.2 ⊙). Clinical examples representing the spectrum of palatal clefts are shown in Fig. 23.3.

Fig. 23.2 appears online only.

Clefts of the secondary palate

Also called incomplete cleft palate, a cleft of the secondary palate may be variable, from an opening in the posterior soft palate to a cleft extending up to the incisive foramen (see Fig. 23.3B,C). There is almost always a separation of the bony shelves of the hard palate, which is variable but may extend anteriorly to the incisive foramen. Most commonly, dentition is normal and symmetric (see Fig. 23.3C).

Submucous cleft palate

Submucous cleft palate occurs when the palate has mucosal continuity but the underlying levator palatini muscle is discontinuous across the midline and longitudinally oriented, similar to the muscle anatomy in overt clefts of the palate.

Calnan's classic triad of a midline clear zone (zona pellucida), a bifid uvula, and a palpable notch in the posterior hard palate is diagnostic of this condition. With contraction of velar musculature, a distinct midline muscle diastasis may be seen (see Fig. 23.3A).

The significance of a submucous cleft may be difficult to assess clinically; the child with submucous cleft palate is often undiagnosed in infancy. In a study screening a large population of schoolchildren in Denver, the overall incidence of submucous cleft palate in the population was found to be 1 : 1200.[38] Another similar cohort study reported that 45–55% of patients with isolated submucous cleft palate were symptomatic with regard to speech, serous otitis media, or hearing loss.[39,40] In a large series of children with submucous cleft palate in Mexico, examination with fiberoptic nasoendoscopy showed about one-third to have velopharyngeal insufficiency.[41] Other attempts to identify risk of speech problems with submucous cleft palate have been problematic because referrals to cleft palate clinics are usually based on the identification of speech issues rather than of the submucous cleft itself. Therefore, an infant identified with submucous cleft palate need not routinely undergo repair because a significant number of individuals with submucous cleft palate will not develop velopharyngeal insufficiency. Rather, these patients should be closely monitored with serial speech evaluations and audiometric surveillance.

Patients who present with velopharyngeal insufficiency and submucous cleft palate on examination require full evaluation, including speech evaluation and endoscopy.[42] Even in the absence of obvious findings on clinical examination, anatomic abnormalities are found in most patients (>90%) at the time of surgery[43,44]; thus, the so-called "occult submucous cleft palate" is simply one that is less obvious on clinical evaluation. There will still be rare patients, however, who have true palatopharyngeal disproportion and present with velopharyngeal insufficiency without any cleft, submucous or otherwise.

Corrective surgical technique for submucous cleft palate is focused on anatomic correction of the velar muscle diastasis. Although pharyngeal flaps and sphincter pharyngoplasty have been proposed as primary means of treatment,[41] most surgeons focus on repair of the abnormal levator muscle position.[45] The Furlow double opposing Z-plasty (see below) is an ideal procedure for patients with isolated submucous clefts and velopharyngeal insufficiency in the absence of 22q deletion syndrome, because there is no width discrepancy to be overcome (Fig. 23.4).[46] This avoids the potential for nasal obstruction and sleep apnea in these patients if a pharyngeal flap is used.

Pierre Robin sequence

Pierre Robin described the triad of micrognathia, glossoptosis, and respiratory distress.[47] Of the children diagnosed with Pierre Robin sequence, 60–90% have cleft palate[48,49]; the palatal cleft is usually isolated to the velum and can be "V" shaped or, more typically, "U" shaped.[50,51] In the past, this has been thought to be secondary to hyperflexion of the head *in utero* with resultant displacement of the tongue between the palatal shelves, preventing their fusion. More recently, extensive analysis of multiple syndromes associated with Pierre Robin sequence has delineated genetic associations, indicating that

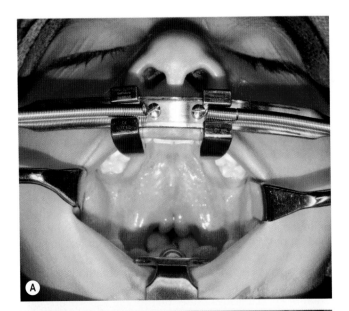

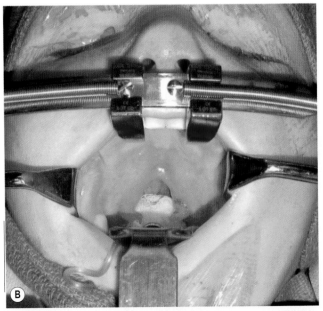

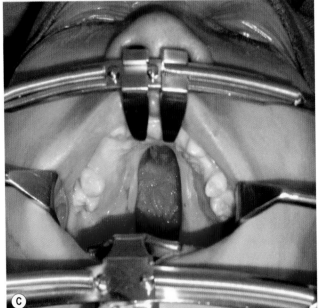

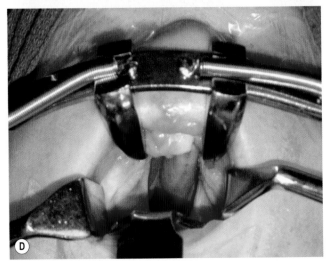

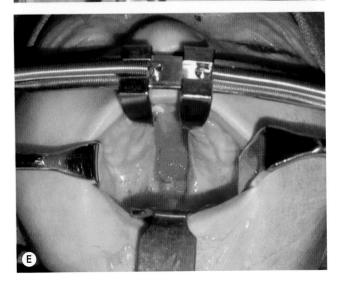

Fig. 23.3 Cleft palate spectrum. **(A)** Submucous cleft palate. **(B)** Incomplete cleft of the secondary palate involving mainly the soft palate. **(C)** Incomplete cleft involving the entire secondary palate extending to the incisive foramen. **(D)** Left unilateral complete cleft lip and palate. Note vomer contiguous with the right maxillary segment. **(E)** Complete bilateral cleft lip and palate. Vomer is straight, in the midline, and separated from both maxillary segments.

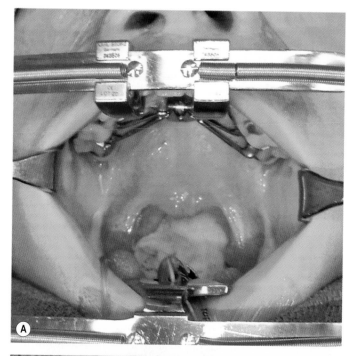

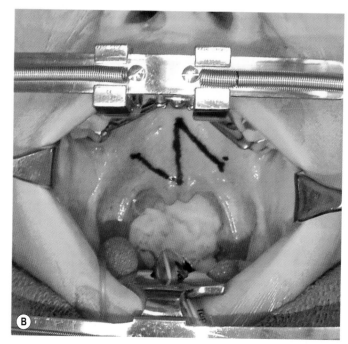

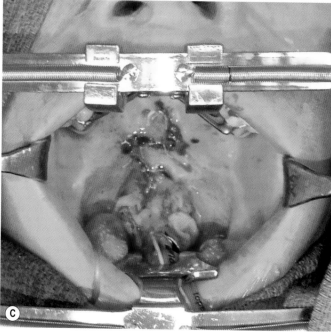

Fig. 23.4 Submucous cleft palate. **(A)** Note bifid uvula and thinning of central palate. On palpation, there is a notch in the posterior hard palate rather than a posterior nasal spine. **(B)** Furlow double opposing Z-plasty repair of submucous cleft palate. **(C)** Appearance of double opposing Z-plasty after repair.

the etiology may not be such a simple mechanical event.[52–54] Infants with Pierre Robin sequence also have increased incidence of associated anomalies, particularly cardiac and renal problems.[55]

Newborns with Pierre Robin sequence may have severe respiratory and feeding difficulty because of the posterior displacement of the tongue. Initial treatment consists of placing the child prone and use of gastric lavage feeding tubes to push the tongue forward.[56] Nasal airways have been used for the same purpose with reported success rates of 80–90%.[57] If these conservative measures fail, surgical management of the airway may be required. A tongue–lip

adhesion has been used as an alternative to tracheostomy and is generally effective.[58,59] More recently, mandibular distraction osteogenesis has been used in neonates with success in averting tracheostomy.[60] Although definitive long-term outcomes with regard to mandibular growth and dental development are not yet available, existing outcomes data do not suggest major deleterious effects of neonatal distraction on mandibular growth and dental development.[61,62] In all cases, if management is focused on the upper airway, bronchoscopy should be performed to rule out any intrinsic subglottic problems (e.g., laryngomalacia) that might necessitate tracheotomy.

Palatoplasty in children with Pierre Robin sequence must be carefully timed with growth of the child, particularly the mandible. There is some controversy about "catch-up" growth of the mandible in children with Pierre Robin sequence; basically, there is good documentation of extra growth in the first year of life,[63,64] but growth is subsequently commensurate with that of normal children. Children with syndromes tend to have less growth than in non-syndromic cases. Late cephalometric evaluation has consistently shown that the children with Pierre Robin sequence have smaller mandibles than normal.[65] Closure of the palate narrows the effective area for respiration and can lead to respiratory distress. If the mandible attains reasonable size in the first year of life, palate repair can still be performed safely before 1 year of age. In the rare patient who has previously undergone tracheostomy, the palate should be repaired before decannulation. The risk of airway compromise after palatoplasty reaches 25%, with an emergent tracheostomy or reintubation rate of 11% at one institution.[66] However, careful preoperative evaluation incorporating the use of polysomnography and upper endoscopy informs palate repair decision-making and minimizes risk.

Syndromes

Multiple malformations or syndromes have been found frequently in cleft patients.[67] Cleft palate without associated cleft lip has been reported to be associated with a syndrome in as many as 50% of cases, while cleft lip and palate together have an incidence of syndromes of about 30%. Van der Woude syndrome is associated with a mutation in the interferon regulatory factor 6 (IRF6) gene that also causes popliteal pterygium syndrome; this is an autosomal-dominant syndrome associated with lower lip sinus tracts ("lip pits"), and has variable penetrance including the full range of cleft lips as well as palates.

Children with cleft palate associated with an identified syndrome must be evaluated thoroughly and have individualized planning and timing of therapy. Infants with a profound developmental delay and severely shortened life span projection should have surgical intervention delayed or should undergo palatoplasty under special circumstances only. In addition, syndromic children may have increased incidence of cardiac anomalies, requiring specific anesthetic and postoperative considerations. Repair of cleft palate in the hope that this will stimulate or allow a severely disabled child to speak gives unreasonable expectations and hope to parents; as noted before, it is critical to explain that palate repair may aid speech production but not speech development. The majority of syndromic infants with cleft palate can attain adequate weight gain and growth with proper nutrition and feeding assistance. Therefore feeding benefit associated with palate repair is often outweighed by the risk of airway compromise and absence of speech-related indications for repair. Palate repair in severely disabled children can lead to altered airway status and obstructed upper airway in those with neuromuscular delay.

22q chromosomal deletion

Velocardiofacial syndrome, which is associated with 22q chromosomal deletions, is diagnosed by fluorescent immunohybridization (FISH). These children have a characteristic "bird-like" facial appearance, velopharyngeal dysfunction, developmental delay, and various cardiac conditions. The same deletion gives rise to DiGeorge syndrome with associated B-cell and immune dysfunction; these children all need appropriate immunology referral and follow-up. Most children with 22q deletions do not have overt cleft palate and may not even have submucous clefts; usually the velar dysfunction is related to absence of movement of an otherwise normal soft palate. This may complicate decision-making regarding surgery for speech in these patients, and soft palate procedures alone are generally not sufficient to correct the velopharyngeal insufficiency.

Growth

At birth, the average weight is the same for cleft and unaffected newborns.[68,69] However, cleft infants have been shown to exhibit poor weight gain in early infancy. Studies observing infants with cleft lip and palate show initial growth retardation by the time they undergo surgical lip repair. When the same children reach the age for palatoplasty, they have significantly lagged on the growth curve. However, longitudinal studies show that after repair of the palate, average growth returns to normal compared with unaffected children by the age of 4 years. Stratification of risk within the longitudinal cohort shows pronounced growth retardation in associated syndromes and also in children with isolated clefts of the secondary palate.[70,71]

Children with orofacial clefting stabilize and continue normal growth to at least 6 years of age, with no statistically significant differences in height and weight when compared to unaffected children. In later childhood, however, average weight and height of children with cleft appear to diminish compared with those of control subjects. In a Danish study of skeletal maturity assessing both body height and radius length as an index of growth in male cleft patients, onset of puberty was found to be delayed on average by 6 months, and the velocity of skeletal growth during puberty was blunted. However, duration of puberty and pubertal skeletal growth were prolonged an average of 1 year, resulting in final attained body height and radius length the same as those of control subjects.[72]

Numerous causes are thought to contribute to these differences in growth patterns. There are certainly feeding difficulties early in life before palate repair,[73] but it has also been suggested that intrinsic growth disturbances may be responsible for slow postnatal growth.[74] The increased frequency of ear and airway infections has been implicated in early growth retardation,[68] as have the multiple operative procedures that these children undergo.[73] Adding more confusion to the etiology is the fact that growth hormone levels may be diminished in cleft children. In summary, any growth disturbance is likely to be of multifactorial origin throughout infancy, childhood, and puberty. Fortunately, families can be counseled that most children attain norms of height, weight, and development.

Feeding and swallowing

The intact palate provides a barrier between the respiratory tract and the alimentary tract. To understand the difficulty cleft infants have with feeding, one must understand the normal role of the palate in sucking and swallowing. Oral intake is divided into two separate activities, generation of suction force (negative intraoral pressure) and swallowing.

For negative intraoral pressure to be produced, the velum seals off the pharynx posteriorly; the lips close anteriorly, and negative pressure is produced by moving the tongue away from the palate and by opening the mandible. This effectively increases the intraoral volume within a closed system, resulting in generation of negative pressure. If the individual is unable to close the nasopharynx or to generate a seal of the lips, or if the palate is not intact at the point of contact with the tongue, negative pressure cannot be produced. This failure of velopharyngeal closure is the basis of difficulty with breast-feeding or normal bottle-feeding in the patient with cleft palate.

Suction on the nipple in a breastfeeding infant is thought to stabilize the nipple position while motion of the tongue against the nipple pushes fluid into the mouth. Ingestion through an artificial nipple is different; infants learn to manipulate the nipple and flow rates by closing the alveolus against the artificial nipple. Tongue motion is primarily used to transfer the bolus to the pharynx for swallowing. In the cleft infant, the communication between the oropharynx and nasopharynx prevents a seal of the tongue against the palate, and negative pressure cannot be generated. Suckling is therefore not productive, and breastfeeding is ineffective.

Most infants with clefts are unable to breastfeed. Infants with clefting limited to the posterior velum can often use posterior tongue position to generate a partial negative seal. The exception to this is the child with Pierre Robin sequence and isolated velar cleft, who can develop respiratory distress or ineffective suction from glossoptosis. Obviously, patients with isolated cleft lip and an intact palate should and do have little difficulty with breastfeeding.

Infants who are unable to breastfeed because of cleft palate have a number of options for feeding. Regimens and devices have evolved to nourish the infant, including specialty nipples such as lamb's nipples, crosscutting of standard nipples, and long soft nipples that place the liquid at the posterior tongue. Special flow bottles such as gravity flow and squeeze bottles allow the caregiver to carefully control the flow rate (Fig. 23.5). The strategy of each technique is low resistance to flow, with controllable flow rate for optimal volume and minimal effort by the infant. All of these techniques are effective, and selection is generally by personal preference and the baby's acceptance of the method. Other key considerations are elevated head positioning during feeding and careful observation of feeding time and volume ingested.[75–78]

Swallowing involves a complex interaction of the tongue and pharynx. Coordinated swallowing is dependent on neuromuscular control and rhythmic coordinated contraction of the tongue and pharynx. Children with clefts generally do *not* have difficulty with swallowing and aspiration unless intrinsic neuromuscular abnormality of the tongue or pharynx is present. It is an error to ascribe aspiration simply to the presence of a cleft palate; indeed, aspiration with swallowing should stimulate an appropriate diagnostic evaluation, including thin barium swallow studies, bronchoscopy, and gastroscopy. Children may cough or sputter with reflux of the ingested material into the nose, particularly if volume or rate of feeding is excessive. During normal deglutition, the tongue moves the food bolus to the pharynx by complex interaction of tongue against palate. When the palate has an open cleft, food may reflux into the nasal passage. Nasal reflux is irritating to the nasal mucosa and can predispose to sinusitis and

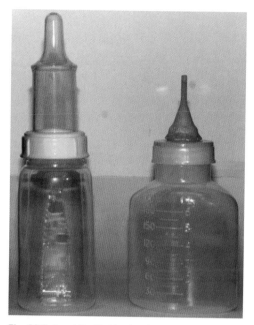

Fig. 23.5 Specialized bottles for cleft palate feeding. Left, Haberman feeder with reservoir in continuity with nipple. Right, Mead–Johnson feeder, which requires squeezing the bottle to improve flow of fluid.

ulceration. In the older child, a persistent communication through a fistula in the palate may result in regurgitation of food through the nose, which is socially unacceptable.

Weight gain and skeletal growth confirm success of the feeding regimen. Once the palate is successfully closed surgically, special feeding methods are generally unnecessary.

Speech

The primary goal of palatoplasty is normal speech. Patients can grow and even thrive, despite feeding difficulties, but speech cannot be normalized if the palate is not repaired. The ability to partition the oropharynx and nasopharynx is crucial for normal speech production. The palate elevates during production of any sounds requiring positive pressure in the oropharynx; the levator palatini is primarily responsible for this movement (Fig. 23.6).

Speech is a complex issue, and many factors may influence speech development in a child with a cleft palate. In addition to the importance of the palate itself, speech development may be influenced by motor or neurologic developmental delay (often seen in syndromes), by hearing, and by environmental stimuli. It is important to distinguish between speech production, which is primarily dependent on normal anatomic function, and speech development, which is influenced more by global developmental issues. Speech production also requires normal articulation, which in turn depends on tongue placement, lip competence, and dental position, all of which may be abnormal in cleft patients.[79]

If palate function is not corrected, velopharyngeal insufficiency results, with speech that is hypernasal, often with hoarse quality due to difficulty in directing airflow through the mouth. When complete closure cannot be anatomically or functionally obtained, compensatory mechanisms for sound production are learned. These are maladaptive patterns that interfere with global intelligibility and include glottal stops

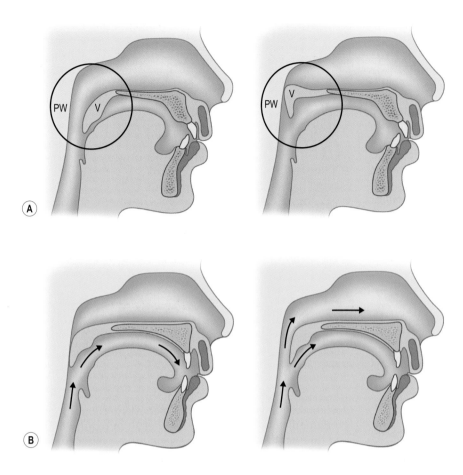

(A)

(B)

Fig. 23.6 (A) In the lateral cephalogram, the soft palate or velum ("V") is shown at rest (above left) and during speech, making contact with the posterior pharyngeal wall ("PW") (above right). **(B)** This line drawing shows the air flow during normal speech (left), with the velum making contact with the posterior pharynx to direct air out the mouth. If the velum is too short or movement is inadequate (right), air can escape through the nose during speech, creating velopharyngeal insufficiency.

and pharyngeal fricatives. In addition, tongue placement for various phonemes is altered to achieve the most normal production of sounds. Eliminating these learned compensatory articulations is difficult, even with the best of speech and language therapy. Compensatory articulations may persist even in the face of a functional palate repair, especially in later repairs or secondary correction of velopharyngeal insufficiency.

Timing of palate repair

The normal palate serves several important functions, all related to functional separation of the oropharynx from the nasopharynx. Whereas the *sine qua non* for palate repair is normal speech, consideration of cleft palate surgery must balance developmental, dentofacial growth, and otologic issues as well.

Speech

The driving force for palatoplasty is the development of normal speech. Two crucial aspects of palatoplasty are important in optimal speech outcome: (1) surgical technique and (2) timing of palate repair. Victor Veau[11] first made the observation of a correlation between age at repair and speech outcome in 1931. He noted that children who had undergone repair before 12 months of age were much more likely to have normal speech than those with repair between 2 and 4 years

of age. Children who underwent repair after 9 years of age had the worst speech outcome. Adults with unrepaired cleft palate (see Fig. 23.3C) have little or no possibility of neuromotor adaptation to a newly repaired palate and unfortunately do not exhibit significant speech gains. Therefore palate repair in adults is indicated for correction of nasal regurgitation alone. The optimal time of palatoplasty still remains scientifically unproven. Confounding variables of technique, surgeon's skill, lack of standardization of speech evaluations, and therapies preclude exact determination of optimal age at repair.[80]

Most would agree that the best speech results are correlated with closure of the palate near the time of the infant's beginning language acquisition, which for the normal-developing child is before 12 months of age.[81,82] Indeed, there is a body of evidence that phonologic development actually begins earlier, at 4–6 months of age.[83,84] Most studies of the timing of palatal repair have looked at secondary outcomes; increased compensatory articulations were shown in one study and increased need for pharyngeal flaps in another when the palate was repaired after 1 year of age. Although repairs before 1 year of age are now common, this is not a rigid chronologic milestone; rather, repair should be related to the child's speech development. Some studies have shown that if correction occurs even as late as 21 months, compensatory maladaptive patterns are infrequent. Despite the absence of hard evidence supporting earlier palate repairs, a growing body of opinion seems to support palate repair around 9–10 months of age for children with apparently normal development.[85,86] Very early repair of the palate (6 months or younger) has been proposed by some surgeons,[87–90] primarily as a means of improving feeding; however, long-term results are lacking for any large cohort of these patients. Prospective longitudinal assessment is currently in progress to attempt to better define the optimal timing of cleft repair.

Maxillary growth

Palatoplasty is generally assumed to detrimentally affect maxillary growth, and evidence in support of this is that cephalometric analysis of adults with unrepaired cleft palate has shown normal maxillary dimensions and growth.[91,92] There is experimental evidence that the lip repair may restrict sagittal growth of the maxilla,[93,94] but in most patients it seems that the palate repair is more significant. Many children with repaired cleft palate display typical findings of transverse maxillary deficiency requiring orthodontic widening of the maxilla once permanent teeth have erupted.

Transverse growth of the maxillary arch is narrowed in comparison with that in non-cleft patients, resulting in typical malocclusion traits of crowding, lateral crossbite, and open bite.[32,95–97] Whether the narrowed arch and maxillary growth inhibition result from surgical scarring[98,99] or intrinsic maxillary underdevelopment remains a matter of debate; most likely it is a combination of the two. There may be a sagittal growth deficiency as well; whereas 35–40% of children will develop an anterior crossbite, as many as 15–20% of children with cleft palate go on to require a Le Fort I maxillary advancement in some series. There is some evidence that the development of crossbite and maxillary hypoplasia may be related to the severity of the original cleft.[100,101]

Although it might seem preferable to wait until a more advanced age for palate repair, given the growth effects on the maxilla, it is far more difficult to establish normal speech in older children after cleft repair than to correct occlusion with a combination of orthodontic treatment and orthognathic surgery.

Treatment/surgical technique

Technical considerations

A number of perioperative considerations must be addressed regardless of the type of repair used. The general health and the developmental status of the child play a role in the timing of the palate repair and are also important for anesthetic and surgical management. Audiology evaluation is routinely obtained preoperatively so that the otolaryngologist can place ventilating tubes in the tympanic membranes if indicated, saving the child an additional anesthetic. Most surgeons use preoperative antibiotics, although consensus is lacking. One recent randomized, placebo controlled study demonstrated a lower fistula rate with the use of additional postoperative antibiotics.[102]

The use of a Ring–Adair–Elwyn (RAE) endotracheal tube facilitates placement of the Dingman gag without kinking the tube. The airway must be assessed constantly for problems; if lower central teeth are present, this can be a source of tube compression against the retractor. The Dingman gag, the most

commonly used instrument for exposure, compresses the tongue and causes ischemia; if it is used for longer than 2 h, significant postoperative tongue swelling can occur. Lidocaine 0.5% and epinephrine 1:200 000 are infiltrated into the palate 7–10 min before incision; use of a 3-mL syringe makes the injection into the hard palate somewhat easier than with a larger syringe. A maximum of 1 mL/kg is used.

Palate repair is performed with the surgeon at the child's head, with use of a fiberoptic headlight or retractor. A rolled towel under the shoulders will extend the neck; it is important to assure that the child does not have any syndromes that predispose to cervical spine anomalies. The use of curved needle holders facilitates suture placement without obstruction of vision.

The most important aspect of surgical anatomy is the location of the greater palatine neurovascular bundle, which emerges through the greater palatine foramen through the lateral posterior hard palate. Incisions on each side are best made with the surgeon's contralateral hand to bevel the incision away from the vascular pedicle. Circumferential freeing of the palatal attachments around the pedicle and gentle stretching of the pedicle out of the foramen can be essential to obtain a tension-free closure of the oral flap.[103] In general, the goal is to obtain complete nasal and oral closure from front to back. This may not be possible in wide clefts, particularly on the nasal surface, or in cases of complete clefts with poorly aligned alveolar segments. The most difficult area for closure, around the junction of the hard and soft palate, is the most common location for fistulas.

Hard versus soft palate closure

It is easier to understand cleft palate surgery by separating techniques used for the hard palate from those used for the soft palate. In general, all techniques use some form of mucoperiosteal flap for the hard palate closure; the soft palate repair emphasizes correction of the abnormal position of the levator palatini muscles. The location of the incision along the cleft margin can be varied to include more or less mucosa to be turned over for nasal lining. In the discussion below, the hard palate techniques are discussed first followed by soft palate closure.

von Langenbeck

Bernhard von Langenbeck introduced the use of mucoperiosteal flaps to close clefts of the secondary palate in the late 1800s. The initial description of the technique involved a simple approximation of the cleft margins with a relaxing incision that began posterior to the maxillary tuberosity and followed the posterior portion of the alveolar ridge. Some variation of the Langenbeck repair is still used commonly for clefts of the secondary palate. Intravelar veloplasty, or repair of the levator palatini muscle, as described below, is added today to reproduce the normal muscle sling (Fig. 23.7).

V-Y pushback (Veau–Wardill–Kilner)

George Dorrance (1877–1949) of Philadelphia realized that a distinct number of patients with cleft would develop velopharyngeal dysfunction caused by inability of the soft palate to touch the posterior pharyngeal wall.[104,105] In fact, he advocated muscle transposition but did so by fracturing the hamulus,

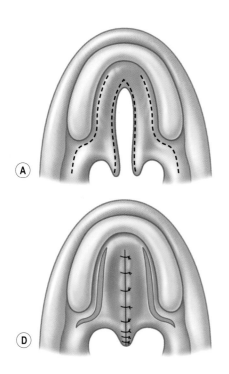

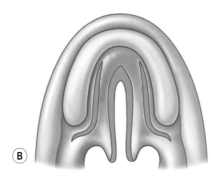

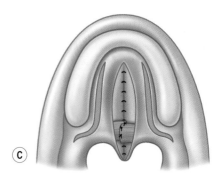

Fig. 23.7 Von Langenbeck repair. **(A)** Relaxing incisions are made behind the alveolar ridge, creating bilateral bipedicle flaps for midline closure. The greater palatine vessels must be preserved. **(B)** The cleft margins are incised in a manner to leave adequate nasal mucosa for complete closure. **(C)** Closure of the nasal mucosa and muscle repair. **(D)** Final appearance.

which he believed would change the vector of muscle contraction and in combination with techniques of Langenbeck would lengthen the palate. He also advocated division of the major palatine neurovascular bundles to assist with the pushback. Thomas Kilner (1896–1964) was important in development of the V-Y palate repair along with Victor Veau and William E.M. Wardill (1893–1960). In addition, he pushed for palate repair at an earlier age, 12–18 months.[106]

The essence of the pushback repair is the central "V" incision on the hard palate that is then closed in a straight line, creating length on the oral side of the closure (Fig. 23.8). The initial description included osteotomy of the posterior hard palate at the greater palatine foramina to release the palatine vessels; circumferential dissection, with release of the periosteum behind the vessels, was subsequently advocated to stretch the vessels, which works as well with less risk of injury

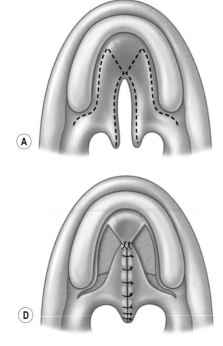

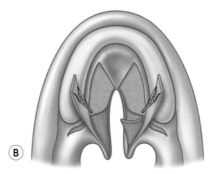

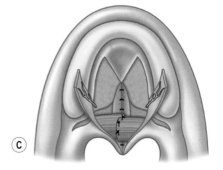

Fig. 23.8 Pushback repair. **(A)** Design of anterior "Y" incision. **(B)** Elevation of bilateral mucoperiosteal flaps based on palatine vessels. The levator veli palatini muscles are freed from the posterior border of the hard palate. **(C)** The muscles are repaired across the midline of the soft palate. **(D)** The "Y" closure creates additional length but also leaves large raw areas bilaterally.

to this vital blood supply.[103,107] The nasal tissue is released and left open; some authors have proposed providing nasal lining, either with septal flaps[108] or with buccal mucosa (Fig. 23.9).[109] The soft palate is addressed with repair of the cleft margins and transverse closure of the levator muscle.

The pushback technique has the advantage of providing increased length for the palate and placing the levator muscle in a more favorable position. Large open areas are left anteriorly and on the nasal surface; as these close by contraction, a good deal of the length gain is lost. Additionally, the contraction of the oral mucosal defects results in loss of maxillary width anteriorly, a situation more difficult to correct than posterior maxillary narrowing. The arch may also be flattened anteriorly, a difficult problem for the orthodontist. The closure

anteriorly in a complete cleft is a single layer of nasal mucosa only, which gives rise to a higher fistula rate in pushback repairs than in other techniques.[110]

Two-flap palatoplasty

Bardach and Salyer[111] originally described a technique of freeing mucoperiosteal flaps from the cleft margins only, arguing that the arch of the cleft would provide the length needed for central closure. This is certainly not a universal finding, and it is probably most applicable in relatively narrow clefts. The more extensive two-flap palatoplasty is a modification of the Langenbeck technique, extending the relaxing incisions along the alveolar margins to the edge of the cleft. This designs flaps entirely dependent on the circulation from the palatine vessels but also much more versatile in terms of their placement. In a complete unilateral cleft, the flap from the greater (medial) segment can be shifted across the cleft and closed directly behind the alveolar margin. This virtually eliminates fistulas in the anterior hard palate.[112]

The soft palate closure is accomplished with a straight line closure in the typical two-flap technique. Intravelar veloplasty is an essential part of this closure (Fig. 23.10).

Vomer flaps

There is confusion about the terminology applied to anterior closure of the nasal mucosa in complete cleft lip and palate. The original vomer flap is described as inferiorly based; an incision is made high on the septum, and the flap is reflected downward to provide a single-layer closure on the oral side. A number of European centers noted a high number of patients with maxillary retrusion, presumably from injury to the vomer–premaxillary suture, as well as a high fistula rate, and changed to a two-layer anterior closure.[113–115]

Similar problems have not been found with superiorly based vomer flaps. This technique involves reflecting the mucosa from the septum near the cleft margin, dissecting only enough to close the nasal mucosa of the opposite side. In bilateral cleft palate, this requires a midline incision along the septum, and two flaps are reflected in each direction. This technique results in a two-layer closure of the hard palate mucosa, with low fistula rates and less effect on maxillary growth.[110]

Intravelar veloplasty

Although Victor Veau first advocated midline reapproximation of the levator palatini muscle, Braithwaite[116] was the first to perform more extensive muscle dissection for posterior repositioning and tension-free approximation. He emphasized careful dissection and freeing of the levator palatini from the posterior edge of the hard palate before approximation in the midline.

Cutting[117] has described a technique of veloplasty that includes division of the tensor palatini tendon at the hamulus and repositioning of the muscle. This method, known as radical levator transposition, requires an extensive dissection of the levator muscle, freeing it from both nasal and oral mucosa (Fig. 23.11). Although there is a reasonable thickness of oral mucosa, the adherence of the nasal mucosa to the muscle makes the dissection difficult on this side and at times results in perforation of the mucosa. Sommerlad described the

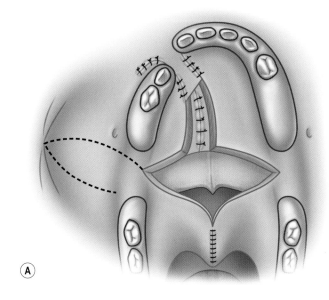

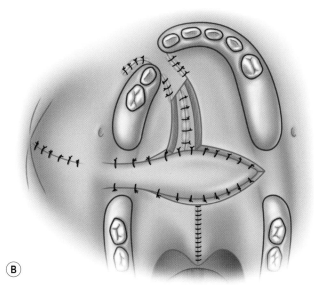

Fig. 23.9 (A) Buccal mucosal flap. Kaplan advocated use of this flap to elongate the nasal mucosa. **(B)** Flap transposed into the nasal surface. In some situations bilateral flaps can be used with the second flap lining the oral surface.

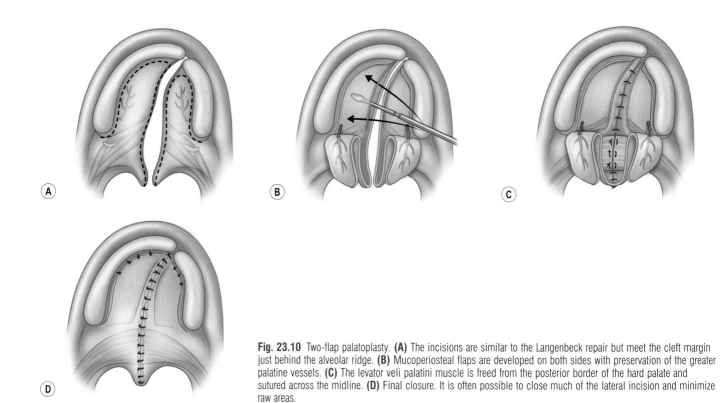

Fig. 23.10 Two-flap palatoplasty. **(A)** The incisions are similar to the Langenbeck repair but meet the cleft margin just behind the alveolar ridge. **(B)** Mucoperiosteal flaps are developed on both sides with preservation of the greater palatine vessels. **(C)** The levator veli palatini muscle is freed from the posterior border of the hard palate and sutured across the midline. **(D)** Final closure. It is often possible to close much of the lateral incision and minimize raw areas.

use of the microscope for dissection of the muscle to reduce injury of the nasal mucosa. The blood supply of the levator veli palatini is derived from the ascending palatine and ascending pharyngeal arteries with generous collateralization.[118] Precise identification of the vascular pedicles is not performed during cleft surgery and significant devascularization of the levator is thought to be uncommon. However, the surgeon should be aware that the majority of the velar blood supply enters from the region lateral to the hamulus, in the space of Ernst, and the region immediately posterior (through which the motor innervation passes as well), and excessive dissection in these areas is probably best avoided. The tensor tendon is

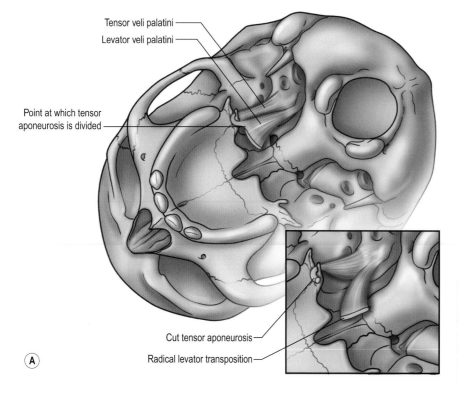

Tensor veli palatini

Levator veli palatini

Point at which tensor aponeurosis is divided

Cut tensor aponeurosis

Radical levator transposition

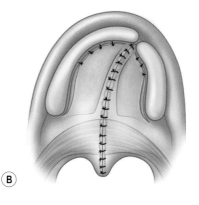

Fig. 23.11 Cutting's radical levator transposition. **(A)** The levator veli palatini is freed completely from the posterior hard palate as well as from nasal and oral lining. The tensor tendon is cut medial to the hamulus to effect a complete release of the muscular sling. **(B)** The muscles are repaired in the midline after being transposed into a horizontal position and situated in the posterior portion of the soft palate.

released just medial to the hamulus, and the levator muscle is overlapped to provide appropriate tension on the repair. This is presumably similar to the muscle overlap accomplished by Furlow's double opposing Z-plasty method. This technique has shown excellent speech outcomes in early evaluations. Both Cutting and Sommerlad[119] have proposed "re-repair" of the levator muscle when primary palatoplasty still results in velopharyngeal insufficiency.

Double opposing Z-plasty (Furlow)

Furlow[120] first described his technique for palate closure in the 1980s, adapting the Z-plasty principle to palatal closure. By alternating reversing Z-plasties of the nasal and oral flaps and keeping the levator palatini within the most posterior flaps, he reported initial early success in both speech outcomes and skeletal growth.

A Z-plasty is developed on both the oral and nasal surfaces of the soft palate but in opposite directions. For both of the Z-plasties, the central limb is the cleft margin, and the posteriorly based flap is designed to include the levator muscle. Furlow recommended that the posteriorly based oral flap be on the left side for a right-handed surgeon because the elevation of the muscle from the nasal mucosa is the most difficult part of the dissection (Fig. 23.12).[121]

This technique addresses closure of the soft palate in a manner that provides complete nasal and oral closure as it re-establishes the levator sling. Because the nasal Z-plasty is placed more laterally, a higher and presumably more functional sling is formed. The theoretical disadvantage of this technique is that it is non-anatomic, in that it completely ignores the small longitudinal uvular muscle, but overall speech results have been comparable to or better than those with other techniques.[122,123]

Although Furlow described the use of relaxing incisions when necessary, Peter Randall and other surgeons at The Children's Hospital of Philadelphia incorporated their use routinely, with elevation of bipedicled mucoperiosteal flaps in their modification of the Furlow procedure.[124] The chief problem may arise in very wide clefts, in which the distance to be traversed by the Z-plasty may be excessive. The anteriorly based oral flap can be joined to the relaxing incision to design an island flap based on the greater palatine vessels and giving considerably greater mobility, although this will shift the closure to the side of the posteriorly based flap. Another alternative is to extend the relaxing incision along the lateral border of the soft palate to allow oral closure and to use acellular dermal matrix for any nasal defects. A third alternative is to employ a straight line closure in wide cases, reserving the Z-plasty as a secondary procedure if needed for speech. The rationale for the latter is that the added length gained with Z-plasty in very wide clefts, come at the expense of increased contracture by secondary healing laterally. As the child grows, adequate soft tissue develops such that secondary Z-plasty of a straight line repair is a relatively easy procedure that results in significant improvement in muscle position and palate function.

Direct comparison of Z-plasty and intravelar veloplasty has not been done controlling for surgeon, cleft type, and other significant variables. A review of published studies showed overall better speech outcomes reported by groups using the Furlow technique or its modifications.[125] However, there is a wide range of reported speech outcomes, and, as discussed above, a number of surgeons have reported excellent speech results using intravelar veloplasty with straight line repairs. Thus, available data to date have not led to a consensus recommendation for either individual technique over the other for all soft palate repairs. The authors'

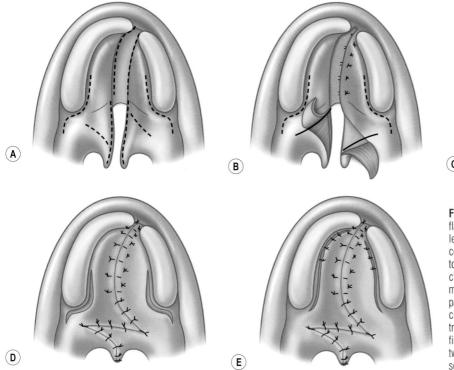

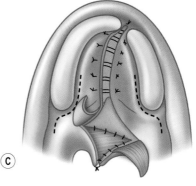

Fig. 23.12 Furlow double opposing Z-plasty. **(A)** The oral flap design is shown with the posteriorly based flap on the left side. If necessary, the relaxing incisions can be continued up to the cleft margin behind the alveolus, similar to the two flap palatoplasty (Fig. 23.10) for the hard palate closure. **(B)** The left-sided oral flap is raised with the levator muscle, the right-sided flap above the muscle. The reverse pattern is planned for the oral side. A vomer flap is shown closing the nasal mucosa anteriorly. **(C)** The nasal flaps are transposed and the anterior oral mucosa closed. **(D)** The final appearance after transposition of the oral flaps. **(E)** A two-flap palatoplasty can be combined with a Z-plasty of the soft palate.

preference for primary repair of complete clefts is to use a two-flap technique for the hard palate combined with a double opposing Z-plasty of the soft palate, or in the case of very wide clefts, a straight line repair with a radical levator transposition (Fig. 23.13). This approach has resulted in a very low fistula rate[126] and excellent speech results.

Two-stage palate repair

The problem of maxillary growth after cleft palate repair has led some surgeons to advocate a two-stage approach to palatoplasty, with earlier repair of the soft palate only and later repair of the hard palate. The general protocol, originally introduced by Schweckendiek and Doz,[127] entailed repair of the soft palate at the same time as the cleft lip repair, around

4–6 months. The hard palate was obturated and repaired at about 4–5 years of age. Earlier ages have subsequently been proposed for hard palate repair, usually around 18–24 months.[128]

The rationale for this approach has been that the hard palate cleft narrows during the time between procedures, requiring less dissection and thus resulting in less maxillary growth disturbance. Although it is appealing on a theoretical basis, numerous studies have shown significantly poorer speech results from these two-stage procedures, with marginal if any salutary effect on the growth of the maxilla.[129–131] As noted before, good speech outcomes become more difficult to achieve with increasing age, whereas most maxillary growth problems can be addressed with orthodontic treatment and, if needed, surgical maxillary advancement.

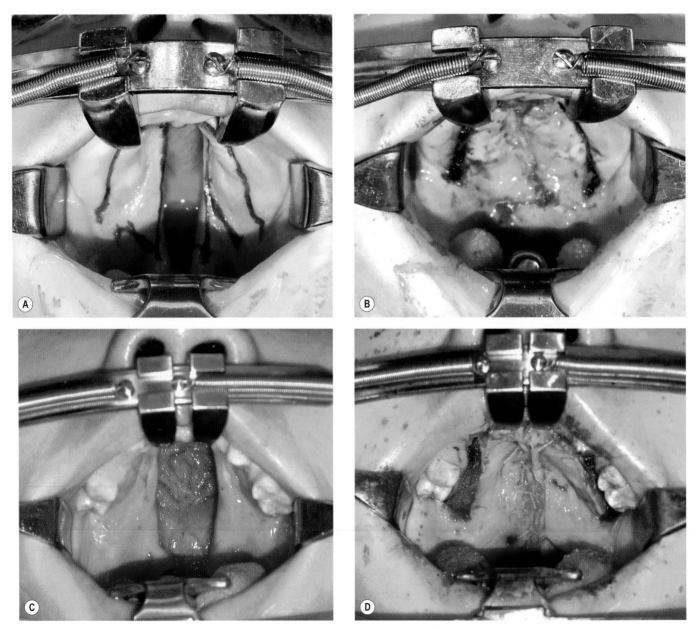

Fig. 23.13 Authors' general approach to technique selection. **(A)** Moderate width complete unilateral cleft lip and palate. **(B)** Two-flap palatoplasty combined with double opposing Z-plasty. The two-flap approach gives maximum mobilization of the mucoperiosteal flaps and is particularly effective for minimizing the occurrence of an anterior fistula. **(C)** Wide cleft of the secondary palate. **(D)** Two-flap palatoplasty with straight line soft palate closure and intravelar veloplasty.

Postoperative care

In the immediate postoperative period, breathing is the critical concern. The child with an open cleft palate has become accustomed to a larger than normal nasal airway, which is virtually occluded after cleft palate repair, especially with the introduction of a small amount of blood or mucus in the nose. Postoperative hypoxemia is not uncommon, but generally resolves after 24–48 h.[132] The use of a traction suture in the tongue during the immediate period after extubation may avoid the need for utilizing any oral devices for maintaining the airway. Some centers use nasal trumpets routinely to improve ventilation. Monitoring with continuous pulse oximetry and minimizing narcotic use will help to avoid catastrophic problems. Acetaminophen 15 mg/kg alternating with ibuprofen 10 mg/kg will usually give adequate pain relief. Recently, use of intravenous acetaminophen has been associated with decreased opioid requirements.[133] Any patient who has had prolonged surgery (over 2 h) with the mouth gag in place should be observed for at least 48 h for tongue edema. Some surgeons routinely release the mouth gag at set intervals throughout the procedure, analogous to releasing the tourniquet during hand surgery.

Children with Pierre Robin sequence are a special group. These and any other children with syndromes that may affect breathing must be observed closely, even in an intensive care unit setting, to be sure that there is no significant respiratory obstruction. Most Pierre Robin children stay additional time in the hospital for this reason.

Bleeding is not uncommon after palate repair. There are inevitably raw surfaces, which may ooze for 12–24 h. Hemostatic rolls (e.g., Surgicel) are sutured into raw areas by some surgeons to reduce postoperative bleeding (see Fig. 23.13B,D). Bleeding can also be reduced by surgery that takes less than 90–120 min because the epinephrine will still have some effect during emergence from anesthesia. Light pressure on the hard palate repair at the conclusion of the procedure will often control bleeding when necessary. The authors have found that application of ice packs to the posterior neck is almost always effective in stopping postoperative bleeding in recovery or on the ward; this is a technique that has not been documented previously but has been used by experienced surgeons.[134]

Postoperative feeding is generally limited to liquids for 10–14 days, to prevent particulate matter lodging in the areas that are left open at the end of the procedure. Reducing or stopping intravenous fluids the morning after surgery causes some thirst, and almost all patients start to take adequate liquids under these circumstances. The parents must learn to time feeding 30 min or so after analgesic administration.

Arm splints may be used as well to prevent children from putting their fingers or, more likely, foreign objects in the mouth.

Outcomes of cleft palate repair

Fistula

Fistula formation is one complication that has been studied in some detail. Fistulas may be a source of persistent nasal air loss even in the face of a functioning soft palate; they are also a source of nasal regurgitation of fluids. In one particularly extensive review of fistulas at a single institution, use of the Furlow repair was shown to markedly reduce fistulas relative to the V-Y pushback or von Langenbeck technique. The width of the cleft was the other factor in this multivariate analysis.[110] Late closure of fistulas may be difficult, especially in the hard palate, and two-layer closure with lining turnover and the use of large mucoperiosteal flaps or facial artery musculomucosal (FAMM) flaps[135] on the oral side are recommended to give the best outcome. Closure of fistulas at the soft–hard palate junction can also be incorporated into double opposing Z-plasty palate-lengthening procedures when indicated for treatment of velopharyngeal insufficiency (Fig. 23.14 ⊕).[136] If there is reason for delay of repair, a palatal plate may aid in obturating a fistula for speech purposes until surgical correction can be achieved.

Fig. 23.14 appears online only.

Speech outcomes/velopharyngeal insufficiency

Normal speech is the primary goal of cleft palate repair. Specifically this refers to the lack of velopharyngeal insufficiency (VPI) and nasal air loss in speech. It can be difficult to interpret some studies, as it is common that "good" and "excellent" results are grouped together, or that the nasality is rated on a numerical scale. In general, it is preferable to look at the presence or absence of nasality and ideally to use a binary outcome measure for analysis.

In the majority of studies in which some form of muscle repair is utilized, good speech results are obtained about 85–90% of the time. These results are in non-syndromic cleft patients; syndromic patients will always have poorer results for a variety of reasons, but their good outcomes may be in the 50–60% range. It appears that width of cleft is related to outcome, as bilateral clefts often have worse speech outcomes, but there have been few studies looking at this in detail.

Some studies have examined the long-term stability of speech outcomes. In some patients, nasality may develop in puberty or later, probably related to involution of the adenoid pad, but this is rare in our experience.

Maxillary growth

Normal maxillary growth is a secondary goal of palate repair. While some orthodontists might contest this, it is much more difficult to correct nasal speech after puberty than to perform a LeFort I maxillary advancement. It is clear that avoidance of large, raw surfaces on the hard palate will improve maxillary growth long term, and that minimizing scar tissue will have a salutary effect as well. However, the use of relaxing incisions has not been shown to independently affect maxillary growth or to induce posterior crossbite.[137] Fistula formation requiring additional procedures will increase scar tissue and often decrease maxillary growth.

The need for maxillary advancement is highly variable, from 10–40% in non-syndromic cleft patients. Because different centers have different surgeons as well as different protocols, it is difficult to tease out the critical differences in practice that might account for these variations in outcome. Wider clefts and bilateral clefts have a higher rate of maxillary hypoplasia, possibly related to greater need for dissection at the time of palate repair.[138]

It is clear that syndromic patients have a higher rate of maxillary hypoplasia, which may well be genetically determined. In our review of van der Woude syndrome, the need for maxillary advancement was about 85% compared to less than 10% in a matched group of non-syndromic unilateral cleft patients.

Conclusion

Cleft palate repair has undergone major changes in the past quarter century. Overall, results have improved as far as speech outcomes; this is probably due to the growth of centers for cleft care as well as to refinement of techniques. The team approach has decreased the number of operations needed to obtain better outcomes as the surgeon has gained knowledge from the other specialists involved in cleft care. The increased application of methods that incorporate reconstruction of the levator palatini muscle has produced much more predictable speech results. Current trends of earlier surgical intervention for cleft palate and presurgical alignment of the dental arches should result in still more predictable outcomes.

 Bonus images for this chapter can be found online at
http://www.expertconsult.com

Fig. 23.2 Kernahan's (left) and Veau's (right) classification of clefts allows for standardized reporting of the severity of both cleft lip and palate.
Fig. 23.14 Palatal fistulas. **(A)** Fistula in hard palate. **(B)** Large mucoperiosteal flap for oral closure. **(C)** Repaired fistula. **(D)** Fistula in anterior hard palate and alveolus. **(E)** Left facial artery musculomucosal (FAMM) flap for oral closure. **(F)** Repaired fistula. **(G)** Fistula at junction of hard and soft palate. **(H)** Fistula closure incorporated into double opposing Z-plasty palate lengthening.

 Access the complete reference list online at   **http://www.expertconsult.com**

14. Huang MH, Lee ST, Rajendran K. A fresh cadaveric study of the paratubal muscles: implications for Eustachian tube function in cleft palate. *Plast Reconstr Surg.* 1997;100:833–842. *Cadaveric dissections were performed to clarify possible ramifications of palatal clefting on Eustachian tube function. Functional hypotheses are drawn from morphological findings.*

44. Kaplan EN. The occult submucous cleft palate. *Cleft Palate J.* 1975;12:356–368.

46. Chen PK-T, Wu J, Hung KF, et al. Surgical correction of submucous cleft palate with Furlow palatoplasty. *Plast Reconstr Surg.* 1996;97:1136–1146. *Sleep apnea is a recognized adverse outcome of pharyngeal flaps performed for velopharyngeal insufficiency (VPI). This report demonstrates that Furlow palatoplasty is a reliable alternative to pharyngeal flaps for the correction of VPI in the context of submucous cleft palate.*

47. Robin P. Glossoptosis due to atresia and hypotrophy of the mandible. *Am J Dis Child.* 1934;48:541–547.

60. Denny AD, Talisman R, Hanson PR, et al. Mandibular distraction osteogenesis in very young patients to correct airway obstruction. *Plast Reconstr Surg.* 2001;108:302–311. *This clinical series correlates airway measurements before and after distraction with functional outcomes. The authors conclude that distraction improves tongue base position such that airway space is effectively increased.*

63. Figueroa AA, Glupker TJ, Fitz MG, et al. Mandible, tongue, and airway in Pierre Robin sequence: a longitudinal cephalometric study. *Cleft Palate Craniofac J.* 1991;28:425–434.

94. Bardach J. The influence of cleft lip repair on facial growth. *Cleft Palate J.* 1990;27:76–78.

117. Cutting C, Rosenbaum J, Rovati L. The technique of muscle repair in the soft palate. *Operative Techniques Plast Surg.* 1995;2:215–222.

120. Furlow LT Jr. Cleft palate repair by double opposing Z-plasty. *Plast Reconstr Surg.* 1986;78:724–738. *Furlow describes his palatoplasty in the context of a 22-patient case series. Optimistic speech outcomes are reported.*

128. Rohrich RJ, Byrd HS. Optimal timing of cleft palate closure. Speech, facial growth, and hearing considerations. *Clin Plast Surg.* 1990;17:27–36.

136. Emory RE Jr, Clay RP, Bite U, et al. Fistula formation and repair after palatal closure: an institutional perspective. *Plast Reconstr Surg.* 1997;99:1535–1538. *The authors report an 11.5% post-palatoplasty fistula rate. Local flaps are advocated to repair these lesions.*

24

Alveolar clefts

Richard A. Hopper and Gerhard S. Mundinger

Access video content for this chapter online at expertconsult.com

SYNOPSIS

- Treatment of the alveolar cleft remains one of the most controversial topics in cleft care.
- Treatment protocols have varied in timing, technique, and selection of graft material.
- Currently the "gold standard" is secondary bone grafting with autogenous cancellous graft at the time of mixed dentition.
- Outcomes of proposed alternate treatments such as gingivoperiosteoplasty, primary bone grafting, and use of inductive proteins need to be compared to documented outcomes of the gold standard.
- Regardless of which technique is employed, coordination and communication between surgeon and orthodontist are essential for success.
- Failed or complex alveolar bone graft sites remain a considerable challenge. These recalcitrant alveolar clefts can benefit from recent applications of distraction osteogenesis techniques.

 Access the Historical Perspective section online at
http://www.expertconsult.com

Introduction

- Compared to soft-tissue repair techniques, surgery on the bony alveolar defect in cleft lip and palate patients is relatively new.
- Early approaches including primary grafting in infancy fell into disfavor due to iatrogenic impairment of facial growth.
- Secondary bone grafting in mixed dentition and primary gingivoperiosteoplasty (GPP) were introduced in the 1960s.
- Secondary bone grafting has become the gold standard for comparison of other techniques.
- Primary bone grafting and GPP remain controversial.

Basic science/disease process

Anatomy of the alveolar cleft

The alveolar cleft is more than a linear gap in the maxillary arch. With soft tissue removed, the cleft is best visualized as a tornado, increasing in size from incisal to apical, becoming widest as it extends into the nasal cavity and distorts the surrounding anatomy (Fig. 24.1). The soft-tissue distortion caused by this skeletal deficiency can be minimized by a correctly performed cleft lip repair, but not completely eradicated. In the patient with an untreated alveolar cleft, the alar base of the nose lacks the bony support of the non-cleft side, and if release of the lateral nasal wall and reconstruction of the nasal component of the orbicularis oris muscle have not been achieved at the primary lip repair, the nasal base will remain attached to the hypoplastic piriform rim, with inferior and posterior malposition.

The fistula between oral and nasal cavities has three distinct boundaries. The nasolabial fistula is located at the apex of the cleft, high up in the labial sulcus, and consists of loose wet labial mucosa transitioning to nasal mucosa. The oronasal fistula extends from the incisive foramen to the alveolar process, and is a transition of attached palatal mucoperiosteum to nasal mucosa. At the corner of these two fistulas, at the alveolar process itself, attached alveolar gingiva is located, which is the only appropriate support lining of erupting teeth. Whichever technique is employed to close the soft tissues of the nasolabial and oronasal fistulas, attached gingival tissue must be present at the anticipated site of eruption to ensure long-term support of the adult teeth.

Dental development

An alveolar cleft is associated with variable anomalies in dental development that must be taken into consideration with presurgical preparation, timing of surgery, surgical technique, and post-surgical orthodontic planning. Anomalies

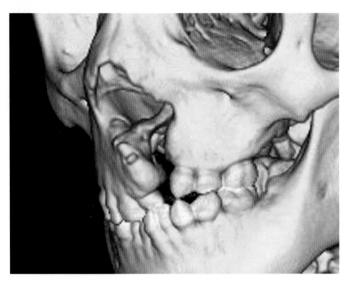

Fig. 24.1 Bony anatomy of an untreated unilateral cleft lip and palate in a 4-year-old. The lateral piriform rim is hypoplastic, increasing the width of the piriform opening on the cleft side, creating a tornado-shaped defect. The maxillary nasal crest is deviated away from the cleft, carrying the bony septum with it. The collapse of the ungrafted maxillary arch is apparent with a lingual crossbite of the lesser segment.

can include the number of teeth (missing teeth, supernumerary teeth), the location (mesial or distal to cleft), the shape (pegged or conical), the size (microdontic), the time of formation and/or eruption, and crown and root malformations.[9,10]

A goal of successful alveolar cleft treatment is to provide a stable supporting environment for eruption of the permanent canine. The adjacent lateral incisor, however, must be taken into consideration prior to surgery with a coordinated surgical–orthodontic plan. The lateral incisor is often missing in complete clefts; however, if present, it can be positioned either mesial or distal to the cleft. Although still debated, many consider the lateral incisor to be supernumerary when distal.[11]

It is important that the patient and family be informed before the bone graft procedure that in many cases a permanent lateral incisor is congenitally absent, will not erupt, or will be extracted as part of the treatment protocol.[12–15] If needed, the lateral incisor is extracted to create space for the permanent canine to migrate and erupt through the newly grafted area. The orthodontist can then perform canine substitution of the lateral incisor if it was absent or not supernumerary.

Diagnosis/patient presentation

Gingivoperiosteoplasty

Prior to undergoing a GPP, the infant with a cleft must be evaluated by the practitioner coordinating the presurgical molding, as well as the surgeon who will be performing the GPP. It must be emphasized that not all infants will be candidates for GPP due to individual variations of anatomy. Some infants with particularly wide unilateral clefts can be "mesenchymally deficient". Compressing and closing the alveolar

cleft with molding and a GPP would unnaturally constrict the arch form. Isolated clefts of the primary palate are also difficult to predict if a GPP is possible. Due to the bony fusion of the secondary palate, the alveolar segments are more resistant to presurgical molding, and in some cases cannot be adequately aligned. Finally, in bilateral complete clefts, it is not always possible to align both sides of the premaxilla with the alveolar segments. In this case, one alveolar cleft can undergo a GPP to convert the arch form to a lesser and greater segment similar to a unilateral cleft. Assessment of parallel alveolar molding can be difficult, and benefits from a team presurgical evaluation (Fig. 24.2). If the alveolar anatomy and presurgical molding outcome are favorable, a GPP can be offered to the family at the same time as the primary lip repair.

Primary bone grafting

Grafting at the time of primary dentition is practiced by relatively few centers, with the most published group being that of Rosenstein and Dado, who have used primary grafting as their approach to the alveolar cleft for over 20 years. Patient selection is based on the family's ability to undertake the staged surgical and orthodontic appliance protocol necessary to maintain arch relationship before and after grafting.[16]

Secondary bone grafting

As the patient is approaching the time of secondary bone graft, the craniofacial orthodontist and surgeon should discuss plans for timing of the graft, the fate of adjacent teeth, and the timing of arch expansion. Any dental morbidity such as poor hygiene or caries should be addressed by a pediatric dentist prior to the surgery. In some cases, primary teeth adjacent to the cleft should be extracted 3–6 weeks prior to grafting in order to ensure a viable mucosal seal of the oral surface of the grafted area. In most cases, however, the teeth can be preserved until the time of grafting to maximize bone retention, avoid an additional procedure, and be extracted at the grafting surgery.

Arch expansion can be performed either before or after the graft surgery. Preoperative arch expansion allows the orthodontist to take full advantage of the mobility of the two or three ungrafted segments of the alveolus to achieve appropriate maxillary anterior and posterior arch width. When the graft is then placed and heals in the expanded cleft, the continuous maxillary arch form has an optimal relationship with the mandible. A collapsed overlapping alveolar cleft can also benefit from expansion by increasing the access and visibility of the surgeon to the fistula at time of operation. The disadvantages of presurgical expansion, however, include overexpansion, such that the alveolar cleft becomes challenging to treat due to simultaneous expansion of the oronasal fistula and resulting excessive tension on any soft-tissue repair. If an expander is in place at the time of surgery and obstructs the site, then replacement of the device with a custom acrylic retention splint at the time of surgery is indicated. Postoperative expansion should wait 6–8 weeks from the date of surgery, and conventional orthodontic movements should not be attempted before the cleft is grafted, but can start within 3 weeks of surgery.

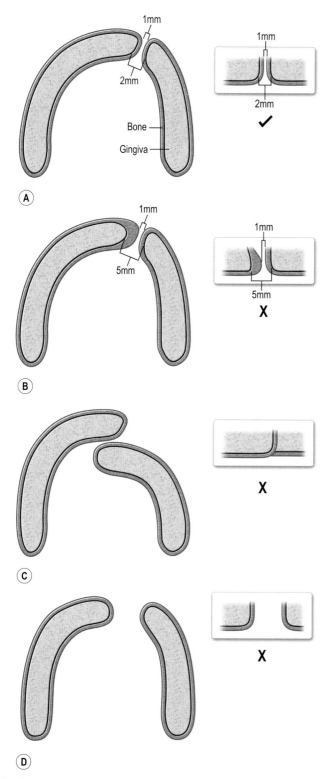

Fig. 24.2 (A) An appropriately molded unilateral alveolar cleft candidate for gingivoperiosteoplasty (GPP). There is parallel alignment of the alveolar cleft edges with a smooth arch form. (B) Gingival hypertrophy in the alveolar cleft is masking a bone gap that is too wide for a GPP. (C) A collapsed arch form not amenable to GPP. Although the edges are touching, the opposing bone segments within the cleft are not aligned for bone formation. (D) A mesenchymal-deficient arch form that should not undergo GPP. If this cleft was approximated with molding followed by a GPP that formed a bone fusion, it would unnaturally constrict the projection of the alveolar arch. Arch expansion with bone grafting of the alveolar gap is the indicated treatment.

Debate continues regarding the appropriate timing of secondary bone grafting. The mixed dentition phase is variable among patients, but typically falls between ages 6 and 11 years. Proponents of grafting early in mixed dentition believe that a stable, healed graft prior to canine eruption results in a superior bone environment (Fig. 24.3). El Deeb et al.[17] found that successful eruption of cuspids though the graft occurred when root formation of the canine adjacent to the cleft was one-fourth to one-half formed at the time of graft placement. Bergland et al.[18] found a higher proportion of graft failures and cases with lower interdental septa when grafting was done adjacent to fully erupted teeth compared to just before eruption. In comparison, Long et al. retrospectively performed detailed periapical radiograph analysis of bone formation and found no significant correlation between final graft success and the amount of canine crown eruption in the cleft at the time of grafting.[19]

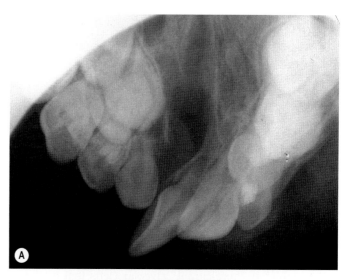

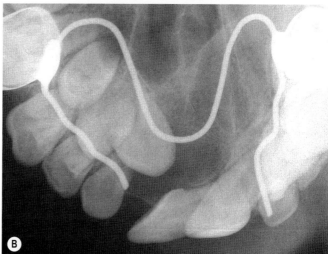

Fig. 24.3 (A) A unilateral alveolar cleft in mixed dentition ready for preoperative arch expansion and secondary bone grafting. The permanent canine is descending but is still covered with bone. The cleft extends from the alveolus up into the piriform cavity. (B) The same cleft after preoperative palate expansion and successful autogenous bone grafting. With the expansion and with orthodontic uprighting of the adjacent central incisor, there will be sufficient bone support and space for the erupting permanent canine.

Bone morphogenetic protein-2

Recombinant human bone morphogenetic protein-2 (rhBMP2) is a mitogen that has been demonstrated to stimulate osteoblastic activity and induce bone nodule formation in animals. It has been approved by the US Food and Drug Administration for clinical use in human spine fusion procedures, and has been shown to decrease nonunion, donor site morbidity, and operating time over autogenous grafting in this population.[20] More recent clinical applications have been on patients undergoing alveolar augmentation and implant placement,[21] and early trials at individual centers for the treatment of alveolar clefts have been completed. The risk–benefit profile of rhBMP2 in these patients remains largely unknown, and elucidation thereof will require further high-quality randomized controlled trials.[22]

Late bone grafting

Some centers have advocated delaying alveolar bone grafting in patients who are known to need a LeFort I osteotomy procedure at skeletal maturity in order to perform both simultaneously. This, however, has largely been abandoned in the presence of an erupting canine, since eruption into a bone graft is felt to provide better bone support and periodontal status.[12]

However, in any cleft center, patients can present in permanent dentition without having had their alveolar cleft treated. In these cases, a combined segmental orthognathic and bone grafting procedure is required. Outcomes of these techniques are not as favorable as grafting in mixed dentition followed by dental eruption into the graft and orthodontic movement.

Alveolar distraction

Successful primary or secondary treatment of the alveolar cleft should obviate the need for alveolar distraction in this patient population. Unfortunately there exist patients with "ungraftable" or "recalcitrant" alveolar clefts that have few options available to them other than undergoing transport distraction osteogenesis (TDO) of alveolar bone.[23] The typical patient who falls into this category has unhealthy, scarred gingiva, a large nasolabial and/or oronasal fistula, and a history of repeated unsuccessful bone grafts with infections and exposure. Another possible presentation is a previously grafted maxilla that has severe vertical deficiency along with scarred mucogingiva preventing additional graft augmentation. In both these cases, TDO is a useful tool to have in the cleft armamentarium.

In the wide "ungraftable" cleft patient (Fig. 24.4), a tooth-bearing transport segment can be slowly moved into the gap, closing the fistula and converting the problem into a narrow cleft amenable to traditional secondary grafting. In the vertically deficient alveolus (Fig. 24.5), a transport segment of superior maxillary bone, with or without prior bone augmentation, can be slowly lowered, leveling the alveolar ridge by gradually bringing the scarred attached gingival tissue along with the advancing bone front.

Factors that may have contributed to previous failed surgeries in patients with "recalcitrant" clefts must be carefully considered to avoid the plan for TDO suffering the same fate. Any dental caries or periapical disease must be addressed to minimize the infection risk during the period when the device

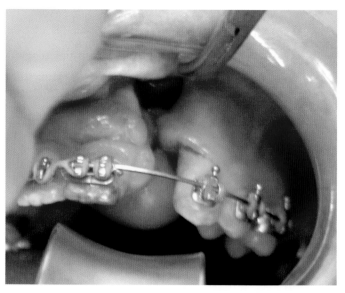

Fig. 24.4 A good candidate for interdental horizontal transport distraction. The patient had undergone three previous attempts at treatment of bilateral alveolar clefts, including transfer of a facial artery musculomucosal (FAMM) flap, seen hanging from the anterior palate. The patient has extensive scarring and a large tornado-shaped oronasal and nasolabial fistula. The recommended treatment was simultaneous closure of the nasal lining using the FAMM flap tissue with transport distraction of a three-tooth segment from the lesser segments, as shown in Fig. 24.10, followed by secondary bone grafting of the residual cleft.

is in place. Alcohol, smoking, and drug abuse must be ruled out, and the expectations on the patient must be discussed and documented. All current distraction devices require activation by the patient or caregiver and frequent follow-up during the period of activation. Therefore, a patient who is considered unreliable, non-compliant, or unable to return to clinic regularly is not a suitable candidate. TDO is currently

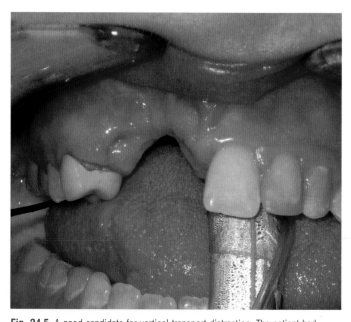

Fig. 24.5 A good candidate for vertical transport distraction. The patient had undergone six previous attempts of alveolar grafting with infection and graft loss. The result was vertical deficiency of the alveolus, loss of the adjacent three permanent teeth, and tight scarred gingival covering. The patient underwent staged cortical grafting and vertical transport distraction, as shown in Fig. 24.12.

reserved for patients past mixed dentition due to the risk to unerupted tooth follicles during the segmental osteotomies. Coordination with the patient's orthodontist or prosthodontist is essential in order to agree upon the desired goals of the procedure and the endpoint of activation. Frequently the treatment plan may include arch expansion or tooth extraction, which should be performed prior to the TDO procedure. Written directions and a device-turning log should be carefully explained to the patient to avoid complications during activation. Dental hygiene must be maintained during activation with perioperative chlorhexidine mouthwash and a soft toothbrush.

Treatment/surgical technique

Gingivoperiosteoplasty

The GPP can be performed at any point of the primary cleft lip repair, but is easiest after all other dissection has been completed, and before repair of the lip elements. The "roof" of the GPP is the repair of the anterior palate (nasal floor) from the nasal sill back to the incisive foramen that is typically done with most modern cleft lip repairs. This is achieved by suturing the inferior edge of the reconstructed lateral nasal wall to a superiorly based mucoperiosteal vomer flap (nasal flap) (Fig. 24.6). The incision along the vomer to create the leading edge of the vomer flap is at the level of the oral–nasal mucosa demarcation. This demarcation is also visible on the opposing lateral nasal wall. The vomer flap vertical dissection is kept to the minimum needed to achieve closure of the nasal floor. After the mucosal incision, most of the vomer dissection can be achieved with an elevator, with the exception of the region of the premaxillary suture, which will require sharp dissection with a small blade. This nasal floor closure separates the nasal from the oral cavity back to the incisive foramen and provides the superior barrier of the guided tissue regeneration tunnel between the alveolar segments.

The "floor" of the GPP tunnel is created by elevating inferiorly based mucoperiosteal flaps from the oral edges of the alveolar cleft (oral flaps). These flaps are contained within the cleft itself, and extend from the labial surface of the alveolus back to the incisive foramen. They are typically 2–3 mm in vertical height, such that when they are inferiorly rotated, they meet across the oral boundary of the cleft and can be sutured together with everting resorbable 5-0 gut or Vicryl sutures.

The attached mucoperiosteum that remains within the alveolar cleft between the superior anteroposterior incision made to create the nasal closure flaps and the inferior one made to create the oral closure is the tissue used to close the anterior border of the GPP. The alveolar cleft can be visualized as a pyramid with the apex at the incisive foramen, where the superior and inferior vomer incisions converge. Anteriorly, these two incisions diverge, creating anteriorly based triangular flaps that are brought out from between the alveolar segments, pedicled anteriorly, and flipped across the cleft, closing the labial border of the GPP (labial flaps). In designing the GPP flaps, the incisions on one side of the cleft are shifted slightly superiorly, so that the labial flap covers the upper half

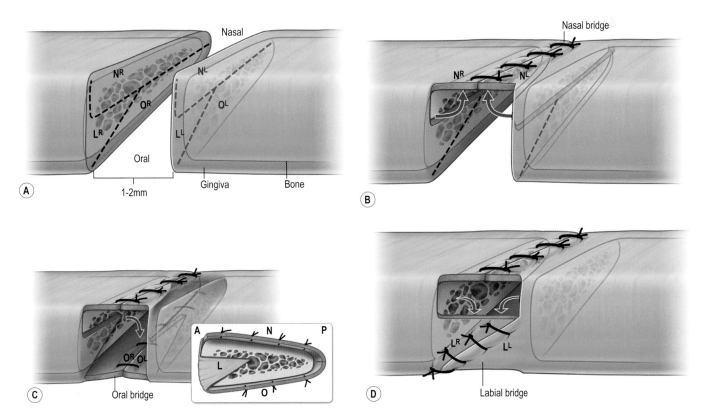

Fig. 24.6 Gingivoperiosteal flap design and elevation for the Millard-type gingivoperiosteoplasty. The dissection is limited to the tissues within the cleft. The flaps are named by the part of the periosteal tunnel they construct. See text for details. L^R, right labial flap; O^R, right oral flap; N^R, right nasal flap; L^L, left labial flap; O^L, left oral flap; N^L, left nasal flap; A, anterior; P, posterior.

of the labial border of the cleft, while on the contralateral side, the incisions are shifted inferiorly for the labial flap to cover the lower half. The superior edge of the upper labial flap is sutured to the lip mucosa, and the inferior edge of the lower labial flap is sutured to the anterior edge of the two oral flaps. In this fashion, a guided tissue regeneration "chamber" is sealed nasally, orally, and labially by mucoperiosteal flaps, and contains two opposing bone surfaces on the mesial and distal walls. It is essential that this end goal is visualized throughout the GPP procedure to ensure that all soft-tissue interference is removed from the alveolar cleft during creation of the flaps, and that the flaps are positioned correctly to direct bone growth across the cleft.

Technical pitfalls of the GPP include: elevation of the flaps in a submucosal instead of subperiosteal plane; inaccurate planning of flaps such that viability of the anteriorly based labial flaps is compromised; and trauma to the flaps from compressive handling with forceps. Frequently, a deciduous tooth follicle is encountered during the flap dissection. Careful sharp dissection between the follicle and the periosteum is required to prevent disruption of dental eruption. If the flaps appear too thin or non-viable during the follicle dissection, the GPP should be aborted and the mucosa replaced.

Primary bone grafting

Protocols for primary bone grafting vary, but typically involve a staged approach of molding the maxillary arch segments in the first year of life followed by stabilization of the maxillary arch with an autogenous bone graft in infancy. In the protocol used by Rosenstein and Dado, a maxillary appliance is used prior to lip repair to align the alveolar segments.[16,24] Following a lip repair at 6–8 weeks of age, the appliance is modified to prevent posterior collapse of arch width while allowing the repaired lip musculature to mold and close the anterior cleft as a "butt joint". Once the cleft is molded to approximation, at around 4–6 months, the segments are stabilized with an autogenous split rib graft. The appliance is continued for 6–8 weeks post-surgery and the palate is closed at or before 1 year of age.

Secondary bone grafting

When performing secondary bone grafting, we recommend chlorhexidine mouthwash and nasal antibiotic ointment in the days before surgery to decrease the bacterial load. The patient is positioned supine with a small support under the posterior iliac crest to facilitate bone graft harvest. There should be two sterile fields to avoid contamination between the oral field and donor field.

We follow a modification of the technique described by Abyholm *et al.*[25] (Fig. 24.7 and Video 24.1 ▶). A superiorly based mucoperiosteal flap is raised off the lesser segment of the alveolus with a back cut into the loose mucosa anterior to Stenson's duct. If the site immediately adjacent to the cleft has sufficient attached gingiva, this is included in the tip of the flap. If not, the attached gingiva of the one or two teeth distal to the cleft must be included in the flap, and when the flap is advanced, the papillae are shifted by one tooth width towards the cleft.

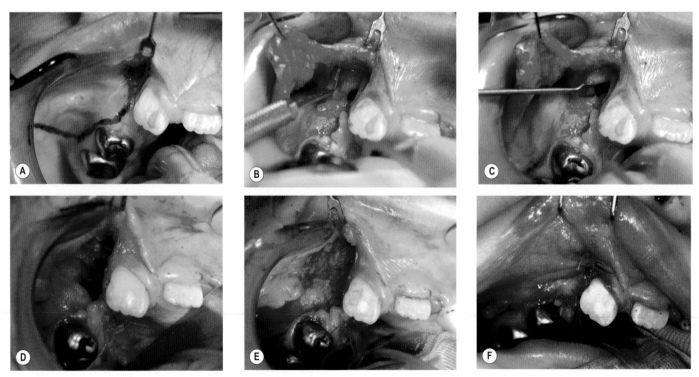

Fig. 24.7 Modified Abyholm technique for secondary bone grafting of a unilateral alveolar cleft. See text for details. **(A)** The superior-based lesser-segment flap for labial surface closure has been marked. The tip is covered with attached gingiva for transfer into the cleft. **(B)** The flap is raised off the lesser segment in a subperiosteal plane and cleft mucosa separated from the labial mucosa with an angled blade. **(C)** The opposing surfaces of mucosa within the cleft have been separated from alveolus to incisive foramen. The superior flaps (hook in place) are used to repair the nasal lining. **(D)** The two reflected superior mucosal flaps have been sutured together to close the nasal fistula and the two inferior flaps closed to repair the oral fistula. **(E)** Cancellous iliac crest bone graft has been packed within the cleft. **(F)** The lesser-segment mucoperiosteal flap is transposed across the labial surface of the graft without tension. The frenum was released secondarily.

The lesser-segment flap is raised in a subperiosteal plane and then mobilized by performing a periosteal release across the undersurface of the flap, parallel to the occlusal surface, approximately 2.5 cm from the inferior edge. Since the periosteum contributes to the perfusion of the flap, the further the release is performed from the edges of the flap, the better. This periosteal release is continued towards the cleft separating the labial mucosa from the cleft mucosa. For this release of labial mucosa, an angled blade is used to undermine the incision at the superior extent of the alveolar cleft labionasal fistula, taking care to cut up into the lip and not towards the nasal floor. This mobilizes the oral mucosa above the cleft along with the lesser-segment flap without violating the nasal cavity (see Fig. 24.7C).

The opposing alveolar cleft mucosal surfaces are then cut from incisive foramen to labial surface of the alveolus, separating them into upper (nasal lining) and lower (oral lining) flaps. The upper mucoperiosteal nasal lining flaps are reflected out of the cleft and up into the piriform aperture and sutured to each other with a small curved needle repairing the labionasal fistula (see Fig. 24.7D). If the space is too tight for a needle, the repair is done through the nose, passing a large needle from the nose into the cleft through one of the lining flaps, and then passing it back from the cleft into the nose through the opposing lining flap and tying the knot inside the nostril. The lower oral lining flaps within the cleft are then reflected down into the mouth, such that they can be closed to each other with everting sutures to repair the oronasal fistula. If the cleft is too wide, then anterior hard-palate tissue is raised as posteriorly based mucoperiosteal flaps pedicled on the greater palatine vessels, and sutured together to close the oral surface of the cleft without tension.

With closure of the oronasal fistula, the graft can now be harvested. Numerous donor sources of bone graft have been described,[26] but iliac crest cancellous bone graft is considered the gold standard (Fig. 24.8). After the skin incision, the dissection proceeds directly down to the cartilage cap of the crest, without any muscle dissection or stripping. The cartilaginous crest is opened as an H-shaped incision to gain access to the underlying cancellous bone. The bone is harvested using a curette or gouge and stored in blood. If a cortical strut is planned to "reconstruct" the pyriform rim and provide a barrier between the graft and nasal lining, it is harvested from the inner table of the ilium. The graft donor site is then packed with gel foam soaked with plain bupivacaine to minimize postoperative pain[27] and the cartilage tightly approximated prior to closing the skin.

If a cortical barrier strut is used, it is placed under the nasal lining repair, resting on the opposing edges of the piriform rim at the superior aspect of the cleft. The graft is then carefully packed into the prepared graft site, using a bone tamp to compress the pieces. If there is graft remaining after filling the cleft from incisive foramen to labial surface and from nasal lining to oral lining, the remaining bone is used to augment the deficient maxillary bone in the region of the cleft-side piriform rim. This onlay graft helps support the alar base of the nose, and can improve symmetry in the unilateral cleft nasal deformity. The lesser-segment mucoperiosteal buccal sulcus flap is then mesially advanced over the labial surface of the graft and carefully secured with fine resorbable sutures to the mesial alveolus and oral palate. The most common site of dehiscence is at the junction of the lesser-segment flap and the oral lining repair, often at the edge of the central incisor crown. Meticulous atraumatic suture technique must be used in this area.

Postoperative care includes gentle oral hygiene with a soft manual toothbrush and antibiotic mouthwash. A mechanical soft diet is followed for 6 weeks. Radiographic preservation of the graft is assessed with a periapical film at 8–10 weeks. If a small portion of the graft site becomes exposed in the early postoperative course, it can often be salvaged with debridement of the exposed bone chip and antibiotic rinses. If the entire graft itself becomes contaminated or purulent, it must

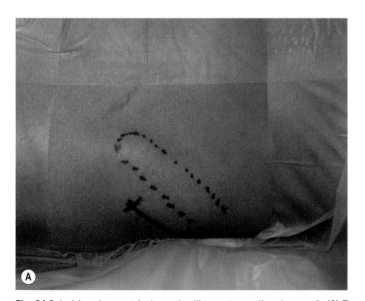
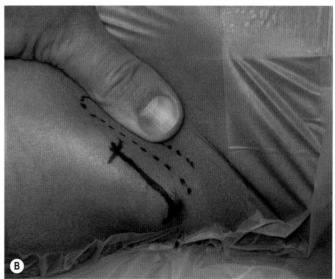

Fig. 24.8 Incision placement for harvesting iliac crest cancellous bone graft. **(A)** The anterior superior iliac spine and crest have been marked in dotted lines. **(B)** Upward traction is placed on the skin over the crest and the incision is marked along the iliac crest such that when the skin is released, the scar will lie off the crest and below the pant line. The incision should be 2 cm behind the anterior superior iliac crest to avoid iatrogenic damage to the lateral femoral cutaneous nerve. Excessive traction or transaction of the nerve will result in meralgia paresthetica.

be removed and the site allowed to heal before attempting a repeat graft.

For bilateral clefts, the same technique is used, but care must be taken to ensure that the U-shaped fistula behind the premaxilla is closed. If this has not been done adequately at the time of the palate repair, an angled blade is used to incise the posterior aspect of the premaxilla transversely, separating the mucosa into oral and nasal components. The nasal lining is repaired as in primary cases. The anterior hard-palate mucosa is then raised as unipedicled mucoperiosteal flaps and sutured to the oral mucosa of the posterior premaxilla. If the vascular supply of the premaxilla is tenuous, then the repair should be staged, doing each graft at different settings. Alveolar cleft repair can be staged with an initial soft-tissue oronasal fistula repair followed by standard bone grafting. A stabilization splint is essential for a bilateral cleft repair, or the mobility of the premaxilla post-surgery will prevent healing of the grafted clefts.

Occasionally at the time of bone grafting, unrestricted overgrowth at the premaxillary suture in patients with bilateral complete cleft lip and palate prevents the orthodontist from achieving the appropriate arch alignment needed for successful grafting. This can be seen in delayed or untreated clefts found in adopted children, when the lack of a repaired oral muscle sphincter did not mold the projecting premaxilla in early childhood. In these rare cases, premaxilla setback is required. This technique involves separating the premaxilla from the vomer and resecting a portion of the vomer and septum, allowing the entire premaxilla to be set back into alignment with the lesser segments (Fig. 24.9 and Video 24.2 ⊙).[28] This procedure carries the risk of necrosis of the premaxilla and loss of the anterior dentition, and should therefore only be performed when other options are not available.

Horizontal TDO of a tooth-bearing alveolar segment

This procedure is typically performed for a recalcitrant alveolar cleft with large oronasolabial fistula. The principle is to create a transport segment by separating an adjacent two- or three-tooth-bearing segment of the distal alveolus from the maxilla without damage to the tooth roots and without violation of the attached gingiva (Fig. 24.10). The distraction device is then applied to the stable maxilla and the transport segment with an anterior/mesial vector, such that when the device is activated, the segment gradually closes the alveolar cleft until it is touching the premaxilla. At this point, the remaining cleft is amenable to standard grafting techniques. The device is then left in place and not activated during the 8- to 12-week consolidation period, during which the generate formed in the distraction gap distal to the transport segment gradually ossifies and stabilizes the transport segment. For large naso-orolabial fistulas, performing the nasal lining closure at the time of the device placement may be easier due to the improved visibility and access via the wide cleft. As the transport segment advances and the cleft and fistula are compressed, the repaired nasal lining will fold on itself and seal any remaining small holes, allowing the secondary grafting procedure to focus solely on closing the oral lining.

Activation of the device is initiated 5 days post-operation at 0.5–1 mm/day. Orthodontic guidance can be provided with brackets and an arch wire as long as the direction dictated by the orthodontic force is not competing with the distraction vector; otherwise, the device footplates and screws will be under strain. When performing simultaneous bilateral distraction for bilateral clefts, care must be taken to control protrusion of the ungrafted premaxilla as the transport segments contact it towards the end of activation (Fig. 24.11). The device can be removed after 8–12 weeks of consolidation with simultaneous secondary grafting of the remaining approximated cleft.

Vertical alveolar TDO

Vertical alveolar TDO is useful for augmentation of a previously grafted cleft when the gingiva or previous surgeries have made augmentation with standard grafting techniques not possible (Fig. 24.12). Ten millimeters of vertical bone height below the maxillary sinus is the minimum required to perform an osteotomy and distraction without prior onlay grafting. If there is no or minimal bone below the maxilla, a cortical graft can be harvested as a separate procedure from the mandible angle, iliac crest, or outer calvarium and rigidly lag screwed as an onlay graft over the planned future osteotomy. The osteotomy and distraction can be performed 2–3 months later, transporting the increased bone volume from the incorporated onlay graft into the defect. The same activation and consolidation protocol for horizontal TDO is followed. During vertical distraction, however, the activation arm can often be covered with a custom temporary prosthesis created by the patient's prosthodontist.

Outcomes, prognosis, and complications

Gingivoperiosteoplasty

Long-term evaluation is now available of the Millard GPP protocol that used the Latham device to narrow the cleft such that a limited subperiosteal GPP could be performed. In evaluating their own patients, Millard et al.[29] found that a bony bridge formed in 63% of unilateral and 83% of bilateral clefts and a very low percentage (3%) required secondary bone grafting. An increase in anterior crossbite was reported in patients treated with GPP, but they did not seem to require orthognathic surgery more frequently than did controls, although the follow-up was admittedly too short to tell definitively.

Others, however, were less optimistic in their evaluations of these same patients. Henkel and Gundlach reported vertical growth disturbance of the maxilla in 42% of patients with unilateral and 40% of patients with bilateral clefts treated with Millard's technique.[30] Berkowitz analyzed the occlusion of these patients and found crossbites in 100% of patients treated with GPP, and he reported more difficulty in treating the crossbite deformity.[31] Matic and Power[32,33] retrospectively reviewed 65 unilateral and 43 bilateral clefts treated with Latham active molding and GPP. The clinical success rate compared to a historical group treated with secondary bone grafting was 41% for unilateral GPP and 58% for bilateral GPP, compared to 88% and 90% respectively for the secondary graft comparisons.

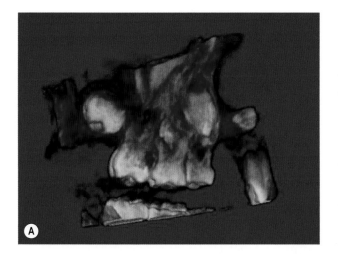

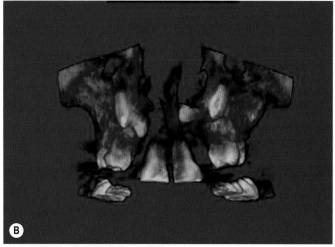

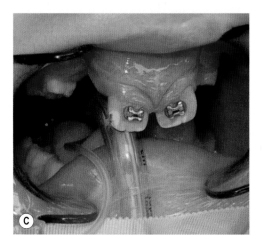

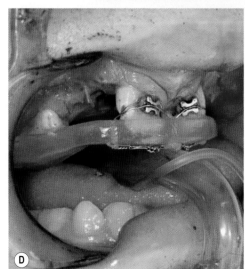

Fig. 24.9 Premaxillary impaction in a 7-year-old bilateral cleft patient with a low premaxillary occlusal plane. **(A)** Preoperative lateral three-dimensional cone beam CT image demonstrating extreme premaxillary position following maximal orthodontic alveolar expansion. **(B)** Preoperative anterior–posterior three-dimensional cone beam CT image. **(C)** Preoperative clinical appearance. **(D)** Following vomer osteotomy, the premaxilla was repositioned 6 mm superiorly based on an anterior gingival pedicle, and secured in place with a customized splint. The bilateral alveolar clefts were repaired as described in Fig. 24.7, and simultaneously bone grafted with iliac cancellous grafts.

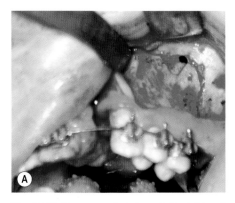

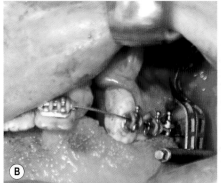

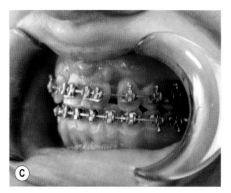

Fig. 24.10 The same patient shown in Fig. 24.4 undergoing horizontal alveolar transport distraction. See text for details. **(A)** An interdental osteotomy has been performed to create a three-tooth segment for transport. **(B)** The internal alveolar distraction device has been placed across the osteotomy. **(C)** Appearance post-distraction, consolidation, device removal, and secondary bone grafting. The patient is now ready for orthodontic alignment and dental restoration.

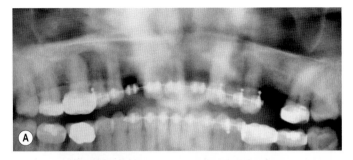

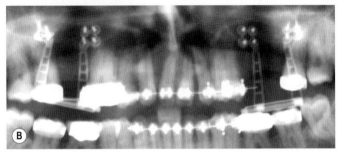

Fig. 24.11 Panorex radiograph of the bilateral transport distraction performed on the patient shown in Figs. 24.4 and 24.10. **(A)** On the left side, the patient had undergone a previous extraction, creating an ideal site for the interdental osteotomy. On the right side, the osteotomy is distal to the third tooth on the segment. **(B)** Post-activation, the canines are now adjacent to the central incisors and the alveolar clefts have been compressed. The distracted osteotomy contains generate tissue that will ossify during consolidation, effectively lengthening the maxillary arch.

Grayson et al.[34] described the use of nasoalveolar molding (NAM) instead of the Latham device to narrow the cleft prior to GPP, with the theory that the more passive "guided molding" of NAM would be less detrimental on future facial growth and dental relationship. In retrospectively examining their cohort at mixed dentition, they reported bone formation in 80% of clefts with 73% not requiring secondary bone grafting.[35,36] In evaluating facial growth, they found no adverse effect on midface growth during mixed dentition, and on repeat analysis up to 18 years of age.[37,38] Continued prospective evaluation of the NAM and GPP protocol at other

institutions will be required to determine if these results can be reproduced.

Primary bone grafting

On self-evaluation of this approach on 20 consecutive patients, Rosenstein et al.[24] reported no cephalometric evidence of impaired growth compared to a similar cohort who did not undergo primary grafting. Hathaway et al., at a separate center, retrospectively evaluated 17 patients who underwent primary grafting, and reported no difference in arch form compared to ungrafted clefts.[39] Ross evaluated cephalograms from 15 cleft centers and reported that grafting in infancy may have a negative effect on both vertical and horizontal midface growth, but it was not clear whether this was any greater than the effect of secondary bone grafting between the ages of 4 and 10 years.[40] The potential increased risk of exposing infants to an additional surgery and anesthesia in the first year of life must be weighed against the possible benefit of avoiding a secondary bone graft procedure in mixed dentition.[41]

Secondary bone grafting

Some of the most commonly used outcome measures for bone grafts are: the Bergland scale,[18] based on interdental height of bone; the bone height index,[42] based on the percentage of bone covering the roots of adjacent teeth; the Chelsea index,[43] measuring position and quality of bone; and the Kindelan bone-fill index,[44] which is a four-point scale of percentage bone infill. All but the last require eruption of the permanent cuspid before they can be used. In addition to the variability of outcome measures, there is wide variation in the literature in timing of evaluation, as well as limitations inherent to plain film analysis such as rotation variability. Some have proposed cone beam computed tomography as a superior method of graft evaluation.[45,46]

In the context of these study limitations, the success rate of secondary alveolar bone grafting in the literature ranges from 70% to 80% in most studies,[42,43,47,48] to over 90% in a few reports.[49–52] Scottish cleft services reported a dramatic increase in graft success from 58%[53] to 76%[54] as a presumed result of a reorganization that decreased the number of surgeons

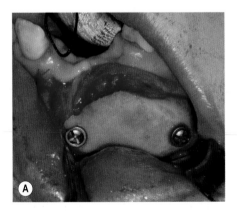

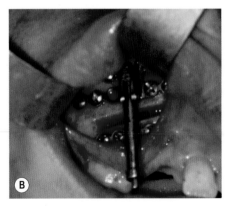

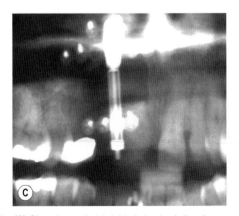

Fig. 24.12 The same patient shown in Fig. 24.5 undergoing vertical alveolar transport distraction. See text for details. **(A)** Since the vertical height of alveolus below the maxillary sinus was less than 10 mm, the site was augmented with an onlay autogenous split calvarial bone graft held in place with lag screws. **(B)** Three months later the lag screws are removed and a rectangular osteotomy is created within the consolidated graft. An internal vertical distractor has been placed across the osteotomy with a vector that will augment the vertical height of the alveolus and simultaneously lower the level of the gingival surface. **(C)** Radiograph of the device post-activation demonstrating alignment of the transport segment with the adjacent gum line. The generated tissue within the superior osteotomy site will consolidate over 2 months.

performing bone grafts and the establishment of nationally followed standard protocols.

Bone morphogenetic protein-2

Although a number of retrospective studies have shown promising results comparing rhBMP2 in combination with various non-autologous bone scaffolds to autologous iliac crest bone grafting for isolated alveolar cleft repair,[55–57] only four prospective randomized trials have been reported.[58–61]

The first randomized trial of 21 skeletally mature patients with a unilateral cleft alveolar defect showed that patients treated with a collagen sponge soaked in rhBMP2 demonstrated improved bone healing, and reduced donor morbidity and cost compared to those filled with autogenous iliac crest cancellous graft.[58] This group did not trial rhBMP2 in growing patients in mixed dentition due to their previous animal studies that demonstrated ectopic bone formation in 1%, as well as the high success rate of conventional autogenous grafting in this age group.

The second randomized trial compared rhBMP2 collagen matrices and iliac crest bone grafting in 16 patients aged 8–12 years with unilateral clefts.[59] This study demonstrated significantly lesser bone height in the BMP group at 1 year follow-up as determined by computed tomography (CT) analysis. Bone filling was equivalent, as was tooth eruption. There was a greater incidence of significant swelling (37.5%) in the BMP group, and 87.5% of patients in the iliac crest group reported postoperative pain. Lengths of stay and surgical costs were not reported in this study.

A more recent follow-up study including patients aged 8–15 years by this center compared three groups (rhBMP2 collagen matrices; iliac crest bone grafting; and GPP) of six patients each.[60] This trial demonstrated equivalency between rhBMP2 and iliac crest bone grafting in terms of bone volume, bone formation, maxillary height, and formed bone density at 12 months as evidenced by CT analysis. Complications, lengths of stay, and surgical costs were not reported.

A fourth randomized trial from Sweden compared rhBMP2 hydrogel to iliac crest bone grafts in 8–11-year-old unilateral cleft patients.[61] In a total of four patients in the rhBMP2 arm, the authors found that an rhBMP2 concentration of 50 µg/mL failed to form bone, while patients receiving hydrogels with an rhBMP2 concentration of 250 µg/mL experienced severe postoperative gingival swelling, leading to premature trial closure. Surgical times and hospital stays were lower in the rhBMP2 group, but not significantly so.

Of note, only the first randomized trial[58] was available for evaluation in a recent Cochrane review.[22] This first study met inclusion criteria and was evaluated as a legitimate randomized controlled trial. It remains unclear if the remaining three trials would meet stringent Cochran Collaboration criteria.

Although rhBMP2 shows promise in reducing healthcare costs and donor site morbidity, cognizance of reported complications of rhBMP2, including ectopic bone formation, bone resorption or remodeling at the graft site, hematoma, neck swelling, painful seromas, and severe gingival swelling, which led to the premature closure of one randomized clinical trial,[61] is paramount. Additional theoretical concerns include carcinogenicity and teratogenic effects.[62] The risk–benefit profile of rhBMP2 in cleft patients will likely remain unknown for the next decade, pending results of additional high-quality randomized controlled trials. Patient selection should, therefore, be based on enrollment in an institutional review board (IRB)-approved trial with appropriate consent and evaluation, including oversight by an independent data safety monitoring board.

Late bone grafting

When an alveolar cleft is bone-grafted before eruption of the cuspid, there is more than 80% chance of success, and the result provides adequate long-term periodontal support. With age, this success rate drops sharply, approaching 50% at 25 years of age.[25,63] Grafting after eruption of permanent dentition also does not correct periodontal defects (i.e., inadequate periodontal ligament), even with subsequent orthodontic movement into the graft.

The goal of grafting in adults is therefore no longer to provide support for erupted teeth, but rather to provide sufficient bone stock for prosthetic placement. In addition, the adult alveolar cleft is typically larger due to the poor health and loss of adjacent teeth. The technique of grafting an adult cleft involves rigid fixation of a corticocancellous graft with either resorbable or titanium fixation. Due to the slower incorporation of this graft architecture, an increased attention to the vascularity of the mucoperiosteal flaps and the nasal closure is essential. The cleft is also minimized by segmental maxillary osteotomies and advancement of the posterior segment into the cleft. In bilateral clefts, staging the surgery may be necessary. Implant placement should take place 3–4 months post-grafting to avoid loss of the graft.

Graft site augmentation

As with all bone, the alveolar graft requires mechanical stimulation to avoid resorption. Eruption of teeth into the graft and orthodontic movement of teeth can both provide this stimulation. In some cases where canine substitution is not performed, the bone graft placed to support the erupting canine may experience an "unstimulated" region adjacent to the central incision due to the missing lateral incisor. In these cases, focal crestal resorption can occur and an alveolar augmentation procedure is required prior to implant placement at skeletal maturity.

Access the complete reference list online at **http://www.expertconsult.com**

1. Brauer RO, Cronin TD, Reaves EL. Early maxillary orthopedics, orthodontia and alveolar bone grafting in complete clefts of the palate. *Plast Reconstr Surg Transplant Bull*. 1962;29: 625–641.
2. Georgiade NC, Pickrell KL, Quinn GW. Varying concepts in bone grafting of alveolar palatal defects. *Cleft Palate J*. 1964;16:43–51.
3. Pickrell K, Quinn G, Massengill R. Primary bone grafting of the maxilla in clefts of the lip and palate: a four year study. *Plast Reconstr Surg*. 1968;41:438–443.
4. Schmid E. Die Annaherung der kieferstempfebei lippen-kiefer. Gaumensplaten: ihre schadlichen folgen und vermiedung. *Forschr Keifer Geisichtschir*. 1955;1:168–180.

5. Schrudde J, Stellmach R. [Primary osteoplasty of defects of the inferior maxillary arch in cleft palate and harelip in infants; preliminary report.]. *Zentralbl Chir.* 1958;83:849–859.

6. Boyne PJ, Sands NR. Secondary bone grafting of residual alveolar and palatal clefts. *J Oral Surg.* 1972;30:87–92. *Landmark article largely recognized as initiating the popularity of secondary bone grafting. Boyne introduced the concept in the 1960s, advocating treatment towards the end of the first decade of life to minimize growth impairment while still supporting eruption of the adult dentition. Most of the described principles are still followed today.*

12. Cassolato SF, Ross B, Daskalogiannakis J, et al. Treatment of dental anomalies in children with complete unilateral cleft lip and palate at SickKids Hospital, Toronto. *Cleft Palate Craniofac J.* 2009;46:166–172. *Retrospective study of 116 children with complete unilateral cleft lip and palate treated since birth. The article quantifies dental anomalies in permanent dentition associated with complete unilateral cleft lip and palate and surveys treatment modalities used to address these problems.*

22. Guo J, Zhang Q, Wu G, et al. Secondary bone grafting for alveolar cleft in children with cleft lip or cleft lip and palate. *Cochrane Database Syst Rev.* 2011;(6):CD008050.

23. Liou EJ, Chen PK, Huang CS, et al. Interdental distraction osteogenesis and rapid orthodontic tooth movement: a novel approach to approximate a wide alveolar cleft or bony defect. *Plast Reconstr Surg.* 2000;105:1262–1272. *Detailed case-based review of interdental transport distraction osteogenesis to treat wide alveolar clefts by the recognized expert.*

36. Sato Y, Grayson BH, Garfinkle JS, et al. Success rate of gingivoperiosteoplasty with and without secondary bone grafts compared with secondary alveolar bone grafts alone. *Plast Reconstr Surg.* 2008;121:1356–1367, discussion 1368–1369. *Most recent retrospective evaluation by the New York University team of GPP outcomes with and without secondary bone grafting. They concluded that GPP alone or combined with secondary alveolar bone grafting results in superior bone levels when compared with conventional secondary alveolar bone grafting alone.*

54. McIntyre GT, Devlin MF. Secondary alveolar bone grafting (CLEFTSiS) 2000–2004. *Cleft Palate Craniofac J.* 2010;47:66–72. *A good discussion article delineating some of the key components associated with quality and outcome of alveolar bone grafting. The authors relate the changes to the Scottish Regional Cleft Programme that increased graft success rate from 58% to 76%.*

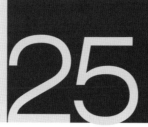

25

Orthodontics in cleft lip and palate management

Alvaro A. Figueroa, Alexander L. Figueroa, Gerson Chinchilla, and Marta Alvarado

SYNOPSIS

- Patients with orofacial clefts are best treated through a team approach.
- Close collaboration between the orthodontist and surgeon is critical during the care of patients with orofacial clefts.
- A developmental approach needs to be undertaken by orthodontists treating patients with orofacial clefts.
- In infancy the orthodontist can support the surgeon with nasoalveolar molding and maxillary orthopedics.
- In the primary dentition stage the orthodontist can correct mild to moderate posterior and anterior crossbites.
- In the transitional dentition the orthodontist prepares the maxillary arch prior to bone grafting and premaxillary repositioning.
- In the full permanent dentition the orthodontist finalizes arch alignment and coordination.
- The orthodontist supports the surgeon during planning, preparation of appliances, and follow-up of patients requiring orthognathic surgery and/or distraction osteogenesis during adolescence.
- The orthodontist works closely with other specialists in pediatric dentistry, prosthodontics, oral, and plastic surgery to rehabilitate the dental, oral, and facial conditions of patients with orofacial clefts.
- The application of new three-dimensional surgical and orthodontic diagnostic and treatment modalities to patients with orofacial clefts is likely to improve treatment outcomes.
- Orthodontic movement of primary and permanent teeth through a recently placed bone graft can enhance osteogenesis.

Introduction

The state of the art for the management of patients with oral facial clefts requires the use of a multidisciplinary approach, as various structures, traditionally treated by several specialists, are involved. In the oral cavity, the cleft affects not only the soft and hard palate, but also the alveolus and dentition. The structural rehabilitation of these patients requires the surgical correction of the soft- and hard-tissue defects, as well as the secondary effects of the cleft on maxillary development, dental support, and dental–occlusal alignment. The role of the orthodontist in cleft management is essential as the orthodontist assists the surgeon during all stages of reconstructive care: in the early stages, with presurgical nasal and maxillary orthopedics; during the transitional dentition stage, with alignment of the maxillary segments and dentition in preparation for secondary alveolar bone grafting; during the permanent dentition and late adolescent years, by obtaining satisfactory dental and occlusal relationships; and, also to prepare the dentition for prosthetic rehabilitation and orthognathic surgery, if required. In addition, it has been the role of the orthodontist to monitor craniofacial growth and dental development, as well as the treatment effects on these patients through the use of roentgencephalometry.

With this approach, the management of the cleft patient has evolved dramatically in recent years. The reason for improved outcomes is based on refinements in primary and finishing surgical techniques, as well as timing and incorporation of other procedures such as presurgical orthopedics, orthodontics, and new prosthetic approaches utilizing resin-bonded prosthesis and/or osseointegrated implants.

It is our experience that patients treated within the context of the multidisciplinary approach can obtain excellent outcomes related to speech, ideal occlusion, satisfactory lip aesthetics, and skeletal balance (Fig. 25.1 ⊕). However, it is the secondary cleft nasal deformity that still gives the patient the "cleft stigmata".

Fig. 25.1 appears online only.

In recent years, new orthodontic and surgical treatment modalities have become available that may further improve outcomes in patients with orofacial clefts. In infancy, this includes the use of presurgical nasoalveolar molding techniques. In the mixed dentition, novel orthodontic–orthopedic approaches to correct maxillary hypoplasia are utilized. Finally, in the permanent dentition, the use of new appliances and dental materials to facilitate orthodontic treatment, along with the application of bone anchorage screws (BAS) to facilitate orthodontic tooth movement, are employed. In addition, the use of distraction osteogenesis to improve the position of the maxilla, in those cases with severe maxillary hypoplasia, has become a well-accepted procedure. The availability of new diagnostic techniques such as digital skull and dental models, three-dimensional (3D) photogrammetry, lower radiation computed tomography (CT) scans, cone beam CT (CBCT), and the development of 3D digital protocols to plan orthognathic surgery, are now at the forefront of current orthodontic and surgical approaches. The efforts towards improvement of orthodontic and surgical treatment strategies developed for non-cleft patients will benefit the challenging problems presented by cleft patients and are a welcome addition to the current treatment protocols. Advances in molecular biology and biotechnology, along with a better understanding of their application, have opened doors to new treatment approaches in medicine and dentistry. These include the clinical use of homologous bone substitutes and application of bone morphogenetic proteins.

In this chapter, some of the new orthodontic and surgical strategies that are of benefit to cleft patients will be presented. The reader is directed to previous publications that deal with the role of the orthodontist in the management of the cleft patient to complement the information presented in this chapter.[1-4]

Infancy

On many occasions, the surgeon is faced with an infant who has a severe cleft with marked distortions of not only the maxillary segments but also the cartilage of the nose. This situation can occur in both the unilateral and bilateral cleft lip and palate patient. Since 1995, we have offered the use of nasoalveolar molding in the treatment protocol of those cleft patients presenting with premaxillary protrusion, hypoplastic columellas, and moderate to severe nasal distortions, following the general principles reported by Grayson and associates.[5-10] These protocols utilize premaxillary and maxillary orthopedics with the additional purposes of not only aligning the maxillary and premaxillary segments, but also to reposition the nasal cartilages prior to lip repair.

Unilateral cleft lip

Evaluation of the cleft nose demonstrates the presence of distorted nasal cartilage with deviation of the nasal tip towards the non-cleft side and severe angulation of the columella also to the non-cleft side. In addition, we have observed that the soft tissues caudal to the lateral nasal cartilage may be hyperplastic and prominent. Repair of the lip under these conditions, even with surgical repositioning of the nasal cartilages, results in a suboptimal nasal morphology, even though the lip repair is satisfactory. It is for this reason that we have now embarked on the process of orthopedic repositioning of the nasal cartilages, columella, nasal tip, and lateral wall of the vestibule in order to provide these patients with the best possible primary nasal reconstruction with less invasive surgical techniques. The procedure of presurgical infant nasal remodeling utilizing a modified intraoral plate was first described by Bennun and co-workers in Argentina.[11,12] Since then, it has been popularized in the US as nasoalveolar

molding by Grayson *et al.*[5-10] The authors have used this technique since 1995 and have made some modifications.[13]

Our technique is as follows: the nasoalveolar molding plate is made utilizing a light-cured orthodontic resin. A loop wire is incorporated to support the nasal conformer (nasal stent), made of light-cured acrylic, to reposition the nasal structures. The nasal stent is covered with soft acrylic to avoid irritation of the delicate tissues of the nasal mucosa. The palatal aspect of the plate is covered with soft-tissue liner in order to obtain perfect adaptation to the maxillary palatal shelves and undercuts created by the cleft (Figs. 25.2 & 25.3 ⊕). An exact fit of the plate is required for adequate retention, especially since we do not rely on external adhesive tape to maintain the plate in position. We utilize denture adhesive cream, after drying the plate and the oral mucosa prior to insertion. The parents are instructed to clean and replace the denture adhesive one to two times per day. Patients return on a weekly basis for adjustments to increase the length of the supporting wire and reshape the nasal stent. While the nasal molding is taking place, selectively grinding acrylic medial to the palatal shelves and adding acrylic lateral to the alveolar processes narrows the distance between the maxillary segments (Fig. 25.4). In addition, facial taping can be utilized to apply transverse pressure to the cleft segments and help with the cleft narrowing and nasal molding process (Fig. 25.5).

Figs. 25.2–25.5 appear online only.

The results expected from this technique include repositioning of the nasal tip towards the non-cleft side with straightening of the columella and equalizing the height on the nasal domes as much as possible. In addition, the nasal stent is adjusted in such a way as to exert lateral pressure on the lateral nasal wall against the hyperplastic soft tissues caudal to the lateral nasal cartilage (see Fig. 25.5). This results in a straighter nose with convex nasal cartilages and flattened hyperplastic lateral wall vestibular tissues.

At the time of surgery, the surgeon will repair the lip with medial repositioning of the base of the nose and narrowing of the nasal domes with tacking of the vestibular tissues to the lateral nasal wall. We believe that this combined effort will provide these patients with better noses that will require less extensive secondary revisions. The outcomes obtained with this technique are consistent and predictable and these variations of the molding technique have been incorporated with favorable results.

In cases that start with severe nasal distortion, we support the nasal molding with postsurgical nasal stents utilizing commercially available removable nasal stents.[13-15] The stent is usually kept in place using facial taping (Fig. 25.6 ⊕) and is maintained for at least 2–3 months or for as long as the patient can deal with it comfortably.

Fig. 25.6 appears online only.

Bilateral cleft lip

The patient with bilateral cleft lip and palate represents the most challenging condition for the reconstructive team. The premaxilla is extremely protrusive, the premaxilla and prolabium can be of variable size, the columella is deficient or almost nonexistent, the palatal clefts are wider than usual, and occasionally, the maxillary palatal shelves are collapsed. In addition, the nasal domes are wide apart, and the tip projection is decreased (Fig. 25.7 ⊕). It has been our experience that, in patients with bilateral cleft lip and palate, with a protrusive premaxilla, it becomes imperative that the premaxilla is repositioned into a more favorable relation with the maxillary segments in order to achieve definitive lip closure with minimal tension. If this is not done, a poor repair or failure with unfavorable consequences may occur. For this purpose, we have successfully utilized premaxillary orthopedics with an intraoral appliance that is retained with denture adhesive and has an elastic strap for premaxillary retraction.[16,17] This approach has allowed the surgeon to close the lip satisfactorily (Figs. 25.8 & 25.9 ●).

Figs. 25.7–25.9 appear online only.

In the bilateral cleft lip and palate patient the approach requires repositioning of the premaxilla prior to the nasal molding technique. For the last 20 years we have used a self-retaining intraoral plate[17] that has been modified from the original design.[16] This modification allows for easy adjustments and fewer frequent patient visits.

Grayson and coworkers[6–8,10] have utilized nasoalveolar molding for bilateral clefts. The appliance was intended to retract the premaxilla as well as molding the nasal cartilage and elongating the columella. Their plate design included retention through extraoral taping and elastics. We have modified the design utilizing our principles of a self-retained appliance[13,16,17] to avoid using facial taping to support the prosthesis. A light-cured resin plate is constructed to which orthodontic buttons or custom-formed wires are attached for retraction of the premaxilla with the elastomeric band. In addition, the plate is relined with soft-tissue conditioner for close adaptation to the palatal tissues. After premaxillary retraction and repositioning are completed, the plate is modified by adding two wires that go into each nasal vestibule. The ends of the wires are bent in a loop and are covered with a light-cured acrylic covered with soft denture lining material (nasal stents). In addition, loops are bent about the level of the superior aspect of the prolabium for attachment of an elastomeric chain that has been covered with a soft-tissue denture liner. The purpose of the elastomeric chain across the prolabium is to hold it down, while the nasal prongs at the end of the wires are gradually elevated, lifting and medially repositioning the nasal domes and, at the same time, elongating the hypoplastic columella (see Fig. 25.8 ●). The plate is used 24 hours a day, is removed daily for cleaning, and is held in position with the aid of a denture adhesive cream. In addition, the palatal aspect of the plate can be modified by adding material on the lateral aspects of the plate and removing acrylic on the medial aspects. This will allow for gentle and gradual repositioning of the maxillary segments, resulting in narrowing of the cleft. This technique has given the surgeon an improved situation for not only obtaining adequate lip repair but also providing a better situation for primary nasal reconstruction with remodeling of the nasal domes and nasal tip and elongation of the hypoplastic columella. The main advantage of this procedure is that it eliminates the need for secondary procedures for columella elongation in the early childhood years. All of the patients in whom this technique has been used have adjusted extremely well to the use of the appliance and the families have been extremely pleased with the results (see Fig. 28.9 ●), as well as with the ease in which the orthopedic phase is carried out.

The described protocol has been well tolerated by patients and readily accepted by parents. This treatment protocol has been used for a few years, and there are not enough long-term data to demonstrate the effects of the technique on the fully developed nasal structures. However, some patients are in the midteen years, and the clinical impression at this time is that they will require less extensive nasal revision procedures at the completion of facial growth (Fig. 25.10 ●).

Fig. 25.10 appears online only.

Primary dentition

Orthodontic treatment at this stage is limited to the correction of certain posterior crossbites and anterior crossbites of mild to moderate degree.

Posterior crossbite

In the cleft patient, posterior crossbites are of both skeletal and dental origin. They are skeletal because the maxillary segments are usually collapsed after cleft palate surgery, especially in the canine region. In most instances, this change in arch form occurs prior to the eruption of the primary canines; therefore, at the time of eruption of these teeth, the maxillary cleft-side primary canine erupts medially to the lower one. In addition, this early relationship causes minor palatal displacement of the maxillary primary canine and labial displacement of the mandibular one.[3] This is an important observation, as this is the reason why cleft patients in the primary dentition rarely have occlusal or functional shifts. Patients in whom an occlusal shift is detected are those who are candidates for either selective tooth grinding or expansion procedures. Expansion can readily be accomplished, but it should be noted that, after it is completed, unless a bone graft is placed, it has to be retained until the time of alveolar reconstruction with a bone graft. For this reason, we prefer to delay transverse expansion in the primary dentition until the patient is older and just prior to secondary alveolar bone-grafting procedures usually undertaken in the transitional dentition.

Anterior crossbite

Anterior crossbite of mild to moderate degree can be managed in the primary and transitional dentition stages utilizing elastic protraction forces delivered through a facial mask.[18–20] However, if it is noted that this crossbite is related to a moderate to severe skeletal maxillary hypoplasia, the patient is best managed with a surgical approach. If it is felt that the maxillary advancement is important at an early age due to its severity, it can be instituted by means of distraction osteogenesis.

Transitional dentition

This is the developmental stage in which a cleft patient, involving the alveolus, will receive the next surgical procedure after lip and secondary palate repair. In most instances, the dentition around the cleft presents severe malposition, limiting surgical access to the alveolar site (Fig. 25.11 ●). For this purpose, the dentition adjacent to the cleft has to be repositioned, preparing the cleft site for the secondary alveolar bone graft. Reconstruction of the cleft alveolus and anterior aspect of the maxilla is deferred until this stage, in an attempt to

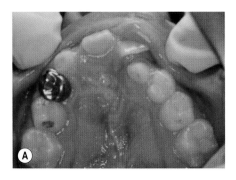
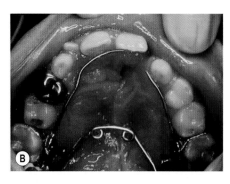
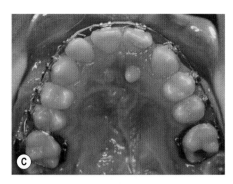

Fig. 25.13 Patient with unilateral cleft lip and palate before orthodontic treatment in preparation for bone grafting **(A)**, during expansion with quad helix expander **(B)**, and after bone grafting with erupted cleft-side canine and peg cleft lateral incisor erupting palatal **(C)**. Note arch alignment after expansion and adequate arch form after expansion, bone grafting, and orthodontics.

minimize the growth restriction resulting from surgical trauma and scarring.[23–25]

Fig. 25.11 appears online only.

If it is determined that the patient requires orthodontic treatment for preparation of the surgical site, it should be initiated based on dental development of the permanent teeth to be moved rather than chronological age.[3,13,26] It is known that cleft patients present with delay of dental development and eruption.[26,27] Orthodontic treatment should not be initiated until the near-complete root development of the incisors, on which orthodontic brackets will be placed (see Fig. 25.11M–O). Adherence to this guideline will result in minimal resorptive changes of the maxillary incisor roots. If the necessary treatment for secondary bone grafting of the maxilla is based on dental development rather than chronological age, a safeguard for the adverse effects of surgery on growth is added. Our own studies[26] indicate that development and eruption of the cleft lateral incisor are markedly delayed when compared with a contralateral incisor (see Fig. 25.11M–O). This observation allows for placement of orthodontic appliances on the remaining incisors while the cleft lateral incisor has not yet erupted. When a viable cleft maxillary lateral incisor is present, this ensures its preservation and adequate bone support for eruption of both lateral incisor and canine after the bone graft.

The expansion of the arch can also be done with this appliance (Fig. 25.12), but occasionally it has to be supported with a maxillary expander. The expander commonly used in our protocol is the quad helix expander (Fig. 25.13). We rarely use a screw expander unless it is observed that the palatal tissues are severely scarred (Fig. 25.14). Fortunately, with the use of more delicate surgical techniques, this latter situation is uncommon.

Fig. 25.12 appears online only.

The expansion required for alveolar bone grafting should provide well-aligned maxillary segments with a minimal increase in the size of the alveolar gap. Wider alveolar gaps are difficult to close using local flaps.[28] In cases in which the clinician determines that the required expansion of the maxilla or repositioning of the premaxilla will create a wider gap between the maxillary segments, expansion and bone-grafting procedures are deferred until adolescence. At this time, the maxillary segments can be surgically mobilized and approximated, allowing for closure with local flaps at the time of final orthognathic surgery.

After the maxillary segments and dentition are placed in their ideal positions, the patient is referred for secondary alveolar bone grafting.[29] Presurgical orthodontics in preparation for this reconstructive stage can be completed within a period of 6–12 months. Immediately prior to the bone graft, all appliances over the palate are removed and the labial aspects of the orthodontic wire are segmentalized for surgical access. In addition, supernumerary or primary teeth in the

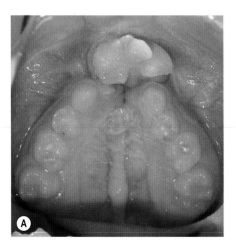
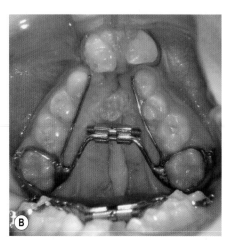
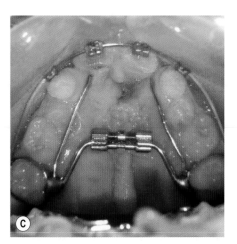

Fig. 25.14 Intraoral views of a patient with bilateral cleft lip and palate with arch collapse **(A)**. A rigid screw expander was used **(B)**. After expansion **(C)**, note improvement on arch form and opening of alveolar spaces in preparation for bone grafting.

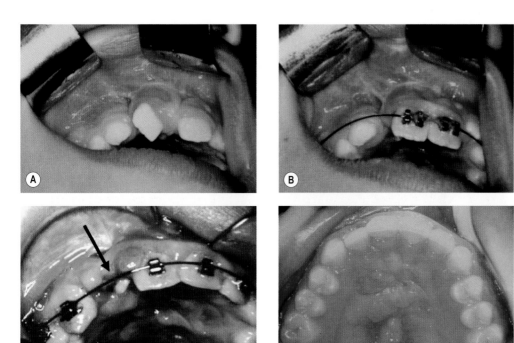

Fig. 25.15 (A–D) Patient with right unilateral cleft lip and palate with permanent maxillary lateral incisor and canine present. After the bone graft the canine erupted with adequate gingival support. The lateral incisor erupted later on spontaneously (arrow) and was incorporated into the dental arch. At the completion of treatment the tooth was cosmetically enlarged.

surgical site are extracted 8–12 weeks prior to surgery. This will provide the surgeon with intact gingival tissues for proper coverage of the bone graft.

The presence of alveolar bone is dependent on the presence of teeth. When the lateral incisor is present, with adequate crown and root anatomy, and in favorable position, every attempt should be made to preserve it. If the lateral incisor erupts through the bone graft, suitable alveolar bone will be available in the alveolar ridge as well as for the erupting canine (Fig. 25.15). If the permanent lateral incisor on the cleft side is missing or needs to be extracted due to its poor anatomy or position (see Fig. 25.11J–O 🌐), then the actively erupting canine could take its place and preserve the reconstructed alveolus.

Orthodontic treatment can be restarted 8–12 weeks after bone graft surgery. As soon as appropriate maxillary arch and dental relations are achieved, the orthodontic appliances are removed and the patient is placed in retention until there is full permanent dentition. Teeth that were severely rotated prior to treatment need to be retained. Absent teeth can be temporarily replaced with a removable prosthetic appliance to improve aesthetics and limit the effects on speech production (see Fig. 25.11P 🌐).

Patients treated with the protocol outlined above complete the preparatory phase of orthodontic treatment in the preteen or early teen years. Patients are followed every 6 months to determine their craniofacial growth and dental development, especially eruption of the maxillary lateral incisor and canine on the cleft side. Occasionally, the maxillary canine is impacted and requires surgical exposure and orthodontic incorporation into the arch as the child is in the full permanent dentition. Impacted or severely malpositioned cleft-side maxillary lateral incisors are usually extracted (see Fig. 25.11J–L 🌐).

Finally, if it is determined that there is anteroposterior skeletal disharmony, the reconstructive team has to decide if it is convenient to do the bone grafting in the transitional dentition or if it should be done in combination with future orthognathic surgical procedures. Patients in whom there is marked tissue deficiency, including maxillary hypoplasia and congenitally missing teeth, are likely candidates for postponement of the traditional approach with secondary alveolar bone grafting, and will be treated later on in the permanent dentition in combination with orthognathic surgery. If it is deemed important to preserve the dentition adjacent to the alveolar cleft, orthodontics are therefore indicated, even in the presence of a skeletal disharmony. The purpose of the orthodontic treatment is then to prepare the dentition for the alveolar bone graft and also to coordinate the maxillary arch to the mandibular arch for future orthognathic surgery that will be performed in the teen years. This approach minimizes the required orthodontic treatment prior to orthognathic surgery in the adolescent years.

Orthodontic tooth movement to regenerate a homologous lyophilized bone graft combined with platelet rich plasma to reconstruct the alveolar cleft: "Chinchilla–Asensio Approach"

Advances in molecular biology and biotechnology now offer the possibility of accelerated healing and tissue regeneration.[30–38] At the Centro Infantil de Estomatología in Antigua, Guatemala some of these new advances for the treatment of cleft lip and palate patients have been incorporated. The use of lyophilized homologous bone combined with autologous platelet rich plasma, in combination with graft stimulation by orthodontic movement of primary teeth adjacent to the cleft (usually primary canine), has shown favorable graft incorporation with excellent clinical outcomes.

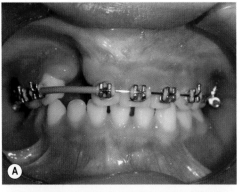

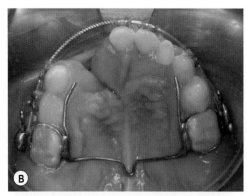

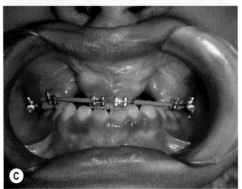

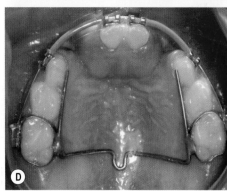

Fig. 25.16 Frontal **(A)** and occlusal **(B)** views of a patient with a complete right unilateral cleft lip and palate in the primary dentition. Note orthodontic brackets in all maxillary primary teeth and transpalatal bar used to maintain the expansion. Frontal **(C)** and occlusal **(D)** views of a patient with bilateral cleft lip and alveolus in the primary dentition. Note orthodontic brackets on the maxillary anterior primary teeth and transpalatal bar used to maintain the expansion.

This unique protocol includes orthopedic and orthodontic alignment of the arch as early as 4 years of age. The bone graft is performed between 5 and 8 years of age; and, 3 months after the graft, orthodontic movement of teeth, adjacent to the grafted site, is initiated to stimulate incorporation of the graft. To date, 66 cases have been treated in this fashion, 54 unilateral and 12 bilateral alveolar clefts with a follow-up of 7 years.

Orthodontic protocol – pre-graft

Pre-graft orthopedics and orthodontics

The orthodontist must assure that the dentition is healthy prior to treatment. Patients can be in full primary dentition or early transitional dentition to initiate the protocol. As indicated previously in the chapter, the objectives of orthopedic and orthodontic treatment at this stage are to align the maxillary segments, correct dental malpositions, improve arch form, and facilitate access to the cleft alveolus at the time of surgery.

Careful assessment is done of the periodontal condition, degree of apical development, root inclination, and proximity of primary and permanent teeth to the alveolar cleft. In younger children, special attention is given to the root status (resorption) of the maxillary primary incisors and primary canine(s) adjacent to the alveolar cleft(s).[26,39–41]

After maxillary arch expansion, a transpalatal arch bar with anterior extensions is used for retention, making sure to keep the extensions off the surgical site. Standard orthodontic brackets of appropriate size (i.e. mandibular incisor brackets) are placed on as many anterior teeth as necessary. Tubes are designed on the transpalatal bar bands of the primary second molars. This set-up provides sufficient stability to the appliance (Fig. 25.16).

Alignment of the maxillary dentition is completed with a series of highly flexible to rigid arch wires. The initial level and alignment process is slowed by replacing arches at no less than at 8-week intervals, preventing possible initiation of rapid root resorption of the primary teeth. Once the patient is in a heavy archwire (rectangular gauge 0.016" × 0.022" or heavier) and the segments stabilized, referral to the surgeon is done. Primary teeth adjacent to the alveolar cleft with root resorption, significant mobility, or caries are extracted at least 2 months prior to the alveolar bone graft surgery to allow gingival tissue healing. Prior to surgery, the orthodontic arch is removed, so as not to interfere with surgical access. In both unilateral and bilateral cases it may be necessary to replace the arch immediately after the procedure.

Surgical protocol

The incision design of Abyholm *et al.* is utilized to access and prepare the alveolar cleft site.[29] Once the nasal floor and palatal aspect of the alveolar cleft are closed, a gelatin plasma membrane is applied to the closed walls of the alveolar cleft. Lyophilized homologous bone, mixed with platelet rich plasma into a malleable and easy to manipulate paste, is applied into the defect. Two additional layers of gelatin plasma membrane are applied over the bone.[31,32,35,36,42] To close the alveolar border, a horizontal mattress suture is used to hold one or two of the fibrin membranes and, in this way, achieve a hermetic seal. After closure, additional liquid plasma is injected into the alveolar cleft site (Fig. 25.17).[32,42]

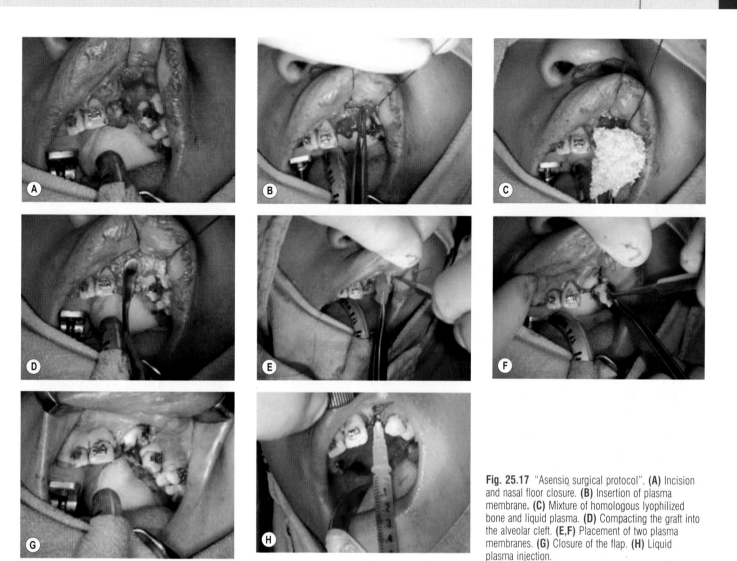

Fig. 25.17 "Asensio surgical protocol". (A) Incision and nasal floor closure. (B) Insertion of plasma membrane. (C) Mixture of homologous lyophilized bone and liquid plasma. (D) Compacting the graft into the alveolar cleft. (E,F) Placement of two plasma membranes. (G) Closure of the flap. (H) Liquid plasma injection.

Orthodontic protocol – post-graft

Patients are evaluated 4 and 20 days after the alveolar bone graft. At 3 and 6 months radiographs are obtained of the site.

Two situations may occur, and are based on the dental development of the patient and the presence of primary and/or permanent teeth, supernumerary, or peg-shaped incisors.

1. The cleft permanent central and lateral incisor, supernumerary, or peg shaped lateral incisor may erupt spontaneously; and, subsequently the maxillary permanent canine also erupts naturally (Fig. 25.18).

2. If the position of the cleft maxillary canine is high in the bone, the primary canine is moved towards and through the recently reconstructed alveolar cleft site. This is done by means of light orthodontic forces (60 grs) with a nickel titanium open spring. The movement of the primary canine through the bone grafts regenerates the newly grafted bone and increases the alveolar ridge bone volume. This is possible due to the ability of the periodontal ligament to generate bone during orthodontic tooth movement.[43–45] Also a supernumerary or peg-shaped lateral with adequate root length can be moved through the bone graft for the same purpose. Moving teeth to regenerate bone is a procedure frequently used in periodontally compromised patients, cases requiring dental implants, and prosthetic rehabilitation[34,35,37,46] (Figs. 25.19, 25.20 & 25.21).

Completing the post-graft orthodontic treatment may take between 6 and 8 months. The total duration of treatment can be between 12 and 18 months, including orthodontics and bone grafting. After this period, patients undergo routine follow-up until they are ready for their final orthodontic treatment in the teen years, as shown later in this chapter.

Outcomes and benefits

To date, 66 patients with alveolar clefts (52 unilateral, 14 bilateral), between 5 and 8 years of age, have been successfully treated with this approach. The average age for bone grafting was 6½ years. Some 52% of the cases underwent bone grafting during primary dentition, and the rest during the early transitional dentition. Although many of the patients were younger than the usual time for traditional secondary alveolar bone grafting, they tolerated the orthodontic treatment surprisingly well. A significant amount of time is spent educating the children and parents on the importance of good oral health, hygiene, and excellent care of their orthodontic appliances.

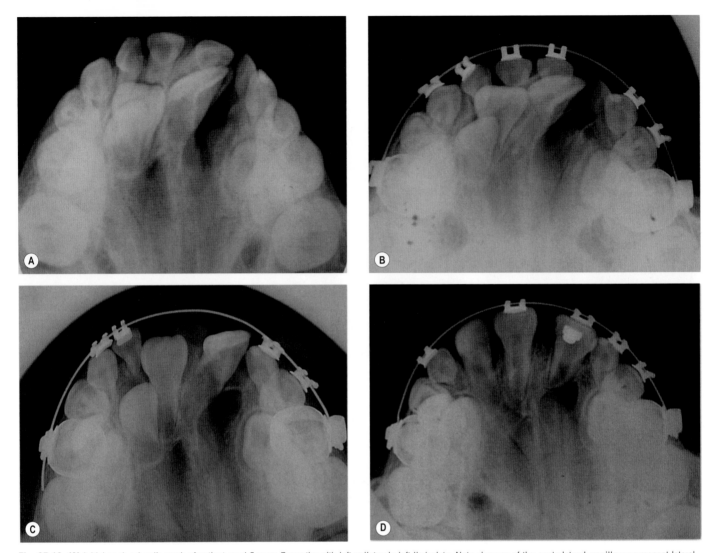

Fig. 25.18 **(A)** Initial occlusal radiograph of patient aged 5 years 7 months with left unilateral cleft lip/palate. Note absence of the contralateral maxillary permanent lateral incisor and rotation of the cleft-side central incisor towards the cleft. **(B)** Six months after alignment of the arch and prior to bone graft. **(C)** After exfoliation of the maxillary primary central incisors, the cleft-side maxillary incisor is erupting into the bone graft with better alignment. **(D)** The occlusal radiograph demonstrates the orthodontic appliance and adequate osseous bridge to support orthodontic dental movement.

The benefits of this approach are numerous, including no harvest site and eliminating donor site morbidity; taking advantage of the osteogenic regenerative capacity of the periodontal ligament during orthodontic tooth movement; providing and maintaining vertical and horizontal alveolar bone level until the permanent teeth erupt; facilitating tooth (lateral incisors and canines) eruption naturally into the reconstructed alveolar bone; allowing the permanent maxillary lateral incisor and/or canine to follow the orthodontic movement of the primary canine, thereby enhancing natural eruption; obtaining closure of the oro-nasal fistula; providing adequate attached gingiva to support dental eruption and periodontal health; and, finally, possibly improving self esteem as young children can attend school without the stigma of a cleft-related malocclusion, especially maxillary anterior dental alignment.

For the protocol to be successful, the maxillary arch needs to be aligned, the alveolar cleft should not be too wide to allow closure with local flaps, and the root of the primary canine (to be moved into the grafted site) needs to be of adequate length (Fig. 25.22A). The vertical height and thickness of the alveolar bone ridge has been measured radiographically to be close to the length of the root of the primary canines (11 mm) and the thickness of its diameter (5–6 mm) (Fig. 25.22B). In addition, biopsies have been obtained in a few cases to uncover canines for faster incorporation of the canine into the arch and have revealed viable trabecular bone (Fig. 25.23).

Available radiographic evidence demonstrates that the primary canine is usually not affected by accelerated root resorption after being moved distances between 5 and 8 mm (Fig. 25.24). The process of radicular resorption and exfoliation is usually no different to that observed in patients without clefts. However, in some cases, premature exfoliation is noted in conjunction with earlier eruption of the cleft side canine.

Other considerations

The possible disadvantages of this approach may include the need to select the patients at a time when the roots of their

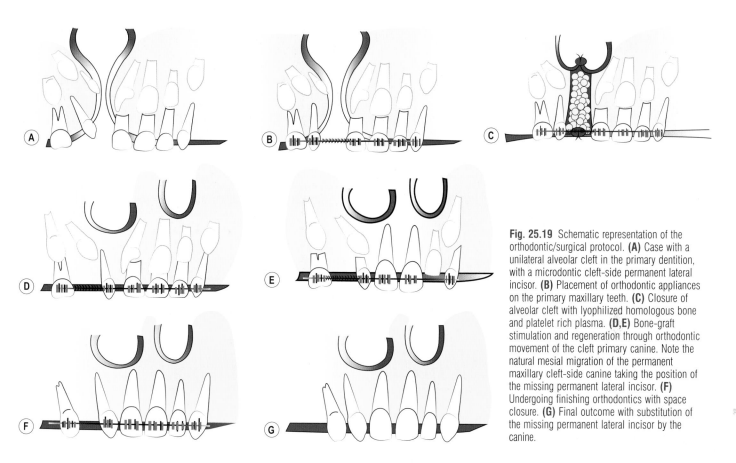

Fig. 25.19 Schematic representation of the orthodontic/surgical protocol. **(A)** Case with a unilateral alveolar cleft in the primary dentition, with a microdontic cleft-side permanent lateral incisor. **(B)** Placement of orthodontic appliances on the primary maxillary teeth. **(C)** Closure of alveolar cleft with lyophilized homologous bone and platelet rich plasma. **(D,E)** Bone-graft stimulation and regeneration through orthodontic movement of the cleft primary canine. Note the natural mesial migration of the permanent maxillary cleft-side canine taking the position of the missing permanent lateral incisor. **(F)** Undergoing finishing orthodontics with space closure. **(G)** Final outcome with substitution of the missing permanent lateral incisor by the canine.

maxillary primary canines are intact. Patients treated under this protocol tend to be younger, therefore appropriate management techniques need to be applied to allow the young patients to accept, tolerate, and cooperate with the orthodontic treatment. Early radiographic examinations and education to referring health professionals need to be conducted. The cost and access to the lyophilized homologous bone and the equipment to process the plasma may affect the decision to use this

technique. However, obtaining plasma is relatively simple for many teams. Once the cost for the processing equipment is covered, the costs are minimal. Homologous lyophilized bone is easily found through medical suppliers.

In patients with wider clefts, the pyriform aperture may require higher bone placement to support the alar base. It is not certain if the bone graft performed in this manner can provide sufficient bone for this purpose. However, if the nasal

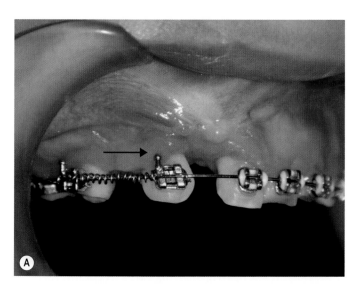
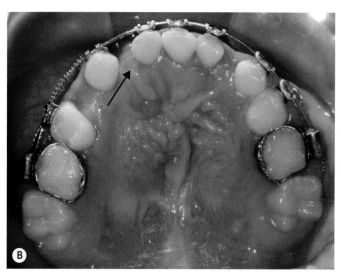

Fig. 25.20 Mesial movement (arrows) of the cleft side primary canine through the recently grafted alveolar cleft in a case missing the permanent maxillary lateral cleft-side incisor. A nickel titanium spring (60 grs) is used to move the tooth. Lateral view **(A)**, occlusal view **(B)**.

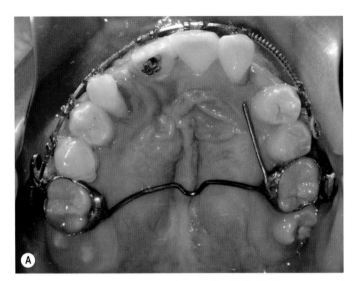
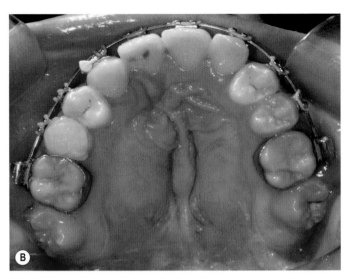

Fig. 25.21 Occlusal views of the case shown in Fig. 25.20. **(A)** After movement of the cleft-side primary canine through the alveolar graft a peg-shaped lateral incisor erupted spontaneously. Note on the left side or non-cleft side the absence of a permanent canine. This tooth required extraction due to an abnormal short root. **(B)** After extraction of the cleft-side peg-shaped incisor the permanent canine erupted spontaneously and was orthodontically moved to the position of the missing maxillary lateral incisor. Note a consolidated and well-aligned maxillary arch.

floor is properly addressed during the primary lip repair, this may not be a factor. Although this approach is used in non-cleft patients to build up bone in preparation for placement of osseointegrated fixtures, it is not known if sufficient bone is created to support a future implant in the alveolar cleft region. However, the main purpose of this early approach is to allow migration of the patient's own teeth and, in this way, eliminate the need for prosthetic replacements.

This approach has been successful in the rehabilitation of the alveolar cleft. Integration of the graft is possibly enhanced by the osteogenic stimulation of the orthodontic movement of the primary cleft canine into the graft, as well as through natural dental eruption of adjacent teeth. It has resulted in satisfactory bone levels in both the vertical and horizontal dimension, as well as adequate levels of attached gingiva and healthy periodontal condition of the teeth adjacent to the

reconstructed alveolar cleft. The functional and aesthetic benefits have been favorable and are demonstrated in the following case with a complete unilateral cleft lip and palate (Fig. 25.25 ⊕).

Fig. 25.25 appears online only.

Permanent dentition

At the time of near complete or complete permanent dentition, the orthodontist must perform definitive orthodontic treatment for the cleft patient. The goals are no different than those for non-cleft patients, but certain conditions must be kept in mind during treatment planning. These include arch length requirements and need for dental extractions in cases of severe crowding; integrity of the dentition and supporting

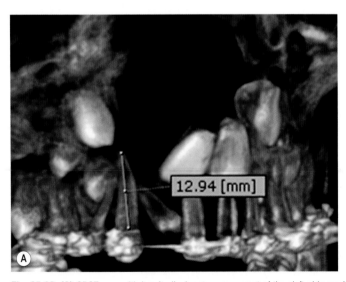
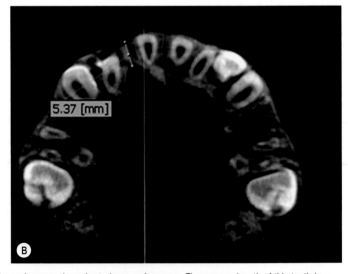

Fig. 25.22 (A) CBCT scan with longitudinal root measurement of the cleft-side maxillary primary canine prior to bone graft surgery. The average length of this tooth is 11 mm. **(B)** Coronal section demonstrating a 5.37 mm anteroposterior width of the bony bridge after bone graft and movement of the primary canine through it. The average bucco-lingual diameter of the canine is 5.5 mm.

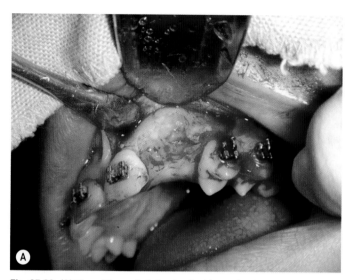
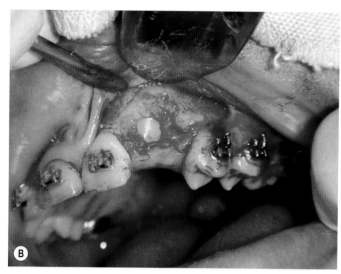

Fig. 25.23 (A) View of the grafted alveolar site 12 months after eruption of adjacent permanent teeth in a case in which the primary canine was moved to stimulate and regenerate the graft. The permanent cleft-side canine had delayed eruption. **(B)** It became necessary to expose it and move into the arch with orthodontic forces. The removed bone was histologically examined and revealed dense well-trabeculated bone.

structures, especially for teeth adjacent to the alveolar cleft; unusual dental positions, such as impactions; dental transpositions; congenitally missing or severely abnormal teeth that may need to be extracted requiring replacement either with a prosthesis or with orthodontic space closure, especially in the cleft region; maxillary and mandibular dental midlines and their relation to the facial midline; and anterior/posterior, transverse, and vertical relationships of the maxilla and mandible to each other and to the face.[1–3,13]

The introduction of new flexible wires and self-ligating appliances permits physiologic forces allowing favorable soft-tissue and bone remodeling responses, especially on those severely malpositioned teeth adjacent to the cleft (Figs. 25.12 & 25.26). Every attempt should be made to complete the case with class I cuspid and molar relationships with ideal overjet and overbite (Figs. 25.1 & 25.27A ●). If the cleft lateral incisor is missing, the clinician must decide if this tooth needs to be replaced with a prosthesis or the space closed with orthodontics or with a combined surgical–orthodontic approach. Prosthetic replacement is usually reserved for those cases in which ideal class I cuspid relationships and overjet and overbite are present. In these cases, if the anatomy of the adjacent teeth to the dental gap is sound, a bonded prosthesis or an osseointegrated fixture can be utilized.[1–3,13,47,48]

In those cases with a missing lateral incisor, in which the maxillary canine has migrated forward and is erupting into the grafted alveolar ridge (see Fig. 25.29), one must consider substituting the lateral incisor with the canine, and moving

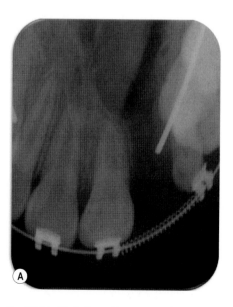
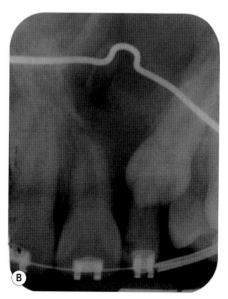
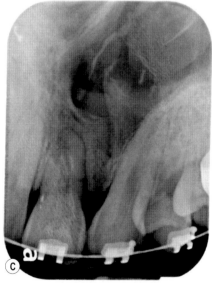

Fig. 25.24 (A) Radiographic sequence demonstrating the alveolar cleft prior to bone graft. Note the primary cleft-side primary canine with a bracket and adjacent to the cleft. **(B)** Orthodontic movement of the primary canine for stimulation and osseous regeneration of the bone graft. Note preservation of the primary canine root and spontaneous mesial migration of the permanent canine. **(C)** Completed movement of the permanent canine into the position of the missing maxillary cleft-side permanent lateral incisor.

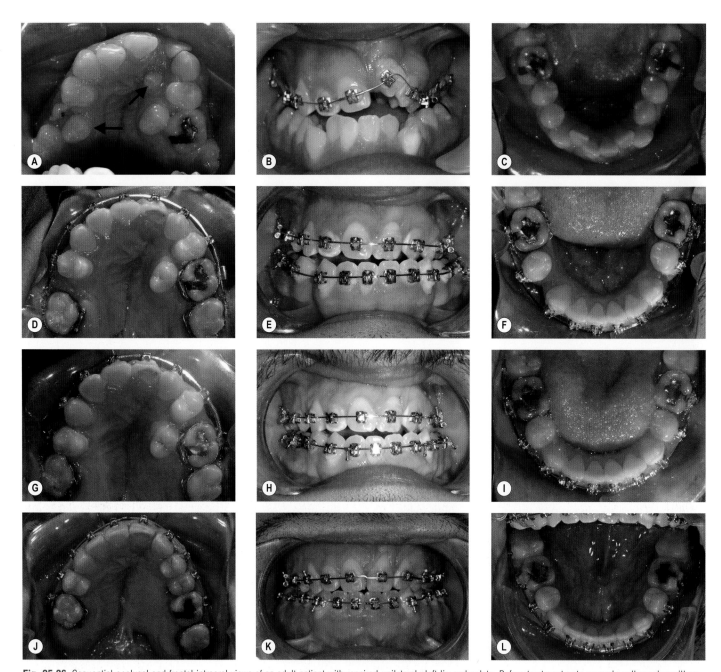

Fig. 25.26 Sequential occlusal and frontal intraoral views of an adult patient with repaired unilateral cleft lip and palate. Before treatment note severely collapsed maxillary arch and crowding in both arches. A peg left maxillary incisor was present. Due to severe crowding dental extractions of teeth number 4, 7, 21, and 28 **(arrows)** became necessary. Highly flexible wires and a self-ligating bracket system were used from the beginning of treatment **(A, B, C)**. Soon after leveling the gingival condition of the maxillary left central incisor was healthy. After further alignment and space closure the gingival condition remained healthy **(D, E, F)**. Space was developed to incorporate tooth number 13 into the arch **(A, D, G, J)**. After dental alignment, the occlusion was corrected with orthognathic surgery and the gingival condition remained healthy **(J, K, L)**.

all the posterior teeth forward. In a non-extraction case, the cleft side will be finished with class II relations; however, if the lower bicuspids were extracted, the cleft-side occlusion should finish with class I relations (see Fig. 25.1 ⊕). In cases with a non-ideal bone graft outcome, the clinician may want to move the canine forward into the grafted site to improve bone morphology, rather than replacing the lateral incisor with an osseointegrated fixture or a prosthesis that might need additional bone grafting. In cases where the canine has migrated forward into the lateral incisor position, and ideal class I molar relations are present, the canine could be replaced

with an osseointegrated implant (see Fig. 25.27). Other considerations include deciding on how to manage the missing cleft-side maxillary incisor, as well as the shape, size, and color of the canine, and the gingival contour in the area of the cleft.[3] If properly planned, both the prosthetic and orthodontic options to manage the missing cleft-side lateral incisor can provide outstanding results (Figs. 25.1, 25.15 & 25.27A ⊕).

In situations where the alveolar cleft is too wide for conventional bone grafting, the clinician may elect to surgically shift the entire cleft-side posterior maxillary segment forward and place the canine in the position of the missing lateral

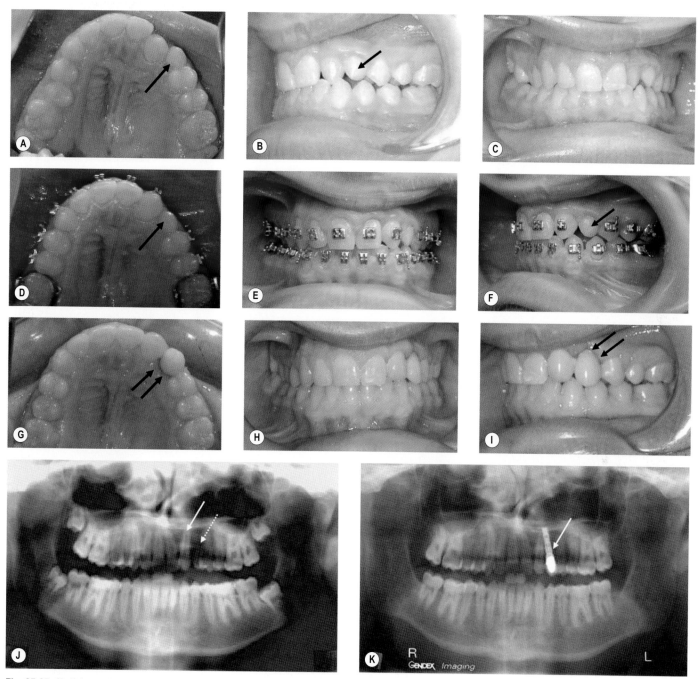

Fig. 25.27 (A–I) Intraoral views of a patient with left unilateral cleft lip and palate, who was missing the cleft-side maxillary lateral incisor, had the maxillary canine substituting the missing incisor, and had a retained primary canine (single arrow). Since ideal posterior occlusion was present, it was decided not to close the space with orthodontics, but to replace the primary canine with an osseointegrated implant (double arrow). Note satisfactory occlusion and aesthetics after treatment. **(J, K)** Note in the pretreatment panoramic radiograph **(J)** the presence of the permanent maxillary left canine in the position of the missing lateral incisor (arrow), and the retained primary canine (dotted arrow). After treatment **(K)**, note replacement of the primary canine with an osseointegrated implant (arrow).

incisor. This assures not only closure of the alveolar defect, but also closure of the dental gap created by the missing cleft-side maxillary lateral incisor.[3,13,49] After bone grafting, it is not uncommon to find that the cleft-side maxillary canine has an unusual eruption path and is impacted. These teeth need to be managed surgically by exposing them so the orthodontist can incorporate them into the dental arch (Fig. 25.28).

In some situations it is necessary to move teeth to close extraction spaces or reposition teeth within the arch to obtain better occlusal relations. In the past, intra-arch movements were difficult as the orthodontist depended on the adjacent teeth and patient cooperation using elastics or extraoral appliances for anchorage control. With the introduction of BAS, also known in orthodontics as temporary anchorage devices, the orthodontist's ability to achieve significant tooth movements has been enhanced.[50] BAS permit anteroposterior and vertical control of a single tooth or group of teeth during orthodontic treatment. The application of BAS is a simple office procedure. After completing the orthodontic treatment, the BAS are simply removed without negative sequelae (Fig. 25.29).

Orthodontic management following the "developmental approach", as outlined above, allows the clinician to take advantage of developmental and growth changes. In addition, it permits the patient and family to recognize the need for distinct phases of orthodontic treatment, which also allows for sufficient phases of rest between stages. This approach assures patient and family acceptance, compliance, and cooperation with the treatment protocol.

Orthognathic surgery and distraction procedures for the cleft patient

Skeletal and dental discrepancies between the maxilla and mandible are not uncommon in cleft patients. These

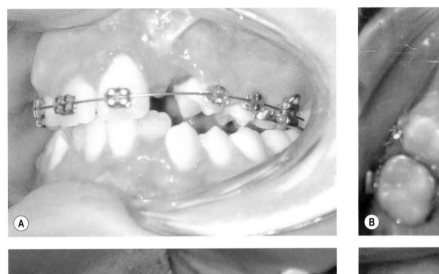

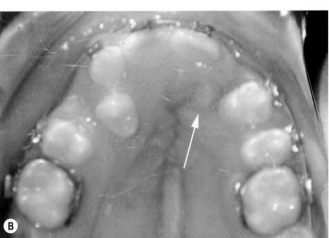

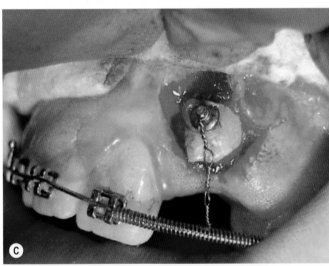

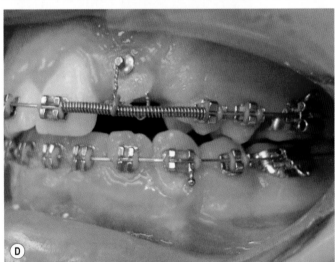

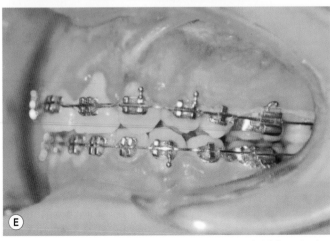

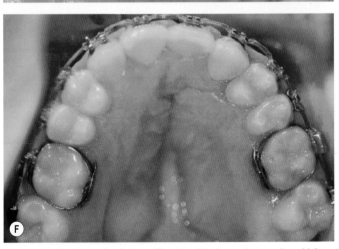

Fig. 25.28 (A–F) Intraoral views of a patient with left unilateral cleft lip and palate that was congenitally missing the right maxillary lateral incisor and a peg-shaped left one (arrow). The peg incisor was extracted, and the right maxillary canine was impacted, and needed surgical exposure so it could be incorporated into the arch. Note satisfactory gingival and occlusal relations obtained after treatment.

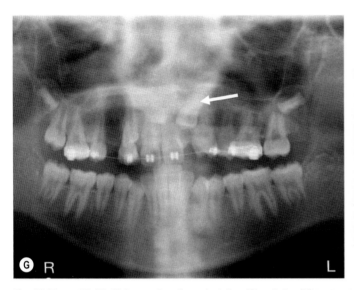

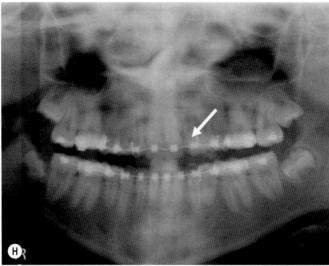

Fig. 25.28, cont'd (G, H) Panoramic radiographs before **(G)** and after **(H)** treatment. Note high position of the left maxillary canine (arrow) and incorporation into the dental arch.

discrepancies can be in the sagittal, transverse, and vertical planes. If the discrepancies are moderate to severe, they are best managed with a combined surgical/orthodontic approach. This approach results in substantial functional and aesthetic improvements in the cleft patient (see Fig. 25.1 ⊕).

It is generally accepted that patients with orofacial clefts have mandibles that are of normal size or slightly smaller.[51] For this reason, in most patients with maxillary hypoplasia, the surgeon may choose to perform sagittal correction with surgery limited to the maxillary bone. In cases where there is

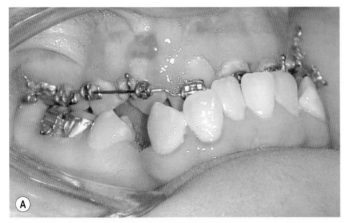

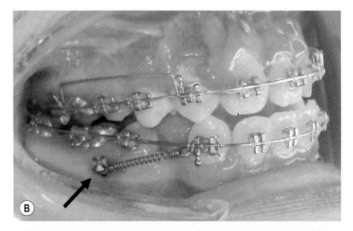

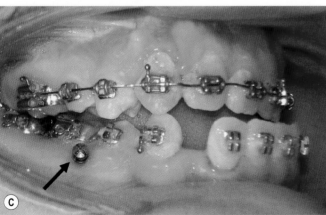

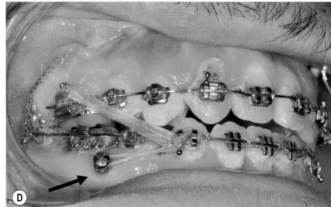

Fig. 25.29 (A–D) Intraoral views of a patient with unilateral right cleft lip and palate with anterior crossbite and severe maxillary and mandibular crowding. Maxillary lateral incisors and mandibular first bicuspids were extracted. After the maxillary arch was consolidated, an anchorage screw (arrows) was used to assist with canine and incisor retraction. Note space closure and correction of the anterior crossbite.

Table 25.1 Values obtained from the virtual planning software representing the desired movements in three dimensions of the various maxillary, mandibular, and dental structures

Point	Name	Anterior/Posterior	Left/Right	Up/Down
ANS	Anterior nasal spine	8.00 mm anterior	1.28 mm left	0.98 mm up
A	A point	7.53 mm anterior	1.09 mm left	1.30 mm up
ISU1	Midline of upper incisor	6.00 mm anterior	0.50 mm left	1.00 mm up
U3L	Upper left canine	6.12 mm anterior	0.54 mm left	1.55 mm up
U6L	Upper left anterior molar (mesiobuccal cusp)	6.19 mm anterior	0.56 mm left	1.92 mm up
U3R	Upper right canine	6.12 mm anterior	0.52 mm left	2.85 mm up
U6R	Upper right anterior molar (mesiobuccal cusp)	6.21 mm anterior	0.55 mm left	3.41 mm up
ISL1	Midline of lower incisor	2.94 mm posterior	4.53 mm right	3.72 mm up
I6L	Lower left anterior molar (mesiobuccal cusp)	1.03 mm posterior	2.15 mm right	0.80 mm up
L6R	Lower right anterior molar (mesiobuccal cusp)	5.11 mm posterior	2.30 mm right	3.72 mm up
B	B point	1.73 mm posterior	5.15 mm right	3.30 mm up
Pog	Pogonion	1.15 mm posterior	5.66 mm right	3.24 mm up

Note 6 mm advancement of the upper incisor and movement of pogonion to the right 5.66 mm.

a skeletal open bite and marked mandibular deficiency or asymmetry, a two-jaw approach must be undertaken. The advantage of this surgical/orthodontic approach is that, with one operation, the reconstructive team can provide the patient with close to ideal occlusal relations, with markedly improved function and aesthetics.

To assure success, close cooperation between the orthodontist and surgeon is required. It is the responsibility of the orthodontist to support the surgeon, so at the time of surgery, adequate occlusal relationships can be obtained. This, in turn, will add stability to the orthognathic procedure.

The planning for orthognathic surgery in the cleft patient is no different to that done for the patient with a non-cleft dentofacial deformity. This includes a detailed clinical examination and collection of pertinent records prior to orthodontic treatment and again before surgery. All patients with palatal clefts who undergo maxillary advancement surgery are at risk for velopharyngeal insufficiency (VPI); therefore, evaluation by the team speech and language pathologist is required before and after surgery to discuss potential risks for and postoperative correction of VPI if necessary. After all the necessary records are obtained, the orthodontist will perform a cephalometric analysis and prediction surgical tracing to determine the required surgical movements. This can be done by hand tracing the X-rays or by using computerized imaging – virtual surgical planning (VSP) and cephalometric analysis. With the introduction of VSP digital 3D software technology, based on CT scans and more recently CBCT, a new approach has been developed to assist surgeons and orthodontists in the planning of craniomaxillofacial surgery.[52–56] This approach utilizes digital data from the scans, which in turn is managed by specialized software to create a 3D virtual model of the craniofacial skeleton. The desired surgical movements can be performed digitally. Based on the digital data, a physical model of the skull or the surgical splints can be constructed through stereolithography. This approach obviates the use of the traditional presurgical planning that included use of a face bow and dental articulators to plan and do model surgery.

Although the traditional approach has provided satisfactory outcomes, it can be inaccurate for complex movements and requires a sophisticated degree of proficiency acquired through experience. Delegation of this approach is not possible, and the surgeon and orthodontist need to spend significant laboratory time to plan surgery and prepare the needed surgical splints.

Significant research and technological developments have permitted accuracy of VSP, especially the incorporation of accurate digital dental models from plaster casts into the maxillofacial model obtained through the CT and CBCT scans.[57–59] As VSP approaches become more familiar and accessible to clinicians, the planning and construction of surgical splints, surgical guides, and the execution of complex maxillofacial surgery required by cleft patients should improve and predictable and successful outcomes should be routinely obtained (Figs. 25.30 & 25.31; Table 25.1). In addition the clinician should be able to delegate significant aspects of the planning and splint fabrication procedures.[60,61] This approach gives the clinician a close approximation of the desired outcome, but they must be aware of the limited knowledge on soft-tissue responses (lip, nose, and velopharyngeal structures) relative to skeletal movement, especially in cleft patients. Additional research on 3D responses of the facial soft tissues after maxillo/mandibular surgery is still needed. It is emphasized that it is the clinician and not the computer that will make the final treatment and surgical decisions. The 3D computerized technological advances of VSP allow the clinician diagnostic evaluation in all three planes of space, providing postsurgical evaluation that was not possible before. These include changes in airway volume after maxillary and mandibular surgery[62–64] and volumetric bone changes after alveolar bone grafting.[65,66]

Recently, however, there has been a resurgence of a "surgery first, orthodontics later" approach.[67,68] The desired approach, especially for the cleft patient, is opposite – "orthodontics first", followed by surgery and finishing orthodontics. Before

Text continued on p. 613

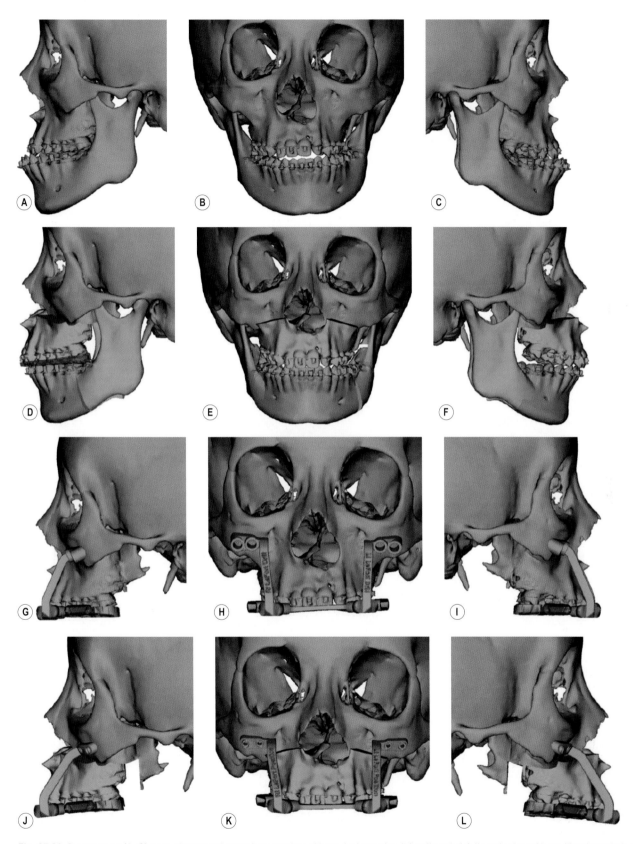

Fig. 25.30 Pre-treatment **(A–C)** three-dimensional scans from a patient with repaired complete left unilateral cleft lip and palate with maxillary hypoplasia and left mandibular asymmetry. A two-piece maxillary Le Fort I advancement (green), with simultaneous bilateral sagittal split osteotomies (blue) for correction of the asymmetry were planned **(D–F)** for the patient. **(G–L)** Orthognathic Positioning System. Virtual design of occlusal based removable drilling guides to place reference holes above the osteotomy line **(G–I)**. The guides will be manufactured with hard resin through stereolithography. The round openings on the guides will be used to place a metal drill guide for exact placement of the landmarks. Using the post maxillary advancement virtual plan, the final positioning guides **(J–L)** are designed and manufactured as indicated above. These guides are longer than the drilling guides as they are made with the maxilla in the advanced desired new position. The smaller perforations on the final guides are used to locate the reference landmarks to assure exact position of the advancement maxilla and also for temporary fixation with bone screws. Once secured, medial rigid fixation is applied with plates and screws, the guides are removed, and the maxillary buttresses are fixated.   *Continued*

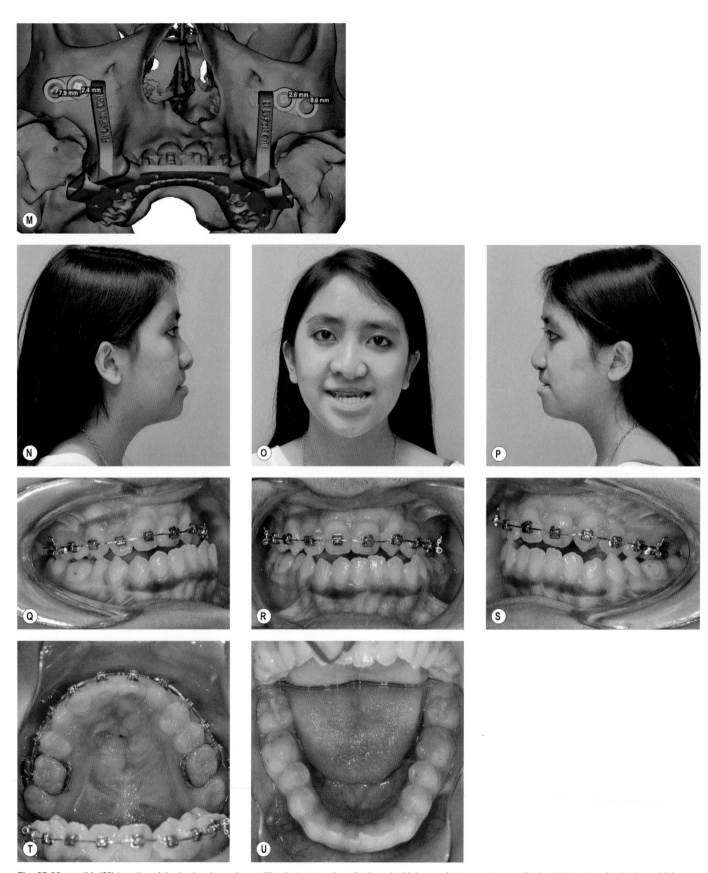

Fig. 25.30, cont'd (M) Location of the landmarks on the maxillary buttresses where the bone is thick enough to support screw fixation. Note values for the bone thickness on the intended reference perforations or landmarks. Facial **(N–P)** and intraoral **(Q–U)** photographs of a 16-year-old female with a repaired left complete unilateral cleft lip and palate after initial orthodontics and alveolar bone graft surgery. Note retrusive upper lip, prominent lower lip, and mandibular skeletal asymmetry to the left. Intraorally, she had anterior and left crossbites, anterior open bite, teeth #5 and 10 were missing, the mandibular dental midline was to the left of the upper one and there was mild lower crowding.

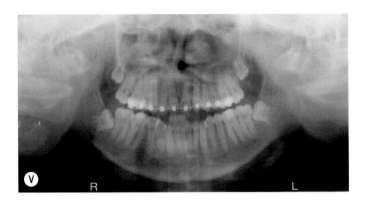

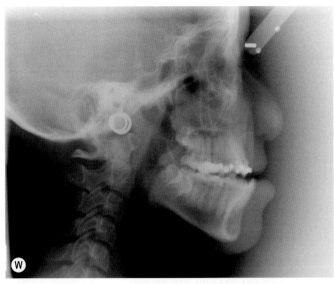

Fig. 25.30, cont'd The panoramic radiograph **(V)** confirms missing teeth #5 and 10 and impacted teeth #17 & 32. The cephalometric radiograph **(W)** reveals maxillary hypoplasia and mild mandibular prognathism.

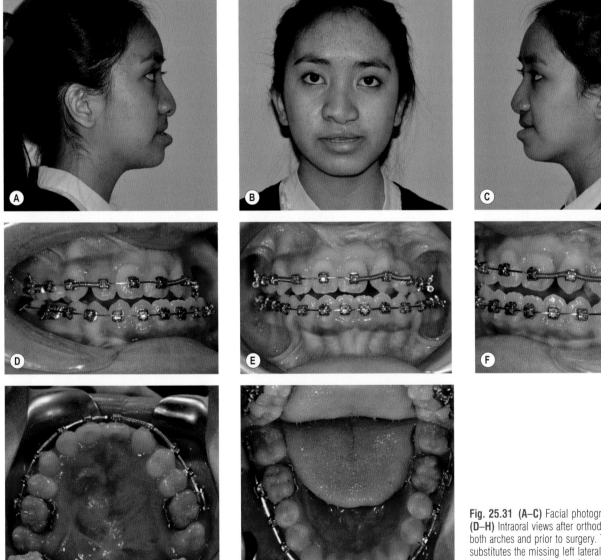

Fig. 25.31 (A–C) Facial photographs prior to surgery. **(D–H)** Intraoral views after orthodontic alignment of both arches and prior to surgery. Tooth #11 substitutes the missing left lateral incisor (#10). Note decompensation of the dentition with worsening of the anterior crossbite. The arches are aligned and coordinated; the mandibular midline is to the left of the upper one.   *Continued*

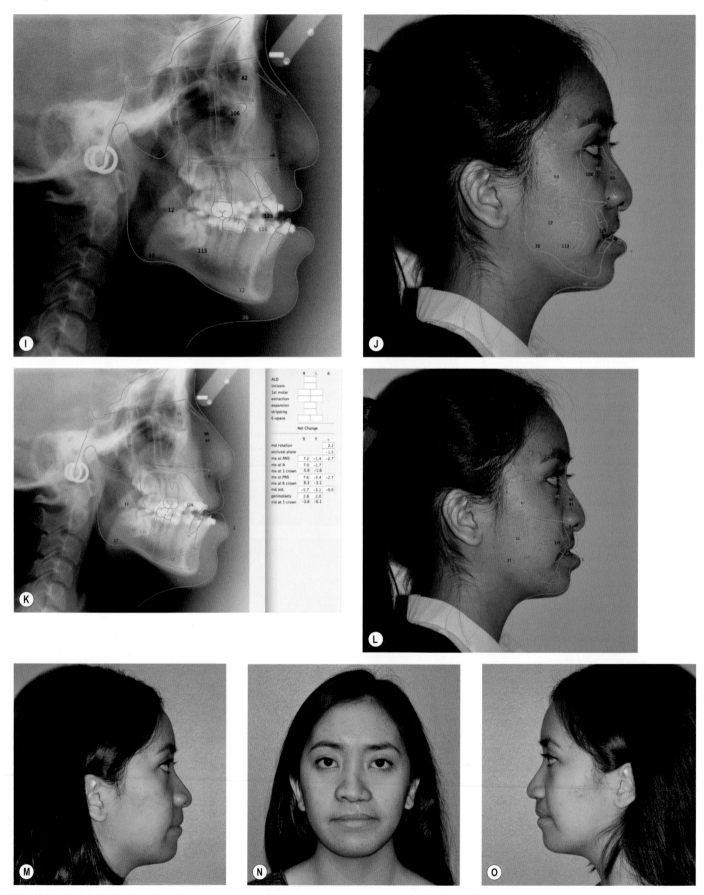

Fig. 25.31, cont'd **(I)** Cephalometric tracing superimposed on the presurgical cephalometric radiograph. **(J)** Prediction tracing demonstrating the planned maxillary advancement, mandibular setback, and genioplasty. Computer generated numbers are seen to the right. **(K)** Note similarity to those obtained during the virtual surgical planning. **(L)** Computer morphing of the lateral facial photograph demonstrating the predicted improved profile facial change. Facial **(M–O)** and intraoral **(P–T)** photographs after surgery. Note improvement of the upper lip retrusion and mandibular skeletal asymmetry. The intraoral photographs demonstrate excellent occlusal relations with correction of the anterior and left crossbites. Clinical results are similar to the virtual and cephalometric plans.

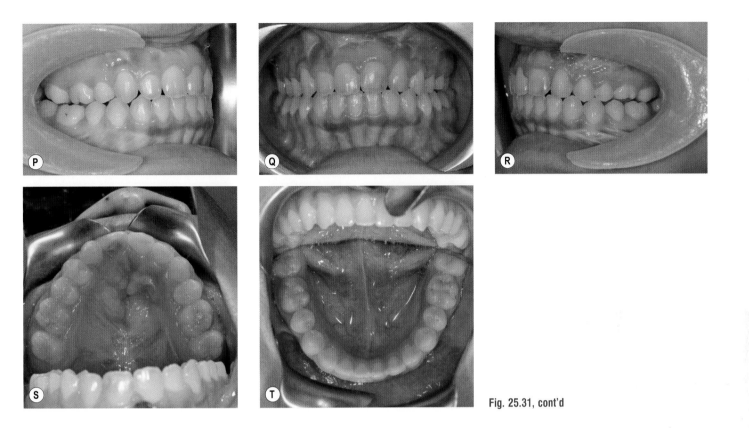

Fig. 25.31, cont'd

surgery, the orthodontist must position all teeth within their supporting basal bones with the maxillary incisors in an ideal position relative to the palatal plane and the mandibular incisors in ideal axial inclination relative to the mandibular plane. Both arches need to be properly coordinated to allow for ideal occlusal interdigitation at the time of surgery. In addition, the orthodontist must create interdental spaces to facilitate instrumentation, if interdental osteotomies are anticipated. The orthodontic appliance is used during the period of intermaxillary fixation and immediately after surgery for postsurgical elastic therapy (Fig. 25.32 ⊕) and detailing of the occlusion. Close cooperation between the orthodontist and surgeon during the planning and initial orthodontic treatment stages should yield favorable occlusal, functional, and aesthetic outcomes (see Figs. 25.1 & 25.32 ⊕).

In patients in whom the maxillary deficiency is severe and where there is substantial scarring or existing pharyngeal flaps, conventional orthognathic procedures are not reliable due to the inherent lack of stability and high relapse tendencies.[69,70] When performing conventional procedures in young patients with severe maxillary hypoplasia, one must wait until adolescence for surgical correction as these techniques rely on rigid fixation that requires substantial bone for placement of the hardware. Further, unerupted tooth buds might be injured during the application of rigid fixation plates. For young patients with severe maxillary deficiency, we have utilized distraction osteogenesis with a rigid external distraction (RED) device, and internal devices for patients with mild to moderate deficiencies. The technique of maxillary distraction utilizing a RED device has been previously described[71–75] and consists of five steps: (1) the fabrication of an intraoral splint that is used to deliver the distraction forces to the maxilla via the teeth; (2) a complete high Le Fort I osteotomy

with septal and pterygomaxillary disjunction; (3) the placement of a cranial halo with an external adjustable distraction screw system; (4) distraction; and (5) rigid and removable retention, as previously presented.

This technique has been applied to young children as well as adolescents and adults, with excellent functional and aesthetic results (Figs. 25.33 & 25.34). The stability of the procedure has been remarkable and superior to that reported for conventional orthognathic surgical approaches.[73,75–78] The soft-tissue changes have also been superior to those reported when conventional orthognathic surgical techniques are used in cleft patients.[79,80] The velopharyngeal mechanism of these patients is minimally affected, especially for those patients having pharyngeal flaps who report improved articulation and resonance. Patients without pharyngeal flaps requiring major advancements can have postdistraction velopharyngeal incompetence requiring treatment with a pharyngeal flap or another type of pharyngoplasty.[81,82] To date, we have not seen negative effects on dental development; although, when performed in children under 6 years of age, we have noted, on occasion, rotation of a permanent second molar tooth bud as a result of increases in posterior arch length or surgical trauma.

Internal devices have been used in patients with less severe maxillary hypoplasia. The device used by the authors is a hybrid device (skeletal and dental anchorage) with the main advantage of not requiring a second operation for its removal. The device has been used successfully, with excellent functional and aesthetic outcomes[83] (Figs. 25.35–25.37 ⊕).

Figs. 25.35–25.37 appear online only.

Maxillary distraction now offers a solution for the difficult cleft maxillary hypoplasia deformity. In addition, the technique has been expanded to other patients with syndromic

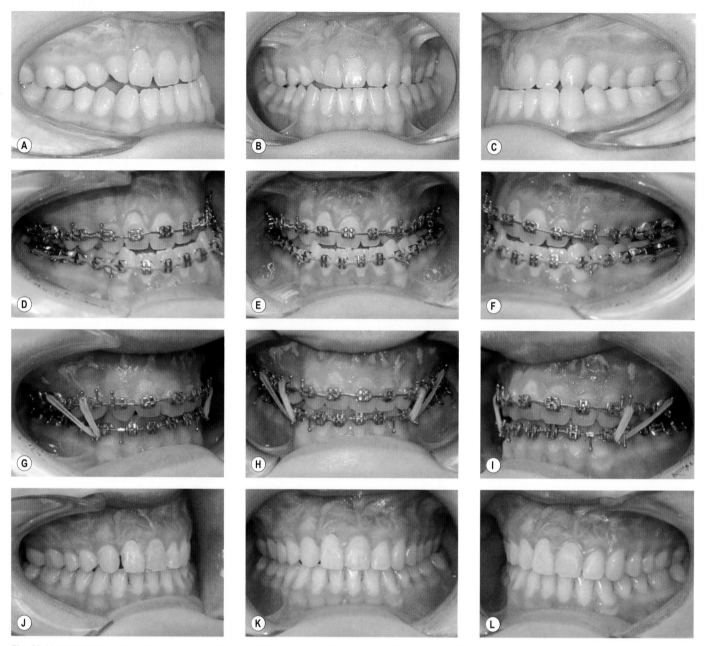

Fig. 25.32 Intraoral views of a patient with right unilateral cleft lip and palate with missing maxillary right lateral incisor and anterior crossbite **(A–C)**. After alveolar bone grafting and orthodontic alignment **(D–F)**, the patient underwent maxillary advancement with midline correction **(G–I)**. Note use of elastics to the orthodontic appliance for fixation and occlusal settling after surgery. After treatment, satisfactory occlusal relations were obtained. Note substitution of the missing right maxillary lateral incisor with the canine, with right class II molar relations and left class I molar and canine relations **(J–L)**.

conditions, such as Apert and Crouzon syndromes, and traumatic deformities.

Growth and orthodontic treatment

It is imperative to recognize that abnormal facial growth will present an added challenge to the reconstructive team. It is understood that cleft patients do have different facial growth patterns than those seen in non-cleft individuals. However, cleft patients have significant growth potential. If

this potential is not negatively affected by the reconstructive procedures required by the patient, it is likely that a favorable outcome will be obtained. Orthodontic treatment will be simplified if minimal growth disturbances affect the patient. Simplification and shortening of orthodontic treatment, which is usually the longest therapeutic intervention for many cleft patients, are desired, as this will decrease the burden of care (e.g., patient, family, provider, public health system, society).

Cleft teams should strive to obtain optimal outcomes by critically assessing their protocols and incorporating proven

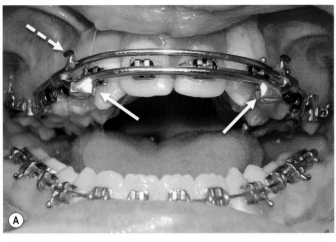
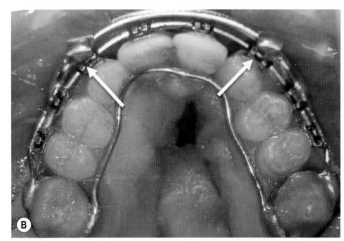
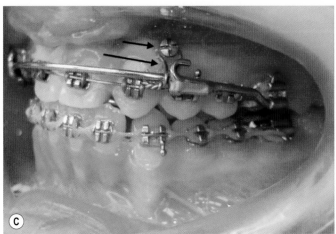
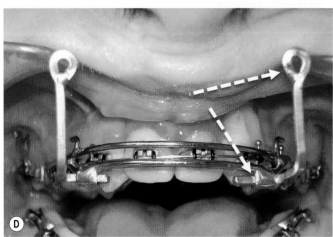

Fig. 25.33 Views of the intraoral splint with removable hooks used for maxillary and midface distraction with rigid external distraction. Note the square tubes (solid arrows) and retention face mask hooks (broken arrow) **(A)**. Occlusal view demonstrating labial and palatal bars soldered to the first molar bands and position of square tubes (arrows) **(B)**. At surgery, bone anchorage screws are placed and suspension wires are dropped to enhance anterior stability of the splint (arrows) **(C)**. Extraoral hooks with traction eyelets inserted through the square tubes of the splint (broken arrows) **(D)**.

strategies to manage their patients. It is accepted that surgery will likely create significant scarring in the infant maxilla, resulting in growth attenuation. Careful attention should be given to those protocols that minimize scarring in the anterior maxilla (i.e., delaying alveolar bone grafting and minimizing palatal scarring by avoiding damage to the maxillary body).[84,85] This, in turn, will result in less need for extended and complex orthodontic procedures. Finally, it should be emphasized that the care of patients with orofacial clefts does not end in adolescence; it will continue through the life of the individual. As patients age, they will undergo the expected soft- and hard-tissue facial changes seen in the non-cleft population. In addition, they may be more susceptible to unfavorable changes due to previous surgeries and the resulting scarring. The maxillary dentition, adjacent to the cleft, is likely more susceptible to periodontal issues due to dental abnormalities (short roots, abnormally shaped crowns), lower than normal bone levels after alveolar bone grafting, previous orthodontic treatment, dental restorations, and issues related to deficient dental hygiene (usually during the early teen years). The cleft team should make every effort to follow patients long-term, in order to advise and remain as a resource, providing additional treatment as it becomes necessary.

Conclusion

The important contribution of the orthodontist to the comprehensive surgical orthodontic management of the cleft patient is illustrated herein. The role of the orthodontist is to support the surgeon with all aspects of craniofacial growth, dental development, occlusion, and treatment planning so that ideal outcomes can be obtained. With the addition of nasal alveolar molding as well as maxillary distraction osteogenesis, the traditional protocols for cleft management have been expanded. In addition, the incorporation of new technological advancements in orthodontics, such as highly flexible orthodontic arch wires, self-ligating orthodontic appliances, BAS, and accessibility to new virtual surgical planning technology and manufacturing, facilitates the required treatment interventions. It is hoped that these innovations will provide clinicians with new strategies for the difficult management of the cleft patient and will provide the patient with outstanding outcomes. The treatment plan of the patient should be developed around the anatomical, functional, and developmental needs of the patient. Close cooperation between the surgeon and orthodontist is imperative for a successful outcome.

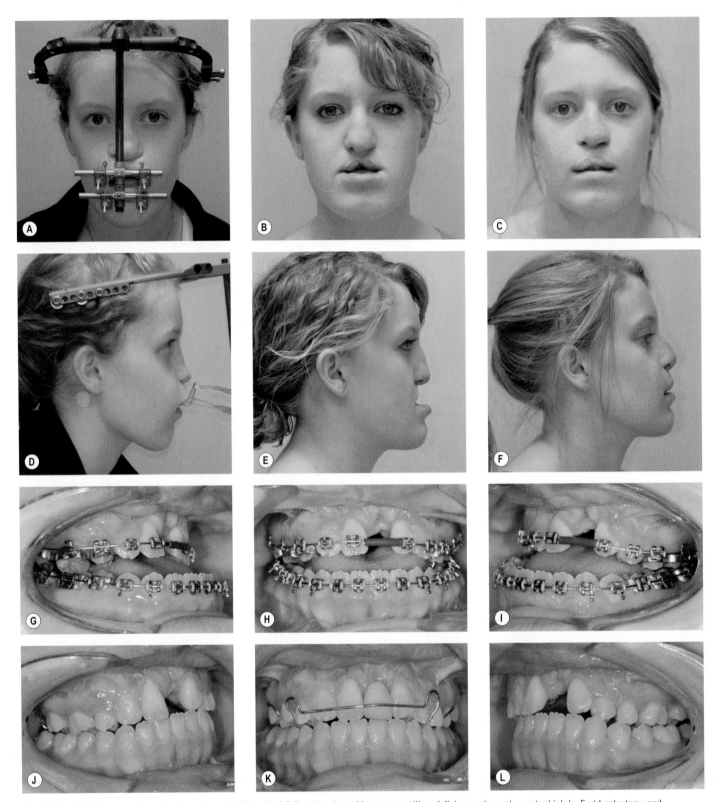

Fig. 25.34 (A–F) Facial photographs of a patient with bilateral cleft lip and palate with severe maxillary deficiency who underwent a high Le Fort I osteotomy and advancement with rigid external distraction **(A,D)**. Before **(B,E)** and after **(C,F)** distraction frontal and profile views. Note dramatic facial balance improvement after treatment. Intraoral views before **(G–I)** and after **(J–L)** distraction. Note severe class III relations before treatment and restoration to a functional and aesthetic occlusion after treatment.

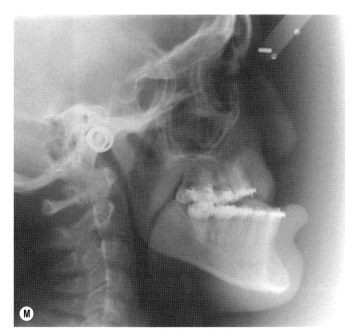 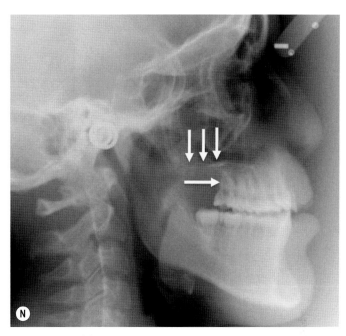

Fig. 25.34, cont'd Before treatment **(M)** note vertical and horizontal maxillary hypoplasia. After treatment **(N)**, the amount of advancement is indicated by the horizontal arrow. The vertical arrows indicate the newly formed bone. Note absence of any fixation hardware, correction of preoperative open bite tendency, as well as anterior dental relations.

Bonus content for this chapter can be found online at

http://www.expertconsult.com

Anterior crossbite
Transitional dentition
Fig. 25.1 (A–I) Facial and **(J–R)** intraoral photographs; **(S–U)** panoramic and **(V–X)** lateral cephalometric radiographs of a patient with unilateral cleft lip and palate. The patient underwent lip and palate surgery in infancy. He had an alveolar bone graft in the transitional dentition. He had a diminutive tooth number 7 that was extracted and substituted with number 6. In late childhood, maxillary deficiency was noted and persisted until adolescence. He had orthodontic preparation of the dentition and underwent surgical maxillary advancement with rigid fixation. His treatment was successful, with satisfactory facial, occlusal, and skeletal outcomes.
Fig. 25.2 Dental cast **(A)** of an infant with unilateral cleft lip utilized to fabricate a palatal plate **(B)** to which a stainless-steel wire **(C)** is attached to fabricate the nasal stent required for molding the nasal structures.
Fig. 25.3 The wire to fabricate the nasal stent is left long **(A)**, measured relative to the height of the nose, and cut and bent, leaving an "adjustment loop" (lower arrow) and a terminal loop (upper arrow) to attach the nasal conformer part of the stent **(B)**. The end of the wire is covered by hard acrylic and lined with soft acrylic to fabricate the nasal stent (arrows) **(C)**. Patient without **(D)** and with **(E)** nasoalveolar molding plate in place.
Fig. 25.4 Facial photographs of a patient with unilateral cleft lip and palate before **(A)**, after nasoalveolar molding and before lip surgery, frontal view **(B)** and worm's-eye view **(C)**. Intraoral views before **(D)** and after **(E)** nasoalveolar molding. Note alveolar and palatal cleft narrowing and improved nasal form after nasoalveolar molding and prior to lip surgery. Frontal facial photograph after nasoalveolar molding and lip surgery **(F)**.
Fig. 25.5 Patient with unilateral cleft lip and palate undergoing nasoalveolar molding **(A)** and with facial taping **(B)**. Note rounding of the alar cartilage around the nasal stent.
Fig. 25.6 After nasoalveolar molding and lip surgery a nasal stent is inserted **(A)** and secured with tape **(B)**. Note base tapes adhering to the cheeks **(A)**, used to secure the nasal stent tape and to prevent skin irritation during frequent tape replacement.
Fig. 25.7 (A) Frontal, **(B)** profile, and **(C)** intraoral photographs of a patient with bilateral cleft lip and palate with protrusive and deviated premaxilla. She

underwent premaxillary repositioning with an intraoral plate **(D)** with an anterior elastomeric chain **(E)**. **(F, G)** Frontal, **(H)** profile, and **(I)** intraoral photographs after premaxillary repositioning and prior to nasal molding. Note reduction of premaxillary asymmetry and protrusion as well as improved nasal form.
Fig. 25.8 After initial premaxillary repositioning, patient with bilateral cleft and palate undergoing nasal molding. Note two nasal stents added to the plate with an anterior elastomeric chain **(A, B)**. While the elastomeric chain is holding the premaxilla and prolabium down and back, the nasal stents elevate the nasal tip, repositioning the nasal domes towards the midline and elongating the columella **(C–E)**.
Fig. 25.9 Frontal, profile, and nasal photographs of a patient with bilateral cleft lip and palate who underwent presurgical nasoalveolar molding treatment and primary lip repair. Comparison of before **(A–C)** and after **(D–F)** nasoalveolar molding photographs illustrate reduction of premaxillary asymmetry and protrusion as well as improvement of nasal asymmetry. A satisfactory lip and nasal repair was obtained soon after lip surgery **(G–I)**. Four years after surgery **(J–L)**, the patient maintains excellent lip line, nose/lip relations, nasal symmetry, and projection.
Fig. 25.10 Long-term follow-up of a patient with unilateral cleft lip and palate treated with presurgical nasoalveolar molding, and only primary lip and palate repair and alveolar bone grafting. Close-up photos of the nose before **(A)** and after **(B)** nasoalveolar molding, and feeding with the nasoalveolar molding prosthesis in place **(C)**. Facial photos before treatment **(D)**, postsurgery at 2 **(E)**, 9 **(F)**, and 16 **(G)** years of age. Note satisfactory outcome with nice lip line and stable nasal symmetry.
Fig. 25.11 Patient with unilateral cleft lip and palate in the transitional dentition prior to orthodontic preparation for alveolar bone grafting **(A–C)**, after orthodontic treatment **(D–F)**, and after bone graft **(G–I)**. Note alignment of the dental arch with a simple segmental edgewise orthodontic appliance. **(J–L)** Occlusal views at similar stages. Note missing lateral incisor and retained primary canine in the cleft area (arrow) **(J)**. This tooth was extracted prior to surgery. Note aligned arch prior to surgery **(K)**. After surgery, the permanent canine erupted through the bone-grafted area (arrow) **(L)**. **(M–O)** Panoramic radiographs at similar stages: note in the pretreatment radiographs **(M,N)** complete apical root development of the maxillary incisors (single arrow),

retained primary canine and missing lateral incisor (dotted arrow), and unerupted maxillary left canine (double arrows). After orthodontics and bone grafting (O), note intact maxillary incisor root apices (single arrow) and maxillary left canine erupting through the bone graft (double arrows). (P) After treatment an interim prosthesis was given to the patient replacing the missing lateral incisor (arrow).

Fig. 25.12 (A–D) Maxillary arch expansion and dental alignment in a unilateral cleft lip and palate patient with severe scarring and collapse. Treatment was achieved in a slow fashion with the use of highly flexible wires and a self-ligating bracket.

Fig. 25.25 (A) Panoramic radiograph of a 6-year-old female patient with complete left unilateral cleft lip and palate in the early transitional dentition stage. She is missing the second right maxillary second bicuspid and has a peg cleft-side permanent maxillary lateral incisor. The cleft-side primary canine had a stainless steel crown and had signs of early root resorption compared to the contralateral canine. This tooth was scheduled for extraction. **(B–E)** Frontal intraoral photographs. **(B)** Pre-treatment view. **(C)** During expansion and maxillary arch dental alignment. **(D)** After arch alignment and eruption of the peg-shaped lateral incisor and prior to the bone graft. **(E)** Orthodontic movement of the peg-shaped lateral incisor through the bone graft. After complete mesialization the patient was placed in retention to allow for eruption of the permanent dentition and finalize orthodontic treatment. **(F)** A year later treatment was re-initiated, the peg-shaped lateral incisor extracted, and the cleft-side permanent canine moved into the position of the lateral incisor. All posterior teeth in that quadrant were moved forward to consolidate the arch. Note adequate gingival tissues and ideal occlusal relations. **(G–J)** Occlusal view of the maxillary arch during various stages of treatment. **(G)** In early transitional dentition prior to treatment. **(H)** Maxillary expander and orthodontic brackets to align the arch and dentition prior to bone graft surgery. Note eruption of the peg-shaped maxillary cleft-side lateral incisor after extraction of the primary canine with stainless steel crown. **(I)** After the alveolar bone graft the cleft-side lateral incisor has been moved through the graft next to the cleft-side maxillary central incisor. Note thickness of the alveolar ridge and transpalatal bar used for retention after expansion. **(J)** Finishing stages of orthodontic treatment after extraction of the peg-shaped maxillary cleft-side lateral incisor and incorporation of the cleft-side maxillary canine in its position. The maxillary arch is well aligned and spaces have been consolidated.

Fig. 25.35 Intraoperative view **(A)** of the placement of a hybrid (bone–dental) internal maxillary distractor for Le Fort I maxillary advancement. Intraoral view **(B)** of the activating arm after incision closure. Note the horizontal arm of the distractor is wired through an intraoral metal splint (arrows). Cephalometric **(C)** and panoramic **(D)** radiographs demonstrating the buttress plates, adjustable and removable vertical stem, and horizontal distractor arm.

Fig. 25.36 After distraction and consolidation the device is removed in the office setting; the horizontal arms are unwired and removed from the vertical stems **(A, B)**. The vertical stem is unscrewed from the buttress plate and removed. The small vestibular wound is left to close spontaneously **(C, D)**.

Fig. 25.37 Before **(A–C)** and after **(D–E)** facial photographs of a patient with right unilateral cleft lip and palate and moderate maxillary hypoplasia who underwent Le Fort I maxillary advancement utilizing an internal adjustable and removable distraction device. Note improvement of facial convexity and lip/nose relations after treatment. Intraoral views before **(G–I)** and after **(J–L)** treatment. Note anterior crossbite and class III relations before treatment. The maxillary canines were used to replace the missing lateral incisors; she was completed with positive overjet and overbite and class II molar relations. Cephalometric and panoramic radiographs before **(M, O)** and after **(N, P)** treatment. Note moderate maxillary hypoplasia and concave profile before treatment as well as the still-erupting second maxillary molars. After treatment the maxilla was advanced, improving the skeletal and soft-tissue profile as well as anterior dental relations. Note continued eruption of maxillary second molars (horizontal arrow) and the buttress plates that remain after the distractor was removed (vertical arrow) after treatment.

⊕ Access the complete reference list online at   **http://www.expertconsult.com**

8. Grayson BH, Santiago PE, Brecht LE, et al. Presurgical nasoalveolar molding in infants with cleft lip and palate. *Cleft Palate Craniofac J.* 1999;36:486–498. *This article introduces the now-widespread concept of presurgical nasoalveolar molding. The authors conclude that nasoalveolar molding eliminates the need for surgical columella reconstruction.*

69. Posnick JC, Dagys AP. Skeletal stability and relapse patterns after Le Fort I maxillary osteotomy fixed with miniplates: the unilateral cleft lip and palate deformity. *Plast Reconstr Surg.* 1994;94:924–932. *This study assesses relapse rates in 35 consecutive patients undergoing Le Fort I osteotomy with miniplate fixation and autogenous bone grafting. The authors found that miniplates do not prevent relapse in this population.*

73. Polley JW, Figueroa AA. Rigid external distraction: its application in cleft maxillary deformities. *Plast Reconstr Surg.* 1998;102:1360–1372.

The authors present the use of rigid external distraction to correct maxillary hypoplasia in patients with facial clefts. Dramatic improvements in skeletal anatomy and soft-tissue deficiencies were observed.

75. Paresi R Jr, Felsten L, Shoukas J, et al. Maxillary distraction osteogenesis. In: Losee J, Kirschner RE, eds. *Comprehensive Cleft Care.* New York: McGraw Hill; 2009:956–968. *This chapter offers a useful review of maxillary distraction in the context of orofacial clefting. Cephalometric evaluation is emphasized.*

82. Guyette TW, Polley JW, Figueroa A, et al. Changes in speech following maxillary distraction osteogenesis. *Cleft Palate Craniofac J.* 2001;38:199–205. *Articulation and velopharyngeal function were assessed before and after maxillary distraction. Metrics included hyper/hyponasality, velopharyngeal passage dimensions, and articulation error.*

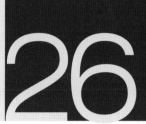

Velopharyngeal dysfunction

Richard E. Kirschner and Adriane L. Baylis

Access video content for this chapter online at expertconsult.com

SYNOPSIS

- Individuals with known or suspected velopharyngeal dysfunction (VPD) are best treated in the context of an interdisciplinary cleft/craniofacial team.
- Diagnosis of VPD requires obtaining a comprehensive patient history, perceptual speech evaluation, physical examination, and appropriate instrumental and imaging studies.
- Successful surgical management of VPD requires precision in diagnosis and individualization of treatment.
- VPD may be the result of velopharyngeal insufficiency, velopharyngeal incompetence, or velopharyngeal mislearning.
- Flexible fiberoptic nasopharyngoscopy should be completed as part of a standard preoperative evaluation to allow for direct visualization of the velopharyngeal mechanism during speech and surgical planning.
- Instrumental assessment of speech should always be interpreted in the context of the results of a comprehensive perceptual speech evaluation.
- Aerodynamic assessment of speech can provide the surgeon with information regarding velopharyngeal orifice size and timing to assist with treatment decision-making and judgment of surgical outcome.
- The primary goal of surgical management is to produce a competent velopharyngeal mechanism for speech while avoiding the complications of nasal airway obstruction.

Introduction

Normal speech is dependent upon the functional and structural integrity of the velopharynx, a complex and dynamic structure that serves to decouple the oral and nasal cavities during sound production. Dysfunction of the velopharyngeal valve (referred to as VPD) may lead to hypernasality, nasal air emission, and compensatory articulation errors, all of which may impair speech intelligibility and lead to stigmatization. There may also be "non-speech" sequelae of VPD including nasal regurgitation. The goal of surgical intervention is to produce or restore velopharyngeal competence while avoid-

ing the complications of upper airway obstruction. Successful surgical management of VPD requires precision in diagnosis and individualization of treatment. Thus, optimization of surgical outcome is critically dependent upon a careful analysis of each patient's history, speech characteristics, structural anatomy, and velopharyngeal dynamics – an analysis best performed with close collaboration between the surgeon, the speech pathologist, and the other members of the cleft/craniofacial team.

Anatomy and physiology of the velopharynx

Anatomy

The velopharyngeal port is defined by the soft palate, or velum, by the lateral pharyngeal walls, and by the posterior pharyngeal wall. Closure of the velopharynx during speech is a subconscious and automated action that is mediated by the motor cortex and that requires the coordinated action of the velopharyngeal musculature. The muscles of the soft palate include the levator veli palatini, the tensor veli palatini, the palatoglossus, the palatopharyngeus, and the musculus uvulae (Fig. 26.1). The levator takes its origin from the petrous portion of the temporal bone and from the medial aspect of the eustachian tube. Its fibers course anteriorly, inferiorly, and medially, inserting into the palatal aponeurosis and decussating with the levator fibers from the opposite side (Fig. 26.2). Contraction of the muscular sling formed by the paired levators is the primary mechanism for velar elevation and closure of the velopharyngeal port, although evidence suggests that the palatoglossus and palatopharyngeus muscles may act as antagonists to the levators to provide fine motor control of velar position during speech.[1,2] The musculus uvulae is a paired intrinsic muscle that likely contributes to velopharyngeal closure both by adding bulk to the dorsal surface of the velum and by contributing to velar stretch.[3–5] It is usually

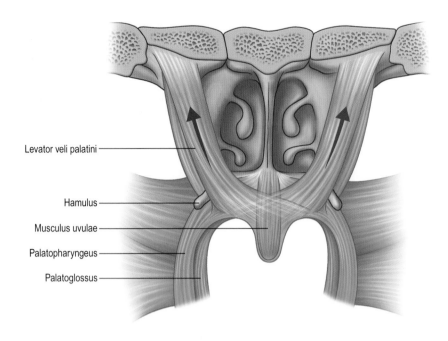

Fig. 26.1 Muscles of the velopharynx.

absent in patients with overt and submucosal clefts of the palate.[6]

The superior pharyngeal constrictor is a broad, thin muscle that takes origin from the velum, the medial pterygoid, and the pterygomandibular raphe, inserting into the median pharyngeal raphe along with the constrictor muscle fibers from the opposite side. Contraction of the superior constrictor may contribute to velopharyngeal closure by effecting medial movement of the lateral walls and anterior movement of the posterior wall of the velopharynx.[7,8] The anatomy of the superior constrictor and its contribution to velopharyngeal closure, however, are highly variable.

With the exception of the tensor veli palatini, which is innervated by the third division of the trigeminal nerve (V_3), all of the muscles of the velopharynx receive motor innervation from the pharyngeal plexus, which is composed of fibers from the glossopharyngeal (IX), vagus (X), and accessory (XI) nerves.[9] Studies have suggested that the facial nerve (VII) may also play a minor role in velopharyngeal motor function.[10,11] It is important to note that, although the functional activity of the velopharyngeal valve during speech and swallowing may be similar, the neurological pathways for these activities are distinct. Velopharyngeal movements for speech are learned, automatized activities that are controlled by the motor cortex,

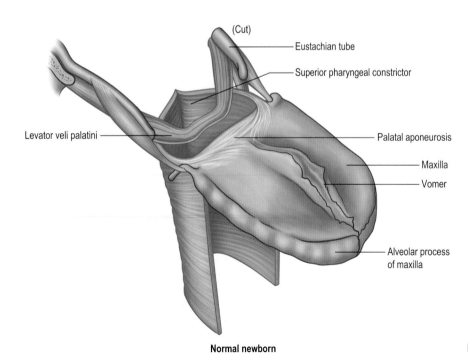

Normal newborn

Fig. 26.2 Schematic of the levator veli palatini.

whereas similar movements for swallowing are primarily involuntary activities that originate from the brainstem.

Physiology

The velopharynx is a complex, three-dimensional valve which serves to uncouple the oropharynx and nasopharynx during speech and swallowing. This section will briefly discuss velopharyngeal function during speech.

It is widely accepted that the levator veli palatini is the muscle that is primarily responsible for velar motion and, hence, for velopharyngeal closure.[12] Fine motor control of velar position may also be governed by the palatoglossus and palatopharyngeus. As noted above, the paired musculus uvulae may play an important role in velar stretch and in filling the gap between the velum and the posterior pharynx during velopharyngeal closure. The relative contribution of the levator and of the superior pharyngeal constrictor to lateral pharyngeal wall movement has been the subject of some debate.

In normal individuals, the velum lifts posteriorly and superiorly during velopharyngeal closure. The normal point of contact with the posterior pharyngeal wall is located approximately three-quarters of the way back on the velum from the posterior nasal spine (Fig. 26.3). The site of velopharyngeal closure is usually at or just inferior to the palatal plane which is typically at or above the level of the first cervical vertebrae (C1), but velar height, as well as the extent of velopharyngeal contact, varies systematically depending upon the phonetic context, speech accuracy, rate, and effort.[13–15]

The contribution of lateral pharyngeal wall movement to velopharyngeal closure varies amongst individuals with or without cleft palate and, as with velar movement, varies with the phonemic task. Maximal lateral pharyngeal wall displacement generally occurs at the level of velopharyngeal contact. Skolnick et al.[16] and Croft et al.[17] have described three basic patterns of velopharyngeal closure observed in normal subjects (Fig. 26.4): (1) coronal, in which closure is effected primarily by velar elevation; (2) circular (with or without Passavant's ridge), in which medial movement of the lateral pharyngeal walls contributes to velopharyngeal closure in near-equal proportion to the velum; and (3) sagittal, in which closure is effected primarily by medial movement of the lateral pharyngeal walls and the velum contacts the lateral walls rather than the posterior wall. Of these, the coronal pattern of closure is observed most commonly in both normal individuals and in patients with VPD. In some individuals, a localized transverse ridge of tissue may be seen to form on the posterior pharyngeal wall during speech. This anterior movement of the posterior pharyngeal wall during velopharyngeal closure was first described by Passavant in 1863[18] and is therefore frequently referred to as "Passavant's ridge". Although some have written that its appearance is always indicative of pathologic velopharyngeal function, Croft et al.[17] have demonstrated that Passavant's ridge may play a role in velopharyngeal closure in both normal speakers and in those with VPD.

Electromyographic studies support the notion that normal velopharyngeal function requires the central coordination of velopharyngeal muscle activity with other articulatory movements.[19] Changes in velar position during sound production represent the end result of a complex interaction of several interrelated variables, including auditory and proprioceptive feedback. Moreover, for a single individual, there may be significant flexibility in the system of sound production such that there may be a limited but variable repertoire of velopharyngeal movements that may produce the same perceived sounds. Despite decades of speech science research, the precise neurophysiology of both normal and abnormal velopharyngeal function remains incompletely understood.

MRI has quickly gained ground as the primary method for studying the anatomy, and emerging physiologic measures, of velopharyngeal structures. Perry et al.[20] and Bae et al.[21] have shown the application of both traditional and 3D MRI for evaluation of velopharyngeal anatomy in persons with and without clefts. MRI has also been utilized to explore sexual dimorphism in velopharyngeal structures as well as how velopharyngeal anatomy and physiology changes over time with growth and aging.[22] Lastly, dynamic MRI during speech is now feasible in the clinical setting as a complementary tool for clinical evaluation of VP function for speech.[23,24]

Basic science/disease process of velopharyngeal dysfunction

Velopharyngeal insufficiency

The first major diagnostic category of VPD is velopharyngeal insufficiency, a term used to denote an anatomic, or structural, defect responsible for inadequate closure of the velopharyngeal valve. Such defects may be congenital, as in cases of cleft palate or congenital velopharyngeal disproportion (i.e., a short soft palate relative to the depth of the pharynx) (Fig. 26.5), or they may be secondary to surgical procedures that alter velopharyngeal anatomy, as in cases of palatoplasty, tumor resection, or adenoidectomy. The most common

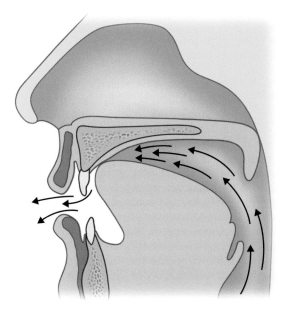

Fig. 26.3 Lateral view of normal velopharyngeal closure for speech during production of an oral pressure consonant.

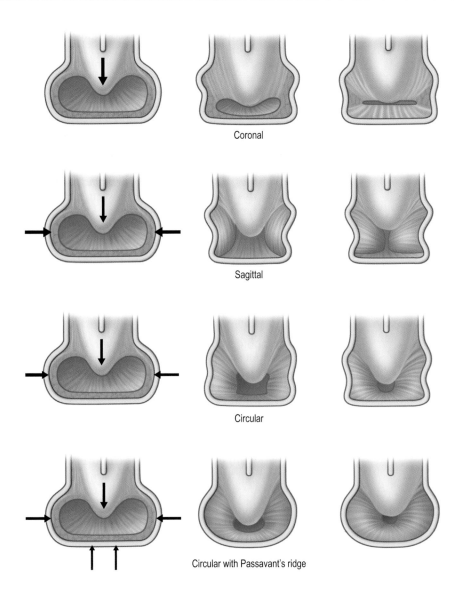

Coronal

Sagittal

Circular

Circular with Passavant's ridge

Fig. 26.4 Types of velopharyngeal closure patterns.

congenital structural defects associated with VPD are cleft palate and submucosal cleft palate. The reported incidence of persistent VPD after cleft palate repair varies widely and is influenced by a large number of variables. In a recent report of long-term outcomes following Furlow palatoplasty, secondary surgery for VPD was only clinically indicated in 8% of children at five years of age.[25] In the absence of an oronasal fistula, however, VPD after palatoplasty is most commonly the result of impaired velar mobility, velopharyngeal disproportion, or a combination of both.

Since adequacy of velopharyngeal closure is largely a function of the ratio of pharyngeal depth to palatal length, patients with a proportionally short palate or deep pharynx may demonstrate incomplete velopharyngeal closure (see Fig. 26.5). Each of these conditions may be the result of either a congenital anomaly or an iatrogenic alteration in velopharyngeal architecture. Cicatricial changes following palatoplasty, for example, may lead to velopharyngeal insufficiency secondary to velar shortening. Congenital differences in skeletal architecture may also play a role in postpalatoplasty VPD. Patients with clefts have been demonstrated to have a broader

nasopharynx than controls, likely the result of alterations in cranial base dimensions.[26–28] Osborne *et al.*[29] and Ross and Lindsay[30] have shown that a higher prevalence of upper cervical spine abnormalities in patients with clefts may result in increased pharyngeal depth. Likewise, platybasia, or flattening of the cranial base angle, may contribute to VPD by increasing pharyngeal depth, and thus the depth-to-length ratio. Ruotolo *et al.*[31] have shown that patients with 22q11.2 deletion syndrome, a condition associated with a high frequency of severe non-cleft VPD, demonstrate several predisposing skeletal and soft-tissue anomalies, including increased pharyngeal depth, platybasia, and cervical spine anomalies.

Velopharyngeal insufficiency may also be caused by postsurgical changes in velopharyngeal anatomy. In young children, velopharyngeal closure is most often velar-adenoidal. Removal of hyperplastic adenoids for the management of nasopharyngeal airway obstruction or chronic otitis media results in an acute increase in pharyngeal depth. In the majority of non-cleft patients, the capacity for velar stretch allows the palate to accommodate for this change. In most cases, postadenoidectomy velopharyngeal insufficiency is transient,

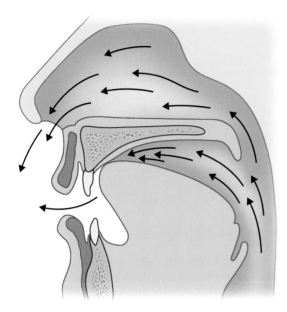

Fig. 26.5 Lateral view of inadequate velopharyngeal closure for speech due to a short soft palate (velopharyngeal insufficiency). The arrows represent the escape of air, pressure, and acoustic energy through the nasal cavity during speech.

and resonance returns to normal within 6–12 months. VPD may persist, however, in a small number of patients, some of whom may have predisposing factors for VPD, including submucosal cleft palate, a short velum, a deep pharynx, or neuromuscular disorders. For patients with these conditions, the adenoids may play a critical role in velopharyngeal closure, and even their normal involution may result in velopharyngeal insufficiency.[12] Careful assessment of velopharyngeal anatomy is therefore essential in all patients prior to adenoidectomy and should be avoided if possible when anatomical factors that predispose to VPD are identified.

In some patients, irregularity of the surface contour of the adenoid pad may interfere with the ability of the velum to achieve complete velopharyngeal closure.[32] In others, enlarged tonsils may intrude between the velum and the posterior pharyngeal wall, resulting in incomplete closure.[33,34] In these cases, the first step in management should be a selective adenoidectomy or tonsillectomy, respectively, as such may be sufficient to solve the problem, obviating the need for any of the surgical procedures later described.

Velopharyngeal incompetence

The second major diagnostic category of VPD is velopharyngeal incompetence. This label is typically reserved for those cases of VPD known or suspected to be due to congenital or acquired neurological and/or neuromuscular causes such as cerebrovascular incidents, traumatic brain injury, brain tumor, abnormalities in muscle tone or function, and degenerative neuromuscular diseases. In velopharyngeal incompetence, there is typically no evidence of any underlying structural abnormality and palatal length is sufficient; however, the function of the velopharyngeal mechanism is suboptimal for speech production and/or swallowing. The speech sequelae of velopharyngeal incompetence are similar to that seen with

velopharyngeal insufficiency, except that many of the individuals also demonstrate other features of dysarthria or other motor speech impairments (e.g., apraxia). Abnormal innervation of cranial nerves IX, X, or XI, or abnormalities in muscle tone/function may result in abnormal timing of palatal elevation which may also exacerbate the perception of hypernasal speech, in excess of that predicted by velopharyngeal gap size alone. In addition, adults with velopharyngeal incompetence, depending on the etiology, frequently exhibit dysphagia and varying degrees of nasal regurgitation.

There are extensive possibilities for neurologic diagnoses that may be associated with congenital velopharyngeal incompetence including, but not limited to, cerebral palsy, myotonic dystrophy, and congenital hypotonia. Asymmetrical velopharyngeal function, such as that typical of patients with hemifacial microsomia, is also a common cause of velopharyngeal incompetency. Acquired or "late" causes of velopharyngeal incompetence may include traumatic brain injury; cerebrovascular accident or brainstem stroke; and progressive diseases such as Parkinson's disease, amyotrophic lateral sclerosis, muscular dystrophies, multiple sclerosis, and other demyelinating diseases.[35–39]

Children and adults with motor speech disorders have also been shown to demonstrate symptoms of velopharyngeal incompetence of varying degrees of severity and consistency. Apraxia of speech (also referred to as developmental apraxia of speech or childhood apraxia of speech, in children) is a neurologic condition resulting in difficulties with speech motor programming and control.[40] Apraxia may be characterized by inconsistent symptoms of VPD such as inconsistent nasalization of vowels or consonants and inconsistent nasal emission. In addition, many individuals with apraxia may exhibit a combination of both inconsistent hypernasality and hyponasality, providing additional evidence of the abnormal coordination of the palate during speech sound production. Younger children with apraxia may demonstrate some overlapping speech features often seen in children with congenital velopharyngeal incompetence of other causes. For example, children with a history of VPD may have a limited inventory of sounds and demonstrate difficulties learning to produce oral consonants in the first few years of life. These children may produce a pattern of compensatory articulation errors (i.e., glottal stop substitutions) or omit sounds completely. Children with apraxia have difficulty with generating the appropriate "motor program" (blueprint) for producing the sequence of motor movements to produce a sound, which is not typical of children with isolated VPD or clefting. The importance of obtaining a thorough speech pathology evaluation to diagnose these conditions differentially is critical for appropriate treatment decision-making.

Lastly, stress velopharyngeal incompetence is a special case of velopharyngeal incompetence for non-speech behaviors. It is most commonly observed in wind musicians given the high pressure demands.[41,42] There may or may not be comorbid hypernasality or nasal emission in speech. In some cases, stress velopharyngeal incompetence may be an indicator of an underlying physical cause of velopharyngeal incompetence, which may have been masked, or very mild, in the past. In some cases, neurologic or structural causes of VPD (e.g., submucous cleft palate) are diagnosed following the presentation of stress velopharyngeal incompetence, further emphasizing the importance of a thorough clinical evaluation of all patients with any form of VPD.[43] Treatment for stress velopharyngeal incompetence may follow a similar course as that for VPD for speech, although there have been reported cases of spontaneous recovery after a period of rest.

Velopharyngeal mislearning

The third, and lesser known, type of VPD involves velopharyngeal mislearning.[44] In this category, the velopharyngeal mechanism appears to be anatomically and physiologically capable of consistent and complete velopharyngeal closure for speech, despite the observation of inconsistent velopharyngeal closure for speech. In this type of VPD, the patient has mislearned how to produce certain speech sounds accurately. The most common example is that of phoneme-specific nasal emission, in which nasal airflow is produced as a complete substitution for an oral consonant, despite adequate velopharyngeal closure ability for other consonants.[45] Clinically, this will often be observed in a child with nasal emission heard on a selected set of sounds, most commonly S, Z, SH, or CH, but not on other sounds such as P, B, T, D, K, G. Another example of velopharyngeal mislearning is the case in which a child produces compensatory articulation errors (e.g., glottal stops) which may prevent or interfere with the achievement of adequate velopharyngeal closure for speech. The velopharyngeal movements during the production of these aberrant speech errors have been shown to be counterproductive (distal versus medial movement of the lateral pharyngeal walls) to the achievement of velopharyngeal closure for speech. A related example is that seen in children with congenital hearing loss with an inability to self-monitor their own speech production, resulting in nasalized speech errors with an otherwise physiologically intact velopharyngeal mechanism.

Velopharyngeal mislearning should be treated with behavioral speech therapy, not surgery. It is critical that a well-trained speech pathologist perform a thorough clinical evaluation to diagnose such conditions differentially in order to make the most appropriate treatment recommendations.

Combined types

In some cases, individuals with craniofacial anomalies and/or clefting may exhibit a combined disorder with evidence of velopharyngeal insufficiency, velopharyngeal incompetency, and/or velopharyngeal mislearning, which poses a diagnostic challenge. Some patients with 22q11.2 deletion syndrome have been shown to demonstrate evidence of a combined type of VPD due to the combination of structural clefting disorders, increased pharyngeal depth, and hypotonia of the velopharynx.[46] Regardless of the type of VPD which is present, a complete and thorough physical exam, clinical speech evaluation, and any necessary instrumental or imaging studies should be completed to confirm the etiology and identify the most appropriate treatment plan.

Diagnosis/patient presentation

Patient history and physical exam

Individuals with known or suspected VPD are best treated in the context of an interdisciplinary cleft palate team. Regardless of age, the clinical examination typically includes a brief history and physical exam, perceptual speech evaluation, imaging and acoustic measures, and team discussion for treatment planning. The following information should be obtained during a patient interview when undergoing evaluation for VPD:

- Current patient/family concerns with speech
- Pregnancy history, complications, medication use, and any exposure to teratogens
- Birth and delivery history and complications
- Primary medical diagnoses (e.g., cleft palate, syndromes, cardiac defects, neuromuscular disease)
- History of any feeding or swallowing difficulties during infancy and any current swallowing concerns, including nasal regurgitation and difficulty with breastfeeding or bottlefeeding during infancy
- History of hearing loss or ear disease, including history of frequent ear infections or effusions
- History of snoring or symptoms of sleep apnea
- Surgical history, including prior tonsillectomy, adenoidectomy, and, if appropriate, cleft-related surgical history and timing
- History of any genetic testing and results
- Family history of cleft lip/palate, nasal speech, speech delay or articulation/pronunciation difficulties, hearing loss, learning disabilities, and medical conditions
- Developmental history
- Speech therapy history.

Every patient, regardless of age, should undergo direct craniofacial and oral examination by the surgeon and speech pathologist with experience in clefting/craniofacial anomalies. The oral exam should be completed in an appropriate examination room and with appropriate lighting. Components of the examination should include an assessment of:

- Craniofacial symmetry
- Oral–facial movement and symmetry
- Dentition and occlusion
- Presence and location of any fistulae
- Presence of signs of submucous cleft palate, including bifid uvula, zona pellucida, and palpate for notch
- Soft palate length, symmetry, and degree of elevation and symmetry during phonation
- Tonsil size and symmetry.

The observations from the physical exam should be interpreted together with the clinical speech evaluation results. For example, if an exam reveals a submucous cleft palate but the patient has normal speech, surgical management would not be recommended. On the other hand, a normal oral exam with clinical speech findings suggestive of severe VPD does not negate the need for physical treatment. The findings from the oral examination may provide hints regarding the source or cause of VPD; however, imaging studies should be completed to confirm the etiology, size/shape, and consistency of the velopharyngeal gap, and to assess the surrounding anatomy of the upper airway.

Perceptual speech evaluation

Perceptual speech assessment is considered the gold standard in the diagnosis of speech disorders of persons with cleft palate and VPD.[47] Additional instrumental assessment and imaging are considered adjunct to the perceptual speech findings, which are the ultimate arbiter of a patient's need for treatment. Perceptual speech evaluation of this patient population should be completed by a speech pathologist with coursework, training, and continuing education in the area of cleft palate and craniofacial anomalies.

During the speech evaluation, the speech pathologist obtains the necessary clinical information regarding the presence and perceived severity of VPD, identifies and describes speech characteristics, determines a suspected etiology, and makes preliminary decisions regarding treatment recommendations to discuss with the team. In addition, the speech pathologist is making diagnostic decisions regarding the presence of comorbid conditions such as articulation disorders, voice disorders, and language difficulties. Box 26.1 provides a list of common speech pathology terminology used for describing the speech characteristics associated with VPD. The most common speech sequelae of VPD include reduced speech intelligibility; articulation disorders ranging from mild to severe articulation disorders (e.g., pervasive use of glottal stop substitutions); reduced intraoral pressure for oral consonants; audible nasal emission or nasal turbulence on oral pressure consonants; hypernasal resonance; possible hoarseness; and decreased loudness.[47–49]

The components of a standard speech evaluation for the assessment of velopharyngeal closure for speech should include an assessment of intelligibility, resonance, voice, and articulation during a spontaneous speech sample, conversation, and/or picture description tasks.[50] A standard reading passage is suggested for use with adolescent and adult patients. Articulation skills should be assessed with standardized measures (i.e., a standardized articulation test), as well as word and sentence repetition tasks (e.g., American English Sentence Sample[50,51]). Oral-only or nasal-only stimuli (e.g., *Buy baby a bib, Pet the puppy, Mama made muffins*, etc.) are also used to assess resonance, nasal emission (audible and inaudible), and pressure for consonants. Special mirrors or listening tubes may also be utilized to evaluate the presence of inaudible nasal emission. The speech parameters are typically rated with five- or seven-point equal-appearing interval scales or other ratio-based scaling methods (e.g., visual analog scales).[47] The Cleft Audit Protocol for Speech-Augmented (CAPS-A)[52] is one rating tool that is now widely used in many cleft centers with adaptations now available for American English as well (CAPS-A-Americleft modification[53]). Audio or video recording of the speech examination should be completed whenever possible for clinical archiving, comparison pre–post treatment, assessment of speech outcome, and for potential research purposes. If clinical symptoms of VPD are present, additional diagnostic testing should follow. Standard speech evaluations for the cleft or VPD population should occur on at least an annual basis and more frequently if there are changing needs (e.g., postsurgery, post-therapy). Speech evaluations after surgical management (e.g., pharyngeal flap) should occur at least 3–6 months postsurgery to allow for adequate time for healing, decrease in postoperative edema, and an initial period in which patients can "practice" speech with their newly modified speech mechanism.

BOX 26.1 Common speech pathology terminology

Intelligibility: perceived amount of speech (i.e., number of words) understood

Resonance: the perceptual balance of oral and nasal sound energy in speech. In speakers with velopharyngeal dysfunction, there is an abnormal escape of excessive nasal sound energy through the velopharyngeal port and into the nasal cavity, which is referred to as hypernasality

Hypernasality: perception of excessive nasal sound energy in speech, typically on vowels, glides (W, Y), and liquid sounds (L, R)

Hyponasality: perception of decreased nasal sound energy in speech, typically on nasal sounds M, N, and usually due to structural obstruction (e.g., enlarged adenoid pad, nasal congestion)

Mixed resonance: combination of both hypernasality and hyponasality perceived by a listener. Cul-de-sac resonance is sometimes considered a form of mixed resonance in which sound energy escapes to the anterior nasal cavity and becomes trapped by some form of nasal obstruction or constriction, such as a deviated septum

Nasal emission: abnormal escape of airflow through the nose during consonant production (can be audible or inaudible). When audible, may also be referred to as nasal turbulence

Compensatory articulation errors: a category of articulation errors typically observed in populations with cleft palate or velopharyngeal dysfunction, believed to result from an active strategy to regulate pressure and airflow for speech. Typically includes a pattern of producing sounds in a posterior place of the vocal tract such as the pharynx or larynx, where pressure and airflow can be "valved" prior to their escape to the level of the velopharynx or oral cavity

Glottal stop substitutions: the most common type of compensatory articulation errors seen in children with cleft palate or a history of velopharyngeal dysfunction, produced by adducting the vocal folds together and abruptly releasing the pressure beneath to create the sound of an oral pressure consonant. Often used as a replacement (substitution) for pressure consonants like P, B, T, D, K, G

Nasal substitutions: the active replacement of oral sounds P, B, T, D with nasal sounds M, N

Active nasal fricative: a learned articulatory behavior in which an oral sound (usually S, SH, CH) is replaced with a voiceless nasal sound (i.e., all airflow is emitted through the nose); this is sometimes accompanied by a nasal grimace

Weak pressure consonants: the perception of decreased pressure in oral consonants such as P, B, T, D, F, resulting from a fistula or velopharyngeal gap, causing these sounds to take on nasalization (e.g., the B sound is perceived as an M, the D is perceived as an N), even though the speaker is accurately attempting to produce the correct sound. Often co-occurs with nasal emission

Sibilant distortions: incorrect tongue placement resulting from faulty learning or malocclusion, resulting in imprecise production of sounds S and Z

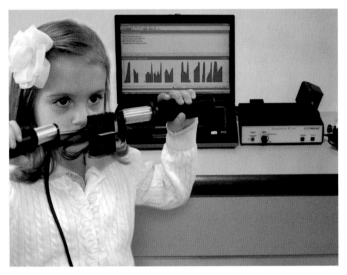

Fig. 26.6 Nasometer II. *(Courtesy of Kay Pentax.)*

Indirect measures of velopharyngeal closure for speech

When clinical speech evaluation suggests the presence of VPD, instrumental assessment of speech and velopharyngeal closure may be useful as an adjunct to perceptual judgments. Instrumental measures can provide confirmation of perceptual judgments and further evidence of the need for intervention, as well as allow for objective pre–post treatment measurements. The most popular clinical tools for indirect instrumental evaluation include acoustic assessment of nasality and aerodynamic testing.

Nasalance is an acoustic index of nasality which has been shown to correlate with perceptual judgments of resonance.[54] Nasalance can be measured using commercially available products such as the Nasometer (Kay Pentax) (Fig. 26.6), Nasality Visualization System (Glottal Enterprises), Nasalview (Tiger DRS), and other similar systems. Nasalance is a ratio of the nasal sound energy divided by the sum of the oral plus nasal sound energy in the speech signal.[54] The patient wears a specialized headpiece with nasal and oral microphones that capture the speech signal while the patient reads or repeats a standardized speech sample (see Fig. 26.6). Automated analysis provides a nasalance score (expressed as a percentage), which is then interpreted against the perceptual speech observations. Nasalance can range from 0 to 100%; higher numbers represent a higher degree of nasality in speech. A variety of normative and "cutoff" scores have been suggested, which are dependent upon the type of speech stimuli used for the nasalance score calculation.[55–58] Surgeons and clinicians should exercise caution in reliance on nasalance scores, however, due to the variety of potential confounding variables that can artificially inflate or reduce nasalance scores. These include nasal turbulence, articulation errors, vocal hoarseness, mixed resonance, and equipment placement variations, which may reduce with the validity of this measure.[58–60] Nasalance should be considered a supplement to the perceptual speech evaluation, *not* a substitute for it.

Pioneered by Warren and colleagues,[61,62] pressure–flow testing was developed to obtain quantitative measurement of intraoral and nasal pressure and airflow, velopharyngeal orifice size, and velopharyngeal closure timing for speech. The schematic in Fig. 26.7 illustrates the type of instrumentation and set-up often utilized for aerodynamic assessment of velopharyngeal closure for speech. Custom-designed and commercially available aerodynamic systems, e.g., PERCI-SARS (Microtronics), offer both clinical and research applications for the assessment of velopharyngeal closure for speech. Warren and others[61–66] suggested the use of the word "hamper" as the speech stimulus for pressure–flow testing because of its /mp/ sound sequence which requires the velopharynx to open and close rapidly. An orifice of 10–20 mm² (or larger) during the /p/ sound of this stimulus has been shown to correlate highly with perceptual observations of hypernasality.[62] Some studies have suggested that even smaller gap sizes may be clinically significant, especially when variations in velopharyngeal timing are also present.[46,64–66] Pressure–flow

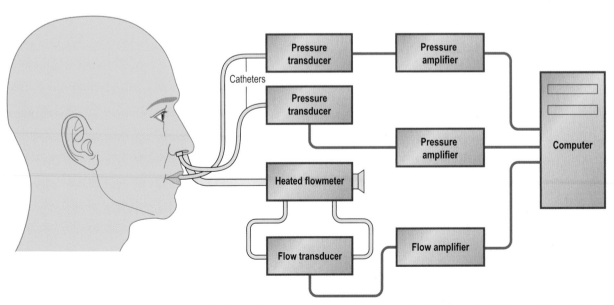

Fig. 26.7 Pressure–flow instrumentation for measuring intraoral pressure, nasal airflow, velopharyngeal orifice size, and velopharyngeal closure timing during speech.

testing provides quantitative data that are easy to interpret for diagnostic purposes. Some pressure–flow systems also offer the ability to use the information for biofeedback purposes for speech therapy. The disadvantages of pressure–flow testing include its cost and increased cooperation required for use with younger children.

Imaging

Imaging of the velopharynx is critical for making the most appropriate treatment decision. It is important for the surgeon to visualize the velopharyngeal mechanism *in vivo* during speech in order to identify or confirm the etiology and extent of the problem, as well as to determine which type of surgical approach will best manage the speech problem. In addition, imaging is helpful for clarifying the status of the adjacent structures of the upper airway which could impact treatment planning, such as the size of the tonsils and adenoid pad. It is important that imaging be conducted with a trained speech pathologist in order to ensure that an appropriate speech sample is utilized, accuracy of speech attempts is interpreted, and diagnostic decisions are accurate. Imaging is best completed when a patient has the ability to produce at least some oral pressure consonants with accurate placement of the articulators and not just compensatory errors, in order to view the "best effort" of the velopharyngeal mechanism during speech.

Static radiographs

A basic lateral cephalometric radiograph obtained at rest (quiet breathing) and during sustained production of sounds, such as /u/ or /s/, is one of the oldest approaches to evaluate the velopharyngeal mechanism[67] (Fig. 26.8). This type of image may be helpful for confirming palatal length and velar stretch, as well as tonsil and adenoid size; however, there is no way of assessing connected speech and the dynamic function of the velopharyngeal mechanism.[68]

Multiview videofluoroscopy (Videos 26.1 and 26.2 ▶)

During multiview videofluoroscopy, a connected speech sample is recorded while motion fluoroscopy records the movement of the velopharyngeal mechanism from multiple angles. The benefit of this imaging approach is that it requires a lower degree of cooperation (as compared to nasopharyngoscopy) and also provides information regarding palatal length, pharyngeal depth, velopharyngeal gap size, and tonsil and adenoid size. Clinicians can examine the velopharyngeal mechanism during connected speech (as compared to static images), which results in increased sensitivity to detect a smaller or inconsistent velopharyngeal gap; however, the radiation dose is higher than that of a traditional static radiograph. In this procedure, barium contrast is often instilled through the nose to help highlight the nasal surface of the velum and posterior pharyngeal wall, to aid in identification of the velopharyngeal gap. Multiple angles can be obtained, including lateral, frontal, base, and Towne's, with the lateral view as the most common.[69] Due to radiation exposure and the availability of other imaging options, videofluoroscopy for speech is becoming less common at many cleft centers.

Nasopharyngoscopy

Nasopharyngoscopy involves the passage of a flexible fiberoptic endoscope into the nasal cavity. Once the scope is positioned slightly above the velopharyngeal port, the view should allow for complete observation of all velopharyngeal structures during speech and swallowing, including anteriorly, the soft palate; posteriorly, the posterior pharyngeal wall or adenoid pad; and laterally, the lateral pharyngeal walls. Nasopharyngoscopy during speech is usually conducted by

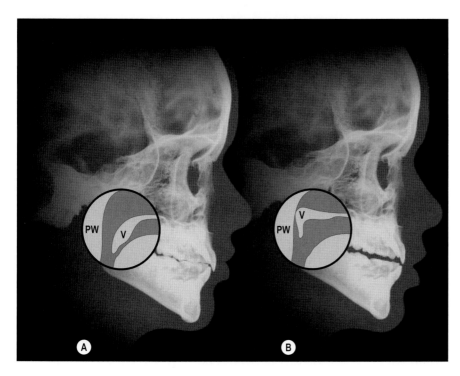

Fig. 26.8 Static lateral cephalometric radiographs of the velopharyngeal mechanism at rest compared with during oral speech. PW, posterior pharyngeal wall; V, velum.

the surgeon, otolaryngologist, or a trained speech pathologist. Regardless, a speech pathologist should be present during the examination to model the correct speech stimuli for the patient to imitate during the procedure and assist with the interpretation of the imaging results. Sufficient cooperation can be anticipated in most 4–5-year-olds, and even some mature 3-year-olds, when they have been shown to be capable of producing a sufficient speech sample. A topical anesthetic and decongestant and scope lubricant are often utilized for increased patient comfort and cooperation.

The scope should be inserted into the middle meatus of the nasal cavity whenever possible, as the inferior meatus may provide a view of the velopharyngeal port but is more prone to artifact based on the viewing angle. The estimated size, shape, and consistency of the velopharyngeal gap can be viewed during speech, and the type of velopharyngeal closure pattern can also be determined (Fig. 26.9). Tonsil and adenoid size can be examined, as well as laryngeal structures, if needed. The benefit of nasopharyngoscopy is the direct view of the velopharyngeal mechanism from above the velopharyngeal port during speech, in color. Nasopharyngoscopy is also better for assessing small velopharyngeal gaps, asymmetrical velopharyngeal function, and velopharyngeal inadequacy persisting post-pharyngeal flap, and is the most direct assessment option for suspected occult submucous cleft palate. Another benefit of nasopharyngoscopy is that it may also be useful for slightly older children, adolescents, and adults, who may benefit from biofeedback during speech therapy (Video 26.3 ▶).

For multiview videofluoroscopy and nasopharyngoscopy, the speech sample should include words and phrases or sentences, which are carefully selected by the speech pathologist so that the patient's best attempts at velopharyngeal closure can be visualized during accurate articulation (and may also be contrasted with the least amount of velopharyngeal closure during nasal sounds or compensatory errors). Imaging exams should be audio- and video-recorded for later review whenever possible. Standard procedures for acquiring, rating, and interpreting videofluoroscopic and nasendoscopic images of the velopharynx during speech have previously been reported.[70]

Two other imaging methods, computed tomographic scans and magnetic resonance imaging (MRI), have been utilized for the assessment of velopharyngeal closure for speech but primarily for research purposes. Dynamic MRI is still in the early stages of translation into the clinical setting for assessment of the velopharyngeal mechanism, with preliminary studies demonstrating the ability to capture the movement of the velopharyngeal mechanism during the phonation of vowels and consonants and limited speech tasks.[71–73]

Treatment/surgical techniques

The primary goal of surgical management is to produce a competent velopharyngeal mechanism while avoiding the complications of nasal airway obstruction, including hyponasality, obligate mouth-breathing, snoring, and obstructive sleep apnea. In all cases, surgical management should be individualized, taking into consideration each patient's velopharyngeal anatomy and function, as well as any comorbid conditions that may influence surgical outcome. All surgical

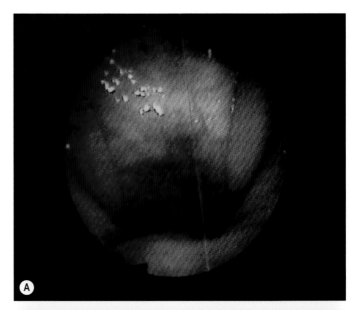

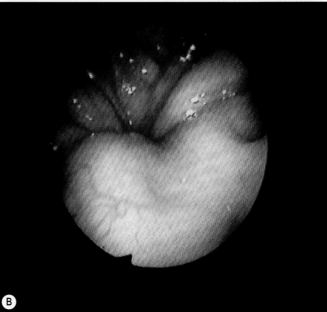

Fig. 26.9 Views of the velopharyngeal port during speech obtained by nasopharyngoscopy. **(A)** Inadequate velopharyngeal closure during speech resulting in a large central gap. **(B)** Complete closure of the velopharyngeal port during speech.

procedures for the management of VPD seek to reduce the cross-sectional area of the velopharyngeal port and/or improve the dynamic function of the velopharyngeal valve. The procedures most commonly used for the management of VPD include Furlow double-opposing Z-palatoplasty, posterior pharyngeal flap, and sphincter pharyngoplasty. Posterior pharyngeal wall augmentation has been used less frequently.

Preoperative evaluation

In order to optimize surgical results while minimizing the likelihood of complications, all patients considered candidates for surgical management should undergo thorough preoperative evaluation. Individualization of surgical management is critical to optimizing surgical outcome. That is, differential management based upon specific anatomic and functional abnormalities allows for selection of the surgical technique most likely to achieve velopharyngeal competence in each patient.

The surgeon should elicit a thorough history, carefully assessing each patient for prior surgery on the palate, velopharynx, tonsils, and adenoids, as stated earlier in this chapter. The presence of associated syndromes and comorbid conditions should be noted, as should a prior history of upper airway obstruction. Appropriate preoperative medical and anesthetic consultation should be obtained. Patients with a history of Pierre Robin sequence, loud snoring, or obstructive sleep apnea should undergo a careful preoperative evaluation of the airway, including polysomnography. In all such cases, stabilization of the upper airway should precede surgical management of VPD.

In addition to the perceptual speech evaluation, careful physical examination should be performed in all patients who may be candidates for surgical management of the velopharynx. Patients should be assessed for stigmata of syndromic diagnoses (e.g., 22q11.2 deletion syndrome) that may influence their management and outcome or those (i.e., Pierre Robin sequence) that may increase their risk for postoperative upper airway obstruction. Intraoral examination yields important information regarding oropharyngeal anatomy. Patients noted to have enlarged tonsils and/or adenoids should undergo tonsillectomy and adenoidectomy prior to posterior pharyngeal flap surgery in order to reduce their risk of postoperative upper airway obstruction. Examination of patients who have undergone prior tonsillectomy, however, may reveal scarring of the tonsillar pillars that may preclude sphincter pharyngoplasty. In patients who have undergone prior palatoplasty, the palate should be inspected carefully for velar dehiscence and oronasal fistulae. Patients with velar dehiscence should undergo re-repair of the palate prior to reassessment of velopharyngeal function and, if necessary, pharyngoplasty. Likewise, fistulae large enough to be of aerodynamic significance should be repaired and velopharyngeal function reassessed. Oropharyngeal examination may also provide useful information in those patients who present with persistent or recurrent velopharyngeal dysfunction after pharyngoplasty. For example, a pharyngeal flap appropriately positioned at the level of velar closure will be difficult to visualize on oral examination. The presence of a pharyngeal flap easily visible on the posterior pharyngeal wall below the palate should raise suspicion that the flap may be tethering the velum and impairing velopharyngeal closure.

In addition, preoperative imaging of the velopharynx is also essential to surgical planning. The diagnosis of VPD should be confirmed by nasendoscopy and/or multiview videofluoroscopy, as earlier described. The site, pattern, and symmetry of velopharyngeal closure should be noted, as should gap size, shape, and location. Imaging further allows the surgeon to assess orientation of the levator fibers, velar anatomy and function, and adenoid and tonsillar size and morphology. Markedly enlarged tonsils or irregularly shaped adenoids may impair velopharyngeal closure in some patients. Preoperative imaging allows the operator to assess the contribution of adenoid or tonsillar abnormalities to VPD, thereby avoiding misguided attempts at pharyngoplasty in patients

for whom adenoidectomy or tonsillectomy is indicated as an initial procedure. Previous research has suggested that when a patient is observed to exhibit a short velum or decreased palatal elevation, but at least an average degree of medial movement of the lateral pharyngeal walls during speech, a pharyngeal flap procedure may be most likely to result in a better speech outcome. On the other hand, if a patient demonstrates average palatal length and elevation with minimal lateral pharyngeal wall contribution to velopharyngeal closure, a sphincter pharyngoplasty may be the more appropriate procedure. Surgeon experience, skill, and preference, as well as any potential concerns with airway obstruction in the patient's history, will also interact with imaging findings as part of the treatment decision-making process.

Furlow double-opposing Z-palatoplasty (Fig. 26.10)

Although originally described for the primary repair of palatal clefts,[74] the Furlow double-opposing Z-palatoplasty incorporates several features that make it an ideal procedure in selected patients with VPD. Transposition of the posteriorly based myomucosal flaps reorients the levator muscles from the sagittal to the horizontal position, thereby reconstructing the levator sling. The Z-plasty design provides for palatal lengthening while avoiding velar shortening that may occur

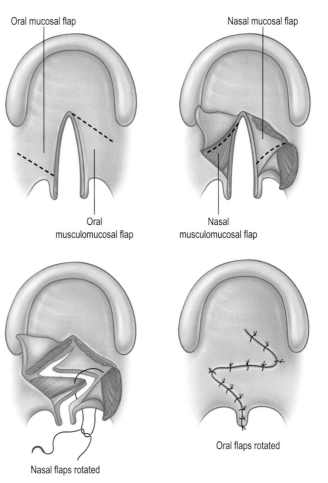

Fig. 26.10 Furlow palatoplasty.

after straight-line closure. Thus, the Furlow Z-palatoplasty is well suited for the management of VPD in patients with an unrepaired submucosal cleft palate and in those who have undergone cleft palate repair without levator reconstruction. The technique is inappropriate, however, for patients in whom the levator muscle fibers are not sagittally oriented, as transposition of the myomucosal flaps would disrupt the anatomically normal or the previously reconstructed levator sling.

The design of the Furlow palatoplasty incorporates mirror-image Z-plasties on the oral and nasal aspects of the velum, such that the posteriorly based flaps contain both mucosa and the attached fibers of the levator veli palatini. In contrast, the anteriorly based flaps contain mucosa and submucosa alone. The Z-plasty design is determined by palatal anatomy, the incisions extending from the hamulus to the junction of the hard and soft palate at the cleft margin on one side and from the base of the uvula to the hamulus on the other. The posteriorly based flap is elevated in the nasal submucosal plane, thereby creating an oral myomucosal flap. Care must be taken to divide the levator fibers completely from the posterior edge of the hard palate in order to allow for complete posterior rotation of the flap and for horizontal repositioning of the levator. The contralateral flap is elevated in the oral submucosal plane, creating an anteriorly based mucosal flap.

The anteriorly based nasal mucosal flap is then developed by incising the nasal mucosa from the base of the uvula to a point just medial to the orifice of the eustachian tube. On the opposite side, the posteriorly based nasal myomucosal flap is incised along the posterior edge of the hard palate, again completely dividing the attachment of the levator to the bone. The nasal flaps are then transposed and sutured in place. Transposition of the oral flaps reconstructs the levator sling and completes the repair.

Several reports confirm the efficacy of the Furlow Z-palatoplasty in the management of VPD in selected patients with unrepaired submucosal cleft palate and with repaired overt clefts. In a series reported by Hudson et al.,[75] 85% of patients with VPD after primary palatoplasty demonstrated normal resonance after conversion to a Furlow Z-palatoplasty. Chen et al.[76] reported that the majority of patients with a velopharyngeal gap of less than 5 mm achieve velopharyngeal competence after Furlow repair, whereas the repair is far less successful when the gap size exceeds 10 mm. D'Antonio et al.[77] reported normal resonance after conversion to a Furlow Z-palatoplasty in six of eight patients with persistent VPD after cleft palate repair. All patients in their series demonstrated a central V-shaped notch in the posterior soft palate, good velar motion, and a "small" velopharyngeal gap.

High success rates for the management of VPD by Furlow palatoplasty have been reported in patients with submucosal cleft palate. As for previously repaired overt clefts, the likelihood of success in patients with submucosal clefts may be related primarily to gap size. Seagle et al.[78] reported that 83% of patients with VPD and submucosal cleft palate achieved velopharyngeal competence after Furlow repair, noting that successful outcomes are far more frequent in those patients in whom gap size measured less than 8 mm. Likewise, Chen et al.[79] reported that 97% of patients with submucosal clefts achieved velopharyngeal competence when gap size did not exceed 5 mm. Studies have confirmed that the Furlow Z-palatoplasty increases palatal length in most patients and have suggested that speech outcome after Furlow repair may

be determined to a large extent by the degree of velar lengthening achieved,[77] an effect that is related primarily to the angles of the Z-plasty design. As noted above, however, the Z-plasty angles are determined not by any specific geometric design, but rather by the underlying palatal anatomy. As velar length decreases, the Z-plasty angles increase, thereby reducing the amount of velar lengthening effectively achieved following transposition of the flaps. Velopharyngeal competence after Furlow Z-palatoplasty, therefore, can be anticipated in the patient with a small velopharyngeal gap and good velar length but may be more difficult to achieve in patients with a large gap and short velum.

Complications after Furlow Z-palatoplasty include bleeding, oronasal fistula, and nasal airway obstruction. Fistula formation can be minimized by ensuring that the repair is completed with minimal tension. When necessary, lateral relaxing incisions should be employed in order to achieve a tension-free closure. Although mild obstructive apnea has been documented in patients following Furlow Z-palatoplasty, such has been noted to resolve in nearly all patients within 3 months of surgery.[80] When compared to patients who have undergone posterior pharyngeal flap surgery for the management of VPD, patients treated by Furlow repair demonstrate significantly lower incidence and severity of upper airway obstruction 6 months or more postoperatively.[81]

Posterior pharyngeal flap (Fig. 26.11)

The creation of midline flaps from the posterior pharyngeal wall represents the oldest surgical technique for the management of VPD. In 1865, Passavant published the first report describing the surgical management of VPD by adhesion of the soft palate to the posterior pharyngeal wall.[82] Schoenborn described the use of an inferiorly based pharyngeal flap in 1875 and of a superiorly based flap a decade later.[83,84] The superiorly based pharyngeal flap was described in the US by Padgett in 1930,[85] and by the middle of the 20th century, the procedure was widely employed as the standard surgical treatment for VPD.

The pharyngeal flap functions primarily as a central obturator of the velopharyngeal port. Closure of the lateral side ports during speech is dependent upon the medial movement of the lateral pharyngeal walls. Hence, this technique is optimally suited for patients with VPD that is characterized by the presence of a central gap and that is associated with good lateral pharyngeal wall motion. To be effective, the pharyngeal flap should be carefully placed at the level of attempted velopharyngeal closure as determined by preoperative imaging. Flaps that have been created too low or that have migrated inferiorly due to postoperative cicatricial changes may tether the velum and interfere with velopharyngeal closure. Patients with an asymmetrical velopharyngeal closure pattern should have flap design altered accordingly.

The width of the pharyngeal flap should be tailored to the functional and anatomic needs of each patient, again as determined by preoperative imaging. That is, patients with large gaps and those with relatively poor lateral pharyngeal wall motion may require a wider flap design in order to achieve velopharyngeal competence. Flap width is dependent not only upon the breadth of the flap itself, but also on the breadth of its inset on the posterior velum. Inset of the flap may be accomplished either by dividing the soft palate in the

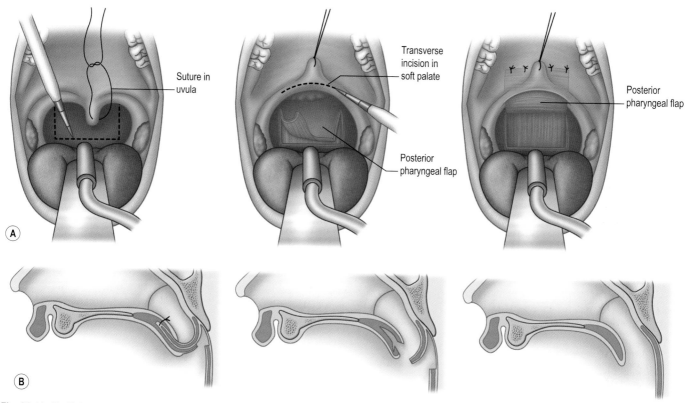

Fig. 26.11 (A, B) Posterior pharyngeal flap.

midline or by dissecting a submucosal pocket through a posterior transverse ("fishmouth") incision. The latter allows for somewhat greater flexibility in the design of flap width and lateral port dimensions.[86] Cicatricial change, or "tubing", of pharyngeal flaps may result in significant flap narrowing and, consequently, in deterioration of velopharyngeal function.[87] Pharyngeal flap narrowing can be minimized, however, by lining the raw surface of the flap with mucosal flaps of velar mucosa or by designing short, broad flaps. In all cases, the need to create wide flaps must be judiciously balanced against an associated increase in the risk of postoperative obstructive sleep apnea.

Careful surgical planning and individualization of flap design are essential to surgical success. Accurate interpretation of reported series is made difficult, however, by the use of different surgical techniques, heterogeneous patient populations, and non-standardized, often unreliable measures of surgical outcome. Argamaso[86] reported that hypernasality was eliminated after pharyngeal flap surgery in 96% of 226 patients. Similarly, normal or borderline sufficient velopharyngeal function was achieved in 97% of 104 non-syndromic patients described by Sullivan et al.[88] Cable et al.[89] reported stability in resonance scores over 14 years of follow-up after pharyngeal flap surgery, suggesting that surgical outcome after pharyngeal flap surgery is durable.

Several authors have expressed concerns regarding the negative impact of pharyngeal flap attachment on midfacial growth. Although several studies have yielded conflicting data, the majority of evidence from large series has failed to demonstrate that attachment of pharyngeal flaps has any significant long-term influence on maxillary development.[90]

Complications of pharyngeal flap surgery include bleeding, dehiscence, and nasal airway obstruction, including obstructive sleep apnea.[91] Rarely, deaths have been reported following the procedure, primarily related to airway compromise.[92] Fraulin et al.[93] reported that predictive factors for complications include the operator, associated medical conditions, concurrent surgical procedures, and an open flap donor site. Of all complications, upper airway compromise occurs most commonly. Nearly all patients experience transient nasal airway obstruction and perhaps mild obstructive apnea in the early postoperative period. The vast majority of patients demonstrate resolution of clinical and polysomnographic evidence of nocturnal upper airway obstruction within several months of surgery, as edema subsides. Wells et al.[94] documented clinical evidence of nocturnal upper airway obstruction in 12 of 111 patients following pharyngeal flap surgery, three of whom required takedown of the flap. Nine of the 12 patients underwent polysomnographic evaluation, and this revealed obstructive apnea in only one patient. Thus, clinical evidence of postoperative nocturnal airway obstruction may not correlate with the presence of apnea. Syndromic patients and those with a history of Pierre Robin sequence may be at greater risk for airway compromise after pharyngeal flap surgery due to the presence of associated functional or anatomic airway abnormalities.[94,95] Similarly, patients with tonsillar enlargement may be at greater risk for postoperative upper airway obstruction and should therefore undergo tonsillectomy at or prior to the time of pharyngeal flap surgery.[96]

Postoperative monitoring of upper airway status, including continuous pulse oximetry, should be considered the standard of care for all patients following posterior pharyngeal flap surgery. For patients at high risk for postoperative airway obstruction, consideration should be given to the use of a nasopharyngeal airway, placed intraoperatively through one of the lateral ports, and to admission to the intensive care unit for overnight monitoring. Patients may be discharged from the hospital once they demonstrate adequate airway stability and oral fluid intake.

Sphincter pharyngoplasty (Fig. 26.12)

In 1950, Hynes[97] first described the technique of pharyngoplasty by transposition of musculomucosal flaps containing the salpingopharyngeus muscles. He later modified the technique to include the palatopharyngeus muscles, noting that success of the technique could be attributed to narrowing of the velopharyngeal port and to augmentation of the posterior pharyngeal wall with bulky, "often contractile" flaps.[98,99] Orticochea[100] stressed the concept of creating a true "dynamic sphincter" in order to achieve velopharyngeal competence. He dissected bilateral palatopharyngeal myomucosal flaps and inset them into an inferiorly based mucosal flap on the posterior pharyngeal wall. Jackson and Silverton[101] later

modified the procedure, eliminating the posterior pharyngeal flap, instead insetting the palatopharyngeal flaps into a transverse incision located higher on the posterior pharyngeal wall.

The surgical technique used most widely today represents a modification of the Hynes pharyngoplasty. Vertical incisions are made anterior to both posterior tonsillar pillars, and the palatopharyngeus muscles are exposed. The longitudinally oriented muscle fibers are carefully dissected from the posterolateral pharyngeal wall, so as to include the entire muscle in each of the flaps. Vertical incisions are then made posterior to the pillars, creating flaps that measure approximately 1 cm in width. On each side, the parallel incisions are joined by a transverse incision at the lowest aspect of the pillar, and the flaps are elevated. The flaps are then rotated medially and inset into a transverse incision that connects the most superior aspect of the medial palatopharyngeal flap incisions.

Riski et al.[102] have stressed the importance of preoperative patient selection and of proper surgical planning for optimizing surgical outcome. Flap inset should be high on the posterior pharyngeal wall at the site of attempted velopharyngeal closure, as determined by preoperative imaging. Since

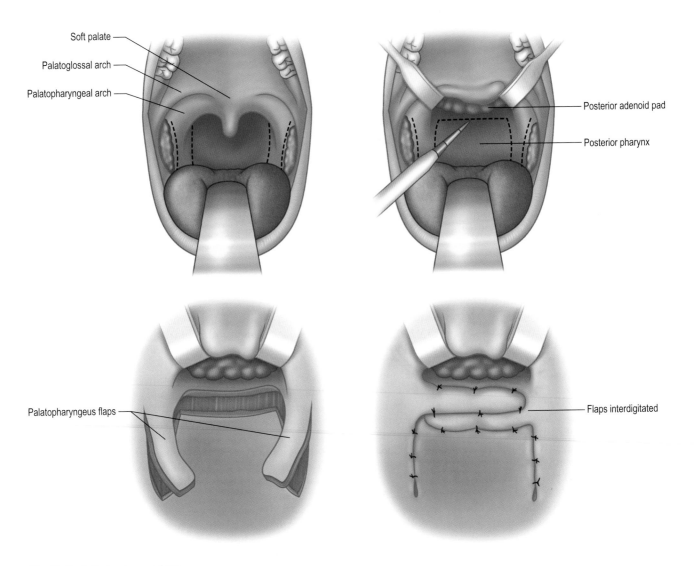

Fig. 26.12 Sphincter pharyngoplasty.

a dynamic sphincter may be achieved in only a subset of patients,[103,104] anatomic factors, such as reduced port size and augmentation of the posterior pharyngeal wall, may be essential to achieving postoperative velopharyngeal competence. In a retrospective review of speech outcome in 48 patients who underwent sphincter pharyngoplasty, Shewmake et al.[105] reported that 85.4% achieved normal resonance. Riski et al.[106] reported that, of 139 patients who underwent sphincter pharyngoplasty, 78% demonstrated resolution of hypernasality and normal pressure–flow measurements. Most surgical failures were the result of the pharyngoplasty being placed too low on the posterior pharyngeal wall. Similarly, Witt et al.[107] noted that 16% of patients required pharyngoplasty revision, although the primary cause of failure was noted to be complete or partial flap dehiscence. In a series of 250 patients, Losken et al.[108] noted a revision rate of 12.8%, noting that persistent VPD after pharyngoplasty was more common in patients with 22q11.2 deletion syndrome. Failure was seen more often in patients with greater nasalance scores and velopharyngeal valve area on preoperative instrumental evaluation.

Several studies have compared speech outcome after posterior pharyngeal flap surgery and sphincter pharyngoplasty. Ysunza et al.[109] reported on 50 patients with cleft palate and residual VPD who were randomized to undergo one or the other procedure, finding no significant difference in the frequency of persistent VPD (12% and 16%, respectively) between the two groups. Similarly, Abyholm et al.[110] reported no significant difference in speech outcome 1 year following posterior pharyngeal flap or sphincter pharyngoplasty in a randomized multicenter trial.

Complications of sphincter pharyngoplasty are similar to those of posterior pharyngeal flap surgery and include bleeding, flap dehiscence, and upper airway obstruction. In a multicenter, prospective randomized trial of 97 patients, Abyholm et al.[110] noted that polysomnographic evidence of obstructive apnea 1 year after surgical management of VPD was rare, with no significant difference between patients undergoing posterior pharyngeal flap surgery and those undergoing sphincter pharyngoplasty. Saint Raymond et al.[111] examined polysomnograms of 17 patients before and after sphincter pharyngoplasty and found that the procedure induced no significant impairment in either the apnea–hypopnea index or the nocturnal oxygen saturation. Despite this, however, there was a notable reduction in slow-wave sleep and an increase in cortical microarousals postoperatively, suggesting that the reduction in nasopharyngeal airway diameter may increase airway resistance sufficiently enough to cause fragmentation of sleep architecture even in the absence of detectable sleep apnea.

Posterior pharyngeal wall augmentation

Augmentation pharyngoplasty, using both autologous tissues and alloplastic materials, has long been used by surgeons to reduce the size of the velopharyngeal orifice in patients with VPD. Long-term results have been variable and have depended upon both patient selection and the choice of augmentation material. Overall, the most durable results have been achieved in patients with good velar motion and relatively small velopharyngeal gap size.

In 1862, Passavant became the first to describe the use of local tissues to augment the posterior pharyngeal wall. In his initial description, he sutured the palatopharyngeal muscles together in the midline. In 1879, he described the use of a pedicled flap of posterior pharyngeal mucosa, rolled upon itself and inset across the posterior pharyngeal wall.[112] After disappointing results, the technique was abandoned. Hynes reported the use of myomucosal flaps containing the salpingopharyngeus (and later the palatopharyngeus) muscles nearly a century later.[97,98] In 1997, Witt et al. reported on the use of a rolled, superiorly based pharyngeal flap for posterior pharyngeal wall augmentation, noting no significant improvement in the speech of 14 patients treated.[113] In contrast, however, Gray et al.[114] reported good results using folded flaps in young patients with good velar motion.

In 1912, Hollweg and Perthes[115] described the use of autologous cartilage grafts inserted through a cervical incision. This procedure was later modified by others utilizing a transoral approach. Although many authors have reported some success with cartilage grafts placed into the posterior pharynx, the results and durability of these procedures have been variable. Denny et al.[116] reported elimination of hypernasality in 25% of 20 patients treated by retropharyngeal bone or cartilage grafts with lesser degrees of improvement seen in another 65%. Follow-up studies of the same cohort of patients, however, failed to document durability of the results achieved. The body of evidence suggests that some degree of graft migration and resorption after pharyngeal augmentation with cartilage appears inevitable. Recent reports have documented improvement in velopharyngeal function following injection of autologous fat into the posterior pharynx in selected patients,[117] although the application and effectiveness of this technique await greater experience and long-term follow-up.

The earliest attempts to augment the posterior pharyngeal wall by injection of exogenous material may have been those of Gersuny, who reported the use of petroleum jelly in 1900.[118] Although the technique achieved some success in improving patients' speech, the technique was associated with several serious complications, including blindness and death. In 1904, Eckstein[119] described injection of paraffin without untoward complications. Blocksma[120] reported augmentation pharyngoplasty using implantable blocks and injectable fluid Silastic. Although he noted improvement of speech in many patients, a high incidence of implant infection and extrusion led him to recommend the use of autologous implants as the preferred method for pharyngeal augmentation. Lewy published a single case report on the use of Teflon injection for the management of VPD in 1965.[121] Bluestone et al.[122] later reported success with Teflon injections in several patents, noting no instances of infection, extrusion, or foreign-body reaction. Smith and McCabe[123] documented complete elimination of hypernasality in 60% of 80 patients who underwent augmentation pharyngoplasty by Teflon injection. Furlow et al.[124] reported successful treatment of VPD by Teflon injection in 74% of 35 patients. Nevertheless, the risk of potentially serious complications has led the Food and Drug Administration to withdraw approval of its use for augmentation pharyngoplasty. Other exogenous materials that have been used to augment the posterior pharyngeal wall in patients with VPD include Proplast and calcium hydroxyapatite.

The majority of evidence suggests that posterior pharyngeal wall augmentation may be successfully used for the management of carefully selected patients with good velar motion and small-gap VPD. In order to be effective, augmentation should be performed precisely at the level of attempted velar contact on the posterior pharyngeal wall as determined by preoperative imaging. To date, no single alloplastic material has been found to be uniformly safe, effective, and reliable, and single type of autologous graft has demonstrated consistent long-term stability. Therefore, augmentation pharyngoplasty should be considered only as a secondary option in carefully selected patients with VPD.

Surgical management in the 22q11.2 deletion syndrome

Velopharyngeal dysfunction in persons with 22q11.2 deletion syndrome (22q11DS) is multifactorial and typically results from a combination of structural and functional causes such as submucous cleft palate, palatopharyngeal disproportion, obtuse cranial base, and/or hypotonia. Optimization of surgical outcomes in this specific patient population requires precision in diagnosis, surgical management, and multidisciplinary team care. Children with 22q11DS tend to have more severe hypernasal speech than that of other cleft and VPD populations. In addition, children with 22q11DS traditionally undergo VPD surgery at slightly later ages than their peers with cleft palate or non-syndromic VPD due to a variety of factors including but not limited to (1) significant ongoing medical issues (e.g., cardiac, airway); (2) delayed expressive language development; and (3) severe articulation disorders, which may interfere with the ability to obtain VP imaging with sufficiently accurate articulation and adequate cooperation for the study.

Non-surgical treatment options

While surgery is the preferred treatment option for most cases of VPD, there may be patient-specific factors which cause non-surgical options to be considered. Prosthetic or behavioral speech treatment may be appropriate for a select set of patients for whom surgery is not possible, not desired, or if the prognosis for surgical outcome is guarded.

Prosthetic treatment

Speech prostheses may be an appropriate treatment option for patients who have an unclear, guarded, or poor prognosis for improvement with surgery, such as (1) when the diagnosis of VPD is unclear based on perceptual speech and/or imaging findings; (2) when the comorbid speech problems make it difficult to determine if surgical intervention will result in meaningful improvement in speech; and (3) when the patient has a known neuromuscular or degenerative condition that has been shown to result in suboptimal surgical outcomes. In addition, the patient may have known medical contraindications to having surgery or have cultural, religious, or other ethical conflicts with surgery. To be a good candidate for prosthetic management, the patient and family must demonstrate adequate compliance and dedication to completing the prosthetic treatment plan, which may require several visits, and be an appropriate dental candidate for fabrication of a speech prosthesis (i.e., demonstrate good dental hygiene).

The palatal lift and the speech bulb are the most commonly used speech prostheses[125] (Fig. 26.13). A pediatric or general dentist, orthodontist, or prosthodontist may fabricate the device, usually with the input from the speech pathologist. A palatal lift is basically a standard orthodontic retainer with an extension posteriorly to "lift" up the soft palate. It is an appropriate treatment option for patients with a soft palate of sufficient length but lacks adequate movement during speech and/or swallowing, such as in cases of velopharyngeal incompetence. A speech bulb is more appropriate for patients with velopharyngeal insufficiency in which the palate is too

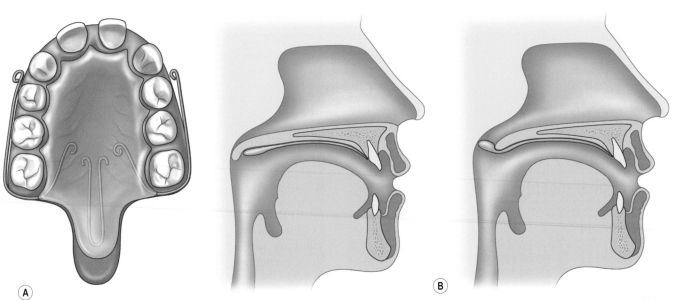

Fig. 26.13 (A) Schematic of a palatal lift (intraoral and lateral view). Note how the lift extends along the oral surface of the velum to lift it to the level of the palatal plane. The length of the palate is sufficient, but in cases of velopharyngeal incompetency, the function of the velopharyngeal mechanism is impaired. The palatal lift places the velum into position to provide adequate closure for speech and swallowing. **(B)** Speech bulb appliance assisting with velopharyngeal closure for speech. Note that the bulb fits up into the velopharyngeal orifice to obturate the velopharyngeal port, as the length of the velum is insufficient to achieve closure independently.

short to contact the posterior pharyngeal wall. The speech bulb is similar to the palatal lift, with an addition of a "bulb" of acrylic material to fill in the remaining velopharyngeal gap during speech. Other types of obturators, without any posterior extension, may also be helpful for temporary or long-term obturation of palatal fistulae.

Behavioral speech therapy approaches

In selected patients with borderline or inconsistent VPD and/or velopharyngeal mislearning, a trial period of behavioral speech therapy may be helpful prior to proceeding with surgical management.[126,127] Speech therapy is always the most appropriate treatment for articulation errors, as surgery cannot change lip and tongue placement for the production of speech sounds. Speech therapy is also the most appropriate treatment for phoneme-specific nasal emission or phoneme-specific nasalization of sounds (velopharyngeal mislearning) as surgery cannot correct these articulation disorders.[128] There are also some behavioral speech therapy methods which may be effective for reducing mild or inconsistent hypernasality or nasal air emission, as well, especially when biofeedback is provided. If one considers the velum to be an articulator, just as the lips and tongue are, the idea of changing the "behavior" of the velum may be a reasonable goal. The patient must then be provided with the right tools and feedback, assuming that the underlying anatomy of the velopharyngeal mechanism otherwise appears intact. The ideal patient for such a treatment trial would have many of the following characteristics:

- Age 6–8 years or older
- Intact cognitive skills
- Intact motor skills
- Adequate attention span and maturity
- Normal hearing and vision
- Good self-monitoring or speech self-correction skills
- At least inconsistent velopharyngeal closure for speech
- At least some accurate articulation skills already in the speech repertoire
- Can demonstrates measurable change within the first few sessions of therapy.

Biofeedback is often a cornerstone of behavioral speech therapy to improve velopharyngeal closure for speech. Biofeedback may be provided through enhanced auditory, visual, or tactile–kinesthetic cues. Patients may benefit from technology that provides information during online speech production about oral pressure, nasal airflow, and nasalance. Nasopharyngoscopy is also a useful biofeedback tool as it allows for direct visualization of the velopharyngeal port and its movement during speech. It can be used for treating learned nasal emission and even glottal stop substitutions in selected patients.[129–131] Lastly, continuous positive airway pressure (CPAP) has been proposed as a treatment modality to improve velopharyngeal closure by "working" the muscles against artificially increased nasal resistance (nasal pressure) during speech for longer durations of time. The first round of CPAP clinical trials has yielded mixed speech outcome results.[132] In contrast, it should be stated that, although the velopharyngeal mechanism is a dynamic muscular system, "oral–motor exercises" of the lips, tongue, and palate have not been shown to be effective for improving long-term speech outcomes. Multiple studies have shown that palatal massage, electrical stimulation, swallowing exercises, blowing exercises, and blowing against resistance (i.e., horn/whistle programs), are not effective for improving speech.[133–135] Overall, significantly more research is needed to identify the most effective behavioral speech therapy approaches for improving velopharyngeal closure for speech.

12. Peterson-Falzone SJ, Hardin-Jones MA, Karnell MP. Anatomy and physiology of the velopharyngeal system. In: Peterson-Falzone SJ, Hardin-Jones MA, Karnell MP, eds. *Cleft Palate Speech*. 3rd ed. St. Louis: Mosby; 2001:69–86.

17. Croft CB, Shprintzen RJ, Rakoff SJ. Patterns of velopharyngeal valving in normal and cleft palate subjects: a multi-view videofluoroscopic and nasendoscopic study. *Laryngoscope*. 1981;91:265–271. *The authors studied 80 control subjects and 500 patients with velopharyngeal dysfunction using direct nasopharyngoscopy and multi-view videofluoroscopy. The incidence of the different patterns of velopharyngeal closure was found to be similar in frequency in both groups. The importance of these patterns is discussed in relation to the surgical management of patients with velopharyngeal dysfunction.*

47. Kuehn DP, Moller KT. Speech and language issues in the cleft palate population: the state of the art. *Cleft Palate Craniofac J*. 2000;37:348–383. *This summary paper covers all aspects of speech language assessment and treatment options relevant to cleft palate and velopharyngeal dysfunction. A review of the anatomy and physiology and instrumental assessment of the velopharyngeal mechanism is also provided.*

48. Peterson-Falzone SJ, Hardin-Jones MA, Karnell MP. Diagnosing and managing communication disorders in cleft palate. In: *Cleft Palate Speech*. 4th ed. St. Louis: Mosby; 2010:221–247.

50. Henningsson G, Kuehn DP, Sell D, et al. Universal parameters for reporting speech outcomes in individuals with cleft palate. *Cleft Palate Craniofac J*. 2008;45:1–17. *The Universal Parameters System (UPS) for rating speech in patients with cleft palate and velopharyngeal dysfunction is discussed. Examples of standard speech stimuli, a rating form, and various rating scales are included.*

61. Warren DW, DuBois AB. A pressure-flow technique for measuring orifice area during continuous speech. *Cleft Palate J*. 1964;1:52–71.

70. Golding-Kushner KJ. Standardization for the reporting of nasopharyngoscopy and multiview videofluoroscopy: a report from an international working group. *Cleft Palate Craniofac J*. 1990;27:337–348. *This manuscript describes a protocol for rating velopharyngeal structures and movement during speech using multiview videofluoroscopy and flexible nasopharyngoscopy. These standards were published as a result of an International Working Group meeting of experts in the field of clefting/velopharyngeal dysfunction and speech pathology.*

76. Chen PK, Wu JT, Chen YR, et al. Correction of secondary velopharyngeal insufficiency in cleft palate patients with the Furlow palatoplasty. *Plast Reconstr Surg*. 1994;94:933–941. *The results of this study demonstrate that a Furlow palatoplasty can satisfactorily correct velopharyngeal dysfunction in carefully selected patients. The most important factor is the size of the velopharyngeal gap.*

The majority of patients with a successful surgical outcome had a velopharyngeal gap less than 5 mm.

98. Hynes W. The results of pharyngoplasty by muscle transplantation in failed "cleft palate" cases, with special reference to the influence of the pharynx on voice production. *Ann R Coll Surg Engl.* 1953;13:17–35.

102. Riski JE, Serafin D, Riefkohl R, et al. A rationale for modifying the site of insertion of the Orticochea pharyngoplasty. *Plast Reconstr Surg.* 1984;73:882–894. *The authors demonstrate the importance of insetting the sphincter pharyngoplasty at the site of attempted velopharyngeal closure. With this modification, successful outcomes were achieved in 93% of patients.*

27

Secondary deformities of the cleft lip, palate, and nose

Edward P. Buchanan, Laura A. Monson, Edward I. Lee, David Y. Khechoyan, John C. Koshy, Kris Wilson, Lawrence Lin, and Larry H. Hollier Jr.

Access video content for this chapter online at expertconsult.com

SYNOPSIS

- How did we get here? What led to this secondary deformity?
  - Spectrum of clefts: type and severity
  - Primary operative techniques
  - Technical expertise/experience
  - Growth
  - Timing of repair.
- Cut as you go.
- Prevention, prevention, prevention.

Introduction

Identifying and treating secondary cleft lip and palate deformities is a challenging endeavor for even the most experienced surgeon. Proper diagnosis involves an understanding of previous operations as well as a thorough physical examination. Surgical timing depends on deformity severity, age of patient, and understanding and willingness of family members.

Examination and evaluation

Children born with clefts of the lip and palate should ideally be cared for by a multidisciplinary cleft team who adhere to the international standards set forth by the American Cleft Palate and Craniofacial Association.[1] The standards set forth by this organization provide for the proper care and follow-up required to achieve successful long-term outcomes. Occasionally, children do not have access to these teams, and their care is performed outside of this standard. If these children are initially treated elsewhere and are referred into a team, there can be secondary deformities related to their initial treatment.

A thorough history, including an understanding of all previous interventions, must be obtained. Often, knowing where the operations occurred will help to understand what was previously done. Many parents are not familiar with repair techniques, but surgeons are often aware of the types of repairs performed in different areas of the world. The physical examination can provide further clues as to what was previously performed. Scars around the nose and lip can alert the examiner to the primary or secondary techniques. Animation can help the examiner understand the status of the underlying orbicularis oris muscle. Intraoral examination may reveal which operations were done on the palate and identify the presence of oronasal fistulas, the status of the levator muscles, the length of the soft palate as well as the presence of alveolar clefts. Intranasal examination will help determine if a primary rhinoplasty was performed, the status of the nasal septum and turbinates, and the patency of the nasal cavity. A proper speech assessment will determine the functionality of the palate and whether more tests need to be done.

Unilateral cleft lip

Secondary unilateral cleft lip deformities are a common occurrence in cleft centers.[2] The etiology of these deformities is varied and can result from any number of contributing factors, including but not limited to continued facial growth, scarring, infection, or inaccurate primary repair.

Secondary deformities frequently require surgical intervention for correction, spanning from minor revision to a complete takedown and re-repair. Many different techniques have been described, depending on the location and severity.[2–6] Proper treatment begins with an accuVrate analysis of the deformities in relation to the involved anatomic structures (Video 27.3 ▶).

A thorough history and physical examination should be performed in a systematic fashion and documented in the medical record. 2D photographs should be performed in a standardized fashion so as to consistently and objectively capture pre- and postoperative data for evaluation and outcomes purposes. When examining the cleft lip deformity, a top down approach is advocated for simplicity's sake. The examiner starts with the nose and ends with the mucosa of the upper lip. Care to evaluate symmetry between the affected and unaffected sides is of major importance. Review of the nose (dorsum, tip, alae, base, and sill), and lip (philtral unit, Cupid's bow, vermilion, and mucosa) should all be done in a systematic fashion. A list of the involved anatomic structures is recorded. Treatment planning should consider the anatomy of all structures involved so that a plan to restore appropriate form and function can be made.

The timing of cleft lip revision depends on the severity of deformity, the age of the patient, and the preference of the patient, family, and surgeon. Deformity severity and functional disability is relevant to surgical timing. If the lip repair is inadequate, affecting the ability to eat or drink properly, impacting speech production, or is socially unacceptable, a revision could be planned soon after evaluation. These findings would represent the more severe cases and not the norm, as most revisions can be delayed until pre-kindergarten years (4 to 5 years of age), or prior to full social integration. This allows for the previous lip surgery scar to fully mature and the opportunity to combine other cleft-related operations if needed, such as speech surgery.

Vermilion/Mucosa

Vermilion notching

Proper alignment and repair of the vermilion is key to creating a symmetric and harmonious appearing lip. To accomplish this, the height of the vermilion on the cleft side should match the contralateral side. If this is not the case, and the vermilion height is less on the cleft side, a vermilion notch will result. The appearance of the lip with a vermilion notch can have the initial appearance of a short lip, but on further inspection, the vermilion discrepancy should be appreciated. The central or lateral incisor on the affected cleft side can be more noticeable than the opposite side. Furthermore, if mucosa is displaced into the vermilion, an area of persistent dry skin will result. This becomes extremely annoying to the patient and noticeable for the family.

Vermilion notching can occur despite a perfectly restored vermilion/mucosal "red line" junction. Scarring along the repair site may result in vermilion notching and may require revision. It is important to appreciate that this deformity is not necessarily a result of a loss or lack of tissue, but may be secondary to abnormal scarring or misalignment of the red line.

This deformity may be prevented by properly choosing the Cupid's bow point on the lateral lip element (Noordhoff's point).[7] An incision placed too laterally compromises an already short lip in the transverse/horizontal orientation. An incision placed too medially compromises the vertical height of the lip and vermilion and also risks losing the white roll. Therefore, adhering to Noordhoff's point during the primary repair is paramount in establishing the correct height of the lip's vermilion.

If lip notching results from scar contracture, a Z-plasty maybe used to break up the scar. Failure to initially repair the muscle or subsequent muscle dehiscence should be appreciated during the preoperative visit and addressed by dissection and re-suturing of the orbicularis oris. This

can help prevent further scar contracture and notching during animation.

Augmentation with autologous fat has been used to correct notching as well as vermilion deficiency in cleft patients. This technique is indicated when the deformity results from soft-tissue discrepancy only.

Mucosal excess

The symmetry of the upper lip can be compromised by an increase in the amount of scar tissue produced, after the original repair, at the level of the mucosa (Fig. 27.1). Scarring at the lip margin can be unpredictable and result in an asymmetric lip. Careful attention to aligning the mucosa directly below the level of the vermilion and up into the gingivobuccal sulcus is important. Furthermore, using a suture that does not cause an excess amount of inflammation can help prevent a large amount of postoperative scarring.

Mucosal thickening is a common occurrence and a hard problem to prevent. Often, mucosal excess develops during

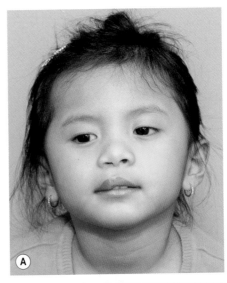

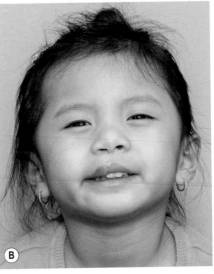

Fig. 27.1 A young female with lateral vermilion fullness. This affects the patient in repose **(A)** with contour changes along the free vermilion border, as well as when smiling **(B)**.

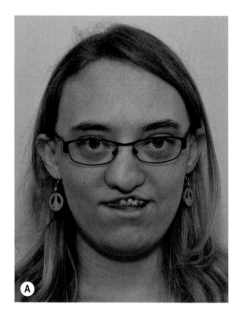
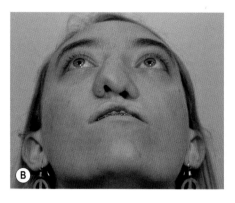
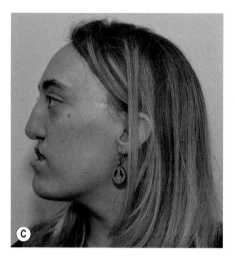

Fig. 27.2 (A–C) Classic secondary cleft lip and nose deformities associated with the unilateral cleft lip, including a short lip deformity, inferolaterally displaced alar base, as well as a depressed nasal tip. She also demonstrates midface retrusion.

the healing process, and not being able to control how much scar tissue will form is frustrating. Excising this mucosa can be a satisfying operation, nonetheless resulting in an unsatisfying experience during the follow-up period. Secondarily, a simple transverse wedge made at the level of the mucosa, inferior to the vermilion mucosal red-line margin, is normally done to achieve balance. If mucosal thickening recurs after revisionary surgery, performing scar therapy and waiting a full year to 18 months for maturation is indicated. Oftentimes, with facial growth, this thickness will "even out" and further revisions may not be required.

Skin

Short lip

The short lip, after a unilateral cleft lip repair, usually results from postoperative scarring, but can result from failing to balance the Cupid's bow (Fig. 27.2). This deformity is one of the most commonly seen and revised given its tendency to distort the normal lip architecture. All straight-line scars can shorten; and, with time, a perfectly repaired cleft lip can shorten and result in an imbalanced repair and "under-rotated" Cupid's bow. Prevention of this deformity can be achieved by "breaking up" the incision during the original repair.

Minor vertical height deficiencies up to 1 mm can be corrected using an elliptical excision of the previous cleft scar at the red–white line.[4,8] Due to the Rose–Thompson effect, this will elongate the lip the necessary 1 mm to match the opposite lip length and balance the Cupid's bow. If a triangular flap repair was initially performed and the lip is moderately short (around 2–3 mm), a Z-plasty just above the white roll can be made to level Cupid's bow and break up the scar. Alternately, an opening incision on the medial lip segment, above the white roll, can be made and a triangular flap from the lateral lip segment can fill the opening incision.[8] Any major discrepancy in vertical height requires complete revision of the lip repair, including adequate release of all lip components from abnormal attachments, "un-bunching" of the lateral lip muscle, precise muscle alignment, and accurate leveling of the

cleft-side peak of the Cupid's bow. The use of permanent or long-lasting resorbable sutures should be considered for muscle repair to relieve tension on the closure and to prevent postoperative scar widening.

Long lip

The appearance of a long lip as a secondary deformity in the unilateral cleft patient is an unusual occurrence. It is more commonly seen after a patient has been repaired with a Z-plasty type repair technique (Fig. 27.3).[8,9] This deformity occurs when the cleft-side height has been overcorrected and there has been overrotation of Cupid's bow.

Minor vertical height excess can be reduced with a horizontal wedge excision along the nasal base. The incision is kept in this groove to prevent any noticeable scarring. Major vertical height discrepancy should be addressed with a complete revision and re-approximation of anatomic structures.

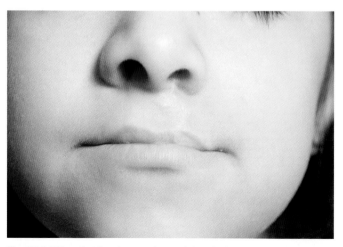

Fig. 27.3 This patient has the scar characteristics of a Randall–Tennison-type cleft lip repair. Her lip demonstrates a nice three-dimensional shape, but the scar runs transversely across the midportion of her lip. This is the primary critique of this repair.

White roll discontinuity

Misalignment of the white roll is another common problem seen in unilateral cleft deformities, and one of the most easily detectable from a conversational distance. A step-off at this level is readily detected by the human eye, given its position at the vermilion–cutaneous junction and its involvement in the harmony of the entire upper lip contour (Fig. 27.4).

In cases of white roll mismatch, a diamond-shaped excision of the white roll scar, extending above and below the roll, will align the white roll. White roll mismatch may be associated with under-rotation or vertical height deficiency of the medial lip segment. Often, excising the scar is enough to lengthen the lip and restore appropriate balance.

Poor scarring

Poor postoperative scarring is an adverse event, which transcends the finest surgical technique and is completely unpredictable. Despite that, there are a few factors believed to be associated with poor scarring, including local wound tension, infection, and genetic predisposition. Measures are made to prevent or alleviate any factors that may contribute to a poor scar. To help relieve any unnecessary tension, complete dissection of involved structures, as well as a strong muscle repair, is performed. This should allow for the skin structures to be easily repaired without undue tension. Aggressive postoperative wound care is done to prevent infection. Scar management is employed to help achieve a thin, flat, and well-blended scar (Fig. 27.5). This is normally done with taping, scar massaging and sun protection. Scar management lasts for 12–18 months, or until the scar has fully matured.

Choice in the type of suture material has been much debated and depends on the preference of the operative surgeon. Permanent sutures need to be removed in 5–7 days to prevent permanent scarring at the sutures sites. Removal usually occurs in the procedure room, requiring another anesthetic exposure. Patients, who get dissolvable sutures, do not need to have their sutures removed; however, sutures must be gone by the 5th–7th day. If they are not, notable scars along the length of the incision can result.

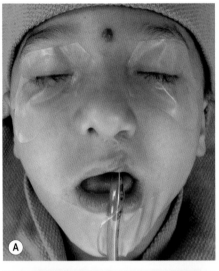
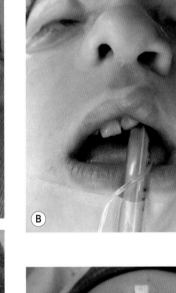
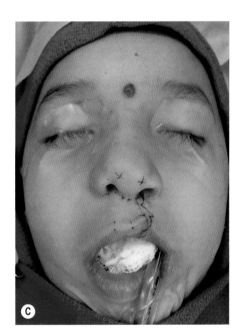
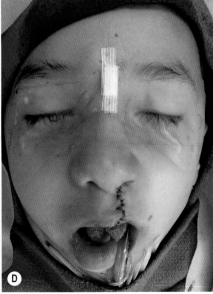
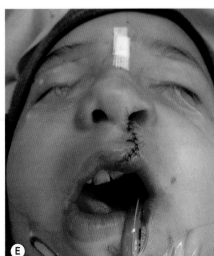

Fig. 27.4 This young man has a notable step-off at the vermilion and significant cleft lip scarring. He also has scarring in to the columella **(A,B)**. Markings were made to realign the white roll and excise the widened scar **(C)**, with the subsequent on-table result **(D, E)**.

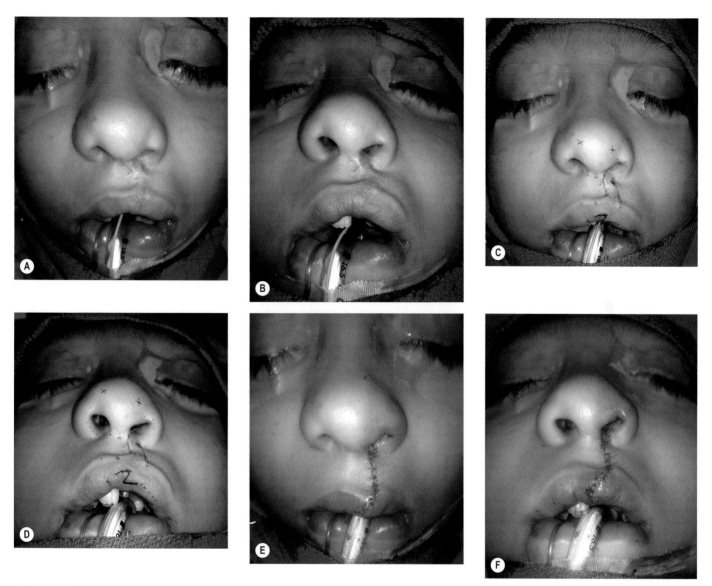

Fig. 27.5 This young man demonstrates hypertrophic scarring, notching and discontinuity of the white roll, as well as vermilion mismatch at the red line **(A, B)**. Surgical intervention required excision of the areas of hypertrophic scarring, as well as Z-plasty-based rearrangement of the red line **(C, D)**. The immediate postoperative outcome is demonstrated **(E, F)**.

Scar location is another important consideration in cleft surgery. Most unilateral cleft lip operations attempt to place the repair scar along the cleft-side philtral column to match the normal side. Some repairs will incorporate a lateral rhinotomy incision to help reposition the alar base. This incision should be approached with caution due to its visibility and potential negative impact it can have on nasal alae growth.

Red or pink scars after surgery are expected and fall within the realm of normal scar maturation. Parents and families should be educated to prepare them for the amount of time it will take for this scar to fade. If, however, the scar begins to get thick, raised, and redder, a hypertrophic scar may be developing, and treatment can include taping and injections. More frequent follow-ups should be made to monitor the progress of the scar.

Unsightly scars can be addressed with scar revision by excising the scar down to underlying muscle and adequately mobilizing skin flaps for tension-free closure. The underlying muscle is assessed at the time of scar revision. If the muscle is scarred or abnormally oriented, then excision and full-thickness revision is advised. If the muscle repair is intact, then muscle imbrication, to reduce tension on the closure, can be performed. It is important to understand that scar revision also shortens an already deficient skin envelope and should be approached with caution to prevent unnecessary shortening.

It is important to assess the position of the alar base during revision. If the alar base is asymmetric, usually posterior and cephalic, the scar revision can facilitate correcting this problem. Access to the alar base and the nasalis portion of the orbicularis oris can be achieved, allowing for repositioning. During any revisionary operation, care to fully assess all other deformities should be performed with a mind towards an overall aesthetic subunit correction.

Muscle

Dehiscence

Failure to properly dissect and repair the muscle at the time of primary repair, or muscular dehiscence after surgery, can lead to lip asymmetry, unnatural animation, imbalance of the nasal bases, and vermilion notching. Muscle continuity can be assessed by evaluating for lateral muscle bulging during animation.

Failure to repair the marginal component of the orbicularis muscle, at the level of the muscle vermilion interaction, can result in notching of the vermilion. Failure to properly identify the nasalis portion of the orbicularis muscle, at the level of the nasal base, can result in an abnormally positioned alae and nasal asymmetry. Careful examination can reveal these very subtle but easy to correct problems.

Lip revision is recommended when muscle dehiscence is suspected. Revision should include complete dissection of the muscle and proper orientation of the nasalis, marginalis, and main portions of the orbicularis muscle. More so than in the primary repair, the use of permanent or long-lasting absorbable suture should be entertained to prevent muscle dehiscence and scar widening.

Bilateral cleft lip

Treatment of patients with secondary bilateral cleft deformities requires an understanding of previous operations, as well as a thorough evaluation of anatomy. Recognition of common deformities will help facilitate the surgical planning process and assist the surgeon during future procedures. Timing of any surgical intervention is dependent upon the severity of the deformity, age of the patient, and the understanding and expectations of the family. There are characteristics specific to the bilateral cleft lip that make secondary deformities distinct from those seen in unilateral clefts, including a paucity of central lip tissue, the size of the columella, and the limited blood supply to the prolabium. It is helpful to think of bilateral cleft lip deformities in terms of issues within the layers of the lip: mucosa/vermilion, muscle, and skin. If these are taken into consideration, a successful secondary correction can be achieved.

As with unilateral clefts, the timing for bilateral lip revisions can be controversial and should be decided by communication with the patient's family. Secondary revisions have both functional and aesthetic components. If significant issues with speech, nasal regurgitation, or socialization exist, revision should be considered sooner than later. If the revision is for aesthetic concerns, then it can be delayed until the patient and family are interested. Revisions should be delayed long enough to allow for maximal scar maturation. Revisions are often delayed until the pre-kindergarten years (age 4–5 years), unless there are functional concerns.

When revising a bilateral cleft lip, diagnosing the deformity and understanding the previous operations is of paramount importance. The nose, upper lip, and gingivobuccal sulcus should be considered in detail. Furthermore, the components of the lip, including skin, mucosa, vermilion, and orbicularis oris, should all be examined and addressed prior to devising the surgical plan. It is important to include the family in the operative plan so they are aware of what will occur.

Vermilion/Mucosa

Vermilion deficiency – whistle deformity

Deficiency of the midline vermilion is primarily associated with bilateral clefts and is the most common form of vermilion deformity. The "whistle deformity" is a result of a number of factors, such as failure to restore normal muscular continuity at the level of the vermilion, failure to properly restore mucosal and vermilion continuity, muscular dehiscence, or severe postoperative scarring. Identification of each of these will help dictate the surgical approach.

Treatment of a whistle deformity is probably one of the most common reasons to revise a bilateral cleft lip (Fig. 27.6). If the whistle deformity is due to vermilion deficiency alone, then a simple vermilion revision re-approximating the vermilion and creating a fuller lip is called for. This sometimes can be done with a simple Z-plasty at the level of the vermilion to break up a previous straight-line scar. If the deformity is due to vermilion deficiency as well as muscle dehiscence, a more in-depth revision should be planned. If the whistle deformity includes scarring of the lip skin, a complete takedown of the previous repair and revision should be performed. This will allow for maximal access to the mucosa, muscle, and skin. In older children, permanent suture muscle repair should be considered to prevent gradual muscle dehiscence and postoperative scar widening.

Vermilion excess

Vermilion excess is commonly seen in patients with bilateral deformities after a Manchester repair. The original Manchester repair incorporated the vermilion from the prolabial segment. Furthermore, the orbicularis muscle sphincter and the anterior gingivobuccal sulcus are not created. This repair usually

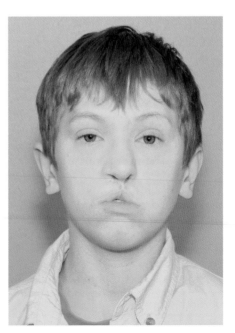

Fig. 27.6 This figure demonstrates the whistle deformity, which is absent apposition between the upper and lower lip centrally.

results in an unsightly, dry, and flaky vermilion at the level of the central tubercle. Furthermore, due to the inherent lack of adequate white roll in the prolabial segment, there is no continuity of the white roll across the upper lip. This deformity becomes apparent from a conversational distance and a constant source of dissatisfaction from patients and families. The vermilion in this area can have a "pressed on" appearance, without the impression of a symmetric and confluent lip (Fig. 27.7). Patients who had a Manchester-type bilateral cleft lip repair will have vermilion from the original prolabial segment within the upper lip.[10] If this is the case, at least the skin and vermilion should be revised. Usually this revision

will also require a more invasive muscle repair, as well as addressing an insufficient gingivobuccal sulcus. Therefore, a complete takedown and revision of the mucosa, vermilion, muscle, and skin is recommended (Video 27.3 ▶). The lateral lip elements need to be brought together at the vermilion, mucosa, and white roll level to create a harmonious and symmetric lip.

Mucosal excess

Excess mucosa and mucosal show with animation is a common problem seen after bilateral cleft lip repair. Creation of the

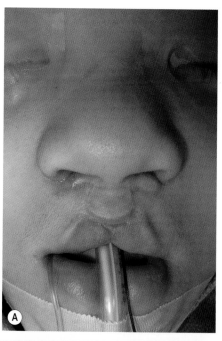
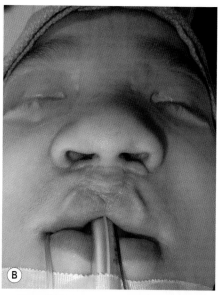
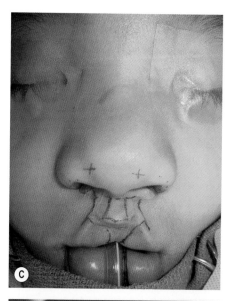
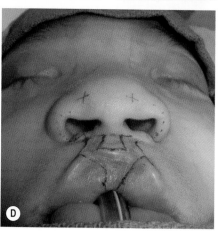
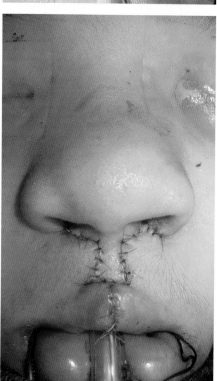
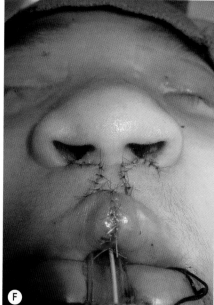

Fig. 27.7 A young male with the classic sequelae associated with the Manchester repair. The central prolabial segments were retained to reconstruct the nasal sills, the white roll, and the central vermilion. He has both a widened philtrum and a discontinuous white roll **(A, B)**. He subsequently underwent revisionary procedure to excise the widened scars as well as excess tissue in the nasal sills **(C, D)**, with the immediate on-table result **(E, F)**.

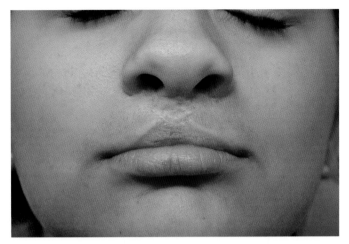

Fig. 27.8 Preoperative image demonstrates correction of a discontinuous white roll from previous bilateral cleft lip repair.

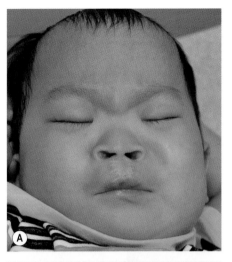

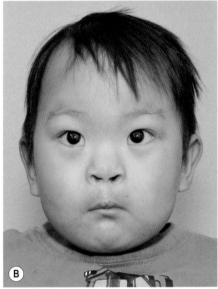

Fig. 27.9 This figure **(A)** demonstrates prominent suture marks associated with previous bilateral cleft lip repair. Subsequent surgical correction required excision and primary revision **(B)**.

anterior gingivobuccal sulcus during the initial repair is paramount to preventing this deformity (Video 27.5 ⊙). Some older techniques did not include creation of this sulcus, and the upper lip was tethered to the premaxilla. If the sulcus is inadequately created, then redundant prolabial mucosa can mask the upper central incisors during animation and repose. If this is the case, a vestibuloplasty is performed. The anterior mucosa of the prolabium is released and sutured to the raw surface of the premaxilla. It is important that the prolabial mucosa is thinned so that it will become adherent to the raw surface of the premaxilla, recreating the attached gingiva, and successfully creating the posterior surface of the gingivobuccal sulcus. A 1–2 mm margin of mucosa is left free to suture to the lateral mucosal lip segments in the depth of the sulcus. The lateral mucosal lip segments create the anterior surface of the gingivobuccal surface.

Skin

Poor scarring

Despite the most perfect surgical technique, a poor lip scar can cause any cleft lip repair to be noticeable (Fig. 27.8). In addition to the usual risk factors, those specific to the bilateral cleft lip patient can include inadequate release and repair of the orbicularis muscle, a protruding premaxilla, and excessive cleft width – all contributing to an excess amount of wound closure tension at the time of repair.

The use of permanent cutaneous sutures, kept in for too long, or dissolving sutures that do not dissolve rapidly enough can result in lip scars that have noticeable crosshatching marks (Fig. 27.9). Assuring that sutures are gone within 5 days will prevent them from causing permanent scars.

As with any unsightly scar, scar revision may be recommended. If the scars are widened or have crosshatch marks, an excision and re-approximation can be performed (Fig. 27.10). An attempt to prevent future scar widening can be considered by imbricating the underlying orbicularis muscle so as to create a tension-free closure at the level of the skin. This can be done with a permanent suture, especially in older children where muscle memory and coordination are well

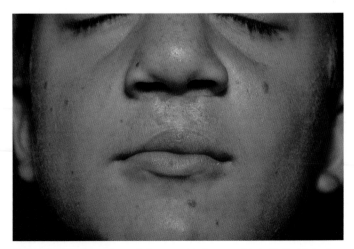

Fig. 27.10 This figure demonstrates scar widening associated with the bilateral cleft lip deformity. Widened scars that were mature would generally be managed with excision and primary closure.

established. Scar revision is rarely done in isolation and usually is involved with correction of other deformities, such as a widened prolabium, white roll mismatch, vermilion asymmetry, or alar base malposition.

Skin deficiency

A tight upper lip can be seen in patients who have had multiple revisions, who have had too much lateral lip skin removed during the initial operation, or who have had prolabial necrosis after repair. Patients undergoing multiple revisions require repeated skin excision to line up landmarks, and this makes the upper lip horizontally shorter compared to the lower lip, giving the upper lip a flat appearance.

The prolabium's blood supply should be respected during surgery to prevent ischemia. After surgical intervention, the prolabium should be pink and perfused to ensure survival. If it appears white, then sutures should be removed to help prevent tissue ischemia. If the prolabium becomes ischemic and necrotic, it will heal as a scar, result in a poor cosmetic outcome, and potentially lead to a short and tight upper lip.

When local options for tissue rearrangement have been exhausted and there is skin deficiency, an Abbe flap may be incorporated (Video 27.1 ▶).[11,12] This procedure is used when there is a loss of tissue from multiple operations or when the prolabium has been discarded. The Abbe flap is being used less frequently given the improvements in primary techniques. It does have the ability to reconstruct the upper lip in all three layers, restoring a normal-appearing Cupid's bow, central tubercle, and philtrum. In addition, it decreases the horizontal size of the lower lip, helping camouflage upper lip deficiency.

When designing the Abbe flap, reconstructing the entire philtral unit should be planned, improving upper lip tightness and providing a balanced facial profile. The flap is transposed from the center of the lower lip and inset into the upper lip. This allows for the recreation of Cupid's bow and the entire philtral unit. Designing this flap slightly smaller than normal will account for stretching of the flap once inset and tension-free closure on the lower lip donor site. The flap is based on the inferior labial artery, which can be divided at least 10–14 days after inset. At the time of flap division and inset, compressing the pedicle prior to division will confirm viability of the flap.

Skin excess

In bilateral cleft lips, the philtrum can progressively widen over time. Growth is the most likely reason for this widening, but scarring and tension have been thought to contribute as well. Contemporary primary repair techniques suggest the prolabium design to be around 1.5–2 mm at the hemi-Cupid's bow and 2–3 mm at the base.[13] These measurements account for the widening that can occur with growth. Given the risk of vascularity with a prolabium of this size, care is exercised to keep the base intact so as to prevent devascularization.

A widened philtrum can be addressed at any point during growth, but usually waiting until final growth is complete is recommended, so as to prevent future revisions. If lip appearance is a significant concern in a growing patient, revisions can be made after consultation regarding future surgeries. When designing the size of the philtral subunit, anthropomorphic studies have evaluated the size of the normal male and female philtrum.[14] These measurements can be incorporated into the surgical plan, but clinical judgment should be exercised as it relates to the final appearance.

Muscle

Dehiscence

Failure to properly dissect and reapproximate the orbicularis oris muscle at the initial repair, as well as postoperative muscle dehiscence, accounts for many secondary bilateral cleft lip deformities. This is diagnosed by lateral lip muscle bulging during animation, representing discontinuity of the muscular sling. Furthermore, failure to appropriately dissect the orbicularis oris muscles from the nasal base can result in widened alar bases. Careful attention should be made to identify and repair the different components of the orbicularis muscle in the upper lip.[15] An attempt to repair the nasalis, the marginal, and main components of the orbicularis oris are important to restoring the normal contour to the upper lip. If the muscle is repaired appropriately, the amount of tension placed on the skin repair is minimal, and this can prevent future scar widening.

If muscle dehiscence is suspected, then re-repair is recommended to achieve normal lip appearance and function. Restoring orbicularis oris continuity is one of the most important components of a successful repair. Determining the different components of the orbicularis muscle during revision is recommended. Permanent or a long-lasting absorbable suture will help prevent postoperative muscle dehiscence and prevent undue tension on the skin closure, helping prevent scar widening.

Cleft palate

Some feel that outcomes in cleft palate surgery have been overlooked, when compared with cleft lip, not only due to the lack of visibility, but also due to poor definitions and inconsistent evaluation methods. Standardization of the evaluation and characterization of speech outcomes is a difficult goal, in part because of the subjective nature of speech evaluation; however, it is a goal that will greatly assist the ability to measure outcomes. Unlike a cleft lip repair, visible for all to see, the results of a cleft palate repair require a more in-depth evaluation. While the goal of cleft palate repair is normal speech and resonance, fistulas and velopharyngeal insufficiency (VPI) can occur. Consistent and accepted definitions of fistula and VPI will help cleft teams communicate more effectively.

Velopharyngeal insufficiency

The diagnosis of VPI, of which hypernasality is one feature, and the recommendation for secondary surgery can be different for every patient and are highly dependent on cleft center. Ideally, children should have at least an annual speech evaluation prior to age six and have any surgery for VPI completed by school age.[16] However, there will be patients who are lost to follow-up, experience involution of adenoids, have maxillary growth or maxillary advancement, and will require work-up and treatment at an older age. A symptomatic fistula can also be a source of nasal air loss and may need to be addressed alone or in conjunction with secondary speech surgery.

Workup and algorithm

Patients who present with continued speech concerns require a thorough work-up by an experienced speech and language pathologist who is a member of the cleft team. A formal speech evaluation will diagnose features of velopharyngeal insufficiency including hypernasality, audible nasal emission, light articulatory contacts, as well as compensatory articulation errors. This evaluation is used to set goals for therapy as well as determine the efficacy of surgical intervention. Nasoendoscopy and videofluoroscopy visualize the pattern of velopharyngeal closure during speech production. Indirect measures, such as pressure flow testing and nasometry, are often completed during a formal speech evaluation. These studies are used as objective measurements to supplement perceptual ratings. Guided by a thorough work-up, the speech pathologist determines if the speech difference is due to a structural problem, and would therefore be aided by a surgical solution, or if the speech difference may be corrected through speech therapy. The speech pathologist will also help to determine which surgical option would be the best, based upon the pattern of velopharyngeal closure.

Outlining the complete speech evaluation for a child with VPI is beyond the scope of this chapter; however, the operative surgeon should understand some basic considerations. First, the patient needs to be mature enough to cooperate and provide an adequate speech sample. For children without significant speech delays, this can typically be done by age 3. Pressure flow and nasometry may be achieved with a very mature and cooperative preschool-aged child. Nasoendoscopy, while our preferred method for imaging, may not yield a representative speech sample until the child is older. Videofluoroscopy can be performed on a child as young as three or four years old, or for those children who will not tolerate nasoendoscopy.

In addition to perceptual and instrumental speech exams, physical examination of the palate during phonation can provide a great deal of information for the surgeon. A palate previously repaired with a straight midline technique, without complete dissection and repair of the levator palatine muscles, will demonstrate a "vaulted V"-shaped pattern of elevation. This is due to the sagittally oriented levator muscles that were never completely dissected from the clefted position and placed in the anatomic transverse orientation. When stimulated (with phonation or a gag), the muscles bulge laterally in the palate with no motion along the midline, resulting in the vaulted V-shaped pattern of palatal elevation. This finding should alert the examiner to the abnormal muscle orientation and help them determine what the most appropriate intervention will be.

Oronasal fistulas can result in significant speech difficulties as well as velopharyngeal insufficiency. A formal speech evaluation can help determine whether a fistula is contributing to any speech abnormalities. Fistulas can be characterized as functional or non-functional. Non-functional fistulas usually do not cause any speech disability and do not require surgical intervention. These fistulas are usually small and are not surgically corrected. As fistulas get bigger, they can cause nasal regurgitation, air escape, and hypernasality (Fig. 27.11).

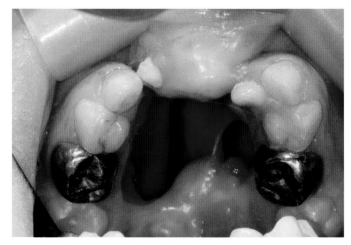

Fig. 27.11 This patient has a large type IV, V, and VI oronasal fistula associated with a bilateral cleft palate. She has constant nasal regurgitation and air escape.

These symptomatic fistulas are considered to be functional and need to be surgically addressed.

Patients who have already undergone secondary speech surgery and still display evidence of VPI are in a more advanced stage of cleft care and will need to have another speech evaluation to help determine the cause of their disability. As before, speech evaluation with objective measures such as pressure flow testing and nasometry as well as imaging should be considered. A thorough intraoral exam should be performed to evaluate the architecture of the soft palate and velopharyngeal structures. A nasoendoscopy is the best way to see the velopharyngeal architecture during phonation. This helps the treating physician understand the limitations of the original cleft palate surgery as well as any other surgeries that have been performed. Videofluoroscopy may have limited benefit in the patient who has already undergone secondary speech surgery, particularly if the suspected defect is very small.

Fistula closure

Closure of palatal fistulas is a significant challenge for the cleft surgeon. Small fistulas can be managed conservatively if they are non-functional or asymptomatic. Fistulas are clinically significant or functional when they lead to nasal air escape (hypernasality and audible nasal emission), speech distortion, or nasal regurgitation of liquids and solids. The published rate of postoperative fistulas varies widely, from 0–70%.[17–19] This is in part due to the lack of a standard classification scheme, which hinders both communication and research efforts. At our institution, we prefer to use the Pittsburgh Fistula Classification System, described by Losee et al., due to its ease of use.[20] The Pittsburgh Fistula Classification System includes seven fistula types: those at the uvula, or bifid uvulae (type I); in the soft palate (type II); at the junction of the soft and hard palates (type III); within the hard palate (type IV); at the incisive foramen, or junction of the primary and secondary palates – reserved for Veau IV clefts (type V); lingual–alveolar (type VI); and labial–alveolar (type VII) (Fig. 27.12).

Fistulas are difficult to repair and have a reported recurrence rate approaching 65%.[21] Many strategies for palatal

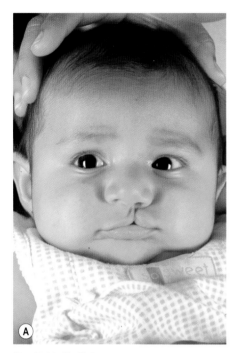

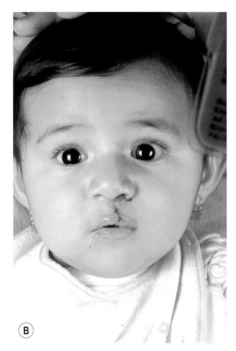

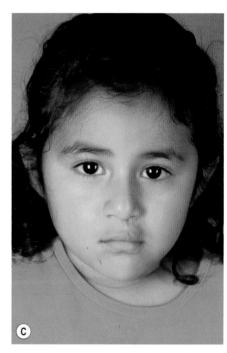

(A) (B) (C)

Fig. 27.12 (A–C) Even with perfect surgical technique, postoperative scarring and inflammation vary, resulting in a broad spectrum of secondary deformities.

fistula repair have been reported over the years, the complexity of which ascends the reconstructive ladder.[21–40] From direct cauterization by Obermeyer in 1967,[41] to an appliance/obturator by Berkman, to the myriad of local flap designs by von Langenbeck to Gabka in 1964, to free conchal grafts by Ohsumi,[25,36,38,41] the options put forth for closure of palatal fistulas have been numerous. Guerrero-Santos and Altamirano popularized the tongue flap in the 1960s and 1970s, which has remained a mainstay at some centers for closure of larger anterior fistulas.[32,42] Multiple pedicle flaps, including the facial artery myomucosal (FAMM) flap, have been described to treat the most difficult anterior fistulas.[23,28,32,42,43] Even free tissue transfer[24,27,31,35,37,38] has been described for when all other modalities have been exhausted. As with many situations in plastic surgery, when there are numerous procedures described, it is often because no one option works universally. The most recent advances in fistula treatment have been the use of acellular dermal matrix (ADM), as described by Kirschner et al.,[33,34] and the use of the buccal fat pad flap.[44]

In general, the larger the fistula, the larger the surgery required to address it. Small local flaps have the inherent problem of utilizing already scarred, stiff tissue that is often friable and difficult to work with due to the constant exposure to regurgitating nasal and oral contents (Fig. 27.13). The well-described procedures such as the FAMM flap and tongue flap have the benefit of bringing in vascularized, unscarred tissue but at the expense of considerable donor site morbidity, technical difficulty, considerable postoperative care, and need for a second surgery (Figs. 27.14 & 27.15). The preferred method at our institution for fistulas of the soft palate only (types I and II) is a direct excision and repair, often in conjunction with a conversion Furlow palatoplasty if the fistula occurs in the presence of velopharyngeal insufficiency.

Fistulas at the junction of the hard and soft palate (type III), and those of the hard palate (type IV) require considerably more than direct excision and closure due to their nature and paucity of malleable local tissue. The local transposition flaps described in various textbooks are often inadequate for complete closure, as the arc of rotation often falls short. If local nasal tissue proves to be inadequate, palatally based hinge flaps or nasal septal flaps may be utilized. Another option, based on the work of Kirschner and Losee et al.,[33,34,45–48] is the use of acellular dermal matrix as an adjunct when local soft-tissue options prove inadequate for a watertight closure (Fig. 27.16). They advocate for use of a thin piece of acellular dermal matrix for *augmenting the nasal lining closure* and have data to support its use in all fistula types, except those of the soft palate only, with a decrease in recurrent fistulas to 3.6%.[33,34,45]

Another option, when local tissue is insufficient for closure of either the nasal or oral lining, is use of the buccal fat pad flap, which has been widely described for closure of palatal defects both in the head and neck literature as well as in the cleft palate literature.[44,49–51] It has several advantages over other options and has become the preferred method for closure of larger fistulas of the hard palate at our institution. It is a simple flap to raise, requires no tedious dissection, is reliable, has minimal donor morbidity, does not require tunneling or a second operation, and can easily reach the midline or the lingual central incisors. Additionally, it is well-vascularized, autologous tissue that epithelializes readily and can be used for either nasal or oral closure.

In the case of fistulas, as in most secondary cleft surgery, prevention is the key. A well-executed primary palatoplasty is the best defense against fistula formation. A tension-free closure and careful postoperative care are crucial in prevention. During the primary palatoplasty, whether it is a two-flap

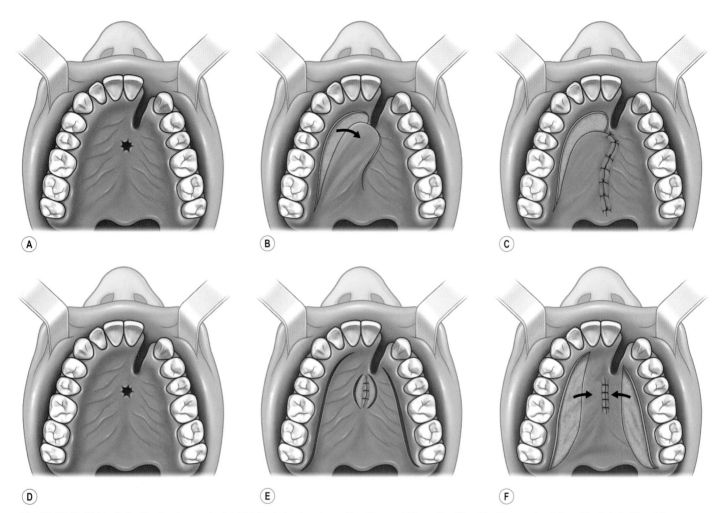

Fig. 27.13 (A–F) The first option for closure of palatal fistulas is local random-pattern tissue, which can be utilized in either a unipedicle or bipedicle fashion. It is important to note, however, that the majority of the peripheral hard palate is granulated mucosa after primary palatoplasty.

procedure with an intravelar veloplasty or a Furlow palatoplasty, care should be taken to include the following elements in order to prevent fistulization: relaxing incisions, complete intravelar veloplasty, total release of the tensor tendon at the level of the hamulus, complete dissection of the neurovascular bundle with optional osteotomy of the bony foramen, meticulous surgical precision to limit unnecessary handling or crushing of the mucosal edges, and diligent postoperative care.

Furlow palatoplasty

The double-opposing Z-plasty, as described by Dr. Leonard Furlow, is one of the first-line treatments in secondary speech surgery.[52] It accomplishes the goals of anatomically overlapping the levator veli palatine muscles in the posterior half of the palate and placing them under maximal functional tension. It lengthens the palate and, due to the nature of the Z-plasty effect, results in narrowing the velopharyngeal port, resulting in a built-in pharyngoplasty. The Furlow is the option of choice for patients with a short but mobile palate, those who have not had a previous complete repair of the levators, and those with a coronal closure pattern.

It is drawn as double-opposing Z-plasties, one on the oral side and one on the nasal side. The posterior flaps, the left/oral side and the right/nasal side, contain the levator muscle as well as the mucosa. The anteriorly based flaps (the right side on the oral surface and the left side on the nasal surface) contain mucosa only. The left-side myomucosal flap is drawn at approximately 60° from the junction of the hard and soft palate medially towards the point where the levator exits the skull base laterally (or the hamulus) (Fig. 27.17). The right-sided mucosal only flap on the oral side is drawn slightly greater than 60° from the junction of the uvula and soft palate towards the hamulus. On the left side the muscle is taken off the posterior edge of the hard palate and dissected laterally and posteriorly, taking care to take down all of the abnormal lateral attachments, until the muscle can be rotated 90° to the skull base and transposed across the midline easily. The nasal Z-plasty on the left side is then incised from the junction of the uvula and soft palate, at a 60° angle, heading towards where the levator exits the skull base and the hamulus. On the right side, the anteriorly based mucosa-only flap is raised to the posterior edge of the hard palate. The levator is then dissected off the posterior edge of the hard palate from medial to lateral. The nasal lining is incised from medial to lateral

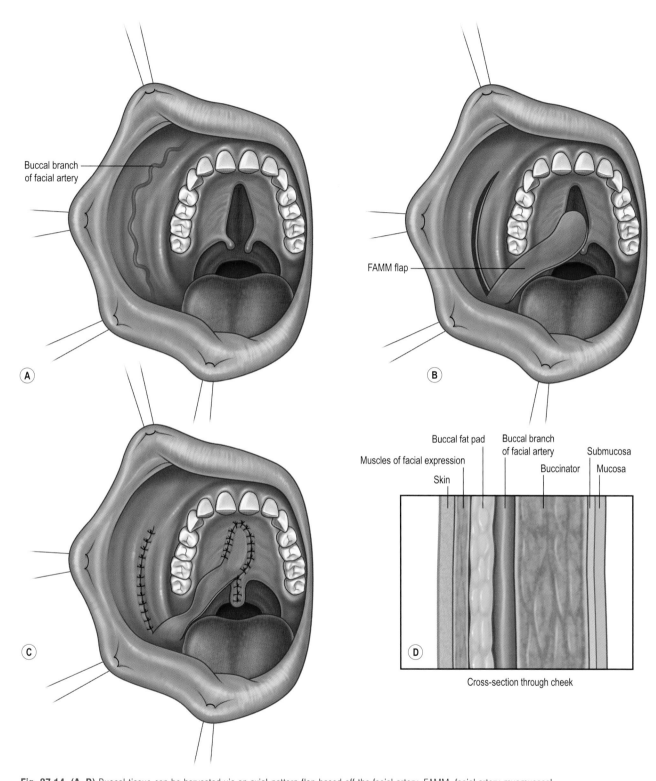

Fig. 27.14 (A–D) Buccal tissue can be harvested via an axial pattern flap based off the facial artery. FAMM, facial artery myomucosal.

from just behind the posterior edge of the hard palate along the trajectory of the levator laterally at a 60° angle; care is taken to leave the levator attached to the nasal lining and to take down all of the abnormal lateral attachments. This incision is made laterally – only as far as needed to adequately

transpose the right-sided posteriorly based musculomucosal flap to be inset into the left side. The nasal limbs can now be transposed and inset. The nasal lining is closed with interrupted absorbable sutures. Some surgeons prefer to perform an intermuscular repair with permanent or absorbable sutures.

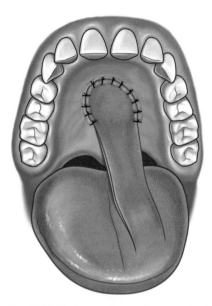

Fig. 27.15 The tongue offers another regional option for palatal fistula repair.

The oral lining is then closed with interrupted absorbable sutures (Fig. 27.18).

A nasal trumpet or tongue stitch is placed for postoperative airway management per surgeon preference. The patient is maintained on a liquid diet for one week postoperatively and then advanced to a soft diet for an additional two weeks.

Posterior pharyngeal flap

The posterior pharyngeal flap (PPF) is a secondary speech surgery (pharyngoplasty) that creates a static bridge of tissue between the posterior free edge of the velum and the posterior pharyngeal wall. The PPF relies on adequate lateral pharyngeal wall motion to achieve velopharyngeal competence. It is ideally suited for patients with sagittal or circular closure patterns.[53] Variations exist in the design of the PPF; however, today most surgeons utilize a superiorly based flap that is lined with the nasal mucosa of the soft palate. An appropriately executed PPF will not be visible on intraoral inspection, as it should be placed at the level of velopharyngeal closure, usually above the palatal plane. Of note, when planning a PPF, especially in children with velocardiofacial syndrome, the surgeon should remember the potential for medially

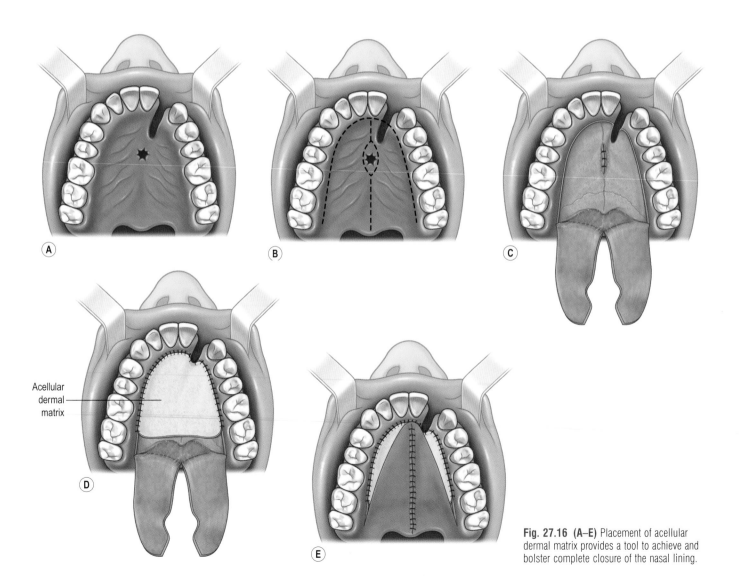

Acellular dermal matrix

Fig. 27.16 (A–E) Placement of acellular dermal matrix provides a tool to achieve and bolster complete closure of the nasal lining.

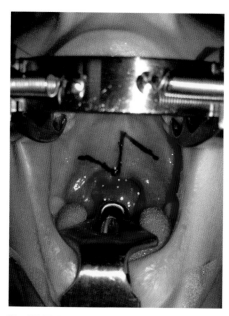

Fig. 27.17 This picture demonstrates the oral-side markings for the Furlow cleft palate repair technique.

displaced internal carotid arteries and should proceed with care.

Surgery begins with splitting the soft palate down the midline and laterally retracting each hemipalate. The extent of the PPF is marked out along the posterior pharyngeal wall, with adequate length to reach the posterior edge of the hard palate. The width of the flap will be determined by the patient's anatomy, the size of the preoperative gap, and the surgeon's preference. Some surgeons place red rubber catheters, nasogastric tubes, nasopharyngeal airways, or any combination of the three, at the time of surgery to assist with sizing of the lateral ports. The superiorly based flap is raised at the level of the prevertebral fascia. The cranial base of the

flap is just above the level of the palatal plane typically and should be placed at the level of predicted velopharyngeal closure. The flap raised from the posterior pharyngeal wall will become the nasal side of the PPF, and the oral lining of the PPF will be the nasal mucosal flaps pedicled at the posterior free edge of the soft palate.

Nasal mucosal lining flaps are then raised from the soft palate and pedicled on the posterior free edge of the velum, taking care to obtain adequate width for lining. The defect in the posterior pharyngeal wall can be partially or completely closed primarily. The flaps are inset with resorbable suture; each stitch is placed and tagged until all are placed. The authors' preferred method is to use 4-0 chromic gut suture with three sutures along the posterior edge of the hard palate, three along the posterior pharyngeal wall, and two on either side for a total of ten sutures in all.

Overnight monitoring in a step down unit with pulse oximetry, a nasopharyngeal airway, and a nasogastric tube is preferred. A full liquid diet for one week and then a soft diet for an additional two weeks is recommended. Due to its static nature, the PPF has a risk of creating obstructive sleep apnea (OSA). Children who have had PPF surgery should be closely monitored, not just in the immediate postoperative period, but throughout growth and development, for signs of OSA.

Sphincter pharyngoplasty

Sphincter pharyngoplasty is a dynamic pharyngoplasty for the treatment of velopharyngeal incompetence, utilizing the palatopharyngeus muscles to decrease the overall size of the velopharyngeal (VP) area. By reducing the transverse diameter, the soft palate is better able to achieve VP competence.

After identifying the posterior tonsillar pillars, a vertical incision is made in the anterior mucosa (between the tonsil and the posterior pillar) and posterior mucosa (between the posterior tonsil and the posterior pharyngeal wall) from the upper third of the tonsil to its inferior pole. The palatopharyngeus muscle is separated from the superior constrictor, and the myomucosal flap is elevated, extending beneath the inferior pole of the tonsil and pedicled superiorly. Care must be taken near the superior attachment to the soft palate where the muscle is innervated. This is performed bilaterally.

At the level of the second cervical vertebrae, a horizontal incision is made on the posterior pharyngeal wall (connecting laterally to the posterior mucosal incision) to receive the resected posterior tonsillar pillars. The horizontal incision must consist of mucosa, intra- and peripharyngeal aponeurosis, and superior constrictor muscular fibers.[54] The sphincter flaps are brought together with sutures along the posterior pharyngeal raw surface. They can be brought together end-to-end or overlapped entirely, depending upon the desired size of the VP port. A central, dynamic opening bounded by the repositioned posterior tonsillar pillars, the soft palate, and the posterior pharyngeal wall is created. If hypernasality is still present after surgery, the VP port size can be secondarily modified by tightening the sphincter flaps.

Posterior pharyngeal wall augmentation

Posterior pharyngeal wall augmentation is another form of pharyngoplasty intended to decrease the velopharyngeal port size by moving the posterior pharyngeal wall closer to the

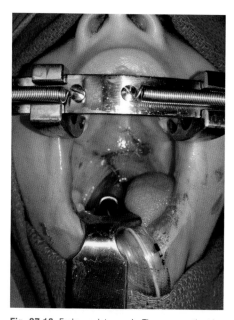

Fig. 27.18 Furlow palate repair. The same patient is presented as in Fig. 27.17.

palate. Augmentation is typically less invasive than other secondary speech procedures because it usually involves injection or insertion of a durable, long-lasting material, not requiring dissection and tissue rearrangement. Many different materials have been described for augmentation, including Vaseline, silicone, cartilage, acellular dermal matrix, and autogenous fat. For very small holes in the velopharynx during phonation, we prefer fat grafting for augmentation.

Fat can be harvested from the abdomen or buttock, depending on the abundance. Most children, during the early school age years, are rather thin and will require a buttock donor site. An abdominal donor site is most commonly used for older children. Manual suction with 10 cc syringes and a large cannula through small access incisions are commonly used. Once harvested, fat can be processed in a number of different ways, in an attempt to increase the vitality of the fat cells.[55] Once harvested and processed, the fat is loaded into syringes for injection. Our standard practice is to perform the procedure with the assistance of the otolaryngology team. A nasoendoscopy is performed at the time of injection, and confirmation of injection is made by both surgeons. The preoperative nasoendoscopy is reviewed prior to the operation and should be readily available for confirmation of injection site. No less than 10 cc of fat is injected per patient to account for graft resorption.[56] Grafting is normally done as an outpatient operation and patients are discharged on pain medication and oral antibiotics. Follow-up speech evaluation is done at 1–3 months after surgery.

Cleft nasal deformity

The cleft nasal deformity involves the skin, cartilage, mucosa, and skeletal platform. Theories regarding the etiology of the deformity have been discussed extensively and continue to be debated. The exact findings have been well measured and documented.[57] An appreciation of the pathologic anatomy in the unilateral and bilateral cleft nose deformity is essential to achieve a satisfactory aesthetic and functional result.

Patients should be thoroughly evaluated with a history and physical exam prior to surgery. Previous surgeries should be reviewed to prepare for possible findings intraoperatively. Patient concerns regarding their nasal airway and nose and lip symmetry should be addressed. Preoperative photographs are taken to document the deformities; they are also helpful when consulting the patient regarding operative goals.

Physical exam of the nose should be done in relation to its position on the facial skeleton. Cephalometric analysis evaluates jaw and chin position and the effect on overall facial balance. These issues should be brought up with the patient and family, and if they are not interested in orthognathic surgery and are happy with the overall facial appearance, an exam centered on nasal shape and symmetry is performed.

Nasal examination should always be performed in a very systematic and repeatable fashion. Gunter diagrams are very helpful for preoperative planning purposes. The secondary cleft nasal deformity is related to what existed at primary repair but altered by any previous surgery. It is important to understand these changes, as it may affect the planned operation.

The unilateral cleft nasal deformity involves the soft tissues and skeleton of the nose (Fig. 27.19). Aberrant muscle insertion results in an imbalance that is influenced by maxillary skeletal hypoplasia.[58] Rather than a horizontal orientation and continuous orbicularis oris across the upper lip, the muscle inserts in a discontinuous manner, into the base of the columella on the non-cleft side. This can create an unopposed force that pulls the columella and caudal nasal septum to the

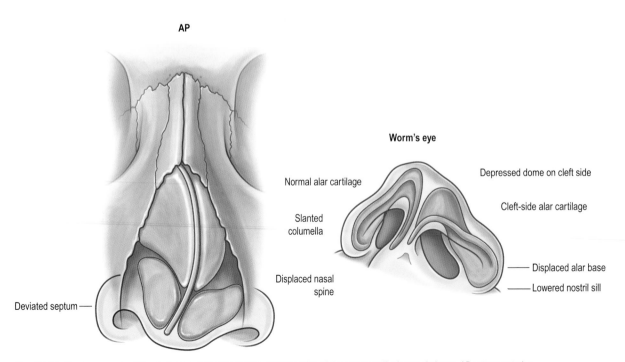

Fig. 27.19 The key aspects of the cleft nose deformity involve abnormalities of the osseocartilaginous skeleton. *AP*, anteroposterior.

AP

Worm's eye

Normal alar cartilage

Slanted columella

Displaced nasal spine

Deviated septum

Depressed dome on cleft side

Cleft-side alar cartilage

Displaced alar base

Lowered nostril sill

non-cleft side.[4] On the cleft side, the orbicularis inserts into the alar base, retracting it laterally, inferiorly, and posteriorly (due to poor maxillary skeletal support) (Fig. 27.20).

The asymmetric nasal tip results from the irregular lower lateral cartilage on the cleft side. While not ubiquitously accepted, the length of the lower lateral cartilage on the cleft side is considered equal to the non-cleft side, primarily differing in shape and position.[59–62] On the cleft side, the medial crus is shorter and the lateral crus is longer with a less defined, wider dome.[6] This results in an underprojected tip defining point when compared to the non-cleft side (see Fig. 27.2).

Deviation of the nasal septum is seen bilaterally. On the non-cleft side, the unopposed pull of the orbicularis oris muscle, as well as the premaxillary ligament, results in caudal septal deviation. However, the premaxillary ligament only affects the caudal septum, permitting bowing of the majority of the septum towards the cleft side. Whether alone or in conjunction with hypertrophied nasal turbinates, the aperture of the internal nasal valve is decreased, resulting in nasal obstruction.[63]

Nasal obstruction at the external nasal valve from the introverted lower lateral cartilage is common. The cephalic edge of the lower lateral cartilage introverts into the vestibule in a posterior inferior direction resulting in a visibly thickened and hooded ala.[64] Attachment of the lateral nasal sidewall to the depressed cleft side piriform results in a vestibular webbing that is visible through the cleft-side nares.

Timing of cleft nasal surgery can be divided into primary, intermediate, and secondary repairs. Studies have disproved the idea that early manipulation of the nasal cartilage interferes with growth.[59] Original experimental studies demonstrated that large submucous resections of the nasal septum affected subsequent nasal and midface growth; however, studies by McComb and Coghlan demonstrated that repositioning the lower lateral cartilage, without cartilage resection, did not interfere with subsequent nasal and midfacial development.[65,66] As a result of this research, primary cleft rhinoplasty today regularly occurs with the initial lip repair.[67] The benefit of early intervention is restoration of nasal shape with the potential for more symmetric nasal growth. However, it is important to note that surgery done at an early age will result in scar tissue likely affecting future surgeries.

Intermediate rhinoplasty

Intermediate rhinoplasty is usually performed before school, between 4 and 6 years old.[68] The goal of surgery is to correct the aberrant position of the cleft-side lower lateral cartilage so that future nasal growth will not exacerbate the cleft nasal deformity. At this time, the surgeon may also perform any minor lip revision, as necessary. Septal surgery should be deferred until post-adolescence so as not to prevent disturbance in nasal growth.[64]

In unilateral cleft deformities, the intermediate rhinoplasty addresses the cleft-side lower lateral cartilage (LLC) as well as any lateral vestibular webbing. An open rhinoplasty approach can be performed to expose the lower lateral cartilages, directly observe anatomic differences, and correct them with suture techniques. Cartilage grafting is not performed at this young age, given the residual growth potential of the nose.[69] If there is lateral vestibular webbing, a V–Y type incision can lengthen the lateral nasal sidewall and advance the lower lateral cartilage forward.[68]

In bilateral cases, the intermediate rhinoplasty addresses the depressed lower lateral cartilages and lengthens the shortened columella.[13,68] This is done via an open rhinoplasty technique where the lower lateral cartilages are exposed through transcolumellar and infracartilagenous incisions. The LLCs are sutured together with a transdomal suture decreasing their angle of divergence and placing them in a more projected orientation.[13] Soft tissue that is commonly found between the dome points of the LLC can be thinned to help achieve better tip projection and definition. The incisions are then closed with plain gut in the vestibule and permanent suture on the columella.

Secondary cleft rhinoplasty – unilateral

Secondary rhinoplasty occurs after facial growth has completed, around 14–16 years old in female patients and 16–18 years old in male patients.[70,71] Surgical techniques rely on well-accepted rhinoplasty principles for unilateral or bilateral cleft nasal deformities.[72–74] The open approach is preferred for better exposure and visualization. Placement of cartilage grafts for support and reinforcement is a major component of

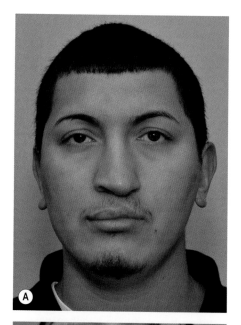

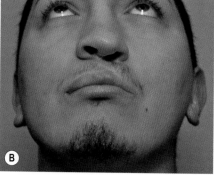

Fig. 27.20 These images **(A, B)** demonstrate classic deformities associated with the cleft nasal deformity. This includes deviated nasal septum and tip, inferolaterally and posteriorly displaced cleft-side alar base, and abnormal nasal sill.

the cleft rhinoplasty operation. Cartilage grafts reinforce the structural support of the nose, allow for improved tip definition, and prevent wound contracture and collapse.

Alar base support is essential for attaining definitive repair and relies on the skeletal foundation of the face. Varying degrees of unilateral or bilateral maxillary hypoplasia are typically present in the cleft patient. Bridging the alveolar cleft with bone graft is often performed prior to eruption of the canine teeth, between the ages of 9 and 11 years (Video 27.2 ▶).[4,75,76] This serves to support, augment, and reposition the alar base. When inadequate support of the alar base is encountered, secondary augmentation using bone, cartilage, and alloplastic implants may be applied. In severe maxillary hypoplasia, maxillary osteotomies and advancement can be used to reconstruct the anterior–posterior dimensions of the face. Advancement should be completed prior to definitive rhinoplasty.[69]

Incision

Cleft rhinoplasty via an open approach allows for direct visualization of nasal structures as well as anatomic reconstruction of abnormal components. Transcolumellar and infracartilagenous incisions are most frequently employed to visualize the lower lateral cartilages as well as the nasal septum. Care should be taken when elevating the columella not to injure the medial crura of the lower lateral cartilages. Superficial dissection should proceed in these areas to prevent injuring these structures. Once the skin has been elevated, the nasal structures can be addressed (Video 27.4 ▶).

The septum

The nasal septum can be approached by separating the medial crura of lower lateral cartilages. The caudal septum is identified, and a subperichondrial dissection can be started, ensuring that the dissection is in the proper plane, validated by the blue appearance of the cartilage. A portion of the septum is harvested to obtain cartilage for grafting as well as to correct deviation causing nasal airway obstruction. A 1 cm dorsal and caudal strut should remain to avoid nasal collapse. Any displacement of the caudal septum should be corrected at this time by release and repositioning in the facial midline. In clefts, there is often a bony septal/vomer spur that needs removal to achieve a patent nasal airway.

The nasal tip

The nasal tip is buttressed using a columellar strut, placed in between the medial crura and sutured in place (Fig. 27.21). The LLCs are advanced and secured to the strut using mattress sutures, obtaining appropriate tip projection (Fig. 27.22).[77] The columellar strut is placed behind the medial crura, so it does not increase the columella width.[78] When the lower lateral cartilages are wide, the tip may benefit from cephalic trimming. Despite this, projection maybe inadequate on the cleft side, and batten grafting with onlay cartilage grafts on the cleft-side LLC can provide better support and shape.[78] Tip defining sutures are placed to reconstitute the dome into a more cephalic position (Figs. 27.22 & 27.23). Onlay shield grafts can augment nasal tip definition, and other grafts can camouflage other tip asymmetries (Fig. 27.24).[78]

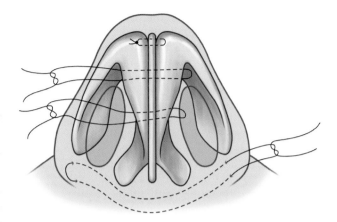

Fig. 27.21 Columellar struts involve the placement of a graft between the medial crura and suturing the structures together using mattress sutures. This improves nasal tip support and projection, columellar length, and nasolabial angle.

Nasal vestibule

Nasal vestibule contracture, resulting from either the primary repair or revisions, is a difficult and common problem encountered during secondary rhinoplasty. Scarring can lead to nostril stenosis and collapse of the external nasal valve. Local tissue rearrangement with healthy tissue can help reconstruct this area and disrupt the constrictive forces. Alternatively, the scar, along with redundant subepithelial soft tissue, may be excised, followed by placement of a bolster to encourage lateral healing.[79] Redundant skin may also be used to line a stenotic vestibule.[80] A laterally or medially based sliding chondrocutaneous flap, harvested using the previous cleft lip scar, can be used for lining vestibular deficits due to its healthy blood supply.[80]

A micronostril is a very difficult problem to correct, and the creation of this deformity during primary repair should be recognized and avoided at all costs. If there is significant constriction of the nostril, and loss of tissue along the nostril sill, the nasal alae should be repositioned. One way to correct this problem is by introducing new skin into the nasal sill with a peri-alar nasolabial transposition flap. This can increase the size of the nostril, reposition the medially displaced alar base laterally, and increase the length of the sill, more accurately matching the opposite side.

Lateral vestibular webbing is a common problem seen in secondary rhinoplasty. A V–Y advancement will move the cartilage–mucosal flap into a more anatomic position. This deformity can be limited during the primary lip repair by releasing the lateral nasal sidewall from the piriform and advancing the alar base to its correct position.

Nasal dorsum

The nasal dorsal root is usually directed toward the cleft side, resulting in tip deviation away from the cleft. Dorsal humps, if present, can be addressed prior to harvesting cartilage grafts from the septum, thereby assuring an adequate 1 cm dorsal septum. The nasal bones are commonly thick and wide; therefore, low-to-low lateral osteotomies in combination with medial to lateral osteotomies superiorly can be performed to

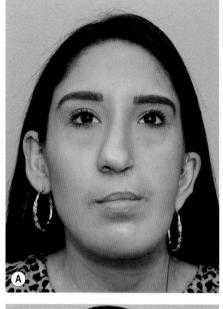

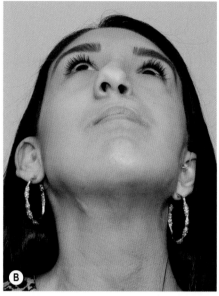

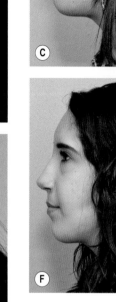

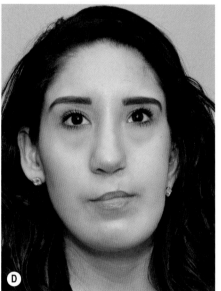

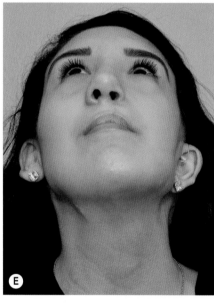

Fig. 27.22 Pre- **(A–C)** and postoperative images **(D–F)** demonstrate improvement in this patient's dorsal aesthetic lines, small dorsal hump, septal deviation, wide boxy tip, nasal tip projection, and nostril shape/symmetry.

reposition the nasal root to the midline and narrow the nasal base width.[78] If this does not adequately narrow the dorsum, a central segment can be removed creating an open roof via paramedian osteotomies. The nasal bones can then be in-fractured to achieve adequate narrowing. If this is done, spreader grafts may be necessary to reconstruct the internal nasal valve.

Nasal alae

Addressing the malpositioned nasal alae is often one of the final stages of secondary rhinoplasty (Fig. 27.25). Often laterally and inferiorly malpositioned, the alae can potentially be in any orientation. With a full-thickness peri-alar incision, the alae can be brought into a symmetric position. The lateral ala can be repositioned using a V–Y advancement along the alar facial groove. The ala can be moved laterally with a lateral skin flap transposition into the nasal floor. Superiorly

positioned alae are dropped by excision of superior lip skin. Skin from the cheek is advanced superiorly to mobilize the inferiorly positioned alae into a more symmetric position.

Bilateral cleft nasal deformity

Components of the bilateral cleft nose often resemble those of the unilateral deformity; however, there is often greater symmetry in the bilateral deformity (Figs. 27.26 & 27.27). The columella can be short or nearly absent with decreased soft tissue between the nasal tip and vermilion border of the lip.[81] The degree of the columellar shortening is related to the extent of prolabial development, cephalic nasal tip rotation, and cleft severity. The lower lateral cartilages have an increased inter-domal distance due to the aberrant muscular insertions, resulting in decreased projection and tip definition.[64] The septum may be midline in incomplete clefts; however, in complete as well as asymmetric bilateral clefts, the septum is

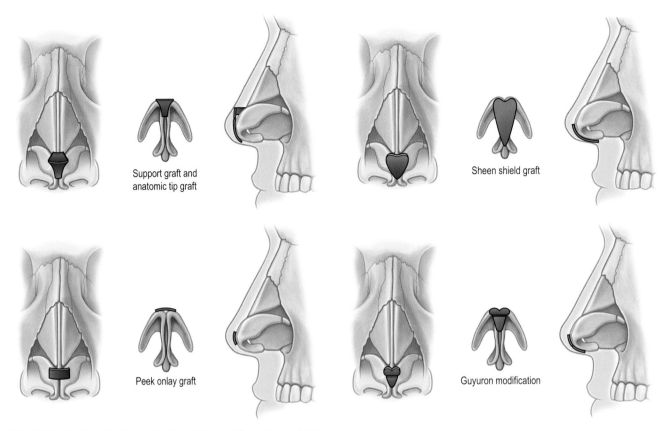

Support graft and
anatomic tip graft

Sheen shield graft

Peek onlay graft

Guyuron modification

Fig. 27.23 Shield grafts allow modification of the nasal tip and infratip lobule.

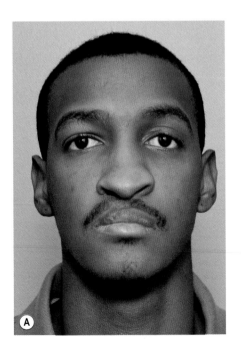

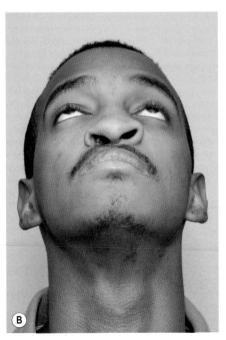

Fig. 27.24 This figure demonstrates another example of common deformities seen with the unilateral cleft nasal deformity. Most significant in this patient is the absent nasal tip projection and wide dorsal aesthetic lines **(A, B)**, which have been improved by performing an open rhinoplasty and osteotomies **(C, D)**.

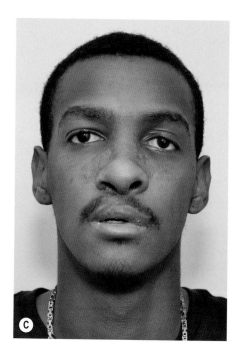

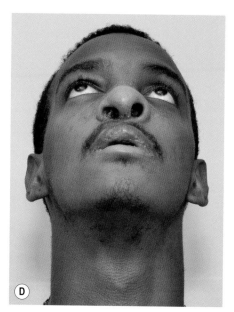

Fig. 27.24, cont'd

often displaced and obstructing. A wide septum is not uncommon and may present as nasal obstruction.

Bilateral deformities require repositioning both LLCs with reshaping techniques and tip suture techniques. Removing the collection of fibrofatty tissue once separating the LLCs helps with tip definition. If the lower lateral cartilages are not strong enough to allow for appropriate projection, a columellar strut as well as onlay grafts can be beneficial.[78] Onlay grafts, or Sheen grafts, provide tip definition for bilateral clefts with typical thick nasal skin. Again, the goal for the

bilateral deformity is to decrease the angle of divergence between the domal points of the LLCs as well as provide a strong columellar framework for tip projection.

The nasal dorsum is usually too wide. Symmetric low to high osteotomies, or lateral low-to-low combined with medial-to-lateral superior osteotomies, are done to narrow the dorsum and create more appropriate dorsal aesthetic lines. A cartilage graft along the nasal dorsum can be considered if these osteotomies do not provide an adequate amount of dorsal narrowing. However, elevating the nasal dorsum will increase the amount of tip projection required – an already challenging task in the bilateral cleft nasal deformity.

Conclusion

Treating patients with cleft lip and palate is a challenging task and should be undertaken by teams specifically experienced

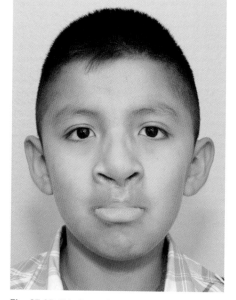

Fig. 27.25 This figure demonstrates hypertrophic scarring associated with bilateral cleft lip repair. Acutely, this might benefit from steroid injections; however, in the mature setting, treatment would involve excision and primary closure.

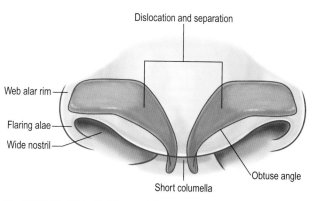

Fig. 27.26 The bilateral cleft nose deformity involves bilateral displacement and distortion of the osseocartilaginous skeleton of the nose. The shortened columella plays a prominent role in the bilateral deformity and must be lengthened in subsequent procedures.

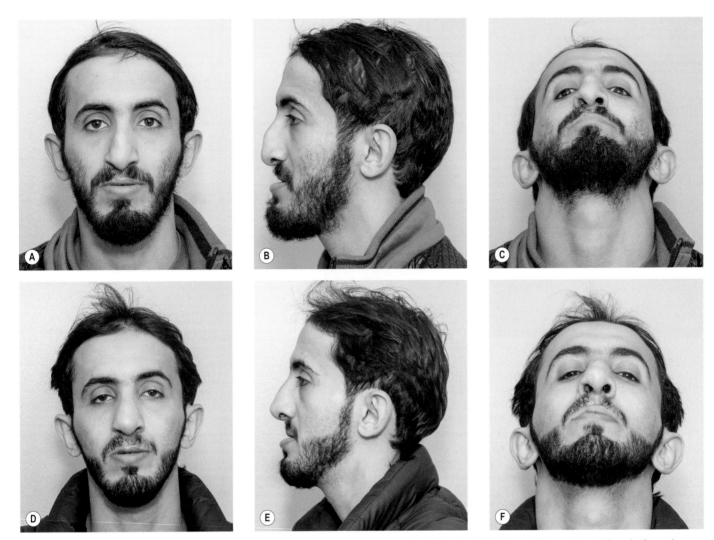

Fig. 27.27 Pre- **(A–C)** and postoperative images **(D–F)** after cleft rhinoplasty demonstrate correction of dorsal aesthetic lines and improved nasal tip projection and symmetry.

in this care. The best treatment for secondary deformities is prevention, with an appropriately performed primary operation. Cleft team care ideally decreases the number of operations by successfully addressing deformities during the original operation. Secondary cleft surgery is ideally mini-mized with this approach. Secondary operations can be technically more challenging and the postoperative outcomes more unpredictable. Centers with dedicated teams, treating patients with clefts on a daily basis, should improve patient outcomes over time.

🌐   Access the complete reference list online at   **http://www.expertconsult.com**

4. Fisher DM, Sommerlad BC. Cleft lip, cleft palate, and velopharyngeal insufficiency. *Plast Reconstr Surg.* 2011;128:342e–360e. *Fisher and Sommerlad provide a comprehensive overview of cleft lip and palate repair in the 21st century. Beginning with a foundation in pathological anatomy of the cleft lip and palate, the authors step through surgical management of the cleft alveolus, lip, and palate. The article details multiple techniques for unilateral cleft lip repair, discussing their origins and aesthetic outcomes in comparison to others. Similar attention is given to techniques of palatoplasty. A discussion of velopharyngeal insufficiency, a measure of success for palate repair, guides the reader in choosing an appropriate reconstructive technique. It is important to consider the outcome most significant to the patient to select the best cleft lip and palate repair.*

5. Stewart TL, Fisher DM, Olson JL. Modified Von Langenbeck cleft palate repair using an anterior triangular flap: decreased incidence of anterior oronasal fistulas. *Cleft Palate Craniofac J.* 2009;46:299–304. *Oronasal fistulas are a frequent complication during primary cleft palate repair with a high rate of recurrence. The authors present a modified Von Langenbeck technique resulting in a fistula rate close to 0%. Their inclusion of an anterior triangular oromucosal flap reflected posteriorly reduces tension for nasal side mucosal closure. At 4 to 8 weeks postoperatively, 0 of 182 patients who had a modified Von Langenbeck had a suspected oronasal fistula. The modification to the common Von Langenbeck technique described provides a substantial reported reduction in oronasal fistula rates for closure of U-shaped fistulas. Even with a growing array of successful techniques for secondary*

fistulas, prevention during the primary cleft repair remains the ideal outcome.

7. Noordhoff MS, Chen YR, Chen KT, et al. The surgical technique for the complete unilateral cleft lip-nasal deformity. *Operat Tech Plast Reconstr Surg.* 1995;2:167–174.

8. Fisher DM. Unilateral cleft lip repair: an anatomical subunit approximation technique. *Plast Reconstr Surg.* 2005;116:61–71. *Fisher presents a technique for repair of unilateral cleft lip based on meticulous adherence to anatomical subunits of the lip. Upon observation of Noordhoff and Thomson's techniques, this repair attempts to place the majority of the scar line along the reconstructed cleft-side philtral column. There is no rotation incision unlike Millard's technique. A total of 144 unilateral cleft lip repairs using the new technique are presented. In the subsequent discussion, major benefits of the technique are presented such as an exact approximation of vertical height on the lateral lip element. This new method of repair has steadily gained use among cleft lip/palate surgeons since its conception.*

13. Mulliken JB. Primary repair of bilateral cleft lip and nasal deformity. *Plast Reconstr Surg.* 2001;108:181–194. *Mulliken set out to describe the advances in bilateral cleft lip repair as well as the movement towards single-stage cleft repairs such as primary nasolabial repair. Bilateral cleft surgical care has lagged behind advances in unilateral cleft care; however, recent surgical advancements have improved bilateral cleft lip and nasal repair to match or overtake unilateral cleft repair. Mulliken describes in-detail the primary nasolabial repair of a bilateral cleft lip and nasal deformity, followed by consideration for anatomical variants such as asymmetric or incomplete bilateral clefts. Objective measurements for weighing surgical revisions are also addressed with a section dedicated to common revisions after primary cleft repair. Lastly, the author comments on the distribution of care and structure of multidisciplinary teams for cleft patients in a rapidly changing healthcare environment.*

14. Farkas LG. *Anthropometry of the Head and Face in Medicine.* New York: Elsevier; 1981. *In the 1980s, Farkas created the first comprehensive atlas of craniofacial surface anthropometry. The atlas outlines a measurement system that is meticulously applied to the identification and layout of anthropometric landmarks on the head and face. The text was immediately useful for anthropological studies but has grown in application to plastic and oral/maxillofacial surgery. Its utility has come to include even medical and clinical genetics. For plastic surgery, Farkas's measurements are critical in preoperative evaluation, surgical planning, and postoperative assessment. This text continues to be the reference for standard and objective measurements in craniofacial surgery.*

17. Bardach J, Morris H, Olin W, et al. Late results of multidisciplinary management of unilateral cleft lip and palate. *Ann Plast Surg.* 1984;12:235–242. *This study describes the status of 45 pediatric patients with history of unilateral cleft lip and palate treated by a multidisciplinary cleft care team. At 14 to 22 years of age, the patients were evaluated for completion of treatment by the comprehensive team, composed of plastic surgery, orthodontics, and speech pathology. It was uncovered that only 16% of patients had completed treatment for all three specialties. Factors including lack of patient cooperation, socioeconomic factors, and changing treatment algorithms were cited as possible culprits for delayed treatment. However, the most significant effect in the authors' opinion was that a multidisciplinary cleft palate team experienced significant delay in overall treatment for patients. With a well-run and organized team providing*

substandard treatment, poor care was certain for patients seeking medical treatment outside multidisciplinary teams.

52. Furlow LT. Cleft palate repair by double opposing Z-plasty. *Plast Reconstr Surg.* 1986;78:724–736. *Furlow proposed a primary cleft palate repair of two opposing Z-plasties across the primary defect. At a time when cleft palate repairs achieved either normal speech production or matched midfacial growth, the proposed opposing Z-plasty repair simultaneously achieved improved speech by palatal muscle mobilization and palatal lengthening to counteract midface hypoplasia. In a series of 22 patients, 90% achieved velopharyngeal sufficiency. Although evidence of crossbite, a criterion for midface growth, was present in 11 of 19 patients, only three had more-than-mild crossbites. The Furlow palatoplasty technique has become a commonplace surgical technique for the primary repair of the cleft palate.*

59. McComb H. Primary correction of unilateral cleft lip nasal deformity: a 10-year review. *Plast Reconstr Surg.* 1985;75:791–797. *In 1985, McComb addressed a long-standing concept of postponing cleft nasal deformity repair until adulthood and facial maturity. The author presented a series of 10 patients now 10 years of age or greater who had combined primary lip and nasal corrections. During primary lip repair, the displaced alar cartilages were elevated to improve symmetry. After ten years of growth, the patients did not present with worse nasal deformities or interference to nasal growth. Additionally, they benefitted from improved nasal appearance during childhood. The evidence showed that surgical intervention of nasal structures did not grossly alter the growth pattern. This study along with many others has helped shift cleft lip and nasal care towards fewer procedures and improved quality of life for pediatric patients.*

72. Mulliken JB. Principles and techniques of bilateral complete cleft lip repair. *Plast Reconstr Surg.* 1985;75:477–486. *In the 1980s, evidence was slowly building to begin cleft nasal repair as early as cleft lip repair. Mulliken described a two-stage repair supporting early cleft nasal deformity correction with nasal repositioning in the second procedure. The author performed the two-stage repair for 15 pediatric patients, presenting follow-up pictures ranging from 1 to 6 years postoperatively. Five principles for successful bilateral cleft lip were discussed: (1) attention to symmetry, (2) primary muscle continuity, (3) prolabial shape and size, (4) central tubercle construction from lateral lip tissue, and (5) early reconstruction of nasal tip and columella. The concepts presented in this text were critical to gradually improving bilateral cleft care to meet satisfactory outcomes of its simpler sibling, the unilateral cleft lip.*

73. Cutting CB. Secondary cleft lip nasal reconstruction: state of the art. *Cleft Palate Craniofac J.* 2000;37:538–541. *Cutting provides a thorough and step-wise review of procedures for secondary cleft lip nasal reconstruction. The article discusses treatment for the skeletal base, nasal dorsal bone and cartilage, nasal tip cartilage, the skin envelope, and the bilateral cleft nose. By altering the skeletal base through a Le Fort I advancement or prosthesis, the lower maxilla can be projected forward without altering nasal dorsum projection. Cutting also describes several techniques for altering nasal dorsal bone and cartilage through single block maneuvers or spreader-strut grafts. The use of cartilage flaps through either Potter or Dibbell's techniques can be used to revise nasal tip projection. The author introduces Tajima's incision as a method to improve the skin envelope of the patient. As the nose is a focal point for facial aesthetics, techniques of secondary cleft nasal repair can provide considerable relief for the patient.*

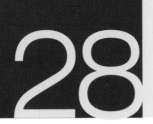

Cleft and craniofacial orthognathic surgery

Jesse A. Goldstein and Stephen B. Baker

SYNOPSIS

- Dentofacial deformities, in particular maxillary retrusion resulting in class III malocclusion, are typical of the cleft lip/palate population. Of patients in this group, 25–30% have midface retrusion severe enough to require orthognathic surgery

- Orthognathic surgery should ideally be performed after facial growth is complete. If surgery is performed earlier, the likelihood is high that additional (though possibly less complicated) surgery may be required when the patient reaches skeletal maturity

- Treatment should favor expansive movements (anterior and inferior repositioning) to achieve class I occlusion rather than contractile movements (superior and posterior repositioning) in order to minimize premature aging.

 Access the Historical Perspective section online at
http://www.expertconsult.com

Introduction

Orthognathic surgery is the term used to describe surgical movement of the tooth-bearing segments of the maxilla and mandible. Candidates for orthognathic surgery have dentofacial deformities that cannot be adequately treated with orthodontic therapy alone. Children with cleft lip and palate as well as certain craniofacial anomalies are especially prone to developing malocclusion. Indeed, where approximately 2.5% of the general population have occlusal discrepancies that warrant surgical correction, 25–30% of patients who undergo surgical correction of cleft lip and palate in infancy will have severe enough midface retrusion to require orthognathic surery.[1] Maxillary hypoplasia resulting in class III malocclusion is the typical deformity seen in patients with cleft and craniofacial deformities, but class II malocclusion, anterior open bites, occlusal cants, and many other dentofacial defor-

mities can also occur. Regardless of the etiology, patient examination and treatment-planning principles remain the same. The goal of orthognathic surgery, therefore, is to establish ideal dental occlusion with the jaws in a position that optimizes facial form and function.

Basic science

Growth and development

Timing of orthognathic surgery in the pediatric patient is key to good and predictable outcomes and is mediated by the development and maturation of the craniofacial skeleton. The foundation of maxillofacial growth relies on a complex interplay between genetic processes and micro- and macroenvironmental factors which must be understood to plan orthognathic procedures on patients with clefts and craniofacial disorders.

The osteogenesis of the maxillofacial skeleton occurs by way of two well-understood processes: intramembranous ossification and endochondral ossification. The cranial vault, upper face, midface, and a majority of the mandible arise from the former mechanism. Although there is a great amount of variability between individuals and genders, skeletal maturation generally progresses in a cranial-to-caudal direction with the cranial vault reaching close to adult size in early adolescence, followed closely by the upper face in the early teen years, the maxilla in the mid-teens, and the mandible in the late teen years (Fig. 28.1).[3]

Dental eruption patterns proceed in a similar stepwise fashion, and the transition from mixed dentition (6–12 years of age) to permanent dentition (12–20 years of age) mirrors the maturation of the maxillofacial skeleton. Indeed, midface and lower face development is, in part, mediated by the budding deciduous and permanent dentition, providing regional signals to the alveolus and stimulating bony deposition. During this period, an alteration of tooth position can, in turn, alter the direction of growth of both the maxilla and

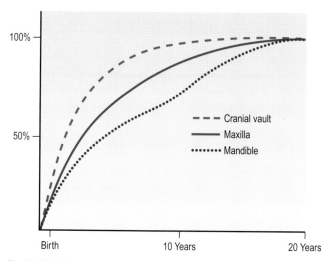

Fig. 28.1 Skeletal maturity of the cranial vault, the maxilla, and the mandible from infancy to skeletal maturity (scaled to 100% of adult size).

mandible. Orthodontists take advantage of this active phase of development through their use of braces, palatal expanders, and various external devices to alter maxillary and mandibular growth trajectories.[4] For this reason, surgical intervention is usually delayed until skeletal maturity is reached and orthopedic movements are no longer effective.

Diagnosis/patient preparation

Preoperative evaluation

The cleft and craniofacial team

The chance of a favorable surgical outcome is optimized if presurgical planning is performed in conjunction with a cleft/craniofacial team which includes plastic surgeons, otorhinolaryngologists, dentists, geneticists, orthodontists, and many others. Speech pathologists, for example, play an integral role in the evaluation of the velopharyngeal mechanism and the potential effects that maxillary advancement may have on speech nasality and articulation. A preoperative video fluoroscopy and/or nasoendoscopy has been shown to yield information that can aid in predicting postoperative hypernasality.

The orthodontist's role in the preoperative evaluation and management is critical. Prior to surgery, the potential surgical candidate requires a comprehensive work-up that includes an analysis of the occlusal characteristics and the age of the facial skeleton, need for presurgical orthodontics, tooth extraction, and possibly even palatal expansion. If orthognathic surgery is attempted before the facial skeleton reaches maturity, the need for revision surgery will be increased because of continued postoperative growth.

The history and physical examination

It is important to obtain a thorough medical, dental, and surgical history from every patient. Systemic diseases such as juvenile rheumatoid arthritis, diabetes, and scleroderma can affect treatment planning. Multiple past cleft and craniofacial surgeries increase the scar burden and may make maxillary advancement surgery difficult. With jaw asymmetries, a history of hyperplasia or hypoplasia from syndromic, traumatic, postsurgical or neoplastic etiologies affects treatment considerations. Each patient should be questioned regarding symptoms of temporomandibular joint disease or myofascial pain syndrome. Motivation and realistic expectations are important for an optimal outcome. It is likewise important for patients to have a clear understanding of the procedure, recovery, and anticipated result. In younger patients, a family discussion in terms they can understand helps to alleviate preoperative anxiety. Orthognathic surgery is a major undertaking, and the patient and family must be appropriately motivated to undergo necessary preoperative and postoperative orthodontic treatment in addition to the surgery itself.

A complete physical exam should be performed on every patient prior to surgery. The frontal facial evaluation begins with the assessment of the vertical facial thirds (trichion to glabella, glabella to subnasale, and subnasale to menton) and the horizontal facial fifths (zygoma to lateral canthus, lateral to medial canthi, and intracanthal segment). The most important factor in assessing the vertical height of the maxilla is the degree of "incisor show" while the patient's lips are in repose. Males should show at least 2–3 mm, whereas as much as 5–6 mm is considered attractive in females. If the patient shows the correct degree of incisor in repose, but shows excessive gingiva in full smile, the maxilla should not be impacted. It is more important to have correct incisor show in repose than in full smile. If lip incompetence or mentalis strain is present, this can be an indication of vertical maxillary excess or retrognathia/retrogenia.

The inferior orbital rims, malar eminence, and piriform areas are evaluated for the degree of projection. These regions often appear deficient in cleft patients, and maxillary advancement is therefore indicated; if they are prominent, posterior repositioning may be necessary. The alar base width should also be assessed prior to surgery since orthognathic surgery may alter this width; which, in turn, may accentuate any asymmetries associated with a cleft nasal deformity. Asymmetries of the maxilla and mandible should be documented on physical examination, and the degree of deviation from the facial midline noted.

The profile evaluation focuses on the projection of the forehead and malar region, the maxilla and mandible, the nose, the chin, and the neck. An experienced clinician can usually determine whether the deformity is caused by the maxilla, the mandible, or both simply by looking at the patient. This assessment is made clinically and verified at the time of cephalometric analysis. The intraoral exam should begin with an assessment of oral hygiene and periodontal health. These factors are critical for successful orthodontic treatment and surgery. Any retained deciduous teeth or unerupted adult teeth are noted. The occlusal classification is determined, and the degrees of incisor overbite and overjet are quantified. The surgeon should assess the transverse dimension of the maxilla, as prior cleft palate repair will often result in transverse growth restriction. If the mandibular third molars are present, they must be extracted 6 months prior to sagittal split osteotomy. Any missing teeth or periapical pathology should be noted, as should any signs or symptoms of temporomandibular joint dysfunction. These issues should be addressed prior to proceeding with orthognathic surgery.

The term "dental compensation" is used to describe the tendency of teeth to tilt in a direction that minimizes dental malocclusion. For example, in a patient with an overbite (Angle class II malocclusion), lingual retroclination of the upper incisors and labial proclination of the lower incisors minimize the malocclusion. The opposite occurs in a patient who has dental compensation for an underbite (Angle class III malocclusion). Thus, dental compensation, which is often the result of orthodontic treatment, will mask the true degree of skeletal discrepancy. Precise analysis of the dental compensation is done on the lateral cephalometric radiographs.

If the patient desires surgical correction of the deformity, presurgical orthodontics will upright and decompensate the occlusion, thereby reversing the compensation that has occurred. This has the effect of exaggerating the malocclusion, but it also allows the surgeon to maximize skeletal movements. If the patient is ambivalent or not interested in surgery, mild cases of malocclusion may potentially be treated by further dental compensation, which may camouflage the deformity and restore proper overjet and overbite. The importance of a commitment to surgery prior to orthodontics lies in the fact that dental movements for decompensation and compensation are in opposite directions, so this decision needs to be made prior to orthodontic therapy.[5]

Patient selection

Identifying the proper patient for orthognathic surgery is a key step to ensuring satisfaction and successful outcomes. This includes amassing considerable data beyond a simple history and physical exam and should be coordinated with other members of the cleft/craniofacial team.

Cephalometric and dental evaluation

A cephalometric analysis and comparison to normative values can help the surgeon plan the degree of skeletal movement needed to achieve both an optimal occlusion and an optimal aesthetic result. A lateral cephalometric radiograph is performed under reproducible conditions so that serial images can be compared. This film is usually taken at the orthodontist's office using a cephalostat, an apparatus specifically designed for this purpose, and a head frame to maintain consistent head position. It is important to be certain the surgeon and orthodontist can visualize both the bony and soft-tissue features in order to facilitate tracing every landmark. Once the normal structures are traced, several planes and angles are determined (Fig. 28.2).

The sella–nasion–subspinale (SNA) and sella–nasion–supramentale (SNB) are the two most important angles in determining the positions of the maxilla and mandible relative to each other as well as the cranial base. These angles are determined by drawing lines from sella to nasion to "A point" or "B point", respectively. By forming an angle with the sella and nasion, this position is referenced to the cranial base. "A point" provides information about the anteroposterior position of the maxilla. If the SNA angle is excessive, the maxilla exhibits an abnormal anterior position relative to the cranium. If SNA is less than normal, the maxilla is posteriorly positioned relative to the cranial base. The same principle applies to the mandible: "B point" is used to relate the mandibular position to the cranial base. The importance of the cranial base

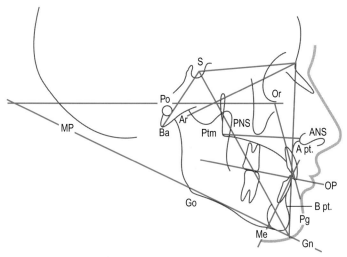

Fig. 28.2 The cephalometric radiograph is used to identify skeletal landmarks used in determining the lines and angles that reflect facial development. These measurements aid in determining the extent to which each jaw contributes to the dentofacial deformity. S, sella turcica, the midpoint of the sella turcica; N, nasion, the anterior point of the intersection between the nasal and frontal bones; A pt, "A point", the innermost point in the depth of the concavity of the maxillary alveolar process; B pt, "B point", the innermost point on the contour of the mandible between the incisor tooth and the bony chin; Ba, basale, the most inferior point of the skull base; Pg, pogonion, the most anterior point on the contour of the chin; Go, gonion, the most inferior and posterior point at the angle formed by the ramus and body of the mandible; Po, porion, the uppermost lateral point on the roof of the external auditory meatus; Or, orbitale, the lowest point on the inferior margin of the orbit; PNS, posterior nasal spine, the most posterior point on the maxilla; ANS, anterior nasal spine, the most anterior point on the maxilla; Gn, gnathion, the center of the inferior contour of the chin; Me, menton, the most inferior point on the mandibular symphysis; MP, mandibular plane, the line connecting the Go and the Gn; OP, occlusal plane.

as a reference is that it allows the clinician to determine if one or both jaws contribute to a noted deformity. For example, a patient's class III malocclusion (underbite) could develop from several different etiologies: a retrognathic maxilla and a normal mandible as is common in cleft patients, a normal maxilla and a prognathic mandible, a retrognathic mandible and a more severely retrognathic maxilla, or a prognathic maxilla and a more severely prognathic mandible. All of these conditions yield a class III malocclusion, yet each requires a different treatment approach. The surgeon can delineate the true etiology of the deformity by the fact that the maxilla and mandible can be independently related to a stable reference, the cranial base. Next, cephalometric tracings are performed.

Cephalometric tracings give the surgeon an idea of how skeletal movements will affect one another as well as the soft-tissue profile. They also allow the surgeon to determine the distances the bones will be moved to achieve the goals of a specific procedure. Different tracing methods using acetate paper are used for isolated maxillary, isolated mandibular, or two-jaw surgeries. Much of the traditional hand cephalometric tracing, however, has given way to computer-aided cephalometric analysis, which allows the surgeon to position the maxilla and mandible electronically on the cephalogram while recording the soft-tissue changes and measuring the degree of repositioning.

Complete dental records, including mounted dental casts, are needed to execute preoperative model surgery and fabricate surgical splints. Casts allow the surgeon to evaluate the occlusion both before and after articulation into proper positions. Analysis of new occlusion gives the clinician an idea of how intensive the presurgical orthodontic treatment plan will be. Casts also allow the clinician to distinguish between absolute and relative transverse maxillary deficiency. Absolute transverse maxillary deficiency presents as a posterior crossbite with the jaws in class I relationship. A relative maxillary transverse deficiency is commonly seen in a patient with a class III malocclusion. A posterior crossbite is observed in this type of patient, raising suspicions of inadequate maxillary width. However, as the maxilla is advanced or the mandible retruded, the crossbite is eliminated. Articulation of the casts into a class I occlusion allows the surgeon to distinguish easily between relative and absolute maxillary constriction.

Model surgery

Using the cephalometric tracings as a guide, the next step is to reproduce the maxillary and/or mandibular movements on articulated dental models. This allows for the fabrication of occlusal splints to be used intraoperatively to guide jaw repositioning in preparation for osteosynthesis. Model surgery begins by obtaining accurate casts of the patient's occlusion. If the surgeon does not have a dental laboratory, the orthodontist will obtain the casts. The success of the technical portion of orthognathic surgery correlates directly with the accuracy of the model surgery and splint fabrication.

Isolated mandibular surgery

It should be noted that if isolated mandibular surgery is being performed, the casts can be hand-articulated into the desired occlusion. The Galetti articulator is a useful tool that allows securing of casts with a screw mount. A universal joint allows the casts to be set in the desired relationship. Surgical splints can then be made from the articulator. If the maximum intercuspal position is the desired postoperative occlusion, a splint may be unnecessary. The surgeon can osteotomize the mandible and secure it into its new position using the maximum intercuspal position as a guide to the new position. The surgeon should always verify the desired postoperative occlusion with the orthodontist prior to surgery.

Isolated maxillary and two-jaw surgery

A "face bow" is a device used to relate the maxillary model accurately to the cranium on an articulator. If a maxillary osteotomy is being performed, one set of models should be mounted on an articulator using the face bow. Two other sets of models are used in treatment planning. Next, an Erickson model block is used to measure the current position of the maxillary central incisors, cuspids, and the mesiobuccal cusp of the first molar. The face bow-mounted maxillary cast is placed on the model block. The maxillary model is then measured to the tenth of a millimeter vertically, anteroposteriorly, and end-on. By having numerical records in three dimensions, the surgeon can reproduce the maxillary cast's exact location, as well as determine a new location. Reference lines are circumferentially inscribed every 5 mm around the maxillary cast mounting. The distances the maxilla will move in an anteroposterior, lateral, and vertical direction have been determined from the previous cephalometric exam. These numbers are added or subtracted from the current values

measured on the model block to determine the new three-dimensional position of the maxillary cast. The occlusal portion of the maxillary cast is removed from its base using a saw. As much plaster is removed from the cast as is necessary to accommodate the new position of the maxilla. Once the model block verifies the maxilla is in its new position, the cast is secured with sticky wax or plaster to the mounting ring. Now it can be placed on the articulator. At this point, the surgeon has a mounting of the postoperative maxilla related to the preoperative mandible. An acrylic splint is made at this point. This splint is called the intermediate splint and is used in the operating room to index the new position of the maxilla to the preoperative position of the mandible. A second mounting with the casts in the occlusion desired by the orthodontist is used to make a final splint that represents the new position of the mandible to the repositioned maxilla. This is fabricated in a manner similar to the splint for isolated mandibular surgery. If the occlusion is good, intercuspal position can be used to position the mandible without the splint.

3D CT modeling

There are several computer-assisted design (CAD) programs that are now commercially available that can assist the surgeon with some or all of the preoperative patient preparation. A computed tomography (CT) scan of the facial skeleton, as well as updated dental casts, are obtained preoperatively. Although conventional helical CT scans with fine cuts through the face are ideal, cone beam CT scans offer a comparable image quality with considerably less cost and radiation exposure ($50\,\mu Sv$ compared to $2000\,\mu Sv$). The program then joins the CT and the dental cast to render a complete three-dimensional model of the facial skeleton. A cephalometric analysis can then be performed as well as simulated movements of the jaws and chin in any dimension. Once the surgeon verifies the osteotomy movements, CAD/CAM (computer-aided manufacturing) technology is used to fabricate surgical splints for the patient. If necessary, 3D models of the patient can be made showing the exact proposed movement (Fig. 28.3). Some systems can actually "wrap" a 2D digital image around the soft-tissue envelope of the 3D CT image, thus replicating a 3D image of the patient's face in color.

In these authors' experience, 3D CT modeling has demonstrated improved accuracy in diagnosis and treatment. The elimination of traditional model surgery saves the surgeon time in patient preparation. Finally, the 3D aspect of this treatment-planning approach enhances the surgeon's ability to predict how osteotomies may affect soft tissue of the face. These advantages facilitate the ability of the plastic surgeon to provide optimal care for these patients.

Developing a treatment plan

Once the data are obtained, the surgeon can determine which abnormalities the patient exhibits and the extent to which these features deviate from the norm. The treatment plan is the application of these data to provide the best aesthetic result while establishing a class I occlusion. The goal is not to "treat the numbers" in an attempt to normalize every patient. The appearance of the soft-tissue envelope surrounding the facial skeleton is the most crucial factor in determining the aesthetic success of orthognathic procedures, and the jaws

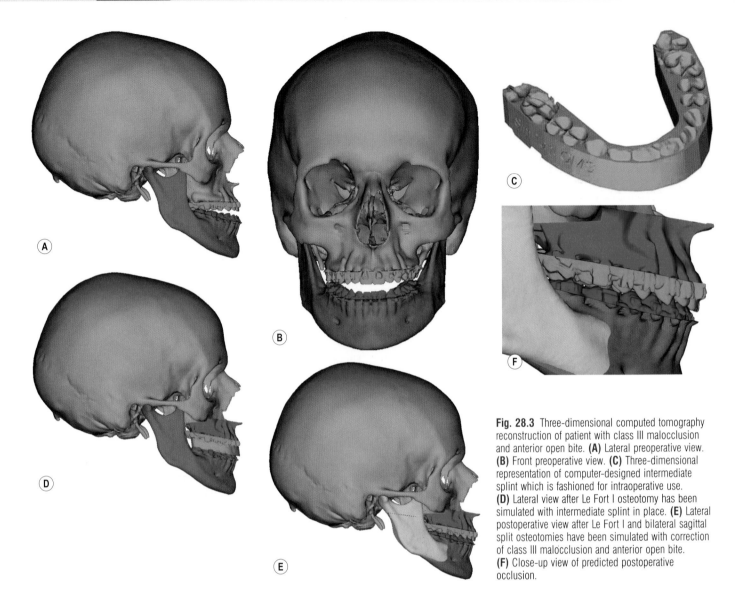

Fig. 28.3 Three-dimensional computed tomography reconstruction of patient with class III malocclusion and anterior open bite. **(A)** Lateral preoperative view. **(B)** Front preoperative view. **(C)** Three-dimensional representation of computer-designed intermediate splint which is fashioned for intraoperative use. **(D)** Lateral view after Le Fort I osteotomy has been simulated with intermediate splint in place. **(E)** Lateral postoperative view after Le Fort I and bilateral sagittal split osteotomies have been simulated with correction of class III malocclusion and anterior open bite. **(F)** Close-up view of predicted postoperative occlusion.

should be positioned so they provide optimal soft-tissue support.

Historically, skeletal movements that expanded the soft tissue of the face were less stable, so posterior and superior movements were preferred. Although these movements were more stable, they resulted in contraction of the facial skeleton with the associated soft-tissue features of premature aging. Since the introduction of rigid fixation systems, osteotomies that result in skeletal expansion have been achieved with a great degree of predictability. An attempt is made to develop a treatment plan that will expand or maintain the preoperative volume of the face. If a superior or posterior (contraction) movement of one of the jaws is planned, an attempt should be made to neutralize the skeletal contraction with an advancement or inferior movement of the other jaw or the chin. It is important to avoid a net contraction of the facial skeleton as this may result in a prematurely aged appearance.

A class I occlusion can be achieved with the jaws in a variety of positions. The goal in treatment planning is to use the data from the patient's examination to predict the location

of the jaws that will optimize the soft-tissue features of the face. By reducing the emphasis on "normal" values and increasing the awareness of soft-tissue effects of skeletal movements, it is realized that skeletal disproportion often leads to a more favorable result.[6]

Treatment/surgical technique

General principles and pertinent anatomy

Several principles have broad application to jaw surgery. Blood loss can be substantial in maxillofacial surgery and even small volumes can have significant clinical implications in the pediatric population. Standard techniques of head elevation, hypotensive anesthesia, blood donation, and the preoperative administration of erythropoietin are useful adjuncts to reduce blood loss, especially in the younger population. Before incisions are made, an antimicrobial rinse is helpful to minimize the intraoral bacterial count. A topical steroid is applied to the lips to reduce pain and swelling associated with prolonged retraction. Intravenous steroids may also be useful to reduce postoperative edema.

The occlusion desired may not be the same as maximum intercuspal position. The splint is useful in maintaining the occlusion in the desired location when it does not correspond to maximal intercuspal position. It is easy for the orthodontist to close a posterior open bite, but very difficult to close an anterior open bite with orthodontic treatment. At the end of the case it is important to have the anterior teeth and the canines in a class I relationship without an open bite.

Guiding elastics are useful postoperatively to control the bite. Class II elastics are placed in a vector to correct a class II relationship (maxillary lug is anterior to the mandibular lug). Class III elastics are applied to correct a class III discrepancy. With rigid fixation, the elastics will not correct malpositioned jaws; they serve only to help the patient adapt to the new occlusion. Minor malocclusions can be corrected with postoperative orthodontic treatment.

Certain skeletal movements are inherently more stable than others. Stable movements include mandibular advancement and superior positioning of the maxilla. Movements with intermediate stability include maxillary impaction combined with mandibular advancement, maxillary advancement combined with mandibular setback, and correction of mandibular asymmetry. The unstable movements include posterior positioning of the mandible and inferior positioning of the maxilla. The least stable movement is transverse expansion of the maxilla. Long-term relapse with rigid fixation has not been demonstrated to be clearly superior to non-rigid fixation in single-jaw surgery. However, in two-jaw surgery, rigid fixation results in less relapse. The judgment of the surgeon will dictate the extent to which the facial skeleton can be expanded without resulting in unacceptable relapse.

The maxilla is associated with the descending palatine artery, the infraorbital nerve, the tooth roots, and the internal maxillary artery. The internal maxillary artery runs about 25 mm from the pterygomaxillary junction, and the descending palatal artery descends into the posteromedial maxillary sinus. The infraorbital nerve exits the infraorbital foramen below the infraorbital rim along the mid pupillary line. The maxillary tooth roots extend within the maxilla in a superior direction. The canine has the longest root and is usually visible through the maxillary cortical bone.

The patient who presents with a cleft lip and/or palatal anomaly will have several anatomic differences when compared to an unaffected patient. The maxilla is typically deficient in both the anteroposterior and vertical dimensions. Because midface retrusion can be significant, it frequently appears that the mandible is prognathic, but it is rare that the mandible demonstrates a true prognathia. It is a relative prognathia secondary to the maxillary deficiency. Finally, because of lesser-segment collapse, the dental midline is often deviated toward the cleft side.

Despite having alveolar bone grafting performed, many cleft patients have deficient or missing bone in the region of the alveolus. Persistent palatal fistulas may be present as well. The lateral incisor is frequently missing in these patients and closure of this space must be taken into consideration at the time of treatment planning. If a large fistula is present in the alveolus, modifications of the Le Fort I procedure can be performed to facilitate a tension-free alveolar closure.

The important mandibular structures that may be injured with the mandibular osteotomy are the mental nerve, the inferior alveolar nerve, and the tooth apices. The third branch of the trigeminal nerve enters the mandibular foramen to become the inferior alveolar nerve. It runs below the tooth roots and exits at the level of the first and second premolars through the mental foramen. The region where it is most medial to the outer cortex is located near the external oblique ridge. This is where the vertical portion of the sagittal split osteotomy is made because it affords the largest margin of error.

Le Fort I osteotomy

The first step in any facial osteotomy is satisfactorily securing the nasal endotracheal tube; our preference is a nasal Ring–Adair–Elwin (RAE) endotracheal tube. The vertical position of the maxilla is recorded by measuring the distance between the medial canthus and the orthodontic arch wire. These vertical measurements are absolutely critical. The maxillary vestibule is injected with epinephrine prior to patient preparation. An incision is made with needle tip electrocautery 5 mm above the mucogingival junction from first molar to first molar. A periosteal elevator is then used to expose the maxilla around the piriform rim and infraorbital nerve. Obwegeser toe-in retractors are held by the assistant at the head of the operating table. As the dissection extends laterally, it is important to remain subperiosteal to avoid exposure of the buccal fat pad. A Woodson elevator is used to initiate reflection of the nasal mucosa, and a periosteal elevator is used to complete the dissection of the nasal floor and lateral nasal wall. A double-balled osteotome is used to release the septum from the maxilla and a uniballed osteotome is used to release the lateral nasal wall. The surgeon can insert a finger on the posterior palate to help feel when the cut is complete. A periosteal elevator is used to protect the nasal mucosa, and then a reciprocating saw is used to make a transverse osteotomy from the piriform aperture laterally until the cut descends just posteriorly to the last maxillary molar and drops through the maxillary tuberosity. The cut should be made at least 5 mm above the tooth apices. This distance is determined from preoperative Panorex radiographs. If cuts are complete, the maxilla is downfractured with manual pressure, or with Rowe disimpaction forceps which fit into the piriform aperture and on the palate to provide increased leverage for the downfracture. Pressure should be applied in a slow, steady, controlled fashion, not in a series of quick movements. If the maxilla is not mobilized with relative ease, the cuts are likely not complete and should be re-evaluated. Scoring the posterior maxillary wall with a 10 mm osteotome may be necessary to aid in downfracture and to prevent an uncontrolled fracture superiorly toward the cranial base. Once the downfracture is complete, a bone hook can be used by the assistant to hold the maxilla down while any remaining bony interferences are removed. The descending palatine arteries will be seen near the posteromedial maxillary sinus. These can be clipped prophylactically without compromising the blood supply to the maxilla (Fig. 28.4). Any rents in the nasal mucosa are repaired at this stage with chromic suture. The splint is then used to place the maxilla in its proper position in occlusion with the mandible. Mandibulomaxillary fixation (MMF) is then applied with 26-gauge wires around

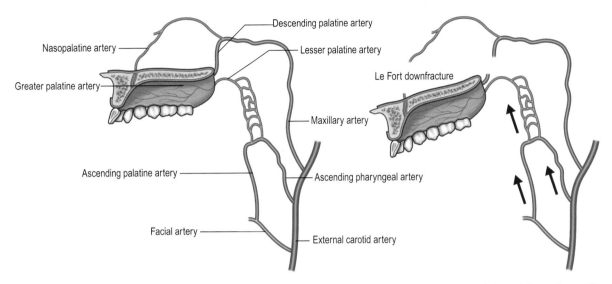

Fig. 28.4 Blood supply to maxilla before (left) and after (right) Le Fort I osteotomy and downfracture. After the nasopalatine and descending palatine arteries are transected, perfusion of the maxillary segment occurs via the lesser palatine artery.

the surgical lugs. The amount the maxilla will be impacted or elongated was determined in the treatment plan. This distance is added or subtracted from the medial canthal–incisor distance to determine the new vertical position of the maxilla. Four 2-mm plates, usually L-shaped, can be used to secure the maxilla. The MMF is released and occlusion verified prior to closure. If the alar base is wide, an alar cinch can be performed to normalize the width. Lip shortening may also result from closure. A V–Y closure at the central incisor can help alleviate this effect.

In patients who require increased cheek projection, a high Le Fort I osteotomy can be performed. This differs in that the transverse osteotomy is made as high as the infraorbital nerve will allow. If further cheek projection is necessary, bone grafts can be added. In the case of inferior or anterior positioning, gaps between the segments greater than 3 mm should be grafted with autogenous bone, cadaveric bone, or block hydroxyapatite. Finally, if simultaneous expansion of the maxilla is necessary, the maxilla can be split into two or more pieces to allow concurrent expansion.

Surgically assisted rapid palatal expansion

Correction of transverse maxillary constriction is common in patients with repaired cleft palates or those with craniofacial syndromes such as Apert or Cruzon syndrome. Such palatal constriction can be addressed in adolescence with non-surgical orthodontic appliances. As the sutures begin to close during late adolescence, relapse rates increase. A multiple-piece Le Fort I osteotomy can be performed to provide simultaneous maxillary expansion, but the degree of relapse is high. In the young adult, the preferred procedure is the surgically assisted rapid palatal expansion (SARPE) procedure. The orthodontist places a palatal expander prior to the procedure. A Le Fort I osteotomy is performed to mobilize the maxilla completely from the upper face. A small osteotome is used to make a thin cut between the roots of the central incisors, and a midline split is completed to the posterior

nasal spine. Separation is verified by activating the device. The maxilla is widened until the gingiva blanches and then is relaxed several turns to avoid ischemia. The SARPE offers the best stability for maxillary expansion in the young adult and older patient. Transverse deficiencies of the mandible can be corrected with a similar technique, that of distraction osteogenesis (DO).

Bilateral sagittal split osteotomy (BSSO)

The endotracheal tube placement and epinephrine injection are carried out in a similar fashion to the Le Fort I osteotomy. The mucosal incision is made with electrocautery about 10 mm from the lateral aspect of the molars and extends from the mid-ramus to the region of the second molar. If insufficient tissue is left on the dental side of the incision, closure is more difficult. A periosteal elevator is used to expose the lateral mandible and the anterior coronoid process in a subperiosteal plane. As the coronoid process is exposed, placement of a notched coronoid retractor may facilitate the dissection. A curved Kocher forcep with a chain can be clamped to the coronoid process and the chain secured to the drapes. To optimize blood supply, subperiosteal dissection is limited to those areas required to complete the osteotomy. A J-stripper is used to release the inferior border of the mandible from the attachments of the pterygomasseteric sling. The eternal oblique ridge and inferior border of the mandible should be exposed. The medial aspect of the ramus is also dissected subperiosteally. The mandibular nerve should be identified. A Seldin elevator is inserted medial to the ramus to protect the nerve. A Lindemann side-cutting burr is used to make a cut on the medial ramus that is parallel to the occlusal plane and extends about two-thirds of the distance to the posterior ramus.

The osteotomy proceeds from medial to lateral until the burr is in the cancellous portion of the ramus. Mandibular body retractors are then placed and a fissure burr, or a reciprocating saw is used to make an osteotomy from the mid-ramus down along the external oblique ridge, gently curving to the inferior border of the mandible. The cuts are verified with an osteotome, and then large osteotomes are inserted and rotated to separate the segments gently. The tooth-baring segment is referred to as the distal segment, and the condylar portion as the proximal segment.

The inferior alveolar nerve should be identified and found in the distal segment. If part of the nerve is located within the proximal segment, it should be gently released with a small curette. After both osteotomies are complete, the distal segment is placed into occlusion and secured by tightening 26-gauge wire loops around the surgical lugs. If a surgical splint is necessary to establish a required occlusion, it is placed between the teeth before MMF wiring. The proximal segments are then gently rotated to ensure they are seated within the glenoid fossa. When each condyle is comfortably seated within the fossa, it is rotated to align the inferior borders of the two segments and secured into position with a clamp. Three lag screws are placed at the superior border of the overlapping segments on each side of the mandible. To ensure that the transbuccal trocar will be placed properly, a hemostat is placed at the proposed screw location and pointed toward the cheek. A small stab incision is made in the skin, and the trocar is placed through the tissue bluntly until the tip enters the oral incision. The trocar is then exchanged for a drill guide, and the 2.0-mm and 1.5-mm drills are used in the lag sequence to make three holes through the overlapping portion of the proximal and distal segments. The screw lengths are measured and the screws inserted. Alternatively, the Dal Pont modification to the BSSO carries the buccal osteotomy anteriorly to the level of the first mandibular molar creating a longer proximal segment which can be fixated without a transbuccal screw. Instead, 2.0-mm plates with monocortical screws are used to fixate the segments after the occlusal splint is placed. The MMF is released, and the mandible is gently opened and closed to verify the occlusion. If a malocclusion is noted, the most likely etiology is that one or both condyles were not seated properly during application of fixation. The fixation should be removed and replaced until the correct occlusion is established. The wounds are irrigated and closed with interrupted 4-0 chromic sutures.

Intraoral vertical ramus osteotomy

A second technique for correcting mandibular prognathism or asymmetry is the intraoral vertical ramus osteotomy. The incision is the same as described above. A subperiosteal dissection is performed from the lateral ramus, and a LeVasseur Merrill retractor is used to hold this tissue laterally. An oscillating saw is then used to make a vertical cut from the sigmoid notch to the inferior border of the mandible. The osteotomy must be made posterior to the mandibular foramen on the medial side. The antilingula is a useful landmark, and is found as an elevation on the lateral mandible, indicating the approximate location of the mandibular foramen. After both sides of the mandible are complete, the distal segment is moved into occlusion, making sure that the proximal segments remain lateral to the distal segments posteriorly. Because rigid fixation is difficult to apply, a single wire, or no fixation at all, is used, and the patient remains in MMF for 6 weeks. This osteotomy can be done from an external approach, but this incision results in a scar on the neck.

Two-jaw surgery

Moving the maxilla and the mandible in one procedure requires osteotomizing both jaws and precisely securing them into position as determined by the treatment plan. If proper treatment planning, model surgery, and splint fabrication are performed, each jaw should be able to be placed into its desired position with precision. In a maxilla-first approach, the mandibular bony cuts are started first but terminated prior to osteotomy completion. The maxillary osteotomy is made, and the maxilla is placed into its new position using the intermediate splint. The splint is used to wire the teeth into MMF, allowing for indexing the new position of the maxilla to the preoperative (uncorrected) position of the mandible. With the condyles gently seated, the maxillomandibular complex is rotated so that the maxillary incisal edge is at the correct vertical height. The maxilla is plated into position, the MMF is released, and the intermediate splint removed. Next the mandibular osteotomies are completed, and the distal segment of the mandible is placed into the desired occlusion using the final splint. If the teeth are in good occlusion without the splint, the final splint may not be necessary to establish the desired occlusal relationship. Wire loops secure the occlusal relationship, and the rigid fixation is completed as previously described.

Genioplasty

Including a genioplasty in the treatment plan can be a powerful adjunct to mandibular movements, either by offsetting soft-tissue collapse secondary to posterior mandibular repositioning or by augmenting anterior mandibular movement. When performed asymmetrically, a genioplasty may also correct for minor mandibular asymmetries.

After adequate local anesthetic infiltration, the mucosa is incised from canine to canine with needle tip electrocautery, 5 mm below the mucogingival junction. The mentalis is transected, being sure to leave enough muscle cuff to allow for reapproximation during closure. Failure to do so can result in a ptotic soft-tissue envelope, or "witch's chin" deformity. Next, the dissection is carried out in a subperiosteal fashion identifying and protecting the mental nerves bilaterally. Using a reciprocating saw, the mandibular midline is gently marked to aid in centric fixation. The transverse osteotomy is made approximately 3 mm below the mental foramina in order to protect the intraosseous course of the mental nerves and the canine tooth roots. The trajectory of the osteotomy can be varied depending on the type of correction required. The mobilized segment is then fixed into the desired position with plates and screws, using the midline mark as a guide. The mentalis is then repaired and the mucosa closed.

Cleft surgery

Orthognathic surgery in cleft lip/palate patients is done similarly to non-cleft patients with the exception of several important modifications that are necessary to maintain blood supply and assist in fistula closure.

In a unilateral cleft lip patient, the standard maxillary incision can be made with little jeopardy to the premaxillary blood supply (Fig. 28.5). Each side of the cleft has an incision made similar to that of the alveolar bone graft incision. This

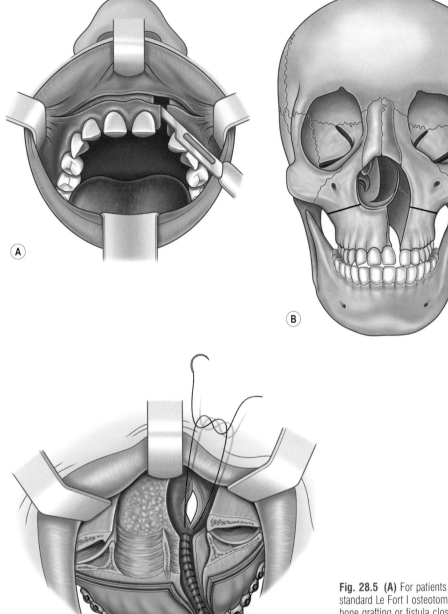

Fig. 28.5 (A) For patients with a unilateral cleft lip, the incision is made similar to a standard Le Fort I osteotomy, except an alveolar dissection is used if supplemental bone grafting or fistula closure is necessary. **(B)** The Le Fort osteotomy allows compression of the maxillary segments if necessary to close a pre-existing fistula. **(C)** Fistula repairs are easier after compression of the segments and exposure of nasal and palatal tissue.

allows for a two-layer closure of the palatal and nasal mucosa. If supplemental bone grafting needs to be done at this time, harvested bone can be placed into the alveolar gap after fixation has been applied. If a wide fistula is present, the surgeon can compress the maxillary segments to reduce the size of the alveolar space. This ensures the soft-tissue closure is under minimal tension and the chance of fistula closure is optimized. The canine may now be adjacent to the central incisor, but the restorative dentist can fabricate a prosthetic crown for the canine to make it look like a lateral incisor.

In the bilateral cleft patient, care must be taken not to make the vestibular incision across the premaxilla. The premaxillary blood supply originates from the vomer and the buccal mucosa. Since the vomer will be split, the majority of blood flow to the premaxilla must course from the premaxillary buccal mucosa. A circumvestibular incision that violates this mucosa will severely jeopardize the blood supply of the premaxillary segment (Fig. 28.6). To minimize the risk of complications, the incision is stopped just lateral to the alveolar cleft on each side. One minimizes reflection of the mucosa from the premaxilla in order to preserve the blood supply. The osteotomy of the premaxillary segment is made from a posterior approach just anterior to the incisive foramen. This allows mobilization of the segment without violation of the buccal mucosa. Similar to the unilateral cleft maxilla, residual fistulae and inadequate alveolar bone may be present. If either is

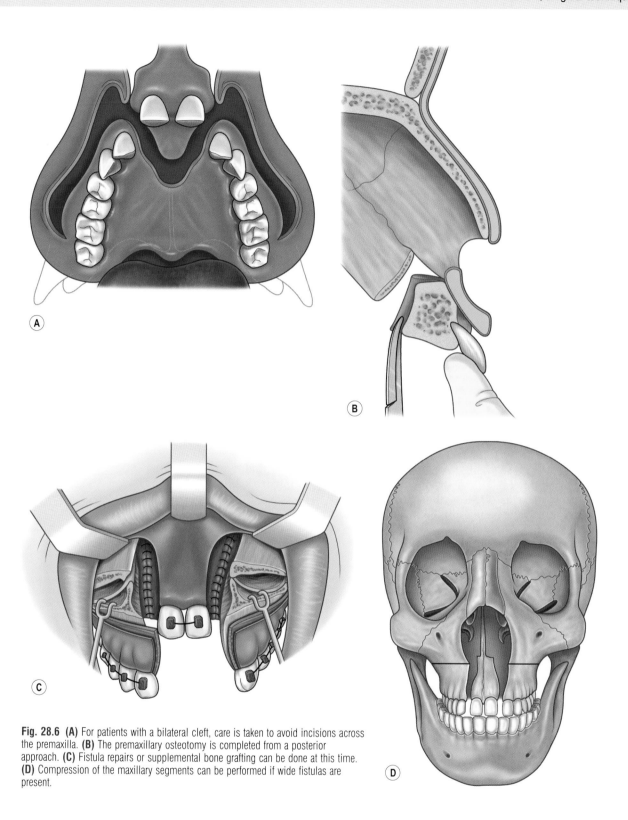

Fig. 28.6 (A) For patients with a bilateral cleft, care is taken to avoid incisions across the premaxilla. **(B)** The premaxillary osteotomy is completed from a posterior approach. **(C)** Fistula repairs or supplemental bone grafting can be done at this time. **(D)** Compression of the maxillary segments can be performed if wide fistulas are present.

identified, it can be corrected by a two-layer mucosal closure and bone grafting into the alveolar defect. If large gaps are present that may jeopardize fistula closure, the segments can be compressed at the alveolar gaps to reduce tension of the repair. Postoperative orthodontics and prosthetic restorations of the teeth can correct almost any postoperative dental aesthetic irregularities.

Once the incision is made, the mucosa is reflected in a subperiosteal plane to expose the piriform aperture, the zygomatic buttress, and the posterolateral maxilla. A reciprocating saw is used to make a high Le Fort I osteotomy in most cases. A high Le Fort I osteotomy is cut horizontally in a lateral direct line from the piriform aperture to the zygomatic buttress. One takes this line as high as possible while staying at least 5 mm below the inferior orbital foramen. A vertical cut is now made from the lateral edge of the horizontal cut and taken to an area about 5 mm above the tooth root apices. The lateral nasal walls are cut with a uniball osteotome and mallet. The vomer and septum can be reached through the lateral maxillary osteotomies so the mucosa remains preserved. The pterygomaxillary junction can be separated with a 10-mm curved osteotome, or the maxillary tuberosity can be cut posterior to the last molar in the arch. The latter choice makes downfracture easier and results in fewer complications. Downfracture is now completed with either digital pressure or application of the Rowe disimpaction forceps. If a wide alveolar fistula is present, the greater and lesser segments can be compressed at the alveolus. The occlusion that would result from segment compression would be evaluated on the dental casts during preoperative model surgery. Any deficiency of alveolar bone can be corrected with supplemental bone grafts after application of fixation, and fistulas can be corrected as well.

The surgical splint is then placed to orient the new position of the maxilla to the mandible. Wire loops (26-gauge) are used to place the patient in maxillomandibular fixation. It is extremely important to make sure the condyles are seated as the maxillomandibular complex is rotated to its new vertical dimension. Generally, cleft patients have vertical maxillary deficiency in addition to the sagittal deficiency. This requires the maxilla to be positioned inferiorly to its new position. If vertical lengthening greater than 5 mm is required, bone grafts are placed between the osteotomy segments to reduce relapse. Rigid fixation is now used to secure the maxilla into its new position. If any instability remains across the maxillary segments, a small plate can be placed across the segments to reduce mobility and maintain the bone graft. Because the osteotomized cleft maxilla results in a multisegment maxilla, the surgical splints are wired in place for 6–8 weeks in order to allow for bone healing.

Distraction osteogenesis

Distraction osteogenesis (DO) is a useful technique to gain large advancements reliably with relatively low rates of relapse. This technique takes advantage of osteoinductive properties of tension and stress across the osteotomy to expand the mandibular or maxillary segment rapidly while allowing the soft tissue to relax over time. Without the need for anatomic reduction or rigid fixation at the time of surgery, DO is often technically easier and faster than traditional orthognathic surgery. Moreover, various methods of distraction allow for precise control in several different vectors to position the osteotomized segment accurately in space with relation to the cranial base and other dentofacial landmarks.

Basic approaches to commonly encountered problems

The following paragraphs outline basic treatment approaches to commonly encountered dentofacial deformities commonly seen in orthognathic patients.

Skeletal class II malocclusion

Conditions such as Treacher Collins syndrome, Stickler syndrome, and Pierre Robin sequence are often associated with

class II malocclusion, which is almost always caused by mandibular retrognathia and is almost always best treated by mandibular advancement (Fig. 28.7). The mandible is small, and forward positioning is an expansile movement that enhances facial form. If the maxilla is also slightly deficient or in an abnormal position, one may consider a bimaxillary advancement to enhance further facial soft-tissue definition,

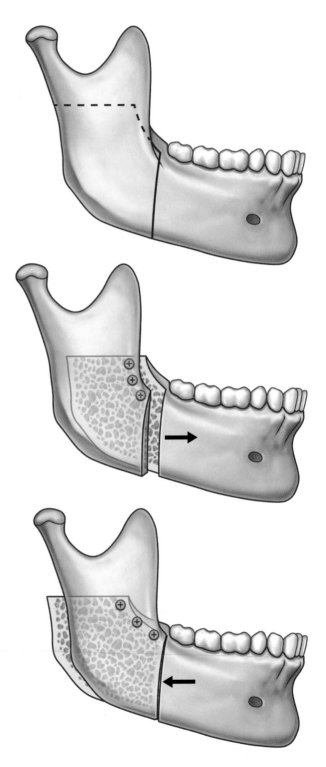

Fig. 28.7 Mandibular sagittal split osteotomies demonstrating mandibular advancement and mandibular setback.

especially in more mature patients. If the malocclusion is minimal and there is little pre-existing dental compensation, one may choose to have the orthodontist intentionally compensate the dentition to correct the occlusion and avoid surgery. In contrast, if the malocclusion appears minimal but there is dental compensation, the skeletal discrepancy will be more significant after the orthodontist decompensates the dentition, and the patient may be a good surgical candidate (Fig. 28.8).

Skeletal class III malocclusion

A class III malocclusion may be treated by advancing the maxilla, posteriorly positioning the mandible, or by combining these procedures. It is important to consider the contributions of the mandible and the chin separately as each may require different treatments to achieve aesthetic goals. If some posterior positioning of the mandible is necessary, one may advance the maxilla to counteract the skeletal contraction produced from posteriorly positioning the mandible. Additionally, the patient may benefit from an advancement genioplasty, counteracting any skeletal contraction occurring from a mandibular setback. As in the class II patient, a minor malocclusion with minimal dental compensation may be corrected with orthodontic treatment alone. In contrast, a minor malocclusion with dental compensation may become a significant malocclusion after dental decompensation, and the patient will be a good surgical candidate. In cleft patients with class III malocclusion, where the maxilla may be scarred from prior interventions, combined Le Fort I advancement and BSSO setback may be necessary even for relatively small degrees of negative overjet (unless maxillary DO is entertained) (Fig. 28.9).

Maxillary constriction

Patients can present with a maxilla that is narrow in a transverse dimension. Maxillary constriction may occur as an isolated finding or as one of multiple abnormalities. Up to about 15 years of age, the orthodontist can usually expand the maxilla non-surgically with a palatal expander. If orthopedic expansion cannot be done, a SARPE can be performed. If the maxilla requires movement in other dimensions, a two-piece (or multipiece) Le Fort I osteotomy can be performed to place the maxilla in its new position while simultaneously achieving transverse expansion (Fig. 28.10).

Apertognathia

An anterior open bite is caused by a premature contact of the posterior molars and is commonly seen in patients with syndromic craniosynostoses such as Apert or Crouzon syndromes. The recommended treatment is a posterior impaction of the maxilla. By reducing the vertical height of the posterior maxilla, the mandible can come into occlusion with the remaining mandibular teeth. Posterior maxillary impaction does not necessarily result in incisor impaction; the posterior maxilla is simply rotated clockwise and upward using the incisal tip as the axis of rotation. Therefore, incisor show should not be affected. If a change in incisor show is also desired, the posterior impaction is performed, and then the whole maxilla can be inferiorly positioned or impacted to its new position (Fig. 28.11).

Vertical maxillary excess

Vertical maxillary excess is typically associated with lip incompetence, mentalis strain, and an excessive degree of gingival show (long-face syndrome). The treatment approach is to impact the maxilla to achieve the proper incisor show with the lips in repose. Impaction, however, may result in skeletal contraction, so the surgeon must consider anterior repositioning of the jaws to neutralize the associated adverse soft-tissue effects. As the maxilla is impacted, the mandible rotates counterclockwise (with respect to a rightward-facing patient) to maintain occlusion. This rotation results in anterior positioning of the chin and is called mandibular autorotation. The opposite occurs if the maxilla is moved in an inferior direction. In this case, the chin point rotates in a clockwise direction, resulting in posterior positioning of the chin point. It is important to note these effects on the cephalometric tracing during treatment planning because a genioplasty may be required to re-establish proper chin position.

Short lower face

A short lower face is marked by insufficient incisor show and/or a short distance between subnasale and pogonion. Treatment is aimed at establishing a proper degree of incisor show. The facial skeleton should be expanded to the degree that provides optimal soft-tissue aesthetics. As the maxilla is inferiorly positioned, resulting clockwise mandibular rotation leads to a posterior positioning of the chin. The surgeon needs to assess the new chin position preoperatively on the cephalometric prediction tracing to determine if an advancement genioplasty will be necessary to counter the effects of mandibular clockwise rotation.

Postoperative care

Postoperative care of patients undergoing orthognathic surgery is paramount to a successful surgical outcome and a satisfied patient and family. Close adherence to an oral hygiene regimen, including regular tooth brushing and chlorhexidine mouth rinses, will minimize the risk of postoperative infection, as will a short course of antibiotics targeted toward common mouth flora. Additionally, steps taken to reduce swelling, including ice, head elevation, and anti-inflammatory medication such as Solu-Medrol, will greatly improve patient comfort. A soft diet for at least the first 3 weeks postoperatively will help reduce the risk of malunion or hardware failure. As well, guiding elastics are usually employed for the first 2–3 weeks.

Outcomes, prognosis, and complications

Accurate assessment of orthognathic surgical outcomes is essential to maintaining safe practices, maximizing patient satisfaction, and effectively evaluating an ever-changing field. Indeed, this importance is echoed in the ways investigators have analyzed postoperative results. These range from measurement tools such as three-dimensional CT scanning and volumetric analyses (used to evaluate postoperative changes in bony and soft tissues immediately and over time) to

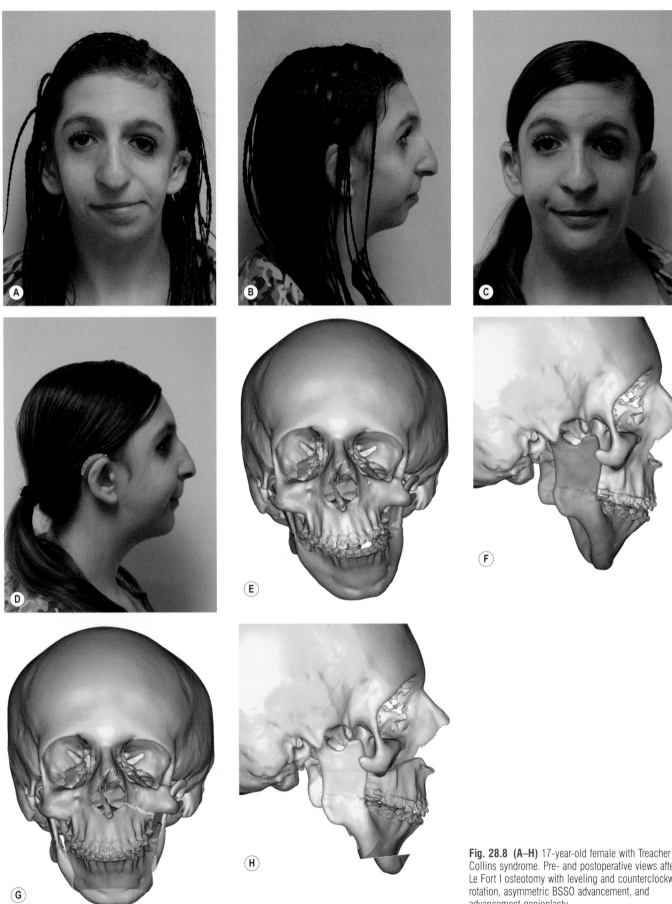

Fig. 28.8 (A–H) 17-year-old female with Treacher Collins syndrome. Pre- and postoperative views after Le Fort I osteotomy with leveling and counterclockwise rotation, asymmetric BSSO advancement, and advancement genioplasty.

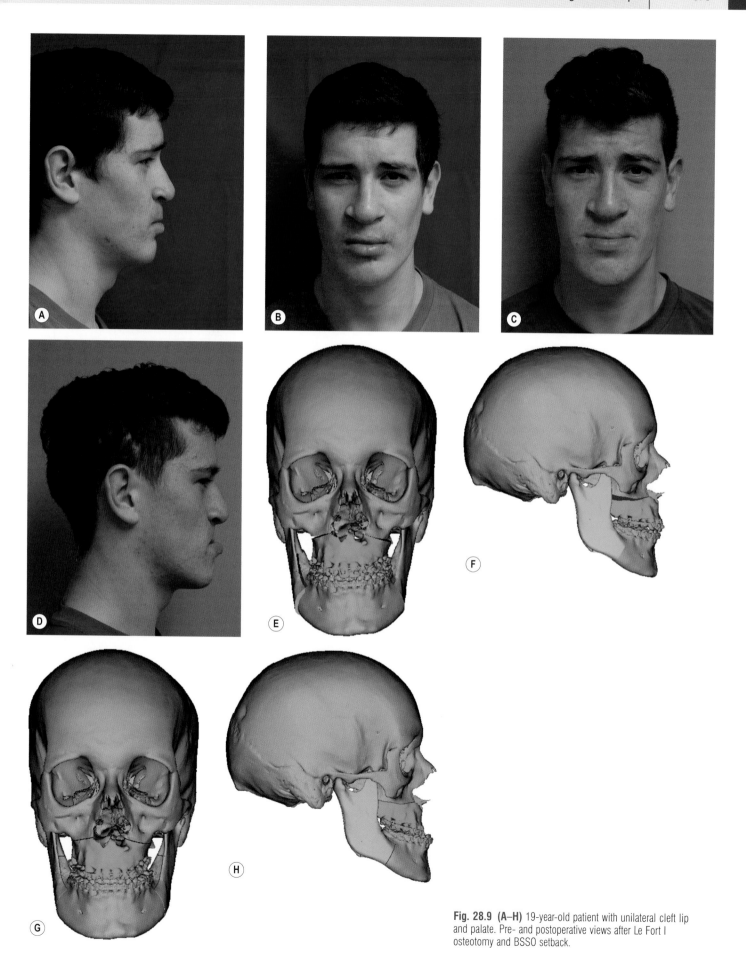

Fig. 28.9 (A–H) 19-year-old patient with unilateral cleft lip and palate. Pre- and postoperative views after Le Fort I osteotomy and BSSO setback.

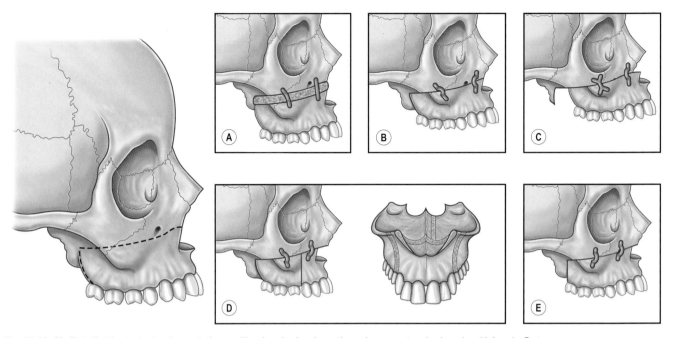

Fig. 28.10 (A–E) Le Fort I osteotomies demonstrating maxillary lengthening, impaction, advancement, setback, and multipiece Le Fort.

questionnaires assessing patient-reported satisfaction scales and quality of life. While there is currently no universally accepted tool to demonstrate patient outcomes after orthognathic surgery accurately and reliably, with reasoned and reasonable expectations on the part of the patient, family, and surgeon alike, orthognathic surgery can result in high levels of satisfaction from both a functional and aesthetic level.

Of particular importance to the cleft and craniofacial population is the effect of orthognathic surgery on speech. It is generally accepted that the etiology of velopharyngeal insufficiency (VPI) in the cleft patient is due to the malalignment or shortening of the palatal musculature, as well as growth, development, and/or surgical sequelae that can lead to abnormal structural relationships. Given the intricate attachment of the muscular apparatus of the velum to the maxilla, it follows that movement of the maxilla can change the preoperative velopharyngeal function.

Janulewicz *et al.* performed a retrospective study of the change in velopharyngeal function of 54 cleft lip and palate patients who underwent maxillary advancement with or without a mandibular setback procedure over a 21-year period.[7] As summarized in Table 28.1, their study shows a decline in competent velopharyngeal function (from 42% to 18%), an increase in both borderline incompetence (from 9% to 22%), and complete VPI (from 13% to 20%). The authors also noted that the quality of speech declined, as evidenced by the increase in overall objective speech score from 2.46 to 4.24 (the higher the score, the worse the speech). In contrast, the authors noted that articulation defects improved, although the improvement did not achieve statistical significance. Preoperatively 84% (46 patients) had at least one articulation defect as compared to 73% (40 patients) postoperatively.

Other published studies have shown similar results or no change in VPI function following jaw surgery. In their study,

Table 28.1 Comparison of preoperative and postoperative speech variables

Total number of patients: 54	Preoperative evaluation % (*n*)	Postoperative evaluation % (*n*)
VP function: competent	42% (23)	18% (10)
VP function: borderline competent	36% (20)	40% (22)
VP function: borderline incompetent	9% (5)	22% (12)
VP function: complete VPI	13% (7)	20% (11)
Normal nasality	40% (22)	40% (22)
Mild hypernasality	18% (10)	29% (16)
Moderate hypernasality	4% (2)	15% (8)
Severe hypernasality	4% (2)	2% (1)
Hyponasality	33% (18)	15% (8)
Reduced sibilant IOAPs	26% (14)	35% (19)
Reduced fricative IOAPs	16% (9)	26% (14)
Reduced plosive IOAPs	6% (3)	22% (12)
Anterior dentition errors	64% (35)	47% (26)
Mean speech score	2.46	4.24

IOAP, intraoral air pressure; VP, velopharyngeal; VPI, velopharyngeal incompetence.
(Reproduced from Janulewicz J, Costello BJ, Buckley MJ, et al. The effects of Le Fort I osteotomies on velopharyngeal and speech functions in cleft patients. *J Oral Maxillofac Surg.* 2004;62:308–314.)

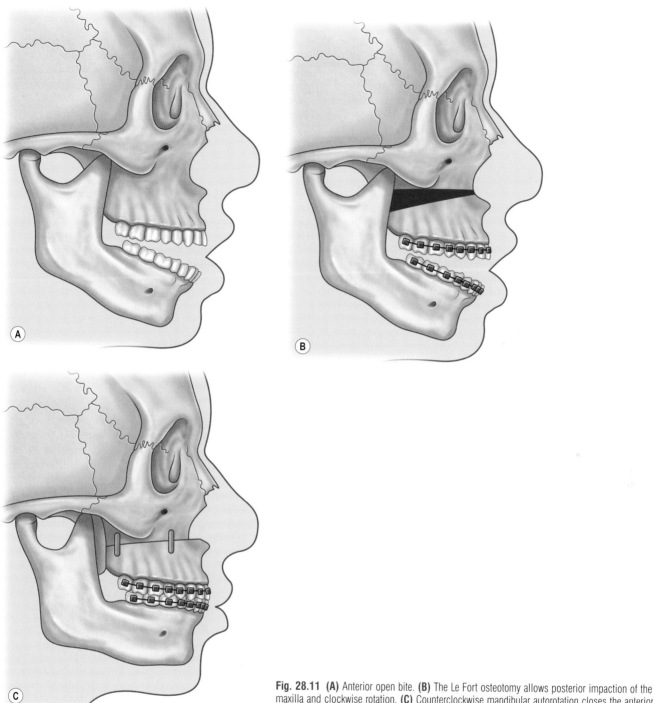

Fig. 28.11 (A) Anterior open bite. **(B)** The Le Fort osteotomy allows posterior impaction of the maxilla and clockwise rotation. **(C)** Counterclockwise mandibular autorotation closes the anterior open bite.

Phillips *et al.*[8] showed that the extent of anteroposterior movement of the maxilla is unrelated to velopharyngeal deterioration and is not a useful predictor. In their study of 26 cleft patients (16 unilateral complete and 9 bilateral complete cleft lips and palates), Phillips *et al.* demonstrated that all patients with perceived hypernasal speech preoperatively had hypernasality after advancement. Furthermore, 9 of 12 patients who had preoperative nasopharyngoscopy showing borderline or inadequate VP closure developed postoperative VPI. Based on these results, Phillips *et al.* conclude that preoperative

assessment can predict postoperative speech and velopharyngeal function.

In summary, it appears that, while a positive effect on articulation might be achieved by orthognathic surgery, it might be at the expense of velopharyngeal function. Further prospective, controlled studies would be helpful in elucidating the relationships between maxillary advancement and speech.

Posnick and Tompson[9] performed a retrospective study evaluating relapse in cleft patients who had undergone orthognathic surgery between 1987 and 1990. They found that there was no significant difference in outcome between patients who had maxillary surgery alone and those who had operations on both jaws. Furthermore, the outcome did not vary significantly with the type of autogenous bone graft used or the segmentalization of the osteotomy. All 35 patients included in the study underwent a modified Le Fort I maxillary osteotomy with varied degrees of horizontal advancement, transverse arch widening, and vertical change. Eleven of the 35 patients also required mandibular surgery, consisting of sagittal split osteotomies. In 13 of 35 patients a pharyngoplasty was in place at the time of maxillary Le Fort I osteotomy. The results of the study are summarized in Table 28.2.

The mean horizontal advancement achieved for the group was 6.9 mm; 5.3 mm was maintained 1 year later (mean relapse 1.6 mm). In 11 of the 35 patients the relapse was less than 1.0 mm. For the 13 patients who had a pharyngoplasty at the time of the Le Fort I osteotomy, the mean horizontal advancement was 8.2 mm immediately after the operation and 6.5 mm 1 year later. Stability of the vertical displacement was also evaluated. No maxillary vertical change was necessary in 12 of 35 patients. The mean vertical displacement of the maxilla in patients who underwent vertical displacement was 2.1 mm; 1.7 mm was maintained 1 year later. The authors concluded that neither horizontal nor vertical relapse was related to the extent of movement. The overjet from the cephalometric radiographs at the 1-year postoperative interval was maintained in all patients, whereas a positive overbite was maintained in only 30 of 35 patients (85%).

Other investigators have found a correlation between relapse and the degree of advancement. To identify factors associated with relapse after orthognathic surgery in the cleft lip/palate patient, Hirano and Suzuki[10] performed a retrospective study on 58 cleft patients who underwent orthognathic surgery over a 10-year period. From their study, they identified the following factors related to relapse:

1. Horizontal advancement: In their series the mean horizontal relapse was 24.1% of the mean advancement. There was significant correlation between extent relapse and advancement. The authors report that complete surgical mobilization of the maxilla is important in preventing relapse.

2. Vertical displacement (inferior positioning): In their study the mean inferior vertical elongation was 3.0 mm with a relapse of 2.1 mm. Based on their study, the authors recommend a 2-mm overcorrection in inferior positioning of the maxilla.

3. Rotation, clockwise or counterclockwise: The authors report that most of their surgical rotation was lost and relapse was seen in both clockwise and counterclockwise rotations. They suggest overcorrection to mitigate the effects of relapse.

4. Type of cleft: Orthognathic surgery in a bilateral cleft patient was more likely to result in relapse, according to their study. They attribute the increase in likelihood of relapse to increased scarring of palatal tissues and multiple missing teeth.

5. Previous alveolar bone grafting: Although studies have reported the value of alveolar bone grafting in establishing stability of advancement and minimizing relapse, the study by Hirano and Suzuki[10] found no association between alveolar bone graft and the rate of relapse in unilateral cleft lip and palate patients.

6. Number of missing teeth: The study by Hirano and Suzuki[10] also found no correlation between the number of missing teeth and relapse although the authors stress that multiple missing teeth can compromise the stability of the occlusion.

7. Type of orthognathic surgery: There was no difference in the relapse rate between patients undergoing maxillary surgery alone and those who underwent two-jaw surgery.

While both relapse and worsening VPI can occur with the movements performed in orthognathic surgery, they are a result of primary deficiencies in the soft tissue due to prior scar formation as well as the underlying deformity and thus are under only limited surgeon control. There are several complications, however, on which the surgeon can have a direct effect.

Improper positioning of the jaws is noted by malocclusion or an obvious unaesthetic result. Special care must be taken to ensure proper condyle positioning during fixation of the mandibular osteotomy. If malocclusion results from improper condyle position during fixation, it must be removed and reapplied. The same is true for improper indexing of the splint. For this reason, it is wise to verify splint fit prior to surgery. Meticulous treatment planning prior to surgery minimizes splint-related problems.

Measures to reduce the chance of an unfavorable mandibular split should always be employed. Removal of mandibular third molars 6 months prior to the osteotomy allows time for sockets to heal, decreasing the chance of a bad split. If the segments do not appear to be easily separating, the surgeon should verify that the osteotomies are complete. Excessive force that could increase the chance of an uncontrolled mandibular split should be avoided. If an unfavorable split occurs, the segments can be plated to re-establish normal anatomy, and the proximal and distal segments can then be secured into the desired position with rigid fixation.

Bleeding may occur from any area, but most commonly from the descending palatine artery in the maxilla. This can be stopped with packing or by placing a hemoclip on the artery. Bone wax is useful for bleeding bony edges.

Nerve damage is rare, but can occur. The nerves associated with these procedures are the infraorbital, inferior alveolar, and mental nerve. If a transaction is witnessed, coaptation

Table 28.2 Patients with unilateral cleft lip and palate undergoing Le Fort I osteotomy with miniplate fixation: mean horizontal/vertical displacement and relapse

Time after surgery	Effective horizontal mean advancement (mm)	Effective vertical mean change (mm)
1 week	6.9 ± 2.6	2.1 ± 2.4
6–8 weeks	6.3 ± 2.6	1.9 ± 2.1
1 year	5.3 ± 2.7	1.7 ± 2.0

(Reproduced from Posnick JC, et al. Cleft-orthognathic surgery: the unilateral cleft lip and palate deformity. In: Craniofacial and Maxillofacial Surgery in Children and Young Adults, Vol. 2, Chapter 34. Philadelphia: WB Saunders; 2001.)

with 7-0 nylon suture is recommended. The patient should be informed that there is approximately a 70% chance of some paresthesia immediately after surgery, but permanent changes are seen in only 25% of patients.

The incidence of nonunion or malunion is rare after surgery. If a malunion occurs, the jaw may need to be osteotomized again to move it into proper position. A nonunion requires secondary bone grafting to establish osseous continuity.

Secondary procedures

The need for secondary procedures in orthognathic surgery is uncommon, especially when careful patient selection and preoperative evaluation are employed. However, orthognathic surgery rarely can completely resolve a significant preoperative dentofacial deformity. Indeed, maxillary and mandibular movements, in addition to altering occlusal relationships and skeletal proportions, may highlight features previously de-emphasized by malocclusion. In such cases, procedures such as rhinoplasty, fat grafting, or malar augmentation may help restore facial harmony.

It is important to realize that underlying issues related to the primary cleft or craniofacial disorder may not be fully addressed with orthognathic surgery. For example, patients with repaired clefts who undergo orthognathic surgery to address a class III malocclusion may still need surgeries to complete their dental rehabilitation. Bone grafting and vestibuloplasty may be as necessary after orthognathic surgery as before.[11] Likewise, in the setting of persistent edentulous spaces, osseointegrated implants which are resistant to orthopedic movements should be utilized only after jaw surgery and postoperative orthodontics have determined final tooth positions.

References

1. DeLuke DM, Marchand A, Robles EC, et al. Facial growth and the need for orthognathic surgery after cleft palate repair: literature review and report of 28 cases. *J Oral Maxillofac Surg*. 1997;55:694–697, discussion 7–8.

2. Obwegeser H. Surgery of the maxilla for the correction of prognathism. *SSO Schweiz Monatsschr Zahnheilkd*. 1965;75:365–374.

3. Enlow EH. Craniofacial growth and development: normal and deviant patterns. In: Posnick JC, ed. *Craniofacial and Maxillofacial Surgery in Children and Young Adults*. Philadelphia: W B Saunders; 2000:22–35. *In this comprehensive chapter, the author provides a detailed account of the development of the craniofacial skeleton, under both normal conditions and in disease states. It highlights the temporal relationship between growth of the cranial skeleton and the facial skeleton as well as the differences among genders and in specific conditions of craniofacial abnormalities.*

4. Mao JJ, Wang X, Kopher RA. Biomechanics of craniofacial sutures: orthopedic implications. *Angle Orthod*. 2003;73:128–135.

5. Tompach PC, Wheeler JJ, Fridrich KL. Orthodontic considerations in orthognathic surgery. *Int J Adult Orthodon Orthognath Surg*. 1995;10:97.

6. Selber JC, Rosen HM. Aesthetics of facial skeletal surgery. *Clin Plast Surg*. 2007;34:437–445. *This article highlights the changing paradigm in orthognathic treatment planning from one based on pure cephalometric analysis to one encompassing an evaluation of the aesthetic facial soft-tissue proportions.*

7. Janulewicz J, Costello BJ, Buckley MJ, et al. The effects of Le Fort I osteotomies on velopharyngeal and speech functions in cleft patients. *J Oral Maxillofac Surg*. 2004;62:308–314.

8. Phillips JH, Klaiman P, Delorey R, et al. Predictors of velopharyngeal insufficiency in cleft palate orthognathic surgery. *Plast Reconstr Surg*. 2005;115:681–686. *This article is a retrospective examination of 26 patients who underwent orthognathic advancement. Assessments of speech and velopharyngeal function before and after orthognathic surgery and the role of nasopharyngoscopy are detailed.*

9. Posnick JC, Tompson B. Cleft-orthognathic surgery: complications and long-term results. *Plast Reconstr Surg*. 1995;96:255–266. *This article is a retrospective evaluation of 116 patients with cleft palate who underwent orthognathic surgery to correct malocclusion. The authors report a mean follow-up of 40 months and describe common complications and outcomes.*

10. Hirano A, Suzuki H. Factors related to relapse after Le Fort I maxillary advancement osteotomy in patients with cleft lip and palate. *Cleft Palate Craniofac J*. 2001;38:1–10. *This article is a retrospective study of 58 patients (42 unilateral cleft and 16 bilateral cleft) who underwent orthognathic surgery to correct maxillary hypoplasia. The authors report a mean follow-up period of 2.5 years. Based on cephalometric and statistical analyses, the authors elucidate factors related to relapse after Le Fort I maxillary advancement.*

11. Baker S, Goldstein JA, Seiboth L, Weinzweig J. Posttraumatic maxillomandibular reconstruction: a treatment algorithm for the partially edentulous patient. *J Craniofac Surg*. 2010;21:217–221.

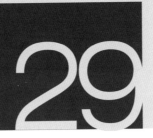

Pediatric facial fractures

Edward H. Davidson and Joseph E. Losee

SYNOPSIS

- Traumas that would likely produce fractures in adults often do not in children due to intrinsic anatomical factors.

- In addition to the unique anatomy of the pediatric patient, future growth and development must be accounted for when addressing these injuries.

- In deciding between operative and non-operative management of pediatric facial fractures, the practitioner is essentially weighing the risk of growth disturbance against the benefit of precise reduction and rigid fixation.

- When indicated, employing less invasive approaches to operative management should be practiced.

 Access the Historical Perspective section online at
http://www.expertconsult.com

Introduction

Facial fractures are relatively uncommon in children. Traumas that would likely produce fractures in adults often do not in children due to intrinsic anatomical factors such as larger fat pads, decreased pneumatization of sinuses, increased skeletal flexibility secondary to more malleable bone stock, and compliant sutures. Parental supervision also prevents many would-be fractures.[1] The same structural characteristics of the pediatric craniofacial skeleton that thwart fracture are responsible for the unique injury patterns that are observed when bony injury does occur. Pediatric facial fracture evaluation begins with the conventional trauma evaluation and proceeds through clinical and radiographic assessment, culminating in conservative or operative management. In addition to the unique anatomy of the pediatric patient, future growth and development must be accounted for when addressing these injuries. A non-operative approach is advised whenever feasible, and long-term follow-up is mandatory to ensure adequate outcomes and inform future practice. The objective of this chapter is to provide the reader with an understanding of the anatomical and growth-related factors that make pediatric craniofacial fracture repair a unique entity and to offer a discussion of specific treatment modalities in this context.

General principles

Epidemiology

Amongst the numerous authors that have catalogued and analyzed their experience with pediatric facial fractures there is consensus that these account for less than 15% of all facial fractures. Frequency increases with age, prevalence is greater in males (2–3:1), and severity of injury also worsens with advancing age and male gender. Motor vehicle collision (MVC), assault, and falls are the most common cause of facial fracture.[2–7] Reportedly, pediatric facial fractures are more prevalent in spring and summer months, present in greater numbers between midnight and noon, and most commonly occur on Sundays and least commonly on Thursdays.[4]

The most common facial fracture in all pediatric age groups is the orbital fracture. However, there is some contention in determining the relative incidence of fracture patterns with many studies having significant selection biases: subjects enrolled or excluded according to admission status (inpatient versus outpatient), necessity of operative management, and treating specialty. To better characterize the full spectrum of pediatric facial fractures, the authors described injury patterns, associated injuries, and outcomes in a large consecutive group of all pediatric patients with facial fractures evaluated in a major children's hospital emergency department from fracture regardless of operative requirements, necessity for hospital admission, or treating service. In this cohort, patients were subdivided into three age groups: 0 to 5, 6 to 11, and 12 to 18 years.[8] Although this stratification was based primarily on dental maturity, additional characteristics are reflected by this division. Children from 0 to 5 years of age are in primary dentition and are more likely to be involved in supervised activity; they also have the highest cranial-to-facial ratio. From 6 to 11 years of age, children are in mixed dentition, enter school, and begin to participate in sports. Patients from 12 to 18 years of age are in permanent dentition, are more independent, and participate in potentially more at-risk activities. Half (48%) of fractures were sustained by patients 12–18 years of age; 6–11-year-olds accounted for 32% of fractures; and children under 5 years of age contributed 20% of fractures.[8] Similar patterns have been observed by other authors.[1–4,9] Although orbital fracture was the most common fracture type for all age groups combined (29.8% of all fractures), fracture type did vary by age at injury. Maxillary, zygomaticomaxillary complex, and nasal fractures were more common in older patients; oblique craniofacial fractures (skull fractures occurring in combination with a facial fracture) were more common in younger patients. Of mandible fractures in the authors' series (n = 179), condylar head and subcondylar fractures were most common (48%).[10] Anatomical distribution varies with age; condylar fracture incidence decreases, while body and angle fractures increase.[11] Nasal fractures are likely often underreported, with many treated in an outpatient setting or going untreated.[12] Midface fractures are uncommon (10.4% of facial fractures in the authors' series), likely secondary to the protection of the midface by the prominent forehead and mandible in children, in addition to the robust anatomy of this region.[8] Zygomaticomaxillary complex (ZMC) fractures are the most common of the rare midface fractures.[1]

The cause of injury also varied by age: violence, assault, and MVC were the most common causes of injury in 12–18-year-olds, while activities of daily living caused the most fractures in 0–5-year-olds.[8] Fifty percent of injuries in abused children involve the head or neck, and facial fractures are seen in 2.3% of abused children.[13] Craniofacial injury is the second most common sport-related injury and is involved in up to 20% of all pediatric sport-related injuries in the United States with 10.6% of craniofacial injuries being sports-related.[14] In the context of MVC, unrestrained children were significantly more likely to sustain facial fractures: 65–70% of children involved in all-terrain vehicle or bicycle accidents were not wearing helmets.[3] In the authors' series, there was a 69%:31% male-to-female ratio. A total of 62.6% of patients were admitted to hospital, and 18.6% to an intensive care unit, data consistent with other reports.[8] The literature regarding operative fixation of pediatric facial fractures is quite diverse, varying from 25 to 78%. Nonetheless, older children require surgery more frequently than younger children.[15]

The authors have also examined the epidemiologic data of pediatric craniofacial fractures secondary to violence, comparing these data to craniofacial fractures sustained from all other causes. Patients with violence-related fractures were more likely to be older, male, and non-white and live in a socioeconomically depressed area. A greater number of patients with violence-related injuries sustained nasal and mandible angle fractures, whereas more patients with non-violence-related injuries sustained skull and orbital fractures.[16]

Associated injuries

Facial fractures are high-energy injuries, and as such are heavily associated with other injuries (up to 88% in some reports).[13] Facial fractures and a depressed Glasgow Coma Score (GCS) show a strong correlation with intracranial hemorrhage and cervical spine fracture. Evaluation for such injuries is recommended in those with facial fractures and an abnormal GCS.[17] In the authors' series, excluding soft-tissue injuries, brain trauma was the injury most commonly associated with facial fractures across all age groups. A total of 55% of patients with facial fractures had associated injuries: 81% of these were considered "serious" and included cardiovascular, cervical spine, or intra-abdominal trauma. Some 47% had neurological injuries (60% of these were concussions), and 3% had ophthalmologic injuries, including blindness. In all, 1.4% died as a result of their injuries.[8] Mechanism of injury contributes to this; there were significantly more associated neurologic injuries in children who sustained a craniofacial fracture due to a non-violent mechanism – specifically, a greater number of subarachnoid bleeds, subdural bleeds, concussions, and comas. Patients in the non-violent group were also more likely to have an injury to a vital organ system; they experienced a greater number of respiratory, abdominal, and musculoskeletal injuries.[16] Nearly one third of pediatric patients with facial fractures in the authors' retrospective series were diagnosed with a concomitant concussion. These data suggest that a higher index of suspicion for concussion should be maintained for patients with skull fractures and potentially orbital and maxillary fractures. Given the possibility of a worse outcome with delayed concussion diagnosis, patients with facial fractures may benefit from more active early concussion screening.[18]

Though soft-tissue injury is presumed to be commonplace with pediatric facial fractures, characterization of injury patterns, influence on management, and any subsequent effect on facial development have not been well investigated.[19] Although uncommon, facial fractures associated with dog bites (1.4% of dog bites) are a significant source of soft-tissue morbidity, often requiring complex surgical repair in over 80% of cases.[20]

Growth, development, and fracture patterns

Craniofacial development is the culmination of a complex and incompletely understood interaction between intracellular processes, intercellular signaling, and environmental influences. Cranial-to-facial ratio decreases with maturity from 8:1

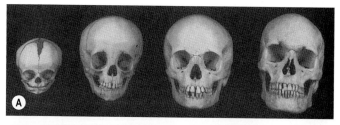
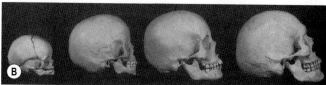

Fig. 29.1 **(A)** Frontal view and **(B)** side view of the growing craniofacial skeleton. Note the decreasing cranial-to-facial ratio and increasing facial prominence. *(Reproduced from Mathes S, Hentz V. Plastic Surgery, 2nd edn. Philadelphia, PA: Elsevier; 2006.)*

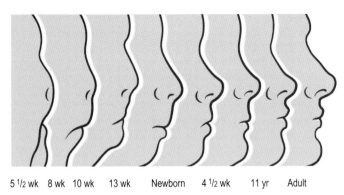

5 ½ wk   8 wk   10 wk   13 wk   Newborn   4 ½ wk   11 yr   Adult

Fig. 29.2 Schematic of growing face, in profile. Note decreased protection of face afforded by cranium and increasing prominence (and exposure to injury) of mandible.

at birth to 2:1 in adulthood (Figs. 29.1 & 29.2).[21] The cranium grows secondary to the brain, which triples in size during the first year of life.[21–24] This is a continuous process that is 25% complete at birth, 75% complete at 2 years, and 95% complete by 10 years. Facial growth is sporadic: it is 40% complete at 3 months, 70% at 4 years, 80% by 5 years, pauses until puberty, and resumes until 17 years of age.[21] The upper face grows secondary to brain and ocular development; midfacial growth follows the development of the nasal capsule and dentition. Orbital growth is complete by 6–8 years, and nasal growth is largely complete by 12–14 years. The majority of nasal growth occurs in two distinct postnatal growth spurts, ages 2–5 years and again during puberty. Additional growth after is usually complete by age 16 to 18 in girls and 18 to 20 in boys, although further growth of the nasal septum may occur up to the age of 25 years.[25] The palate and maxilla achieve two-thirds adult size by 6 years.[26] At birth, the mandible is formed by two bones joined by cartilage at the symphysis, ossifying within the first year of life. The majority of permanent teeth erupt by 12 years of age. The gonial angle becomes increasingly acute, the ramus and body enlarge, and the distance between the dentition and the inferior mandibular border increases. Cortical bone replaces tooth buds as the primary component of mandibular volume. The inferior alveolar nerve is displaced superiorly to rest midway from the superior and inferior mandibular borders. The mental foramen migrates to rest ultimately beneath the first or second permanent premolar.[27]

The decreased bone mineral content of the infant skull yields increased tolerance to force without fracture; fractures that do occur are more likely to be incomplete, greenstick fractures. In addition to mineralization, sinus pneumatization and dental eruption are responsible for the evolving craniofacial load-bearing capacity and subsequent fracture patterns (Figs. 29.3 & 29.4). The maxillary sinus is aerated at 12 years of age; the frontal sinus is not aerated until adulthood. Oblique craniofacial fractures precede the Le Fort patterns seen in adulthood as an incompletely pneumatized frontal sinus transmits energy directly from the site of impact to the supraorbital foramen and then to the orbit and zygoma. In one large study, Le Fort fractures were only seen in patients greater than 10 years of age.[9] Forehead fractures in children may develop into growing skull fractures (documented in 0.6–2% of pediatric skull fractures).[28] These lesions develop secondary to brain pulsations transmitting through occult dural disruptions and driving a growing bony diastasis resulting in a

leptomeningeal cyst or "hernia". Another consequence of the underdeveloped frontal sinus is an increased incidence of isolated orbital roof "blow-in" fractures.[29] Blindness also occurs with increased frequency due to the direct transmission of force to the orbit.[29] Trapdoor fractures are more common secondary to greater bony elasticity.[30] Children tend to have fractures without enophthalmos or vertical orbital dystopia (VOD), likely secondary to more robust supporting structures existing in this population. Enophthalmos and VOD require composite injury to bone, ligaments, and periosteum allowing for an increase in intraorbital volume (Fig. 29.5).

Isolated midface fractures are rare in children as this region is shielded by the prominent forehead and mandible.[31] Palatal splits are more common secondary to incomplete ossification of the hard palate. These injuries represent significant potential for growth disturbances secondary to the presence of growth centers in the maxilla and nasal capsule and because the midface is retruded relative to the cranium at this age.[32,33] Incomplete zygomaticofrontal (ZF) suture union leads to fracture dislocations characterized by inferior displacement of the zygoma and orbital floor, further contributing to oblique fracture patterns.[26] Oblique fracture patterns are also encouraged by the underdevelopment of the midface skeleton and major buttress systems. Until 10 years of age, the underdeveloped maxillary sinus transmits force to the

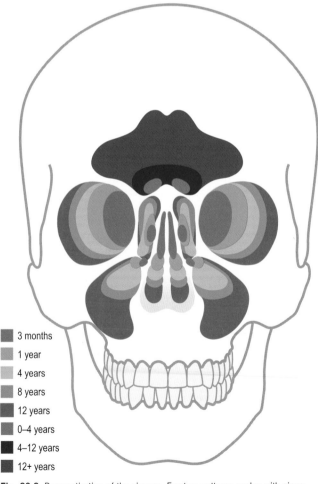

■ 3 months
□ 1 year
□ 4 years
■ 8 years
■ 12 years
■ 0–4 years
■ 4–12 years
■ 12+ years

Fig. 29.3 Pneumatization of the sinuses. Fracture patterns evolve with sinus development.

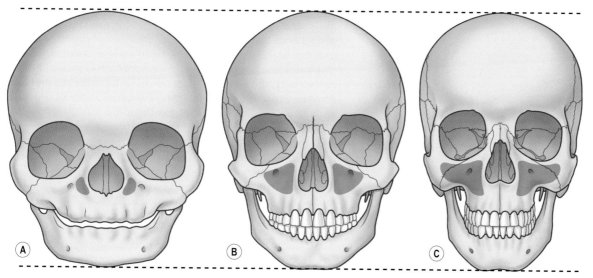

Fig. 29.4 (A–C) Development of the maxillary sinuses. The maxillary sinus plays an important role in determining how traumatic force will be transmitted through the midface.

alveolus, resulting in alveolar fractures instead of Le Fort I fractures. In the immature skeleton, Le Fort IIs are replaced by unilateral naso-orbito-ethmoid (NOE) fractures. Le Fort IIIs are replaced by multifragment oblique craniofacial fractures (Figs. 29.6–29.8).[9]

The less mineralized, more compliant pediatric mandible is more resistant to comminuted fractures. Condylar head and subcondylar fractures are seen more frequently in children due to incomplete ossification and a relatively weak condylar neck (Figs. 29.9 & 29.10). While certain regions of the mandible are classically highlighted as growth centers (e.g., condyles and lingual tuberosity), condylectomy and differential masticatory strain studies point to a more diffuse, dynamic process by which morphological change proceeds via coordinated bone deposition and resorption.[27] Heightened awareness of potential growth disturbance and temporomandibular joint (TMJ) ankylosis is, however, justified in the setting of condylar fractures given an incomplete understanding of these injuries' implications.

Diagnosis and presentation

The importance of a consistent approach to evaluating the patient with craniofacial trauma cannot be overemphasized. The first step in treating acute craniofacial injuries is ensuring that the primary and secondary surveys have been completely addressed. The craniofacial surgeon's most direct interaction with this process will likely be in assuring a secure airway in cases where anatomy has been severely distorted. Given the documented incidence of associated injuries, particularly neurological, and the usual inability to cooperate with a thorough physical exam, it is the author's opinion that pediatric patients with facial fractures benefit from routine CT scans of the skull, face, and mandible. Periocular injuries benefit from the formal evaluation by the ophthalmology service.

Infants are obligate nasal breathers, and their nasal airway is relatively narrow and thus easily obstructed.[34] Meticulous hemostasis must be achieved given a child's relatively

decreased blood volume and ability to mask significant losses with normotension prior to rapid decompensation.[34,35] Hypothermia is also more likely to be problematic given a child's increased surface area-to-volume ratio.[34] A systematic physical exam is performed. Eyelid hematoma, hearing loss, hemotympanum, and cranial nerve (CN) palsy may herald skull base fractures. Exophthalmos and inferior globe displacement may represent a supraorbital or roof fracture. Ptosis may be present secondary to levator paralysis. Orbital trauma will likely be accompanied by periorbital ecchymosis and subconjunctival hematoma. Extraocular muscle restriction may cause diplopia (Figs. 29.11 & 29.12). Forced duction is required to rule out muscle entrapment in obtunded patients. Superior orbital fissure syndrome (internal and external ophthalmoplegia (CN II, IV, VI paralysis), proptosis, and CN V paresthesia) and orbital apex syndrome (superior orbital fissure syndrome with blindness secondary to CN II involvement) must be emergently addressed (Fig. 29.13). Gaze limitations – even if other clinical signs and symptoms are minimal and radiographic studies are equivocal – may represent entrapment in an entity termed the "white-eyed blowout fracture".[36] In naso-orbito-ethmoid fractures, a bowstring test (palpation of the bony medial canthal attachment on lateral distraction of the lower eyelid) will assess the integrity of the medial canthal tendon. Intraorbital distance is assessed to exclude traumatic telecanthus.

Maxillary mobility and malocclusion may represent midface fractures. ZMC fractures may be accompanied by upper buccal sulcus hematoma, epistaxis secondary to a fractured maxillary sinus, a preauricular depression, cheek flattening, or lateral canthal dystopia. Impingement of a depressed zygomatic arch on the coronoid process may yield trismus. Medial displacement of the lateral wall with subsequent decrease in orbital volume may yield exophthalmos (Fig. 29.14). Nasal deviation, compressibility of the nasal dorsum, and septal hematoma must be appreciated on exam. Nasal airway obstruction may represent septal hematoma.

Signs and symptoms consistent with mandible fracture include malocclusion, drooling, trismus, decreased maximal

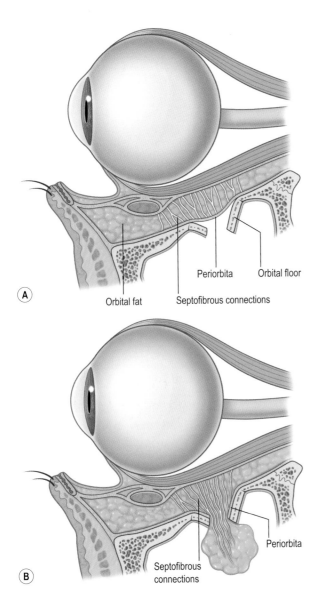

(A)

Periorbita   Orbital floor

Orbital fat   Septofibrous connections

(B)

Periorbita

Septofibrous connections

Fig. 29.5 Sagittal section of the orbit. **(A)** Orbital floor fracture with preserved orbital volume secondary to intact periorbita. **(B)** In contrast, the herniation of orbital contents secondary to disrupted periorbita in association with a floor fracture. It is the injury depicted in **(B)** that is required for enophthalmos or vertical orbital dystopia.

incisive opening, discomfort on mandibular excursion against symphyseal pressure, and dental step-off. The TMJ can be evaluated by palpating the external auditory canal while ranging the jaw. Certain patterns of malocclusion are associated with specific fractures. Anterior open bite often results from bilateral condylar/subcondylar fractures secondary to loss of posterior mandibular height and premature molar contact. Unilateral posterior condylar/subcondylar fracture may result in contralateral open bite. Mandible fractures must trigger suspicion for cervical spine fractures given the proximity and high-energy nature of these injuries.

Treatment

Certain principles may be applied to the management of all pediatric craniofacial fractures. In deciding between operative and non-operative management of pediatric facial fractures, the practitioner is essentially weighing the risk of growth disturbance against the benefit of precise reduction and rigid fixation. In the immature craniofacial skeleton with minimally displaced fractures, a conservative approach is logical. For the older child approaching skeletal maturity with significantly displaced fractures, treatment is similarly straightforward with open reduction and internal fixation (ORIF). However, these two scenarios represent "tails of the bell-shaped curve" with "black and white" decision-making. Most practitioners are faced with a very large "gray area" in between, representing the vast majority of pediatric facial fractures – specifically, the conundrum of "what to do" with the minimally displaced fracture in the immature craniofacial skeleton.

The younger the patient, the higher the threshold for operative intervention. If operative intervention is pursued, while it is critical to visualize fracture lines adequately, periosteal stripping should be minimized as, in accordance with Moss and Salentijn's "functional matrix" principle, stripping may adversely affect growth and development.[37] Growth disturbances are felt by some to be minimized by using absorbable plating systems in skeletally immature patients. A 10-year retrospective review of 44 patients demonstrated resorbable plates and screws can be an effective fixation method for facial fractures in children in the primary and mixed dentition periods. Whether used for plate fixation of fractures of the tooth-bearing region of the mandible, a bone-anchored method of mandibulomaxillary fixation (MMF), or in the very low load-bearing upper and midface regions, they provide adequate stability for the rapid bone healing of youth. The blunt tips of the screws and their eventual resorption theoretically offer decreased risk to developing teeth and nerve structures or ongoing facial growth and eliminate long-term foreign body retention. No delayed foreign-body reactions or inflammation has been seen with the resorbable polymers used in this patient series.[38]

For mandible fractures, the authors have championed the safe and efficacious use of arch bars in patients during primary and mixed dentition as a challenge to conventional teaching. A cohort of 23 pediatric patients with mandible fractures were successfully treated with the aid of arch bars. There were no periodontal defects, tooth avulsions, or disturbances to permanent dentition noted with regard to arch bar use.[39]

While some surgeons favor delaying intervention of facial fractures until swelling resolves, others note the pediatric craniofacial skeleton's enhanced healing: loose fragments may adhere within 3–4 days of injury.[26] Converse advocated prompt repair in the 1960s.[40] The authors maintain that if the decision is made to operate, this should be done early so long as the degree of swelling is not prohibitive.

Outcomes, prognosis, and complications

Outcomes and complications in pediatric facial fractures are understudied. A broad range of complication rates in the literature (2.6–21.6%) implies vague documentation of these injuries.[9,41,42] Photographic, radiographic, and functional documentation over time is essential in developing literature to inform our ongoing treatment of these potentially life-altering

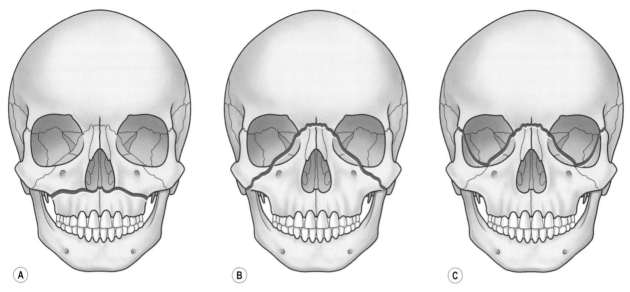

Fig. 29.6 These are the classic Le Fort fracture patterns described in adult craniofacial fractures: **(A)** Le Fort I; **(B)** Le Fort II; **(C)** Le Fort III. Children exhibit distinct fracture patterns, as described in the text and demonstrated in Figs. 29.7 and 29.8.

injuries. Meaningful outcomes analysis in this field is dependent on improved standardization of data collection.[43] To this end, the authors have introduced a classification system to facilitate the clear characterization and discussion of adverse outcomes in these injuries.[44] Type 1 adverse outcomes are intrinsic to the fracture itself (i.e., blindness following orbital fracture, tooth loss following mandibular fracture). Type 2 adverse outcomes are directly secondary to surgical management (i.e., ectropion following subciliary incision, enophthalmos following orbital fracture repair). Type 3 adverse outcomes are those subsequent to the fracture itself, its treatment, and/or the subsequent altered growth and development – such as the development of a class II malocclusion many years following mandibular fracture (Table 29.1). Specifically, whether the subsequent mandibular hypoplasia and class II malocclusion were the result of the mandibular fracture, its treatment with ORIF, or an inherent growth issue that would have resulted in such a malocclusion despite sustaining a fracture.

Infection, nonunion, and malunion are rare in comparison to adults; secondary to increased osteogenesis; less frequent indications for open reduction; and a lower frequency of severely displaced fractures in children.[15] Metallic cranial hardware may pose a direct hazard to growing children as it may translocate intracranially secondary to ectocranial bone deposition and endocranial bone resorption (Figs. 29.15 & 29.16).

Growth outcomes

Growth disturbance secondary to facial trauma is an incompletely understood phenomenon. Furthermore, establishing whether it is the initial trauma, the subsequent management, or contributions from both affecting facial growth remains equally uncertain. Mustoe *et al.* concluded that closed reduction of nasal fractures is not deleterious for growth.[45] Invasive rhinoplasty is similarly benign according to Ortiz-Monasterio and Olmedo.[46] Other authors express significant concern for

subsequent growth effects.[47,48] Complete resection of the septum, as in hypertelorism correction, is well documented to have devastating effects on the growth and development of the midface.[49] Severe bony and cartilaginous central facial injury has been suggested to result in growth and developmental anomalies in up to 40% of patients.[21] However, this does not represent an undisputed consensus in the literature. Schliephake *et al.* examined 12 patients who had suffered midface fractures during their childhood, and no correlation was found between the age, the severity of injuries, surgical treatment, and resulting deformities.[50]

The contribution of hardware to growth retardation is not clear. Laurenzo *et al.* examined the effects of soft-tissue manipulation, rigid microplate fixation, and multiple osteotomies on the growing midface in rabbits. Disturbances in craniofacial growth were produced by rigid plate fixation as well as *de novo* by trauma, independent of fixation.[51] Other groups, however, have demonstrated regional bone growth compensation that may overcome local growth restriction in response to craniomaxillofacial bone planting in infant rabbits, such that there is no long-term impairment.[52,53] Berryhill *et al.*

Table 29.1 Authors' classification system for adverse outcomes in pediatric facial fractures

Classification	Definition	Example
Type 1	Intrinsic to fracture	Loss of permanent tooth with mandible fracture
Type 2	Secondary to intervention	Marginal mandibular nerve injury during open reduction, internal fixation of mandibular fracture
Type 3	Subsequent to growth and development	Asymmetric mandibular growth after condylar fracture

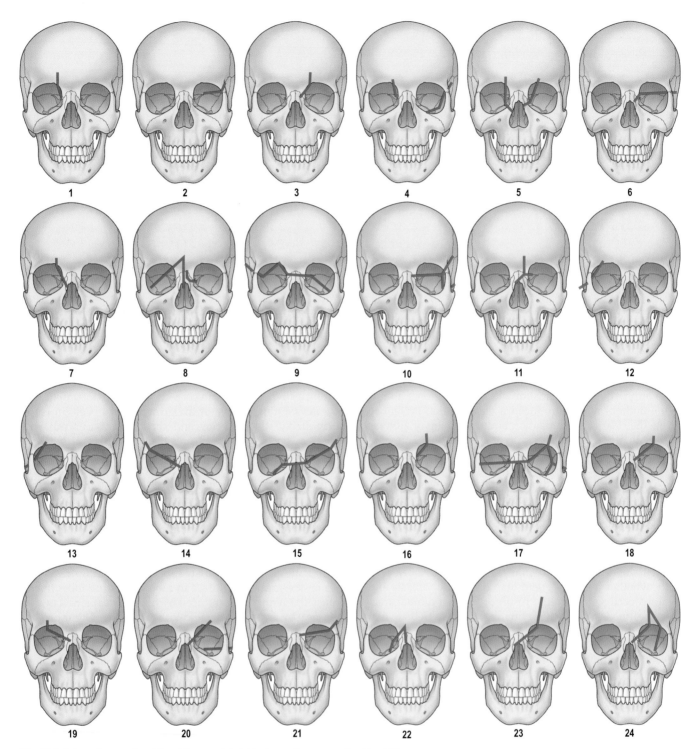

Fig. 29.7 Schematic examples of the oblique craniofacial fracture patterns encountered in children.

reported 6 of 96 children with facial fractures undergoing ORIF to have experienced delayed or restricted growth. As they state, however, it is impossible to separate the developmental effects of fixation from other intrinsic and extrinsic factors.[54] At an average of 3 years after treatment, the authors' cohort of mandible fractures did not demonstrate growth disturbances.[10] In severe midface trauma, however, the authors have described clinically significant impairment in growth in up to 86% of cases.[19]

Secondary procedures

Imola *et al.* provide a useful overview of secondary procedures that may be required in managing craniofacial fractures.[55] Soft-tissue deformity and the evolution of a scarred soft-tissue envelope are the single greatest barriers to optimal outcomes. Poorly reduced fractures may require osteotomy and repeat ORIF. Traumatic telecanthus may require

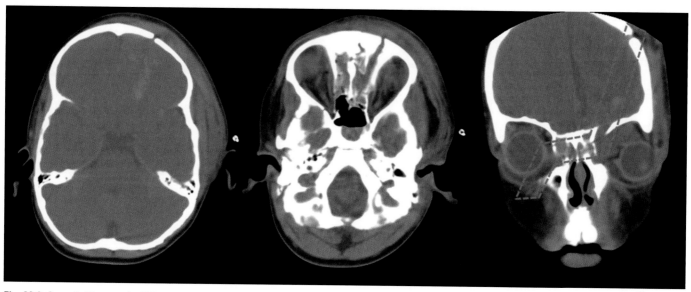

Fig. 29.8 Computed tomography (CT) scans in the axial plane demonstrate an oblique fracture at the level of the cranium (left) and cranial base (center). Right, the CT scan represents a sagittal reconstruction of the same patient, with the course of the oblique fracture outlined in red.

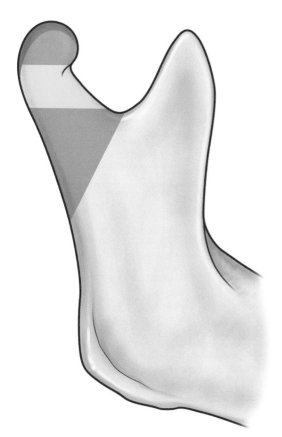

Fig. 29.9 Anatomical vocabulary pertaining to the mandibular condyle. The condylar head is green (except its articular surface, which is blue), the condylar neck is yellow, and the subcondylar region is orange. Vague terminology in reference to these structures often causes confusion in the clinic and in the literature.

transnasal fixation; if the medial canthus must be reinserted, it is essential to ensure sufficiently superior and posterior positioning. Dorsal nasal deficiency may exacerbate the appearance of telecanthus, and this may also be surgically addressed. Mandibular growth disturbances may necessitate advancement genioplasty or distraction. Secondary correction of enophthalmos requires anterior globe repositioning, reduction of the orbital contents, and/or osteotomy and repositioning of skeletal components. VOD may require four-wall osteotomies for optimal results.[55] Diplopia may occur secondary to extraocular muscle dysfunction and/or globe malposition; the inferior rectus and superior oblique are the muscles most commonly involved. Growing skull fractures require dural repair and cranioplasty. Hardware removal may be indicated to minimize growth disturbances, to avoid risks associated with transcranial migration, or if the hardware is causing discomfort or aesthetic concern. Initial conservative approaches to nasal trauma is often practiced to mitigate iatrogenic impact on growth, albeit in the knowledge that definitive septorhinoplasty will likely be required to restore form at skeletal maturity.

Cranial base and skull fractures

Diagnosis and presentation

In children, between 10% and 30% of head injuries result in skull fracture. It is important to remember that for the growing child prior to development of a frontal sinus, forehead trauma could result in skull and cranial base fractures. Patients must be evaluated for evidence of fracture displacement, cerebrospinal fluid (CSF) leak, intracranial hematoma, deformed facial contour, frontal-lobe contusion with mass effect, and growing skull fracture. These may be indications for operative management.

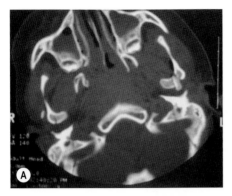

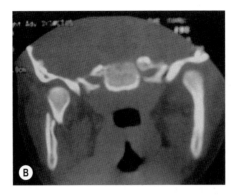

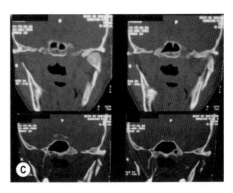

Fig. 29.10 **(A)** Axial computed tomography scan demonstrating condylar head fractures. **(B)** Coronal view of a condylar neck fracture. **(C)** Serial coronal views of a subcondylar fracture. *(Reproduced from Mathes S, Hentz V.* Plastic Surgery, *2nd edn. Philadelphia, PA: Elsevier; 2006.)*

Treatment

Pediatric skull fractures remain distinct from their adult counterpart with a greater capacity to heal and remodel such that the majority of pediatric skull fractures can be managed conservatively.[56,57] The authors performed a retrospective review of 897 pediatric patients with a skull fracture. Of these patients, 86% were treated non-operatively. The remaining patients were grouped according to the indication for their surgical intervention; 6.5% underwent repair of the fracture

for fracture elevation, frontal sinus repair, open fracture debridement, or cosmetic repair; 7.5% required intervention for treatment of a traumatic brain injury including hematoma evacuation, external ventricular drain (EVD) placement, or decompressive craniectomy.[57]

Goals of cranial base and skull fracture repair include protection of the neurocapsule, dural reconstruction and control of CSF leaks, prevention of infection, and aesthetic restoration of craniofacial contour. A functioning sinus capable of adequate drainage through growth and development must be achieved. A coronal incision allows for craniotomy and ORIF (Figs. 29.17–29.19). After exposing fractures with subperiosteal dissection, fracture fragments must be removed to inspect the underlying dura. Epidural hematomas are evacuated, and dural lacerations are repaired by the pediatric neurosurgical team. The bone fragments are then replaced and fixated. Caution must be exercised in manipulating frontal–temporal orbital fractures given the proximity to the

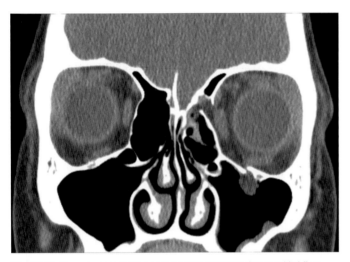

Fig. 29.11 Coronal computed tomography scan demonstrating an orbital floor fracture with an entrapped inferior rectus muscle on the patient's left side.

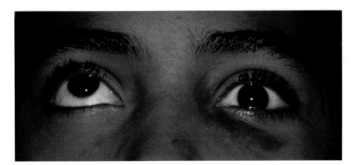

Fig. 29.12 Patient with an entrapped left inferior rectus. He is being instructed to "look up", but is unable to do so with his left eye due to the entrapped inferior rectus.

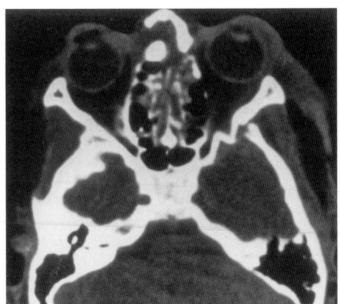

Fig. 29.13 Superior orbital fissure (SOF) syndrome may well result from the injury demonstrated in this axial computed tomography scan, in which a left frontal–temporal–orbital fracture has collapsed the SOF. *(Reproduced from Mathes S, Hentz V.* Plastic Surgery, *2nd edn. Philadelphia, PA: Elsevier; 2006.)*

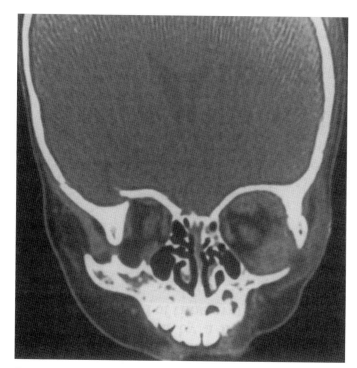

Fig. 29.14 Coronal computed tomography scan demonstrating a right frontal–temporal–orbital fracture. The lateral orbital wall is compressed medially, decreasing orbital volume and resulting in exophthalmos. *(Reproduced from Mathes S, Hentz V. Plastic Surgery, 2nd edn. Philadelphia, PA: Elsevier; 2006.)*

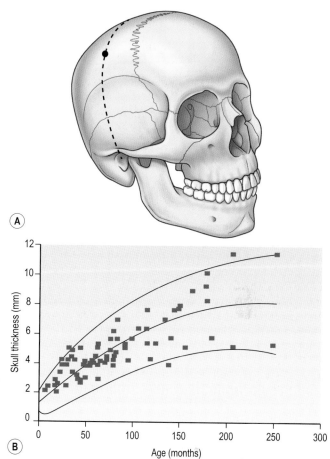

Fig. 29.15 (A, B) The skull increases in thickness with craniofacial development in a relationship reported by Pensler and McCarthy. *(Redrawn from Pensler J, McCarthy JG. The calvarial donor site: an anatomic study in cadavers. Plast Reconstr Surg. 1985;75:648.)*

middle meningeal artery. For patients mature enough to have a frontal sinus, Rodriguez *et al.* present a useful algorithm of approach.[58] If the nasofrontal duct is obstructed, obliteration or cranialization is indicated (see Fig. 29.18). Advantages of cranialization over obliteration include wide exposure of the injured area and single-stage elimination of the sinus as a potential focus of infection. If the duct is traumatized but still patent, nondisplaced anterior and posterior table fractures can be carefully followed. Severely displaced anterior table fractures can be reconstructed. If the frontal sinus is preserved, serial CTs must be followed to ensure proper sinus development and adequate drainage, and the nasofrontal ducts may be stented via an endonasal approach. The presence of a CSF leak directs management decisions regarding frontal sinus fractures.[59] Leaks are observed for 4–7 days of bed rest, possibly with lumbar drain, and cranialization is performed if the leak persists. If the leak stops and the nasofrontal duct is unobstructed, the sinus may be preserved. In the case of an autocorrected leak with an obstructed duct, anterior table ORIF is accompanied by "partial obliteration" (use of fracture fragments to obliterate only the nasofrontal duct and the base of the frontal sinus) following complete removal of sinus mucosa. For the patient with a minimal to moderate isolated anterior table fracture with cosmetic concerns only, the authors have reported on a single 11-year-old patient with a depressed frontal sinus fracture who was a candidate for surgical repair. The patient chose no treatment, and at 1-year follow-up the fracture was entirely remodeled – presumably secondary to ongoing development and the complete pneumatization of the immature frontal sinus.[56]

For the immature patient, cranial bone loss is a difficult problem, especially in children too old (over 2 years) to spontaneously regenerate large calvarial defects, yet in whom split calvarial grafts are unreliable due to an underdeveloped diploic space.[60,61] This is controversial, however, as several authors have described split calvarial grafts in young children, even those less than 1 year of age.[62–64] It is the authors' belief that despite the technical ability to split calvarial bone, the concern lies in the quality of the bone product obtained for reconstruction. Significant donor site morbidity (infection, pain, hemorrhage, and nerve injury) in up to 8% of patients, as well as low tissue yield, limits the usefulness of autogenous

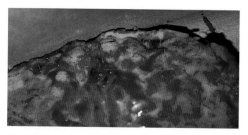

Fig. 29.16 Endocranial surface of a calvarial bone flap demonstrating transcranial migration of metallic hardware in a pediatric patient. *(Reproduced from Guyuron B, Erikkson E, Persing J, et al. Plastic Surgery: Indications and Practice. Philadelphia, PA: Elsevier; 2008.)*

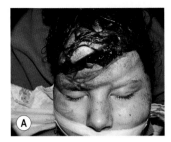
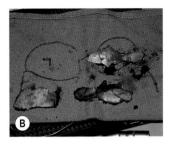
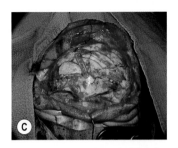
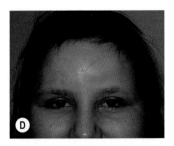

Fig. 29.17 **(A)** Frontal bone fracture after a motor vehicle collision. The bone fragments are mapped out as shown in **(B)** before they are reconstructed with absorbable plates, as in **(C)**. **(D)** The 6-month follow-up result. *(Reproduced from Guyuron B, Erikkson E, Persing J, et al. Plastic surgery: indications and practice. Philadelphia, PA: Elsevier; 2008.)*

bone grafts.[65] Bone substitutes are limited by a lack of biocompatibility and susceptibility to infection.[66] In patients with favorable wound conditions, the authors favor a bilaminate construct composed of intra- and extracranially placed bioresorbable mesh with interposed demineralized bone matrix mixed with bone dust and chips.[67] The authors are cautiously optimistic that a potential future role may exist for protein therapy in pediatric craniofacial reconstruction.[68,69] The role of prophylactic antibiotics in pediatric skull fractures remains unclear.

Outcomes, prognosis, and complications

These injuries may be complicated by CSF leak, meningitis, sinusitis, mucoceles, mucopyoceles, or brain abscesses. CSF leaks usually resolve spontaneously within 1 week; if the leak persists, a 5–7-day lumbar drain trial should precede operative intervention.[70,71] A cranial base fracture with an occult dural disruption may lead to a "growing skull fracture" secondary to cerebral pulsations enlarging even innocent-appearing cranial base fractures. Growing skull fractures complicate 0.03–1% of skull fractures and usually occur in patients younger than 3 years of age.[72,73] Missed growing skull fractures may lead to gliosis, lateral ventricular dilation, cerebral herniation, pulsatile exophthalmos, and VOD.[28]

In the authors' series, of those patients undergoing surgical intervention for cranial and skull base fractures, 42% experienced complications, of which 24% were surgery related and 76% were related to the initial trauma. These included wound infection, painful hardware, and CSF leaks.

Orbital fractures

Diagnosis and presentation

The clinical diagnosis of pediatric orbital fractures may be complicated by the difficulty of achieving a complete examination in an uncooperative patient. When there is any suspicion of fracture or neurological injury, CT scanning should

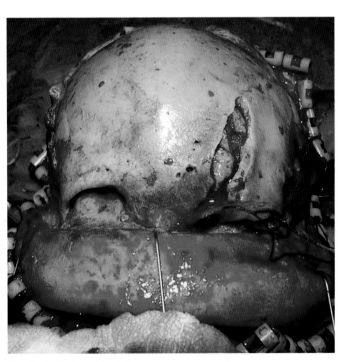

Fig. 29.18 Fracture of frontal bone.

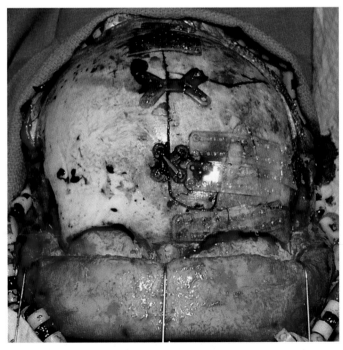

Fig. 29.19 The fracture shown in Fig. 29.18 has been reconstructed according to the method depicted in Fig. 29.17.

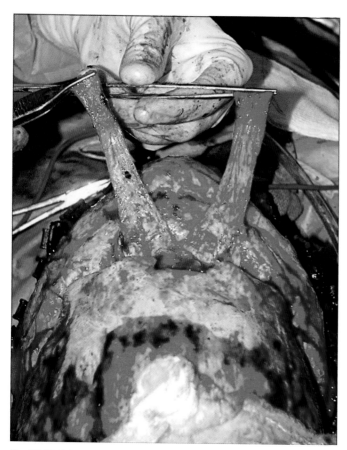

Fig. 29.20 Galeal flaps pedicled at the level of the brow have been raised to line the reconstructed anterior cranial base. A maneuver such as this is required to ensure that a barrier is in place to protect the intracranial contents from "the outside world". *(Reproduced from Guyuron B, Erikksson E, Persing J, et al. Plastic Surgery: Indications and Practice. Philadelphia, PA: Elsevier; 2008.)*

faster than the soft tissues can recoil, and the bony edges of the fracture incarcerate the trapped soft tissue, strangulating it. As well, for those children who do have phenotypically "adult-like" orbital fractures resulting in bony displacement and defect, resulting enophthalmos and VOD are less likely to occur, possibly due to more elastic and robust orbital periosteum and supporting ligaments (Fig. 29.20).[76]

Treatment

In the absence of entrapment or acute globe malposition (enophthalmos and/or VOD), orbital fractures in children are otherwise treated non-operatively; the predictors of late enophthalmos described for adults may be less relevant in children due to the hypothesized resistance of ligaments and periosteum to tearing, thereby preventing expansion of intraorbital volume and possibly guiding subsequent bone healing.[76–81] Stronger supporting structures may render open reduction, internal fixation (ORIF) less necessary in these fractures. The authors analyzed operative necessity in the context of a three-group orbital fracture classification system (*n* = 81): type 1, pure orbital fractures (limited to the orbit without extension to adjacent bones); type 2, craniofacial fractures (oblique fractures extending from the skull into the orbital roof and face); type 3, orbital fractures contributing to described patterns (impure blowout, ZMC, NOE) (Table 29.2).[76] Type 1 fractures were non-operative (88%) unless there was evidence of acute enophthalmos, VOD, or muscle entrapment on forced duction. Type 2 fractures were managed conservatively and tracked with serial scans until an absolute operative indication was encountered (17% were ultimately operative). Type 3 fractures were more likely (72%) to require operative intervention because of the functional disability secondary to enophthalmos and/or VOD. Overall, 23 (28.3%) orbits were managed operatively.[76] Success with this conservative strategy is evidenced by a low rate of adverse outcomes.

The goals of orbital fracture treatment include the restoration of globe position and the correction of diplopia. If ORIF is necessary, some authors have opined that the

ensue. In 1965, Soll and Poley published a paper on 4 young patients with a history of orbital trauma with minimal evidence of injury on imaging. During surgery, they noted orbital tissues trapped within linear or wedge-shaped floor fractures. This report was the first to demonstrate that the internal orbital fractures in children are different than those in adults. Whereas adults have comminution, pediatric orbital fractures, with children's more flexible bones, tend to sustain linear and/or trapdoor fractures.[74] In 1998, Jordan and colleagues coined the term white-eyed blowout fracture. They are white-eyed because there is no subconjunctival ecchymosis.[36] The eye looks uninjured; however, the patient will have severe restriction of gaze secondary to entrapped tissue in a fracture line that may be so small that there is no CT evidence of a fracture, but the involved rectus muscle is not within the orbit, instead being found within the sinus; so-called "missing muscle syndrome".[75] This is often associated with the oculocardiac reflex (bradycardia, nausea and syncope) and is an absolute indication for urgent surgical intervention. The mechanism by which these injuries occurs is an increase in intraorbital pressure from the traumatizing force, which creates a linear or trapdoor fracture of the bony floor or wall. As the fracture opens, the periorbital soft tissues are pushed through the open space. Because the bones in children are elastic, the bone snaps back into position very quickly, much

Table 29.2 The authors' orbital fracture classification system	
Type 1	**Pure orbital fractures**
1a	Floor fractures
1b	Medial wall fractures
1c	Roof fractures
1d	Lateral wall fractures
1e	Combined floor and medial wall fractures
Type 2	**Craniofacial fractures**
2a	Growing skull fractures
Type 3	**Orbital fractures associated with common fracture patterns**
3a	Fractures of the floor and inferior orbital rim
3b	Zygomaticomaxillary fractures
3c	Naso-orbito-ethmoid fractures
3d	Other fracture patterns

transconjunctival approach to the orbit is preferred secondary to good cosmesis and a lower risk of ectropion. If lateral exposure is necessary, a subciliary or mid-lid incision with lateral "crow's foot" extension avoids the lateral cantholysis that may be necessary with a transconjunctival incision and affords generous exposure extending to the lateral–superior orbital rim/orbit. If medial exposure is necessary, a transcaruncular approach is performed, often obviating the need for a coronal incision. A gingival buccal sulcus incision can be added if necessary. Herniated tissues are reduced from the fracture, the fracture is cleared of debris, and stable foundations for fixation and grafting are identified (in the pediatric population, this being autologous bone and/or resorbable mesh).

In adults, because of the thinness of the bony orbital walls, the bone usually shatters when injured, so one cannot simply reduce the bones of the orbit. The bones are missing or non-usable. Sheets of bone or another biomaterial are required to replace the bony walls to restore the pretrauma anatomy. With linear or trapdoor fractures in the pediatric patient, however, once the soft tissues have been carefully removed from the fracture, the defect may not require reconstruction. If the defect has been made larger or a residual defect exists, reconstructing it with whatever biomaterial the surgeon chooses may be necessary.[82] Particularly for the pediatric population, there are advocates for resorbable implants. Typically, this involves the use of a material made of a polymer of polylactic and polyglycolic acid. These implants all resorb over one or more years. Theoretically, the implant leaves a sheet of fibrous tissue, allowing support of the globe that is sufficient once the implant has resorbed, and published studies have not shown problems with enophthalmos once the implant is gone.[81] Alternatively, split calvarial grafts can be used (Fig. 29.21). Some surgeons suggest that over time these can remodel to recapitulate normal anatomy and growth. In the case of repair of orbital floor fractures, irrespective of the implant used, placement along the orbital floor behind the vertical axis of the globe to recreate the convexity or upward bulge of the maxillary sinus is important to maintain the anterior position of the globe.[82,83] The implant should be secured to prevent mobility and/or extrusion. In the operating room, immediately after reconstruction, the surgeon should evaluate globe position; and a slightly overcorrected, proptotic appearance to the eye is the hallmark of an anatomic reconstruction, owing to edema induced by surgery. However, there should be no vertical asymmetry (hyperglobus) of the reconstructed globe, because this will not change as the edema resolves. Care must be taken to resuspend midface soft tissues when closing the incisions.

Outcomes, prognosis, and complications

As with adults, potential complications include retrobulbar hematoma, orbital cellulitis, lid malposition, persistent enophthalmos and persistent diplopia.[84] Retrobulbar hematoma is an uncommon but potentially vision-threatening complication that presents with worsening pain, proptosis, internal ophthalmoplegia, impairment, or loss of the pupillary reflex. Management necessitates orbital decompression with urgent lateral canthotomy and cantholysis as well as adjunctive pharmacologic treatment with mannitol, acetazolamide, corticosteroids, and timolol. Orbital cellulitis is also rare but may be more common if there is evidence of concomitant paranasal sinusitis at time of fracture or operative repair. Periorbital pain, erythema, and edema warrants treatment with intravenous antibiotics and surgical drainage of any abscess. If left untreated, it can lead to blindness, cavernous sinus thrombosis, meningitis, or cerebral abscess. There is no evidence that routine antibiotic prophylaxis affects risk. Lid retraction/ectropion and entropion are a risk of any incision in the lid with a higher risk of ectropion seen with subciliary incisions. This may be temporary and respond to lid massage and closure exercises if mild. If persistent, repair is not easily remedied and may involve canthopexy, mucosal grafts, and skin grafts. Some orbital fractures will result in diplopia due to initial edema or trauma to the orbital contents, similarly seen in the early postoperative period. Persistent postoperative diplopia, despite adequate surgical correction, may necessitate strabismus surgery. Enophthalmos can be measured objectively by exophthalmometry or subjectively by noting posterior displacement of the globe on worm's-eye view, asymmetry of the upper eyelid creases, and asymmetry in the distance between ciliary margin and superior and inferior limbus.[76] Enophthalmos can sometimes be corrected by orbital floor or wall bone grafting, but may require osteotomies and bony relocation and possibly lateral or medial canthal adjustment.

In the authors' series, 10.7% of isolated orbital fractures suffered adverse outcomes: type 1: 3.6%; type 2: 3.6%; and type 3: 3.6%. Three patients with isolated orbital fractures had enophthalmos, all less than the clinically significant threshold of 2 mm. Persistent diplopia did not occur in the authors' series but was reported to be as high as 36% in a study by Cope et al.[76,85]

Nasal and naso-orbito-ethmoid fractures

Diagnosis and presentation

Children's noses are structurally different from the adult nose. The pattern of injury follows this underlying anatomy. In very young children, nasal fractures are uncommon because of the underdeveloped nasal bones. Instead, the projecting soft tissues of the anterior nose are composed of compliant cartilages. These easily bend during facial trauma. Blunt force is

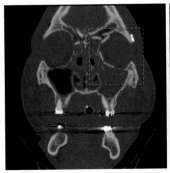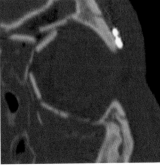

Fig. 29.21 Coronal computed tomography scan demonstrating orbital reconstruction with split calvarial grafts (the image on the right is a magnified view of the area outlined in red in the image on the left).

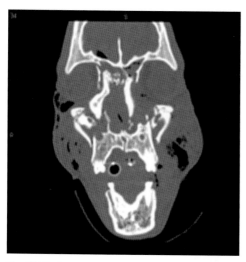

Fig. 29.22 Coronal computed tomography scan demonstrating bilateral naso-orbito-ethmoid fractures with their requisite "central fragments".

dissipated across the maxilla and its buttresses. Subsequently, this results in widespread generalized edema. However, septal cartilage dislocation can result in acute airway obstruction and cause long-term growth disturbances. Children younger than 2 years tend to have flexible bones, making greenstick fractures more common. After the age of 2 to 3 years, increased bone mineralization makes greenstick fractures less common.[86,87]

Patients should be evaluated for subjective nasal airway obstruction and assessed for nasal deviation, compressibility of the nasal dorsum, lacerations, crepitus, edema, tenderness, depression, and deviation, or widening of the nasal base. Adequate internal examination requires a nasal speculum. Attention should be directed to an evaluation of the septum to rule out associated hematoma, fracture, or obstruction.

NOE fractures are characterized by posterior and lateral displacement of the nasal bones and medial orbital rims, with fractures of the medial orbital walls and ethmoids. A free medial orbital rim segment containing the insertion of the medial canthus (the "central fragment") (Fig. 29.22) results in traumatic telecanthus. Even if not immediately apparent, telecanthus may develop 7–10 days after trauma. Other typical deformities suggesting NOE fracture include a shortened nose with upturned tip and saddle nose deformity with blunted dorsal nasal projection. The lack of a well-developed frontal sinus in young children decreases this region's ability to absorb blunt force and act as a "crumple zone", resulting in force being directed into the supraorbital bar, basilar skull, and intracranially. Hence, heightened suspicion of intracranial injury is mandatory in a child with NOE fractures.[86,87]

Treatment

Septal hematomas warrant immediate intervention with an incision through the mucoperiosteum. If bilateral septal incisions are made, overlap must be avoided as septal perforation may result. Dead space may be eliminated with septal quilting sutures or internal splints to compress the mucoperichondrium to the septal cartilage.

Non-displaced or minimally displaced nasal fractures may be externally splinted. In the case of a displaced fracture,

closed reduction may be inadequate secondary to insufficient release of tension on the septum, cartilages, and bony pyramid. However, aggressive open treatment in children has significant potential to affect facial growth adversely. Therefore a closed reduction is usually offered to children with definitive open management delayed until skeletal maturity. Uncomplicated injuries to the nasal septum (i.e., septal cartilage dislocations from the maxillary crest) can also be managed in a closed fashion.

Pediatric patients, given their ability to heal more quickly, need reduction sooner, typically 3–7 days after injury.[87–90] Several authors have, however, demonstrated no significant differences in outcomes of airway obstruction and cosmesis between pediatric nasal fractures treated early and those with relatively delayed treatment.[91,92]

Septorhinoplasty following trauma in pediatric patients should arguably be reserved for severely displaced fractures, nasal obstruction resulting in sleep apnea, chronic mouth breathing (causing malocclusion), and chronic refractory sinus disease. Specific to the pediatric patient undergoing nasal surgery is the discussion that the expected benefits of an early intervention have to outweigh the possibility of iatrogenic inhibition of nasal growth. It should also be made clear that the short-term postsurgical improvements may diminish with future nasal growth and that revision surgery is a possibility. Intuitively, surgery should be less aggressive in younger children.[25] Another important caveat for pediatric patients is that a septoplasty can be safely performed as long as the surgeon avoids the growth center at the nasal spine of the maxilla.[87]

Pediatric NOE fractures are treated as in adults, and intercanthal distance must be restored to age-specific norms (Table 29.3) by reduction of the medial orbital rims. If necessary, the medial canthal tendons are reattached with transnasal wires passing superior and posterior to the posterior lacrimal crest (type 2 and 3 NOE fractures of the classification of Markowitz et al.).[93] A cantilever bone graft is employed to restore the nasal dorsal height. Complicated NOE fractures are exposed by coronal, inferior orbital rim, and gingival buccal sulcus incisions. As with pediatric septorhinoplasty, because of ongoing growth, children with NOE fractures may have a higher likelihood of requiring additional secondary surgery.[86] A high index of suspicion for intracranial injury must be maintained for fractures extending to the anterior skull base.

Outcomes, prognosis, and complications

Nasal fractures may result in an appearance deformity or functional airway obstruction. Nasal deviation may result

Table 29.3 Age-specific norms for interorbital distance (IOD)	
Age	**Normal interorbital distance**
Newborn	10–15 mm
2-year-old	20 mm
12-year-old	25 mm
Adult	35 mm
Radiographically: IOD = dacryon to dacryon. Clinically: IOD = Medial intercanthal distance (MICD) − (4–6 mm).	

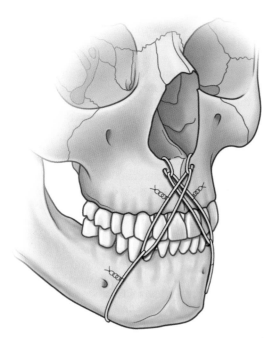

Fig. 29.23 Creative mandibulomaxillary fixation strategies are often required in children.

from cartilaginous warping or incomplete reduction. An untreated septal hematoma may yield septal thickening or perforation, and ultimate saddle-nose deformity. Excessive callous formation and bony overgrowth may lead to a dorsal hump. As previously stated, these may require secondary septorhinoplasty. As such, long-term follow-up with postoperative examination and photographic documentation is essential. There are few long-term follow-ups to address possible growth disturbances after pediatric NOE fractures.

One review included 20 patients who sustained midface fractures with an NOE component. Eight (40%) of these patients required further surgery for various deformities; of these, 6 required additional bone grafting to the nasal dorsum and canthal repositioning, 1 required further frontal bone recontouring, and 1 had midface hypoplasia.[21] One study reports a 5% rate of late lacrimal obstruction after ORIF of NOE fractures. This is managed with dacrocystorhinostomy.[94] In the authors' series, 21.7% of nasal fractures exhibited adverse outcomes (type 1: 8.7% and type 3: 17.4%) consisting of persistent nasal deformity or airway obstruction.[8] Secondary corrective surgery should be delayed until after skeletal maturity unless clinically significant nasal airway obstruction is present.

Maxillary, zygomaticomaxillary complex and midface fractures

Diagnosis and presentation

Clinical symptoms and signs of these midfacial fractures are similar to adults; however, because of the aforementioned small paranasal sinuses and unerupted tooth buds in children, midface fractures of the classical Le Fort patterns are unusual. Examination of the patient may reveal palatal, vestibular, and

periorbital ecchymosis, edema, oral mucosa and conjunctival hemorrhage, and flattening, widening, and elongation of the middle third of the face. Assessment of facial contour, including dental arches, palate, nasal bridge, forehead, zygomaticofrontal, and zygomaticomaxillary sutures, may reveal tenderness, malocclusion or mobility suggestive of fracture. Confirmation with CT imaging is the gold standard especially given that Greenstick fractures arise in higher frequency in children and are otherwise of increased difficulty to detect.[95,96]

Treatment

Treatment of pediatric midface fractures again is similar to in the adult and must aim to achieve satisfactory reduction and sufficiently stable fixation to permit bone healing whilst avoiding disturbance to future growth.

Non-operative management is indicated for minimally displaced and greenstick midface fractures, especially in younger children. Conservative management in such cases is characterized by soft diet and regular re-examination until fracture healing.

Displaced and unstable fractures require either closed reduction and splinting with mandibulomaxillary fixation (MMF) or ORIF. The requirements for both the rigidity and length of fixation are less than those of adults. Incompletely developed dentition can render arch bars difficult to apply, often requiring creative strategies such as circum-mandibular wiring and piriform suspension wiring (Figs. 29.23 & 29.24). Arch bars, despite conventional teaching, can, however, be safely employed during primary and mixed dentition.[39] Depending upon the patient's age, shorter courses of MMF are acceptable; some authors advocate fixation for 1 week or less,[1] followed by dental elastics in the very young.

When ORIF is necessary, the operator must avoid injuring developing tooth buds when plating the facial buttresses. Furthermore, resorbable plating systems are gaining increasing popularity for their perceived decreased risk of resultant growth disturbances compared with their permanent

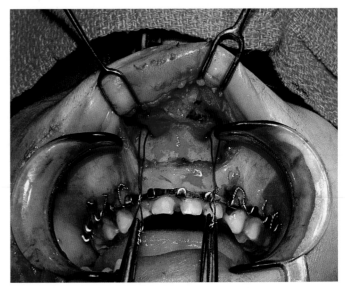

Fig. 29.24 Drop piriform wires being placed for mandibulomaxillary fixation in a pediatric patient. *(Reproduced from Guyuron B, Erikkson E, Persing J, et al. Plastic Surgery: Indications and Practice. Philadelphia, PA: Elsevier; 2008.)*

counterparts. Otherwise, strategies of ORIF of midface fractures replicate those practiced in adults. Operative goals in ZMC fracture management, therefore, include resolution of orbital injury (VOD, enophthalmos), correction of malocclusion, and the restoration of appearance (malar flattening). The zygoma is aesthetically responsible for the malar eminence, and an inferiorly displaced zygoma may displace the lateral canthus via its attachment to Whitnall's tubercle. Access to the ZF suture may be gained through a subciliary incision, a subconjunctival approach with lateral cantholysis, or the lateral portion of an upper lid blepharoplasty incision. Additional exposure is obtained with an upper buccal sulcus incision. Some authors have reported that medially impacted large fragment fractures may be addressed through an upper gingival buccal sulcus incision alone with exposure of the anterior face of the zygoma, fracture reduction, and confirmation of orbital floor continuity with endoscopy via the maxillary sinus.[31] It is generally accepted that adequate reduction at the lateral wall of the orbit or the greater wing of the sphenoid is essential to proper reconstruction; reduction must also be achieved at the lateral orbital rim/ZF suture, inferior orbital rim, and the zygomaticomaxillary (ZM) buttress. Fixation is then performed sequentially at the ZF suture, the inferior orbital rim, and the ZM buttress. The operator must ensure that orbital volume and morphology are not altered by the initial injury or the reduction, and floor reconstruction may be required in the procedure.[34]

Outcomes, prognosis, and complications

Maxillary fractures may result in nasolacrimal obstruction or malocclusion. Adverse outcomes following ZMC fracture repair include persistent infraorbital nerve (V2) hypothesia, enophthalmos, VOD, facial widening, malar flattening, canthal deformity, and ectropion secondary to lower lid approaches. Zygomatic–coronoid ankylosis may occur after severe zygomatic fracture.[31] Pediatric patients undergoing MMF may be particularly vulnerable to malnutrition which is best avoided by thorough nutritional counseling, proper education, and resource availability.

The authors have followed a cohort of children suffering from midface fractures over time in a long-term growth and development study. Severe pediatric midface trauma (i.e. involving orbital fractures and at least half the midface buttresses) was found to often result in compromised bone growth and permanent facial deformity. Surgical intervention to restore projection and realignment is a necessity in these massive injuries, which are rare. The relative contribution of injury pattern and severity, as well as operative management, on growth and development remains unclear.[19]

Mandible fractures

Diagnosis and presentation

Children with mandibular trauma are at risk for airway compromise. Airway obstruction must first be addressed with repositioning, suctioning, or finger sweep (to remove any blood, loose teeth or foreign bodies, etc). Maneuvers such as jaw thrust, anterior traction, or a tongue stitch may also be adopted. Ultimately, endotracheal intubation or establishment

of a surgical airway may be necessary. Cervical spine and head injury must also always be considered and be evaluated for with clinical examination and CT imaging as appropriate.

Lacerations, ecchymosis, and edema may herald underlying fractures locations. Classically, a submental laceration is suggestive of a superiorly orientated midline force and possible injury to the condyles. Paresthesias in the distribution of the inferior alveolar nerve can result from body fractures. Lingual and buccal paresthesias can also occur in displaced fractures. The patient should be asked about how his or her bite feels and about pain, particularly. Drooling and trismus may be seen in association with mandible fractures. Bimanual examination of the mandible can reveal bony step-offs. Palpation of the temporomandibular joints at the external auditory canal during jaw movement may disclose a displaced condylar head or crepitation. External auditory canal bleeding and ecchymosis can also occur. Thorough intraoral exam must also be performed to assess occlusion and any dental injury. Panorex was historically considered to be the imaging modality of choice, although this has now largely been superseded by CT imaging. The most fundamental aspect of diagnosis and the need for intervention is determination of any subjective malocclusion.[97]

Treatment

Goals in the management of mandible fractures include the preservation or restoration of normal occlusion and the achievement of bony union while minimizing potential growth disturbance and injury to developing tooth follicles. For the immature skeleton, the exfoliation of primary teeth and subsequent ability to remodel the jaws, as well as the possibility of future orthodonture, favors the acceptance of minor occlusal discrepancies, rather than aggressive treatment (i.e., ORIF) to restore "perfect" occlusion, in the child with mixed dentition.

Nondisplaced fractures

Nondisplaced or minimally displaced mandibular fractures with normal occlusion in young children may be treated with jaw rest and immobilization with a "jaw bra" and/or cervical collar and liquid diet with regular re-examination until healed.[11] Minor malocclusions after fracture healing can be managed with orthodontics. Dentoalveolar fractures can often be managed conservatively with occlusive splinting, arch bars, or bonded wires in combination with soft diet, good oral hygiene, and mandible rest. Many pediatric patients are in mixed dentition; aside from wear facets, preinjury dental records are the surgeon's only ally in establishing preoperative occlusion. Occlusive splints can be fabricated based on these materials. If necessary, MMF may require creativity in children (see Figs. 29.23 & 29.24) but can be safely practiced.[39]

Condylar fractures

Assuming preserved occlusion, the operative indications for condylar fractures are more controversial. The pediatric condyles are regarded as growth centers, sensitive to disruptions of blood supply and morphology with resultant susceptibility to ankylosis and altered mandibular development.[98] Intracapsular injuries should be managed conservatively to minimize growth disturbance and TMJ ankylosis; the pediatric mandible

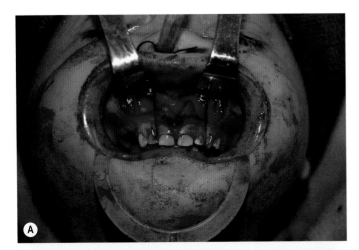

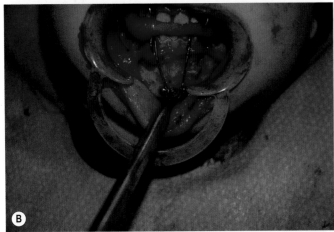

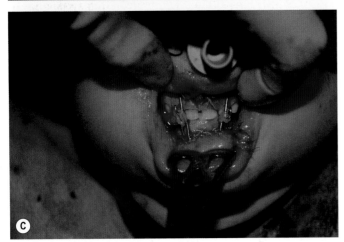

Fig. 29.25 Custom IMF hooks allow for range of motion at the TMJ with rigid fixation of parasymphyseal fracture in combined condylar and parasymphyseal fractures.

has the potential to undergo restitutional remodeling (condylar head regeneration). Unilateral condylar neck fractures are often adequately managed with closed reduction, arch bars, and contralateral elastics. Bilateral condylar neck fractures with a loss of posterior height and resultant anterior open bite may require a more aggressive approach. In younger children, these fractures can be managed with closed reduction and external fixation (MMF for 2–3 weeks). Some argue for a more aggressive approach to dislocated condylar neck fractures in

older children since the condyles are less likely to regenerate in children greater than 7 years of age and may require eventual osteotomy and cartilage grafting for TMJ function and normalization of occlusion.[99,100] In the case of bilateral neck fractures in the older patient, ORIF of one side is reasonable, with a short course of intermaxillary fixation. Other indications for open management include a foreign body in the TMJ, failure to normalize occlusion with closed management, and a condyle displaced into the middle cranial fossa. Every effort should be made to avoid open management for intracapsular fractures, high condylar neck fractures, coronoid fractures, and any fracture in which there are no barriers to motion and baseline occlusion is preserved.[11,101] Condylar head fractures themselves are treated with a short course of rest followed by physical therapy (such as gum chewing). A condylar head fracture in the presence of another mandible fracture is an indication for ORIF of the other fracture to allow for early TMJ motion. Of the 96 consecutive patients in the authors' series, 53% underwent operative management.[10] For combined condylar and parasymphyseal fractures, the most common bilateral mandible fracture combination, rigid fixation of the parasymphyseal fracture whilst allowing range of motion at the TMJ, can be achieved with customized IMF hooks (Fig. 29.25).

Displaced fractures

For displaced fractures with malocclusion requiring open treatment, existing lacerations and an intraoral approach should be utilized whenever possible. Given the immature mandible's ability to remodel under masticatory forces, as well as its amenability to orthodontic manipulation, it is wise to accept imperfect reduction and occlusion in order to preserve developing tooth follicles. Interosseous wiring of the mandibular border and a dental bridle wire and/or a short course of MMF may be adequate to maintain reduction (Fig. 29.26). If internal bony fixation is necessary in young patients,

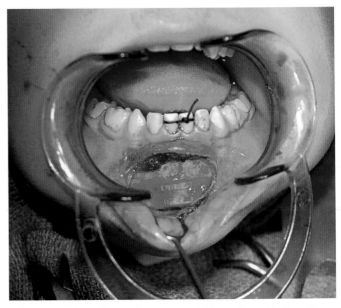

Fig. 29.26 Circumdental suture functions as a bridle wire in combination with an inferiorly placed monocortical adsorbable plate for a symphyseal fracture in a child. *(Reproduced from Guyuron B, Erikkson E, Persing J, et al. Plastic Surgery: Indications and Practice. Philadelphia, PA: Elsevier; 2008.)*

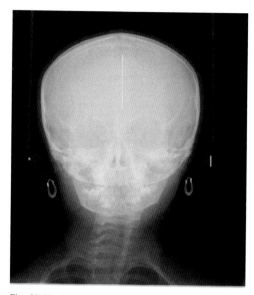

Fig. 29.27 Cephalogram of a patient 2 years after a left mandibular body fracture. The left mandibular ramus, angle, and body demonstrate decreased growth relative to the contralateral side.

was of functional significance. Type 1 outcomes were seen in 20% of operative patients and in 0% of conservatively managed patients ($P = 0.05$), type 2 outcomes were seen in 13.3% of operative patients and in no conservatively managed patients ($P = 0.115$), and type 3 outcomes were seen in 66.7% of operative patients and in 45% of conservatively managed patients ($P = 0.402$).[10] In another reported series, patients were at most risk for growth disturbances and facial asymmetry if they sustained mandibular fractures between 4 and 7 years of age and least likely to have growth sequelae if they were injured prior to 4 years of age (children greater than 11 years of age experienced an intermediate rate of growth disturbance) (Fig. 29.27). The authors of this series explain this age distribution by positing that children in the youngest group have better condylar blood flow, allowing for regeneration and avoidance of growth disturbances; moreover, they note that the majority of mandibular growth spurts occur at either end of their 4–7-year-old age group.[103]

monocortical screws should be utilized and hardware should be placed at the inferior mandibular border to avoid injury to developing tooth buds. Alternatively, resorbable plating systems can be used.[102]

Outcomes, prognosis, and complications

Mandible fractures may be complicated by growth disturbances or functional impairment such as malocclusion, trismus, or TMJ ankylosis. Marginal mandibular nerve injury may result from surgery. In the authors' series of 215 mandible fractures in 120 patients, each child undergoing surgery had a 63% chance of an adverse outcome as compared to 17% in children receiving conservative therapy. However, none of the adverse outcomes recorded (i.e., limited TMJ opening, persistent pain)

Conclusions

The craniofacial skeleton undergoes a dramatic structural and topographical metamorphosis as it matures from the infant to the adult state. The neonatal skull is profoundly different from its adult counterpart and therefore responds to traumatic forces with unique injury patterns. Specific functional and aesthetic criteria must be met in reconstructing the various regions of the pediatric craniofacial skeleton. These objectives must be achieved with strategies that properly balance respect for future growth. Craniofacial development, along with the resilience of the pediatric skull and supporting structures, often facilitates a less invasive approach to managing these complex injuries. Key principles of facial fracture management, unique to the pediatric population, include recognizing the potential for growing skull fractures, determining intervention for orbital fractures upon clinical rather than radiologic findings, and accepting mild malocclusion in pediatric mandibular fractures.

Access the complete reference list online at **http://www.expertconsult.com**

4. Ferreira PC, et al. Pediatric facial fractures: a review of 2071 fractures. *Ann Plast Surg.* 2016;77:54–60. *This large series describes nearly 1500 pediatric facial fracture patients over a 20-year period. Fracture patterns, demographics, and associated injuries were assessed.*

10. Smith DM, et al. 215 mandible fractures in 120 children: demographics, treatment, outcomes, and early growth data. *Plast Reconstr Surg.* 2013;131:1348–1358. *A 10-year study outlining management principles for pediatric mandible fractures.*

11. Smartt JM Jr, Low DW, Bartlett SP. The pediatric mandible: ii. management of traumatic injury or fracture. *Plast Reconstr Surg.* 2005;116:28e–41e.

19. Davidson EH, et al. Severe pediatric midface trauma: a prospective study of growth and development. *J Craniofac Surg.* 2015;26:1523–1528. *This prospective cephalometric study highlights the effect on growth and resultant facial deformity from severe pediatric midface trauma and the need for new methods of management.*

27. Smartt JM Jr, Low DW, Bartlett SP. The pediatric mandible: I. A primer on growth and development. *Plast Reconstr Surg.* 2005;116:14e–23e.

28. Havlik RJ, Sutton LN, Bartlett SP. Growing skull fractures and their craniofacial equivalents. *J Craniofac Surg.* 1995;6:103–110, discussion 111–112.

44. Losee J, Chao M. Complications in pediatric facial fractures. *Craniomaxillofac Trauma Reconstr.* 2009;2:103–112.

58. Rodriguez ED, Stanwix MG, Nam AJ, et al. Twenty-six-year experience treating frontal sinus fractures: a novel algorithm based on anatomical fracture pattern and failure of conventional techniques. *Plast Reconstr Surg.* 2008;122:1850–1866. *An extensive clinical experience is distilled into a practical, clearly presented algorithm for the clinical management of frontal sinus fractures*

76. Losee J, Afifi A, Jiang S, et al. Pediatric orbital fractures: classification, management, and early follow-up. *Plast Reconstr Surg.* 2008;122:886–897.

93. Markowitz BL, Manson PL, Sargent L, et al. Management of the medial canthal tendon in nasoethmoid orbital fractures: the importance of the central fragment in classification and treatment. *Plast Reconstr Surg.* 1991;87:843–853. *This landmark paper introduces a clinically relevant classification scheme for management of nasoethmoid orbital fractures.*

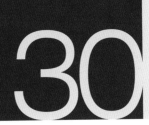

Orbital hypertelorism

Eric Arnaud, Giovanna Paternoster, and Syril James

SYNOPSIS

- Hypertelorism is not a disease in itself; it is just a symptom which may belong to various conditions.
- It is mainly present in facial clefts but may accompany faciocraniosynostosis, where craniosynostosis has to be corrected independently before 1 year of age.
- Surgical treatment of hypertelorism can be undertaken after age 4 and preferably before age 8 (at completion of cerebral growth and before frontal sinus growth).
- The technique of correction depends upon the degree of interorbital distance and on the occlusion.
- According to the degree of interorbital distance, the technique is based on a two-, three-, or four-wall mobilization, through a subcranial or a transcranial approach.
- If the occlusion is normal, the osteotomy is a box-shift type; if the occlusion is angulated, a facial bipartition osteotomy and medialization of the two hemifaces are performed.
- Rhinoplasty is best performed at the end of growth: it represents one of the most important morphological improvements of the whole therapeutic sequence.
- Minor additive procedures contribute to the completion of the result: epicanthus correction, medial and lateral canthopexy, and fat grafting in the temporal region.
- Intellectual development in patients with facial clefts is usually good.

Introduction

Craniofacial malformations are disorders that affect both the cranium and the face. In faciocraniosynostoses, the facial maldevelopment is associated with craniosynostosis (premature fusion of one or several sutures). In facial clefts, the major anomaly affects the face and is occasionally associated with a cranial problem. Hypertelorism is not a disease in itself; rather, it is a symptom or associated finding which accompanies some craniofacial conditions. Hypertelorism is defined by the abnormal increase in the interorbital distance (between the bony orbits). The abnormality may be symmetrical or asymmetrical.

In embryonic development, the development of the face occurs early, between the fourth and eighth weeks of gestation. When one observes that the midportion of the face develops immediately anterior to the forebrain, it is obvious that there is a close relationship between the face and the brain. Lateral to this midline prominence, paired elements appear: the nasal placodes and the maxillary processes. These structures merge in the midline whilst the frontonasal prominence is displaced in a cephalic direction. This prominence narrows to form the bridge and root of the nose. The developing eyes present as optic vesicles "outpouching" from the brain and are initially positioned far laterally. The optic vesicles move closer together as the frontonasal prominence narrows. Simultaneously, the tip of the nose is derived from the paired medial elements, as the paired maxillary and mandibular processes fuse to form the lower part of the face. Clefts of the midline craniofacial structure occur when this delicate sequence of events is disrupted.

 Access the Historical Perspective section online at
http://www.expertconsult.com

Basic science and disease process

If the frontonasal prominence remains in its embryonic position, the optic placodes cannot migrate toward the midline, and this results in orbital hypertelorism, often associated with various anomalies of the forehead and nose. It had been said that "the face predicts the brain", and the importance of the centrofacial anomaly appears to parallel the forebrain defect.[1] Conversely, interrupted development of the medial prominence may lead to an absence of midline structures with excessive narrowing, such as cyclopia or ethmocephaly.

Hypertelorism alone is a mild degree of this sequence at the orbital level.

The associated maxillary anomalies seen with hypertelorism consist mainly of insufficient anterior growth in the upper maxilla, resulting in maxillary retrusion. Since the face is physiologically underdeveloped in infancy, facial anomalies may be more apparent later in childhood when facial growth is completed.

There is little known of the genetics of craniofacial malformations, likely due to the limited number of cases. As major facial clefts are rare, most of our knowledge of the pathogenesis of these malformations is based on studies of the formation of cleft lip and palate. Nevertheless, the role of heredity is obvious in the more frequent clefts of the lip, palate, and the lateral aspects of the orbit.

Radiation, infection, and maternal metabolic imbalances, which can be involved in cleft lip, have not been reported to be responsible for craniofacial malformations. Drugs and chemicals such as tretinoin, thalidomide, corticosteroids, and even aspirin are known to be responsible for malformations; and, while facial development occurs early in pregnancy,[2] mothers may ingest various drugs while unaware of being pregnant. Causal environmental and hereditary factors probably play varying epigenetic roles in the formation of particular malformations.

Various systems of classification have been proposed for craniofacial clefts; two of them are of special value when assessing craniofacial anomalies. These are the "median facial clefts" and the Tessier classification, an orbitocentric cleft classification.

Diagnosis of hypertelorism and patient presentation in facial clefts

Median facial clefts

Median facial clefts can be divided into two categories: those presenting with a deficiency of tissue and missing parts and those without lack of tissue but presenting with a widening malformation.

Midline tissue deficiency malformations are almost always linked with a forebrain deficiency. The term "arrhinencephaly" has been used, but holoprosencephaly, a name proposed by De Myer et al.,[1] better reflects the lack of median tissues. On the basis of this brain–facial linkage, and including some concepts of Cohen and associates, the holoprosencephalic malformations present with hypotelorism, as opposed to hypertelorism.[3]

In contrast with the previous group, near-normal to excess tissue midline disorders do not have a high correlation between the facial anomalies and the underlying brain. The deformities can range from a notch in the upper lip and a widened nose to the most severe form of midline cleft. The term "frontonasal dysplasia", suggested by Sedano et al. for this group of anomalies,[4] is used widely, especially amongst geneticists. Frontonasal dysplasia and holoprosencephaly are therefore at opposite ends in this system of classification of midline anomalies.

This classification does not take into account all the asymmetrical and paramedian anomalies. For easier definition and treatment implications, the authors use the Tessier classification, which is based on surgical experience.

Tessier classification of facial clefts

In the Tessier classification,[5] the orbit is the reference landmark, common to both the cranium and the face. The clefts, numbered from 0 to 14, rotate around the orbit and follow constant lines through the skeleton and soft tissues (Fig. 30.1). Clefts can be mostly cranial if they run upward from the eyelid (7–14) or mostly facial if they run downward from the palpebral fissure (0–6). They are craniofacial if the upper and lower pathways are connected.

The following combinations can be clinically observed: 0 and 14, 1 and 13, 2 and 12, 3 and 11, and 4 and 10. This concept of additive facial and cranial clefts equaling 14 is helpful when examining the patient and often allows identification of malformation along its entire length, above and below the orbit. The severity of the cleft is highly variable and can range from a slight soft-tissue indentation to a complete open cleft. The soft-tissue and skeletal clefts are, on the whole, superimposable. However, a detailed description of the soft-tissue defect, in relation to the skeletal cleft, is more reliable, because the skeletal landmarks are more consistent. The Tessier

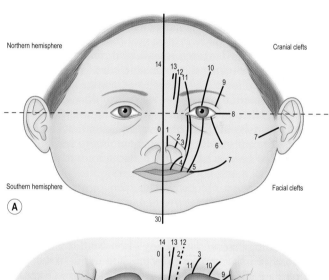

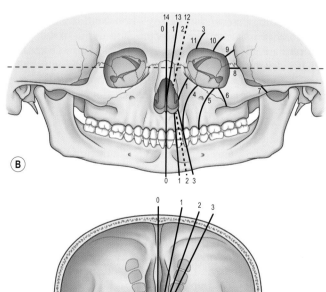

Fig. 30.1 (A–C) Tessier classification.

classification defines the 0–14 cleft as a midline widening, present in frontonasal dysplasia.

Unilateral and bilateral forms of clefting are found in various combinations, mainly asymmetrical when bilateral. Three-dimensional computed tomography has greatly facilitated diagnosis, whilst magnetic resonance imaging explores the brain, looking for an associated malformation. Stereolithographic models, constructed from computed tomography images, are also available and may be useful for diagnosis and surgical planning as these malformations are uncommon and rarely identical.

Some isolated facial clefts, such as those affecting the lateral aspect of the face in Treacher–Collins syndrome (bilateral 6, 7, and 8 clefts), do not present any surgical interest for the neurosurgeon. The central and paramedial clefts affecting the face and cranium are of neurosurgical interest, as the cranium is the means of access for surgical correction.

Diagnosis of hypertelorism and patient presentation in faciocraniosynostosis

Hypertelorism is not the main feature of faciocraniosynostosis, and is variable in its presentation.[6] When mild, it is frequently left untreated; however, when more noticeable, it can be addressed through a separate surgical step. Depending on the dental occlusion, and particularly the horizontal position of the upper maxillary arch, the treatment of hypertelorism will vary between an orbital shift and a facial bipartition. The timing of treatment is variable according to the pathology; however, in the authors' experience, skull expansion for craniosynostosis treatment should precede hypertelorism correction.[7,8]

Crouzon's syndrome

Described by Crouzon in 1912,[9] this syndrome involves only the face and cranium and is not associated with other anomalies elsewhere on the limbs or trunk. The fundamental dysmorphology is an underdeveloped midface presenting with exorbitism secondary to insufficient depth of the orbits, hypoplasia of the malar bones, and a class III malocclusion. Hypertelorism may be present but is usually mild. The nose is short. Brachycephaly is usually present; however, scaphocephaly, plagiocephaly, or even a cloverleaf skull may be present. With an extended classification, the association of facial retrusion and craniosynostosis might be named as a related Crouzon's anomaly. Commonly, the diagnosis of Crouzon's syndrome is difficult to make during the first year of life, even if brachycephaly is obvious. It is often difficult to know whether the midface will be affected, even on radiological examination. Midface retrusion and exorbitism appear later in life. In some cases, however, the diagnosis is evident at birth.

Severe maxillary retrusion may produce airway obstruction with mandatory mouth breathing. There is a great variability of expression, and both severe and mild forms can be observed in the same family.

The strategy of treatment of faciocraniosynostosis is either two-staged[10–12] (fronto-orbital first, then facial advancement later) or a frontofacial monobloc advancement,[13–15] preferably with distraction.[16] Whenever present, the hypertelorism might be corrected around 4–5 years of age, usually with an orbital

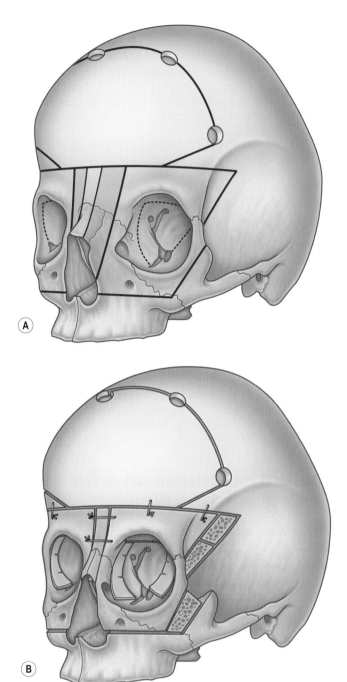

Fig. 30.2 Box-shift mobilization of orbits. **(A)** Before mobilization of the orbits. **(B)** After mobilization of the orbits.

shift (Fig. 30.2), because in Crouzon's disease, the maxillary arch is normal (at least in the horizontal dimension).

Pfeiffer's syndrome

Described by Pfeiffer in 1964, this syndromic entity is an association of faciocraniosynostosis and anomalies of the hands and feet. The brachycephaly induced by bicoronal synostosis is often asymmetrical and is associated with midface retrusion secondary to maxillary hypoplasia. Hypertelorism is often present in this syndrome. The thumbs and great toes are broad with a varus deviation and may be associated with soft-tissue syndactylies, the latter being difficult to diagnose early in life. Some severe forms exist, with marked perinatal frontofacial retrusion resulting in visual and respiratory problems. This condition is sometimes associated with a cloverleaf skull.

The strategy of treatment is similar to that for Crouzon's, but Pfeiffer's syndrome is often more severe than Crouzon's, with a higher tendency to relapse after surgical advancement.

Apert's syndrome (acrocephalosyndactyly)

First described by Apert in 1906,[17] this syndrome is easy to recognize because of the associated syndactylies of the hands and feet. The severity of syndactyly is scored according to Cohen and Kreiborg.[18] Type 1 is syndactyly of the central three digits, type 2 is syndactyly of digits 2–5, and type 3 is syndactyly of all five digits.

The craniofacial involvement is always marked at birth, in contrast with that in Crouzon's, with brachycephaly (sometimes asymmetrical) associated with facial retrusion. Both coronal sutures are fused, although some rare cases present with unilateral coronal synostosis or without any synostoses (4 cases without synostoses in our series). The hypertelorism and the anterior open bite add to the distinction from Crouzon's disease. In fact, the maxillary alveolar arch is higher than the posterior part of the palate. Another main difference with Crouzon's is the frequent sagittal dehiscence of the sutural system with the forehead frequently remaining wide open during the first year of life; this contributes to the abnormally wide forehead and face in this syndrome. Associated abnormalities of the central nervous system are more frequent than in other syndromic craniosynostoses. The exception is Chiari-like malformations, which are common in Crouzon's but, due to premature fusions of the lambdoid sutures, are uncommon in Apert's.[19] Because of these patients' divergent frontal plane, bipartition procedures are more adapted to correct Apert's-associated hypertelorism. Nevertheless, skull expansion (either anterior or posterior) is performed first, usually before 1 year of age to address the craniosynostotic skull.

Craniofrontonasal dysplasia

In the group of craniofacial dysplasias (see discussion of median facial clefts with frontonasal dysplasia, below), some cases present with a bicoronal craniosynostosis, including a subgroup called craniofrontonasal dysplasia. There is a brachycephaly, often marked, associated with the facial anomalies of frontonasal dysplasia, which include hypertelorism, broad nasal bridge, and bifid nose; soft-tissue syndactyly may also be present.

Craniofrontonasal dysplasia is far more common in females than in males, consistent with its X-linked inheritance. In the authors' series, 36% of cases were familial, and 91% of patients were females.

Patient selection

Orbital shift or bipartition?

The choice between orbital shift and bipartition is mainly linked to a series of factors:

- The maxillary arch: if the maxillary arch is narrow and inverted with the incisors being higher than the molars,

bipartition is the operation of choice because it widens the maxilla and improves the angle of the upper dentition. On the other hand, if the maxillary arch and occlusion are normal, it is preferable to avoid an interpterygomaxillary disjunction.
- The axis of the orbits: if the axis is normal, a horizontal mobilization is satisfactory; if the orbits are laterally and downwardly oblique, bipartition is required.
- The nasal fossae: if they are narrow, bipartition and medialization of the upper face improve the airways by enlarging the lower part of the face.
- Extent of the hypertelorism: bipartition is the operation of choice in the most severe cases, whereas orbital shift is indicated for more limited displacements.
- The bipartition procedure can also be used to get access to a lesion of the cranial base. Some midline clefts are associated with an encephalocele of the ethmoidosphenoidal area. After midline splitting, easy access to the encephalocele can be obtained.

Treatment/surgical technique

Surgical principles in facial clefts

Tessier's breakthrough collaboration between plastic and neurological surgery allowed him to conceptually minimize the surgical border existing between the face and the skull and dramatically enhance the surgical treatment of upper facial clefts.[20] Tessier demonstrated that the frontocranial route was a good approach to access the nose and orbits and that frontocranial problems can be treated simultaneously with facial problems. The fear of contamination from the facial cavities was so great among neurosurgeons in 1967 that, for their first case, Tessier and his neurosurgical colleague, Guyot, placed a dermal skin graft on the dura of the anterior cranial fossa after it had been elevated, voluntarily sacrificing both the olfactory nerves. A few months later, they performed the combined craniofacial approach. By 1970, a one-stage procedure to address the orbits from superior and inferior approaches was considered safe, and the olfactory nerves could be preserved.[21] Preliminary disinfection of the nasal cavities, dissection of the mucosal domes and their immediate repair if opened, preservation or perfect repair of dura, changing of instruments if passing through the facial cavities, and perioperative antibiotic therapy were preventive measures that helped to avoid infection, osteitis, and meningitis.

There are two ways to mobilize the orbits when correcting orbital hypertelorism. The treatment planning varies according to the severity of the hypertelorism, the maxillary structure, and the age of the patient. An orbital shift can simply be performed in cases of normal or subnormal dental occlusion. In cases of restricted transverse maxillary structures, mobilization of both hemifaces (necessitating a facial bipartition) can be performed to correct the hypertelorism and the arched palate at the same time.

The classic approach described by Tessier et al. in 1967[20] consisted, after removal of the enlarged medial portion, of an en bloc mobilization of the orbits medially, the lower horizontal cuts being situated below the infraorbital rim, through the malar bone and the maxilla. In Tessier's protocol, especially

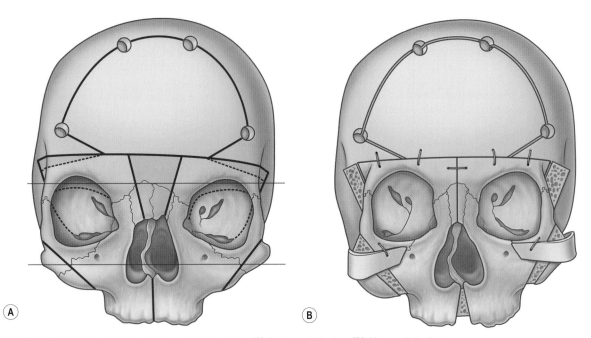

Fig. 30.3 Medialization of the two hemifaces after bipartition. **(A)** Before medialization. **(B)** After medialization.

in adult patients, a supraorbital bar is kept in place in order to ensure stability of the mobilized orbits.[22]

Bipartition, proposed by van der Meulen[23,24] and developed by Tessier,[25,26] represents a mobilization of the two hemifaces (Fig. 30.3). Instead of cutting below the orbits, the surgeon makes the osteotomies through the zygomatic arch, the pterygomaxillary junction, and medially through the palate. The medial resection must have a "V" shape because there will be an element of rotation, along with a narrowing on the midline. The rotation allows for widening of the maxillary arch and the nasal fossae and also for changing the axis of the orbits, which have a lateral slant.

Surgical techniques in facial clefts

Principles

The two main aims of surgery for this condition are to bring the orbits closer together and to create a nose of normal appearance. The basic anatomical anomaly is an increase in both the interorbital distance and the nasal bones whilst the glabellar region is much wider than normal. The enlarged portion of the midline structures is removed, and, after mobilization of the orbits, the nasal skeleton is adjusted with the help of a bone graft if more dorsal projection is needed (Fig. 30.4).

This combined approach allows the surgeon to move the orbits and repair bony anomalies of the fronto-orbitonasal complex. Orbital displacement is key to the treatment of major craniofacial clefts. The orbit can be moved on a horizontal, vertical, anterior, or posterior axis to correct all anomalies. Reconstruction of a missing orbital roof or part of the forehead, canthopexies, and correction of soft-tissue problems can be performed simultaneously.

Not all hypertelorisms are symmetrical, and asymmetrical cases are more complex to correct. The cranial base is also asymmetrical, and so the different distortions must be carefully evaluated by computed tomography three-dimensional

reconstructions. Sometimes both orbits have to be moved in different directions.[26,27]

The age at operation is important. If there is a cranial cleft, it is better to wait for the median frontal defect to ossify before surgery is scheduled. The neurosurgical approach is by means of a frontal bone flap. Its lower part depends on the variable elevation of the orbital rim, often including elevation of one side and transverse displacement on the opposite side.

Soft-tissue anomalies, such as skin excess, may be treated initially by sagittal resection or can be postponed as this tissue may contract over time. Another reason to delay midline skin resection is that dorsal nasal bone grafting, which is almost mandatory to achieve adequate nasal correction, requires some degree of skin excess.

In minor cases, a limited procedure with one- to three-wall mobilization may suffice.

Infrafrontal correction of hypertelorism

In the least significant hypertelorisms (less than 35 mm interorbital distance), a single medial wall mobilization can be undertaken. This procedure can be performed through a limited subciliary incision, but the authors prefer a coronal approach unless medial skin excess makes a nasal incision mandatory. The thin bone of the medial wall of the orbit can be easily in-fractured (Fig. 30.5).

In selected cases presenting with mild symmetrical hypertelorism (35–40 mm), large frontal sinuses, and a high pituitary sella, the supraorbital rim and roof of the orbits can be left in place with mobilization of the other three walls.[20,28–31] However, this method is less effective for the correction of the orbital distance than the box-shift osteotomy. This subcranial approach can be used in a horizontal shift or a bipartition whenever the cribriform plate is high enough. Raveh and Vuillemin[32] used this inferior intracranial approach, cutting the orbital roof and the ethmoidal cells from below, without a frontal craniectomy. They claimed to have good control of

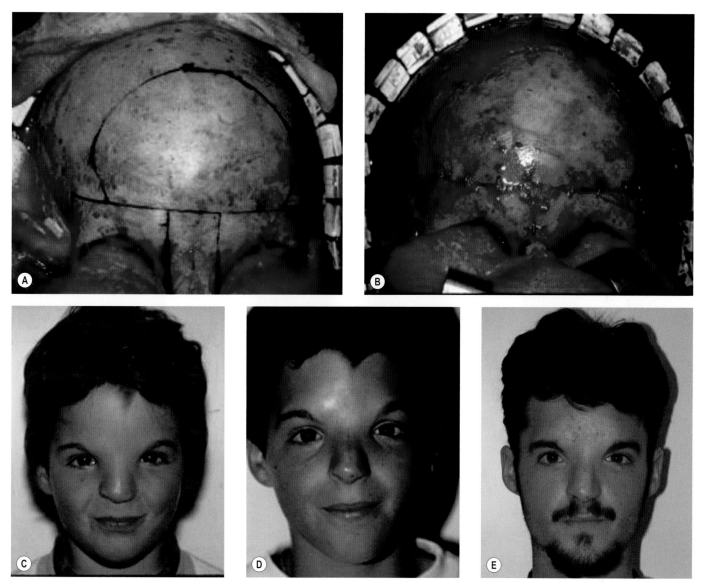

Fig. 30.4 Box-shift osteotomy for midline cleft. **(A)** Before osteotomy: note both lateral spurs, avoiding the need for supraorbital bar. **(B)** After medial shift. **(C)** Age 5 years, before treatment. **(D)** Age 6 years, after operation. **(E)** Age 21 years.

the dura and a shorter recovery period due to less aggressive surgery.

The periorbital regions are widely dissected through a coronal approach and subciliary incisions. The osteotomies are performed posteriorly enough to keep a wide bony platform that will push the globe medially. Medially, the nasal mucosa is dissected from under the nasal bones through a

retrograde approach. A trephine hole can be created from above to improve access for the interorbital resection, allowing the nasal bones to be lifted and affording control of the superior medial wall segments. Should a dural tear occur, a frontal flap can be elevated for intracranial repair. The rest of the osteotomies are performed as in the intracranial approach. The mobilization must be carefully performed because the

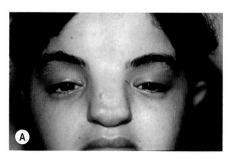
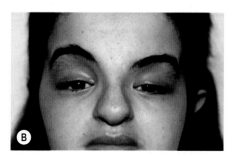
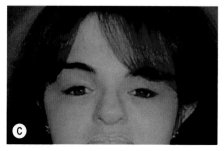

Fig. 30.5 Three-wall medialization osteotomy (horizontal shift). **(A)** Before treatment at age 7 years. **(B)** After operation. **(C)** At age 21 years.

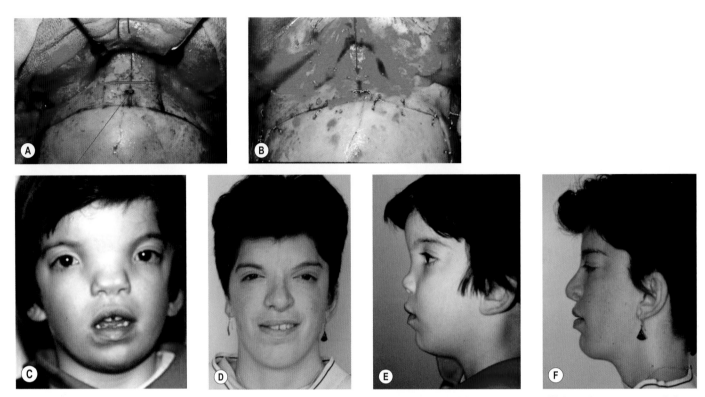

Fig. 30.6 Box-shift osteotomy for midline cleft. **(A)** Before osteotomy: note maximum width of bony resection. **(B)** After medial shift. **(C)** Front view at age 4 years before treatment. **(D)** Front view at age 25 years. **(E)** Lateral view at age 4 years before treatment. **(F)** Lateral view at age 25 years.

three-wall bony orbit is fragile. Stabilization is performed medially with stainless-steel wires. Repositioning of the nasal bones and control of the canthi are performed last before closure.

Box-shift osteotomies (symmetrical orbital hypertelorism)

When the interorbital distance is greater than 40 mm (Fig. 30.6), the neurosurgical approach is critical because it allows access to the orbital roof and the central ethmoidosphenoidal area. Only in rare circumstances, and in older patients, is it possible to move the lower three-quarters of the orbits and remove the excess width of the central nose below the cribriform plate while leaving the roof of the orbits intact. This extracranial approach is only possible if the cribriform plate is very high and the deformity is minimal.

Like most craniofacial teams, the authors prefer to use the frontal approach to have a clear view of the anterior cranial fossa; this also facilitates dura repair if necessary. In hypertelorism, anomalies of the midline often exist and good exposure is essential for dural control. Of note, duplication of the crista galli apophysis is not uncommon.

Frontal craniectomy

Frontal craniectomy allows access to the orbital roofs and medial structures. The design of the frontal craniectomy must be carefully planned by the craniofacial surgeon. The lower limit is of importance. Some surgeons, following Tessier's technique, prefer to keep a bridge of bone intact at the lower part of the forehead between the frontal flap and the mobilized orbits to maintain stability. If this is to be performed, the

supraorbital rim to be preserved is about 1 cm in height; the preserved frontal bridge also measures 1 cm, and the lower limit of the frontal craniotomy must be at least 2 cm above the orbits. Many craniofacial surgeons, including the authors, do not preserve this horizontal band; the lower limit of the craniectomy with this approach is 1 cm above the orbits. This approach facilitates access to the anterior cranial fossa. An anteroposterior landmark and a stable point of fixation are fundamental. For these reasons, the authors preserve a low lateral spur of frontal bone, with the frontal craniotomy flap taking an upward angle at about the middle of the orbits (see Fig. 30.2).

The frontal flap must be elevated with care as anomalies are frequently encountered (e.g., a very deep groove for the longitudinal sinus or a thick, or even bifid, crista galli). After the frontal flap has been elevated, careful dissection of the dura from the orbital roofs and from the edge of the greater wing of the sphenoid bone and the adjacent part of the temporal fossa is performed. The central region around the cribriform plate is the most challenging portion of the dissection. If the cribriform plate is normal or only moderately altered, the resection necessary to decrease the distance between the orbits is performed in the ethmoidal cells on either side of the cribriform plate. Sometimes, the cribriform plate is highly abnormal with the olfactory grooves widely separated and running close to the medial walls of the orbits. In these cases, sacrifice of the olfactory nerves is unavoidable during a large medial resection.

Meticulous repair of the dura is mandatory after resection of the olfactory nerves. A periosteal patch is often useful to reinforce the closure. The central resection is performed by the craniofacial surgeon who has previously dissected the nasal mucosal domes by proceeding cephalad from below the nasal bones. The paranasal osteotomies are performed vertically at a slightly divergent angle. The transverse posterior osteotomy is then performed. It is usually made in front of the crista galli if the olfactory nerves are intact. In the most severe cases, this osteotomy is performed posteriorly, removing most of the ethmoid bone. The medial resection is lifted *en bloc*, and the nasal mucosal domes are exposed. If they are not intact, immediate suturing of the nasal mucosa is performed.

Osteotomies of the orbit

Next, the osteotomies are performed through the orbital roof, lateral orbital wall, and posteromedial wall. The lower osteotomies vary according to whether orbital shift or bipartition is being performed. The orbits are then brought together and contact is established in the midline. All the interposing elements, such as an enlarged superior nasal septum or residual posterior ethmoidal cells, must be removed. The dura must be carefully protected during these maneuvers. After the orbits are rigidly fixated in the midline by wires or miniplates, the neurosurgical portion of the procedure is almost complete. Dural integrity and hemostasis are ensured in the anterior and temporal cranial fossae, and the frontal bone flap is secured back in place.

Bone grafts from the cranial vault are needed to close the gaps in the orbital walls and often to build up the nasal dorsum. Sometimes, in adolescents and adults, it is possible to split the frontal bone flap and use the posterior aspect for bone grafts. More often, it is necessary to take bone grafts from the cranial vault. Specifically, a thick, straight 5-cm segment is necessary for nasal reconstruction. It is convenient to take these bony pieces posterior to the frontal flap. In the authors' practice, bone dust from the burr holes and small residual bony fragments are mixed with fibrin glue and used to occlude the vault defects after the graft removal.

The optic nerve is not straight; it has laxity that allows it to follow the displacement of the eyeball. Even a significant displacement is well tolerated by the optic nerves. To permit a good medial displacement of the eyeball, it is essential that the medial wall of the orbit is also displaced towards the midline. If the osteotomy is too anterior, there will be a step effect, limiting the displacement of the ocular globes.

A secondary rhinoplasty will most likely be necessary to achieve an optimized aesthetic result.

Bipartition with intracranial approach (large symmetrical hypertelorism with arched palate)

This technique varies slightly from the box-shift, but many surgical steps are identical. Differences are as follows (see Fig. 30.3):

- V-shape resection of bone at the nose
- absence of osteotomy in the maxilla at the lower limit of the orbit
- osteotomy at the pterygomaxillary junction
- the medialization part of the upper face creates an opening at the palatal level (Fig. 30.7).

Asymmetrical cases

Asymmetrical cases are more difficult to correct than symmetrical ones. Sometimes each orbit must be moved in different directions whilst on other occasions only one of the orbits is involved in the planned displacement. The cranial base is also asymmetrical; the various distortions must be carefully evaluated by computed tomography with three-dimensional reconstructions. Paramedian clefts create a situation in which the affected orbit is displaced laterally and inferiorly to a variable degree. A defect in the frontal bone is often associated. The orbit may be reduced in size (anophthalmia or microphthalmia). Various anomalies of the maxillary and nasal portion of the face may also be associated.

After the anomaly has been evaluated and classified according to the Tessier system (see previous discussion), a plan of treatment is devised. The correction must be planned from top to bottom; that is, the frontal and orbital regions must be reconstructed first. In most cases, a bilateral asymmetrical correction is required. The neurosurgical approach is by means of a frontal bone flap, its lower limit being carefully planned because of the variable reconstructions of the

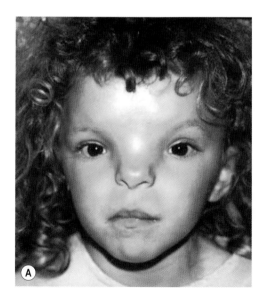
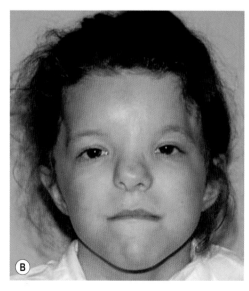

Fig. 30.7 Hypertelorism correction by bipartition for a frontocranial dysplasia. **(A)** Before treatment at age 4.5 years. **(B)** After treatment (observe temporal hollowness, to be corrected secondarily).

supraorbital rim, often including elevation on one side. Transverse movement only is performed on the affected side. In the paramedian clefts, the ethmoidal region is asymmetrical and dural elevation should be performed with care. After the orbits are properly positioned, the frontal bone flap is adjusted and wired into place.

Sometimes only one orbit is displaced, usually inferiorly, with one globe inferior to the other; this condition is defined as orbital dystopia. In these situations, displacement of the entire orbit *en bloc* is the solution. Partial maneuvers such as elevation of the roof and placement of bone grafts on the floor usually produce disappointing results. This *en bloc* displacement of the orbit requires a frontal flap to gain access to the roof. This frontal flap can be unilateral and corresponds to the width of the orbital osteotomy. The frontal segment removed to permit elevation of the supraorbital rim is utilized as a bone graft placed below the orbit to maintain the elevation and fill the resultant bony gap.

In some cases of asymmetrical clefting, an asymmetrical bipartition has been used.

Timing and indications for surgery in faciocraniosynostosis

Without early treatment, intracranial hypertension can lead to optic atrophy and visual loss in craniosynostosis. This is observed mainly in Crouzon's syndrome and in oxycephalies. In the series of Hôpital Necker Enfants-Malades, papilledema was observed in 35% and optic atrophy in 10% of Crouzon's cases. In the other syndromes, papilledema was observed in only 4–5% and no optic atrophy was observed.[19] Because of these risks, and as previously mentioned, strategic management of faciocraniosynostosis usually demands at least a two-stage procedure[7,8,11,12] followed by later refinements. The skull is operated upon first and the face secondarily. Apert's syndrome is definitely the most difficult to treat and might require the largest number of additional procedures.

Orbits

In Necker's experience, the surgical treatment of the associated hypertelorism is delayed until after the frontal advancement and after 4 years of age.[7,8] This strategy provides a thick enough skull bone to perform stable fixation after mobilization of the osteotomized segments. The choice between the orbital shift and the facial bipartition depends on a series of factors:

■ The maxillary arch: if the maxillary arch and occlusion are normal, it seems preferable to avoid an interpterygomaxillary disjunction, and box-shift osteotomies are sufficient; this is the case in Crouzon's and Apert's. Conversely, if the maxillary arch is narrow and inverted, the incisors being higher than the molars, bipartition is the operation of choice because it widens the maxilla and improves the angle of the upper dentition.

■ The axis of the orbits: if the axis is normal, a horizontal mobilization is satisfactory. If they are laterally and downwardly oblique, bipartition corrects these anomalies.

■ The nasal fossae: if they are narrow, bipartition improves the airways, especially if a narrowing in the upper part of the face is associated with a widening of the maxillary arch.

These three criteria are all present in Apert's, and therefore bipartition is the procedure of choice for these patients. The bipartition can be performed with a facial Le Fort III advancement as a combined second step, sometimes by means of osteodistraction. In cases of a Le Fort III osteotomy combined with bipartition and distraction, we would use the combination of internal and external distraction devices (Fig. 30.8).

Face

Le Fort classically described three types of maxillary disjunction depending on the transversal level of the facial fractures. Since the surgical facial advancements approximately reproduce these fracture lines on the face, Tessier gave the names of Le Fort I, II, and III to the facial osteotomies. Although Gillies was the first to perform a facial advancement in the late 1940s,[33] Tessier[10] really developed the Le Fort III type of advancement, his lines of osteotomies being deeper than those of Gillies, located behind the lacrimal apparatus. The facial advancement is usually of the Le Fort III type.

Patients who have previously undergone forehead advancement normally have facial retrusion to a variable degree. As a rule, we prefer to delay the facial advancement until there is permanent dentition and a stable occlusive relationship can be achieved. When the deformity is moderate, there is no difficulty in convincing the patient and the

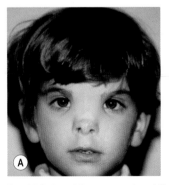
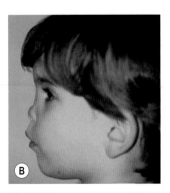
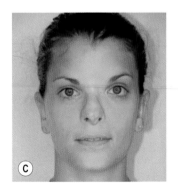
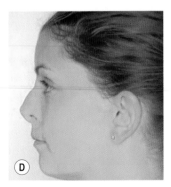

Fig. 30.8 Box-shift osteotomy for midline cleft. **(A)** Before osteotomy: front view at age 4 years. **(B)** Before osteotomy: lateral view at age 4 years. **(C)** Front view at age 23 years after augmentation rhinoplasty (observe good quality of midline nasal scar for skin excess). **(D)** Lateral view at age 23 years after augmentation rhinoplasty (nasal revision to be performed for hump removal).

family to wait. In patients with more severe deformity, the social and psychological pressure is high, as well as the demands of the family and often the child. In most severe cases, difficulties in chewing and breathing as well as significant inferior exorbitism are also present. In these situations, after a warning that another operation (usually a Le Fort I) will be necessary after permanent dentition is in place, we perform a facial advancement.

In Apert's, the advancement will be combined with a facial bipartition, as mentioned earlier. This procedure is performed before final dentition has erupted; therefore no attempt to correct the open bite is made.

Surgical technique of hypertelorism correction in faciocraniosynostosis

Because faciocraniosynostoses are essentially characterized by backward displacement of the forehead and midface, both having to be moved forward, this condition can be treated by advancing the forehead and the face either separately or simultaneously, possibly in combination with the correction of the hypertelorbitism. The classical management includes an initial anterior skull remodeling and, later, a facial advancement as a second step, as detailed previously. In cases where early frontofacial advancement is performed, the hypertelorism is corrected secondarily.[7,8]

Hypertelorism correction by bipartition in combination with Le Fort III osteotomy (Figs. 30.9 and 30.10)

The combination of hypertelorism and maxillary anomalies makes the facial bipartition the logical operation in treating Apert's syndrome. This may be combined with a distraction if indicated.

Coronal approach

The scalp is incised after subcutaneous infiltration with epinephrine solution; the incision follows the scar of the previous skull expansion if present. Exposure of the calvarial vault in the subgaleal or supraperiosteal plane might be complicated by scar tissue and bony dehiscence. Complete dissection of the periorbita is conducted in the subperiosteal plane. Exposure of the root of the nose, as well as the lateral walls of the orbits and the zygomatic arches, is performed after undermining both temporalis muscles.

Subcranial osteotomies

The lower three-quarters of the orbits, the nose, the malar bones, and the upper maxilla are to be mobilized. Bony cuts are performed with a reciprocating saw in a bilateral manner. The lateral cut of the orbit is usually started at the frontozygomatic junction, then continued on to the floor of the orbit to reach the sphenomaxillary fissure. Care must be taken to avoid cutting through the lower orbital rim with an anteriorly based osteotomy so as not to fracture the inferior orbital wall in a shallow, distorted orbit. The zygomatic arch is easily transected. The root of the nose is horizontally sectioned while a 3-mm cranial buttress is maintained. A medial V-shaped resection is then performed; the osteotomy is extended downward to the medial wall of each orbit, taking care to be posterior enough to avoid disruption of the medial canthus. Finally, a bilateral pterygomaxillary disjunction is made from above through the pterygoid fossa, with a finger inside the mouth to control the position of the chisel.

An epinephrine solution is also infiltrated under the palatal mucosa. A medial bony cut might be necessary through a small mucosal opening behind the incisors. This will allow for rotation of the two hemipalates. At this point the two hemifaces are free enough to be mobilized independently. A combined movement of upper medialization and inferior lateralization allows the rotation of both hemifaces to correct the hypertelorism and the down-slanting of the eyelids.

Osteosynthesis and grafts

Osteosynthesis with metallic wires or miniplates is necessary in the orbital region at the lateral junction of the orbital wall and at the zygomatic arch in order to maintain the advancement. Bone grafts, usually taken from the outer table of the parietal calvaria, are mandatory at the root of the nose and in the upper part of the lateral orbital walls. The grafts at the frontozygomatic junction are triangular, whereas two quadrangular grafts, like two parts of the roof of a house, are required at the root of the nose. Bone grafts might be useful to fill the gaps at the lateral orbital walls to prevent enophthalmos if a significant advancement is performed at the Le Fort III level.

An archbar is anchored on the teeth with metallic wires to maintain stability at the maxillary level.

Closure of the scalp is conducted in the usual manner after the temporal muscles have been transposed anteriorly to fill the temporal defect created by the medialization of the lateral walls of the orbits.

If distractors are used for a combined advancement, a few technique modifications would be employed:

- The nose and lateral aspects of the frontozygomatic regions would be grafted but not rigidly fixated.
- In case of external distraction, the pulling wires would preferably be at the pyriform apertures (Fig. 30.9).
- In case of internal distracters, a transfacial pin would be useful for fixation of both hemifaces (Fig. 30.10). Internal distracters may be left as consolidators for a longer period of time (3–4 months).

Postoperative care

Like all major transcranial craniofacial procedures, postoperative care depends on the procedure itself and its implications for systemic homeostasis. Close monitoring is best achieved in a specialized pediatric intensive care unit for at least the first 24 hours. It is not uncommon in our experience that the degree of postoperative airway edema may dictate a prolonged intubation extending up to 3 or 4 days. After such a delay, it is likely that the acute phase of the initial swelling, sometimes impressive after 48 hours at the eyelid level but also in the airway, has nearly, if not completely, resolved. A conservative approach to the airway may avoid unwanted reintubation after an early extubation. This is a significant risk after bilateral hemifacial medialization, even if this procedure enlarges the airway at the base of the nose.

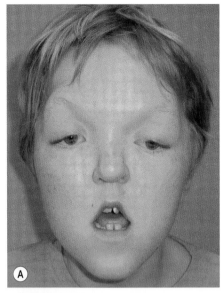

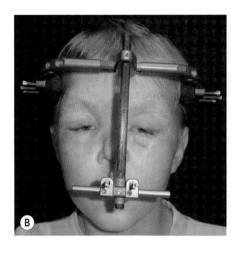

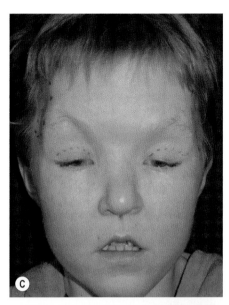

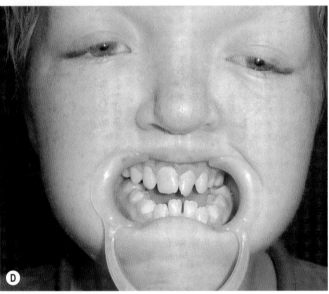

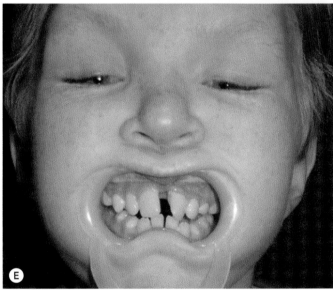

Fig. 30.9 Le Fort III with bipartition and external distraction in an Apert patient aged 11 years (observe gap between incisors) before orthodontic treatment. **(A)** Front view before surgery. **(B)** Front view with external distractor in place. **(C)** Front view after surgery (observe normalization of eyelid cants). **(D)** Occlusion before surgery. **(E)** Occlusion after surgery.

Postoperative bleeding secondary to the various osteotomy lines must be carefully monitored, especially in the context of pre- and intraoperative blood loss and possible resultant coagulopathy. Prophylactic antibiotic therapy is usually not extended beyond 48 hours according to guidelines for an invasive craniofacial procedure with exposed contaminated spaces (ethmoidal sinus, frontal sinus if present).

The prophylactic preoperative tarsorrhaphy is left in place until after successful extubation. The tarsorrhaphy will protect the cornea from ulcer formation and reduce potentially severe chemosis (conjunctival edema). When a box-shift osteotomy has been performed, the subciliary stitches are best removed at day 3 and replaced by Steri-Strips. Sutures from a midline excess skin excision are removed at day 5 like any other facial closure, unless a subcuticular intradermal running suture has been placed.

Prevention of complications remains a key issue in the postoperative period.

Outcomes, prognosis, and complications

Possible complications may be separated into acute and delayed occurrences. As previously mentioned, acute complications must be vigilantly prevented during the initial postoperative period:

- Excessive bleeding, mainly related to a coagulopathy induced by important preoperative transfusion, is a risk.
- Cerebrospinal fluid leakage through the nose is not uncommon and may require lumbar drainage if

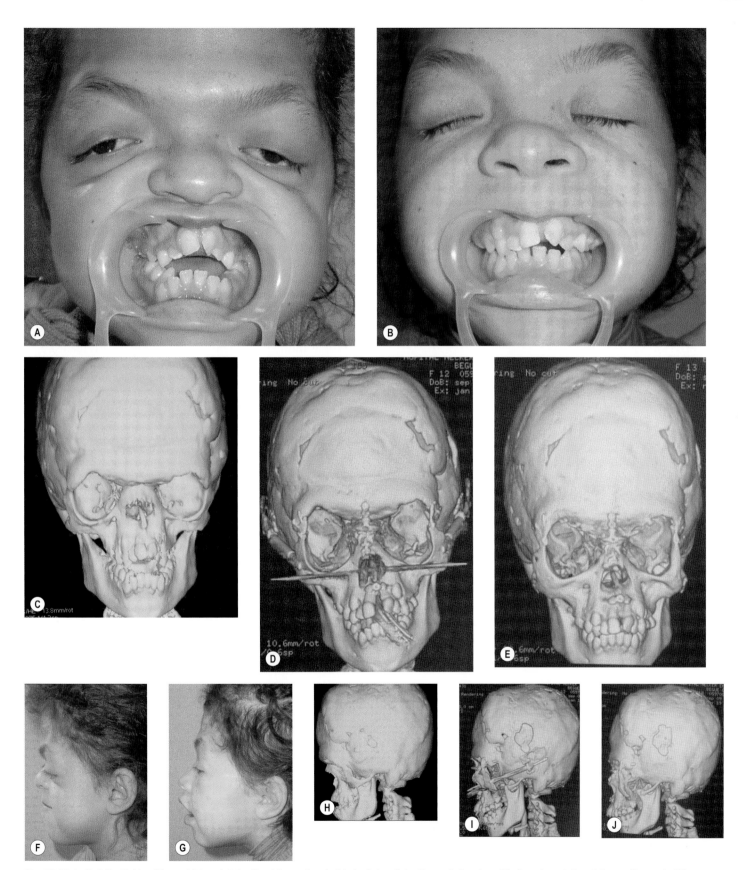

Fig. 30.10 Le Fort III with bipartition and internal distraction (observe transfacial pin during distraction period) and modification of angulation of the maxillary arch. **(A)** Front view before. **(B)** Front view after procedure. **(C)** Computed tomography (CT) scan before Le Fort III (observe retrusion of the midface). **(D)** CT scan during distraction with transfacial pin. **(E)** CT scan after distraction and removal of distractors. **(F)** Lateral view before advancement. **(G)** Lateral view after advancement. **(H)** Lateral CT scan before advancement. **(I)** Lateral CT scan during distraction with internal devices. **(J)** Lateral CT scan after distraction.

persistent after 3 days of lumbar punctures. Rhinorrhea represents a risk of meningitis and can be avoided by careful dissection in the retroglabellar region.

- Infection linked to an insufficient cranialization of the frontal sinus (if a frontal sinus was present at the time of surgery to require cranialization). This may be best prevented by operating early after the age of 4 years, when the frontal sinus has usually not yet developed. Infection may arise anywhere from a few days to a few months postoperatively.

- Ophthalmological complications such as keratitis or chemosis are best prevented by the initial tarsorrhaphy. Blindness represents an exceptionally rare but dramatic complication, and all patients should be warned accordingly. The possibility of a postoperative strabismus is more common, and care should be taken to sufficiently medialize the medial orbital walls posterior to the osteotomies so as to avoid a step-off that may impinge on the medial rectus muscles. Failure to carry the medialization far enough posteriorly may also contribute to an insufficient medialization of the globes despite a satisfactory medialization of the bony orbits.

- In the long term the most important complication is an insufficient correction. This is most likely to occur not by relapse, but by soft-tissue relaxation, especially at the medial canthi. To this extent the medial canthus fixation tends to be disappointing and frequently necessitates a secondary correction (Fig. 30.11). The secondary rhinoplasty greatly contributes to the aesthetic outcome, but must be delayed until adulthood.

- Temporal hollowing is not uncommon, especially if the hypertelorism correction is the second major procedure after a cranioplasty or after a bipartition, which tends to deepen the temporal fossa.

Secondary procedures

Soft-tissue problems are more complex to treat than bony irregularities.

Some craniofacial malformations involve only the skeleton, e.g., mild symmetrical orbital hypertelorism, orbital dystopia, frontal or malar asymmetries, and malposition. Correction can be achieved through hidden approaches, such as bicoronal or vestibular incisions, or through palpebral infraciliary approaches, all of which leave almost invisible scars.

Temporal hollowness can be addressed by fat grafting according to the Coleman technique. Repeated treatments may be necessary.

Excess skin can be adjusted and will retract. After correction of moderate hypertelorism, the excess skin of the glabellar region and dorsum of the nose retracts with the help of good undermining and a bone graft to lift the dorsum of the nose. Possible future soft-tissue correction must be considered in the initial treatment plan such that skeletal access is achieved without sacrificing potential cutaneous flap options. For example, if a frontal skin flap is planned, the design of the coronal incision may have to be altered to avoid violating the future pedicle.

It is usually much easier to reconstruct the skeleton than to correct soft-tissue deficiencies. All the resources of plastic surgery can rarely achieve a perfect contour with minimal scars. The authors briefly consider the primary soft-tissue problems encountered in major congenital craniofacial malformations at the end of this chapter.

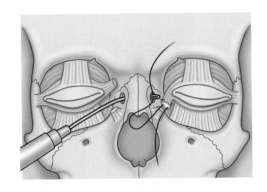

(A)

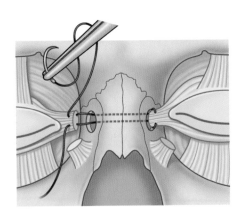

(B)

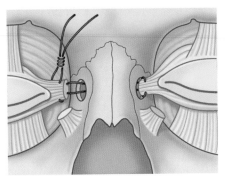

(C)

Fig. 30.11 (A–C) Secondary correction of medial canthus disinsertion.

Regardless, the final rhinoplasty will be the most important element of the definitive aesthetic result.

Refinements in hypertelorism correction (in clefts or craniosynostotic patients)

Irregularities are frequent in the frontal region, the nose, and the temporal fossae. Refinements may be performed early or delayed until the completion of craniofacial growth, after 15 years of age. Techniques to obtain a satisfactory contour have classically included bone remodeling, bone grafting, and the onlay of biomaterials. More recently, fat grafting as described by Coleman has proven useful to correct minor anomalies such as temporal hollowing.

Soft-tissue refinements are aesthetically relevant for the final result and may be divided into several subcategories, as follows.

Canthus correction

During the surgical correction of hypertelorism, it is preferable to maintain the bony attachment of the medial canthus. In so doing, one avoids the need for medial canthus reattachment, which is always possible but is sometimes unreliable in the long term. Even when the medial canthal ligament is preserved, if the medial bony resection is 2 cm, the postoperative intercanthal distance may be reduced by only 1 cm, demonstrating 50% efficacy at the soft-tissue level. It might be necessary to reinsert the medial canthal ligaments under increased tension (with a transnasal technique: see Fig. 30.11) and correct an epicanthal fold (easily achieved with Y–V plasty or a Del Campo technique (asymmetric Z-plasty).[34]

The lateral canthus is less well defined and it is easily repositioned with a lateral suspension, if necessary, at the end of the craniofacial procedure. If this correction proves insufficient in the long term, a lateral canthopexy may be performed secondarily through a small lateral incision.

Scalp and eyebrows

Hairline distortion is frequently observed in craniofacial clefts and reflects the continuity of the cleft at the scalp level. Hair growing down on to the forehead can be removed. Unwanted hair can be incorporated into a frontal skin resection that facilitates exposure, or excision may be achieved secondarily. Eyebrows can be clefted or displaced. Differential repositioning of the forehead and scalp can correct eyebrow displacement, usually by lowering the high side.

Nose

In symmetrical hypertelorism presenting with an excess of skin at the level of the nasal dorsum, it is advisable to avoid the easy solution of midline skin excision. Some of these median scars do very well with time and become hardly visible, but others stretch, become pigmented, and are very prominent. It is therefore better to count on skin retraction, as previously discussed.

If there is a cleft affecting the nose, it should be corrected at the time of the craniofacial procedure to utilize the relative excess soft tissue obtained by the undermining performed around the nose. A cleft can be closed by reapproximation of tissues with plasties at the alar margins, but if there is a tissue deficiency, various nasal flaps should be considered. The excess skin existing on the upper part of the nose can be transferred to the lower part.

In some cases, the nose is very distorted and the shortage of skin is obvious from the start. The frontal area is the best zone from which to obtain the missing skin. On other occasions, correction of the hypertelorism creates an excess of soft tissue at the level of the forehead that can be used as a frontal flap. Sometimes, a preliminary frontal skin expansion may be necessary to provide the required soft tissue. The potential need for nasal reconstruction should be carefully considered early in the planning process as the usually preferred coronal approach may require modification if soft-tissue recruitment becomes necessary in this context.

Eyelids and orbits

Clefts of the eyelids primarily involve the lower eyelid and are addressed during the midface reconstruction, as are oculonasal clefts. The craniofacial clefts discussed in this chapter may also result in pathology of the orbits.

If there is anophthalmia or microphthalmia, the bony orbit does not develop to its normal size. The preferred treatment is a progressive enlargement of the conjunctiva,[35,36] but conformers are very difficult to place; intraorbital expanders are much more efficient and can produce an almost normal growth of the orbit with a prosthesis fitted afterwards. Nevertheless, this orbital expansion is difficult to execute and requires very close follow-up. If orbital expansion fails or is not attempted, a micro-orbit must be faced. This orbit should first be placed in proper position, vertically and horizontally, in relation to the other orbit. It can then be surgically enlarged by expanding the whole circumference. Access to the orbital roof is obtained with a localized frontal craniotomy, as for an orbital dystopia. The secondary soft-tissue work of creating a good cavity capable of retaining an ocular prosthesis, and building up the short, retracted eyelids with auricular composite grafts, is often more difficult and time-consuming than the skeletal work.

Oculomotor disorders

Numerous conditions in craniofacial surgery may present with oculomotor disorders, especially when hypertelorism is apparent. The rule is to perform the bony work first and secondarily to address any oculomotor disorders that are present. Further discussion of the treatment of oculomotor disorders is beyond the scope of this chapter.

Recurrences of hypertelorism

In our experience, hypertelorism recurrences are not frequent if the repair has been performed after 4 years of age, at the completion of skull growth. This recurrence rate would be different if the hypertelorism were corrected earlier; for instance, at 1 year of age the brain is still undergoing significant growth which might counteract medialization of the orbits. An exceptional circumstance of orbital hypertelorism relapse has been encountered with an interorbital encephalocele which had recurred because of ventriculoperitoneal shunt dysfunction. The encephalocele acted as an interorbital expander that progressively enlarged the tissues between the orbital cavities.

Conversely, the inherent lack of growth in faciocraniosynostosis may produce relative relapse of any associated maxillary retrusion, but this finding does not require further revision.

Careful analysis with three-dimensional computed tomography helps tremendously in planning for precise bony work.[37] Nevertheless, minor primary undercorrection of hypertelorism is more frequent than actual recurrence, despite satisfactory bony work. This finding underscores the importance of soft-tissue refinements, especially with regard to nasal correction, which will eventually determine the success of the clinical outcome. In older patients, nasal deformity may not only be the presenting chief complaint; it might also be the final and most important step of the surgical correction.[38,39]

Craniofacial surgery is teamwork

It is obvious from the congenital craniofacial malformations discussed in this chapter that the only possible approach to these patients is via a craniofacial team. Once the team members have examined the patient, and with the invaluable help of modern imaging, a plan of treatment is drawn up by the plastic surgeon and the neurosurgeon to incorporate all the morphological and functional aspects of the correction. These operations are too complex to be performed without significant previous experience with the problems involved. Such experience can only be obtained if these operations are performed in a limited number of specialized centers.

🌐 Access the complete reference list online at   **http://www.expertconsult.com**

5. Tessier P. Anatomical classification of facial, craniofacial and lateofacial clefts. *J Maxillofac Surg.* 1976;4:69.

7. Marchac D, Renier D, Broumand S. Timing of treatment for craniosynostosis : a 20 year experience. *Br J Plast Surg.* 1994;47:211–222. *The authors report their extensive experience in this 983-patient series. With early diagnosis, brachycephalies are corrected between 2 and 4 months of life; other craniosynostoses are addressed in the second half of the first year of life.*

9. Crouzon O. Dysostose craniofaciale héréditaire. *Bull Soc Med Hôp Paris.* 1912;33:545–555.

10. Tessier P. Osteotomies totales de la face: Syndrome de Crouzon, syndrome d'Apert, oxycephalies, scaphocephalies, turricephalies. *Ann Chir Plast.* 1967;12:273.

13. Ortiz-Monasterio F, Fuente del Campo A, Carillo A. Advancement of the orbits and the midface in one piece, combined with frontal repositioning for the correction of Crouzon's deformities. *Plast Reconstr Surg.* 1978;61:507–516. *The authors advocate composite advancement of the orbits and midface in addition to frontal advancement for the management of Crouzon's syndrome. They caution that, while they are optimistic, their data do not have sufficient follow-up to demonstrate the longevity of their results.*

16. Arnaud E, Marchac D, Renier D. Reduction of morbidity of frontofacial advancement in children with distraction. *Plast Reconstr Surg.* 2007;120:1009–1026. *This is a prospective analysis of 36 patients undergoing monobloc distraction for faciocraniosynostosis. The authors assessed their outcomes and concluded that their use of internal distraction reduced the risks inherent to monobloc advancement.*

17. Apert E. De l'acrocephalosyndactylie. *Bull Soc Med Hop Paris.* 1906;23:1310.

19. Renier D, Sainte-Rose C, Marchac D, et al. Intracranial pressure in craniostenosis. *J Neurosurg.* 1982;57:370–377. *Pre- and postoperative intracranial pressure (ICP) measurements were taken in 23 craniosynostosis patients. Elevated ICP normalized after surgery. A correlation was noted between elevated ICP and lower cognitive testing.*

21. Converse JM, Ransohoff J, Matthew E, et al. Ocular hypertelorism and pseudohypertelorism. Advances in surgical treatment. *Plast Reconstr Surg.* 1970;45:1. *This review begins with a discussion of the definition of hypertelorism and associated diagnoses. A detailed survey of corrective procedures follows.*

22. Tessier P. Experience in the treatment of orbital hypertelorism. *Plast Reconstr Surg.* 1974;53:4.

31

Craniofacial clefts

James P. Bradley and Henry K. Kawamoto Jr.

SYNOPSIS

- Congenital craniofacial clefts are abnormal disfigurements of the face and cranium occurring in a variety of patterns and varying degrees of severity.

- Craniofacial clefts are thought to occur spontaneously, except for syndromes with clefting combinations numbers 6, 7, and 8, like Treacher Collins syndrome or hemifacial microsomia.

- If normal embryologic neuroectoderm migration and penetration do not occur, the epithelium breaks down to form a facial cleft. The severity of the cleft is proportional to the failure of penetration by the neuroectoderm.

- Tessier's numeric classification from number 0 to number 14 (facial clefts = numbers 0–8 and cranial clefts = numbers 9–14) offers a descriptive, easy-to-understand system for rare craniofacial clefts and is treatment-oriented.

- Median craniofacial dysplasias consist of hypoplastic (tissue deficiency), dysraphia (normal tissue but clefted), and hyperplastic (tissue excess) malformations.

- During infancy (3–12 months), functional problems, soft-tissue clefts, and midline cranial defects (e.g., encephaloceles) may be corrected.

- In older children (6–9 years), midface and orbital reconstruction with bone grafting or a facial bipartition may be performed.

- At skeletal maturity orthognathic and soft-tissue remodeling are offered as final corrective procedures.

Introduction

Congenital craniofacial clefts are abnormal disfigurements of the face and cranium with deficiencies, excesses, or even a normal (but separated) amount of tissue occurring along linear regions.[1–4] Of all congenital facial anomalies, craniofacial clefts are among the most disfiguring. They may be seen in a variety of patterns and varying degrees of severity. Although at first glance they appear to defy definable patterns, most craniofacial clefts occur along predictable embryologic lines.[5] Craniofacial clefts may be either unilateral or bilateral, and one cleft type can manifest on one side of the face, while a different type is present on the other side.

Classifications of craniofacial clefts

These craniofacial malformations are rare and have multiple variations and a spectrum of severity. For diagnostic and treatment purposes, the use of similar terminology describing embryologic maldevelopment, genetic etiology, or anatomic landmarks is beneficial. Organization of the seemingly heterogeneous clefting malformations is necessary for both morphogenetic understanding and knowledge of surgical anatomy for treatment. Therefore, orderly systems of classification have been described.[1–4]

The American Association of Cleft Palate Rehabilitation (AACPR) separated craniofacial clefts into four categories based on pathologic location: (1) mandibular process clefts; (2) naso-ocular clefts; (3) oro-ocular clefts; and (4) oroaural clefts.[6] First, mandibular process clefts group malformations of the mandible and lower lip. Second, naso-ocular clefts include malformations located between the nasal ala and the medial canthus. Third, oro-ocular clefts consist of clefting anomalies connecting the oral cavity to the orbit between the medial and lateral canthus. Fourth, oroaural clefts describe anomalies involving the region from the oral commissure to the auricular tragus. Subsequent to the AACPR classification, Boo-Chai made modifications based on surface anatomic landmarks, including skeletal components.[7] The oro-ocular clefts were subdivided into two types, the oromedial canthus and orolateral canthus, with the infraorbital foramen as a reference point.

The Karfik classification has an embryologic and morphologic basis and is divided into five groups: (1) group A: rhinencephalic malformations; (2) group B: anomalies of the first and second branchial arch; (3) group C: orbitopalpebral malformations; (4) group D: craniocephalic malformations (e.g., Apert and Crouzon syndromes); and (5) group E: atypical deformities from congenital tumors, atrophy, hypertrophy, and true oblique clefts which cannot be related to any embryologic fusion line.[8] Group A, the rhinencephalic malformations, was further divided into two subtypes: group A1, axial malformations derived from frontonasal prominence, and group A2, paraxial malformations adjacent to the nasal region. Group B, anomalies of the first and second branchial arch, was also further divided into two subtypes: group B1, composed of the lateral otocephalic malformations (craniofacial microsomia, Treacher Collins syndrome, Pierre Robin sequence, and auricular malformations) and group B2, including the mandibular midline malformations.

The Van der Meulen classification used the term "dysplasia" since some of the malformations did not represent true clefts.[9] The defects were labeled by the name of the developmental area (facial processes and bones) that is involved. The malformations are believed to occur before or during the fusion of the facial processes, but before the start of ossification (Fig. 31.1).

Median craniofacial clefts require special consideration because of variation in malformations and deformations. With tissue agenesis and holoprosencephaly at one end (the hypoplasias), and frontonasal hyperplasia and excessive tissue (the hyperplasias) at the other end, median anomalies with normal tissue volume occupy the middle portion of the spectrum.[10] Noordhoff *et al.* limited the term "holoprosencephaly" to cases of alobar brain and preferred the term "dysplasia" rather than "dysgenesis".[11] Thus, for clarification, median craniofacial dysplasias have been organized and divided into:

I. median craniofacial hypoplasia (tissue deficiency or agenesis)
II. median craniofacial dysraphia (normal tissue volume but clefted)
III. median craniofacial hyperplasia (tissue excess or duplication).

Under each division further subclassification is used to describe the specific anomalies of the number 0–14 clefts (Table 31.1).

I: Median craniofacial hypoplasia (tissue deficiency and/or agenesis)

A. Holoprosencephalic spectrum (alobar brain)

1. Cyclopia: described as a single eye in a single orbit. Arrhinia exists with proboscis often located above the single orbit. Microcephaly is also a component.
2. Ethmocephaly: severe hypotelorism exists but the orbits are separate anatomically. Again, arrhinia is present; however, the proboscis is located in between the orbits.
3. Cebocephaly: moderate to severe hypotelorism is noted. There is a proboscis-like rudimentary nose in a more typical nasal position.
4. Primary palate agenesis: the primary palate, including the premaxillary segment and associated midline structures, is absent or severely deficient. Hypotelorism is seen.

B. Median cerebrofacial hypoplasia (lobar brain)

In this condition, midline facial hypoplasia and midline cerebral malformations exist. Unilateral or bilateral cleft lip and palate may be present.

C. Median facial hypoplasia

Midline facial hypoplasia exists without gross cerebral involvement. Unilateral or bilateral cleft lip and palate may again be present.

D. Microforms of median facial hypoplasia

Microform variants of median facial hypoplasia may occur when there are mild deficiencies from maldevelopment of the median facial structures. Unilateral or bilateral cleft lip and palate can also be found. This group also includes:

1. Binder syndrome or anomaly (maxillonasal dysplasia) patients have characteristic flat nasomaxillary facial region with deficient or absent nasal spine and a negative overjet from class III anterior incisor relationship.

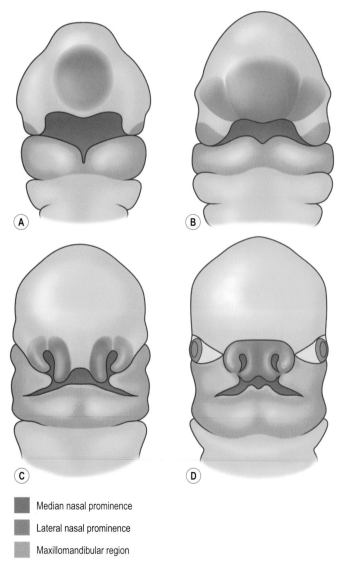

Median nasal prominence

Lateral nasal prominence

Maxillomandibular region

Fig. 31.1 Embryology of the face. Illustration depicting facial development at **(A)** 27 days; **(B)** 33 days; **(C)** 39 days; and **(D)** 46 days with migration of median nasal prominence, lateral nasal prominence, and maxillomandibular region.

Table 31.1 Classification of median craniofacial dysplasia

Subclassification	Description
I. Median craniofacial hypoplasia	Tissue deficiency.
A. Holoprosencephalic spectrum (alobar brain)	*Single holistic brain* with midline facial hypoplasia or agenesis. Four subclassifications: cyclopia, ethmocephaly, cebocephaly, primary palate agenesis.
1. Cyclopia	1. Single eye in a single orbit, arrhinia with proboscis often located above the single orbit and microcephaly.
2. Ethmocephaly	2. Severe hypotelorism but separate orbits. Arrhinia with proboscis located in between the orbits.
3. Cebocephaly	3. Severe hypotelorism. Proboscis-like rudimentary nose.
4. Primary palate agenesis	4. Premaxillary segment missing of hypoplastic.
B. Median cerebrofacial hypoplasia (lobar brain)	*Separate lobes* to brain but with midline cerebral malformation; midline facial hypoplasia.
C. Median facial hypoplasia	Midline facial hypoplasia without gross cerebral involvement.
D. Microforms of median facial hypoplasia	1. Binder anomaly (maxillonasal dysplasia).
	2. Central maxillary incisor anomaly.
	3. Absent upper lip frenulum.
II. Median craniofacial dysraphia	Normal tissue volume but clefted.
A. True median cleft	Isolated cleft of the upper lip or abnormal split between the median globular process. It can be an incomplete or complete form.
B. Anterior encephalocele	Cystic malformation in which central nervous structures are abnormally displaced or herniated through a defect in the cranium.
III. Median craniofacial hyperplasia	Tissue excess or duplication. All forms of excess tissue starting from just thickened or duplicated nasal septum to the more severe forms of frontonasal dysplasia.

2. Abnormalities of the maxillary central incisors: three variants of this include:
   (a) absent central maxillary incisors
   (b) single maxillary central incisor
   (c) hypoplastic central maxillary incisors.
3. Absence of upper lip frenulum.

II: Median craniofacial dysraphia

Median craniofacial dysraphia describes a midline anomaly that has normal tissue volume, but clefting or an abnormal separation of midline structures is present. Within the spectrum of median craniofacial dysplasia there is a group of malformations which have normal tissue volume but have abnormally split (true median cleft lip) or displaced (encephalocele). This group is better placed as median tissue defects midway between hypoplasia and hyperplasia.

A. True median cleft

A true median cleft may manifest as an isolated cleft of the upper lip, "0 cleft", not associated with either hypoplasia or hyperplasia. Alternatively, a true median cleft may have tissue deficiency or agenesis, e.g., absent nasal septum. A true median cleft may also occur with tissue excess, e.g., duplicated nasal septum. With median craniofacial dysraphia a true median cleft has separated, but there is a normal tissue amount. The upper lip deformity is a true median cleft lip with a split between the median globular processes. This is opposed to a "false" median cleft with agenesis of the globular processes. With the true median cleft the separation

passes between the central incisors. The cleft may continue posteriorly as a cleft of the primary and/or secondary palate. When the cleft encroaches into the interorbital region, orbital hypertelorism may be seen.

B. Anterior encephaloceles

An encephalocele is a cystic congenital malformation in which central nervous system structures have herniated through a defect in the cranium in communication with cerebrospinal fluid pathways. They occur between normally developed zones, where a weakness permits brain to escape. The mass further pushes surrounding fields apart.

Anterior encephaloceles are divided into frontoethmoidal and basal groups. In frontoethmoidal encephaloceles, the defect occurs at the junction of the frontal and ethmoidal bones (the foramen cecum).[12] Nasoethmoidal encephalocele is considered a Tessier number 14 cleft or frontonasal dysraphia in Mazzola's morphological classification. Basal encephaloceles are associated with a defect at or behind the crista galli and, in some cases, they may protrude through a defect in the sphenoid bone and are called trans-sphenoidal encephalocele.[13]

III: Median craniofacial hyperplasia (tissue excess or duplication)

This spectrum of anomalies includes all forms of excess tissue starting from just thickened or duplicated nasal septum towards the more severe forms of frontonasal dysplasia.

"Frontonasal dysplasia" was the most widely known of these types of hyperplasias.[14] Objections are raised about the terminology of this condition. Typically, the term "dysplasia" refers to the whole spectrum of abnormal tissue development starting from tissue agenesis and hypoplasia all the way to the other extreme of hyperplasia and excess tissue.

The basic defect of median craniofacial hyperplasia is not known. Embryologically, if the nasal capsule fails to develop properly, the primitive brain vesicle fills the space normally occupied by the capsule, thus producing anterior cranium bifidum occultum and leading to morphokinetic arrest in the positioning of the eyes and nostrils, which tend to maintain their relative fetal positions.[15,16] Experiments have shown that a reduction in the number of migrating neural crest cells results in these multiple defects.[17,18]

Other nasal findings may range from a notched broad nasal tip to completely divided nostrils with hypoplasia and even absence of the prolabium and maxilla with a median cleft lip. In addition, variable notching of the ala is described. Occasionally, associated abnormalities include accessory nasal tags, low-set ears, conductive hearing loss, mild to severe retardation, basal encephalocele, and agenesis of the corpus callosum. Importantly, a high incidence of ocular abnormalities is described. More distant anomalies include tetralogy of Fallot, absence of the tibia, and others. When hypertelorism is severe or when extracephalic anomalies occur, mental deficiency appears to be more likely and more severe.[14,15,17]

The Tessier classification of craniofacial clefts was described in 1976.[1] This classification has proven to be the most complete and has withstood the test of time. This insightful classification was based on the extensive personal experience by Tessier in the anatomy laboratory, in the operating room, and from his embryologic knowledge. The terminology is uniform, and the characterizations of specific features are detailed. It is also reproducible by clinicians evaluating craniofacial clefts. In addition, the classification links the clinical observations with underlying skeletal deformity documented by preoperative three-dimensional (3D) computed tomography (CT) scan imaging and confirmed during surgery. Correlation of the clinical appearance with the surgical anatomic findings improves the clinical utility of this system for the craniofacial surgeon. Distinctive features such as Tessier craniofacial clefts are described below.

Epidemiology and etiologic factors

The true incidence of craniofacial clefts is unknown because of their rarity and because of the difficulty in recognizing sometimes subtle physical findings in mild malformations. However, the incidence of craniofacial clefts has been estimated at 1.4–4.9 per 100 000 live births.[1–3] The incidence of rare craniofacial clefts compared to common cleft lip and palate malformations may range from 9.5 to 34 per 1000.[3]

Most rare craniofacial clefts occur sporadically. However, the role of heredity in the causation of rare craniofacial clefts seems to occur in Treacher Collins syndrome and in some familial cases of Goldenhar syndrome. A dominant gene defect (TCOF-1) causes Treacher Collins syndrome.[19] Although penetrance is somewhat variable, the malformation is very consistent. In a TCOF-1 gene knock-out animal model, regional massive cell death affected crest cell mesenchymal

migration and resulted in zygomatic abnormalities. Constriction limb deformities (amniotic band syndrome) have also been associated with rare facial clefting. Coady et al. found a statistically significant association between craniofacial clefts and limb ring constrictions.[20]

Based on animal and human clinical studies, many environmental factors have also been shown to cause facial clefts. These investigations produced four major categories: (1) radiation[21,22]; (2) infection[23,24]; (3) maternal metabolic imbalances[25]; and (4) drugs and chemicals.[26] A considerable number of drugs and chemicals have teratogenic potential, but few have been shown to cause craniofacial malformations in humans. Some medications, including those containing retinoic acid, are being looked at as a cause of facial malformations.[27]

Although the teratogenic potential of drugs and their effect on facial development are known, the critical phase of embryologic differentiation and development occurs when a mother may be unknowingly pregnant. Teratologists are confronted with the problem of multiple factors acting on numerous pathways and have no simple answer that universally explains the formation of a particular cleft.

Embryologic craniofacial development

The understanding of normal morphogenesis occurring in the embryo and fetus allows the clinician to describe and classify craniofacial clefts of infants and adults. Likewise, the study of rare craniofacial clefts lends clues to facial and neuroembryology. A traditional summary of normal facial development and newer understanding of genetically determined development zones of the face based on neuroembryology is outlined below.

The three primary germ layers, ectoderm, mesoderm, and endoderm, are the basis for tissue and organ formation.[28] In the third week of gestation, the primitive tissues of the trilaminar embryo give rise to notochordal and prechordal mesoderm. Simultaneously, the rostral ectoderm differentiates to form highly specialized neural crest cells, which are responsible for the ultimate development of the brain and midline facial structures.[29] The ectoderm forms a neural plate with bilateral folds which conjoin into a neural tube. During closure of the neural tube, neural crest cells (mesenchyme) migrate into underlying tissue, forming pluripotential stem cells. The embryonic prominences of the face are formed by the migration of these neural crest cells. A segmental pattern of ventral migration of neural crest, termed rhombomeres, provides the precursors of cartilage, bone, muscle, and connective tissue of the face and head.

Any defect in the quantity and quality of this migrating ectomesenchyme is manifest as a craniofacial malformation from severe holoprosencephaly to minor clinical stigmata of craniofacial clefts like dimples or skin tags.[30] Another cause for arrested development causing dysplasias and dystopias (the abnormal formation and location of structures) is abnormal development or involution of embryologic arteries.[31]

Starting at the fourth week of gestation, the face assumes a recognizable form.[32] Between 4 and 8 weeks of gestation the crown–rump length increases from approximately 3.5 mm to 28 mm. The double-layer stomodeal membrane creates the opening for the primitive mouth. An overhanging frontonasal prominence represents the superior border of the stomodeum.[2] Five prominences (the frontonasal and paired maxillary and mandibular) formed by neural crest migration surround the stomodeum (see Fig. 31.1). The frontonasal prominence is formed by neural crest cells migrating ventrally from the mesencephalic region and contributes to the frontal and nasal bones. The maxillary and mandibular prominences are formed by more caudally located migrating neural crest cells that encounter pharyngeal endoderm in their ventral migration around the aortic arches.

Optic vesicles appear from lateral invaginations of the diencephalons and induce lens placodes in ectoderm and neural crest migration to form the sclera. Defective optic vesicle formation results in microphthalmos, or anophthalmos. The movement of this optic tissue from lateral to medial results from the narrowing frontonasal prominence and expansion of the lateral face. Inadequate transition of the eyes produces hypertelorism, and overmigration produces hypotelorism or even median cyclopia.[33]

During the sixth week, the medial nasal processes enlarge and coalesce in the midline. The nasal placodes arise from ectodermal tissue inferolateral to the frontonasal prominence and cephalad to the stomodeum. Nasal placodes invaginate into the face to form nasal pits and elevations at the margins produce a horseshoe-shaped median and lateral nasal prominences. The caudal extensions of the medial nasal processes, the globular processes, are united with the developing maxillary processes to form the upper lip. The medial nasal process gives rise to the nasal tip, the columella, the philtrum, and the premaxilla. The nasal alae are derived from the lateral nasal processes. The frontonasal process contributes the bridge and the root of the nose.

The posterior aspect of each nasal pit is separated from the oral cavity by an oronasal membrane. Failure of this membrane to disintegrate normally leads to choanal atresia.[34] The paired median nasal processes merge with the frontonasal prominence to form the majority of the frontal process. These structures gradually enlarge and superiorly displace the frontonasal prominence. During the sixth week, the two median nasal processes coalesce in the midline, and their most caudal limbs, the premaxillary prominence, expand above the stomodeum. The nasal tip, philtrum, columella, cartilaginous septum, and primary palate are derived from these paired median elements. Cephalad to the medial nasal process, the frontonasal process persists to form the nasal dorsum and root. Elevation of the lateral nasal prominence creates the nasal alae. Defects during this development may be midline and produce arrhinia or a bifid nose.

The maxillary processes are paired mesodermal masses that lie cephalad to the mandibular arch and ventral to the optic neuroectoderm. These triangular masses enlarge, separate from the mandibular arch, and then migrate ventrally. The maxillary process ultimately coalesces with the mesoderm of the globular processes to form the upper lip. The cheek, maxilla, zygoma, and secondary palate are also derived from the maxillary processes. Between the maxillary prominence and lateral nasal prominence a depression exists with a solid rod of epithelial cells.[35] The ends of this rod form a connection from the nasal pit to the conjunctival sac (nasolacrimal duct). With inadequate neural crest cell migration a fissure within the line of this duct may persist as an oblique facial cleft.

The stomodeal aperture is reduced by migrating mesenchyme fusing the maxillary and mandibular prominences to form the oral commissures. Inadequate neural crest cells result in macrostomia while excessive tissue produces microstomia or macrostomia. The mandibular prominence lies between the stomodeum and the first branchial groove, which delineates the caudal limits of the face. The paired free ends of the mandibular arch enlarge and converge ventrally during the sixth week. The lower lip and mandible are developed from this arch. Paired lateral pharyngeal elevations of the arch unite to form the anterior portion of the tongue.

The external and middle ear are also formed during the sixth week of gestation. The tragus and the crus of the helix are derived from three hillocks at the caudal border of the first branchial arch. The malleus and incus of the middle ear are also formed by the first branchial arch. The remainder of the external ear is formed from three hillocks on the cephalic border of the second branchial arch. The stapes of the middle ear is also formed by the second branchial arch.

During a short 4-week period, there is a coordination of cell migration, cellular interaction, and apoptosis. Failure of this intricate program will result in clefts that will usually fall along predictable embryonic lines.

Failure of fusion

Two theories exist that describe how embryologic failure or errors result in craniofacial cleft malformations. First, the "fusion failure" theory suggests that clefts are created when fusion of facial processes fail.[36] Second, the "failure of mesodermal penetration" theory implicates the lack of mesoderm and neuroectoderm migration and penetration into the bilaminar ectodermal sheets as the cause of craniofacial clefts.[37] Although most of the current knowledge is based on animal cleft lip and palate studies, rare craniofacial clefts may be produced by similar mechanisms.

The "failure of fusion" theory, proposed by Dursy in 1869 and His in 1892, purported that the free edges of the facial processes unite in the central region of the face.[35] As various processes fuse, the face gradually forms. When epithelial contact is established between opposing facial processes, mesodermal penetration completes the fusion. Dursy suggested that the upper lip is created when finger-like advancing ends of the maxillary process and the paired global process unite. He asserted that disruption of this sequence results in craniofacial cleft anomalies.

Proponents of the mesodermal penetration theory believed that the finger-like ends of the facial processes do not exist. Warbrick[38] and Stark and Ehrmann[39] suggest that the central facial processes are composed of bilamellar sheets of ectoderm. This bilamellar membrane is bordered by epithelial seams, which delineate the principal processes. During development, the mesenchymal tissue migrates and penetrates this double-layered ectoderm, called the "epithelial wall". Caudal to the stomodeum, the lower face is formed by the branchial arches. The arches consist of a thin sheet of mesoderm, which lies between the ectodermal and endodermal layers. The neural crest cells of neuroectodermal origin, which arise from the dorsolateral surface of the neural tube, migrate under the ectoderm and supplement the mesoderm of the frontonasal process and branchial arches.[40] Most of the craniofacial skeleton is believed to be formed by these neural crest cells. If neuroectoderm migration and penetration do not occur, the epithelium breaks down to form a facial cleft. The severity of the cleft is proportional to the failure of penetration by the neuroectoderm. Unfortunately, the precise nature of the proposed mechanisms in the formation of rare craniofacial clefts is not known. Nevertheless, the concepts of fusion and mesodermal penetration provide an understanding of the problems of the rare craniofacial cleft.

Neuromeric theory

Newer understanding of neuroembryology suggests that a direct relationship exists between the development of the nervous system and those structures to which its contents are dedicated. The neural tube is conceived as a series of developmental zones within the central nervous system.[41,42] Six prosomeres provide a Cartesian system to organize the tracts and nuclei of the prosencephalon (forebrain). The mesencephalon (midbrain) and rhombencephalon (hindbrain) are subdivided into two mesomeres and 12 rhombomeres, respectively. Each of these neuromeres is defined by a unique overlap of several genetic coding zones along the axis of the embryo. In the hindbrain and caudally to the coccyx these neuromeric units are defined by the Homeobox series of genes (Hox genes). In the forebrain, a more complex series of genes is used, such as Sonic hedgehog (Shh), Wingless (Wnt), and Engrailed (En).

The unique "barcode" for each neuromeric zone is shared with all cells exiting from a particular level to form the mesoderm and endoderm of the embryo. For example, the Hox gene which codes for the rhombomeres 2 and 3 (which make up the first pharyngeal arch – PA1) is shared with the mesoderm that makes up those arches. This same Hox gene is also shared with the neural crest cells which subsequently move into the mesodermal "zones" of PA1. The migrating neural crest cells then provide the instructions for differentiation into the appropriate facial tissues. Thus, all the bones and soft tissues of the face can be thought of as genetically determined "fields" with defined cellular content and a fixed position in space. With the folding of the embryo, these fields are placed into their correct topologic positions and a three-dimensional form results.

This system permits the "mapping" of the face into developmental zones with distinct spatial origins in their precursor tissue units. The midline mesoderm of the nasal and ocular fields is of different origin, innervation, and blood supply from all surrounding mesodermal elements. When all the developmental zones are accounted for, the occurrence of craniofacial clefts is nothing more than an orderly progression of deficiency states in the precursor fields, resulting in varying degrees of absence of soft-tissue functional matrix or underlying bone. The anatomic and clinical observations of Tessier and his classification system are exactly compatible with this map. Variations include (1) clefts number 2 and 3 fall within the same zone (cleft number 3 being more posterior) and (2) clefts number 4 and 5 represent varying degrees of involvement in the same zone of the maxilla. Tessier's classification system has been widely adopted by surgeons and other clinicians and has stood the test of time. However, geneticists and embryologists have been slow to embrace his numeric organization of craniofacial clefts because it could not previously be understood by existing theories of embryologic developmental. The consistency of these newer neuroembryologic theories with Tessier's classification of craniofacial clefts reinforces the importance of Tessier's descriptions. With progression of the neuromeric theory, the value of Tessier's organization of rare craniofacial clefts should become apparent to embryologists and geneticists.

Patient selection

Distinctive features of Tessier craniofacial clefts

Tessier developed a classification for rare craniofacial clefts based on his anatomical and operative observations and experiences (Fig. 31.2A,B). The clefts are numbered from 0 to 14, follow well-defined zones of the face and orbit, and correlate with embryologic developmental maps (Fig. 31.2C). The numbered clefts relate soft-tissue clinical features to underlying bony involvement verified by operative findings and more recently preoperative 3D CT assessments.

The eyelids and orbits define the horizontal axis dividing the face into upper and lower hemispheres. Tessier used these landmarks, because the orbit belongs to both the cranium and the face. Thus, the orbit separates the numbered cranial clefts from the facial clefts. In addition, the following combinations of numeric clefts are often clinically observed: 0 and 14, 1 and 13, 2 and 12, 3 and 11, 4 and 10, 5 and 9, and 6 and 8. Clefts 5–9 are considered lateral clefts, because they pass lateral to the infraorbital foramen. Tessier cleft number 7 is the most lateral craniofacial cleft.

The clinical expression of the craniofacial cleft is highly variable. Tessier reported that the soft-tissue and skeletal components were seldom affected to the same extent. Skeletal landmarks are more constant and reliable than the soft-tissue landmarks. Typically, facial clefts located medial to the infraorbital foramen had greater soft-tissue involvement than clefts found lateral to the foramen. By contrast, facial clefts located lateral to the infraorbital foramen had greater bony disruption than clefts found medial to the foramen. Finally, bilateral forms of the clefts are found in varying combinations, often creating an asymmetric malformation.

The craniofacial clefts, as described below, use the Tessier classification to relate soft-tissue features to underlying skeletal involvement. The severity of involvement of regional structures influences the therapeutic strategy. The order of description below consists of facial clefts from medial to lateral followed by cranial clefts from lateral to medial.

Number 0 cleft

The number 0 cleft has been called median craniofacial dysraphia, centrofacial microsomia, frontonasal dysplasia, median cleft face syndrome, or holoprosencephaly; but, for accuracy, it is the facial manifestation or lower half of "median craniofacial dysplasia", as described above.[43,44] Patients with this midline facial cleft may have a cranial extension or a number 14 cleft. As mentioned above, the number 0 Tessier craniofacial clefts are unique in that there may be a deficiency, normal, or excess tissue. With tissue agenesis and holoprosencephaly at one end (the hypoplasias), and frontonasal hyperplasia and excessive tissue (the hyperplasias) at the other end, median anomalies with normal tissue volume occupy the middle portion of the spectrum.

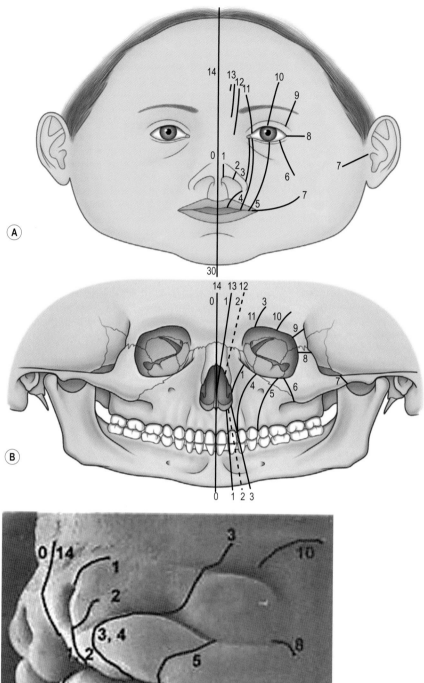

Fig. 31.2 Tessier classification of craniofacial clefts. Soft-tissue landmarks are outlined in **(A)**; skeletal locations of numeric clefts are depicted in **(B)**. Facial clefts are numbers 0 through 7, and cranial clefts are numbers 8 through 14. Mandibular midline facial cleft is number 30. **(C)** Embryology correlation to Tessier facial clefts: Tessier-numbered craniofacial clefts are shown correlating with growth center junctions in this 45-day-old fetus.

Median craniofacial hypoplasia (deficiency of midline structures)

A deficiency may manifest as hypoplasia or agenesis in which portions of midline facial structures are missing (Fig. 31.3). This developmental arrest may range from the mildest form of hypoplasia of the nasomaxillary region and hypotelorism to a severe form of cyclopia, ethmocephaly, or cebocephaly. The subcategories (see Table 31.1) demonstrate that the severity of facial anomalies correlate well with the severity of brain abnormality and mental retardation. A CT scan of the brain can differentiate between alobar and lobar brain anomalies and clarify the spectrum of holoprosencephalic patients. Clinically it may be important to distinguish among patients

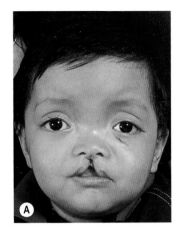

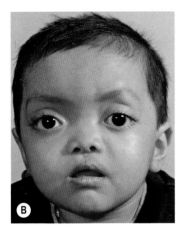

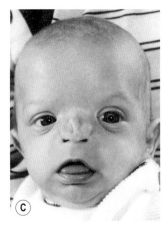

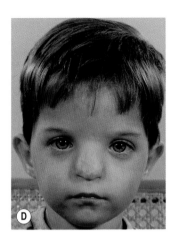

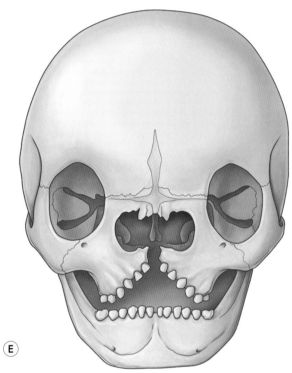

Fig. 31.3 Number 0 cleft. **(A,B)** Patient with a true median cleft lip, cleft palate, hypertelorbitism, and sphenoethmoidal encephalocele (not seen). **(A)** Preoperative view. **(B)** Postoperative view after median cleft lip repair. **(C,D)** Patient with excessive midline tissue manifested by bifid nose and an accessory band of skin on the nasal dorsum. **(C)** Preoperative view. **(D)** Postoperative view after initial nasal surgery. **(E)** Illustration of skeletal involvement demonstrates separation between the central incisors, widening of the nasal region, and orbital hypertelorism.

with poor brain differentiation who may die in infancy from those with a better prognosis.

Soft-tissue deficiencies

Soft-tissue deficiencies with Tessier 0 clefts include the upper lip and nose. Agenesis or hypoplasia may result in a false median cleft lip and absence of philtral columns. When a wide central cleft exists, it typically extends the length of the upper lip and up into the nasal floor (see Fig. 31.3A,B). With nasal anomalies, the columella may be narrowed or totally absent. The nasal tip may be depressed from lack of septal support. The septum may often be vestigial with no caudal attachment to the palate. Dental abnormalities may include absent central maxillary incisors, single maxillary central incisor, and/or hypoplastic central maxillary incisors.

Skeletal deficiencies

Skeletal deficiencies range from separation between the upper central canines to absence of the premaxilla and a cleft of the secondary palate (see Fig. 31.3C). Nasal deficiency may include partial or total absence of the septal cartilage and even nasal bones. The bone defect may extend cephalad into the area of the ethmoid sinuses and result in hypotelorism or cyclopia. Nasomaxillary deficiencies like these may be seen in Binder syndrome.

Median craniofacial dysraphia (normal tissue volume but clefted)

These Tessier 0 clefts placed between the hypoplasias and hyperplasias have normal tissue volume but are abnormally split (true median cleft lip) or displaced (encephalocele).

Soft-tissue involvement

When an isolated cleft of the upper lip is not associated with tissue deficiency (e.g., absent nasal septum) or tissue excess (e.g., duplicated septum) it is considered a "true" median cleft lip. With a true median cleft lip there is a split between the median globular processes, whereas with a false median cleft lip an agenesis of the globular processes may occur. An encephalocele is a cystic congenital malformation in which central nervous system structures herniate through a defect in the cranium in communication with cerebrospinal fluid pathways.[45] They occur between normally developed zones, where a weakness permits the brain to escape the cranial space. The mass may further push the developmental fields apart.[42]

Skeletal involvement

When the true median cleft passes between the central incisors, the cleft can continue posteriorly as a midline cleft palate. When the cleft encroaches into the interorbital region, hypertelorbitism may occur. Anterior encephaloceles are divided into basal and frontoethmoidal groups. In frontoethmoidal encephaloceles, the defect occurs at the junction of the frontal and ethmoidal bones (the foramen cecum).[12] Basal encephaloceles are associated with a defect at or behind the crista galli and, in some cases, they may protrude through a defect in the sphenoid bone.

Median craniofacial hyperplasia (excess of midline tissue)

This spectrum of midline anomalies includes all forms of excess tissue starting from just thickened or duplicated nasal septum (see Fig. 31.3C) towards the more severe forms of frontonasal dysplasia.

Soft-tissue midline excess

Soft-tissue midline excess tissue may be manifested in the lip with broad philtral columns or a duplication of the labial frenulum. The nose may be bifid with a broad columella and mid-dorsal furrow. The alar and upper lateral cartilages may be displaced laterally.

Skeletal excess

Skeletal excess in a widened number 0 facial cleft can be seen as a diastema between the upper central incisors. A duplicate nasal spine may exist. A characteristic keel-shaped maxillary alveolus is seen. Anterior teeth are angled toward the midline creating an anterior open bite. Central midface height is shortened. The cartilaginous and bone nasal septum is thickened or duplicated. The nasal bones and nasal process of the maxilla are broad, flattened, and displaced laterally from the midline. Ethmoidal and sphenoidal sinuses may be enlarged, contributing to symmetrical widening of the anterior cranial fossa and hypertelorism. The cribriform plate is low, and the breadth of the crista galli is exaggerated. The body of the sphenoid is broadened with displacement of the pterygoid plates away from the midline.

Number 1 cleft

This paramedian facial cleft was first delineated by Tessier.[1] Van der Meulen *et al.* nominated this cleft as a type 3 nasoschisis nasal dysplasia.[9] The number 1 facial cleft continues cranially as a number 13 cleft.

Soft-tissue involvement

The number 1 cleft, similar to the common cleft lip, passes through the cupid's bow and then the alar cartilage dome. Notching in the area of the soft triangle of the nose is a distinct feature (Fig. 31.4A). The columella may be short and broad. The nasal tip and nasal septum deviate away from the cleft. Soft-tissue furrows or wrinkles may be present on the nasal dorsum if the cleft extends in a cephalic direction. The cleft is evident medially to a malpositioned medial canthus, and telecanthus may result. With a cranial extension as a number 13 cleft, vertical dystopia is present.

Skeletal involvement

A keel-shaped maxilla exists with the anterior incisors facing toward the cleft creating an anterior open bite. An alveolar cleft is rare but would pass between the central and lateral incisors. This paramedian cleft separates the nasal floor at the pyriform aperture just lateral to the nasal spine (Fig. 31.4C). The cleft may extend posteriorly as a complete cleft of the hard and soft palate. Extension of the cleft in a cephalad direction is through the junction of the nasal bone and the frontal process of the maxilla. The nasal bones are displaced and flattened. Ethmoidal expansion leads to hypertelorism. Also, there is asymmetry of the greater and lesser sphenoid wings, the pterygoid plates, and anterior cranial fossa.

Number 2 cleft

Soft-tissue involvement

This other paramedian facial cleft also may begin in the region of the common cleft lip. However, the nasal deformity is in the middle third of the alar rim and distinguishes the number 2 cleft (Fig. 31.5). In the number 2 cleft, the ala is hypoplastic, whereas in the number 1 cleft, the ala is merely notched at the dome, and in the number 3 cleft, the alar base is displaced. The lateral aspect of the nose is flattened, and the dorsum is broad. The eyelid is not involved; the cleft passes medially to the palpebral fissure. Although the medial canthus is displaced, the lacrimal duct is usually not involved. If the cleft continues in a cephalad direction as a cranial number 12 cleft, then distortion of the medial brow is noted.

Skeletal involvement

The number 2 cleft begins between the lateral incisor and the canine. It extends into the pyriform aperture, lateral to the septum and medial to the maxillary sinus. A hard- and soft-palate cleft may occur. The nasal septum may be deviated away from the cleft. The cleft distorts the nasal bones as it passes between the nasal bones and the frontal process of the maxilla. Ethmoidal sinus involvement may result in orbital hypertelorism. Asymmetry of the greater and lesser sphenoid wings and anterior cranial base is present.

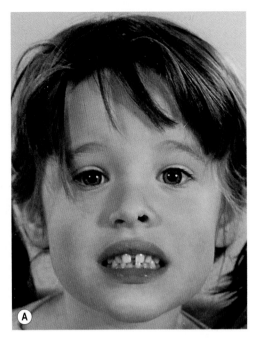

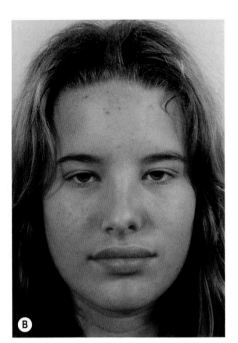

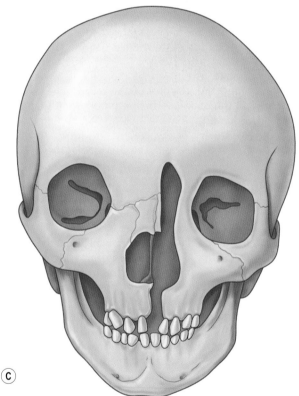

Fig. 31.4 Number 1 cleft. **(A)** Patient with notched left alar dome and orbital dystopia. **(B)** Same patient at maturity after left soft triangle reconstruction with composite graft. **(C)** Skeletal involvement is through the piriform aperture just lateral to the nasal spine and septum. The orbit is displaced laterally.

Number 3 cleft

The number 3 cleft is the most common of the Tessier craniofacial clefts. Morian reported the first case and later classified this as a Morian type I cleft.[46] It is also referred to as a Tessier oro-naso-ocular cleft. The cephalad continuation of the cleft is a number 11 cleft. In contrast to a common cleft lip and palate, a number 3 cleft has the following: (1) an equal distribution between males and females and (2) an

occurrence of one-third on the right, one-third on the left, and one-third bilateral. When bilateral clefting occurs, a number 4 or 5 facial cleft may be seen contralateral to the number 3 cleft.

Soft-tissue involvement

The number 3 cleft begins similar to a number 1 and 2 cleft, passing through the philtral column and floor of the nose.

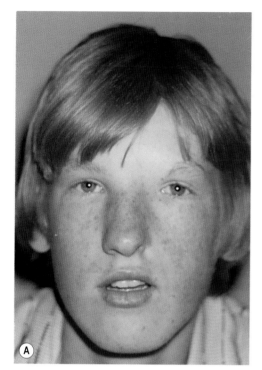

may occur directly on to the cheek instead of into the nasal cavity.

The medial canthus is inferiorly displaced and may be hypoplastic. Colobomas of the lower eyelid are medial to the inferior punctum. In mild forms, colobomas may be the only obvious evidence of this cleft. In mild cases it is important to check a CT scan for bony involvement and maintain an index

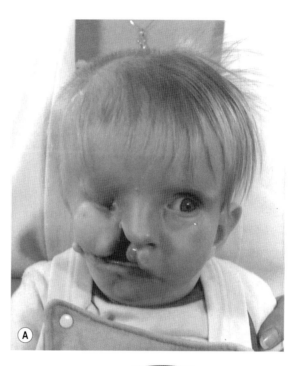

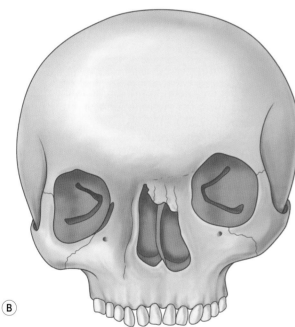

Fig. 31.5 Number 2 cleft. **(A)** Patient with hypoplasia of the middle third of the right nostril rim causing the appearance of alar base retraction. The lateral nose is flattened. The medial border of the eyebrow is also distorted as evidence of a number 12 cranial cleft. There is also orbital dystopia and displacement of the right medial canthus. **(B)** Skeletal involvement shows deformity of the piriform aperture and nasal bone.

Deficiency of tissue between the alar base and lower eyelid results in a shortened nose on the affected side. The cleft passes between the medial canthus and the inferior lacrimal punctum (Fig. 31.6A). The lacrimal system, particularly the lower canaliculus, is disrupted. Blockage of the nasolacrimal duct and recurrent infections of the lacrimal sac are common. The inferior punctum is displaced downward, and drainage

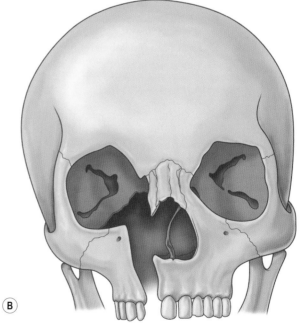

Fig. 31.6 Number 3 cleft. **(A)** Patient with complete form has a right cleft lip and palate and severe shortening of tissues between the right alar base and medial canthus. The right nasal ala is displaced superiorly, the medial canthus is displaced inferiorly, and the nasolacrimal system is disrupted. **(B)** Skeletal involvement is between the lateral incisor and the canine extending up through the lacrimal groove. The cleft creates a direct communication among the orbital, maxillary sinus, nasal, and oral cavities.

of suspicion for disruption of the lacrimal system. Involvement of the globe is rare, but microphthalmia may occur. Typically, the eye is malpositioned inferiorly and laterally. Injury to the eye, including corneal erosions, ocular perforation, and loss of vision, may result from desiccation unless the globe is protected.

Skeletal involvement

Osseous characteristics of this facial cleft include involvement of the orbit and direct communication of the oral, nasal, and orbital cavities (Fig. 31.6B). The cleft begins between the lateral incisor and the canine. In contrast to the number 1 and 2 facial clefts, the anterior maxillary arch is flat in the number 3 cleft. The number 3 cleft disrupts the frontal process of the maxilla and then terminates in the lacrimal groove. In the severest form, the cleft is bilateral and skeletal disruption is significant. With bilateral cases the contralateral facial cleft may be a number 4 or 5 cleft. There may be narrowing of the ethmoid and sphenoid sinuses. Both the orbital floor and anterior cranial base are displaced inferiorly.

Number 4 cleft

The number 4 cleft occurs lateral to the nose and other median facial structures. The cleft has been called meloschisis (separation of cheek). Dick reported the first case in the English literature and von Kulmus may have recorded the initial description in Latin in 1732.[47] The cleft has also been classified or referred to as oro-ocular (AACPR), orofacial cleft,[1] and medial maxillary dysplasia.[1,44] The cranial continuation of the cleft is the number 10 cleft. For unilateral number 4 facial clefts it is estimated that a distribution exists for right to left side of 2 to 1.3 and a distribution exists for male to female of 2.5 to 1. In contrast, bilateral cases occur in equal numbers of males and females. Bilateral cases are associated with contralateral craniofacial clefts numbers 3, 5, and 7.

Soft-tissue involvement

As opposed to numbers 1, 2, and 3 facial clefts, the number 4 cleft begins lateral to Cupid's bow and the philtral column and medial to the oral commissure (Fig. 31.7A). The orbicularis oris muscle is located in the lateral lip element with no muscle centrally. The cleft passes lateral to the nasal ala. Although the ala is not involved and the nose is intact, it is displaced superiorly. Bilateral involvement pulls the nose upward (Fig. 31.7B). The cleft extends through the cheek and into the lower eyelid lateral to the inferior punctum. The lower eyelid and lashes may extend directly into the lateral aspect of the cleft. The medial canthus and nasolacrimal system are normal. The globe is typically normal, but microphthalmia and anophthalmos may be seen.

Skeletal involvement

Skeletal involvement is usually less extensive than the number 3 cleft. The alveolar cleft begins between the lateral incisor and the canine (Fig. 31.7C). The cleft extends lateral to the pyriform aperture to involve the maxillary sinus. The medial wall of the maxillary sinus is intact. A confluence exists between the oral cavity, maxillary sinus, and

orbital cavity but not the nasal cavity. The cleft then passes medial to the infraorbital foramen. This landmark defines the boundary between the medial number 4 facial cleft and lateral number 5 facial cleft. The number 4 cleft terminates at the medial aspect of the inferior orbital rim. With an absent medial orbital floor and rim, the globe may prolapse inferiorly. In bilateral cases the medial midface and premaxilla are protrusive. The sphenoid body is asymmetric, and pterygoid plates are displaced but the anterior cranial base is unaffected.

Number 5 cleft

This facial cleft is the rarest of the oblique facial clefts. It has been called the oculofacial cleft II, Morian III cleft, a lateral maxillary dysplasia, or an oro-ocular type II cleft (AACPR classification).[1,48] The cephalad progression of the number 5 cleft is the number 9 cleft. One-quarter of cases are unilateral, one-quarter of cases are bilateral, and one-half of cases are combined with another facial cleft.

Soft-tissue involvement

The number 5 facial cleft begins just medial to the oral commissure and courses along the cheek lateral to the nasal ala (Fig. 31.8A,B). The cleft terminates in the lateral half of the lower eyelid. Although the globe is typically normal, microphthalmia may occur.

Skeletal involvement

The alveolar cleft begins lateral to the canine in the region of the premolars. In contrast to the number 4 cleft, the number 5 cleft then courses lateral to the infraorbital foramen and terminates in the lateral aspect of the orbital rim and floor (see Fig. 31.8A,C). The cleft is separated from the inferior orbital fissure. The maxillary sinus may be hypoplastic. Prolapse of orbital contents through the lateral orbital floor defect into the maxillary sinus causes vertical orbital dystopia. The lateral orbital wall may be thickened and the greater sphenoid wing abnormal. The cranial base is normal.

Number 6 cleft

This zygomaticomaxillary cleft represents an incomplete form of Treacher Collins syndrome. It was nominated a maxillozygomatic dysplasia by Van der Meulen et al.[44] Similar and often more severe cleft facial features are seen in Nager syndrome. Nager syndrome patients also may have radial club deformities of the upper extremities.

Soft-tissue involvement

The cleft is often identified as a vertical furrow, due to hypoplastic soft tissue, from the oral commissure to the lateral lower eyelid (Fig. 31.9A). This line of hypoplasia runs through the zygomatic eminence along an imaginary line from the angle of the mandible to the lateral palpebral fissure. The lateral palpebral fissure is pulled downward. The lateral canthus is displaced inferiorly. This may create an appearance of a severe lower lid ectropion and an antimongoloid slant. Colobomas appear in the lateral lower eyelid and mark the cephalic end of the cleft.

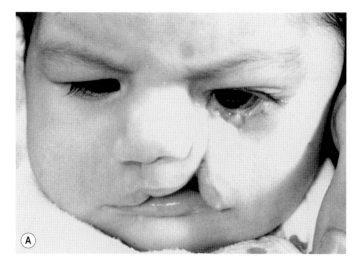

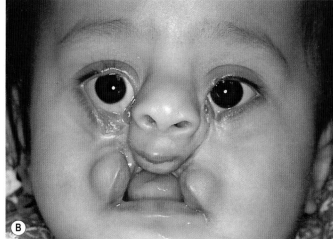

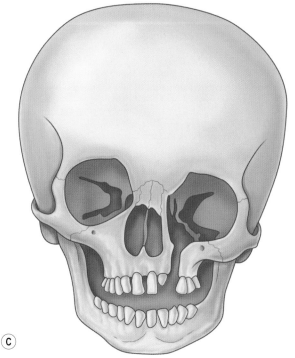

Fig. 31.7 Number 4 cleft. **(A)** Patient with left-side cleft that begins lateral to Cupid's bow and terminates in the lower eyelid medial to the punctum. **(B)** Bilateral clefting of the upper lip lateral to Cupid's bow and malar extension lateral to the nose up to the lower eyelids with asymmetric involvement. **(C)** Skeletal involvement begins between the lateral incisor and canine and extends through the maxilla between the infraorbital foramen and the piriform aperture. The orbit, maxillary sinus, and oral cavities communicate.

Skeletal involvement

The number 6 facial cleft is along the zygomaticomaxillary suture separating the maxilla and zygoma (Fig. 31.9B). There is no alveolar cleft, but a short posterior maxilla may result in an occlusal tilt. Choanal atresia is common. The cleft enters the orbit at the lateral third of the orbital rim and floor. It connects to the inferior orbital fissure. The zygoma is hypoplastic with an intact zygomatic arch. There is narrowing of the anterior cranial fossa. The sphenoid is normal.

Number 7 cleft

This temporozygomatic facial cleft is the most common craniofacial cleft. Other descriptive terms of this cleft include craniofacial microsomia, hemifacial microsomia, otomandibular dysostosis, first and second branchial arch syndrome, auriculobranchiogenic dysplasia, hemignathia and microtia syndrome, oroaural cleft (AACPR), a group B1 lateral otocephalic branchigenic deformity, and zygotemporal dysplasia.[48–51] Goldenhar syndrome (oculo-auriculo-vertebral spectrum) is an autosomal-dominant more severe form additionally with epibulbar dermoids and vertebral anomalies.[52] The number 7 cleft is also seen in Treacher Collins syndrome. The incidence is approximately 1 in 5600 births. There is a slight (3:2) male predominance and bilateral involvement.

Soft-tissue involvement

The cleft begins at the oral commissure and runs to the preauricular hairline. The intensity of expression varies from a mild broadening of the oral commissure with a preauricular skin tag to a complete fissure extending toward the microtic ear (Fig. 31.10). Typically the cleft does not extend beyond the anterior

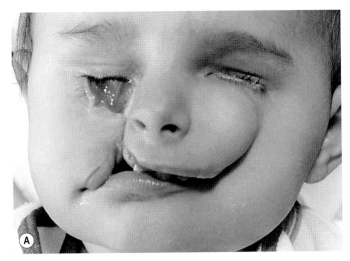

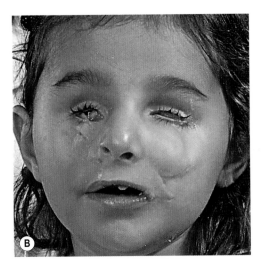

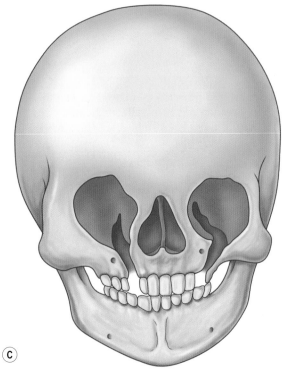

Fig. 31.8 Number 5 cleft (left) and number 4 cleft (right). **(A)** This patient demonstrates bilateral facial clefts: The number 5 cleft begins just medial to the oral commissure and extends up the lateral cheek to the middle of the eyelid, while the more medial number 4 cleft begins lateral to Cupid's bow and extends up to the medial third of the lower eyelid. **(B)** Postoperative view of same patient after repair of bilateral clefts. **(C)** Skeletal involvement in the number 5 cleft (left) begins at the premolars and extends lateral to the infraorbital foramen, while the number 4 cleft begins between the lateral incisor and canine and passes medial to the infraorbital foramen.

border of the masseter. However, the ipsilateral tongue, soft palate, and muscles of mastication (cranial nerve V) may be underdeveloped. The parotid gland and parotid duct may be absent. Facial nerve weakness (cranial nerve VII) may be present. External ear deformities range from preauricular skin tags to complete absence. External ear and middle-ear abnormalities have been documented by Longacre et al.,[51] Grabb,[53] and Converse et al.[54] Preauricular hair is usually absent in patients with craniofacial microsomia. Patients with Treacher Collins syndrome often have preauricular hair from the temporal region pointing to the oral commissure. The ipsilateral soft palate and tongue are often hypoplastic.

Skeletal involvement

Osseous anomalies in a number 7 cleft include a wide range. The skeletal cleft passes through the pterygomaxillary junction. Tessier believed that the cleft is centered in the region of the zygomaticotemporal suture. The posterior maxilla and mandibular ramus are hypoplastic in the vertical dimension, creating an occlusal plane that is canted cephalad on the affected side. The coronoid process and condyle are also often hypoplastic and asymmetric, contributing to a posterior open bite on the affected side. The zygomatic body is severely malformed, hypoplastic, and displaced. In the most severe form, the zygomatic arch is disrupted and is represented by a small stump. The malpositioned lateral canthus is caused by a hypoplastic zygoma that results in the inferiorly displaced superolateral angle of the orbit. Occasionally, severely deforming number 7 clefts can cause true orbital dystopia. The abnormal anterior zygomatic arch continues posteriorly as a normal zygomatic process of the temporal bone. The cranial base is asymmetric and tilts causing an abnormally positioned glenoid fossa. The anatomy of the sphenoid is

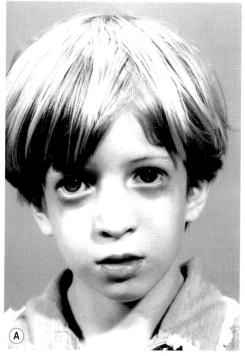

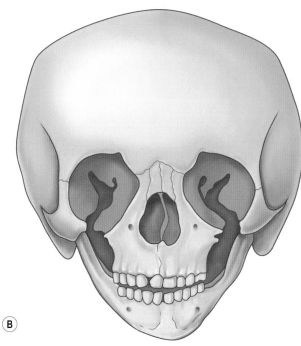

Fig. 31.9 Number 6 cleft. **(A)** Patient with an incomplete form of Treacher Collins syndrome shows bilateral linear malar hypoplasia. **(B)** Skeletal involvement occurs in the region of the zygomaticomaxillary suture. The zygoma is hypoplastic.

abnormal, and there can be a rudimentary medial and lateral pterygoid plate.

Number 8 cleft

This frontozygomatic cleft located at the lateral canthus is the equator of the Tessier craniofacial time zones (Fig. 31.11). It is the temporal continuation of the orolateral canthus cleft (AACPR), the commissural clefts of the ophthalmo-orbital disorders, and zygofrontal dysplasia.[44] The number 8 cleft

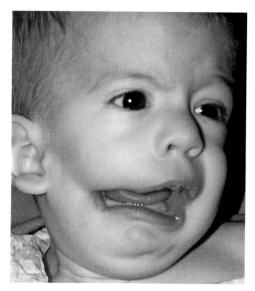

Fig. 31.10 Number 7 cleft. Patient with a complete fissure of the right oral commissure which extends toward the external ear, resulting in macrosomia. *(Courtesy of D Hurwitz)*

divides the facial clefts from the cranial clefts. The number 8 cleft rarely occurs alone but is usually associated with other craniofacial clefts. It appears to be the cranial extension of the number 6 cleft. The bilateral occurrence of the combination of numbers 6, 7, and 8 craniofacial clefts is unique. Tessier believed that this pattern of clefts best describes Treacher Collins syndrome (Fig. 31.12). Infants with Goldenhar syndrome will typically have more soft-tissue involvement, while those with Treacher Collins syndrome tend to have more severe bony abnormalities.

Soft-tissue involvement

The number 8 cleft extends from the lateral canthus to the temporal region. A dermatocele may occupy the coloboma of the lateral commissure. Occasionally hair markers can be seen

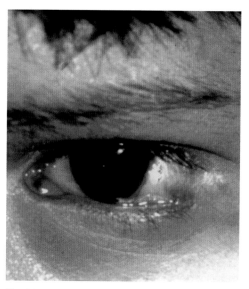

Fig. 31.11 Number 8 cleft. In this patient's left eye the lateral commissure of the palpebral fissure is obliterated by a dermatocele. This cleft separates the facial and cranial clefts.

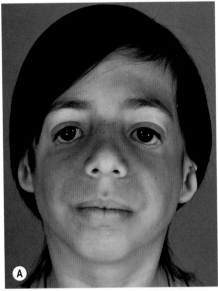

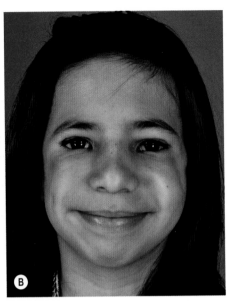

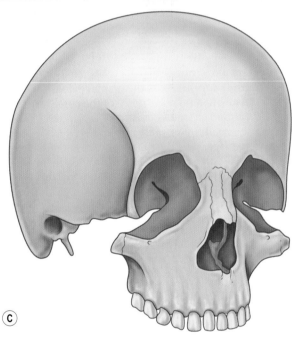

Fig. 31.12 Combination number 6, 7, and 8 cleft. **(A)** Patient with Treacher Collins syndrome demonstrates malar hypoplasia and antimongoloid slant to palpebral fissure. **(B)** Postoperative image after malar reconstruction with cranial bone grafts and eyelid reconstruction with lid switch flaps. **(C)** Skeletal involvement in the complete form includes absence of the zygoma, lateral orbital wall (greater wing of sphenoid provides remaining portion of the lateral wall), and lateral orbital floor.

along a line between the temporal area and the lateral canthus. The soft-tissue malformation presents as a true lateral commissure coloboma (dermatocele) with absence of the lateral canthus. Abnormalities of the globe, in the form of epibulbar dermoids, are also often present, especially in Goldenhar syndrome.

Skeletal involvement

The bony component of the cleft occurs at the frontozygomatic suture. Tessier noted a notch in this region in patients with Goldenhar syndrome (combination number 6, 7, and 8 clefts). In the complete form of Treacher Collins syndrome (combination number 6, 7, and 8 clefts) the zygoma may be hypoplastic or absent and the lateral orbital wall missing (see Fig. 31.12C). Thus, the lateral palpebral fissure's only support is the greater wing of the sphenoid and downward slanting occurs. With

this defect there is soft-tissue continuity of the orbit and temporal fossa.

Number 9 cleft

This upper lateral orbit cleft is the rarest of the craniofacial clefts. The number 9 cleft begins the medial movement through the cranial clefts. This defect was nominated frontosphenoid dysplasia by Van der Meulen.[44] It is the cranial extension of the number 5 facial cleft.

Soft-tissue involvement

The number 9 cleft is manifested by abnormalities of the lateral third of the upper eyelid and eyebrow. The lateral canthus is also distorted. In the severe form, microphthalmia is present (Fig. 31.13). The superolateral bony deficiency of the

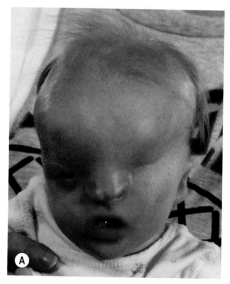

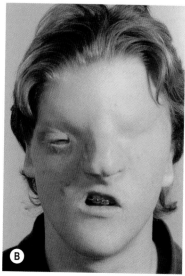

Fig. 31.13 Number 9 cleft. **(A)** Patient with left-side rare number 9 cleft through the superolateral orbital roof with anophthalmia. **(B)** Same patient at maturity after nasal and orthognathic reconstruction.

orbits allows for a lateral displacement of the globes. The cleft then extends cephalad into the temporoparietal hair-bearing scalp. The temporal hairline is anteriorly displaced, and a temporal hair projection is often seen in the number 9 cleft. Furthermore, a cranial nerve VII palsy in the forehead and upper eyelid is common.

Skeletal involvement

The bony defect of the number 9 cranial cleft extends through the superolateral aspect of the orbit. Distortion of the upper part of the greater wing of the sphenoid, the squamosal portion of the temporal bone, and surrounding parietal bones may be present. This hypoplasia of the greater wing of the sphenoid results in a posterolateral rotation of the lateral orbital wall. The pterygoid plates may be hypoplastic. There may be a reduction in the anteroposterior dimension of the anterior cranial fossa.

Number 10 cleft

This upper central orbital cleft has also been classified as a frontal dysplasia group.[44] The number 10 cleft is the cranial extension of a number 4 cleft.

Soft-tissue involvement

The number 10 cleft begins at the middle third of the upper eyelid and eyebrow. The lateral eyebrow may angulate temporally (Fig. 31.14A). The palpebral fissure may be elongated with an amblyopic eye displaced inferolaterally (Fig. 31.14B). The entire upper eyelid may be absent in severe forms (ablepharia). Colobomas and other ocular anomalies may be present. Frontal hair projection may connect the temporoparietal region to the lateral brow.

Skeletal involvement

The bony component of the number 10 cranial cleft occurs in the middle of the supraorbital rim just lateral to the superior orbital foramen (Fig. 31.14C). Often an encephalocele occupies the defect through the frontal bone and a prominent bulge is observed in the forehead. The orbit may be deformed with a lateroinferior rotation. Orbital hypertelorism may result in severe cases. The anterior cranial base may also be distorted.

Number 11 cleft

This upper medial orbital cleft is the cranial extension of the number 3 cleft. Van der Meulen included this malformation in the frontal dysplasia group.[44]

Soft-tissue involvement

The medial third of the upper eyelid may show involvement with a coloboma. The upper eyebrow may have a disruption evident which extends up to the frontal hairline (Fig. 31.15). A tongue-like projection at the medial third of the frontal hairline may also be identified.

Skeletal involvement

The number 11 cleft may be seen as a cleft in the medial third of the supraorbital rim if it passes lateral to the ethmoid bone. If the cleft passes through the ethmoid air cells to produce extensive pneumatization then orbital hypertelorism is seen clinically. The cranial base and sphenoid architecture, including the pterygoid processes, are symmetric and normal.

Number 12 cleft

The number 12 cleft is the cranial extension of the number 2 cleft.

Soft-tissue involvement

The soft-tissue cleft lies medial to the medial canthus, and colobomas extend to the root of the eyebrow. There is a lateral displacement of the medial canthus with an aplasia of the medial end of the eyebrow. There are no eyelid clefts. The forehead skin is normal with a short downward projection of the paramedian frontal hairline (Fig. 31.16A).

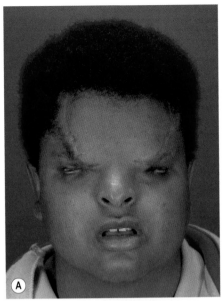

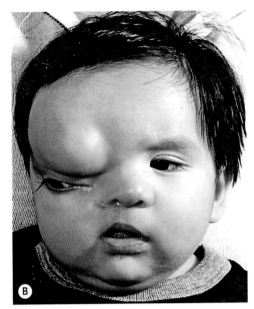

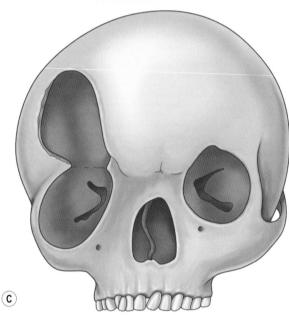

Fig. 31.14 Number 10 cleft. **(A)** Patient with bilateral cleft in the center of the left superior orbital rim and microphthalmia. **(B)** Patient with fronto-orbital encephalocele in the mid right forehead that fills the void from the cleft defect. The right globe is displaced downward. **(C)** Skeletal defect and asymmetric hypertelorism are demonstrated on the right.

Skeletal involvement

The number 12 cleft passes through the flattened, frontal process of the maxilla (Fig. 31.16B). It then travels superiorly, increasing the transverse dimension of the ethmoid air cells, producing orbital hypertelorism and telecanthus. The frontal and sphenoid sinuses are also pneumatized and enlarged. The remainder of the sphenoid and frontal bones are normal. The frontonasal angle is obtuse. The cleft is located lateral to the olfactory groove, thus the cribriform plate is normal in width. Encephaloceles have not been observed with this cleft. The anterior and middle cranial fossae are widened on the cleft side, but otherwise normal.[55]

Number 13 cleft

The number 13 cleft is the cranial extension of the paramedian, facial number 1 cleft (Fig. 31.17).

Soft-tissue involvement

There is typically a paramedian frontal encephalocele, which is located between the nasal bone and the frontal process of the maxilla. The soft-tissue cleft is medial to intact eyelids and eyebrows. The medial end of the eyebrow, however, can be displaced inferiorly. A V-shaped frontal hair projection can also be seen.

Skeletal involvement

Changes in the cribriform plate are the hallmark of a number 13 cleft. The paramedian bony cleft traverses the frontal bone, then courses along the olfactory groove. There is widening of the olfactory groove, the cribriform plate, and the ethmoid sinus, which results in hypertelorism. A paramedian frontal encephalocele can cause the cribriform plate to be displaced inferiorly, leading to orbital dystopia. Unilateral and bilateral

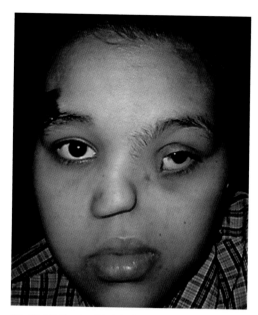

Fig. 31.15 Number 11 cleft. Patient with coloboma in medial third of left upper eyelid extending through the medial third of the eyebrow.

forms of the number 13 cleft exist, similar to most of the other craniofacial clefts. When the cleft is bilateral, some of the most extreme cases of hypertelorism can be seen.[2]

Number 14 cleft

The number 14 cleft occurs in the midline forehead and cranium as an extension of number 0 clefts. As in the number 0 clefts or median craniofacial dysraphia, described above, there may be a tissue deficiency, tissue excess, or normal amount of tissue but clefted in some way.

Soft-tissue involvement

Similar to its facial counterpart, the number 14 cleft can be produced as an agenesis or an overabundance of tissue. When agenesis occurs, orbital hypotelorism is generally seen. Included in this group of craniofacial malformations are the holoprosencephalic disorders, which include cyclopia, ethmocephaly, and cebocephaly (Fig. 31.18A). The cranium is typically microcephalic, and there is hypotelorism. A complete absence of midline cranial base structures can occur, causing the orbits to coalesce. Malformations of the forebrain are usually proportional to the degree of facial abnormality. An extensively involved number 14 cleft can severely handicap the newborn, and life expectancy is usually limited from hours to months.

At the other end of the spectrum, hypertelorism is associated with the number 14 cleft (Fig. 31.18B). The terms frontonasal and frontonasoethmoid dysplasia were used by Van der Meulen to categorize this group.[44] Lateral displacement of the orbits can be produced by midline masses such as a frontonasal encephalocele or a midline frontal encephalocele (Fig. 31.18C,D). Cohen *et al.* thought that the basic fault in embryologic development lies in the malformation of the nasal capsule, and the developing forebrain remains in a low position.[56] A morphokinetic arrest of the normal medial movement of the eyes occurs and the orbits remain in their widespread

fetal position. Flattening of the glabella and extreme lateral displacement of the inner canthi are also seen. The periorbita, including the eyelids and eyebrows, are otherwise normal. A long midline projection of the frontal hairline marks the superior extent of the soft-tissue features of this midline cranial cleft.

Skeletal involvement

The frontal encephalocele herniates through a medial frontal defect. The caudal aspect of the frontal bone is flattened, giving the glabellar region a flattened and indistinct position.

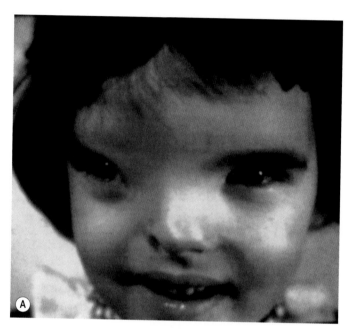

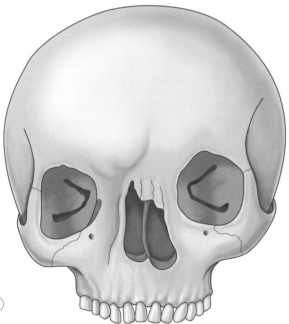

Fig. 31.16 Number 12 cleft. **(A)** Patient with right cleft has orbital hypertelorism and a disturbance of the left medial eyebrow. **(B)** Skeletal involvement of right-side clefting through the frontal process of the maxilla displacing the orbit laterally and hypertelorism results.

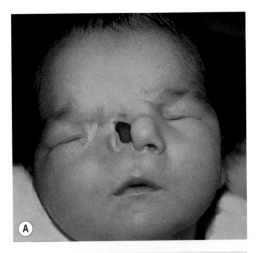

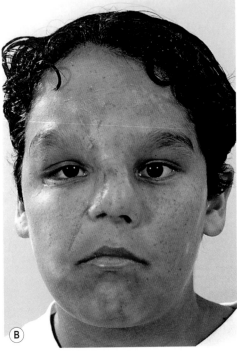

Fig. 31.17 Number 13 cleft. **(A)** Patient with a right cleft which begins cleft through the right alar dome (number 1 cleft) and extends to the frontal bone to cause right-sided telorbitism. **(B)** Postoperative image after corrective facial bipartition and nasal reconstruction with forehead flap.

No pneumatization of the frontal sinus is evident; however, the sphenoid sinus is extensively pneumatized. The crista galli and the perpendicular plate of the ethmoid are bifid, and there is an increased distance between the olfactory grooves (Fig. 31.18E). When the crista galli is severely enlarged, preservation of the olfactory nerve is often not possible during the surgical correction of hypertelorism. The crista galli and ethmoids are widened and caudally displaced. Consequently, the cribriform plate, which is normally located 5–10 mm below the level of the orbital roof, can be caudally displaced up to 20 mm.[57] The greater and lesser wings of the sphenoid are rotated and result in a relative shortening of the middle cranial fossa. The anterior cranial fossa is upslanting, causing a harlequin eye deformity on plain radiographs.

Number 30 cleft

The median cleft of the lip and mandible, first described by Couronne, are extremely rare with less than 100 cases reported.[58] These median clefts of the lower lip and mandible are caudal extensions of the number 14 cranial cleft and number 0 facial cleft (Fig. 31.19). The number 30 clefts include mandibular process clefts, midline branchiogenic syndrome, and intermandibular dysplasia.

Soft-tissue involvement

Soft-tissue involvement of this midline cleft may be as mild as a vermillion notch in the lower lip. However, often the entire lower lip and chin may be involved. The anterior tongue may be bifid and attached to the split mandible by a dense fibrous band. Ankyloglossia and total absence of the tongue have been reported with midline mandibular clefts. The anterior neck strap muscles are often atrophic and replaced by dense fibrous bands which may restrict chin flexion.

Skeletal involvement

Skeletal involvement is typically a cleft between the central incisors extending into the mandibular symphysis. This anomaly is thought to be caused by failure of fusion of the first branchial arch. However, associated neck anomalies are felt to be caused by failure of fusion of other lower branchial arches. The hyoid bone at times is absent and the thyroid cartilages may fail to form completely.

Number 31 cleft

The paramedian cleft of the lip and mandible are even more rare than the median lower jaw clefts. Despite Dr. Tessier's vast experience, he did not evaluate a patient with a lower jaw paramedian cleft and, thus, did not complete his numbering system. For these newly described lower jaw paramedian clefts the numbering system counts up from number 30. Number 31 clefts involve the lower lip and mandible just adjacent to the midline (Fig. 31.20).[59,60]

Soft-tissue involvement

Soft-tissue involvement may be a vermillion notch or depression in the lower lip just off the midline. A linear scar and skin tag may also be noticed to the left or right of the median lip and chin.

Skeletal involvement

Skeletal involvement may involve alveolar notching between the central incisor and lateral incisor. The cleft may also extend further into mandible in this parasymphyseal region.

Number 32 cleft

This other paramedian lower lip and mandibular cleft is located just lateral to the number 31 cleft. The number 32 cleft involves a lower lip defect approximately halfway between the midline and oral commissure (Fig. 31.21).

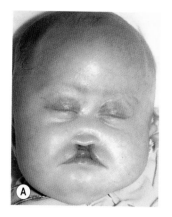
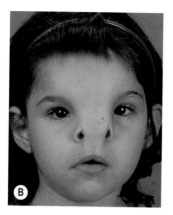
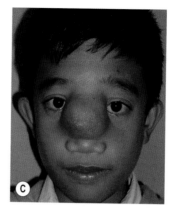
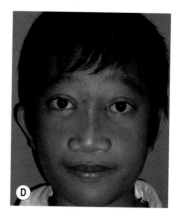

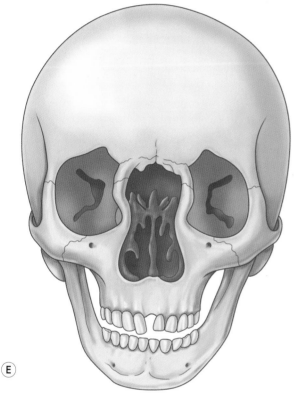

Fig. 31.18 Number 14 cleft. **(A)** Patient with number 14 cleft, holoprosencephaly, a form of median craniofacial hypoplasia (tissue deficiency). **(B)** Patient with number 14 cleft, frontonasoethmoidal encephalocele, a form of median craniofacial dysraphia (normal tissue but clefted). **(C)** Patient with number 14 cleft, craniofrontonasal dysplasia, a form of median craniofacial hyperplasia (excess tissue). **(D)** Postoperative image after corrective encephalocele repair, medial orbit repositioning, and nasal bone grafting. **(E)** Skeletal involvement shows displacement of the frontal process of the maxilla, the nasal bones, and medial orbital walls laterally. This large defect is often occupied by an encephalocele.

Soft-tissue involvement

Soft-tissue involvement may be a vermilion depression and regional attenuation or hypoplasia of the orbicularis oris in the lower lip halfway between the midline and oral commissure.

Skeletal involvement

Skeletal involvement may involve alveolar notching lateral to the lateral incisor or extend into the mandible parasymphyseal region just medial to the mental foramen.

Number 33 cleft

The number 33 cleft is lateral to the number 32 cleft and may be associated with other severe facial deformities like Goldenhar (oculoauriculovertebral) syndrome. Severe malocclusion may be seen because of the mandibular separation near the molar region (Fig. 31.22).[61]

Soft-tissue involvement

Soft-tissue involvement may be a vermilion notch or depression in the lower lip just medial to the oral commissure.

Skeletal involvement

Skeletal involvement may involve alveolar notching or complete separation in the area of the premolar just posterior to the mental foramen and anterior to the first molar.

Summary

The clinical expression of craniofacial clefts is highly variable and ranges from a mild, barely noticeable *forme fruste*

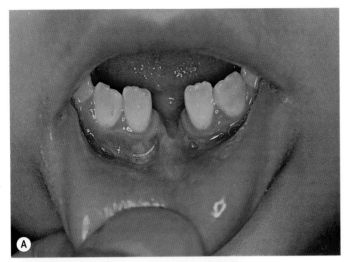

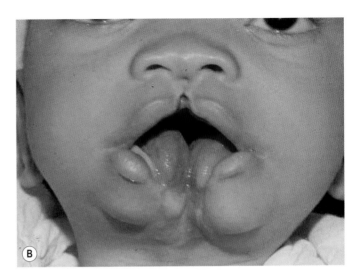

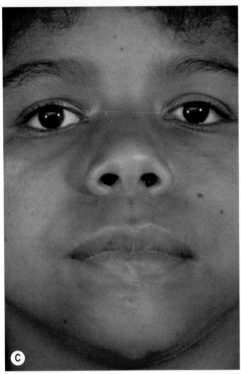

Fig. 31.19 Number 30 cleft. **(A)** Close-up intraoral view of patient with number 30 cleft showed dental separation of central incisors and bony cleft. **(B)** Preoperative view of patient with number 30 cleft with a deep tongue groove and fusion to the clefted mandible. **(C)** Postoperative view of same patient with number 30 midline mandibular cleft after skeletal and soft-tissue repair. *(Courtesy of Cassio Raposo do Amaral, MD.)*

(microform) to a disfiguring, complete defect of skeletal and soft tissue. Tessier's description of craniofacial clefts based on bony and soft-tissue landmarks provides a classification which can be validated by neuroembryology. Craniofacial clefts, far from being considered oddities, will allow plastic surgeons in the future to refine and understand the developmental architecture of the face.

Treatment

Treatment of craniofacial clefts

Standardized treatment plans are not always possible because of the variety of craniofacial clefts and levels of severity. However, guiding principles are helpful in determining the

proper timing and stages for corrective surgery.[2–4] If there are functional problems, like ocular exposure, or airway problems, or if the malformation is severe, then surgery should be performed early. If the malformation is mild, surgery should be delayed. During infancy (3–12 months), soft-tissue clefts and midline cranial defects (e.g., encephaloceles) may be corrected. Midface and orbital reconstruction with bone grafting may be performed in older children (6–9 years). Orthognathic procedures are delayed until skeletal maturity (14 years or greater).

Surgical techniques used for correction of craniofacial clefts depend upon the anatomic regions that are involved. For timing and general corrective protocols, the deformities may be grouped into (1) midline and paramedian clefts (numbers 0–14, numbers 1–13, 2–12, or other combinations); (2) oro-naso-ocular clefts (numbers 3–11, 4–10, 5–9); and (3) lateral

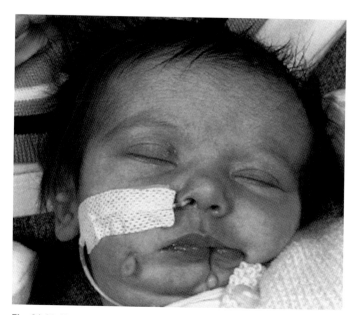

Fig. 31.20 Number 31 cleft. Left side paramedian lower lip cleft just off the midline with a full-thickness break in the vermilion, a linear skin scar and a chin skin tag. *(Courtesy of Steve Wall, MD.)*

clefts including constellation of numbers 6, 7, and 8 clefts like Treacher Collins syndrome of craniofacial microsomia.

First, for midline clefts, proper diagnosis into median craniofacial hypoplasia (tissue deficiency), median craniofacial dysplasia (normal tissue volume but separated), or median craniofacial hyperplasia (tissue excess) is helpful for proper treatment planning. Midline clefts may have symmetrical deformities like bifidity of the nasal cartilages or symmetrical hypertelorbitism, while paramedian clefts manifest asymmetry with unilateral nasal notching or horizontal and vertical orbital dystopia. For the upper lip, correction of cleft defects involves aligning the white roll and vermillion, and restoring

muscular continuity as in a common cleft lip repair. Microform variations may be corrected with intraoral muscle repair, Z-plasty of the white roll, and no cutaneous scar (Fig. 31.23). For lateral clefts, lip reconstruction is performed with a rotation-advancement repair.

For the nose, a median cleft correction may be done in early childhood with a primary rhinoplasty used to unify bifid nasal cartilages after excision of intervening fibrofatty tissue. For paramedian defects, the nose is reconstructed with cartilage grafts or composite skin-cartilage grafts, particularly for asymmetries and soft triangle notching. Alar retraction may be corrected with local rotation flaps or Z-plasty flaps. Secondary nasal reconstruction may be performed with a septoplasty or even cantilevered cranial bone grafts. Correction of

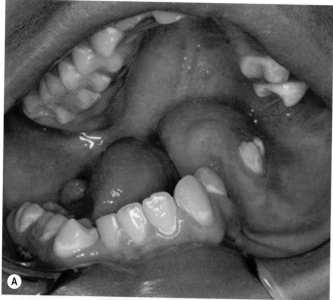

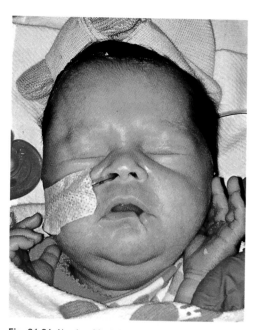

Fig. 31.21 Number 32 cleft. Left side paramedian cleft of the lower lip and skin midway between the midline and left oral commissure.

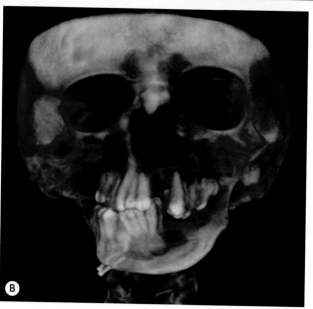

Fig. 31.22 Number 33 cleft. **(A)** Intraoral view of paramedian mandibular cleft between premolar and first molar with redundant gingiva. **(B)** 3D cone beam CT scan shows osseous defect in left side mandibular body but with inferior border intact.

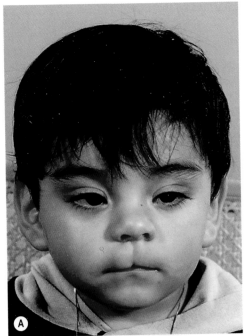

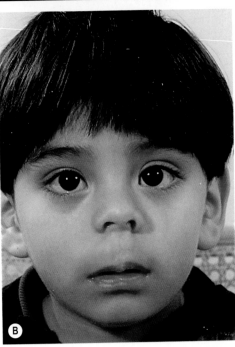

Fig. 31.23 Number 0 cleft correction. **(A)** Preoperative frontal view of patient with midline incomplete cleft lip. **(B)** Postoperative frontal view of patient after intraoral repair of orbicularis oris muscle without cutaneous scar.

duplication of the nasal septum should be reserved until the end of nasal growth.

For orbital dystopia, correction with an orbital box osteotomy has been described for these deformities; however, a facial bipartition allows for more versatility, especially in patients with mixed dentition when occlusal correction is not paramount. A facial bipartition requires bilateral monobloc osteotomies: in the anterior zygomatic arch, lateral orbital wall, orbital roof, medial orbital wall, orbital floor, pterygomaxillary buttresses, and septum (during the midface

down-fracture). Anterior encephalocele reduction and cranial base bone graft may be necessary before midline fixation (Fig. 31.24).[62] For these large anterior encephaloceles, subsequent cleft palate repair may require a pharyngeal flap for nasal lining. With paramedian (numbers 1–13, 2–12) clefts, vertical adjustment of a facial bipartition segment may be necessary to correct vertical, as well as horizontal, orbital dystopia (Fig. 31.25). For these procedures, the misaligned occlusal plane is usually temporary and correctable. Subsequent medial canthoplasty may also be necessary.

Second, for oro-naso-ocular clefts (numbers 3–11, 4–10, 5–9), the original descriptions for correction of the soft-tissue component of these clefts involved the use of Z-plasty flaps. These flaps were designed to lengthen the foreshortened distance between the medial canthus and nasal alar base on the affected side. Presently, flaps are designed to respect aesthetic units by leaving scars along aesthetic lines (Fig. 31.26).[55] For repair, complete dissection of the cleft is necessary. Small orbital floor bone graft or bone graft matrix may be used to fill the cleft defect and separate the orbit from the maxillary sinus. A banner flap from along the median nasal sidewall may be rotated into a subciliary incision beneath the affected lower eyelid, and a transnasal medial canthopexy may be performed. Both vertical and horizontal orbital dystopia may be corrected with a facial bipartition (Fig. 31.27). Abnormal canthal anatomy should be addressed with a medial and/or lateral canthopexy. The goal during mid-childhood is orbital correction even if malocclusion is not corrected or temporarily made worse. Oro-naso-ocular clefts may also present with large encephaloceles from cranial defects (Fig. 31.28). In these cases a staged approach in infancy may be appropriate for optimal correction. Of note, for the lateral lip cleft repair (numbers 4 and 5 clefts), the intervening tissue between the philtral column and lateral cleft should be excised.

The third treatment group, the lateral craniofacial clefts (numbers 6, 7, and 8) include the constellation of clefts like Treacher Collins syndrome and craniofacial microsomia. For the oral commissure (as in cleft number 7), macrostomia may affect feeding, saliva control, and speech acquisition and should be addressed at an early age. The oral commissure should be corrected for symmetry and fall approximately below the medial canthal vertical line. Orbicularis oris muscle fibers should be reoriented and interlaced at the neo-oral commissure, and the cleft should be closed in a straight line. The medial aspect may be closed with a small Z-plasty so that the vertical limb is along the nasolabial fold. For the lower lip (as in cleft number 30), a vertical excision with bilateral extensions (not crossing the labiomental fold) with a layered closure is performed.[63]

For mandibular reconstruction (as in cleft combinations 6, 7, and 8 in both craniofacial microsomia and Treacher Collins syndrome), costochondral grafts may be used for severe deformities, and distraction osteogenesis for moderate deformities in mid-childhood (6–8 years).[64] For mild maxillary deformities resulting in an occlusal cant, correction can wait until adulthood with a Le Fort I osteotomy with or without a concomitant mandibular procedure.

Surgical correction of the periorbital region is necessary in many craniofacial clefts. For the eye, urgent intervention is necessary if the eye is exposed and at risk of corneal ulceration. However, early reconstructive procedures for globe protection must be balanced to allow enough eye opening to

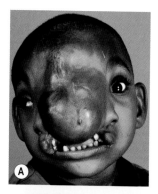

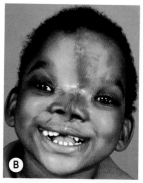

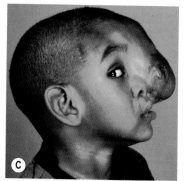

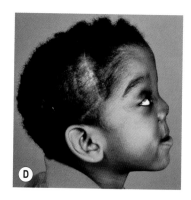

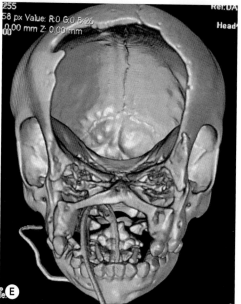

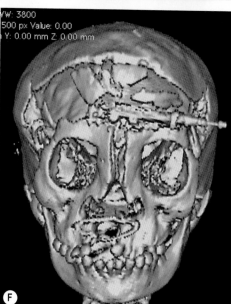

Fig. 31.24 Number 0–14 cleft correction. **(A,B)** Frontal views of patient with Tessier numbers 0–14 craniofacial cleft. **(A)** Preoperative image demonstrating large midline frontonasal encephalocele. **(B)** Postoperative image after gradual orbital contraction procedure and median cleft lip and nose repair. **(C,D)** Lateral views of patient with Tessier numbers 0–14 craniofacial cleft. **(C)** Preoperative image demonstrating the anterior displacement of the encephalocele with functional problems of independent ocular movement and drooling. **(D)** Postoperative image after corrective procedures. Functional improvements in ocular, oral competence, and speech were noted. **(E)** Preoperative three-dimensional computed tomography scan with large central osseous defect and 81-mm interdacryon distance. **(F)** Postoperative image after orbital contraction (midline device in place) with interdacryon distance narrowed to 17 mm.

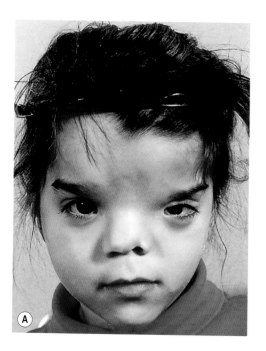

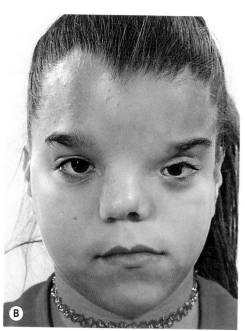

Fig. 31.25 Number 2–12 cleft correction. **(A)** Preoperative view shows left nasal alar cephalad malposition, orbital dystopia, and hairline malformation. **(B)** Postoperative view after facial bipartition and medial canthoplasty. Future nasal correction will be needed.

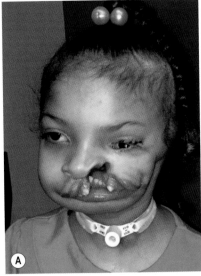
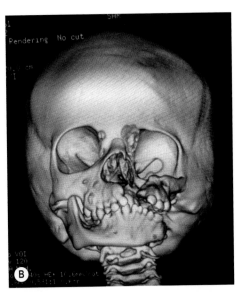
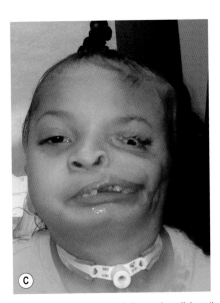

Fig. 31.26 Number 3 cleft correction. **(A)** Preoperative view shows wide left cleft lip and plate and shortening between the notched alar base and distorted medial canthus. Left-side cleft number 7 and number 8 are also present. **(B)** 3D CT scan reveals left-side skeletal defect with unification of orbital, maxillary sinus, nasal, and oral cavities. **(C)** Postoperative view after left-side downward rotation of nose, medial transnasal wire canthopexy, medial upper to lower lid switch flap, and cleft lip repair. Future cleft palate, macrostomia repair, and ear reconstruction will be needed.

prevent deprivation amblyopia. For the eyelid, "lid switch" transposition flaps are used for skin/muscle deficiencies. Palatal grafts may be used for lower lid conjunctival lining. The orbit may be reconstructed with cranial bone grafting to restore orbital continuity and correct dystopia. Accurate repositioning of the medial canthus may be performed with transnasal wiring. Lateral canthopexies are sometimes needed to achieve symmetry. Correction of number 8 (lateral eye) clefts are performed with Z-plasty flaps. For the lacrimal apparatus, disruption of the canalicular system may be corrected with Silastic stents or formal dacryocystorhinostomy.

Outcomes and complications

Proper timing and technique of staged corrective procedures will minimize perioperative complications and long-term sequelae. If early functional problems like globe exposure are not addressed, then corneal ulceration and blindness may result. Likewise, speech problems may develop, as in more common cleft lip and palate deformities. Complications may occur for specific soft- or hard-tissue correction because of the difficult nature of these procedures.

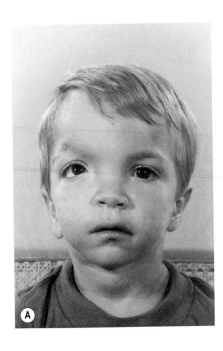
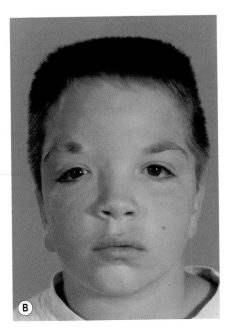

Fig. 31.27 Number 10 cleft correction. **(A)** Preoperative view shows right vertical and horizontal orbital dystopia with notching of midlateral brow. **(B)** Postoperative view after facial bipartition and downward rotation of midlateral brow.

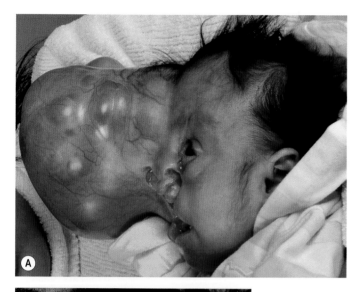

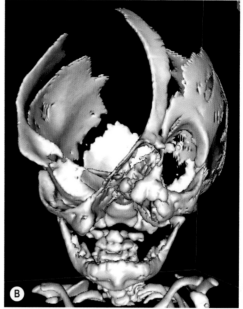

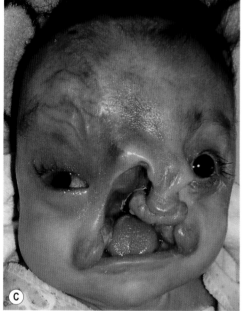

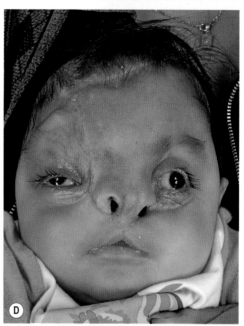

Fig. 31.28 Number 3–10 cleft correction. **(A)** Preoperative left lateral image demonstrated a large right frontoencephalocele. A right-side numbers 3 and 10 and a left-side number 3 craniofacial cleft were present. **(B)** Computed tomography scan revealed significant bony defect of the right fronto-orbital region, encephalocele cyst, and bony deformity. **(C)** After the first procedure of encephalocele repair and right fronto-orbital reconstruction, the patient showed improvement but still had orbital and facial cleft deformities. **(D)** Postoperative frontal images after bilateral cleft lip repair and right nasoforehead rotation and medial canthal repositioning. Future reconstructive procedures will be necessary.

Summary

Craniofacial clefts are highly variable and range from mild (barely noticeable) *forme fruste* (microform), to disfiguring, complete defects of the skeletal and soft tissue. Tessier's description of craniofacial clefts based on bony and soft-tissue landmarks provides a classification which has been validated by neurometric theory of neuroembryology. For corrective surgery, guiding principles are helpful in determining the proper timing and stages, like addressing functional problems (ocular exposure, airway problems) early. General corrective protocols may be grouped into (1) midline and paramedian clefts (numbers 0–14, 1–13, 2–12); (2) oro-naso-ocular clefts (numbers 3–11, 4–10, 5–9); and (3) lateral clefts (numbers 6, 7, 8, like Treacher Collins syndrome of craniofacial microsomia).

1. Tessier P. Anatomical classification of facial, cranio-facial and latero-facial clefts. *J Maxillofac Surg.* 1976;4:69–92. *Tessier introduces his now ubiquitous classification scheme for craniofacial clefts in this account. Cleft position is described in reference to the orbit.*

2. Kawamoto HK Jr. The kaleidoscopic world of rare craniofacial clefts: order out of chaos (Tessier classification). *Clin Plast Surg.* 1976;3:529–572.

3. Kawamoto HK Jr. Rare craniofacial clefts. In: McCarthy JG, ed. *Plastic Surgery*. Philadelphia: Saunders; 1990:2922–2973.

4. Bradley JP, Kawamoto HK. Rare craniofacial clefts. In: Grabb WC, Smith JW, eds. *Plastic Surgery*. Philadelphia: Saunders; 1990:2922–2973.

5. Carstens MH. Functional matrix repair: a common strategy for unilateral and bilateral clefts. *J Craniofac Surg.* 2000;11:437–469.

9. Van der Meulen JC, Mazzola R, Vermey-Keers C, et al. A morphogenetic classification of craniofacial malformations. *Plast Reconstr Surg.* 1983;71:560–572. *The authors describe a new classification scheme for craniofacial clefts. Pathogenesis and cerebral involvement are emphasized.*

10. Allam K, Wan D, Kawamoto HK, et al. The spectrum of median craniofacial dysplasia. *Plast Reconstr Surg.* 2011;127:812–821. *Midline craniofacial malformations are further defined from an embryological perspective. The authors separate these entities into hypoplasias (tissue deficiency), dysraphias (normal amount of tissue, but clefted), and hyperplasias (tissue excess).*

11. Noordhoff SM, Huang CS, Lo LJ. Median facial dysplasia in unilateral and bilateral cleft lip and palate: a subgroup of median cerebrofacial malformations. *Plast Reconstr Surg.* 1993;91:996–1005. *A group of patients characterized by midface anomalies without cerebral involvement is identified. Topics ranging from anatomical considerations to growth potential are addressed.*

55. Longaker MT, Lipshutz GS, Kawamoto HK Jr. Reconstruction of Tessier number 4 clefts revisited. *Plast Reconstr Surg.* 1997;99:1501–1507.

57. Tessier P. Orbital hypertelorism. 1. Successive surgical attempts, material and methods, causes and mechanisms. *Scand J Plast Reconstr Surg.* 1972;6:135–155. *Orbital hypertelorism is described. An extensive case series informs observations on diagnosis and management.*

Nonsyndromic craniosynostosis

Patrick A. Gerety, Jesse A. Taylor, and Scott P. Bartlett

Access video lecture content for this chapter online at expertconsult.com

SYNOPSIS

- Craniosynostosis is the pathologic fusion of one or more cranial vault sutures, usually resulting in an abnormal head shape.
- Nonsyndromic craniosynostosis occurs in a sporadic, non-familial fashion, in the absence of an associated genetic syndrome.
- The fused cranial suture results create a cranial deformity, with areas of restricted growth and compensatory bossing, as well as the potential for functional and organic issues (increased intracranial pressure (ICP) being the most significant).
- Diagnosis entails a clinical examination and computed tomography (CT) corroboration. The optimal timing of treatment is during infancy, between 6 and 9 months.
- Conventional open techniques and new modalities (including springs and distraction osteogenesis) can be entertained.
- The choice of operation depends on the specific suture fused and the degree of dysmorphology. In general, the technical surgical goals entail releasing the area of sutural fusion, repositioning the bone in an anatomic but overcorrected location, eliminating secondary compensatory changes, filling in osteotomy gaps with bone dust slurry, and closing the soft tissue relatively tension-free.
- The physiologic goal is to mitigate functional problems (e.g., intracranial hypertension and developmental delay, optic disc atrophy, and strabismus).
- Complications can be divided into early or late events.
- Secondary revisions may be necessary involving either the soft tissue, bone, or both.
- On rare occasions, the complete intracranial procedure must be repeated. However, major morbidity and mortality are exceedingly uncommon in the modern approach and management of craniosynostosis.

Introduction

Craniosynostosis is a disease involving the early and pathologic fusion of any of the cranial sutures, most often one of the six major sutures. This early fusion results in recognizable patterns of abnormal head shape. In the absence of a known heritable or genetic syndrome as well as other medical problems, it is termed nonsyndromic. This is in contrast to a number of other genetic syndromes, which cause suture fusion as well as other craniofacial abnormalities (see Chapter 33: Syndromic craniosynostosis). Nonsyndromic patients most often present with the fusion of only one suture, but there are instances in which multiple sutures have fused. The incidence of nonsyndromic craniosynostosis is approximately 1 in 2500 live births.[1] These patients represent approximately 80% of cases of craniosynostosis, and this incidence is approximately 10 to 50 times more common than syndromic causes (e.g. Apert and Crouzon syndromes). Sagittal craniosynostosis occurs most frequently while lambdoid synostosis occurs least frequently. A review of the experience at the Children's Hospital of Philadelphia in 2008 suggests that the relative incidence of metopic synostosis has been increasing particularly relative to diagnoses of unicoronal synostosis.[2] This finding has been reported by other groups as well, demonstrating that sagittal synostosis is approximately twice as common as metopic and four times as common as unicoronal.[3,4] The etiology of nonsyndromic craniosynostosis is unknown but it is believed to be multifactorial.

Basic science

Nonsyndromic craniosynostosis has an uncertain etiology, but a host of factors have been identified that may cause or contribute to the premature fusion of cranial sutures. It has been theorized that suture fusion may either be a primary event innate to the suture's biology or a secondary event due to external factors.

There are known cases of inherited and familial nonsyndromic craniosynostosis. Autosomal dominant inheritance is present in approximately 10% of cases. Coronal and metopic suture fusion has a greater likelihood of being familial than sagittal (10% vs 2%). Some data have suggested that rising paternal age may contribute to the increasing incidence of metopic synostosis. Several syndromes (Muenke, Saethre–Chotzen) have variable expressivity and may have a mild phenotype. Thus, they may be assumed to be non-syndromic upon presentation. In fact, these patients are affected by FGFR3 or TWIST mutations. Any patients who present with possible familial pattern of craniosynostosis should receive a genetic consultation for counseling and possible testing.

The cranial sutures play a critical role particularly early in life by allowing significant cranial deformation during birth, allowing expansion for rapid early brain growth, and for controlling complex signaling to lead overall calvarial growth and maturation. The precise etiology of nonsyndromic cranio-synostosis and the underlying cranial suture biology remain poorly understood. Animal model experimentation has lead to a greater understanding of the complex nature of sutures. The sutures represent a complex interaction of tissues (dura, bony front, mesenchymal tissue, periosteum), and within this organ are complex molecular signaling and growth processes.[5] Several important molecules have been identified, including transforming growth factor beta (TGFB), bone morphogenetic proteins (BMP), TWIST, MSX2, and fibroblast growth factor receptors (FGFR).[6] While all of these molecules can be shown experimentally to affect suture fusion, their precise role in the nonsyndromic patient remains unknown.[7] Gene regulation and the products of these genes are clearly different in abnor-mally fused versus open sutures.[8] Sophisticated genetic analysis continues to emerge on possible genetic contribution to nonsyndromic craniosynostosis.[9]

Environmental factors have been shown to affect suture fusion. This is best illustrated by diagnoses of craniosynostosis in which cranial growth has been externally restricted or in which cerebral/cranial growth does not occur normally. Uterine shape (bicornuate), intrauterine position (breech), large fetal size, and multiple gestations have all been associ-ated with premature suture fusion and its sequelae. These external forces apparently cause or increase the risk of prema-ture suture fusion. This concept has been validated in experi-mental and animal data. Lack of outward forces from brain growth or restricted growth of other areas of the cranium are also thought to contribute to craniosynostosis. Cranial base growth restriction has long been theorized as a cause for adjacent suture fusion and craniosynostosis. Similarly, improper brain growth may also impart abnormally low forces on the cranial sutures causing premature fusion.

In addition to mechanical forces, other environmental risk factors have been identified to increase the risk of nonsyn-dromic craniosynostosis. Maternal smoking, white maternal race, advanced maternal age, gestation at high altitude, use of nitrosatable drugs (e.g., nitrofurantoin), paternal occupation (e.g., agriculture, forestry), fertility treatments, endocrine abnormalities (e.g., hyperthyroidism), and warfarin ingestion during gestation have all been linked to craniosynostosis.[10–12]

Patient presentation and diagnosis

Craniosynostosis may be diagnosed at or immediately follow-ing the birth of a baby. The parents or pediatrician will often notice a distinctly abnormal head shape and will be referred to a craniofacial or neurosurgeon. In contrast, patients with deformational (positional) plagiocephaly often present later in life between 4 and 7 months of age.[13] These two diagnoses are often confused by healthcare providers.

A complete history should be obtained including prenatal information (birth position, multiple gestation, duration of gestation), affected parents or siblings, the presence of any other identified anomalies, and achievement of milestones. In older children and adults, elevated intracranial pressure (ICP) may lead to symptoms such as headaches, visual disturbances, lethargy, and vomiting. In neonates and infants these symp-toms are difficult to elicit. An ophthalmologic exam can identify papilledema, a sign of elevated ICP, and should be obtained in all patients with suspected craniosynostosis.

Physical examination will nearly always make the diagno-sis.[14] The exam should focus on head shape, ear position, orbital shape and symmetry, fontanelles, cranial sutures, and measures of cranial morphology (head circumference, cephalic index; Table 32.1). Patterns of specific suture fusion are char-acteristic and have classically been described using Virchow's law.[15] This concept describes cranial growth as perpendicular to sutures. When sutures fuse abnormally, compensatory growth occurs parallel to the fused suture. This produces characteristic craniofacial patterns. The patterns of individual suture fusion diagnoses can be seen in Fig. 32.1 and are described in detail below.

Deformation (positional) plagiocephaly is almost entirely a non-surgical diagnosis, and a full discussion is beyond the scope of this chapter.[16] However, it is critical to include in this discussion because it also results in a characteristic head shape and is often confused with craniosynostosis. Craniofa-cial surgeons are often consulted on, provide counseling for, and coordinate care of patients with deformational plagio-cephaly (positioning, positional aids, helmet orthotics).[17] The successful campaign to reduce the rates of sudden infant death syndrome (SIDS) by promoting back sleeping in infants has lead to an observed rise in deformational plagiocephaly.[18–20] The characteristic deformity involves occipital flattening that is often asymmetric with the ipsilateral ear displaced anteri-orly. This diagnosis can be confused with lambdoid cranio-synostosis; a comparison of these two diagnoses can be seen in Table 32.2. Another significant contributor to deformational plagiocephaly is torticollis which may either precede (and thus cause) or result from deformational plagiocephaly.[21]

The most sensitive and specific diagnostic test for cranio-synostosis is computed tomography (CT) with three-dimensional reconstructions. This allows the visualization of all sutures as well as an examination of ventricular morphol-ogy, brain stem position (Chiari), and midline brain abnor-malities (corpus callosum). Radiologic signs of increased ICP may also be identified. The characteristic "thumb-printing" or

Table 32.1 Cephalic index (CI).	
The ratio of biparietal diameter (BPD) and fronto-occipital diameter (FOD). The measurements are taken where the distances are maximum. CI = BPD/FOD × 100	
Cephalic index	**Cranial morphology**
<76	Scaphocephaly or dolichocephaly
76–81	Normocephaly
>81	Brachycephaly

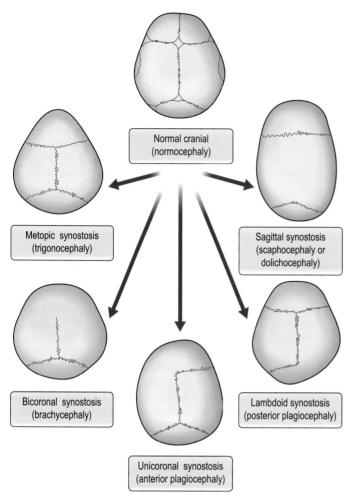

Fig. 32.1 Characteristic skull shape depending on sutural involvement in craniosynostosis.

"copper-beaten" patterns, when evident on 3D scan or the scout film, suggest raised cranial pressure[22] (Fig. 32.2). Similarly, axial cuts can show loss of gyral folding and blunted cisternae along the endocranial surface, consistent with the brain expansion against an immobile, restrictive cranial vault. The CT scan also may aid in surgical planning and serves as a baseline study to compare against postoperative changes. This may also be used as data for virtual surgical planning.[23] Concern has arisen in the last decade of the deleterious effects of ionizing radiation particularly in young children.[24] This has lead institutions such as our own to use dose-reduction protocols and to avoid CT scans when possible including for routine postoperative results.

Patterns of altered head shape develop when one or more of the six major sutures of the cranium fuses prematurely (sagittal, metopic, coronal, lambdoid). These patterns are now described in detail and can be visualized in Fig. 32.1. There are other minor cranial sutures, which may also fuse prematurely but are beyond the scope of this chapter.

Sagittal synostosis develops following fusion of the midline, sagittal suture (Fig. 32.3). This restricts bitemporal growth and promotes anteroposterior expansion resulting in a characteristic "boat-shaped" head. This deformity is alternately referred to as dolichocephaly or scaphocephaly. Cephalic index (CI), the ratio of bitemporal distance (BPD) to fronto-occipital distance (FOD), is the most common measurement used in assessing scaphocephaly. CI is normally 76–82 and in sagittal synostosis typically measures <76. On exam, the sagittal suture may be palpated as a bony ridge, and one or both fontanelles may have closed. The head shape can be affected by variable fusion of the sagittal suture (i.e. entire, anterior, posterior). Fusion of the anterior sagittal suture contributes to significant frontal bossing. Similarly, an occipital bulge results from involvement of the posterior sagittal suture. Varying degrees of frontal or occipital prominence can occur

Table 32.2 Differentiating deformational plagiocephaly from lambdoid and unicoronal craniosynostosis.

	Flat forehead	Flat occiput	
	Unicoronal synostosis (UCS)	Unilateral lambdoid synostosis	Deformational plagiocephaly
Primary feature	Ipsilateral forehead retrusion	Ipsilateral occipital flatness	Ipsilateral occipital flatness
Compensatory changes	Contralateral forehead may be bossed No change in occiput	Ipsilateral mastoid bulge (canted skull base) Ipsilateral forehead, no change or recessed	Ipsilateral forehead may be bossed Contralateral forehead may be retruded
Ipsilateral ear position	Anterior and superior	Varied Posterior and inferior	Varied Anterior
Periorbital region	Ipsilateral Wide palpebral fissure Higher retruded supraorbital rim, brow Harlequin on X-ray	Usually unaffected in anatomic head position	Usually unaffected May have contralateral retrusion of fronto-orbital zygomatic region
Nasal radix	Deviated towards affected side	Midline in anatomic head position	Midline
Head shape from above	Ipsilateral forehead retrusion	Trapezoid	Parallelogram
Incidence	Rare	Very rare	Common

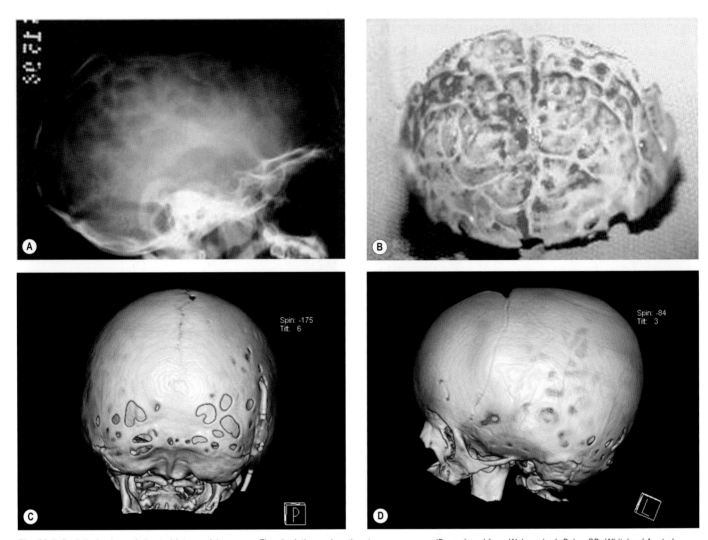

Fig. 32.2 Radiologic signs of elevated intracranial pressure. Thumbprinting and moth-eaten appearance. *(Reproduced from Weinzweig J, Baker SB, Whitaker LA, et al. Delayed cranial vault reconstruction for sagittal synostosis in older children: an algorithm for tailoring the reconstructive approach to the craniofacial deformity.* Plast Reconstr Surg. *2002;110:397–408.)*

depending on the extent and location of synostosis along the sagittal suture.

Metopic synostosis results in a characteristically "keel"-shaped forehead and triangular head shape termed trigonocephaly (Fig. 32.4). In contrast to the other cranial sutures, the metopic suture normally fuses by 8 months,[25] so mild head shape abnormalities detected in late infancy do not necessarily warrant aggressive diagnostics and surgery. The other features of metopic synostosis include bitemporal narrowing, parietal expansion, supraorbital and lateral orbital retrusion, and hypotelorism. The orbital morphology of metopic synostosis is a teardrop shape with the apex pointed toward the metopic suture. Metopic synostosis is also associated with midline brain aberrations, and one report suggests a higher than usual concomitant presentation of Chiari I malformation.[26] Severity of metopic synostosis is fairly variable. While some think of metopic ridge as the most mild form of the disease, it does not share the orbital and other features of true synostosis. The severity may be measured by the degree of supraorbital retrusion, trigonocephaly, and biparietal narrowing. The frontal angle is the angle between

two lines drawn from nasion to pterion on axial cuts of a CT scan. Normal is >104 degrees and severe is <89 degrees. Frontal stenosis measures the severity of biparietal narrowing and is the ratio of interparietal distance to the intercoronal distance.[27] Persing et al. have described two different severities of metopic synostosis; this delineation may also help guide treatment.[28]

Unicoronal synostosis (UCS) has in the past been called "anterior plagiocephaly". Because this term can be confusing, most surgeons now advocate specifying the suture when discussing a diagnosis of craniosynostosis. Plagiocephaly is a generic term denoting an asymmetric flattening of part of the head. This occurs in positional plagiocephaly, unicoronal synostosis, and lambdoid synostosis (see Table 32.2). This confusing terminology is still often encountered in the literature. UCS results in an asymmetric head shape with contrasting ipsilateral and contralateral effects (Fig. 32.5). Ipsilaterally, anterior growth of the forehead is restricted, resulting in a flattened forehead and supraorbital rim with temporal deficiency. The ipsilateral orbital dysmorphology can be quite significant, with a taller and narrower orbit that

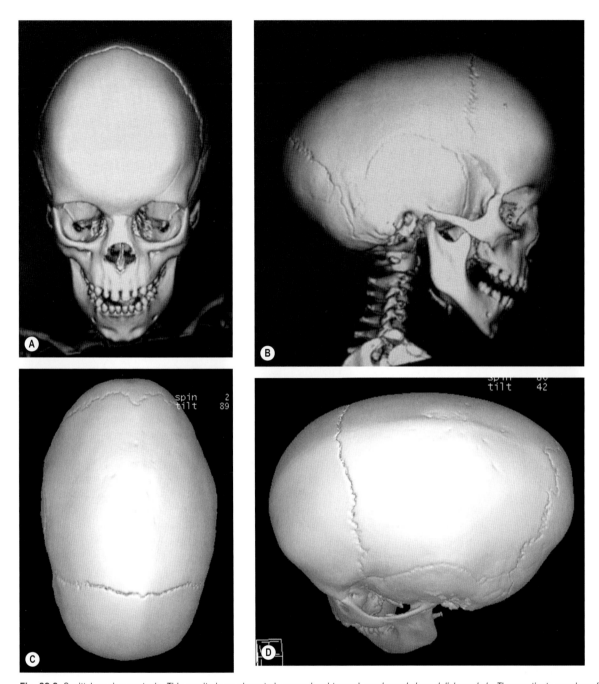

Fig. 32.3 Sagittal craniosynostosis. This results in an elongated, narrow head termed *scaphocephaly* or *dolichocephaly*. These patients may have frontal and/or occipital prominences.

produces the appearance of a raised eyebrow and wide-open eye in contrast to the contralateral side. This results in the harlequin deformity, defined by the orbital shape with a peak in the superolateral aspect. Contralaterally, compensatory overgrowth occurs, producing forehead bossing. The ipsilateral ear is typically positioned anterior and superior secondary to normal contralateral anteroposterior (AP) growth. The effects of UCS can be seen in twisting of the middle and lower thirds of the face with the nasal root moving ipsilaterally. When present, the chin deviates to the unaffected side secondary to changed position of the glenoid fossa.[29] The posterior head shape is typically unaffected. This

normal posterior shape should signal that the process is not positional plagiocephaly, however these two diagnoses may be coincident.

Bicoronal synostosis results in a symmetric head shape (Fig. 32.6). This diagnosis is much more likely to occur in the setting of a syndrome or familial inheritance. Lack of AP growth causes remarkable bossing and expansion of the parietal skull resulting in a large biparietal diameter (BPD). The head shape is termed brachycephaly.[30] This leads to a blunted forehead and supraorbital ridge. In certain cases, there can be a compensatory increase in parietal height causing turribrachycephaly (tall flat head).

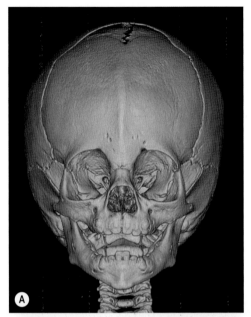

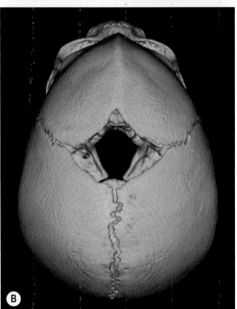

Fig. 32.4 Metopic craniosynostosis. This results in a triangular or keel-shaped head termed *trigonocephaly*. Important features are bitemporal narrowing, hypotelorism, and a teardrop-shaped orbit. The point of the teardrop is superomedial and points towards the fused metopic suture.

Unilateral lambdoidal synostosis is a rare diagnosis (1 in 40 000 live births[31]), which results in a posteriorly based asymmetric head shape. The pattern of deformity is often compared and contrasted with that of positional plagiocephaly (see Table 32.2). It has traditionally been characterized by ipsilateral occipital flatness, posteriorly displaced ear, and mastoid bulging. In the past, there was also belief that compensatory frontal bossing arose in the contralateral forehead, providing an overall trapezoid head shape when viewed from above[32] (Fig. 32.7). This trapezoid shape was in contrast to the parallelogram shape commonly found in deformational plagiocephaly. Clinically, the altered ear position can be quite

variable and in some instances can be anteroinferiorly displaced making ear position an unreliable feature.[33] The consistent features of lambdoid synostosis are in reality ipsilateral occipital flattening and notable contralateral parieto-occipital bossing. This posterior abnormality can translate into a degree of facial asymmetry but this is variable.

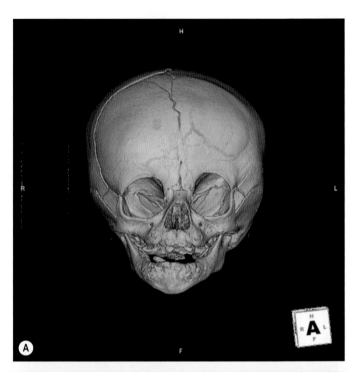

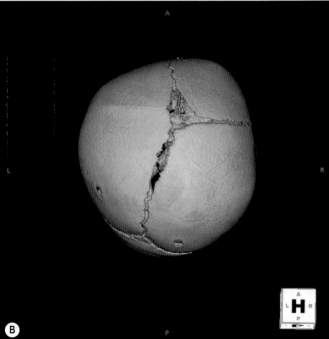

Fig. 32.5 Unicoronal craniosynostosis. This results in an asymmetric head shape termed *anterior plagiocephaly*. Important features include ipsilateral forehead and supraorbital retrusion, a tall ipsilateral orbit with wide-open eye, and nasal root (radix) which deviates toward the affected suture. Contralaterally there is compensatory forehead bossing. The chin deviates away from the affected suture.

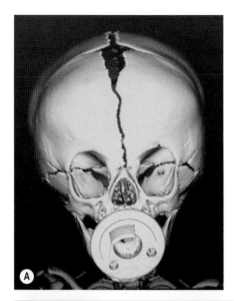

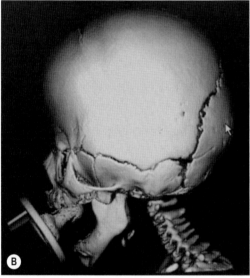

Fig. 32.6 Bicoronal craniosynostosis. This results in a head shape with a shortened fronto-occipital dimension termed *brachycephaly*. This features bilateral supraorbital retrusion. The entire forehead may be retrusive with excessive backwards slope. The vertex and cranium may be tall termed *turricephaly* or *turribrachycephaly*.

Patient selection

The treatment of craniosynostosis, like other craniofacial disorders, requires a multidisciplinary team approach. In particular, the craniofacial surgeon will work with neurosurgery, genetics, ophthalmology, audiology, child psychology, the child's pediatrician, and other specialists during the course of diagnosis and treatment. Because of specific gene mutations (FGFR, TWIST) and the presence of syndromic patients, these patients should be offered genetic counseling. The presence of other findings, familial pattern, bicoronal synostosis, multiple sutures, and other unusual presentations warrant a genetics evaluation. A fundoscopic exam by a neuro-ophthalmologist is required to assess for papilledema. Their exam can also reveal baseline visual information and identify preoperative

strabismus. Neurosurgeons are key partners during the entire process. The neurosurgeon is an intraoperative participant in the care of these patients and preoperatively evaluates the status of the brain parenchyma and associated abnormalities (e.g., hydrocephalus, Chiari malformation).

The fundamental goals of surgical treatment are two-fold: (1) to relieve abnormally high intracranial pressure (ICP) and allow room for normal brain growth and (2) to produce an aesthetic head shape. Patients with mild head shape abnormalities, partial fusion of one suture, and no indication of elevated ICP may be candidates for observation. In contrast, patients with clear evidence of elevated ICP, who are most often those with severe head shape abnormalities, should receive operative correction.

Intracranial hypertension remains a challenging topic. At extreme levels, elevated ICP can lead to blindness. There is literature to suggest that, when unabated, it contributes to developmental delay, even at lower levels. ICP poses a

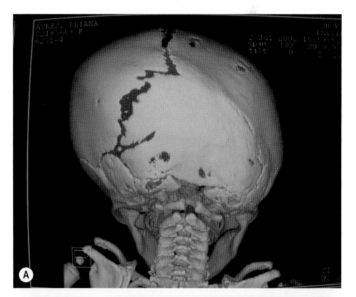

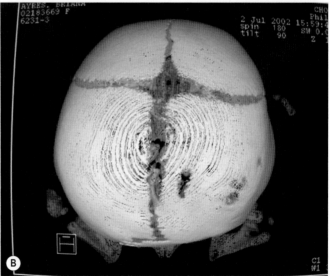

Fig. 32.7 Lambdoid craniosynostosis. This results in an asymmetric head shape termed *posterior plagiocephaly*. This results in ipsilateral occipital flattening and a pathognomonic ipsilateral mastoid bulge. Contralaterally the occipital and frontal regions may have a compensatory bulge.

challenge because no non-invasive exam to date provides an excellent corollary to an invasive intracranial measurement of ICP.[34] A fundoscopic exam revealing papilledema is suggestive of elevated ICP, but approximately 80% of infant patients with elevated ICP do not have papilledema.[35] There are endocranial indications on CT scan such as copper beaten pattern, thumbprinting, and scalloping, as well as blunted gyri that suggest elevated ICP (see Fig. 32.2). Several technologies have attempted to bridge the gap but remain unproven. In nonsyndromic patients, the incidence of elevated ICP is thought to be between 10 and 20%.[36]

Timing of surgery depends upon technique. For vault remodeling procedures such as fronto-orbital advancement and posterior vault remodeling, most surgeons agree that between the ages of 6 and 9 months is ideal. The brain is growing rapidly which will provide internal molding force postoperatively, the cranial bone has matured to allow for hardware but is still malleable for shaping, and the anesthetic risk is lower. Newer techniques such as spring-mediated cranioplasty or strip suturectomy are better performed at between 3 and 4 months of age. The timing of surgery is believed to be a balance between decreasing the neurocognitive impact (early surgery) and decreasing the need for secondary/revisional surgery (later surgery).

Surgical technique

Cranial vault remodeling procedures require a high level of specialization and are best performed in a pediatric hospital with specialists in pediatric anesthesia, critical care, and neurosurgery. Traditionally the chief cause of mortality with cranial vault remodeling was related to blood loss. This has lessened with appropriate recognition and maneuvers by both the surgical and anesthesia teams. There is a rare risk of air embolism, which is assessed by cardiopulmonary status and end-tidal CO_2 recordings.[37] Invasive hemodynamic monitoring (arterial line) is required. Cross-matched blood products should be available and in the room before the start of the case.

Blood loss and its sequelae are the most important consideration during cranial vault operations. Blood loss must be reduced, hemodynamics must be carefully monitored, and resuscitation (often with blood) must be appropriate. Efforts to limit blood loss are individual to surgeons but include hemostatic peri-incisional ("blocking") sutures, Raney clips, Colorado-tip electrocautery, and epinephrine containing tumescent.[38] Most routine blood loss occurs during the skin incision, so these steps may help to limit this. These techniques cause a variable amount of alopecia, which must be recognized.[39] Other sources of routine blood loss are exposed soft tissue, bone perforating venous emissaries, and osteotomies. Careful avascular dissection, bone wax, and low operative times can reduce blood loss from these factors. After craniotomy, the dura may be covered with hemostatic agents such as Surgicel and Floseal. Unexpected and catastrophic bleeding most often occurs if a dural sinus (sagittal, occipital, and transverse sinuses) is injured. This must be treated with rapid surgical hemostasis and resuscitation. Medical adjuncts, specifically anti-fibrinolytic agents, have been used in craniosynostosis surgery. The most common are aminocaproic acid and

tranexamic acid; and data in other invasive pediatric surgeries supports that estimated blood loss, need for transfusion, and volume transfused are lower when these agents are used.[40,41] In order to avoid transfusion, some surgeons have advocated preoperative treatment with erythropoietin which appears to also have an excellent safety profile.[42,43] Numerous techniques have been used to attempt to avoid or decrease the amount of blood transfusion during these case. The literature appears to demonstrate, however, that modern use of blood transfusion is very safe.

Positioning is supine for anterior procedures and prone in a cerebellar headrest for posterior procedures. A modified prone position ("sphinx") may be used for simultaneous anterior and posterior cranial vault remodeling.[44] The authors prefer a staged approach in such cases if possible, to minimize blood loss, and to give more complete access to a single anatomic site (and therefore a more complete correction), rather than a somewhat limited access to two anatomic areas. A coronal incision is required for most cranial vault remodeling procedures. This typically begins just above the ear aligned with the helical root or tragus. The design is non-linear (e.g. zigzag, sinusoidal) to avoid a conspicuous scar and distorting scar contraction.[45]

The choice of procedure is dependent upon the specific suture involved, the degree of deformity, and the age at presentation. Procedures for each deformity are discussed in depth below. The procedures can be divided into several broad categories: conventional vault remodeling, suturectomy, distraction osteogenesis, and spring-mediated cranioplasty. An endoscope can be employed to decrease incisional size and to directly visualize dural dissection. The aim of vault remodeling is to correct the deformity with a degree of overcorrection. In contrast, the goals of suturectomy are to allow the growing brain to remodel the skull (often with the assistance of helmet therapy).[46,47] Inevitably bony gaps will be created, and these are treated with either split calvarial graft when possible or, as the authors do, with bone shavings (curved Safescraper; Meta, Reggio Emilia, Italy) (Fig. 32.8).

Stabilization of repositioned bone segments is obtained using interposition bone grafts, sutures, and resorbable plates and screws. The objective is to create a stable construct but not to restrict brain growth and subsequent skull expansion. Titanium or metallic plates are not utilized in infants undergoing cranial remodeling for fear of transcranial migration and growth restriction[48–50] Limited incision and endoscopic techniques for suturectomy use different, smaller incisions and no fixation.

Sagittal synostosis

The treatment of sagittal synostosis has undergone significant evolution in the past 20 years. There remains a significant amount of disagreement about how to surgically correct these patients.[51] Traditionally, open vault remodeling was used to reshape the scaphocephalic head. In 1998, Jimenez and Barone reported the use of endoscopic strip craniectomy.[52] This procedure reduced the soft-tissue exposure using the endoscopic approach. The sagittal suture is removed and barrel stave osteotomies are made in the parietal skull to accomplish transverse widening. Around the same time in the late 1990s, spring mediated cranioplasty (SMC) was first reported by Lauritzen.[53] This procedure involves using wire to create

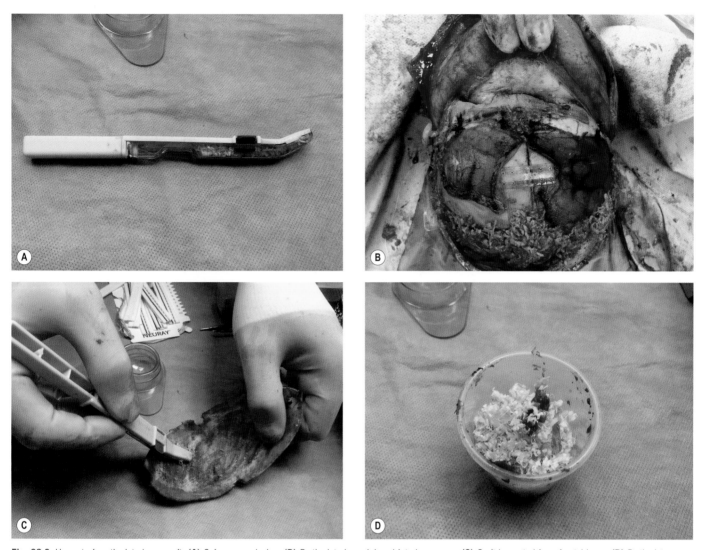

Fig. 32.8 Harvest of particulate bone graft. **(A)** Safescraper device. **(B)** Particulate bone inlayed into bony gaps. **(C)** Graft harvested from frontal bone. **(D)** Particulate shavings collected.

springs that slowly cause bitemporal widening. This technique has been adopted in numerous centers, and most surgeons agree that it is not efficacious if applied after 4 months of age.[54–56] This technique necessitates a second operation to remove the springs.

Conventional vault remodeling is still used, particularly in patients treated at an older age (>8 months). Some surgeons advocate for single stage total vault reconstruction,[57] while other surgeons (the authors included) prefer a staged approach – posterior and then anterior reconstruction +/− fronto-orbital reconstruction as necessary (Figs. 32.9 & 32.10). One well-described technique for cranial vault reconstruction is the *pi procedure*.[58] This involves two parallel parasagittal ostectomies of the two parietal bones, connected with a transverse ostectomy, located behind the coronal suture, and extending to the temporal region (resembling the Greek symbol for pi). The frontal bone and the remaining fused sagittal suture are approximated with sutures or plates to produce fronto-occipital shortening. This shortening produces the desired biparietal/bifrontal widening. The pi procedure has the advantage of being one stage and possibly keeping

more bone vascularized than some total cranial vault procedures, but may not produce as much correction of CI as other procedures and does not address orbital deformities. There are numerous other forms of vault remodeling that differ in the pattern and rearrangement of cranial bone segments to accomplish correction.

In the authors' institution the algorithm for the treatment of sagittal synostosis was previously based on the deformity but used only conventional vault reconstruction.[59] Their current algorithm is to use spring-mediated cranioplasty in patients under 4 months of age and after that to use staged vault remodeling (Figs. 32.11 & 32.12). In a meta-analysis of studies comparing techniques, the authors found that conventional vault remodeling produced a small but statistically significant better correction of cephalic index than strip suturectomy. We found the vault remodeling produced an equivalent correction to spring-mediated cranioplasty. Perioperative measures such as operative time, blood loss, hospital stay, and cost were significantly lower for strip suturectomy and spring cranioplasty though.[60] Spring-mediated cranioplasty is discussed below in detail.

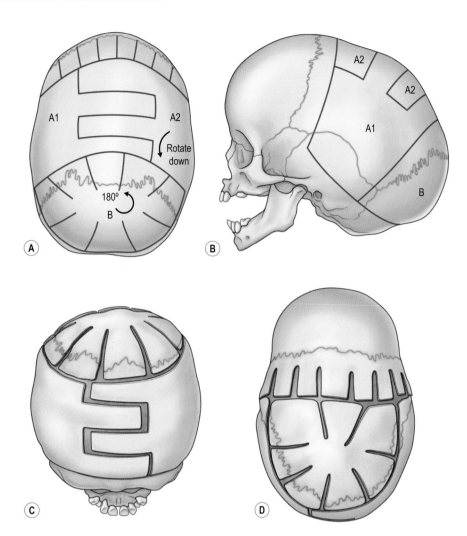

Fig. 32.9 (A–D) Posterior vault remodeling for sagittal craniosynostosis. Markings for osteotomy demonstrate tongue-in-groove pattern of pieces A1 and A2 at vertex that will be widened and switched to the occiput. The occipital segment "B" is radially scored and used to create a lowered vertex. Anteriorly barrel stave osteotomies are used to blend anterior and posterior. The postoperative configuration can be seen.

Metopic synostosis

The primary objective in surgically correcting metopic synostosis involves anterior cranial vault expansion that corrects bitemporal constriction and triangular head appearance.[29] The intent is to round the forehead shape and to widen and advance the supraorbits improving hypotelorism and orbital retrusion.

Most surgeons treating metopic synostosis use some form of frontal orbital advancement. This technique has been in use for nearly 50 years, though it has undergone significant refinement.[61,62] The current iteration at our institution entails splitting the fronto-orbital bar in the midline and interposing a bone segment to increase the bitemporal and interorbital distance (see Figs. 32.10 & 32.13). The new construct exhibits a more obtuse endocranial angle, witnessed by advancement and expansion of the lateral rims and temporal region. This bandeau is held in place by sutures at the zygomaticofrontal and nasofrontal regions and temporally with resorbable plates. Relapse and collapse of the bandeau are prevented with sutures, resorbable plates, and key interposition bone grafts at the temporal region advancement and with notched grafts in the orbit. The widening and advancement are performed in an overcorrected manner in anticipation of loss of bandeau growth potential and continued cranial

growth overall.[62] A clinical example of this can be seen in Fig. 32.14.

Other modalities have been used to treat patients with metopic synostosis. These include endoscopic strip craniectomy followed by helmeting,[47] spring-mediated cranioplasty,[63] and distraction osteogenesis.[64] No large case series or long-term data for these patients exists, so their efficacy remains unknown. In their series, Jimenez and Barone reported on 50 infants with metopic synostosis treated with suturectomy and showed it to be only 43% effective.[47] In addition to new techniques, there continues to be significant disagreement about which patients require surgical correction.[65]

Unicoronal synostosis

In unicoronal synostosis (UCS), the patient is asymmetric with an ipsilateral retrusive forehead and supraorbital rim, as well as an ipsilateral orbit that is too tall. Contralaterally the forehead may have a compensatory bulge. Therefore, the primary goals of treatment on the ipsilateral side are to advance the forehead and supraorbital rim anteriorly (Fig. 32.15). Similar to metopic synostosis, the most effective method for immediate and reliable correction of the UCS deformity remains fronto-orbital advancement. A bifrontal or unifrontal advancement may be performed, depending on the

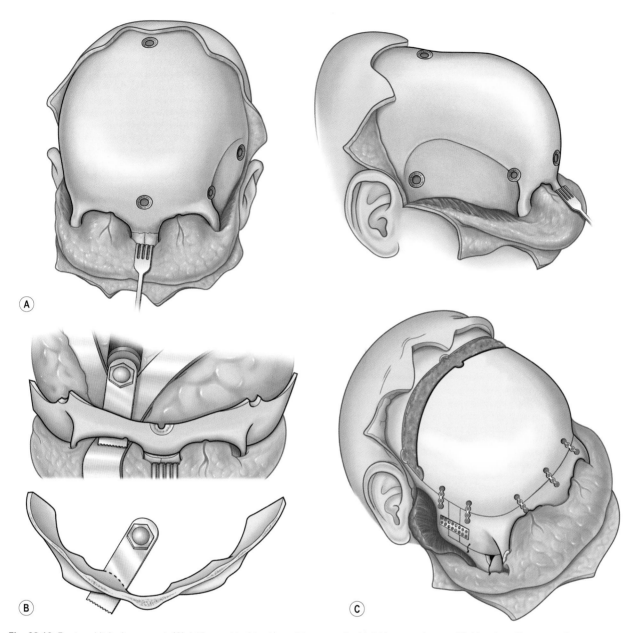

Fig. 32.10 Fronto-orbital advancement. **(A)** A bicoronal incision is used to expose the frontal bones and supraorbital bandeau. The temporalis muscle may be incorporated into the scalp flap (shown) or raised separately. **(B)** After removal of the frontal craniotomy, the supraorbital bandeau is removed. The bandeau is then fixated into an anteriorly advanced position and the frontal bone is replaced. The patient's anatomy and the surgeon's preference dictate alterations to the width and shape of both the frontal bone and bandeau. **(C)** Completed fronto-orbital advancement. *(Redrawn from an illustration by Dr. David Low.)*

severity of the deformity.[66] This approach allows correction of the ipsilateral orbital deformity and reshaping of the ipsilateral and contralateral forehead. A bilateral craniotomy is typically necessary coupled with advancement of the ipsilateral or bilateral supraorbital bandeau (see Fig. 32.15 for a clinical example). In general, correction is possible with an ipsilateral bandeau movement. The bandeau is planned as a very straight osteotomy 2 cm above the supraorbital rim. The movement is a widening with bone graft between the two bandeau segments (typically 5 mm) to accommodate the difference in orbital width as well as an advancement forward into an overcorrected position, typically 6 to 7 mm. The objective of the fronto-orbital advancement is to position the supraorbital rim 12–13 mm anterior to the cornea. An 8–15-mm magnitude

of bandeau advancement is usually required on the affected side. There are several techniques and modifications attributed to the fronto-orbital advancement, depending on the correction sought and the severity of the deformity[67] (see Fig. 32.13). Simultaneous to repositioning the orbital rim, the ipsilateral forehead is advanced, the orbital height may be reduced, and the contralateral forehead is recessed or contoured as necessary. A canthopexy may be performed to lower the affected side lateral canthus if an upward slant is present. Some advocate including the nasal bones in continuity with the frontal bar and uprighting the nasal radix deviation with a closing wedge osteotomy. Others feel the nasal root deviance corrects by adolescence with the lack of continued "pull" toward the fused suture.[68]

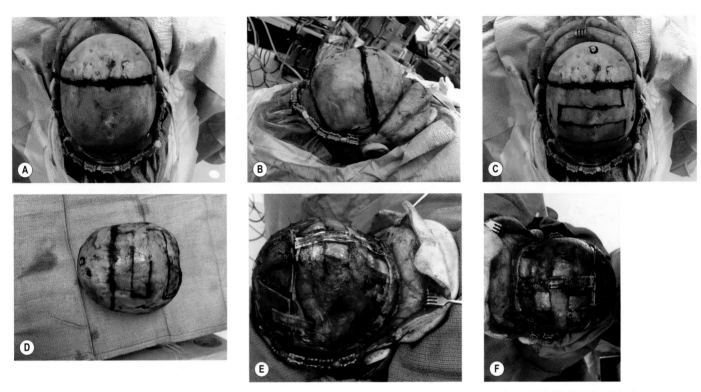

Fig. 32.11 Posterior cranial vault remodeling for sagittal craniosynostosis. Intraoperative depiction of similar expansion as Figure 32.9. **(A, B)** Patient is in the prone position. A large posterior craniotomy has been marked. **(C)** The widening cuts are added to the markings – this can guide the placement of burr holes. **(D)** The large craniotomy specimen on the back table. If necessary the neurosurgeon can remove this in two pieces. **(E, F)** The vertex has been rotated to the occiput and widened via the tongue and groove pattern. This is fixated with resorbable plates and suture. The original occiput has been radially cut and flattened to accomodate the vertex.

Minimally invasive techniques (distraction osteogenesis, spring-mediated cranioplasty) have been proposed and attempted, but these techniques have not yet matured to the point that they produce a reliably efficacious result. Jimenez and Barone used endoscopic suturectomy followed by helmet therapy in a series of UCS patients and found that the success rate was 43%.[47]

Bicoronal synostosis

In contrast to UCS, bicoronal synostosis involves much less asymmetry. This entails largely a forward movement of the supraorbital bandeau and forehead. This is accomplished via bifrontal craniotomy with a bilateral bandeau. Current techniques involve a bifrontal craniotomy and creation of a bilateral frontal bandeau. The anterior dimension is advanced, creating greater forehead prominence, and the supraorbital rim is positioned ahead of the corneal zenith. The width is narrowed by creating a midline endocranial flexion or a median ostectomy of the repositioned frontal bones. In bicoronal synostosis the height of the skull may also be increased (turribrachycephaly), and this can be addressed by barrel staves and greenstick fracture of the posterior parietal or occipital bones.[30]

Lambdoid synostosis

Lambdoid synostosis is a very rare diagnosis. If the deformity is present but mild, patients may be treated with an open broad synostectomy with barrel staves and outfracture of the ipsilateral occipital bone. The correction is prone to relapse because of infant back sleeping, therefore semi-rigid (resorbable) fixation must be used to avoid this. Older infants and children with more severe dysmorphology require treatment by cranial vault remodeling. We recommend a switch cranioplasty with occipital bar advancement[33,69] (Fig. 32.16). The posterior vault bone flap is hemisected, and each half is transposed to the opposite side and rotated 90–180° to achieve a best fit. These are fixed anteriorly with resorbable plates and bone gaps are filled with bone shavings. A number of other posterior vault reconstruction procedures have also been described to correct lambdoid synostosis.[70]

Endoscopic strip craniectomies and molding therapy have been advocated by some in young infants. In a small number of patients there was reported improvement in head circumference and head shape symmetry, but this data is limited.[71,72]

Emerging considerations

Spring-mediated cranioplasty

Spring-mediated cranioplasty (SMC) uses simple springs to apply force across an osteotomy. It is similar to distraction osteogenesis in pushing apart two bony segments, but once in place the spring is not manipulated as a distractor is. This concept was first shown to be experimentally effective in rabbits by Persing et al.[73] Lauritzen et al. were the first to demonstrate this technique clinically.[53] SMC has been demonstrated for numerous craniosynostosis diagnoses including metopic,[63,74] bicoronal,[63] sagittal,[63] and multisuture synostoses.[75]

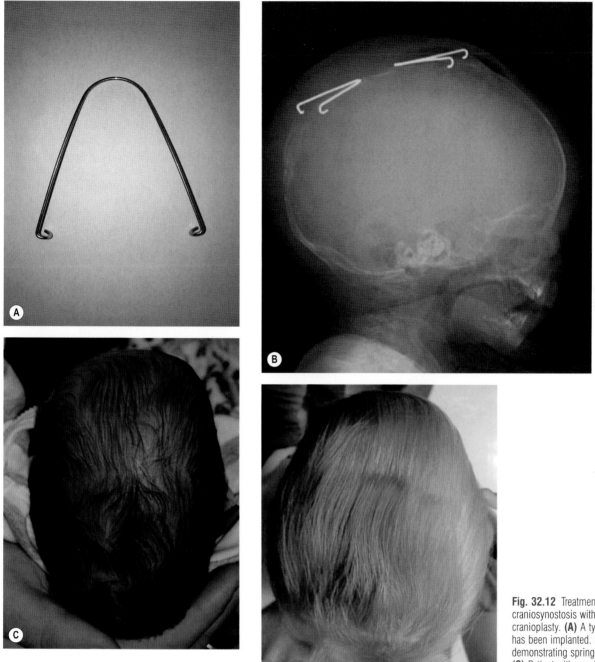

Fig. 32.12 Treatment of sagittal craniosynostosis with spring-mediated cranioplasty. **(A)** A typical spring before it has been implanted. **(B)** Cephalogram demonstrating spring placement. **(C)** Patient with scaphocephaly preoperatively. **(D)** Patient postoperatively with excellent head shape correction.

SMC has gained widest usage for sagittal synostosis in nonsyndromic cases, and, in many institutions, this has now become the standard treatment in patients who present before 4 months of age (see Fig. 32.12). The literature now contains comparative data from several groups[54,55,76–79] as well as systematic reviews.[56,60] To date, the largest series, by David *et al.*, reports on 75 patients. This study demonstrated equivalent correction of cephalic index (CI) as calvarial vault remodeling while showing improved perioperative markers such as blood loss, operative time, transfusion requirement, and length of hospital stay with a nearly four-year follow-up period. This technique is now used routinely at the authors' institution, and in their series they demonstrated similar findings.[56] The authors' patients were on average 4.6 months old. The operative time for placement was 90 minutes with an average blood loss of 85 mL. Importantly, the average hospital stay is only 2.2 days. It is important to recognize that this technique requires a second surgery for spring removal, and in the authors' series this operation required 45 minutes with a blood loss of 45 mL and a hospital stay of 0.9 days. Additionally, the authors' systematic review of the comparative literature showed that for SMC operative time is halved, blood loss

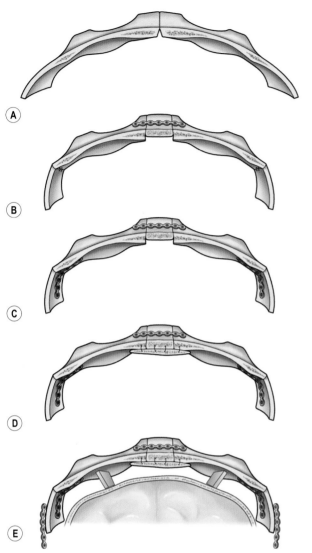

Fig. 32.13 Metopic synostosis bandeau reshaping. **(A)** The bandeau is split in the midline to permit widening. **(B)** A bone graft and a resorbable plate are typically used to stabilize widening. **(C)** The temporal tabs from the zygomaticofrontal suture (ZF) and posteriorly are reshaped to correct the abnormal geometry of the bandeau. This is often supported by endocortical resorbable plates. **(D)** Additional stabilization of the midline is achieved with bone grafts secured by suture or wire. This may be particularly important because of thickness differences between the bandeau of and harvested cranial bone graft. **(E)** The advanced position of the bandeau is further supported by stabilizing bone grafts at the orbital roof resorbable plates and bone grafts at the temporal tabs.

is four-fold lower, length of stay is halved, and cost is approximately one-third when compared to calvarial vault remodeling.[60] Importantly, the correction of cephalic index was found to be equivalent.

SMC is typically used for patients up to ages 6 or 7 months. After this time, cranial development requires a greater widening with greater forces than springs can provide. This typically necessitates calvarial vault reconstruction or distraction osteogenesis with rigid semi-buried distractors. In our institution patients currently undergo spring placement at 3–4 months of age. Springs for this technique are usually bent in-house. An FDA-approved stainless steel wire is used. The diameter is typically 1.3 mm (18 gauge). Average spring force is between

6 and 12 N – we have chosen higher forces over time. Average spring expansile distance is 5 to 7 cm from a compressed position to a relaxed position. Fabrication is typically performed using a purpose-built wire bender. This wire is bent to produce a gentle U-shape, and the ends are bent into 3 mm hooks for bony attachment. The opening force of the compressed spring is then verified using a digital force gauge.[56,80]

Surgery is done in supine position. Two small (5 cm) transverse incisions are at each fontanelle. Through these incisions the sagittal suture and a surrounding strip of cranium (1.5 cm) are removed using an ultrasonic device (Sonopet; Stryker, Kalamazoo, MI, USA). In general, endoscopic visualization of the dura is not necessary. Small notches are made with a rongeur to accommodate the footplates of the springs. Two springs are then placed – one anterior, one posterior. If midvault correction is inadequate after placement of two springs, a third is added. Morselized bone graft is placed in the osteotomy particularly deep to the springs. Plain radiographs are obtained postoperatively, and spring removal is planned for 4 months later.

Cranial vault distraction osteogenesis

Distraction osteogenesis (DO) in the craniofacial skeleton was popularized by McCarthy for mandibular distraction.[81] This technique uses rigid hardware to slowly separate bone causing intervening bone formation. The use of DO has expanded to the midface and the cranium. The largest role that DO now plays in craniosynostosis is in syndromic patients to expand the posterior vault – posterior vault distraction osteogenesis (PVDO) (Fig. 32.17) The advent of distraction has allowed a new paradigm of treatment for some patients with craniosynostosis. This approach has been advocated by several groups[82–85] where PVDO is used early to expand intracranial volume protecting the brain during its high growth period followed by FOA for aesthetic normalization as needed. DO has a number of purported advantages which include ability to gain greater changes in length or volume than traditional reconstruction as well as decreased perioperative morbidity. A recent study from our institution demonstrated that PVDO produces nearly double the intracranial volumetric increase as frontal orbital advancement.[86] Surgeons continue to believe that markers of operative and perioperative morbidity are better with PVDO compared to traditional open calvarial vault reconstruction (CVR); however, there have only been head-to-head studies that demonstrate equivalence. Taylor et al. showed no difference in blood loss, operative time, transfusion requirement, and length of stay.[87]

The disadvantages of DO are primarily that the bone of very young infants is too soft and too thin to withstand the application of hardware and the forces during distraction. Furthermore, with metallic hardware, a second procedure is required for removal and possible plating of the distracted segments. A review by Losee et al. demonstrated that in the limited literature that is available on this topic, complication rates are substantial. In their review of 11 studies and 86 patients, they found a complication rate of 35.5% (12.5–100%). These complications include cerebrospinal fluid (CSF) leak, infection, wound dehiscence, and hardware failure; however, no reports included significant morbidity or mortality.[88] The largest series of PVDO by Johnson et al. reaffirms this high complication rate, reporting a 61% complication rate.[89] Many

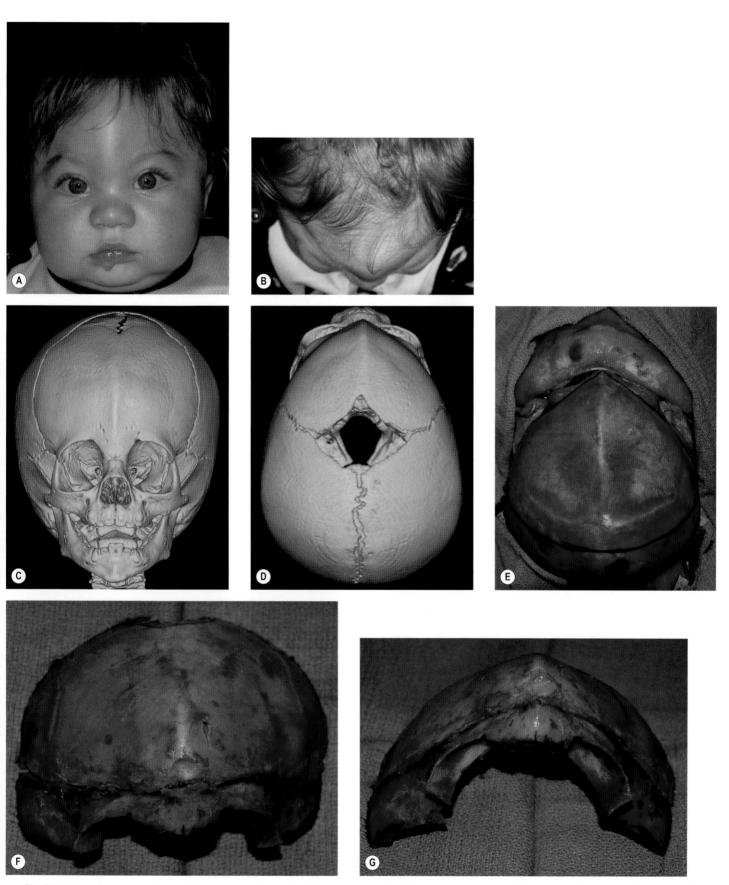

Fig. 32.14 Example of treatment of metopic synostosis with frontal orbital advancement. **(A, B)** Preoperative photographs. **(C, D)** Preoperative computed tomography (CT) scans. **(E)** Large bifrontal craniotomy marked just posteriorly to the coronal sutures. **(F, G)** Frontal bandeau and frontal craniotomy before widening and reshaping.

Continued

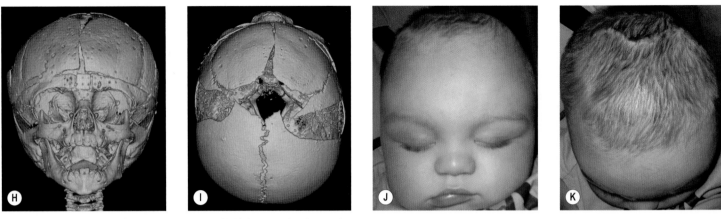

Fig. 32.14, cont'd **(H, I)** Postoperative CT scans. **(J, K)** Postoperative photographs.

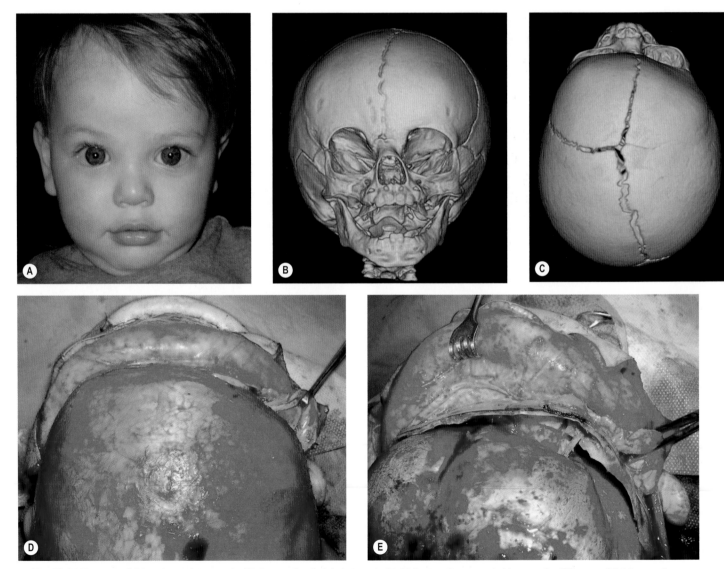

Fig. 32.15 Treatment of right unicoronal synostosis. **(A)** Preoperative frontal photograph. **(B, C)** Preoperative computed tomography (CT) scans. **(D)** Intraoperative: craniotomy and hemi-bandeau. **(E, F)** Intraoperative: bandeau positioning and overcorrection.

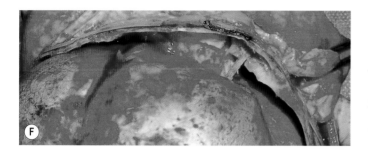

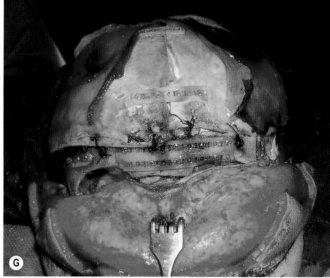

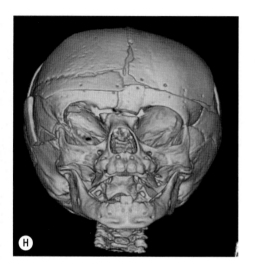

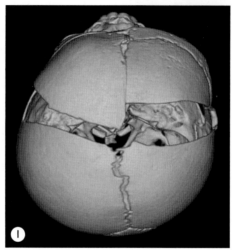

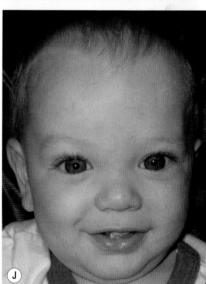

Fig. 32.15, cont'd (G) Intraoperative: fixation with resorbable plates. (H, I) Postoperative CT. (J) Postoperative photograph.

of these complications are related to the semi-buried nature of distraction devices.

There has also been use of DO in single suture nonsyndromic craniosynostosis. This was pioneered in Asia for fronto-orbital advancement. DO has also been used to expand most other cranial suture fusion patterns. Hirabayashi *et al.* first reported the clinical use of distraction for fronto-orbital advancement in an infant with brachycephaly.[90] A multitude of examples have since been reported, including for single suture involvement, multisuture synostosis,[91] and both syndromic and nonsyndromic children. DO has been used to treat metopic,[92] unicoronal,[64,93,94] and lambdoidal[95] synostosis. The future may bring advances that expand common use of DO for other synostosis. There may be a potential to remove the distractor arm non-invasively, obviating the need for an additional operation as has been demonstrated in distractors mounted on absorbable foot plates.[96]

Postoperative care

In general, all patients undergoing primary cranial vault surgery should be admitted to the ICU postoperatively. In the authors' institution this also includes minimally invasive surgery such as spring-mediated cranioplasty. This allows for close monitoring of hemodynamic and neurologic status. Recovery should be targeted with the goal of oral intake as soon as possible. Blood products are given as needed for hemodynamic instability or blood loss anemia. Pain control in infants is typically multimodal and includes oral/rectal/intravenous acetaminophen as well as oral/intravenous narcotic when needed. Perioperative antibiotics are administered for 72 hours. There is no data in the literature to support a specific antibiotic regimen for these patients, but the rates of surgical site infections are very low in reported series. The

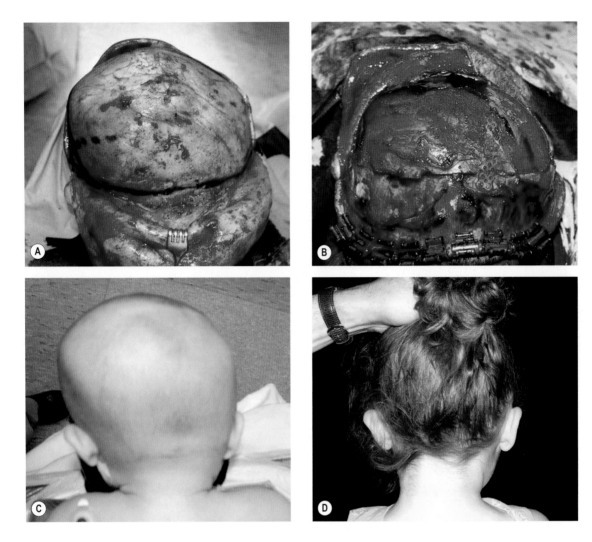

Fig. 32.16 Treatment of lambdoid synostosis. **(A, B)** Switch cranioplasty and occipital bar advancement. **(C, D)** Before and after head shape, from posterior.

craniofacial dressing is removed on the second postoperative day. Output from the subgaleal drain is monitored, emptied, and recorded regularly. Typically the drain is removed on the third postoperative day, regardless of output quantity, so long as the drainage is serosanguinous. In cases where the drainage is clear, and/or known dural tears or CSF leaks are present, a trial of clamping or removing the Jackson–Pratt (JP) drain from suction, alternating with restoration of suction, can be pursued. This prevents continual active suction of CSF and encourages the dural defect to close.

Parents are advised that, although not usually present immediately postoperatively, significant periorbital edema will ensue, peaking on the second or third postoperative day, in infants who have undergone frontal reconstruction. Children who have undergone posterior reconstruction, and were positioned prone, are likely to have periorbital edema immediately postoperatively from prolonged positional dependence. Measures to minimize postoperative edema include gentle dissection along anatomical planes, intraoperative local injection of steroid periorbitally, and systemic administration of corticosteroids.[97–99] In the past, a 3D head CT was routinely obtained postoperatively. This pattern has changed in light of more experience and evidence of the harmful nature of the associated ionizing radiation in children. In very young patients the CT scan also may require an anesthetic, and for

these reasons the authors' philosophy has shifted to an "only when necessary" mentality. For the purposes of teaching and learning, many prior examples are available. The child is typically discharged from the hospital on the third or fourth postoperative day. The first follow-up visit takes place at 3–4 weeks, with subsequent visits typically at 12 weeks, 6 months, 1 year, and annually or biennially thereafter.

Outcomes

Outcomes in craniosynostosis surgery can be broadly separated into three categories: measures of perioperative safety, cognitive and developmental effects, and aesthetic results.

Perioperative complications

Complications may occur in the operating room or in the immediate postoperative period. These can be serious – deaths after vault remodeling have been reported. However, reported complication rates, including at the authors' institution, are very low. In their series, the authors reported a major complication rate of 1.1% and a minor complication rate of 3.5% in 746 patients with nonsyndromic single suture synostosis.[100] Bleeding during surgery and afterward is the most

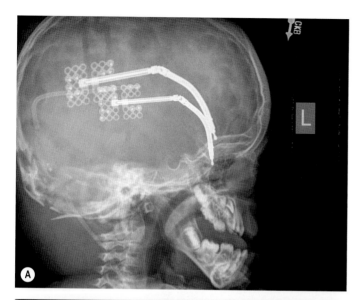

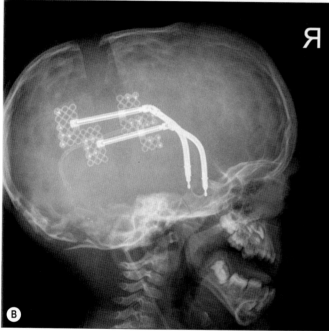

Fig. 32.17 Posterior vault distraction osteogenesis (PVDO). **(A)** Skull X-ray immediately after surgery demonstrates hardware before distraction has begun. Note the anteriorly oriented activation arms and the presence of a VP shunt. The precise position of the distractors is influenced by the shape of the skull and presence of obstacles such as a shunt. Typically they are fairly lateral. **(B)** Skull X-ray after full activation of 30mm distractors. A shelf in the occiput has been mitigated by low barrel stave outfracturing at the initial operation.

common problem encountered. As discussed above, a number of measures are taken to limit blood loss and a number of strategies are used to resuscitate patients. At the authors' institution, 2 units of cross-matched whole blood and 1 unit of packed red blood cells are reserved for each patient, and infusion is begun when incision is made. All of these efforts are made to avoid hypovolemia, shock, and coagulopathy. Typically upon closure most bleeding has subsided and does not continue. Postoperative bleeding may occur and may be in the form of ongoing drainage in a closed suction drain, a hematoma below the scalp flap, or in more serious cases a

subcranial or parenchymal hemorrhage (epidural, subdural, intraparenchymal). The patient's hemodynamic status, urine output, and neurologic exam must be watched closely in the ICU in the early postoperative period (48 to 72 hours). Mental status changes or seizures prompt an emergent head CT scan to investigate for hemorrhage and if confirmed would likely prompt an emergent return to the operating room for evacuation. Complete blood count and coagulation laboratories should be closely monitored with a low threshold for clotting factor and platelet replacement if necessary. Implementing an evidence-based protocol for transfusion can limit the patient's exposure to blood products, as the authors have done at their institution.[101]

Rare reports of optic nerve injury or infarction can lead to blindness following cranial vault reconstruction. One reported case indicated a delayed presentation, after discharge from the hospital, thought to be an ischemic bilateral optic nerve injury predisposed by prolonged prone position and blood loss.[102]

Infection is also a risk. This may include surgical site infection, line infections, osteomyelitis of bone grafts, and meningitis. All of these infections occur at low rates in this patient population. The risk for meningitis may be increased by dural injury intraoperatively with subsequent cerebrospinal fluid leak. If recognized, dural injuries should be repaired. Osteomyelitis of repositioned bone plates is a rare, but potentially devastating, complication associated with cranial vault remodeling.[103] Thankfully these infections are also extremely rare. Infection is more apt to occur in older children where sinus boundaries are crossed. If recognized early, limited debridement and administration of both parenteral and local (e.g., catheter irrigation) antibiotics can eradicate the infection and encourage bone healing. With late presenting or more widespread infection, significant debridement and ostectomy may be required, leaving spans of unprotected dura. This frequently necessitates long-term antimicrobial therapy and staged reconstruction of the calvarial vault.

Neurocognitive outcomes

The precise impact of nonsyndromic craniosynostosis on both unrepaired and repaired patients is unknown.[104–106] This represents a challenge for research because of the longitudinal nature of the follow-up that is required. Early studies were beset with methodologic problems including lack of controls and poor testing modalities. But evidence is now mounting in young children and school-age children that cognitive deficits are present even after early correction of nonsyndromic craniosynostosis. Speltz and colleagues have studied this topic extensively in a multi-institutional fashion. In 2015, they published a study examining single suture craniosynostosis patients compared to a control group into school age (age 7).[107] The findings of this study show that craniosynostosis patients score lower on all intelligence tests used (IQ 2.5 to 4 points lower, 0.25–0.5 SD), are more than twice as likely to have learning delay, and 42% have learning disability compared to 33% in the control group. Subgroup analysis shows that the differences between the patients and controls are larger in the patients with unicoronal and lambdoid synostosis. This paper does not draw conclusion about the cause of these delays. Importantly, the control patients are well matched in terms of gender, age, and parental intelligence. The actual differences in scoring may in reality be wider because craniosynostosis patients receive specialized assistance at higher rates than control patients. The argument has been made that early correction of craniosynostosis may lead to better neurocognitive outcomes, but in this study the patients underwent correction at 7.4 months of age. Other data has failed to show significant differences between cases and control.[107] Birgfeld *et al.* examined the impact of anesthetic duration using the Bayley Scales of Infant Development.[106] This study demonstrated that increased anesthetic exposure is associated with decreased neurodevelopmental outcomes and that non-sagittal synostoses perform worse than sagittal. A systematic review in 2014 demonstrated that of the 33 studies evaluated, most found decreased intelligence in patients with single suture craniosynostosis.[108]

Persing *et al.* have also made significant recent contributions to this literature. In a study of nonsyndromic sagittal craniosynostosis (n=70), they found that patients treated later (after 12 months) fared significantly worse in terms of IQ compared to those patients treated earlier. The group who was treated at less than 6 months of age had the best IQ scores and the lowest rates of learning disabilities.[109] In another similar study there was a suggestion that cranial vault remodeling produced better intelligence than a less invasive technique (strip suturectomy).[110]

Understanding the neurocognitive effects in nonsyndromic craniosynostosis remains a challenge. The role of surgery in mitigating intelligence losses and behavioral problems is unknown. This is further complicated by emerging data that volatile anesthetics may have long-lasting negative neurocognitive impacts as well.

Aesthetic outcomes

The aesthetic results of craniosynostosis reconstruction are related to the balance of final bony position at the time of surgery and ultimate craniofacial growth as the patient matures to adulthood. In addition to this, resorption of bone grafts and incomplete ossification of bony gaps may lead to additional contour irregularities. The Whitaker classification

---

BOX 32.1 **Whitaker classification for surgical revision**

I. Excellent result, no revisions necessary

II. Satisfactory result, soft-tissue revision indicated

III. Marginal result, bony irregularities present, requiring contouring with bone grafts or alloplast/osteobiologicals

IV. Unacceptable result, repeat craniotomy and/or fronto-orbital reshaping necessary

(Reproduced from Whitaker LA, Bartlett SP, Schut L, et al. Craniosynostosis: an analysis of the timing, treatment, and complications in 164 consecutive patients. *Plast Reconstr Surg.* 1987;80:195.)

(Box 32.1) was developed to broadly classify the aesthetic outcomes of this diverse group of patients. The classification is stratified based on increasing need for revision: I, excellent result, no revision necessary; II, satisfactory result, soft-tissue revision indicated; III, marginal result, bony irregularities present, requiring bony contouring; IV, unacceptable result, repeat craniotomy and/or fronto-orbital reshaping necessary.[111] The term relapse has been used for these Whitaker IV patients, but the situation is likely more complex. These patients more likely were both undercorrected at the time of initial surgery, and their continued cranial growth may have also been negatively impacted by surgery. In a review of nonsyndromic patients from the authors' institution, it was found that while only 3.4% were Whitaker class IV with greater than one year follow-up, over 35% were Whitaker class III. This analysis confirmed that overcorrection leads to improved long-term outcomes though the exact degree of overcorrection is still unknown. Temporal hollowing and supraorbital retrusion were a vast majority of the defects[112] (Fig. 32.18). Teenagers and adults are understandably resistant to major operative revision of a suboptimal result from infancy. Therefore, it is critical to continue to follow results to maturity and to refine techniques that ensure high-quality outcomes. Our analysis suggests that reoperation rates are a poor surrogate for aesthetic outcomes.

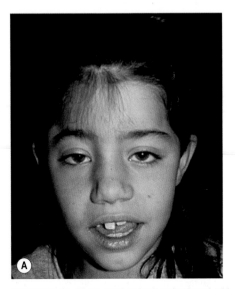 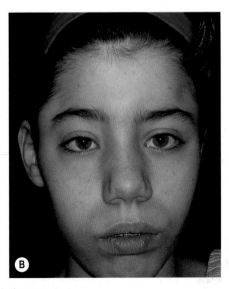 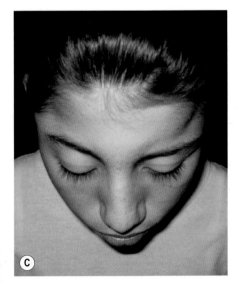

Fig. 32.18 **(A–C)** Temporal hollowing after frontal orbital advancement.

When craniosynostosis surgery is done before the age of one year, many bony gaps will reossify via edgewise and dural osteogenesis. Despite this, sizeable full-thickness cranial gaps may occur in these patients. The authors' preferred method for filling these gaps at the time of primary surgery has evolved to cranial bone shavings. Anecdotally this appears to have decreased dramatically the number of sizeable defects.[113] In older children there is the concern that these full-thickness gaps may put the child at risk for traumatic brain injury. Such injuries in craniosynostosis have never been reported, but it remains a concern. For that reason it is the authors' practice to repair the larger gaps with titanium mesh cranioplasty. This is often combined with revision contouring. In general, split calvarial grafts are no longer used for this purpose. Contour irregularities are typically treated with bone cement (see below).

Besides cranioplasty for incompletely ossified cranial gaps and contouring for bony irregularities (often at the interface of reconstructed bone grafts), there are also patients who have essentially outgrown their original repair. This is likely a combination of continued craniofacial growth outside of the operated area and a loss of growth potential within the reconstruction (e.g. the supraorbital bandeau and frontal bone).[72] This small number of patients with a Whitaker IV result have guided the philosophy and debate regarding proper techniques in craniosynostosis surgery. Good arguments can be made for avoiding a disruption of future growth potential by using minimally invasive techniques (spring-mediated cranioplasty, strip suturectomy with helmeting); however, long-term outcomes are largely not available for these newer techniques. For conventional vault reconstruction, many advocate for overcorrection. This applies to each of the suture fusion patterns. In metopic synostosis, the supraorbital bandeau should be over-widened and over-advanced. The frontal bone (forehead) is similarly widened and advanced in continuity with this. Unicoronal synostosis should be treated similarly particularly if one avoids operating on the unaffected (contralateral) orbit. In staged vault reconstruction for sagittal reconstruction, the biparietal diameter should be overcorrected particularly in the first stage posterior vault operation when the child is an infant. Practically speaking, it must be recognized that the soft-tissue envelope may not tolerate extreme overcorrection. This has forced instances in which disassembly and reduction of the expanded skeleton must be performed to allow for skin closure. The observation that a higher rate of results requiring revision occur in patients who had their first surgery at a young age (<6 months) has prompted a call for delaying initial surgery.[57,72,114] This desire is tempered by a concern for adequate room for brain development and the avoidance of potential elevated ICP.

The reports of long-term outcomes in terms of Whitaker classification vary widely as do the rates of reoperation. In a recent review at the authors' institution, 207 patients with nonsyndromic craniosynostosis were examined, with an average follow-up of 6.2 years after surgery. It was found that a majority of patients (55%) were Whitaker I, but importantly 35% were Whitaker III. This is a significant number of patients, and the study also revealed that deformities such as supraorbital retrusion were more likely with longer follow-up.[112] This number of Whitaker III results was quite similar to our prior report on specifically metopic craniosynostosis with 178 patients and 5.8 years of follow up.[115] As with many other studies, the number of Whitaker IV patients was very low (1.5-3%). The reoperative rates for these studies was approximately 11%.

Two other long-term aesthetic problems are coronal scar widening and temporal hollowing after fronto-orbital procedures. The coronal scar may widen and, as previously discussed, is made less conspicuous through use of a non-linear pattern. To avoid widening, a careful galeal closure must be performed though with a large advancement and continued rapid growth of a young patient it may be inevitable. Scar revisions are well tolerated and may be done at any point. Temporal hollowing is a controversial issue and is likely the result of a combination of temporal muscle and underlying cranial bone abnormalities. The temporalis muscle, when disrupted during exposure, may be inadequately resuspended, malpositioned (i.e. not advanced with the bandeau), or injured during dissection resulting in atrophy. The handling of the muscle by surgeons is variable, with some preferring to dissect it separately and others elevating the muscle within the scalp as a unit, ensuring suspension upon closure.[116–118] Cranial bone morphology certainly plays some role in temporal hollowing as well. In patients with unicoronal craniosynostosis, this is likely related to the preoperative morphology as well as to a deficiency of growth following frontal orbital advancement. Strategies for treating temporal hollowing include soft-tissue augmentation with fat grafting, onlay cranioplasty to augment bony insufficiency, and temporalis muscle resuspension or some combination thereof. While fat grafting has been used to mask this hollowing, the superficial fat content does not appear to be different in patients with unicoronal synostosis.

Secondary procedures

In general, revision surgery is guided by the desires of the patients and their parents. Revision of cranial deformities are divided into two groups – redo surgery and contouring. Redo surgery is fairly uncommon and is based on the principles utilized during primary correction. In general contouring surgery allows for the treatment of any cranial gaps and the repair of bothersome contour irregularities or slight undercorrections. As mentioned above, the authors' choice for cranioplasty is typically titanium mesh. This material is rarely infected, though it has been reported to infrequently erode through the scalp. For smoothing and minimal correction, the authors' preference is the addition of bone cement (Cranios; Synthes, Solothurn, Switzerland). This is fast-setting calcium phosphate cement. It must be used under strict sterile conditions, and it should only be used as a very thin contouring substance. Contamination and infection can be catastrophic with bone cement necessitating difficult explant procedures. Additionally when applied too thickly, the cement in the long term can fracture and deform. When used correctly and encountered years later, the cement will have maintained its form and may become vascularized by ingrowth.[119]

Scar revision can be performed at any time by excision, either as a singular procedure, or frequently whenever the coronal incision is reopened to address deeper bony contour irregularities. A wide, hairless scar can be noticeable and bothersome, especially when hair is worn short or is thin in caliber. Closure under tension, from a significant osseous advancement, and genetic propensity contribute to thick unaesthetic scars. Attempts to avoid unsightly scars on initial closure include a trichophytic closure, and limited use of both electrocautery and compressive scalp clips, though despite the best efforts, scarring remains unpredictable.

Fat-grafting techniques can serve to camouflage hollow areas or depressions. Most commonly, temporal concavities can be observed following fronto-orbital advancement procedures as a result of bony deficiency.[120] Though not addressing the tissue type responsible for the problem, fat grafting is a less invasive technique to provide bulk and improve contour in these areas.[121] The principal issue relates to its unpredictability, in terms of how much resorbs. Patients may require several repeat rounds of fat injections. Depression of medial epicanthal folds may be witnessed following trigonocephaly correction. This can be alleviated by using an onlay bone graft to the depressed nasal radix (effectively tenting up the medial soft tissue).

Periocular surgery is another category of revision after craniosynostosis repair. This falls into the broad categories of brow position, lid position/function, canthal position, and extraocular muscle imbalance. Asymmetric brow position may be addressed as a secondary procedure. The practitioner should recognize that underlying bone asymmetries may contribute to the differential brow position (relatively raised or lowered). For instance, supraorbital ridge retrusion and flattening of the forehead may position the brow higher (akin to the original deformity in UCS). In these instances, bony augmentation of the supraorbital region will aid in properly positioning the brow. Soft-tissue brow-lifting procedures are numerous in the aesthetic literature. Common effective procedures include rotation of the coronal flap away from the side of desired lift and bone fixation and suture techniques.[122,123] A combination of addressing the underlying bony support and soft-tissue browpexy techniques should be employed to correct brow position effectively. There are several techniques to perform canthopexy for differential angulation of the lateral canthal position (most typically seen in UCS).[124] This may be performed at the time of the initial fronto-orbital reshaping, but it is controversial as to whether a canthopexy is always necessary. As a delayed procedure, the canthopexy technique could involve osseous wiring, deep and superior to the zygomaticofrontal suture.[125] Other suture approaches have been reported and involve the lateral canthal tendon or lateral palpebral commissure and periosteum of the internal lateral orbital rim.[126] Strabismus surgery and ptosis repair are outside the scope of this chapter; however, they may be necessary and are typically performed by the ophthalmologist member of the craniofacial team.

🌐 Access the complete reference list online at   **http://www.expertconsult.com**

2. Selber J, Reid RR, Chike-Obi CJ, et al. The changing epidemiologic spectrum of single-suture synostoses. *Plast Reconstr Surg.* 2008;122:527–533. *This series relied upon approximately 800 patients with nonsyndromic synostosis to derive epidemiologic patterns. There was a relative increase in metopic patients and a relative decrease in unicoronal patients. These findings are corroborated by other similar series.*

40. Basta MN, Stricker PA, Taylor JA. A systematic review of the use of antifibrinolytic agents in pediatric surgery and implications for craniofacial use. *Pediatr Surg Int.* 2012;28:1059–1069. *This systematic review examined the available literature for evidence on the efficacy of blood loss reducing agents in use for craniosynostosis surgery. Antifibrinolytics reduced blood loss and transfusion volume but did not demonstrate increased risk for adverse outcomes.*

43. Naran S, Cladis F, Fearon J, et al. Safety of preoperative erythropoietin in surgical calvarial remodeling: an 8-year retrospective review and analysis. *Plast Reconstr Surg.* 2012;130:305e–310e.

47. Jimenez DF, Barone CM. Early treatment of anterior calvarial craniosynostosis using endoscopic-assisted minimally invasive techniques. *Childs Nerv Syst.* 2007;23:1411–1419.

54. David LR, Plikaitis CM, Couture D, et al. Outcome analysis of our first 75 spring-assisted surgeries for scaphocephaly. *J Craniofac Surg.* 2010;21:3–9.

57. Fearon JA, McLaughlin EB, Kolar JC. Sagittal craniosynostosis: surgical outcomes and long-term growth. *Plast Reconstr Surg.*

2006;117:532–541. *A series of approximately 40 patient surgically treated for sagittal synostosis. The series provided long term measurements of head shape and growth with an average follow up of 4.7 years. The paper finds relapse of cephalic index over time and suggest impaired growth over time.*

63. Lauritzen CGK, Davis C, Ivarsson A, et al. The evolving role of springs in craniofacial surgery: the first 100 clinical cases. *Plast Reconstr Surg.* 2008;121:545–554. *A series of 100 patients treated with spring assisted expansion. This demonstrated a 5% rate of reoperation for additional expansion and a low rate of hardware failure.*

100. Tahiri Y, Paliga JT, Wes AM, et al. Perioperative complications associated with intracranial procedures in patients with nonsyndromic single-suture craniosynostosis. *J Craniofac Surg.* 2015;26:118–123.

107. Speltz ML, Collett BR, Wallace ER, et al. Intellectual and academic functioning of school-age children with single-suture craniosynostosis. *Pediatrics.* 2015;135:e615–e623. *This series compared the IQ/intellectual outcomes of 182 single suture craniosynostosis patients to 183 controls. Patients were evaluated preoperatively and at 18 months, 36 months, and 7 years. This study demonstrates decreased measures of IQ and other specific cognitive abilities in craniosynostosis patients in school age.*

112. Taylor JA, Paliga JT, Wes AM, et al. A critical evaluation of long-term aesthetic outcomes of fronto-orbital advancement and cranial vault remodeling in nonsyndromic unicoronal craniosynostosis. *Plast Reconstr Surg.* 2015;135:220–231.

Syndromic craniosynostosis

Jeffrey A. Fearon

SYNOPSIS

- Syndromic craniosynostoses are defined by having coexisting anomalies aside from fused cranial sutures.
- Treatment paradigms are best designed according more to phenotype than genotype.
- The avoidance of neurocognitive delays requires a focus on the prevention of sleep apnea, chronic elevations in intracranial pressure, and a reduction in anesthetic lengths and numbers.
- The management of the syndromic craniosynostoses are best relegated to dedicated craniofacial teams, comprised of experienced subspecialists.

 Access the Historical Perspective section online at
http://www.expertconsult.com

Introduction

Craniosynostosis is a condition resulting in the anomalous fusion of one or more cranial sutures. When just one suture is affected, this may be referred to as "isolated craniosynostosis". Syndromic craniosynostosis signifies the presence of additional anomalies occurring in embryologically distinct areas outside of the skull. As a general rule, infants presenting with single sutural synostoses will not have a syndrome, while those with multiple sutural craniosynostosis are more likely to have a syndrome. However, some syndromes have been described in association with only a single sutural synostosis, and various patterns of multiple sutural fusions (also known as "complex craniosynostoses") may occur in the absence of a recognized syndrome. Most syndromes have been eponymously named after the physician(s) describing the condition; however, many may also be referred to by slightly more descriptive names such as the acrocephalosyndactylies: type 1 (Apert), type 2 (Crouzon), type 3 (Saethre–Chotzen) and type 5 (Pfeiffer). The syndromic craniosynostoses are relatively uncommon and of all the anomalies treated by craniofacial surgeons, they can present some of the greatest treatment challenges. The optimal care of patients with these unusual syndromes is best relegated to experienced craniofacial teams, comprised of multiple subspecialists. By virtue of their increased experience level, and the capability to coordinate care across specialties, such teams can both reduce the total number of operative procedures that affected children must endure, as well as maximize outcomes.

Basic science/disease process

As the field of craniofacial genetics has matured, a more complete picture of the molecular basis for the syndromic synostoses is emerging. Today, over 150 different craniosynostosis syndromes have been described.[14] The majority of syndromic craniosynostoses are the result of FGFR-related mutations, which are primarily autosomal dominant.[15] In addition to the more commonly encountered Apert, Crouzon, and Pfeiffer syndromes, other FGFR-related craniosynostosis syndromes include Muenke, Crouzon with acanthosis nigricans, Jackson–Weiss, and Beare–Stevenson (Table 33.1). Among the non-FGFR mutations are Boston-type craniosynostosis (MSX2), the Philadelphia type, and Saethre–Chotzen (Twist 1). All the FGFR-associated craniosynostoses are gain-of-function mutations, and while MSXS is also a gain-of-function mutation, the TWIST mutation represents a loss of function.[16] Notably, the TWIST mutation has been reported to occur in association with an increased incidence of breast and renal cancers; however, a subsequently published multicenter Australian study failed to support these earlier findings.[17–19]

The majority of infants born with one of the syndromic craniosynostoses will present with bilateral coronal craniosynostosis, either in isolation or associated with other sutural synostoses. In addition, there may be variable effects on the development of the midface, as well as the hands and feet. It has been noted that some genes expressed in craniofacial

Table 33.1 FGFR-related craniosynostoses

Syndrome	Percentage caused by FGFR1 mutations	Percentage caused by FGFR2 mutations	Percentage caused by FGFR 3 mutations
Muenke			100%
Crouzon		100%	
Crouzon with acanthosis nigricans			100%
Jackson–Weiss		100%	
Apert		100%	
Pfeiffer type I	5%	95%	
Pfeiffer type II		100%	
Pfeiffer type III		100%	
Beare–Stevenson		<100%	
FGFR2 isolated coronal synostosis		100%	

(Adapted from Robin NH, Falk MJ, Haldeman-Englert CR. FGFR-related craniosynostosis syndromes. *Gene Reviews*. www.genetests.org)

development are also expressed in limb development.[20,21] One of the more commonly encountered syndromic cranio-synostoses is Crouzon syndrome, which is notable for the presence of phenotypically normal hands and feet. Pfeiffer syndrome is recognizable by the presence of enlarged thumbs and halluces, and Apert syndrome may be easily identified by the associated complex syndactylies of the hands and feet. As the field of molecular genetics has developed, many surgeons have hoped that gene testing could provide specific and accurate diagnoses for each of the phenotypically unique craniofacial syndromes. Thus far, this has proven to not be the case. Not only can the same mutation cause different syndromes, different mutations may be associated with the same syndrome.[22,23] For example, identical mutations have been noted in individuals with Crouzon syndrome, Pfeiffer syndrome, and Jackson–Weiss syndrome, suggesting that unlinked modifier genes, or epigenetic factors, are playing an important role in determining the final phenotype.[24,25] Apert syndrome has been shown to result from at least two separate amino acid missense substitutions in almost all cases: Ser252Trp or Pro253Arg. The Ser252Trp mutation has been reported to occur slightly more commonly and is associated with an increased incidence of palatal clefting, while the Pro253Arg mutation is more often associated with a more severe form of syndactyly.[26,27] Through use of the amplification refractory mutation system, the paternal origin of these mutations for Apert, Crouzon, and Pfeiffer syndromes has been demonstrated, along with a correlation to paternal age.[28–30] Moreover, within syndromes there can be significant phenotypic variability. For example, Pfeiffer syndrome has been phenotypically subclassified into three separate types based on the appearance of the skull: type I is described as the "classic Pfeiffer" and represents a milder presentation, type II is notable for a cloverleaf (or Kleeblattschädel) skull deformity,

and type III is reserved for the most severely affected children. Apert syndrome has also been shown present with different skull configurations: type I describes a split metopic suture without any significant turricephaly, type II infants have a closed metopic suture with moderate turricephaly, and type III is notable for severe turricephaly, similar to a type III Pfeiffer skull shape.[27] In spite of these differences, no specific genetic mutations have yet been noted to correlate with each of these described phenotypes.[31]

Diagnosis/patient presentation

Knowledge of how skull growth is affected by each sutural fusion (with radial growth inhibition occurring in the region of the fused suture and compensatory growth occurring in the remaining open sutures) will enable the astute examiner to correctly diagnose which of the skull sutures are fused.[32] Palpation of open fontanels, and any congenital or acquired skull defects, can provide insight into potential elevations in intracranial pressure. For example, if dura is constantly bulging through the fontanel, if a raised collar of bone is palpable around the fontanel ("volcano sign"), or if multiple unexpected skull defects are noted, these may all be indicators for raised intracranial pressure (Fig. 33.1). It is also important to frequently follow serial head circumference measurements early in life to monitor for the potential development of hydrocephalus, which can be ascertained by progressive upward deviations in the growth curve. The eyes are assessed for the degree of proptosis and the ability to achieve adequate lid coverage, sufficient to prevent conjunctival desiccation. The globes are monitored for further forward displacement with the infant crying, such that the upper eyelid might be potentially trapped behind the globe. When identified, this is best treated with creation of semi-permanent intramarginal adhesions. The palate is examined for possible clefting, and the noise of breathing is assessed with the child recumbent. Further differentiation between syndromes can often be determined by an examination of the fingers and toes.

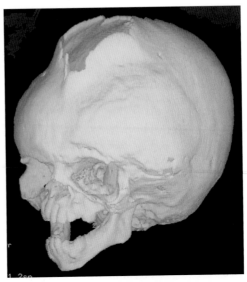

Fig. 33.1 A raised collar of bone is palpable around the fontanel ("volcano sign"), one of many indicators for raised intracranial pressure.

Table 33.2 Clinical findings in selected FGFR-related syndromic craniosynostoses

Syndrome	Skull shape	Midface	Hands and feet
Apert	Moderate to severe brachycephaly with occasional severe turribrachycephaly	Moderate hypoplasia	Pan-syndactylies of hands and feet (thumbs can be free, and partial syndactylies of small fingers and toes may occur)
Crouzon	Brachycephaly	Mild to moderate hypoplasia	Generally unaffected
Muenke	Unilateral or bilateral brachycephaly	Mild to none	Variable carpal and tarsal fusions
Pfeiffer type I	Brachycephaly	Moderate	Broad thumbs and halluces. Variable limited syndactyly
Pfeiffer type II	Cloverleaf skull deformity with pan-synostoses	Moderate	Broad thumbs and halluces. Variable limited syndactyly
Pfeiffer type III	Pan-synostoses with marked turricephaly	Moderate to severe	Broad thumbs and halluces. Variable limited syndactyly

Table 33.2 lists identifying characteristics for the more commonly presenting syndromes. The most important aspect of the initial examination is the assessment for potentially acute impediments to life, such as an airway obstruction or feeding impairment (inadequate intake, reflux, aspiration, etc.). Concerns for intracranial pressure, while important, usually take a secondary role in this initial evaluation. This is because early in life the remaining open sutures are likely effective in compensating for those that are fused.

With regard to initial testing, if there are any suspicions for airway compromise (history for snoring, increased noise of breathing noted during the examination, significant midfacial hypoplasia), the first test performed should be polysomnography. Children with syndromic craniosynostosis can develop either obstructive or central sleep apnea. Most commonly, affected infants will present with obstructive sleep apnea. The cause for this obstruction may be multifactorial but is most often directly related to a three-dimensional midfacial hypoplasia. In addition to maxillary recession there is elevation of the floor of the nose (from a failure of palatal descent), along with palatal narrowing, which correspondingly reduces the size of the nasal passages. The resultant airway compression is different from a true choanal atresia, which is defined by a congenital persistence of tissues separating the nose from the mouth. This reduction in nasal airway aperture is best left untreated because of the dismal success rates that have been observed following any early surgical intervention.[33] Other causes for airway obstruction include tracheomalacia, tracheal stenosis (especially with type II Pfeiffer syndrome), reactive airway disease, and gastroesophageal reflux (anti-reflux medication should be considered for all syndromic infants).[34] It is more unusual to see central sleep apnea in infants with syndromic craniosynostosis. This is because this symptom is usually the result of an acquired Chiari I deformation that causes brain stem compression. With growth, there may be progressive tonsillar herniation, leading to worsening central sleep apnea. Aside from Chiari deformations, central apnea may less commonly occur from general elevations in intracranial pressure. More often, central apneas are seen to arise in children with severe obstructive apnea. These are likely spurious central apneas, which typically disappear when the obstruction is treated. Feeding issues are commonly seen in conjunction with airway obstruction, and when associated with neuromuscular immaturity, silent aspiration may result;

therefore, swallowing studies may be indicated. When obstructive sleep apnea is identified, more conservative treatments include use of continuous positive airway pressure (CPAP) masks and tonsilloadenoidectomies (although the efficacy of this procedure is currently unclear). Some surgeons have reported performing frontofacial advancements in infancy; however, there is currently no evidence to support the efficacy of these early interventions. Therefore, such treatments must be considered as falling outside of the current mainstream of care.[35,36] On the other hand, temporary tracheotomies have been attributed to lowering mortality rates for the more severe patterns of syndromic craniosynostosis and should be considered in all infants and younger children who have failed the more conservative therapies.[34] The incidence for airway compromise can increase with age as the midfacial hypoplasia becomes more progressive.[37]

In addition to airway management, the second critical area of focus for any child with syndromic craniosynostosis is the avoidance of raised intracranial pressure, which can significantly increase with age. Commonly, physicians begin the work-up of any infant with an abnormal skull shape by ordering a CT scan. While such studies can provide a clear assessment of patterns of sutural fusion, it has been shown that for the single sutural synostoses, an accurate diagnosis can be made solely on the basis of a careful physical examination.[38] More importantly, it is not possible to diagnose elevations in intracranial pressure by these scans. Some believe that chronic elevations in intracranial pressure may result in observable changes in the skull radiographs, such as imprinting ("copper-beaten", and/or thinning of the bone); however, there are no supportive studies to confirm this relationship, nor does this finding appear to correlate with intelligence.[39] It is common to see enlarged ventricles on scans of children with syndromic craniosynostosis, but this finding alone does not indicate the need for ventricular peritoneal shunting. The determination of whether or not a child with syndromic craniosynostosis might require shunting is often best determined by serial head circumference measurements. Unfortunately, the clinical determination of elevated intracranial pressure is an extremely challenging endeavor. There have been no published studies evaluating either the specificity or sensitivity of any of the often-cited clinical signs for raised intracranial pressure. Currently, it is unknown exactly how high or for how long intracranial pressure needs to be elevated before there are irreversible adverse effects on cognitive function. Nevertheless, some attempts to determine the presence of potentially elevated intracranial pressure must be made. Studies using direct measurement techniques suggest that when more than one suture is fused (even when there is a normal skull volume), intracranial pressure is more likely to be elevated.[40–42] Given the invasive nature of direct intracranial pressure testing, it is not reasonable to perform serial testing in every child with syndromic craniosynostosis. Instead, secondary assessments for raised pressure are used, such as the physical assessment of fontanels or other skull defects (to assess dural tension), serial head circumference measurements (to look for changes along the growth curves), fundoscopic examinations (to assess for papilledema), reversed visual evoked potentials, optical coherence tomography, and MRI scanning (to monitor for decreasing ventricular size, enlargement of the optic nerves, or progressive tonsillar herniation).[42–48] While a high specificity for the association between papilledema and raised intracranial pressure has been reported, the sensitivity for this test has been shown to be quite low, especially in children under 8 years of age.[47,49] Although it might seem intuitive that progressive skull malformations might correlate with increased intracranial pressure and developmental issues, this relationship has thus far not been supported by retrospective single sutural synostosis studies.[50,51] In addition to the need for evaluating a child for potential airway compromise and raised intracranial pressure, there are additional anomalies that must be considered. The association between cerebellar tonsillar herniation and syndromic craniosynostosis was first described over 30 years ago; since that time, studies have shown that these Chiari malformations are an acquired defect and are likely exacerbated by ventriculoperitoneal shunting.[52–54] Chiari malformations have been observed to occur fairly commonly in Apert syndrome, often in Crouzon syndrome, and almost always in the more severe presentations for Pfeiffer syndrome.[27,34,44,55] For this reason, the magnetic resonance imaging (MRI) scans are probably the single best imaging modality for infants with syndromic synostosis, because of its superior imaging of the hindbrain. This screening test should be considered in all children with syndromic craniosynostosis because, when present, Chiari malformations may lead to disordered swallowing, syringomyelia, symptomatic, or even potentially fatal central sleep apnea. Sequential scans can assist with the diagnosis of hydrocephalus, which sometimes does not become evident until after an initial skull expansion procedure. Additional testing may include a cardiac echocardiogram when murmurs are detected, because of the reported elevated incidence of these anomalies among the syndromic craniosynostoses, particularly atrial and ventricular septal defects.[56] Finally, consideration needs to be given to an upper gastrointestinal series with a small bowel follow-through evaluation for a potential malrotation, which appears to be more common in Pfeiffer syndrome, but may also occur in Apert syndrome.[34]

In formulating a lifelong treatment strategy for any child with syndromic craniosynostosis, it is critically important to remain focused on maximizing development through the prevention of avoidable neurocognitive loss by (1) avoiding prolonged periods of hypoxia and (2) avoiding prolonged periods of raised intracranial pressure. The initial management of any child born with one of the syndromic craniosynostoses typically involves more medical than surgical management. As the affected infant moves farther along the severity continuum, the likelihood for airway compromise may increase, as does the potential for feeding issues.

Patient selection

The determination of which operation should be done, and when it is best to perform this procedure, cannot be decided on a syndrome-by-syndrome basis; instead, these decisions need to be based on phenotypic presentation. It is useful to recognize that the syndromic synostoses actually represent a continuum of birth defects. At one end of this *syndromic craniosynostosis spectrum* would be the isolated bilateral coronal craniosynostoses (without any associated midfacial hypoplasia, and only minimally impaired cranial growth), and at the other end would be the severely constricted Kleeblattschädel skull deformities and complete pan-synostoses with extremely deficient midfacial growth, and associated severe airway anomalies (Fig. 33.2). Appreciating where each child falls on this continuum allows surgeons to apply treatment algorithms specific to the encountered problems.

The timing for the initial surgical intervention for any of the craniosynostoses has not been well studied. With respect to addressing the compromised skull growth, the two primary goals of treatment are to improve appearance and to prevent sustained elevations in intracranial pressure (sufficient to impact cognition). Implicit among these goals is the ability to accomplish them as safely, and with as few procedures, as possible. It is tempting to believe that early surgery needs to be performed to release the skull and reduce intracranial pressure. However, it is more likely that early surgery impairs growth than improves growth. Studies examining long-term calvarial growth following single sutural corrections have shown that growth is not normal postoperatively.[57–61] Considering the rapid development of the brain in infancy, delaying surgical intervention offers the potential to achieve better longer-term results. Early surgical intervention must contend with the reduced mechanical rigidity of the thin infant skull, which can impair the ability to achieve any significant enlargement of the calvaria and limit the ability to accomplish any notable improvements in appearance. Moreover, earlier surgical interventions have the disadvantage of the rapidly growing brain quickly occupying any obtainable increase in intracranial volume. It is important to consider the question: if surgery is performed in the first few months of life, how long can the result be expected to last? Conversely, one must also consider if inappropriate delays in surgical intervention might potentially result in preventable visual or developmental losses.[43,45] Studies measuring intracranial pressure in children with craniosynostosis suggest that elevated pressure is more likely to be encountered when multiple sutures are fused, that elevated pressures may inversely correlate with mental function, and that surgery can successfully reduce intracranial pressure.[40–42] While is it certainly more important to focus on the prevention of developmental delays than it is to just treat an intracranial pressure number, developmental levels are much harder to measure. Studies examining the relationship between development and surgical timing reveal conflicting conclusions. Some suggest that earlier surgery (under 1 year of age) is associated with higher IQ or other developmental

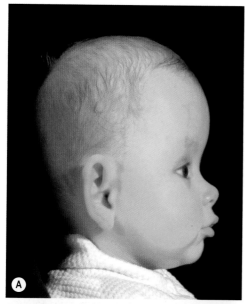

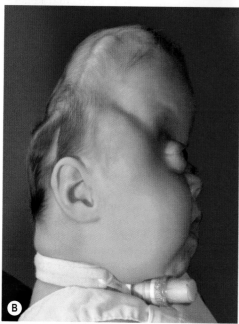

Fig. 33.2 The *syndromic craniosynostosis spectrum* can vary from isolated bicoronal synostosis as seen in Muenke craniosynostosis **(A)** to the pan-synostoses that may be seen in association with Pfeiffer syndrome **(B)**.

scores.[62–64] However, other studies suggest no such correlation between timing and development.[65–67] Further confusing this issue is that all these contradictory studies are retrospective and likely impacted by unintended biases. Given the absence of well-designed studies, surgeons must currently use their best judgment in determining how long it is safe to delay surgical enlargement of the skull. The number of fused sutures, the presence of widely patent decompressing sutures, and the degree of the presenting skull deformity are all factors that may influence the timing for skull decompressions. When concerns for intracranial pressure elevations are low, it is most likely that the older the child is at the time of surgery, the better the long-term morphologic result.

Treatment/surgical technique

Of all the congenital craniofacial anomalies, the syndromic craniosynostoses can present some of the greatest treatment challenges. The aforementioned goals of treatment (normalization of function and appearance) need to be accomplished as safely and with as few operations as possible. The management of the syndromic craniosynostoses requires a team of dedicated specialists and is ideally reserved to those centers that have both a focused interest in these complex problems and sufficient expertise to provide safe and efficient care. Underscoring the challenges of treating the more severe syndromic craniosynostoses are the significant mortality rates that have been described within this subpopulation (reportedly, as high as 66 to 85%).[68,69] The timing for skull surgery, and the selection of the ideal operative procedure, are best based on the phenotypic severity. For those children on the milder end of the syndromic craniosynostosis spectrum (mild brachycephaly or a decompressed skull with a split metopic or sagittal suture), the author will delay surgery until the open bony defects have closed or the dura begins to become tense. As the degree of skull deformity progresses along this severity continuum, progressive turricephaly will be noted. If allowed to progress beyond a moderate stage, the increased skull height can be exceedingly difficult to later correct; therefore, significant turricephaly can be considered a relative indication for earlier surgical intervention. In the author's practice, the first surgical procedure to address impaired skull growth for any child falling along the mild to moderate end of the syndromic craniosynostosis spectrum typically involves enlargement of the anterior fossa. An increase in intracranial volume is accomplished by bringing the supraorbital bandeau as far forward as possible, while simultaneously reducing the associated turricephaly. Surgery performed in children under 9 months of age, who present with more severe growth restrictions, is made more challenging because of the inherent weakness of the thinner skull bone. Further complicating the need to achieve a sustainable correction in younger infants are the observations that any degree of accomplished enlargement is rapidly filled by the expanding brain and the early recurrence of brachycephaly. For these reasons, and because of the potential to achieve a greater degree of expansion when moving larger surface areas of skull bone, some surgeons have advocated for initial posterior decompressions, instead of anterior advancements, and more recently performing these advancements utilizing distraction techniques.[70-72] Although skull distraction procedures have the potential to provide a greater degree of expansion than with remodeling, the requirement for two operative procedures (one to place the device and the other to remove it) and the likelihood for higher complication rates (from mechanical problems) need to be taken into consideration. In addition, because of the relative softness of bone in infancy, the distraction devices may produce undesirable skull deformations adjacent to the device–bone interfaces. One comparative study has shown that distraction did not appear to provide any advantages with respect to either accomplished skull enlargement or the ability to eliminate the need for later subsequent enlargement procedures, so further comparative studies will be needed to better define the roll for distraction.[73]

While there are a number of important factors that need to be assessed in determining if the initial skull expansion should occur anteriorly or posteriorly, one important consideration is the presence or absence of an acquired Chiari deformation. This condition has been reported to affect almost 30% of children with Apert syndrome, 70% of children with Crouzon syndrome, and up to 100% of the children with the more severe Pfeiffer presentations.[27,34,44,55] When identified, a low posterior fossa enlargement with decompression of the foramen magnum might be indicated.[74] It would seem that when these decompressions are performed under a year of age, it might be more likely that these releases will offer only transient benefits because of the potential for the subsequent bony regrowth. Therefore, some believe that posterior skull enlargements should be held in abeyance when possible, pending the development of a symptomatic Chiari deformation. Another consideration in determining whether or not to perform an anterior or posterior decompression is a child's long-term aesthetic appearance. It is well recognized that following any remodeling procedure occurring during growth, removed bone flaps can develop subsequent irregularities over time. One long-term strategy preferred by the author is to preserve a section of posterior parietal bone so that this unaltered smoother section of bone can be exchanged for the irregular frontal bone at skeletal maturity, bringing the benefit of a lifelong aesthetically pleasing forehead. If the posterior skull is surgically altered during infancy, especially when distraction is used, this strategy for aesthetic reconstruction is lost. For this reason, the author prefers to initially treat most children with syndromic craniosynostosis with an anterior procedure, ideally delayed until sometime after a year of age, in order to take advantage of the structurally stiffer bone that will allow for a larger and more stable advancement. Although some surgeons have described the use of molding helmets in treating the syndromic craniosynostoses, the author believes that there is no role for the use of these molding helmets because of their mechanism of action (constricting growth in some areas to direct brain growth to alter the skull shape in other areas) seems counterintuitive in treating a condition that may be associated with raised intracranial pressure.

Multiple techniques have been described to enlarge the frontal fossa in children with syndromic craniosynostosis; most utilize some form of a supraorbital bandeau of varying lengths. Once cut, the bandeau can be advanced into the desired location, and the frontal bone is reattached. The exact positioning of the bandeau is critical, for as the bandeau goes, so goes the rest of the reconstruction. Some surgeons prefer to use a horizontally short bandeau, which extends laterally only as far as the lateral orbital rim (Fig. 33.3).[7,62,75] This particular bandeau design lacks any inherent stability; therefore, very rigid osseous fixation is required in order to stabilize the advancement. Use of a longer horizontal bandeau design, with a tenon-type tongue-in-groove joint that extends posteriorly across the temporal bone, can result in greater inherent stability (Fig. 33.4).[76-78] However, a careful analysis of the deformity resulting from coronal synostosis will reveal that in addition to supraorbital recession, there is also supraorbital elevation. Therefore, the ideal vector for bandeau advancement may not be the simple forward horizontal movement that is often suggested.[79] Instead, the supraorbits need to be repositioned in both a forward and an inferior direction. There

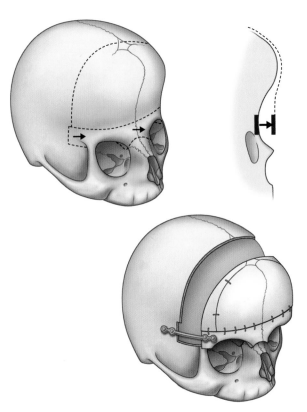

Fig. 33.3 Enlargement of the anterior fossa may be performed utilizing a horizontally short bandeau. This technique requires use of a plating system in order to provide lateral stability. However, significant advancements with this osteotomy design may result in an increase in temporal hollowing.

are numerous potential variations on bandeau designs that can be employed to three-dimensionally overcorrect the observed displacement.[80] For example, for simple isolated bilateral coronal craniosynostosis, a stair-step osteotomy can be used to advance and stabilize the bandeau (Fig. 33.5). However, when there has been compensatory overgrowth of the frontal/temporal region, custom osteotomies can be used to narrow the bandeau while simultaneously advancing and lowering the supraorbits (Fig. 33.6). The frontal bone can also be removed without designing a true bandeau (and also without cutting into the frontal sinuses, avoiding contamination of the surgical field), and then repositioned, or replaced with another bone flap, in both a more forward and inferior position via temporal insets (Fig. 33.7).

When faced with a more deformed skull shape resulting from pan-craniosynostosis, consideration should be given to performing a mid vault decompression at an earlier age (preferably after 6 months of age). This approach spares the aesthetically important forehead for later subsequent advancement, at a time when the bone is thicker and more amenable to creation of a stable construct. The low posterior skull is also left intact, in order to prevent scarring, should a later Chiari decompression be required. The mid vault decompression procedure requires removal and replacement of the parietal bones, with a special focus on those areas of abnormal compression (Fig. 33.8). This procedure can be demanding as keels of bone are often encountered that may extend deeply into the sulci of the brain (Fig. 33.9). It also is important to recognize that as a result of the associated skull base compression,

Finally, for all anterior cranial vault advancements performed in early childhood, especially for children with significant preoperative orbital proptosis, consideration should be made for the placement of absorbable suture temporary tarsorrhaphies to prevent devastating postoperative chemosis that may lead to corneal injury and blindness.[34]

The second important area of focus in treating children with syndromic craniosynostosis is the midface. Significant airway compromise can result from the associated midfacial hypoplasia; therefore, affected patients need to be followed both clinically and with serial polysomnography. The determination for the ideal time to surgically advance the midface is predicated on the development of one of two indicators. The first is obstructive sleep apnea that is not amenable to any less invasive correction (i.e. medication, adenotonsillectomies, and use of a continuous positive airway pressure masks at night). Although there are published reports of midfacial advancement in infancy, these early interventions at best can be expected to provide only transient benefits given the subsequent impairments in growth, and therefore cannot be recommended by the author.[35,36,82] Multiple studies have

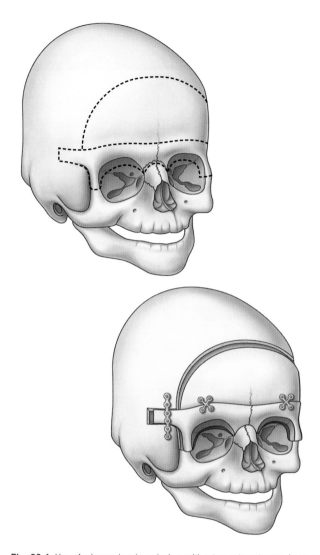

Fig. 33.4 Use of a longer bandeau design, with a tenon-type tongue-in-groove joint, provides inherent stability and may offer a smoother transition into the temporal region. A potential problem with this particular osteotomy design is that it does not inferiorly reposition the supraorbit, which is always necessary with coronal synostosis.

venous hypertension may ensue producing enlarged transosseous veins, typically most prominent in the low central occipital region (Fig. 33.10). These dilated veins should ideally be preserved, as ligation has been cited as the cause of a subsequent postoperative mortality.[81] One caveat to the admonition to avoid early posterior decompressions is for infants noted to have severe Chiari deformations in the presence of ventriculoperitoneal shunts. This particular combination may be one indication for early decompression of the foramen magnum. This is because shunt failures in children with severe Chiari deformations can be devastating, causing brainstem strokes, even death. The performance of any procedure at this early stage of growth means that a subsequent cranial vault enlargement will almost certainly be needed before the child has reached 18 months of age. Frequent clinical evaluations for potential elevations in intracranial pressure, as well as monitoring for the development of an acquired Chiari malformation, need to be performed on a routine basis.

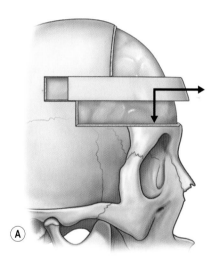

(A)

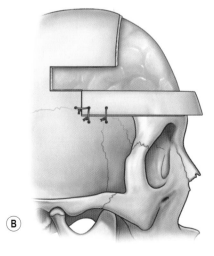

(B)

Fig. 33.5 A stair-step osteotomy can be used to advance and stabilize the bandeau. This design permits both a forward advancement and a simultaneous inferior repositioning of the bandeau.

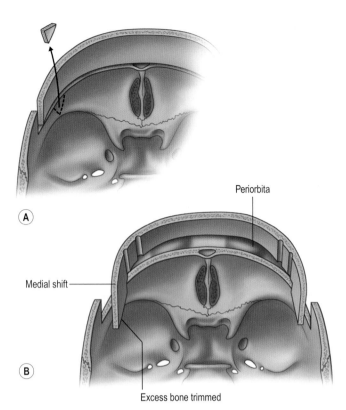

Fig. 33.6 When there is an anomalous increase in frontotemporal width, skull base osteotomies can be performed, which are designed to narrow the bandeau while simultaneously advancing and lowering the supraorbits.

shown that midfacial growth is arrested following frontofacial procedures, and it has also been reported that obstructive apnea may recur following midfacial advancements.[37,83–86] Therefore, for younger children presenting with obstructive sleep apnea refractory to more conservative measures, the author favors placement of a temporary tracheostomy until age 6 or later, at which time a midfacial advancement can be safely and effectively performed. The second indication for a midfacial advancement is based on the child's psychosocial development and issues with self-perception. Currently, the author prefers to delay midfacial advancement whenever possible to sometime around age 8 or 9. At this time, it has been shown to correlate with the ability to avoid the need for a subsequent secondary advancement.[37]

While numerous different osteotomy patterns have been described for advancing the hypoplastic midface, it is possible to subdivide all of these into one of two groups: those requiring intracranial exposure and those that do not. Among those procedures involving a breach of the intracranial space, the most commonly used frontofacial advancement is the "monobloc", which was first described by Ortiz-Monasterio *et al.* (Fig. 33.11).[87] This procedure has the advantage of simultaneously advancing both the midface, and the anterior cranial fossa, theoretically saving the child an operative procedure. Another variation of the frontofacial advancement is the facial bipartition (Fig. 33.12).[88–91] Although initially described for the treatment of hypertelorism, the bipartition has been utilized for advancing the midface while simultaneously reducing intraorbital distance and sagittally bending the midface. The second type of midfacial advancement is the subcranial

approach, which utilizes the Le Fort III osteotomy (Fig. 33.13). In skeletally mature patients, the Le Fort III can be combined with a Le Fort I level osteotomy, which permits simultaneous forward advancement of the midface, with vertical lengthening of the lower maxilla, and the normalization of occlusal relationships (Fig. 33.14). While there is no unanimity among surgeons as to which is the best technique for advancement, currently most surgeons appear to prefer the subcranial Le Fort III approach for a number of reasons: the indications for enlarging the anterior cranial fossa and advancing the midface rarely correspond temporally, the midface usually requires a differential advancement (typically, 2 to 3 times further forward than needed for the forehead), and because the reported complication rates for frontofacial advancements are higher than subcranial advances, likely related to the created connection between the sinuses and the intracranial space.[92]

One of the earliest challenges facing surgeons performing midfacial advancements in children was the inability to obtain, and then maintain, a reasonable advancement. This difficulty led a number of surgeons to explore the use of distraction osteogenesis. Currently, two general types of

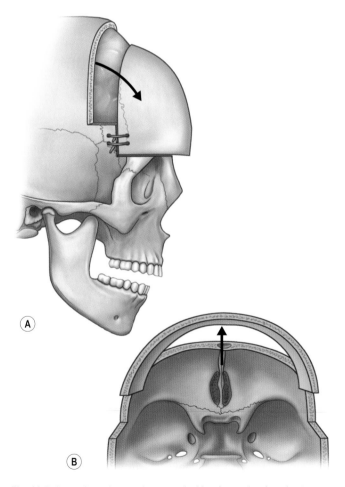

Fig. 33.7 As an alternative to using a standard bandeau, a low frontal osteotomy can be performed to remove almost the entire frontal bone. This bone segment is then repositioned (or rotated 180°) and inset in a more anterior and inferior position. This particular design permits preservation of frontal sinus (avoiding potential contamination) and is particularly useful when the lower bandeau is of poor quality.

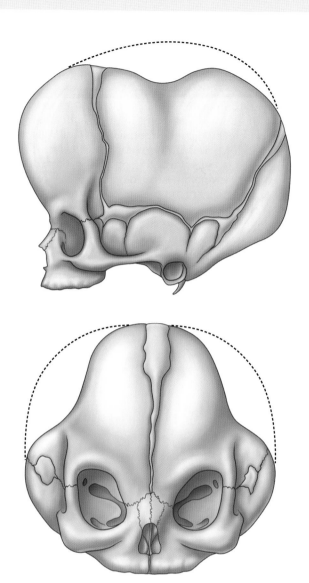

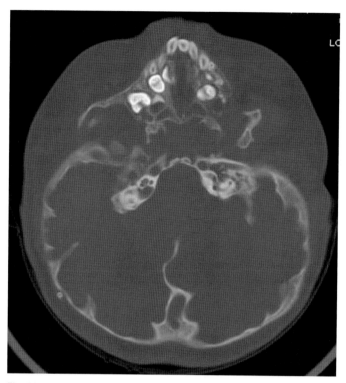

Fig. 33.9 Posterior keels of bone, which extend deep into dural invaginations, can be expected in patients with pan-synostoses, particularly Pfeiffer syndrome.

Fig. 33.8 A mid vault cranioplasty can effectively decompress infants affected with pan-synostosis. This procedure entails careful removal and replacement of the abnormally indented parietal bones.

distraction techniques are being utilized: laterally based semi-buried distraction devices and centrally based external halo devices (Figs. 33.15 & 33.16).[35,93–98] Of these two techniques the centrally based halo distraction offers the advantages of providing a better correction of the central dish-face deformity, while permitting manipulation of the distraction vector after the device has been placed.[96] The halo distraction Le Fort III has also been shown to have lower published complication rates (including being used to salvage semi-buried device failures).[96,99] The ideal distraction vector is best determined by considering final desired position of the malar eminences, as well as the need for dorsal nasal lengthening. When the midface is vertically shortened in addition to being recessed, the distraction vector should not be designed to normalize occlusal relationships. The correction of the vertical maxillary hypoplasia needs to be delayed until the eruption of secondary dentition, at which time either an isolated Le Fort I or a Le Fort III with a Le Fort I can be performed in order to accomplish the required vertical facial lengthening.[96]

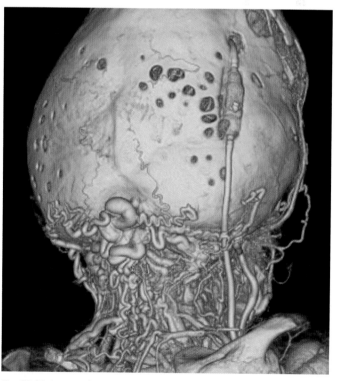

Fig. 33.10 Low, posteriorly draining enlarged transcranial veins are commonly seen with the more severe phenotypic presentations of Apert and Pfeiffer syndrome. Ideally, these vessels should be preserved in order to avoid potentially life-threatening brain edema.

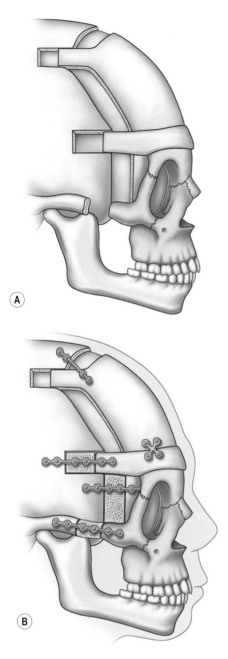

to minimize blood loss, and resultant volume shifts, can substantially contribute to a smoother postoperative recovery. With increased surgical experience, operative times can be reduced along with complications. Moreover, techniques such as preoperative erythropoietin administration, intraoperative blood recycling, tranexamic acid infusions, the judicious use of bone wax, and meticulous electrocautery may all help to minimize the need for perioperative blood transfusions.[103–105] Experienced surgeons will pace the operative procedure in such a way that permits anesthesiologists to ensure the maintenance of adequate blood volumes. Postoperatively, "third space" volume shifts occur secondary to changes in capillary permeability leading to the accumulation of fluid in the enlarged intracranial epidural "dead space" and the subgaleal space, as well as the rest of the body. These volume shifts may be exacerbated by the use of postoperative subgaleal drains (which the author prefers not to use). Hemoglobin levels will generally fall over the first few postoperative days, prior to reaching equilibrium a number of days later. As the estimated blood loss approaches a majority of the patient's

Fig. 33.11 The monobloc frontofacial advancement simultaneously enlarges the anterior cranial fossa and advances the midface. However, this procedure does result in a connection between the sinuses and the intracranial cavity, necessitating placement of some biologic barrier (i.e., pericranial flap) to separate these two spaces, or use of distraction techniques.

Postoperative care

Both cranial vault remodeling and midfacial advancement procedures in children with syndromic craniosynostosis can be accompanied by moderate to massive amounts of intraoperative blood loss, which may be further challenged by impaired airways.[100–102] As a result, the postoperative care of patients with these conditions requires comprehensive pediatric anesthetic and intensive care management. The ability

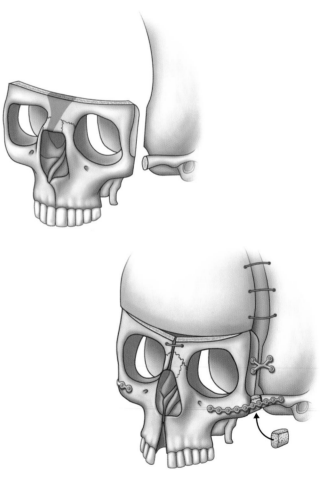

Fig. 33.12 The facial bipartition splits the midface through a combined intracranial and extracranial exposure. This permits simultaneous midfacial advancement, reduction in the intraorbital distance, and sagittal bending of the face. This procedure also results in a connection between the sinuses and the intracranial cavity, necessitating placement of some biologic barrier (i.e., pericranial flap) to isolate these two spaces.

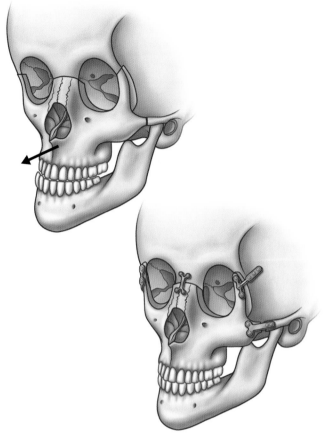

Fig. 33.13 The traditional Le Fort III osteotomy is a subcranial procedure that advances the midface as a single segment. Lateral orbital Z-plasties help to stabilize the advancement.

calculated total blood volume, it is important to monitor for potential dilutional coagulopathies. Disturbances in acid–base balance can also be expected from intraoperative hypoperfusion-associated anaerobic metabolism (resulting in lactic acid production), which can be exacerbated by hypoventilation immediately following extubation (especially with subsequent narcotic administration). If this acidosis is treated with sodium bicarbonate, a secondary hypokalemia (from the intracellular transport of potassium) may result.[106] Some argue that it is better to let this early acidosis self-correct without intervention, as perioperative hypoventilation abates and normal ventilation ensues, permitting the more rapid loss of carbon dioxide. It is also important to closely follow the patient's overall mental status, in order to monitor for the potential development of an intracranial hematoma or for the syndrome of inappropriate antidiuretic hormone (which, when identified, is best initially treated with a restriction in free water intake).[107,108] For those children undergoing midfacial advancements, airway monitoring is critically important. Protocols for managing airway compromise need to be established and available for ready implementation, when indicated.

Outcomes, prognosis, complications

Measuring treatment outcomes in syndromic craniosynostosis is a challenging endeavor, considering that the goals of surgery (the prevention of developmental delays and the normalization of appearance) are outcomes that are difficult to quantify. A number of centers have examined the need for secondary procedures following an initial craniosynostosis correction, and reoperative rates between 2–13% have been reported.[58,77,109,110] One study, specifically examining reoperative rates in the syndromic synostoses, has cited a reoperative rate of 37%, with an average 6-year follow-up.[111] Currently, there are no published outcome studies examining

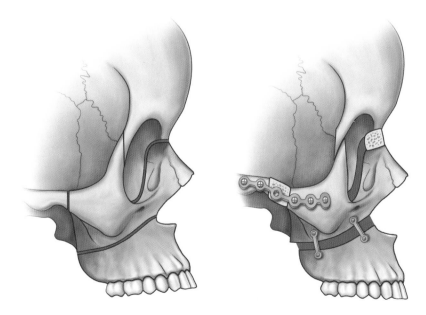

Fig. 33.14 The Le Fort III with a Le Fort I is a two-piece mid facial advancement that permits vertical facial lengthening and idealization of the dental occlusion, while independently repositioning the malar eminences.

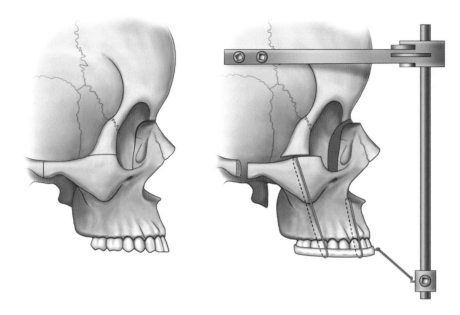

Fig. 33.15 The halo distraction Le Fort III utilizes low lateral orbital straight-line osteotomies and offers the potential for significantly greater maxillary advancements. This technique permits vector changes postoperatively, during the advancement phase.[37,83,85]

reoperative rates at skeletal maturity, and general experience suggests that most children require multiple procedures. A number of factors might be expected to influence the need for a secondary (or tertiary) cranial vault remodeling: the age of the initial operation (with earlier interventions increasing this risk), the degree of growth inhibition (partially syndrome related), the success of the procedure, and the criteria used to determine the need for a secondary procedure. There are also no long-term outcome assessments measuring cognitive function. However, with respect to Apert syndrome, one study has suggested a correlation between early surgery and higher IQ scores while another larger study found no such correlation.[27,112]

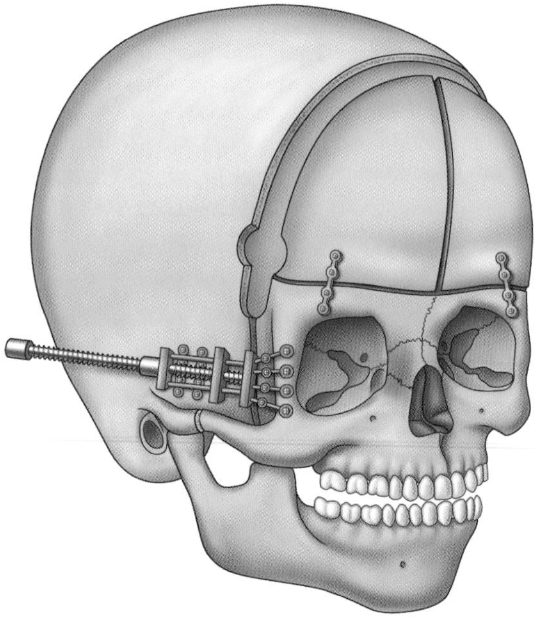

Outcomes have been evaluated following Le Fort III halo distraction, and these studies have documented postoperative skeletal stability without relapse; although following distraction, no further forward growth of the maxilla has been noted.[37,83,85] While some studies have measured improvements in airway diameter following Le Fort III distraction, only one has assessed changes in postoperative ventilation (measured by pre- and postoperative polysomnography), and this study confirmed improvements in airway gas exchange.[83,113,114] While few studies have tried to assess treatment outcomes, complication rates have been more extensively examined. Infection rates following cranial vault remodeling procedures have been reported between 2.5% and 6.5%, with secondary procedures and longer operative times cited as potential risk factors.[115–117] A number of retrospective studies have examined mortality rates following intracranial procedures. These reports suggest an experience-related decline in mortality rates following intracranial expansions, with incidences falling from 2.2% to currently around 0.1%.[118–123]

Secondary procedures

Aside from the two major procedures typically required for treatment of the syndromic craniosynostoses (cranial vault remodeling and midfacial advancement), a number of adjunctive procedures may be necessary. While the use of intracranial hypertelorism corrections in patients with syndromic craniosynostosis has been described, the author has found these types of corrections generally unnecessary.[124,125] Most children with syndromic craniosynostosis will develop only moderate increases in intraorbital distance, falling short of satisfying the usual requirements for directed orbital translation.[126] When a vector for midfacial advancement is selected that appropriately lengthens and raises the nasal dorsum, these changes significantly decrease the perception of telorbitism, eliminating the need to consider additional orbital movements.

Fig. 33.16 Semi-buried lateral facial distraction devices can be used to advance either a subcranial Le Fort III osteotomy or a monobloc (pictured). These devices do not permit vector changes during distraction and may exacerbate a central "dish-face" deformity.

All children affected with Apert syndrome, and rarely some with Pfeiffer syndrome, require treatment for their associated syndactylies, and numerous techniques for digital separation have been reported.[127,128] The author prefers a two-staged approach to separate all ten fingers and toes; however, this comprehensive treatment paradigm does require a dedicated team approach.[129] As the skeletal growth approaches completion, digital osteotomies may be required to correct developing clinodactyly and improve function.

With the completion of facial growth, an isolated Le Fort I may be necessary to maximize occlusal relationships, as well as to vertically lengthen the midface. Following this orthognathic procedure, subsequent malar augmentation can be achieved with the placement of allogenic implants, mitigating the need for a repeat Le Fort III.

Finally, most children with syndromic craniosynostosis will benefit from a reconstructive rhinoplasty at skeletal maturity in order to smooth the nasal dorsum and to correct the "beak deformity" that results from a congenital displacement of the lower lateral cartilages. In addition to rotating the alar cartilages into a more normal relationship, cephalic rotation of the tip and dorsal augmentation may benefit nasal airflow.

⊕ Access the complete reference list online at **http://www.expertconsult.com**

2. Goodrich JT, Tutino M. An annotated history of craniofacial surgery and intentional cranial deformation. *Neurosurg Clin N Am.* 2001;12:45–68, viii.

7. Marchac D. Radical forehead remodeling for craniostenosis. *Plast Reconstr Surg.* 1978;61:823–835. *This classic article marks the progression from treating craniosynostosis with strip craniectomies to a true remodeling procedure. It was also one of the earliest to depict a frontal bandeau.*

11. Gillies H, Harrison SH. Operative correction by osteotomy of recessed malar maxillary compound in a case of oxycephaly. *Br J Plast Surg.* 1950;3:123–127. *This is the first description of a Le Fort III-type osteotomy for advancing the midface. Although his osteotomy lines did not actually follow the "true" Le Fort III pattern, this report is the first to attempt to advance the "whole face and palate".*

13. Tessier P. The definitive plastic surgical treatment of the severe facial deformities of craniofacial dysostosis. Crouzon's and Apert's diseases. *Plast Reconstr Surg.* 1971;48:419–442. *It is likely that patients presenting with Apert and Crouzon syndrome were the real catalyst that spurred Tessier to develop techniques upon which the foundations of craniofacial surgery were built. This article describes some of Tessier's early forays into treating these rare anomalies.*

30. Moloney DM, Slaney SF, Oldridge M, et al. Exclusive paternal origin of new mutations in Apert syndrome. *Nat Genet.*

1996;13:48–53. *This article is one of the first to describe the comprehensive care of patients with Pfeiffer syndrome and details a more updated approach to treating the syndromic craniosynostosis.*

34. Fearon JA, Rhodes J. Pfeiffer syndrome: a treatment evaluation. *Plast Reconstr Surg.* 2009;123:1560–1569.

66. Mathijssen I, Arnaud E, Lajeunie E, et al. Postoperative cognitive outcome for synostotic frontal plagiocephaly. *J Neurosurg.* 2006;105:16–20. *This paper is the earliest description of a combined "orbitofacial advancement", which was later to become known as the monobloc advancement.*

79. Jackson IA, Munro IR, Salyer KE, Whitaker LA. *Atlas of Craniomaxillofacial Surgery.* St. Louis: C.V. Mosby Company; 1982.

80. Fearon JA. Beyond the bandeau: 4 variations on fronto-orbital advancements. *J Craniofac Surg.* 2008;19:1180–1182.

93. Bradley JP, Gabbay JS, Taub PJ, et al. Monobloc advancement by distraction osteogenesis decreases morbidity and relapse. *Plast Reconstr Surg.* 2006;118:1585–1597.

105. Dadure C, Sauter M, Bringuier S, et al. Intraoperative tranexamic acid reduces blood transfusion in children undergoing craniosynostosis surgery: a randomized double-blind study. *Anesthesiology.* 2011;114:856–861.

34

Craniofacial microsomia

Youssef Tahiri, Craig Birgfeld, and Scott P. Bartlett

SYNOPSIS

- Patients with craniofacial microsomia (CFM) require the care of a skilled multidisciplinary clinical team.
- Phenotypic features of CFM are highly variable. While the three structures most commonly affected include the auricle, mandible, and maxilla, abnormal development can occur in any of the derivatives of the first or second branchial arches.
- During the evaluation of CFM, it is essential to assess for retroglossal airspace narrowing and obstructive sleep apnea via endoscopy and sleep studies, particularly in bilateral cases.
- Distraction osteogenesis (DO) of the mandible should be considered in neonates and infants with CFM who exhibit severe respiratory compromise and who may otherwise require a tracheostomy.
- Vectors of mandible distraction (vertical, oblique, or horizontal) should be planned according to treatment goals.
- In cases of severe mandibular hypoplasia, staged procedures with grafting (non-vascularized or vascularized bone) should be performed, often followed by DO.
- If two-jaw surgery is to be performed for CFM, a two-splint (intermediate splint) technique is used and the technique is usually deferred until skeletal maturity has been achieved.
- Orthodontic monitoring is important throughout the years of growth and development. Interventions are especially important during and after the distraction process to prevent undesired movements (i.e., anterior open bite, lateral shift) and in the period surrounding two-jaw surgery.

Introduction

Craniofacial microsomia (CFM) involves a spectrum of congenital malformations of craniofacial structures that arise from or are intimately related to the first and second branchial arches: the mandible, maxilla, external and internal ear, orbit, temporal bone, facial soft tissue and muscles, and the facial nerve[1] (Fig. 34.1). These malformations result in differences in facial aesthetic appearance and various functional difficulties with feeding, hearing, airway anatomy, facial expression, speech, and globe protection. Given the broad spectrum of severity of presentation, the care of patients with CFM should be approached in a multidisciplinary craniofacial team setting that includes plastic surgeons, craniofacial surgeons, microsurgeons, otolaryngologists, ophthalmologists, pediatricians, feeding specialists, psychologists, speech therapists, and nursing.

Basic science/disease process

Incidence

Craniofacial microsomia represents one of the most common congenital malformations of the head and neck, second only to cleft lip and palate.[2,3] CFM has an incidence estimated and raging from 1:642 to 1:26000.[4–8] The majority of CFM cases occur in a sporadic fashion; however, the presence of CFM in successive generations may suggest the presence of various modes of genetic inheritance.

CFM may be unilateral or bilateral. Although bilateral hypoplasia has been noted in 5–30% of cases, when present, it is generally asymmetric.[9,10] Patients diagnosed with unilateral involvement often have subtle abnormalities of the ear, mandible, or orbit on the contralateral side. The higher ratio of bilateral involvement in more recent reviews may be due to an increased appreciation/documentation of subtle contralateral soft-tissue anomalies, such as macrostomia, cheek hypoplasia, preauricular skin tags, etc.

Although many studies have demonstrated a right-sided and male predominance, others have found equivalent right/left and gender distributions. For instance, Grabb reported a male predominance, with a male-to-female ratio of 63:39,[5] and Rollnick[11] reported a similar ratio of 191:103. The clinical series of Horgan et al.[12] reported an equal sex ratio of 59 males to 62 females.

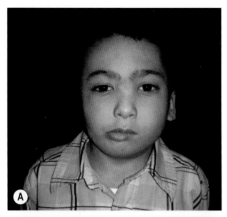

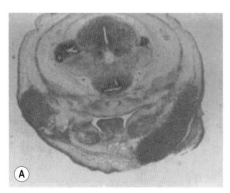

Fig. 34.1 A 5-year-old boy with right craniofacial microsomia. **(A)** AP view highlighting the facial asymmetry, soft-tissue deficiency on the right side, orbital dystopia, mandibular asymmetry, and right macrostomia. **(B)** Right lateral view demonstrating right anotia/microtia and again soft-tissue deficiency.

Embryology of the structures involved

The first branchial arch (mandibular arch) gives rise to the maxilla, mandible, zygoma, trigeminal nerve, muscles of mastication, connective tissue of the face, and a minority of the external ear (tragus, root of helix, superior portion of helix). The second branchial arch (hyoid arch) gives rise to the stapes, styloid process, portions of hyoid bone, facial nerve, facial musculature, and the majority of the external ear (inferior portion helix, antihelix, antitragus and lobule).[13–16]

During the first trimester all branchial arches have their own artery arising from the aortic arch.[16,17] The first aortic branch supplies the first branchial arch and the second supplies the second branchial arch. In the third week of gestation, the internal and external carotid arteries develop from the third branchial arch, while the first and second aortic arch become less necessary. The remnant of the second aortic arch is the stapedial artery, which forms the anastomosis between the internal and external carotid arteries in the fourth week of gestation. During this week the stapedial is the main blood supply for the first and second branchial arches. In the fifth week the stapedial artery atrophies and disappears and around day 40 of gestation the external carotid artery supplies the blood for the first and second branchial arches.[15–17]

Etiology

The etiology of CFM remains unclear but is probably heterogeneous among individuals, with variable contributions from extrinsic and intrinsic factors. It has been thought primarily to be associated with vascular perturbation, teratogen exposure, neural crestopathy, or a combination of the three.

The first hypothesis raised involves a vascular disruption in the development of the first and second branchial arches during the first 6 weeks of gestation. Poswillo[18–20] reproduced in mice some of the phenotypic anomalies seen in CFM phenotype by administering teratogens (triazine) that caused a hematoma of the stapedial artery and resulted in local and regional necrosis (Fig. 34.2). The wide spectrum of resulting facial anomalies was felt to be caused by the vascular injury, the resulting tissue necrosis, and its inability to regenerate. Although a "stapedial artery hemorrhage etiology" is attractive because the vessel is a second branchial arch derivative, a causative association between the bleeding and the deformities has not been made. The hemorrhages occurred 14 days after administration of the teratogen, and there was no clear temporal relationship between the hemorrhage appearance and the associated phenotypic deformity. When mice are exposed to triazine later in development (10 days of gestation), all animals developed deformities; however, only a third showed evidence of a hematoma. The authors concluded that triazine has a direct teratogenic effect and the stapedial

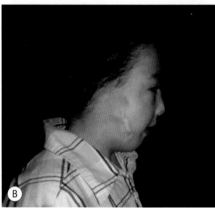

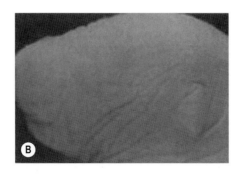

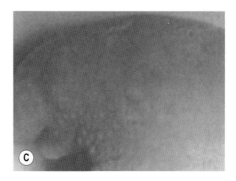

Fig. 34.2 Mouse phenocopy of craniofacial microsomia induced by the administration of triazine. **(A)** Histologic section of the head showing bilateral hematomas. The smaller one is in the ear region (right), and the large one encompasses the ramus and angle of the mandible (left). **(B)** Normal ear–jaw relationship at full term in the normal animal. **(C)** The diminutive helix and abnormal mandible in the unilateral craniofacial microsomia phenocopy. *(Reproduced from Poswillo D. The pathogenesis of the Treacher Collins syndrome [mandibulofacial dysostosis]. Br J Oral Surg. 1975;13;1.)*

artery findings were simply a side effect. In contrast to those described by Poswillo, these animals demonstrated more evidence of bilateral deformities and inner-ear anomalies. Moreover, rats exposed to etretinate, a retinoic acid derivative, show deformities comparable to the first and second branchial arch syndromes. This finding is consistent with the finding that neural crest cells express large amounts of retinoic acid-binding proteins. Furthermore, when retinoic acid is administered early in development, it interferes with cell migration. When administered later in gestation, however, retinoic acid kills ganglionic placodal cells, resulting in a deformity similar to mandibulofacial dysostosis (Treacher Collins).

On the other hand, intermittent occlusion of the internal carotid system of fetal sheep late in gestation has been shown to result in deformities similar in appearance to CFM. The vascular disruption hypothesis, therefore, cannot be excluded.

In an effort to evaluate associations between the individual deformities associated with CFM in a large cohort of patients, Tuin et al.'s study[21] revealed significant associations between deformities of the orbit, mandible, and soft tissue. Nerve involvement and ear deformity were significantly associated as well as nerve involvement and soft-tissue deficiency. A higher degree of deformity of the individual OMENS components demonstrated that the mandible, orbit, and soft tissue on the ipsilateral side were associated with the presence of macrostomia. Thus, they hypothesized that the embryologic origin of the structures involved in CFM could explain the findings in this study. The degree of deformity of the different structures derived from the first branchial arch are significantly associated. These first arch abnormalities include orbital deformity (since the lower orbital rim is formed by the zygoma and maxilla), mandibular deformity, and macrostomia, resulting from the mal-fusion of the mandibular and maxillary process of the first branchial arch. However, the facial nerve and the majority of the ear (85%) develop from the second branchial arch. Their findings demonstrate that these structures, mainly derived from the second branchial arch, are also significantly associated. Additionally, the degree of facial nerve involvement as well as the severity of the ear deformity are also correlated.[21]

Studies have suggested a fundamental role for genetic transmission in some patients.[22] Autosomal dominant and recessive transmission patterns have been described in families with features of CFM, and a positive family history of 50% has been observed in a large series of cases. This etiologic heterogeneity, along with variability in penetrance and expression, could account for the wide phenotypic spectrum seen in CFM. Recently, studies in mice showed inactivation or the allelic reduction of Edn1, Ednra, Dlx5, Dlx6, Gsc, Pitx1, and Gbx2, all of which result in a proximal defect of the developing mandible or of the middle and external ear, which is also characteristic of CFM. Support of a genetic etiology of CFM has come from both animal and human studies. A transgenic mouse model for CFM with an insertional deletion on mouse chromosome 10 has been described with an autosomal-dominant mode of transmission and 25% penetration. The affected animals display low-set ears, unilateral microtia, and jaw asymmetry, without evidence of middle-ear abnormality.

Various human genetic studies have documented a positive family history in 9.4% of 32 probands, 21% of 57 probands, 26% of 88 probands, and 44% of 82 probands. Kaye et al.[23] performed segregation analysis on 74 families of probands

with CFM and rejected the hypothesis that genetic transmission is not a causative factor. The evidence favored autosomal-dominant inheritance; however, recessive and polygenic models were not distinguishable. Despite the suggestion of autosomal-dominant transmission, they found only a 2–3% overall recurrence rate in first-degree relatives. This figure compares to the 10% recurrence risk in first- and second-degree relatives reported by the same group in an earlier study of 294 individuals with CFM.

Studies on the incidence and expression of craniofacial anomalies in twins have provided insight into the etiology of CFM. Mulliken's group[24] described 10 twin pairs with CFM. Only one of the pairs, who were monozygotic, was concordant for the anomaly. Other twin studies have noted a high level of discordance of CFM among monozygotic twins.

To summarize, the exact etiology of CFM is still a matter of debate. This clearly heterogeneous entity is likely to involve multiple factors, including genetic anomalies with various intrinsic modifiers to extrinsic insults such as teratogens or vascular events.

Terminology

Since its earliest descriptions by Canton[25] and Von Arlt[4] in 1861 and 1881, respectively, a variety of names have been adopted for this anomaly. These include craniofacial microsomia,[26] hemifacial microsomia,[26] first and second branchial arch syndrome,[5,27] otomandibular dysostosis,[28,29] auriculobranchiogenic dysplasia,[30] intrauterine facial necrosis,[31] lateral facial dysplasia,[32] hemignathia and microtia syndrome,[27] necrotic facial dysplasia,[33] oto-mandibular-facial dysmorphogenesis,[34] mandibular laterognathism,[35] oculoauriculovertebral spectrum,[36] and facioauriculovertebral malformation complex.[37] This extensive list attests to the difficulty of satisfactorily labeling the breadth of malformations defining this syndrome. Indeed, as Longacre et al. noted: "The prominent feature of these dysplasias is their variability."[38]

Pathology

Orbit

Variable abnormalities of the ipsilateral zygomatico-orbital region are a common finding. The orbit can be of a smaller size and/or can have an abnormal position. These anomalies can occasionally lead to orbital dystopia (see Fig. 34.1A). Moreover, periocular abnormalities may range from mild inferior displacement of the lateral canthus and/or palpebral fissure to microphthalmia/anophthalmia. In rare instances, colobomas of the iris or upper lid with absence of the eyelashes may also be noted.[39]

Mandibular deformity

The mandible has long been considered the "cornerstone" of craniofacial microsomia and is always involved to a degree.[40,41] Mandibular hypoplasia may range from mild hypoplasia or flattening of the condylar head to complete agenesis of the condyle, ramus, and glenoid fossa (Fig. 34.3). A wide array of temporomandibular joint abnormalities results from the variable mandibular hypoplasia, leading to deformities ranging from mild malpositioning with aberrant cranial base

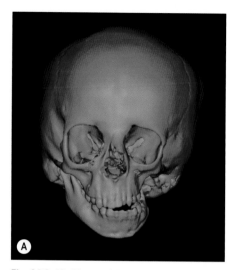 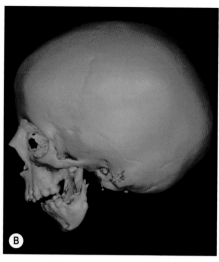 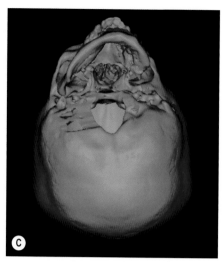

Fig. 34.3 3D CT scan of the head and face of a CFM patient with a severe left mandibular deformity that includes an absent ramus and condyle coronoid as well as a smaller body compared to the contralateral side. **(A)** AP view. **(B)** Left lateral view. **(C)** Worm's eye view.

articulation to complete obliteration. The mandibular body may also be reduced in all dimensions, frequently with an increase in the size of the gonial angle.[42] Steinbacher et al.[43] sought to volumetrically evaluate and characterize the mandible in CFM compared with controls, and to assess for Pruzansky score correlation. As expected, with increasing Pruzansky severity, hemimandibular and proximal segment volumes declined. The hemifacial dentate segment also proved significantly diminished, corresponding to the degree of proximal volume loss.

Maxillary deformity

Historically, it was believed that the mandibular deformity was associated with a maxillary hypoplasia.[44] It was accepted that the maxillary hypoplasia in combination with mandibular deficiency frequently results in dental malocclusion and, depending on the severity of the maxillomandibular deficiency, an upward occlusal cant to the affected side.

A recent study by Wink et al.[45] shed new light on the maxillary deformity in craniofacial microsomia. In evaluating volumetric differences as well as linear measurements between bony structures in the affected side vs. the unaffected side on the same patients, they found little or no relationship between the mandibular and maxillary deformity. Their results demonstrated an absence of any notable midface bone and sinus volume loss in patients. Two-dimensional cephalometric analyses of the maxillary segmentation models also showed no statistically significant differences between the mean values for maxillary width, depth, and height within all severity groups.

While analysis of the measurement ratios (ipsilateral/contralateral) of all volume and linear measurements across severity groups found a statistically significant difference among mandibular volumes, there was no statistically significant difference in the ratio of maxillary bone volume when grouped by degree of mandibular deformity.

Those findings suggest that the maxillary anomaly is not a true volumetric deficiency. The maxillary cant observed is secondary to vertical growth inhibition by the pathologically small mandible.

Those findings were confirmed by Song et al.[46] who demonstrated that the occlusal disharmony is due to an anomaly of the alveolus and teeth, with no differences noted between the affected and unaffected sides with regards to maxillary shape and volume.

Ear

It is not surprising that auricular and/or preauricular malformations are fundamental if not mandatory features of this syndrome since portions of the external/middle ear and mandible share a common embryologic origin.[47] When present as isolated findings, auricular malformations such as microtia or preauricular malformations such as skin tags or sinuses may represent the mildest form of craniofacial microsomia. Auricular malformations seen in CFM are as diverse as those demonstrated by the syndrome's other component features. The ear anomalies associated with CFM can be categorized into external ear malformations (e.g., microtia), middle ear malformations and atresia, and the presence of branchial remnants and sinus tracts.[5,47] Although the presence of branchial remnants in isolation is generally not considered part of the CFM spectrum, the existence of isolated microtia is often considered a component of CFM as the risk factors and affected tissues are similar.

Hypoplasia of the external ear can range from mild effacement of auricular architecture to complete auricular agenesis and external auditory canal atresia. In severe cases, the only observable evidence of external ear development is represented by a primitive auricular remnant and located caudally and ventrally (Fig. 34.4), while in very rare instances, no remnant is observable. Variable hypoplasia of middle ear structures is also a common feature. External and middle ear dysplasia may result in hearing loss, predominantly conductive in nature, in up to 75% of patients.[48] The severity of the external ear deformity may predict the degree of middle ear involvement.

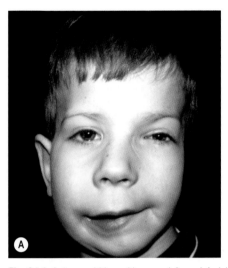
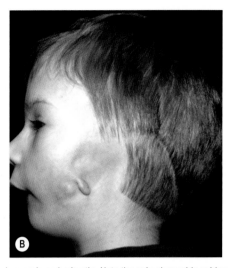
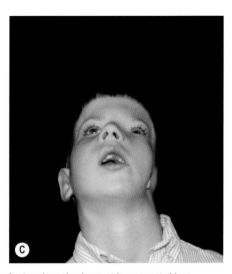

Fig. 34.4 A 4-year-old boy with severe left craniofacial microsomia and microtia. Note the only observable evidence of external ear development is represented by a primitive auricular remnant located caudally and ventrally. **(A)** AP view. **(B)** Left lateral view. **(C)** Worm's eye view.

Nervous system

A wide variety of cerebral anomalies exist in CFM[22] and may include ipsilateral cerebral hypoplasia, hypoplasia of the corpus callosum, hydrocephalus of the communicating type and obstructive type, intracranial lipoma, and hypoplasia and malformation of the brainstem and cerebellum. Other associated abnormalities include cognitive delay, epilepsy, and encephalographic findings suggestive of epilepsy.

Cranial nerve abnormalities are frequent in CFM and can include arhinencephaly of the unilateral and bilateral type, unilateral agenesis and hypoplasia of the optic nerve with secondary changes in the lateral geniculate body and visual cortex, congenital ophthalmoplegia and Duane retraction syndrome, hypoplasia of the trochlear and abducens nuclei and nerves, congenital trigeminal anesthesia, and aplasia of the trigeminal nerve and motor and sensory nucleus.

The most common cranial nerve anomaly is facial paralysis secondary to agenesis of the facial nerve in the temporal bone or hypoplasia of the intracranial portion of the facial nerve and facial nucleus in the brainstem.[49,50] The facial nerve (CN 7) can be affected in craniofacial microsomia to varying degrees. Upper nerve function, lower nerve function, or total nerve function can be compromised. In rare instances, the hypoglossal nerve (CN 12) and trigeminal (CN 5) can also be affected.

Soft tissue

Variable deficiency of facial soft tissues contributes greatly to the phenotypic spectrum of craniofacial microsomia. The deficiencies may involve the skin, subcutaneous fat, and neuromuscular tissues. This deficiency is mostly evident in the malar and masseteric region of the face as well as in the region of the external ear, orbit, and the temporal region (Fig. 34.5). Lack of soft-tissue bulk contributes to a characteristic malar flattening and temporal hollowing that is best appreciated when viewed from a submental perspective.

Moreover, this appearance may be accentuated by hypoplasia involving the muscles of mastication including the temporalis, masseter, and medial and lateral pterygoids, leading also to an impairment of the masticatory muscle function on the affected side.

Macrostomia

Macrostomia, or clefting through the oral commissure (Tessier number 7 cleft), and hypoplasia of the parotid gland may also be present.[51] This may vary from a minor deformity ending medial to the anterior border of the masseter, to a severe cleft through all structures, and terminating in the external auditory canal.

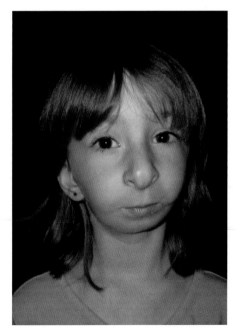

Fig. 34.5 A 7-year-old female with left CFM (bilateral view). Note the facial asymmetry and the significant soft-tissue deficiency on the left side.

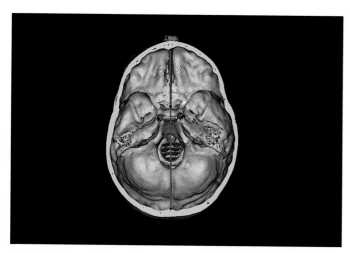

Fig. 34.6 Mean cranial base axis angulation in patients with HFM (blue) and controls (red) differed by less than one degree. This difference was found to be statistically insignificant.

Cranial base

Studies have found notable correlation between cranial base and facial asymmetry, with several authors documenting that cranial base asymmetry contributes to facial asymmetry.[52–61] This association was based on the fact that the anterior and middle cranial fossae of the cranial base articulate with the face and, as such, may affect, or be affected by, alterations in facial morphology.

Paliga and associates[62] used craniometric measurements to characterize the endocranial morphology of the anterior and middle cranial fossae in patients with CFM. The results of their study indicate that there is minimal to no deviation of the anterior cranial base angle, and absent or minor asymmetry of the endocranium in patients with CFM, implying that endocranial asymmetry is not the origin of facial dysmorphology seen in hemifacial microsomia (HFM) (Fig. 34.6).

Tongue dysmorphogenesis

Tongue dysmorphologies in craniofacial microsomia, although usually mild, are frequently overlooked. Tongue dysmorphogenesis, ranging from mild asymmetry to severe hypoplasia, may contribute to the feeding and speech difficulties encountered in this patient population. Chen et al.[63] reported a positive correlation of the tongue, soft tissue, and mandible anomalies, pointing to a common error early in gestation or an interdependence of adjacent growth centers.

Palatal anomalies

Ipsilateral palatal anomalies including weakness or paralysis of the velum have been found in patients with CFM. If significantly affected, velopharyngeal insufficiency can result and surgery (pharyngoplasty) required to obtain normal speech. One study identified 50% of CFM patients having hemipalatal paresis with 14% having overt velopharyngeal insufficiency.[64]

Extracraniofacial anomalies

A vast range of associated extracraniofacial anomalies has been reported in the craniofacial microsomia literature, including skeletal, cardiac, renal, gastrointestinal, and pulmonary malformations.[11,12] For instance, the constellation of hemifacial hypoplasia, epibulbar lipodermoids, and vertebral anomalies, including fused and/or hemivertebrae, defines one of the subsets of CFM named Goldenhar syndrome[7] (Fig. 34.7). Once considered a variant of hemifacial microsomia, Goldenhar syndrome is now widely considered to be part of the CFM continuum.[65–68]

Natural history of the disease

Whether the deformity found in CFM is progressive or static remains unclear.[69–76] Longitudinal clinical studies performed by Kaban et al.[69] suggest that restricted growth of the mandible has a role in the progressive distortion of both the ipsilateral and contralateral craniofacial skeleton. Conversely, both Polley et al.[70] and Kusnoto et al.[71] concluded that growth of the affected side of the mandible parallels growth of the unaffected side, including both ramal height and body length.

Ongkosuwito et al.[72] completed a comprehensive longitudinal study evaluating growth in CFM patients. Their group compared linear ramal height growth curves for children with unilateral CFM (non-operated mandible) to the Dutch normal population. They compared orthopantomograms (OPTs) from 84 patients with unilateral CFM with a control set of 2260 OPTs from 329 healthy individuals, determining mandibular ramal distances. They demonstrated a clear ramal height difference between CFM patients (both affected and unaffected sides) and the control group; however, the growth increase over time was the same in both groups. This significant ramal height difference also occurred within CFM patients between affected and unaffected ramal heights. Furthermore, their results demonstrated a similar constant increase over time, but a clear difference in ramal height between the "mild" and "severe" HFM groups.

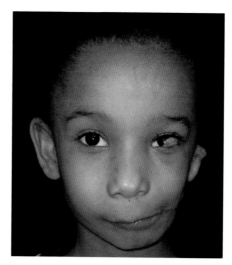

Fig. 34.7 A 4-year-old female with left craniofacial microsomia (specifically Goldenhar syndrome) with left epibulbar dermoid.

Diagnosis/patient presentation

Differential diagnosis

The differential diagnosis of facial asymmetry includes Romberg syndrome, facial lipodystrophy, temporomandibular joint ankylosis, postradiation deformity, condylar hyperplasia, and hemifacial hypertrophy. Treacher Collins syndrome or severe orbitofacial clefts can also be confused with bilateral CFM; however, the deformed ramal and condylar findings so characteristic of CFM are not present.[77]

Postnatal trauma or an infection affecting the condyle and condylar cartilage can result in decreased mandibular growth, leading to a secondary effect on the growth of the surrounding ipsilateral craniofacial skeleton. However, unlike postnatal deformities, CFM is characterized by soft-tissue deficiency, external ear malformations on the affected side as well as more widespread involvement of the skeleton, including the temporal bone, mastoid, and skull base. Moreover, the anomalies seen in patients with CFM are always present at birth. Minimal diagnostic criteria for CFM have been suggested by Cousley and Calvert[78] as "(1) ipsilateral mandibular and ear defects or (2) asymmetric mandibular or ear defects in association with either (a) two or more indirectly associated anomalies or (b) a positive family history of CFM. Indirectly associated anomalies were defined as those 'not normally related either in terms of developmental fields or function'".

Classification systems

The development of clinically useful classification systems is a dilemma confronting all fields of medicine. The optimal categorization for any disorder is a system that is easily performed, reproducible between evaluators, and helpful in predicting treatment and prognosis.

In a classic article published in the late 1960s, Pruzansky segregated the mandibular anomalies of craniofacial microsomia into three grades (types I through III) of increasing hypoplasia based largely on the morphology of the ramus and condyle.[34] The assumed normal and unaffected contralateral hemimandible formed the basis of comparison in all types. It should be noted that the Pruzansky classification (as later modified by Kaban and colleagues)[75] is replicated exactly, with a minor modification in nomenclature, in the mandibular portion of the OMENS classification system.

The most comprehensive classification scheme is the OMENS (Orbital Mandible Ear Nerve Soft tissue) classification, later modified to the OMENS+ to include extracranial manifestations (Fig. 34.8). In the words of Cohen[67]: "The OMENS classification of hemifacial microsomia...is a welcome addition to the literature on the subject." This system was developed by Vento et al. in 1991.[41] They evaluated 154 patients with CFM and substratified each of five anatomical manifestations of CFM according to dysmorphic severity on a scale from 0 to 3. The five anatomical manifestations each constitute one letter of the acronym: orbital asymmetry, mandibular hypoplasia, ear deformity, nerve dysfunction, and soft-tissue deficiency. This system quantifies the mandibular malformations using Kaban's modification of the Pruzansky system, and allows for detailed characterization of the orbital, auricular, facial nerve, and soft-tissue deficiencies to assign a severity score. Scoring

was done on the basis of conventional radiographs including posterior/anterior, lateral, submental, and panoramic views, and physical examination and photographs.[40,75] The pictorial representation of the OMENS+ system was described by Gougoutas et al.[79] and consists of illustrations of the spectrum for each malformation. This allows the clinician to rate the severity and assign a classification score by circling the appropriate diagram for each feature and can be easily incorporated into the patient's medical record.

Scoring of the orbital deformity reflects orbital size and position. The latter, when abnormal, is marked with an arrow indicating superior or inferior displacement.

Scoring within the mandible category is done so on the basis of radiographs and uses the system of Pruzansky, later modified by Kaban[75] (Table 34.1, Fig. 34.9):

Type I: All mandibular and temporomandibular joint components are present and normal in shape, but are hypoplastic to a variable degree.

Type IIA: The mandibular ramus, condyle, and temporomandibular joint are present but are hypoplastic and abnormal in shape.

Type IIB: The mandibular ramus is hypoplastic and markedly abnormal in form and location, being medial and anterior. There is no articulation with the temporal bone.

Type III: The mandibular ramus, condyle, and temporomandibular joint are absent, and the lateral pterygoid muscle and temporalis, if present, are not attached to the mandibular remnant.

Scoring of external ear anomalies uses the systems of Marx[80] and Meurman,[81] with the addition of the grade 0 category meant to reflect the absence of any observable external ear malformation.

Scoring within the facial nerve category groups, the zygomatic and temporal branches into one group and the buccal, marginal mandibular, and cervical branches into another, thus

---

Table 34.1 Pruzansky classification of mandibular deformity with Kaban, Padwa, and Mulliken modification.

Type	Description
I	All mandibular and temporomandibular joint components are present and normal in shape but hypoplastic to a variable degree.
IIa	The mandibular ramus, condyle, and temporomandibular joint are present but hypoplastic and abnormal in shape.
IIb	The mandibular ramus is hypoplastic and markedly abnormal in form and location, being medial and anterior. There is no articulation with the temporal bone.
III	The mandibular ramus, condyle, and temporomandibular joint are absent. The lateral pterygoid muscle and temporalis, if present, are not attached to the mandibular remnant.

(Adapted from Kaban LB, Padwa BL, Mulliken JB. Surgical correction of mandibular hypoplasia in hemifacial microsomia: the case for treatment in early childhood. *J Oral Maxillofac Surg.* 1998;56:628–638.)

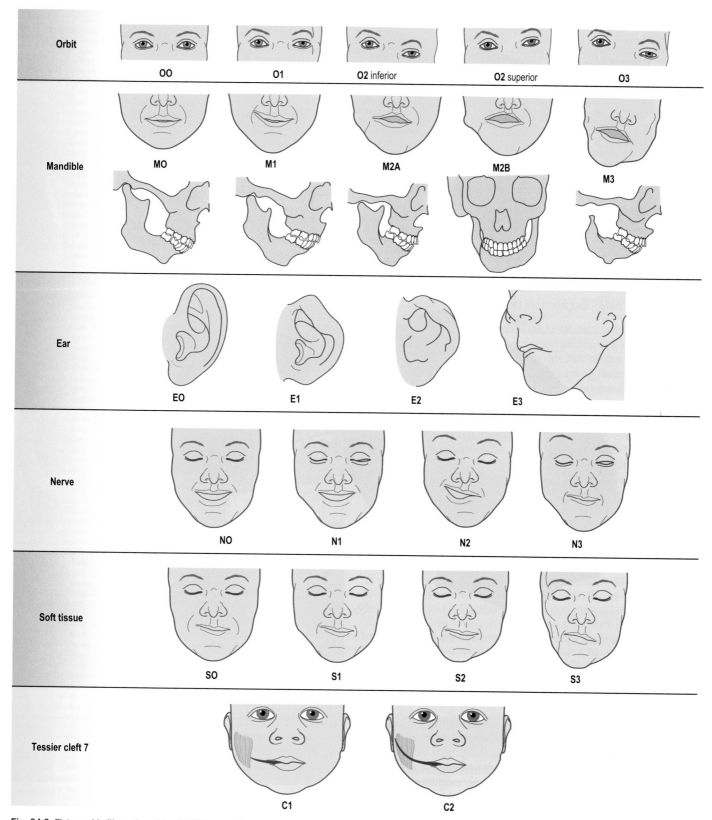

Fig. 34.8 Pictographic illustration of the OMENS+ classification.

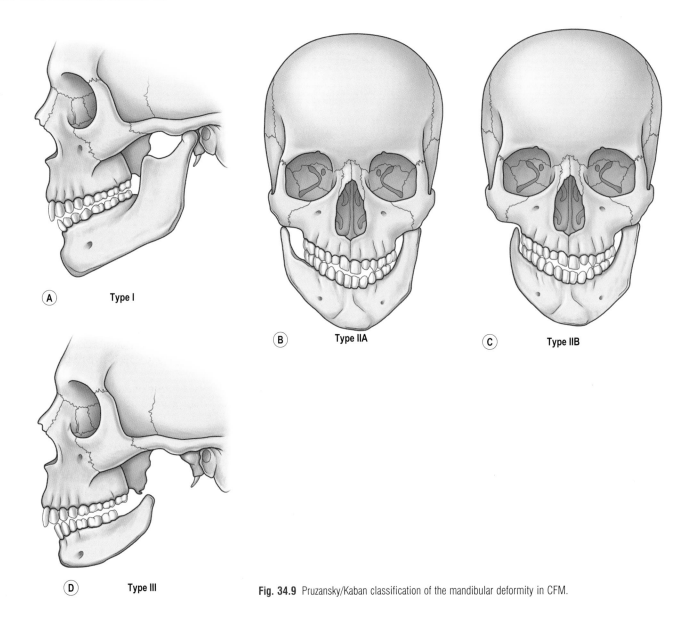

(A)   Type I

(B)   Type IIA

(C)   Type IIB

(D)   Type III   **Fig. 34.9** Pruzansky/Kaban classification of the mandibular deformity in CFM.

divides facial nerve involvement into upper and lower halves. The absence of nerve involvement with pan-hemifacial paralysis has a respective category.

Finally, scoring of soft-tissue deficiencies uses a modified version of the system developed by Murray and colleagues[3] and grades subcutaneous/muscular deficiency as either absent, mild, moderate, or severe. Classification for each side of the face is done separately in cases of bilateral CFM.

To include significant extracraniofacial anomalies, the OMENS classification was modified by Horgan *et al.* in 1995[12] to allow for the optional addition of a plus sign (OMENS+) to denote the presence of those associated extracraniofacial anomalies.

Moreover, criticism has centered on the system's definition of orbital dystopia. Cousley and Calvert[78] suggested that this definition needs to be further refined so as to clarify the amount of radiographic evidence needed to classify the orbit as abnormal in both size and position (O_3 designation). A final suggestion, also by Cousley,[82] calls for the expansion of the auricular category to include both middle ear and

preauricular defects. Additionally, this system does not account for or describe the often-associated lateral facial cleft (macrostomia) nor the tongue or palatal dysmorphology.

Despite these criticisms, the OMENS system represents a very accessible, flexible, comprehensive, and largely objective means of classifying the range of abnormalities constituting the spectrum of CFM. The grading systems within each category encompass the full range of dysplastic severity, defining each anatomical malformation in a very simple and reproducible manner. The use of a numeric classification also serves to objectify, within limits, the many inherently subjective features of this disorder and in doing so aids in the analysis of this population within and between institutions.

Bartlett and associates developed an anatomical classification utilizing 3D computed tomography (CT) scans with the hope of better capturing the wide spectrum of disease and guiding treatment, specifically of the mandibular deformity. The findings of an initial survey suggest that the grading system of the mandibular deformity in CFM based on conventional radiographs and that application of the Pruzansky/

Table 34.2 Bartlett classification of the CFM mandibular deformity

Type		Diagnostic features	Anticipated treatment
0	Normal	Normal	None
1	Mild deformity	Mandible **mildly hypoplastic**, condyle in normal position	Orthodontics or combined orthognathic surgery and orthodontics in adolescence
2	Moderate deformity	Mandibular ramus **moderately deficient vertically**, condyle functional	Childhood distraction osteogenesis
3	Severe deformity, adequate mandibular body	**Condyle and ramus rudimentary/absent**, adequate mandibular body bone stock	Non-vascularized (e.g. costochondral) bone graft
4	Severe deformity, inadequate mandibular body bone stock	**Condyle and ramus rudimentary/absent**, inadequate mandibular body bone stock	Vascularized (e.g. free fibular) bone flap

Kaban classification to 3D CT scans have shown low inter-rater reproducibility.[83] They proposed and validated a classification system that incorporates both diagnostic criteria based on 3D CT scans and corresponding treatment modality(s) based on the severity of deformity[84] (Table 34.2). Each hemimandible is characterized as normal (T0), mild (T1), moderate (T2), or severe (T3 and T4). Type 1 is distinguished from type 0 if the mandible shows noticeable hypoplasia, relative to the contralateral side in hemifacially-affected patients. Type 2 is distinguished from type 1 if the ramus shows sufficient vertical deficiency to anticipate an ipsilateral cross-bite or overjet of more than several millimeters in childhood, but with a condyle that permits functional articulation. Type 3 is distinguished from type 2 by a ramus–condylar complex that is either absent or rudimentary to the degree that it would not likely be functional even if lengthened. Type 3 is distinguished from type 4 by a mandibular body that has sufficient bone stock to support a costochondral graft neocondyle construction, as opposed to requiring a free fibular flap (see Table 34.2).

Broader, more complex, and occasionally nebulous classification systems have also been developed that encompass multiple features of the CFM spectrum.

For example, in 1963, Longacre et al.[38] divided CFM patients into two groups displaying either unilateral or bilateral facial microsomia. These two groups were then further subdivided into four classes of increasing facial deformity. The facial characteristics that defined each class were not specified.

In 1965, Grabb[5] segregated CFM patients into one of six groups defined by varying combinations of skeletal and soft-tissue deficiencies. Rollnick et al.[11] have also developed a mixed feature classification comprised of five groups, each with microtia as the fundamental feature. Edgerton and Marsh.[8] divided patients into four groups based on the "dominant dysplasia" (mandible, soft tissue, ear, composite). Finally, one last classification system of note, developed by David et al.,[85] is modeled after the tumor, node, metastasis (TNM) grading system of malignant tumors.[86]

At the current time, the Pruzansky/Kaban classification remains the most commonly used system, but with the advent of technology, it is expected that it will be displaced by a 3D CT-based system in the future.

Cephalometrics

In addition to CT and cone beam scans, cephalograms are an often-used tool in evaluating facial skeletal structures.

The classic lateral cephalogram provides information on maxillomandibular relationships, as well as the deviation of the bone and soft-tissue profile from documented norms. The posteroanterior and basilar cephalograms are equally important in assessing patients with CFM in that they allow documentation of the facial midline and the degree of facial asymmetry in three dimensions, when combined with the lateral view.

Grayson et al. described the technique of multiplane cephalometry.[87] With lateral, coronal, and basilar radiographs, skeletal landmarks can be identified in three coronal and three axial planes and used to construct an estimation of the midline for each plane. These midlines are compared with the mid-sagittal plane, which is determined by relatively stable bilateral structures such as the occipital condyles, the center of the foramen magnum, and the medial axis of the spheno-occipital synchondrosis. By use of this technique, a phenomenon termed warping can be observed within the skeleton of the patient with CFM. The midline constructs deviate progressively laterally as one passes anteriorly from the skull base to the piriform rim in the coronal plane and inferiorly from the orbits to the mandible in the axial plane.

Computed tomography

CT, including cone beam imaging, has become the primary diagnostic and evaluation tool for all patients with CFM. Unlike cephalography, it does not suffer from superimposition of skeletal landmarks, and both bone and soft tissues can be imaged. Axial and coronal cuts provide detailed information regarding bone and soft-tissue asymmetry, as well as the severity of malformation throughout the entire craniofacial skeleton.

Because data derived from the CT scan are computer-based, programs can be written to present the information in any number of formats, including three-dimensional (3D) CT and multiplanar reformation. 3D CT images provide a visual summary of the underlying skeleton, which can be viewed and analyzed at any angle. These images can also be easily shared with patients and families, and may be very helpful when discussing possible treatment plans. Another useful manipulation of CT data is multiplanar reformation (CT/MPR), or DentaScan, which processes axial CT scan information to obtain true cross-sectional images and panoramic views of the mandible and maxilla similar to a Panorex. This is invaluable when imaging tooth follicles in relation to available bone stock in the immature patient, who is too young for conventional dental imaging and in whom mandibular distraction is planned.

Cone beam CT scan technology allows detailed imaging of the maxillomandibular complex at reduced cost, radiation exposure, and time as compared to conventional helical CT scans.

Magnetic resonance imaging

With the improved accuracy of CT scans, magnetic resonance imaging (MRI) adds little information not obtained by CT scan and does not provide the precision of CT when it comes to assessing bone. On the other hand, it may be helpful in imaging brain and other soft tissues in CFM patients with severe deformities.

Endoscopy

In patients with respiratory insufficiency or sleep apnea, endoscopy is indicated to document the site of obstruction. In bilateral CFM, and occasionally in unilateral CFM, there can be significant tongue-based airway obstruction that can lead to life-threatening retroglossal narrowing secondary to mandibular deficiency. Endoscopy can also visualize the remainder of the tracheobronchial tree to rule out other sites of obstruction.

Sleep studies

In patients with symptoms of obstructive sleep apnea, sleep studies (polysomnography) can define the degree of the respiratory dysfunction. Polysomnography, along with the interpretation of clinical symptoms and endoscopic findings, can be invaluable in determining whether surgical intervention (i.e., mandibular distraction) is indicated.

Photography

Baseline photography should be obtained using standardized lighting and head positioning with lips at rest. Standardized records should include full face, submental vertex, bird's eye, lateral, oblique smile, and occlusal views. Functional facial nerve views are also requisite. The development of 3D camera systems provides a helpful tool for quantitatively documenting the deformity and recording volumetric and contour changes following surgical interventions; it is also an important component of the preoperative planning process.

Treatment/surgical technique

Tracheostomy/gastrostomy

In the neonatal period, tracheostomy can be a lifesaving maneuver in patients with severe respiratory distress, but the need for this treatment modality has been lessened in recent years with the introduction of mandibular distraction. Some newborns requiring perinatal endotracheal intubation can successfully tolerate extubation several days later as they mature. However, if extubation is not possible, the need for mandibular distraction or tracheostomy must be considered (Fig. 34.10). In severe cases of CFM (more dysmorphic forms

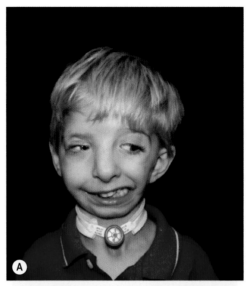
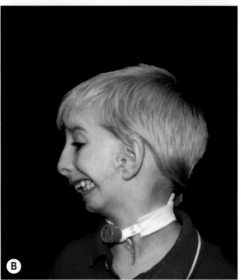

Fig. 34.10 A 4-year-old with severe left CFM. He benefited from a tracheostomy in the neonatal period because of severe respiratory distress. **(A)** AP view. **(B)** Left lateral view. After costochondral rib grafting to the left mandible, he was successfully decannulated.

of type III mandibular deformity), in which mandibular distraction cannot be performed, tracheostomy may be necessary.

For infants with severe swallowing/eating problems, a gastrostomy is indicated to improve the nutritional status of the child and to provide the calories essential for growth and development. The nutritional problem is often compounded by the increased energy requirements associated with respiratory insufficiency.

Commissuroplasty

Clefts of the lip and/or commissure (Tessier VII clefts of macrostomia) are typically repaired in infancy to increase feeding efficiency.[88]

Commissuroplasty, or closure of the lateral facial cleft, is indicated in patients with macrostomia or a true lateral facial cleft. Multiple techniques have been described. To be effective they must (1) normalize the oral commissure position, (2) reconstruct the orbicularis oris, and (3) minimize scar and create normal vermillion structures.

Vermilion and oral mucosal flaps are designed after the position of the projected oral commissure is determined. The flaps are approximated and sutured with resorbable sutures. The orbicularis muscle stumps are skeletonized and closed in a vest-over-pants fashion with resorbable sutures. The cutaneous closure may incorporate a Z-plasty designed to simulate the nasolabial fold (Fig. 34.11).

Nerve palsy management

When facial nerve palsy is identified, it is important to determine if the patient with CFM can protect and lubricate the

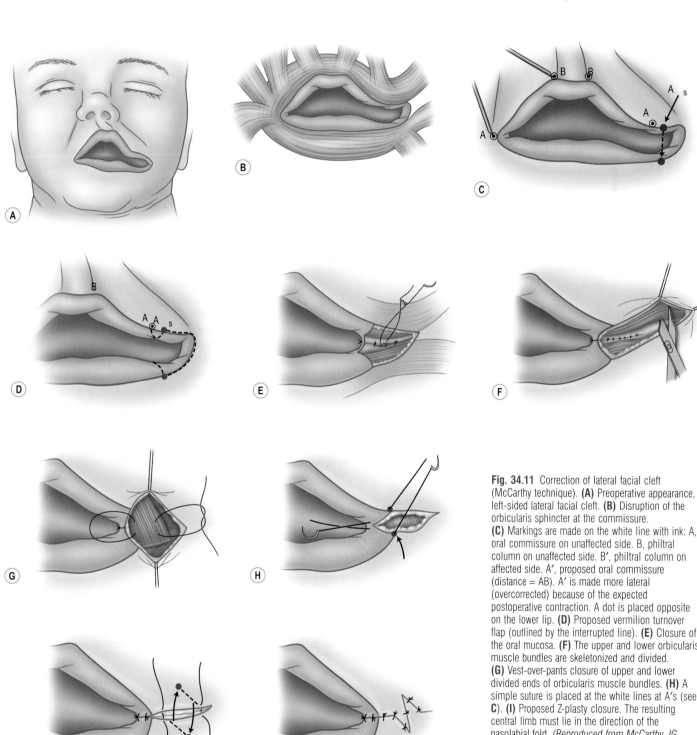

Fig. 34.11 Correction of lateral facial cleft (McCarthy technique). **(A)** Preoperative appearance, left-sided lateral facial cleft. **(B)** Disruption of the orbicularis sphincter at the commissure. **(C)** Markings are made on the white line with ink: A, oral commissure on unaffected side. B, philtral column on unaffected side. B′, philtral column on affected side. A′, proposed oral commissure (distance = AB). A′ is made more lateral (overcorrected) because of the expected postoperative contraction. A dot is placed opposite on the lower lip. **(D)** Proposed vermilion turnover flap (outlined by the interrupted line). **(E)** Closure of the oral mucosa. **(F)** The upper and lower orbicularis muscle bundles are skeletonized and divided. **(G)** Vest-over-pants closure of upper and lower divided ends of orbicularis muscle bundles. **(H)** A simple suture is placed at the white lines at A′s (see **C**). **(I)** Proposed Z-plasty closure. The resulting central limb must lie in the direction of the nasolabial fold. *(Reproduced from McCarthy JG, Grayson BH, Hopper RA, Tepper OM. Craniofacial microsomia. In: Neligan PC, Gurtner GC, Warren RJ, et al (eds). W B Saunders. 2012; Volume 3, Section II, Chapter 36:761–791.)*

cornea. If not, eye drops, lubricant, taping, or a surgical procedure (i.e., tarsorrhaphy, gold weight, eyelid tendon sling) should be considered. Exposure keratitis can eventually lead to corneal scarring and permanent blindness.

Patients who cannot move their mouth (i.e., smile) due to deficiencies of the buccal and marginal mandibular branches should be offered a facial reanimation procedure. Functional muscle transfer remains the gold standard for facial reanimation.

One technique involves the transfer of the temporalis muscle. The temporalis muscle can be detached from the coronoid and advanced to the commissure[89] or flipped over with a fascial extension to provide movement of the lateral mouth.[90] The advantages of this technique include ease of surgery, ease of recovery, and reliability of establishing movement. The disadvantages include weak strength of pull, limitations on vector of pull, and the need to activate cranial nerve V to stimulate a smile.

Facial reanimation, with a functional muscle transfer, can also be accomplished using a two-stage approach with a cross-face nerve graft and muscle free flap.[91] This is the most common procedure performed. In the first stage, a sural nerve graft is harvested and attached to the cut end of a redundant buccal branch on the functioning side. The graft is then passed through the upper lip to the paralyzed side of the face, where it sits until axonal ingrowth has occurred (at a rate of 1 mm/day). In the second stage, the nerve is biopsied to confirm the presence of myelin; then a muscle free flap is harvested and brought to the face. The muscle is attached to 4 points: the commissure, the upper lip, the lower lip, and the zygomatic arch in a direction that mimics the smile vector on the contralateral normal side. Microscopic anastomosis of the vein, artery, and nerve are then performed.[90] The gracilis muscle is the most commonly used muscle. This approach allows for creation of a spontaneous smile in a vector that resembles more closely the unaffected side. The disadvantages include length of surgery, recovery time, and need for microsurgical skills.[92]

The timing of reanimation surgery must be based on the patient's needs and planned around other surgical interventions. It is preferable to perform microtia reconstruction and major craniofacial and/or orthognathic surgery prior to undertaking facial reanimation surgery.

Mandibular reconstruction

CFM patients with a normal but hypoplastic ramus, condyle, and temporomandibular joint (Pruzansky/Kaban types I and IIA mandibular deformity) retain accurate function and position of the temporomandibular joint. Treatment of these patients can consist of mandibular lengthening by distraction osteogenesis or conventional osteotomy.[93] In type IIB and III patients, both function and position of the temporomandibular joint are inadequate, often requiring reconstruction of the mandible to improve function.[94,95]

Patient selection

The approach of each patient is on an individual basis. The treatment of choice should be based on the patient's needs and wishes, but also based on both the quantity and quality of bone stock present and the architecture of the temporomandibular joint. The goal of treatment in each patient is to achieve appropriate symmetry and occlusion with an adequate aesthetic outcome. One should aim for alignment of the maxillary and mandibular dental midlines with the mid-sagittal plane as well as a correction/leveling of the mandibular cant and a restoration of facial symmetry.[95]

Based on these anatomical features, several techniques have been described with which to approach the hypoplastic mandible. Reconstruction, however, is dependent on the degree of ramus and condyle deficiency, with autogenous bone grafting and distraction osteogenesis representing the two most common approaches used.

Surgical intervention for patients with Pruzansky type I mandibular deformity (Bartlett type 1) is often postponed until skeletal growth is complete. In mild cases, the occlusal relationship can be managed with orthodontics. However, in more severe type I cases, orthognathic surgery may be necessary to improve an occlusal cant and facial symmetry. It is then important to assess the dentofacial relationship and determine whether the patient needs unilateral or bilateral mandibular advancement/rotation, or if double jaw surgery is warranted.

Since patients with Pruzansky type IIA (Bartlett type 2) mandibular deformity have a present but smaller condyle, ramus, and sigmoid notch with a glenoid fossa in a satisfactory position, those patients often require some form of vertical lengthening of the mandible. This can be done with either distraction osteogenesis or an osteotomy and interposed bone graft performed after skeletal maturity.

Treatment of patients with Pruzansky type IIB (Bartlett type 3) mandibular deformity remains controversial and varies depending on the degree of severity. Distraction osteogenesis as well as rib grafting have been used alone or in combination for the treatment of these patients.

On the other hand, patients with severe Pruzansky type III (Bartlett type 4) mandibular deficiencies require, at a minimum, bone grafting to create a functional ramus and condyle unit and to restore mandibular height and facial symmetry.

Orthognatic surgery

When indicated, traditional maxillomandibular orthognathic surgery can be a useful tool in the armamentarium of the craniofacial surgeon treating the skeletally mature patient with CFM. The mandibular osteotomies include the bilateral sagittal split of the ramus and the vertical or oblique osteotomy of the ramus.

Obwegeser[96] combined the Le Fort I maxillary osteotomy with bilateral sagittal split of the mandibular ramus and genioplasty to ensure leveling of the occlusal plane and establishment of the optimal occlusal relationships (Fig. 34.12). The Le Fort I osteotomy is repositioned, according to preoperative plans, and rigid skeletal fixation is achieved with plates and screws. The sagittal split and vertical or oblique osteotomies allow repositioning of the tooth-bearing mandibular segments. Fixation is achieved with either lag screws or plates. Genioplasty, usually in three planes, completes the procedure.

Careful planning is essential. The occlusal cant observed in unilateral CFM results from a primary reduction in the vertical dimension of the mandible and a secondary reduction of

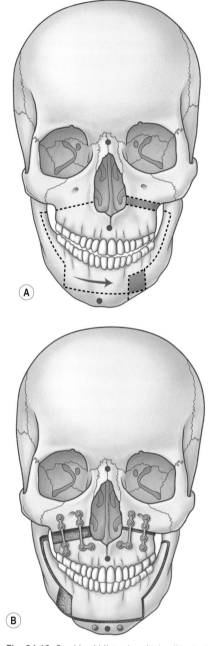

(A)

(B)

Fig. 34.12 Combined bilateral sagittal split osteotomy of the mandible, Le Fort I osteotomy, and genioplasty (Obwegeser). **(A)** Lines of osteotomy. The large dots illustrate the deviation of the craniofacial midline, and the arrow designates the desired direction of movement of the mandible (and maxilla). The shaded areas represent those portions of the maxilla and the buccal cortex of the mandible to be resected. Note the area of resection and impaction of the maxilla on the less affected side. **(B)** After bone grafting of the maxillary defect and rigid fixation of the Le Fort I segment. Lag screws are used on the mandibular rami and genioplasty segment. *(Reproduced from McCarthy JG, Grayson BH, Hopper RA, Tepper OM. Craniofacial microsomia. In: Neligan PC, Gurtner GC, Warren RJ, et al (eds). W B Saunders. 2012; Volume 3, Section II, Chapter 36:761–791.)*

the maxillary vertical dimension.[45] Moreover, superimposed on this growth abnormality, some patients may also show facial findings characteristic of the long-face or short-face syndrome, as manifested by excessive or deficient maxillary gingival exposure at rest or on smiling. The ultimate goals of orthognathic surgery include the correction of the occlusal

cant while at the same time optimizing the lip–incisor relationship.

Mandibular distraction osteogenesis

Distraction osteogenesis has become a valuable tool for augmentation of hypoplastic bony structures using autologous tissue. Distraction osteogenesis was initially described by Ilizarov,[97] then applied to the craniofacial skeleton by Snyder[98] and popularized by McCarthy.[99] Mandibular distraction osteogenesis (MDO) has several distinct advantages over costochondral grafting. MDO increases the vertical length of the mandible, produces greater bone stock and improves soft-tissue asymmetry. Other benefits include shorter operative times, less blood loss, greater vector control of advancement, and the ability to lengthen the mandible at a younger age as bone grafts are not always necessary. MDO can be used to treat type IIa and IIb mandibles (Bartlett type 2), and combined with a bone graft for treatment of type III mandibles (Bartlett types 3 and 4). Variables to control while performing MDO procedure include the vector orientation, the type of device to use, and finally an internal or external approach.[100–111]

The vector of advancement should be based on the mandibular shape.[112] In some mandibular deformities (Figs. 34.13 & 34.14), a vertical vector alone is often adequate, while in others a more obliquely oriented vector to treat the vertical and horizontal ramal deficiency is often required.

Both single and multivector external devices (Fig. 34.15) and semi-buried internal devices (Fig. 34.16) are available; each has unique benefits and deficiencies.[113] External devices allow greater freedom to mold the regenerate by changing the vector of distraction after the osteotomy is made. Additionally, pin placement requires little bone stock, which allows for accurate placement of the devices in hypoplastic mandibles and with minimal disruption of the periosteum. However, the external devices create unsightly scars, dislodge easily, significantly alter the patient's appearance during MDO, and are prone to pin site infections. Internal devices are less visible, create less scarring, and are less prone to trauma and infection. Since the vector cannot be altered once the device is fixated, greater preoperative planning is necessary with internal devices. They also require an additional surgery to remove unless a resorbable system is selected.

The authors' preferred technique for vertical mandibular distraction is as follows:

Through an intra-oral gingival–buccal incision, the ramus and posterior body are exposed in the subperiosteal plane, and landmarks (coronoid, antegonial notch) are noted. The site of the corticotomy/osteotomy is then identified and the vector for distractor placement is noted. Preoperatively, this has been determined based on radiographs and occlusal analysis: a primarily sagittal vector when there is little vertical shortening; an oblique vertical vector when there is both a vertical and a sagittal deficiency; and finally, a vector obtuse to the mandibular plane when occlusal relations are normal sagittally, and a vertical elongation without sagittal advancement is needed.

A conventional or ultrasonic saw is then used to perform complete osteotomies of the lateral anterior and posterior cortices leaving the medial cortex intact. The distractor is then placed. For an internal distractor, a pocket is dissected and an exit point is created inferior to the mandible on the cervical skin. The distractor is then fixated using transbuccal screws. The final medial corticotomy is then completed with a saw or osteotome.

If an external distractor is used, two percutaneous pins are placed on each side of the osteotomy before it is completed. The distractor is then placed and the medial corticotomy is completed.

The device is then activated to be certain a complete separation of bone occurs, especially through the medullary bone since it has been minimally osteotomized. Once completeness

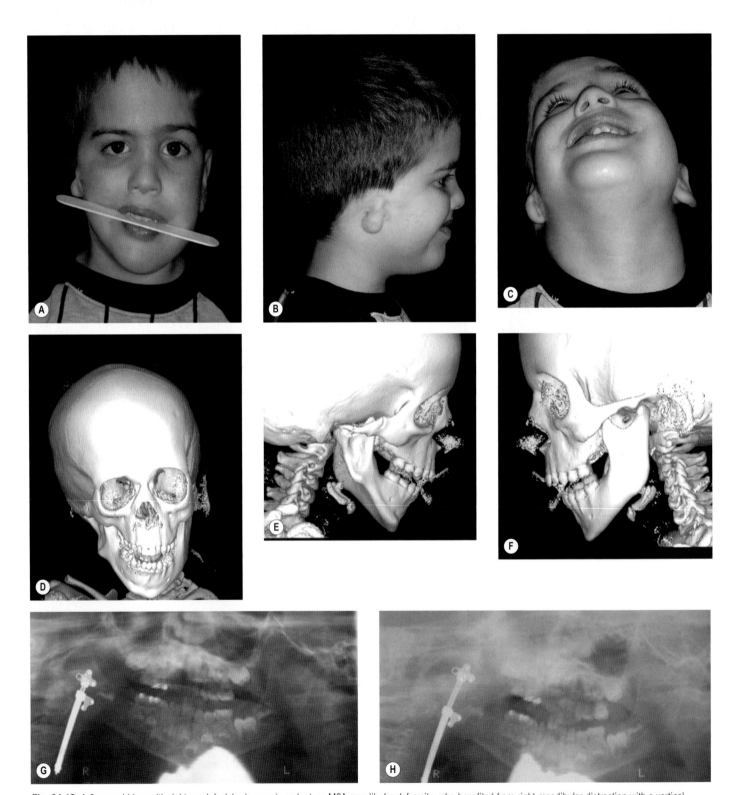

Fig. 34.13 A 6-year-old boy with right craniofacial microsomia and a type M2A mandibular deformity, who benefited from right mandibular distraction with a vertical vector. **(A)** Photograph, AP view, significant right upper cant. **(B)** Photograph, right lateral view. **(C)** Photograph, worm's eye view. **(D)** 3D CT scan, AP view. **(E)** 3D CT scan, right lateral view. **(F)** 3D CT scan, left lateral view. **(G)** Radiograph, AP view, 3 days postoperative. **(H)** Radiograph, AP view, 2 weeks postoperative.

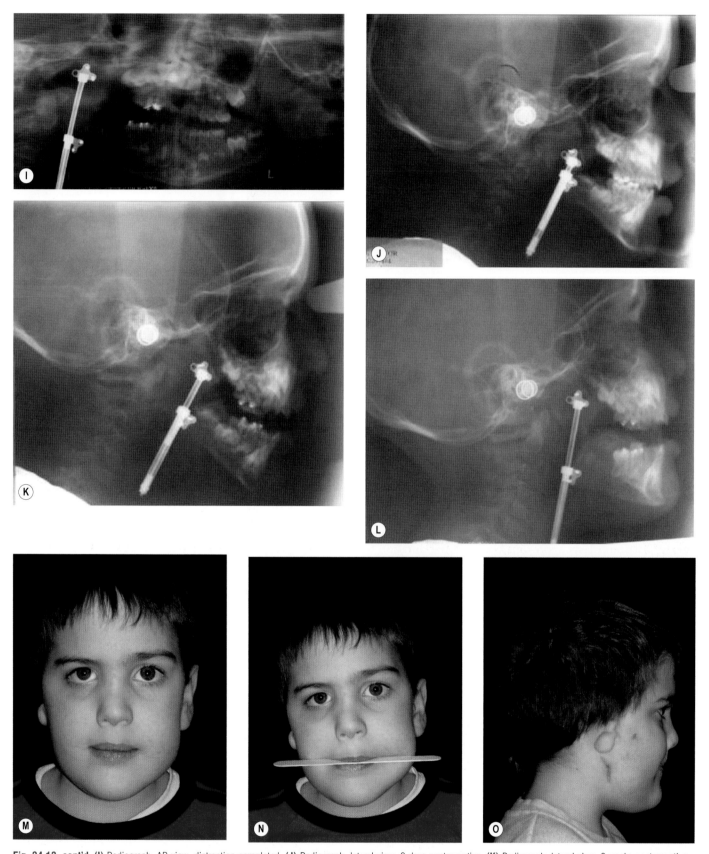

Fig. 34.13, cont'd (I) Radiograph, AP view, distraction completed. **(J)** Radiograph, lateral view, 3 days postoperative. **(K)** Radiograph, lateral view, 2 weeks postoperative. **(L)** Radiograph, lateral view, distraction completed. **(M)** Postoperative photograph, AP view. **(N)** Postoperative photograph, AP view, notice the correction of the cant. **(O)** Postoperative photograph, lateral view.

Continued

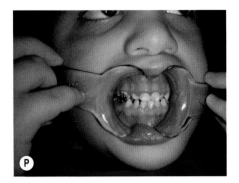

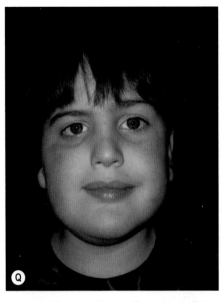

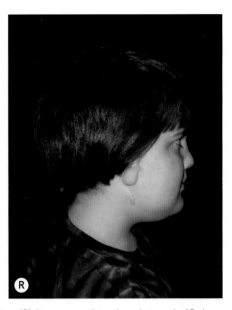

Fig. 34.13, cont'd (P) Intra-oral photograph demonstrating adequate alignment of the maxillary and mandibular arches. **(Q)** 3 years post-distraction, photograph, AP view. **(R)** 3 years post-distraction, photograph, right lateral view.

of the osteotomy is confirmed, the device is returned to its initial position and the soft tissues closed in layers.

Following a latency period of 2 to 5 days (depending on the age of the patient), the distraction phase is started at a rate of 1 mm per day. Patients are followed up weekly with X-rays to confirm the device functionality and distance of distraction. The endpoint of distraction is determined by clinical examination, aiming for alignment of the maxillary and mandibular dental midlines with the mid-sagittal plane as well as a correction/leveling of the mandibular cant and a restoration of facial symmetry. Following distraction, a consolidation period starts and lasts approximately twice the duration of the distraction phase.

Coordination between the surgeon and the orthodontist is critical. Distraction techniques create an open bite once the mandible is lengthened. To prevent relapse, this open bite must be maintained until the maxillary dentition can be brought down to create a stable occlusion. This occurs quickly in children aged 4 to 6 years and may require little management. During mixed dentition, however, the open bite is often managed through occlusal splints or tooth-borne or bone-anchored orthodontics. The maxilla may require concomitant movement with the mandible using bimaxillary distraction after skeletal maturity or a Le Fort I is performed at the time of distractor removal.

After the periods of distraction and consolidations are completed, the distractor is removed. For external devices, this requires disassembly and pin removal, whereas for an internal device, a secondary removal procedure is required.

Bone/cartilage grafting

Gillies described the first costochondral graft for temporomandibular joint (TMJ) reconstruction in 1920.[114] Since then, multiple autogenous grafts such as clavicle and sternoclavicular joint,[115] fibula,[116] iliac bone[117] and metatarsal bone[118] have been described for TMJ reconstruction, particularly in

the CFM patient population with mandibular hypoplasia. However, autogenous costochondral rib graft remains the method of choice for mandibular/TMJ reconstruction in children with Pruzansky/Kaban type IIB and III mandibular hypoplasia (Bartlett type 3).

The authors' preferred technique[95] (Fig. 34.17) is as follows:

Preoperatively: Costochondral grafting for mandibular reconstruction is offered to children with Pruzansky/Kaban type IIB and III mandibular hypoplasia, significant occlusal abnormalities, and facial asymmetry. The goals of the procedure are to reconstruct a new ramus and pseudocondyle with the rib graft, placing it in a pocket that abuts the cranial base, subsequently creating a pseudoarthrosis at the cranial base with an adequate soft-tissue envelope. The authors aim for alignment of the maxillary and mandibular dental midlines with the mid-sagittal plane as well as a correction/leveling of the mandibular cant and a restoration of facial symmetry. No overcorrection is desired since our technique relies on subsequent costochondral rib graft growth. Preoperatively, the orthodontist works with the surgeon to plan the final mandibular position utilizing stone models, radiographic analysis and clinical assessment. Based upon this model surgery, the orthodontist creates a prefabricated occlusal splint using stone models. A large posterior open bite is inherently created on the affected side as a result of ramus elongation, leveling the mandibular cant and bringing the chin point to the mid-sagittal plane. Early in the practice of the senior author, when no on-site orthodontist was available, the splint was made intraoperatively using polymethylmethacrylate. Of note, the prefabrication of the occlusal splint may also be planned virtually using 3D CT technology.

Intraoperatively: After satisfactory nasotracheal anesthesia is obtained, a 4 cm submandibular incision is made on the affected side approximately 1.5 cm below the mandibular angle. Dissection is performed down to the platysma, which is divided after we verify with a nerve stimulator the absence of marginal mandibular nerve fibers. Lifting the platysma

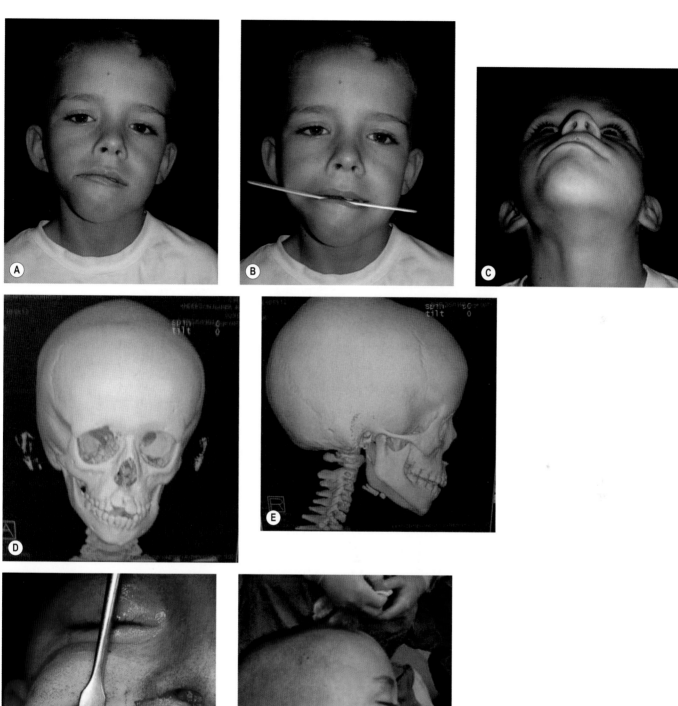

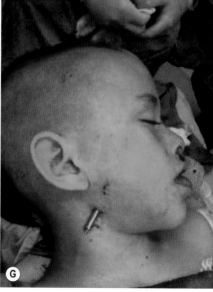

Fig. 34.14 A 5-year-old boy with right craniofacial microsomia and a type M2A mandibular deformity, who benefited from right mandibular distraction with a vertical vector. **(A)** Photograph, AP view.
(B) Photograph, AP view, significant right upper cant.
(C) Photograph, worm's eye view. **(D)** 3D CT scan, AP view. **(E)** 3D CT scan, right lateral view.
(F) Intraoperative intra-oral photograph demonstrating the osteotomy and placement of the distractor.
(G) Intraoperative photograph demonstrating distractor in place. *Continued*

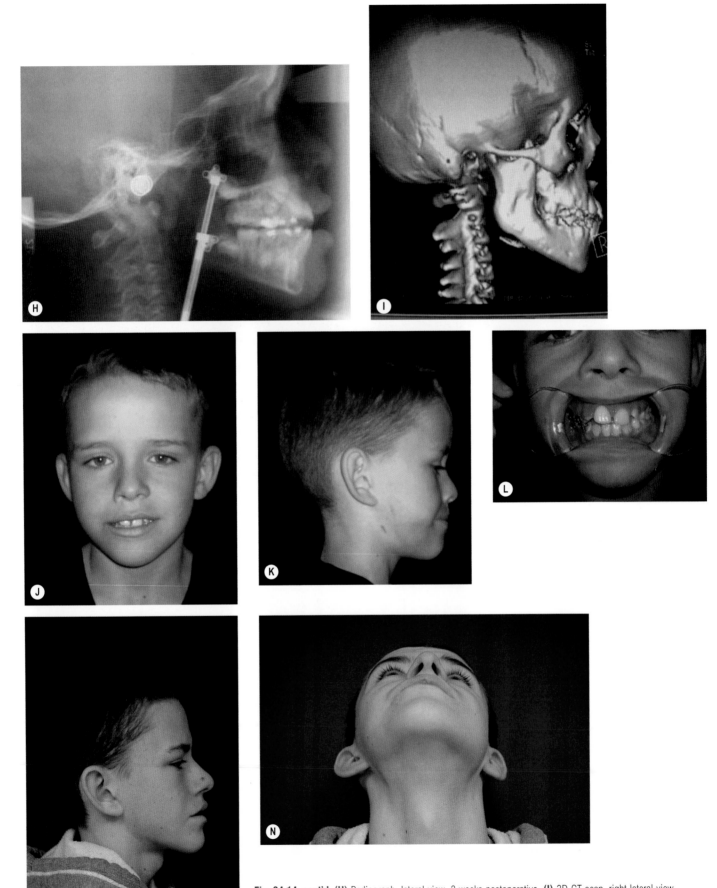

Fig. 34.14, cont'd **(H)** Radiograph, lateral view, 3 weeks postoperative. **(I)** 3D CT scan, right lateral view, demonstrating adequate regenerate after distraction. **(J)** Photograph, AP view, 2 months after removal of distractor. **(K)** Photograph, right lateral view, 2 months after removal of distractor. **(L)** Intra-oral photograph demonstrating adequate alignment of the maxillary and mandibular arches. **(M)** 9 years post-distraction, photograph, right lateral view. **(N)** 9 years post-distraction, photograph, worm's eye view.

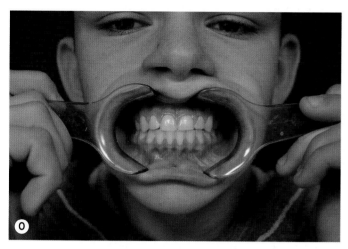

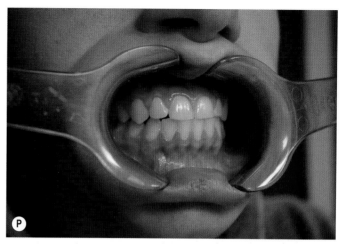

Fig. 34.14, cont'd (O) 9 years post-distraction, intra-oral photograph, AP view, demonstrating adequate alignment of the maxillary and mandibular arches. **(P)** 9 years post-distraction, intra-oral photograph, ¾ view.

superiorly, dissection is carried down to the mandibular border. The periosteum is incised with the cautery and a wide subperiosteal dissection of the mandible is performed.

Blunt dissection is then performed superiorly, in the subperiosteal plane, always staying deep to the facial nerve, until a pocket that abuts the cranial base is created. The zygomatic process of the temporal bone and the zygomatic arch, if present, can be felt laterally to the pocket, which will host the costochondral rib graft. Using a bone hook under the chin, the mandible is brought forward and toward the unaffected side to correct the retrognathia and align the maxillary and mandibular midlines with the mid-sagittal plane. Utilizing the prefabricated occlusal splint, the patient is put into maxillary–mandibular fixation (MMF) using IMF screws and 2-0 cross-connecting wires.

A rib graft is simultaneously harvested from the ipsilateral 6th or 7th costal cartilage through a small transverse incision.

After splitting the rectus muscle fibers, the osteocartilaginous junction is exposed. Using a Doyen rib dissector to strip soft tissues, dissection is carried medially and laterally to the osteocartilaginous junction. Laterally, the periosteum is incised and dissected from the bone up to the osteocartilaginous junction where the periosteum is preserved. Medially, the perichondrium is preserved for approximately 1 to 1.5 cm of the osteocartilaginous junction in order to facilitate adherence of the cartilage to the bone and growth at the osteocartilaginous junction. The graft is then harvested from the rest of the rib using the knife. The cartilaginous head of the rib graft is rounded off with a knife to give it the desired dimension, ranging approximately from 0.5 to 1 cm in height (Fig. 34.18).

With the mandible displaced anterior and inferior, as much as allowed by the contralateral temporomandibular joint and local soft tissues, the rib construct is placed in position,

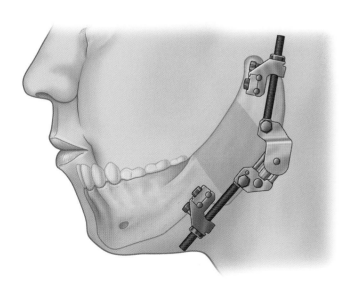

Fig. 34.15 Schematic drawing of an external mandibular distraction device.

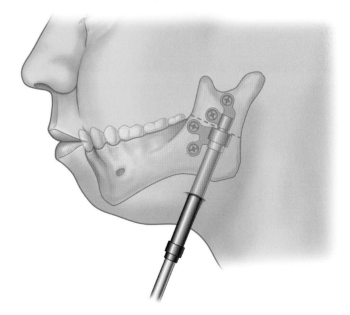

Fig. 34.16 Schematic drawing of an internal/semi-buried mandibular distraction device.

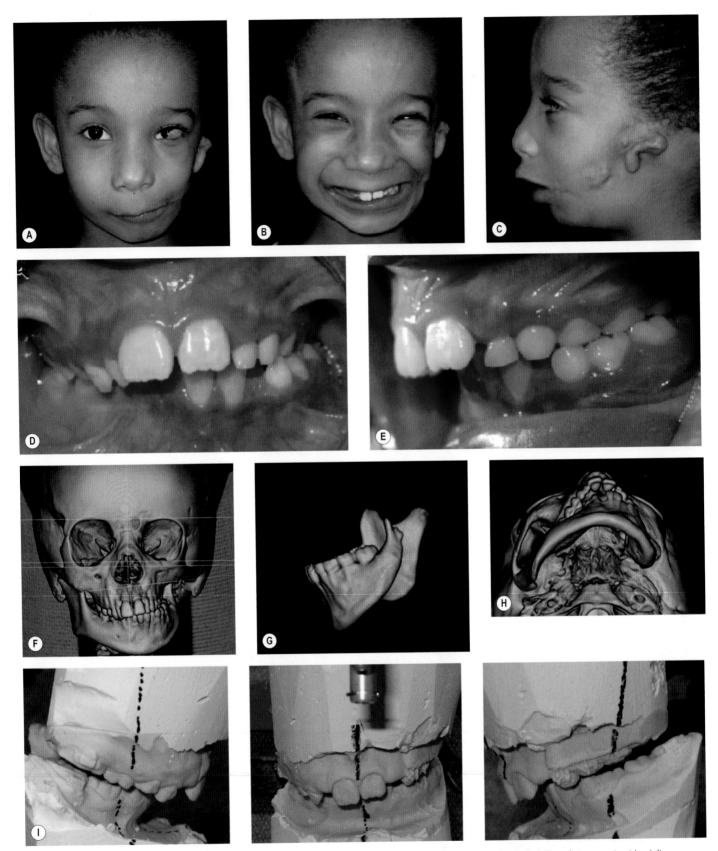

Fig. 34.17 A 6-year-old female with Goldenhar syndrome and type 3 left mandibular deformity. She benefited from costochondral rib graft to reconstruct her left hypoplastic mandible. **(A)** Photograph, AP view (note left epibulbar dermoid and macrostomia). **(B)** Photograph, AP view, patient smiling. **(C)** Photograph left lateral view (note left microtia). **(D)** Intra-oral photograph highlighting the malocclusion and cross-bite, AP view. **(E)** Intra-oral photograph left lateral view. **(F)** 3D CT scan, face, AP view. **(G)** 2D CT scan, mandible, left lateral view. **(H)** 3D CT scan, face, worm's eye view. **(I)** Preoperative stone models, right lateral, AP, left lateral.

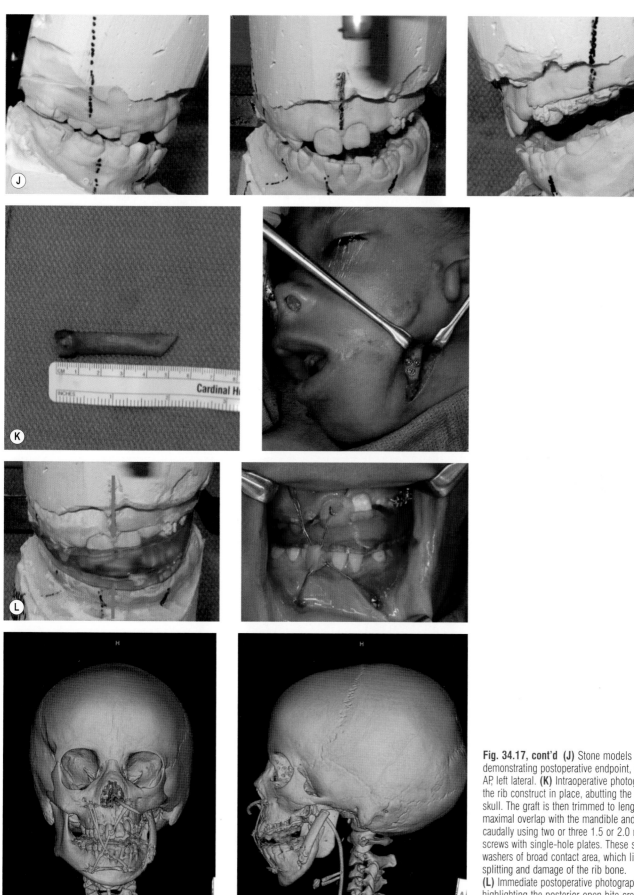

Fig. 34.17, cont'd (J) Stone models demonstrating postoperative endpoint, right lateral, AP, left lateral. **(K)** Intraoperative photographs with the rib construct in place, abutting the base of the skull. The graft is then trimmed to length to allow maximal overlap with the mandible and fixated caudally using two or three 1.5 or 2.0 mm titanium screws with single-hole plates. These serve as washers of broad contact area, which limits splitting and damage of the rib bone.
(L) Immediate postoperative photograph highlighting the posterior open bite created and maintained with a splint. **(M)** Postoperative 3D CT scan AP and lateral views. *Continued*

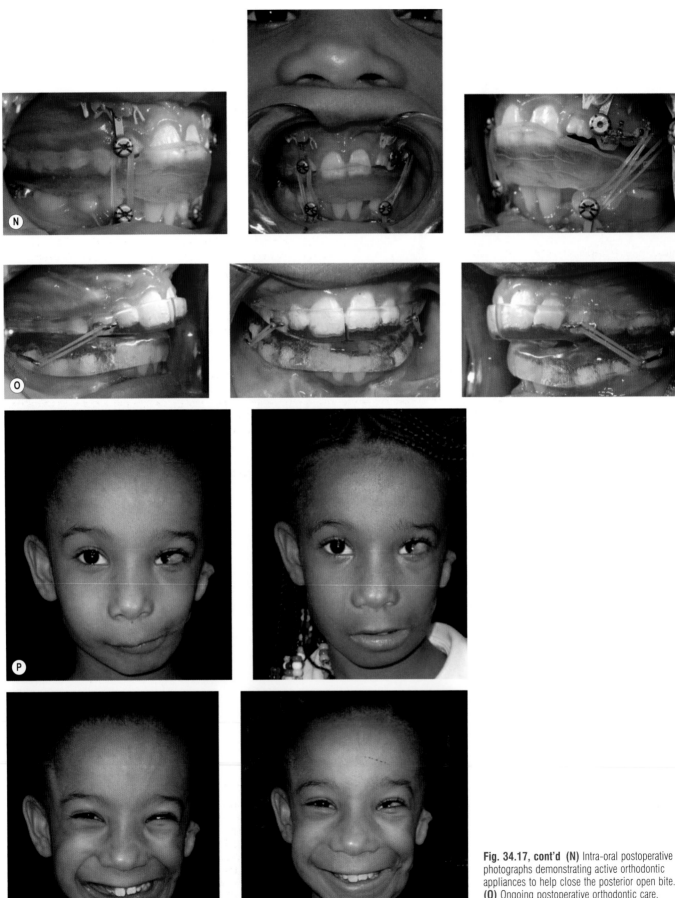

Fig. 34.17, cont'd (N) Intra-oral postoperative photographs demonstrating active orthodontic appliances to help close the posterior open bite. **(O)** Ongoing postoperative orthodontic care. **(P)** Preoperative and 2 years postoperative comparison. **(Q)** Preoperative and 2 years postoperative comparison (smiling).

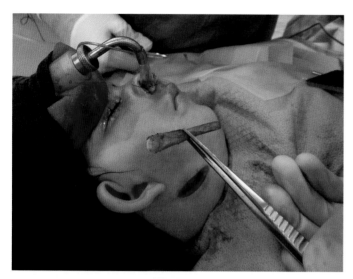

Fig. 34.18 Costochondral rib graft harvested from the ipsilateral 6th or 7th rib. The perichondrium is preserved for approximately 1 to 1.5 cm of the osteocartilaginous junction. The head of the rib graft is then rounded off with a knife to give it the desired dimension (approx. 0.5 cm).

abutting the base of the skull. An expected overlap of the caudal portion of the rib graft and the mandible is observed. The graft is then fashioned to allow maximal overlap with the mandible and fixated caudally using two or three 1.5 or 2.0 mm titanium screws with single-hole plates (Fig. 34.19). These serve as washers of broad contact area, which limits splitting and damage of the rib bone. Maximal bone-to-bone contact is secured to facilitate osteosynthesis, allowing early loading at 3 weeks postoperatively.

The donor and recipient sites are then irrigated and closed in layers. Patients remain in MMF for 3 weeks at which time they are released in the operating room and tested for graft stability. They are then started on an active range of motion protocol, which includes regular food, soft in texture. Physiotherapy may be advised.

Timing: The authors recommend, when feasible, to perform this procedure in patients older than 5 year of age. The quality of the rib graft in patients less than 5 years of age is suboptimal; the rib graft may be very small and thin, thus increasing the risk of splitting and poor fixation.

Postoperative orthodonture

The technique presented here inherently creates a posterior open bite on the affected/reconstructed side. The mandibular reconstruction levels the mandibular cant and corrects its position, but the maxillary cant remains secondary to prior vertical growth inhibition by the pathologic mandible. Careful orthodontic management to postoperatively close the posterior open bite is critical to the success of the procedure and restoration of functional occlusion. In this phase, the authors orthodontically correct the maxillary occlusal cant via vertical elongation of the affected side while maintaining the leveled mandibular occlusal plane. Several techniques have been described for how to achieve these goals. Interarch elastics in conjunction with fixed orthodontic appliances,[119–124] temporary anchorage devices,[120,121] and/or occlusal splints[121–123] have all been used in this series for selectively extruding the

maxillary teeth on the affected side. Age and stage of dental development are the key factors in determining which orthodontic therapies are most appropriate for the patient.

Combination of treatments

In the setting of mandibular reconstruction with rib graft of type 2B and 3 hypoplastic mandibles, distraction osteogenesis is a useful tool to use if the costochondral graft does not grow sufficiently. The use of distraction in conjunction with costochondral rib grafting has been described in various reports in the literature.[98,125–129] The high complication rate (62.5%) initially reported by Corcoran *et al.*[125] in their series of 8 patients and a high nonunion rate (33%) reported by Stelnicki *et al.*[126] seems to be attributed to the fact that their initial distraction osteotomy was performed across the grafted rib. Wan and the UCLA group[129] recently published their series of 17 cases of mandibular reconstruction with costochondral rib grafting in conjunction with mandibular distraction. Mandibular distraction was performed at the three possible locations: within the native mandible (n=4, 25%), at the mandible–rib graft junction (n=3, 19%) and within the rib graft (n=9, 56%). They reported a significantly higher complication rate in patients who underwent distraction at the mandible–graft junction. There was only one complication noted at each of the two other sites of distraction, while all cases of distraction at the mandibular–rib junction had complications. The difference in the embryology of the rib graft (endochondral ossification) and the mandible (intramembranous ossification) creating some form of instability at their junction was the hypothesis raised by Bradley *et al.*[129]

The authors recommend that the distraction osteotomy be performed at the level of the native mandible, slightly mesial

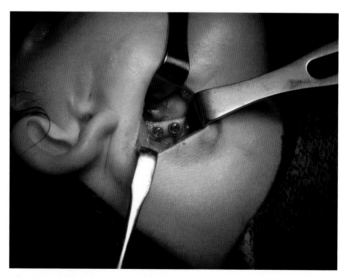

Fig. 34.19 With the mandible forward and down as much as allowed by the contralateral temporomandibular joint and local soft tissues, the rib construct is placed in position, abutting the base of the skull. An expected overlap of the caudal portion of the rib graft and the mandible is observed. The graft is then trimmed to length to allow maximal overlap with the mandible and fixated caudally using two or three 1.5 or 2.0 mm titanium screws with single-hole plates. These serve as washers of broad contact area, which limits splitting and damage of the rib bone. Maximal bone-to-bone contact is then secured to facilitate osteosynthesis, allowing early loading at 3 weeks postoperatively.

to the mandibular–rib graft junction. One may say that, in some cases, the mandibular–rib graft junction may be imperceptible due to union; thus, efforts should still be made to perform distraction at a site mesial to the junction. The results of a previous study published by Tahiri *et al.* demonstrated that distraction osteogenesis was successful at correcting the mandibular asymmetry in cases where the rib grafting may be insufficient in the long term because of inadequate growth of the rib or bone graft resorption (Fig. 34.20).

Orbital reconstruction

Orbital reconstruction in patients with CFM typically involves either bony or soft-tissue surgery. Stimulation of the visual cortex in infants to avoid amblyopia is of prime importance. Moreover, epibulbar dermoids and eyelid colobomas may require treatment to prevent disruption of the visual axis and protection of the cornea, respectively.[130,131] Early protection of the cornea can prevent exposure keratitis.

Typically, orbital bony reconstruction for asymmetry is corrected only if severe and typically is postponed until the orbital growth is complete, which is approximately at age 4 or 5 years. Orbital repositioning can be approached simply with a simple split calvarial bone graft or in more severely asymmetric cases with a 4-wall box osteotomy performed via an intracranial approach. The orbital box can be mobilized in various directions and then fixated into a symmetric position with the contralateral orbit. Cranial surgery can also be performed simultaneously if needed. Such cases are, however, infrequent.

Soft-tissue reconstruction

The reconstructive techniques described below can be used for a patient with a soft-tissue deficiency in isolation or with underlying bony asymmetry.

Fat grafting

Structural fat grafting has revolutionized the way many conditions are treated, including CFM.[132,133] This technique requires (1) fat harvest from the abdomen, flanks, thighs, or buttocks, (2) purification, and then (3) injection of small aliquots (<0.1 cc) in multiple planes within the areas of facial deficiency. The benefits of fat injection are precision of delivery, minimal scarring, and minimal donor-site morbidity. Additionally, the small aliquots do not disrupt the connecting ligaments of the face, so the fat is less likely to droop or disrupt normal facial movement. Some report improvement in the texture and appearance of the overlying skin. The downside of this technique is resorption. One can expect 30 to 80% of the injected fat to resorb depending on location. This necessitates multiple fat grafting procedures. It is preferable to coordinate fat injection procedures with other procedures throughout childhood to minimize recovery and provide improvement in facial symmetry during the developmental years of school age and adolescence.

Microvascular free flap

An adipofascial free flap is the best way to provide a large amount of soft tissue in a single surgical procedure for patients with severe deficiencies.[134,135] Free flap selection includes scapular, parascapular,[136] groin,[137,138] omentum,[139] anterolateral thigh (ALT),[140] and deep inferior epigastric perforator (DIEP), among others. Because adipofascial free flap transfer can provide such augmentation, it may be necessary to follow this with a debulking procedure.[141] Other drawbacks include donor-site morbidity and scarring, length of procedure, and the need for microsurgical skills. This approach is generally performed after the skeletal anomalies of CFM have been corrected.

Dermal fat graft

A dermal fat graft is another way of providing some soft tissue in a single surgical procedure for patients with mild to moderate deficiencies. However, dermal fat grafts are somewhat prone to resorption and may need additional augmentation procedures.[141]

Auricular reconstruction

Ear reconstruction will vary based on the severity of the deformity. When faced with only a mild effacement of the auricular architecture with mild hypoplasia of the ear with all auricular structures being present (E1), surgical treatment involves cartilage folding, scoring, or weakening techniques to restore normal shape and anatomy.[142] On the other hand, when the hypoplasia is more severe (E2 and E3), an auricular reconstruction with a new framework is created in either an autologous fashion or alloplastic fashion.

Autogenous reconstruction

Autologous reconstruction involves the use of the patient's own rib cartilage to create the new auricular framework. The procedure includes the harvest of the costal cartilage grafts, the carving of the framework, placement of the graft, transposition of the lobule, and the creation of a postauricular sulcus.[143–153]

Burt Brent[154] described a four-stage approach, which has been modified to three stages using costal cartilage grafts from the contralateral synchondrosis of ribs 6 and 7 and the cartilage of rib 8.[149] Stage 1 is performed after age 6 years when the ear has reached 85% of its adult size and adequate cartilage is available.[155] The rim of the 6th rib is preserved to minimize the chest wall deformity. A crescent of cartilage is banked in the scalp in a position posterior to the reconstructed ear to be used later as a "wedge" cartilage. A template is traced from the contralateral ear and a pocket is dissected to place the framework in harmony with facial features and symmetrically with the opposite ear. The plane of dissection of the pocket is between subdermal plexus and temporoparietal fascia. The position of new ear is made symmetrical with the opposite side using the lateral canthus, alar rim, and oral commissure as landmarks. Remnant cartilage is discarded. Stage 2 involves lobule transposition and the surgeon creates a postauricular sulcus with the "wedge" cartilage, a scalp advancement, and use of a skin graft in stage 3.

On the other hand, the Nagata technique involves a two-stage approach.[145–148,156] Patients are not generally treated until age 10 years and with a chest circumference of at least 60 cm to ensure adequate cartilage is present for an adult-sized construct. Cartilage from ipsilateral ribs 6, 7, 8, and 9 are harvested in the subperichondrial plane to allow regrowth and

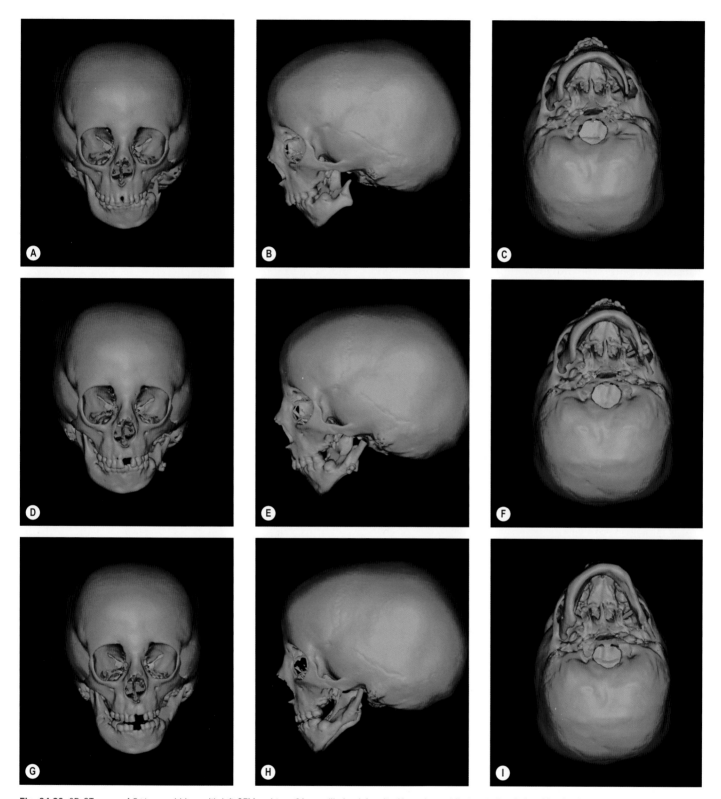

Fig. 34.20 3D CT scans of 5½-year-old boy with left CFM and type 3A mandibular deformity. He underwent first costochondral grafting for the ramus reconstruction. Due to the lack of growth of the graft, he underwent successfully unilateral mandibular distraction osteogenesis (DO). **(A)** Preoperative AP view. **(B)** Preoperative left lateral view. **(C)** Preoperative worm's eye view. **(D)** AP view following costochondral rib grafting. **(E)** Left lateral view following costochondral rib grafting. **(F)** Worm's eye view following costochondral rib grafting. **(G)** AP view following DO. **(H)** Left lateral view following DO. **(I)** Worm's eye view following DO.

minimize donor-site deformity. In stage 1, a three-dimensional construct is carved, placed, and the lobule is then transposed. Nagata's framework already incorporates the tragus, thereby eliminating another stage. Cartilage from the 6th and 7th costal cartilage is used for the base frame, the 8th costal cartilage is used for the helix and the crus helicis, while the 9th costal cartilage is used for the superior and inferior crus as well as the antihelix. Stage 2 involves ear elevation and creation of auriculocephalic sulcus. In this stage, the construct is elevated using a cartilage graft wrapped in temporoparietal fascia. This is generally covered with a split skin graft taken from the scalp.

Alloplastic reconstruction

Various materials have been used for alloplastic ear reconstruction with mixed results.[157–161] Porous polyethylene's inert nature and pore size provides the best safety profile and allows for some tissue ingrowth. John Reinisch popularized this technique. He has provided good long-term follow-up with acceptable morbidity and is to be recommended.[158] It is available in two prefabricated constructs of various sizes, which can be matched to the contralateral ear, secured, and covered with a temporoparietal fascia flap followed by skin grafts. Benefits include rigidity of construct, lack of donor site morbidity, and the ability to reconstruct younger, smaller patients. Criticisms include extrusion and infection, though some report none of these problems.[158,159,161]

Conclusion

The phenotypic expression of craniofacial microsomia relates to the complex, three-dimensional deformity of the underlying craniofacial skeleton. Patients with CFM may display airway obstruction, feeding difficulties, malocclusion, visual impairment, hearing disorders, speech and language delays, and socialization challenges because of their craniofacial anomalies. For these reason, patients with CFM often require complex, multidisciplinary, staged treatment plans.

Access the complete reference list online at   **http://www.expertconsult.com**

3. Murray JE, Kaban LB, Mulliken JB. Analysis and treatment of hemifacial microsomia. *Plast Reconstr Surg.* 1984;74:186–199.

6. Poswillo D. The pathogenesis of the first and second branchial arch syndrome. *Oral Surg Oral Med Oral Pathol.* 1973;35:302–328.

34. Pruzansky S. Not all dwarfed mandibles are alike. *Birth Defects.* 1969;1:120–129.

41. Vento AR, LaBrie RA, Mulliken JB. The O.M.E.N.S. classification of hemifacial microsomia. *Cleft Palate Craniofac J.* 1991;28:68–76.

70. Polley JW, Figueroa AA, Liou EJ, Cohen M. Longitudinal analysis of mandibular asymmetry in hemifacial microsomia. *Plast Reconstr Surg.* 1997;99:328–339.

79. Gougoutas AJ, Singh DJ, Low DW, Bartlett SP. Hemifacial microsomia: clinical features and pictographic representations of the OMENS classification system. *Plast Reconstr Surg.* 2007;120:112e–120e.

83. Wink JD, Goldstein JA, Paliga JT, et al. The mandibular deformity in hemifacial microsomia: a reassessment of the Pruzansky and Kaban classification. *Plast Reconstr Surg.* 2014;133:174e–181e.

95. Tahiri Y, Chang C, Tuin J, et al. Costochondral grafting in craniofacial microsomia. *Plast Reconstr Surg.* 2015;135:530–541.

99. McCarthy JG, Schreiber J, Karp N, et al. Lengthening the human mandible by gradual distraction. *Plast Reconstr Surg.* 1992;89:1–8, discussion 9.

126. Stelnicki EJ, Hollier L, Lee C, et al. Distraction osteogenesis of costochondral bone grafts in the mandible. *Plast Reconstr Surg.* 2002;109:925–933, discussion 934–935.

Hemifacial atrophy

Peter J. Taub, Kathryn S. Torok, and Lindsay A. Schuster

SYNOPSIS

- Initially described in the writings of Dr. Caleb Hillier Parry.
- Exact etiology of PHA is not well understood, but is felt to have a strong autoimmune and neurogenic component.
- The initial clinical manifestations include both cutaneous findings and subcutaneous atrophy.
- Other forms of lipoatrophy are usually not localized to the face.
- The surgical treatment options currently offer the largest amount of tissue with excellent safety.
- Secondary procedures should be part of every treatment protocol.

 Access the Historical Perspective section online at
http://www.expertconsult.com

Introduction

Idiopathic progressive hemifacial atrophy (PHA), also termed Parry–Romberg syndrome, occurs in school-aged children with a slight female and no racial predominance.[19,20] PHA is typically characterized by slow progressive unilateral atrophy of the skin and soft tissue of the face, with deeper involvement of the underlying muscles and osteocartilaginous structures resulting in both aesthetic and functional orofacial issues. PHA is usually restricted to one side of the face, though bilateral facial involvement has been reported, and hemiatrophy of the ipsilateral extremity (arm and/or leg) and trunk is not uncommon (Fig. 35.1).[21] It is likely multifactorial in its etiopathogenesis; however, there is an autoimmune basis provided by histologic evidence of a lymphocytic neurovasculitis (skin and brain);[5,19,22] abnormalities on brain imaging consistent with an inflammatory and/or vasculitic process; and laboratory findings in the sera (autoantibodies), and the CSF (oligoclonal bands).[22,26]

Though controversial in the literature, PHA is considered to be on the same spectrum of disorders as its companion disease, "en coup de sabre" (ECDS), French for "like the cut of a sword", which describes the indentation of the scalp and forehead of these patients.[27] Both PHA and ECDS are considered to be subtypes of localized scleroderma, linear scleroderma affecting the head,[28] with "typical" PHA having more subcutaneous and bone atrophy (less obvious cutaneous findings) and ECDS having a hyperpigmented sclerotic cutaneous linear band with associated alopecia. *Some consider ECDS to be a subtype of PHA, and it is controversial if these two diagnoses are "one of the same" and a spectrum of the same disease process.* Many patients with linear scleroderma affecting the head (face and/or scalp) have a mixture of the two conditions (Fig. 35.1).[19,29,30] When investigated, both PHA and ECDS had the same amount of extracutaneous clinical manifestations[19,31,32] such as dental, eye, and neurologic involvement, further supporting that these conditions are on the same spectrum. Treatment often depends on the clinical assessment of the disease activity state. If cutaneous or extracutaneous manifestations appear to be advancing or show evidence of inflammation (as opposed to fibrosis), then systemic therapy with immunosuppression is warranted.[33,34] This can be followed by surgical intervention when deemed in the inactive state.

Basic science/disease process

The exact etiology of PHA is not well understood, but is felt to have a strong autoimmune and neurogenic component. Certain histologic findings have supported a combination of the two, which may be best described as a lymphocytic neurovasculitis.

Autoimmune process

PHA is a likely variant of the autoimmune disease "localized scleroderma", specifically the subtype of linear scleroderma

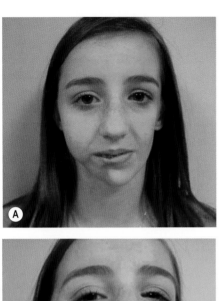

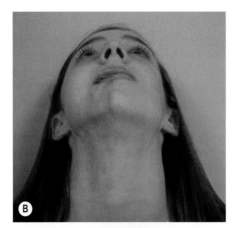

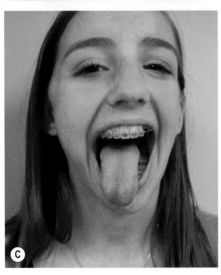

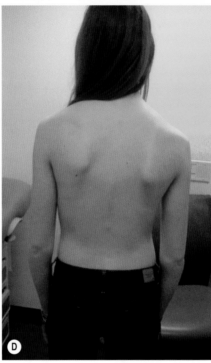

Fig. 35.1 (A,B) A 14-year-old girl with long-standing linear scleroderma of the head, both Parry–Romberg subtype (left hemifacial atrophy) and cutaneous en coup de sabre features (affecting her right lower face/neck). **(C)** She also has hemitongue atrophy, skewed palate, malocclusion, and other dental abnormalities. **(D)** Further examination supports hemiatrophy of right shoulder, upper back, and chest.

that affects the head (en coup de sabre, ECDS). It is often hard to differentiate these two entities, as ECDS often leads to atrophy of subcutaneous tissue and facial bones, causing hemifacial atrophy later in the disease course. Besides the clinical appearance, other etiologic, histologic, and clinical manifestations are similar between PHA and ECDS, which lend support to the theory of different spectra of the same disease. Both share similar characteristics, including age of onset, female preponderance, neurologic involvement, lymphocytic infiltrate on biopsy, and a clinical course of evolution for several years followed by stabilization. Positive autoantibodies, such as anti-nuclear, anti-histone, and anti-single-stranded DNA antibodies, which are found in ECDS, have also been demonstrated in "classic" PHA (hemifacial atrophy without sclerodermatous skin changes).[24,35,36]

Histologic findings

The histologic findings in PHA and ECDS are similar, though there are a few differences. PHA refers to idiopathic

progressive hemifacial atrophy usually without significant cutaneous involvement compared with ECDS, in which cutaneous findings of hyperpigmented and/or sclerotic linear markings are expected. However, skin biopsies performed in patients with idiopathic PHA that had no apparent cutaneous findings demonstrated a cellular infiltrate similar to localized scleroderma. A perivascular infiltrate of mononuclear cells, mostly lymphocytes and monocytes, has been demonstrated in the dermis,[19] with a particular focus surrounding the dermal neurovascular bundles, termed "lymphocytic neurovasculitis" by Mulliken and colleagues.[5] Under electron microscopy, degenerative alterations of the vascular endothelia were also documented. These findings suggest an autoimmune disease process similar to that of localized scleroderma.

There are a few histologic differences noted between ECDS/localized scleroderma and PHA. Although the dermal collagen fibrils appear more closely packed in patients with PHA,[5] they are not as homogenized and fragmented as seen in localized scleroderma. The elastic fibers are preserved and dermal appendages (hair follicles and sebaceous glands) are hypoplastic in PHA compared with the destruction of elastic fibers and atrophy of dermal appendages seen in ECDS.[37,38]

Neurogenic process

Several clinical manifestations support a neurogenic origin of PHA. The distribution of facial atrophy typically follows a dermatome of the *trigeminal nerve*, being unilateral in 95% of the cases and only rarely crossing the midline. Pensler *et al.* reported the initial distribution of atrophy among the divisions of the trigeminal nerve in 41 patients with PHA to be 35% in V1, 45% in V2, and 20% in V3, with eventual progression of disease to involve 65% in V1, 80% in V2, and 50% in V3.[5] Neuritis of the trigeminal nerve is suggested by several patients experiencing episodes of pain in the involved area prior to the onset of tissue atrophy.[39] An internet survey of 205 PHA patients by Stone *et al.* reported 46% of responders experienced facial pain.[20] The dermal lymphocytic infiltrate centered around neurovascular bundles in the dermis on histology also supports a neurologic target. Though most patients with PHA do not experience facial sensory, sympathetic, or parasympathetic dysfunction, some do experience peripheral facial nerve palsy, ocular motor palsy, and optic neuritis.[31,40]

Another theory involving the nervous system is the *hyperactivity of the sympathetic nervous system*, specifically inflammation of the superior cervical ganglion, causing features of PHA. Experimental animal studies support this hypothesis. Resende *et al.* ablated the superior cervical ganglion of rabbits, cats, and dogs and observed clinical features consistent with PHA within 30 days, such as localized alopecia, keratitis, enophthalmos, hemifacial atrophy with slight bone atrophy.[41] Moss and Crikelair also observed similar findings in an experimental rat model after unilateral cervical sympathectomy.[42]

Clinical, radiological, and CSF laboratory findings of patients with PHA highly support that the disease affects the *central nervous system*, likely in an autoimmune fashion. The clinical manifestations of CNS involvement are found in approximately 8–20% of the patients with PHA (same as that found in ECDS).[19] These are usually expressed as seizures, chronic headaches, and/or optic neuritis, and less commonly as neuropsychiatric disorders, deterioration of intelligence, and/or ischemic stroke. When brain imaging is performed in symptomatic patients, abnormalities such as atrophy and calcinosis are common, with up to 63% of 49 patients evaluated by Kister *et al.* having multiple or diffuse brain lesions on MRI.[31] A recent PHA cohort study evaluating abnormal brain imaging[30] noted that the most common finding was white matter T2 hyperintense lesions. Although found more heavily on the ipsilateral side of the face and scalp with subcutaneous atrophy, these lesions were present bilaterally in the majority, supporting a "regional inflammatory process". This is not found in other lateralizing neurocutaneous syndromes, such as Sturge–Weber syndrome,[43] which will more strongly lateralize to only the ipsilateral side, supporting a more developmental etiology, whereas PHA is considered acquired and likely an autoimmune process.

Lumbar puncture analysis of CSF reveals findings consistent with an inflammatory process, demonstrating oligoclonal bands and elevated IgG levels.[44] Further evidence supporting inflammation of the CNS are histologic findings of brain biopsies of PHA patients, which demonstrate the same changes as seen in the ECDS form of localized scleroderma: chronic perivascular lymphocytic inflammation with some vessels showing intimal thickening and hyalinization.[45]

Infection hypothesis

As in most autoimmune diseases, infectious agents have been postulated as an etiologic agent in PHA. The development of clinical disease manifestations has been noted to follow viral or bacterial infections. The most notorious suspect for both PHA and ECDS was *Borrelia burgdorferi*.[46,47] However, further studies have not substantiated this finding.[48,49] The viral infections indicated, such as Epstein Barr virus, correlate to the typical exposure to these infectious agents in first and second decades of life. However, they are more likely coincidental rather than etiologic factors.

Trauma

The role of trauma inducing PHA is quite controversial; however, in several patients a specific history of trauma to the affected area is elucidated, especially following tooth injury or extraction.[50,51] In a self-report survey of 205 patients with PHA, 12% reported injuries they thought could be directly related to their disease onset.[20] There have not been any standardized epidemiologic studies to verify this hypothesis.

Epidemiology

The incidence of PHA is not well defined but is tightly associated with that of the ECDS subtype of localized scleroderma, since many reviews reporting and summarizing these diseases are combined together.[5,36,52] The incidence of localized scleroderma is approximately 3 per 100 000 people, with a prevalence of 50 per 100 000 people. Of those with localized scleroderma, approximately 40% have the linear subtype; of this, only 30% affect the face and/or scalp, termed "en coup de sabre" (ECDS).[53] Therefore, an estimated incidence of 5 per 1 000 000 people and prevalence of 8 per 100 000 people is calculated for PHA. There is no racial predilection of PHA. There is a slight female predominance with most studies having female to male ratios between 2.2:1 and 3:1. The median age of onset for most studies is 10 years old with a general range of 5–15 years of age, which is consistent with ECDS.[54] Most cases of PHA are sporadic; however, a few familial cases have been reported.[7]

Clinical manifestations

The *initial* clinical manifestations include both cutaneous findings and subcutaneous atrophy. A recent survey of initial symptoms reported by 49 patients with PHA demonstrates 37% having hyperpigmentation or darkening of the skin, 22% having a hypopigmented spot or streak of skin, 6% with alopecia of the scalp, medial eyebrow or eyelashes, and 24% noticed an "indentation" signifying subcutaneous atrophy (Fig. 35.2).[55] The subcutaneous atrophy typically evolves first on the cheek or temple, and later extends to the brow, angle of mouth, and/or neck.[56] Later in the disease course, atrophy or growth arrest of the underlying bone and cartilage can occur, causing further facial deformity. Facial muscles may become atrophic, but they tend to maintain their

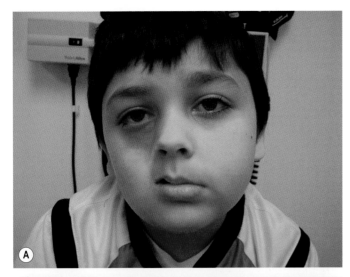

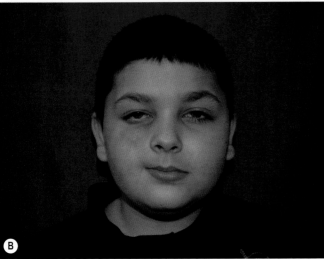

Fig. 35.2 (A) An 8-year-old boy with right hemifacial atrophy demonstrating absence of the medial lower eyelashes and a hyperpigmented lesion of the cheek with associated subcutaneous atrophy. **(B)** The patient 3 months postoperative, after two treatments with autologous structural fat grafting.

normal function. The disease typically progresses slowly over several years (2–10 years) and then tends to enter a stable phase.[50,56]

Cutaneous and subcutaneous involvement

Cutaneous color changes are a common finding in PHA. The discoloration is often described as a "bluish" or dark red, and is commonly mistaken for a bruise that does not heal (Fig. 35.3). This is thought to reflect increased vascularity during the active or inflammatory phase of the disease.[57] At times, the initial blue, violaceous, or erythematous phase is short and goes unnoticed, leaving behind post-inflammatory hyper- or hypopigmentation. These dyspigmentations are typically distributed in a dermatomal distribution along the trigeminal nerve.[5] If the skin lesion becomes fibrotic or atrophic and forms a well-demarcated linear depression (groove) in a frontoparietal or hemifacial distribution, it is considered to be more "classic" ECDS morphea or scleroderma of the head (Fig. 35.4).[58]

For many patients with ECDS after skin and subcutaneous induration and atrophy, the deeper tissues become involved, leading to the development of hemifacial atrophy. Therefore, the end result of ECDS appears the same as PHA without sclerodermatous changes. Cutaneous disease damage parameters include dyspigmentation (both hyperpigmentation and hypopigmentation), dermal atrophy (signified by shiny skin and visible veins), subcutaneous atrophy (described as a flattening or concavity of the subcutaneous tissue), and skin thickening/fibrosis at the center of the lesion.[59] Several skin appendages reside in the dermis, including sweat glands and hair follicles; therefore, alopecia of the scalp, eyebrow, and eyelashes is not uncommon.[60] Pensler *et al.* evaluated the severity of disease damage (in regard to subcutaneous atrophy) using multivariate analysis in a group of 42 patients with PHA, and found it not to be significantly influenced by trigeminal nerve distribution, side of face, age of onset, or extent (surface area) of the disease process.[5]

Musculoskeletal involvement

The facial musculature undergoes atrophy and thinning, mostly affecting the masseteric muscles, tongue (see Fig. 35.1C), and palatal muscles, though function is usually

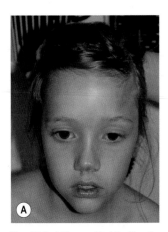

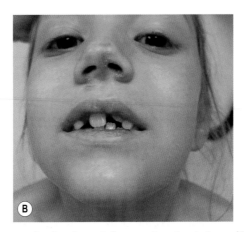

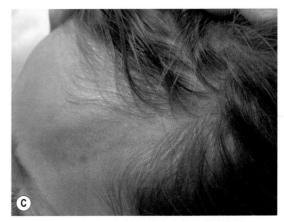

Fig. 35.3 A 7-year-old girl with active en coup de sabre, demonstrating an erythematous lesion on **(A)** the nose, **(B)** philtrum, and **(C)** left forehead.

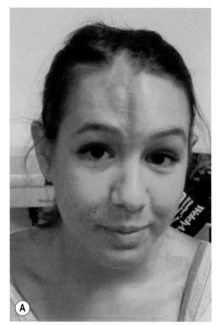

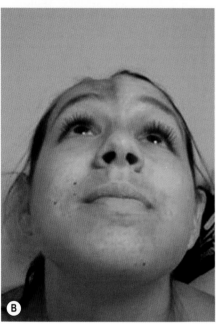

Fig. 35.4 (A,B) A 13-year-old girl with typical en coup de sabre lesion affecting the forehead and scalp with resultant skull depression.

can develop. Although enophthalmos is common when PHA involves the V1 distribution, the radiographic measurements of the skeletal orbit are normal, and the enophthalmos is more related to the atrophy of the periorbital subcutaneous tissues rather than skeletal hypoplasia.[5]

Central nervous system involvement

Central nervous system manifestations occur in approximately 8–21% of the patients with PHA and include seizures, hemiparesis, migraine headaches, neuropsychiatric disturbances, ischemic stroke, and intellectual deterioration.[19,20,31,52,54] These same manifestations and frequency of CNS involvement are reported in association with ECDS. Most patients have CNS symptoms years after the onset of cutaneous or subcutaneous findings, with a mean of 4.3 years, though a minority (approximately 16%) will have neurologic symptoms preceding cutaneous/subcutaneous involvement.[31]

The most common CNS manifestation is localization-related seizures. In a literature review cohort of 54 patients with PHA and/or ECDS that experienced neurologic symptoms, by Kister *et al.*, 73% experienced epilepsy, 33% in whom seizures were described as being refractory to medications.[31] In comparison with other autoimmune disorders of the CNS, such as multiple sclerosis, the brain lesions of PHA (and ECDS) appear to be more epileptogenic.[61] Supporting this notion are the findings of a recent PRS/ECDS cohort study of 88 subjects with the history of having a seizure – all of these patients had cortical or subcortical white matter T2 hyperintensities.[30] In contradiction to MS, focal CNS neurologic symptoms were uncommon in PHA, with only 11% of patients upon presentation and 35% of patients overall reported to have focal deficits (excluding facial palsy). The literature review of 54 cases by Kister *et al.* reported neuropsychiatric symptoms in 15% of the cases and headaches in 35%.[31] Stone's internet survey of 205 patients with PHA demonstrated that 46% of the patients reported anxiety; 10% reported depression with a Hospital Anxiety and Depression score (HADS) >8; and 52% reported migraine headaches.[20]

In those experiencing neurologic symptoms, brain imaging is often abnormal. In Kister's review, 49 of the 54 patients with PHA had an MRI performed, and 90% revealed an abnormality. In each patient, at least one T2 hyperintensity was observed, mainly in the subcortical white matter, followed by corpus callosum, deep gray nuclei, and brainstem (Fig. 35.5).[31] Other abnormalities detected on MRI are intraparenchymal calcifications and brain atrophy. Blaszczyk *et al.* reported an association between calcifications and focal epilepsy.[52] Brain atrophy has been observed and varies from being very focal and related to adjacent subcutaneous atrophy to more widespread, involving an entire cerebral hemisphere, but as with cutaneous disease, respects the midline and typically does not cross over to the opposite hemisphere.[31] MRI findings of cerebral atrophy and encephalomalacia did associate with the presence of seizures in a recent cohort study. There is no direct correlation between the degree of severity of skin and subcutaneous involvement and brain lesions, and several patients with PHA are neurologically asymptomatic, in spite of visible brain lesions.[62] The disease course of the neurologic and dermatologic manifestations also did not seem to correlate in two recent longitudinal cohort studies, which performed repeat imaging and neurologic assessment.[30,63] The

preserved. The degree of skeletal hypoplasia of the afflicted side of the face is dependent upon the age of onset, with those younger than the age of 10 years at onset having the highest risk.[39] It is hypothesized that the facial skeleton does not undergo atrophy, such as the subcutaneous tissue, but likely fails to develop (hypoplastic) during this period of bony growth, due possibly to the adjacent inflammatory and atrophic process of the overlying skin and subcutaneous tissue. The maxilla and mandible are most often involved, with both sagittal and vertical undergrowth, causing cosmetic and dental abnormalities, vertical undergrowth of the ramus, and a deficiency in posterior facial height results in hypoplasia of the mandible. Since hypoplasia of either maxilla and/or mandible is unilateral, profound tilting of the occlusal plane

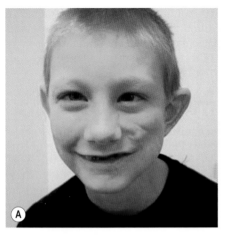
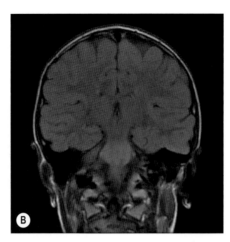
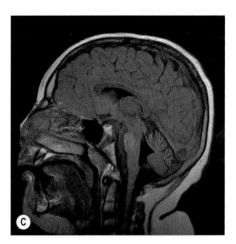

Fig. 35.5 (A) A 7-year-old boy with a 4-year history of PHA developed slurred speech and ataxia. **(B,C)** MRI of the brain demonstrated new T2 prolongation signal of the pons and cerebellar atrophy.

percentage of patients with PHA or ECDS that are neurologically asymptomatic with brain lesions is unknown given the small cohort studies, which do not routinely image all patients with these conditions.

In Kister's cohort of 54 patients, 20 had an MRA or cerebral angiogram performed, eight (40%) of which had vascular abnormalities consistent with vasculitis. Of these cases, biopsy-proven low-grade cerebral vasculitis was observed in three cases.[31] Brain biopsies of other select cases have found brain parenchymal inflammation with a perivascular lymphocytic cuffing.[45] Sclerosis, fibrosis, and gliosis of brain parenchyma, meninges, and vasculature have also been reported.[64] CSF findings in PHA/ECDS also support an inflammatory process by demonstrating oligoclonal bands and elevated IgG levels.[44]

Ocular involvement

A variety of ocular abnormalities have been associated with PHA, including alterations of the adnexal structures, anterior or posterior segments of the eye and the optic nerve. The frequency of involvement is unknown; however, a large portion of those in Kister's study and those in Stone's internet survey report eye findings, 29% and 46%, respectively, with uveitis, optic neuritis, and globe retraction being the most common.[31] Significant enophthalmos, principally due to soft tissue atrophy, is demonstrated in the majority of patients with facial atrophy in the first trigeminal nerve distribution.[5] Ocular muscle paralysis, ptosis, Horner syndrome, heterochromia iridis, and dilated fixed pupil have been reported. Inflammatory conditions of the eye have also been demonstrated, including uveitis (anterior and posterior), episcleritis, keratitis, choroiditis, and papilledema.[65,66] A careful ophthalmologic examination using a slit-lamp is recommended in patients with PHA and/or ECDS to assess for an inflammatory-fibrotic process, which may be arrested by immunosuppressive therapy.

Oral involvement

The soft tissue and craniofacial skeletal involvement of PHA can significantly affect the appearance and function of the

oral–facial complex. The tongue and upper lip on the affected side of the face are often markedly atrophic. The maxilla and mandible may be underdeveloped (hypoplastic), resulting in malocclusion and altered dentition. As a result of jaw hypoplasia, there is often a unilateral posterior crossbite and occlusal canting, and an abnormally skewed high arched palate may also be observed (Fig. 35.6). As the active stage of PHA coincides with the period of root formation and the eruption of permanent teeth, deficient root development and delayed tooth eruption are noted to occur.[67]

Radiographically, the teeth may have atrophic roots causing delayed tooth eruption, but affected teeth are clinically vital.[68] A total of 35% of 201 PHA patients in one survey complained of difficulty opening or closing the jaw, or of jaw pain.[20] Other reported oral characteristics of the disease include: rigid lips; lip incompetence/extra-oral exposure of teeth on the affected side; tongue sclerosis; limited mandibular movements; alteration of the position of the mandibular condyle in relation with the fossa; mandibular joint restriction (pseudoankylosis);[69] tooth root dilacerations;[70] chin point deviation to the affected side and, rarely, angular chelitis;[71] and absent parotid and submandibular glands.[68] One multi-center study of 16 patients reported that the main odontostomatologic complications were: malocclusion (94%); overgrowth tendency of the anterior lower third of the face (82%); gnathologic alterations (69%); dental anomalies (63%); skeletal asymmetry (56%); bone involvement (50%); and temporomandibular joint involvement (19%).[72] The patient in Fig. 35.5 depicts several of these oral–facial characteristics. Early orthodontic referral is important, as treatment during the phase of active facial growth and dental development facilitates the goal of optimized functional and cosmetic outcome.

Laboratory findings and prognostic indicators

A review of the literature and case series demonstrate that initial laboratory testing of inflammatory markers for disease activity assessment to be of limited use with only approximately 10% of the patients having an elevated white blood cell or eosinophil count, and 20% having an elevated sedimentation rate.[73] Autoantibodies, on the other hand, are quite

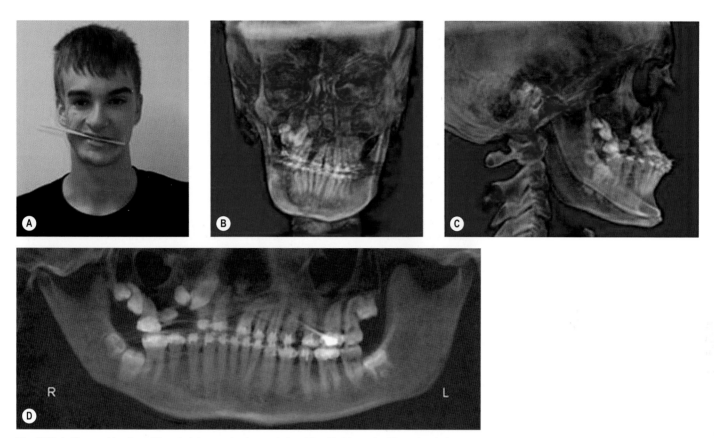

Fig. 35.6 A 15-year-old patient with orofacial anatomic characteristics of hemifacial atrophy. The patient is in orthodontic therapy to prepare for orthognathic surgical correction of the maxillary-mandibular occlusal cant and mandibular ramus height discrepancy. **(A,B)** Occlusal cant and chin point deviation to affected side. **(B–D)** Short mandibular ramus on affected side, asymmetric mandibular planes. **(C,D)** Maxillary right canine impaction, absent root formation, and lack of eruption of maxillary right premolars. Dilacerated maxillary right 2nd molar root. Impacted mandibular right 2nd molar.

common, with anti-nuclear antibody (ANA) positivity in 40–50% of the cases, demonstrating nucleolar, speckled, and homogenous staining patterns.[24,73] Specific antibodies to extractable nuclear antigens have also been found including anti-single stranded DNA (ss-DNA), anti-histone, anti-double-stranded DNA, anti-centromere, and anti-Scl-70 antibodies. Although these antibodies reflect autoimmune disease as an etiologic agent for PHA, they are not specifically associated with active or inactive disease. However, two of the antibodies, ss-DNA and anti-histone antibody, have been correlated to disease severity and progressive disease features, such as larger surface area of the lesion and continued spreading of the lesion in those with ECDS/PHA.[25]

Differential diagnosis

The main two entities included in the differential diagnosis of PHA are congenital hemifacial or craniofacial microsomia (CFM) and the ECDS subtype of localized scleroderma. CFM is present at birth and includes diminution in the size of face on the involved side, but it is not progressive like PHA. In contrast, ECDS is difficult to distinguish from PHA, and there are many that argue they are variants of the same disease rather than two distinct entities, as noted earlier. As ECDS results from an active stage, atrophy of the skin, subcutaneous tissue and bone is morphologically identical to that of the atrophy seen in PHA. *Some would categorize the hemifacial atrophy resulting from ECDS as a subtype of PHA.* A few possible differentiating features that are more distinct to ECDS, when compared with "classic" PHA, are scalp and forehead involvement, and induration of the skin and subcutaneous tissues during the acute phase. However, this is not clear as histologic evidence supports a similar lymphocytic infiltration in both entities, as well as shared neurologic and ophthalmologic features. There is considerable overlap between the two entities, with 30–40% of patients being classified as having coexistent ECDS and PHA (see Fig. 35.1).[19,31] In addition, there are several patients with PHA in association with different subtypes of localized scleroderma affecting other parts of the body besides scalp and face, such as deep, generalized, and plaque morphea (Fig. 35.7).[35]

Other forms of lipoatrophy are usually not localized to the face, such as lipodystrophy from congenital diseases such as Progeria, Dunnigan syndrome, and Kobberling syndrome. Other identified causes of widespread lipoatrophy are endocrine disorders, such as hyperthyroidism and diabetes; other autoimmune diseases, such as systemic sclerosis and dermatomyositis; and drug-induced atrophy, the most notorious being the protease inhibitors for the treatment of HIV. Other craniofacial conditions present with bone hypoplasia (i.e., hemifacial microsomia); however, these syndromes are associated with clinical features distinct from PHA.

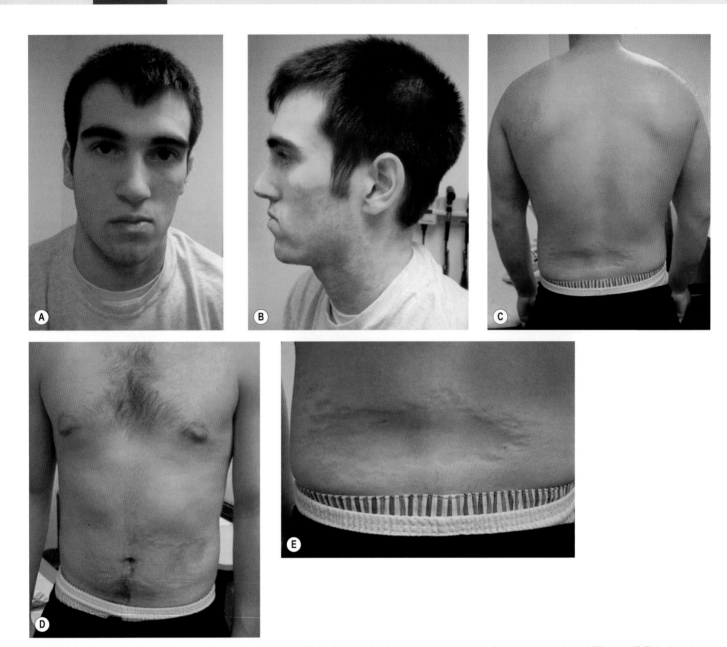

Fig. 35.7 A 17-year-old patient with progressive hemifacial atrophy, **(A)** involving the left face with coexistent generalized plaque morphea of **(B)** neck, **(C,E)** back, and **(D)** abdomen.

Patient selection

When selecting appropriate patients and options for treatment, several factors need be considered. These include: (1) the age of the patient; (2) the nature and the complexity of the deformity (i.e., which tissue types are affected); (3) the presence of associated disorders and conditions; (4) patient's understanding of the problem and what are the options for treatment; and (5) the timing for surgery.

Of these factors, the timing of the surgery is particularly important. It has been generally assumed that reconstructive surgery is best done only after the disease has "burned itself out"; and this could involve waiting as long as up to several years following what looks like the end of progression of the disorder. However, the literature also suggests

that earlier treatment with vascularized tissue, such as a free flap, is possible and that doing so may stop further tissue wasting (i.e., it may interrupt the progression of the disease). However, at this time, the more accepted opinion is to wait until the disease has run its course. Most importantly, treatment of this disorder is determined by the patient's individual deformity, ranging from mild to moderate to severe.

In the mild disease deformity, injectable materials, of which there are now many, may be sufficient to correct the deformity. For both mild and moderate deformities, the use of fat injections (structural fat grafting) has a significant role, as do buried dermal fat grafts. These can be used in more severe deformities as well, often as an adjunct to surgery. However, in the severe deformities, free tissue transfers are an option. In all deformities, combinations of buried materials, injected materials, and free tissue transfers in some combination all have a role to play.

When dealing with free tissue transfers, the original use of muscle and/or myocutaneous flaps, although generally satisfactory, were found to be bulky. Omentum, which also has a place as a free tissue transfer, has the downside of requiring an abdominal exploration and is somewhat harder to fix in place in the facial area. Consequently, fasciocutaneous flaps have become the present choice for free tissue transfer, and several have been described. These include the groin, the anterior lateral thigh, and the SIEA – with consideration being given to suiting the tissue transfer to the needs of the deformity. However, the commonest free tissue transfers now used are those based on the circumflex scapular pedicle, as these allow bulk and pliability as well as better fixation. These flaps can be taken in various combinations including the use of bone if needed.

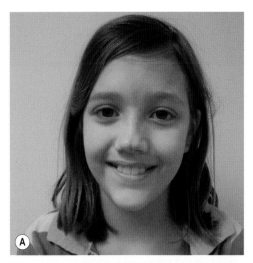

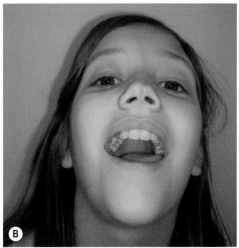

Fig. 35.8 (A,B) The 7-year-old girl pictured in Fig. 35.3, 3 years after initial immunosuppressive therapy with prednisone and methotrexate and continued low-dose therapy.

Treatment/surgical technique

Role of immunosuppression

In patients with PHA that have any cutaneous features of localized scleroderma, such as erythema/purple hue, induration, dyspigmentation or thickness/fibrosis, or the appearance of a demarcated line that is deepening as in ECDS, they should be considered candidates for immunosuppressive therapy. Patients with these features treated with immunosuppression, typically corticosteroids in combination with a disease-modifying agent such as methotrexate, have been found to have cessation of disease progression and reversal/improvement of disease damage (Fig. 35.8). For example, hyperpigmented skin becomes lighter; sclerotic skin softens; subcutaneous atrophy is less noticeable with some "filling in" of fat; hair growth is observed in areas of alopecia; and tongue atrophy is less dramatic.[74–77] Many PHA patients with neurologic manifestations, such as seizures and optic neuritis, have shown benefit from immunosuppressive therapy, and some of these manifestations have flared after weaning off therapy.[34] After a period of 3–5 years on immunosuppressive therapy and continued improved or stable examination and clinical findings, immunosuppression is weaned off as the disease is felt to have stabilized at that point. After an observation period of stable disease off medications, typically 1 year, then it is felt "safe" for surgical intervention.

Non-surgical intervention

Oral rehabilitation

Osseous defects are usually seen when the atrophy manifests before 15 years of age. Fronto-maxillary defects are seen in onset before 5 years of age and mandibular defects when the onset is between 5 and 15 years of age, and later onset (>15 years of age) has almost exclusively soft tissue changes.[78] Accordingly, oral rehabilitation options relate to the stage of onset and nature of anatomic involvement. Orthodontic treatment options include: (1) Phase 1 orthodontics, often to manage crossbite correction with orthopedic expansion of the maxillary mid-palatal suture and dental eruption guidance; (2) functional appliance therapy while the disease is in its active phase and facial skeletal growth is occurring; and/or (3) allowing for the disease progression and facial/skeletal growth to complete before addressing the resultant malocclusion with definitive combined orthodontic and orthognathic surgical intervention. Comprehensive oral/dental rehabilitation also includes prosthodontic treatment to replace missing or compromised dentition.

Orthodontic functional appliance therapy is the application of an oral appliance designed to alter the neuromuscular environment of the orofacial region to improve occlusal development and/or craniofacial skeletal growth.[79] Typically, these muscular forces are generated by altering the mandibular position sagittally and vertically, resulting in orthodontic and orthopedic changes. The period of treatment efficacy correlates with active jaw growth. Despite a long history of use (dating from the 1930s), there continues to be much controversy relating to functional appliance use, method of action, and effectiveness.[80]

The objective of functional appliance treatment in growing patients with PHA is maintenance of parallelism of the facial planes, specifically bilateral symmetry of mandibular ramus height and resultant mandibular plane. The intention of treatment is to stimulate condylar growth of the affected side in a vertical direction to obtain equal vertical development of the mandible and minimize progressive atrophy of facial growth.[67,81] Published case reports discuss the use of a removable orthodontic appliance with an acrylic bite block interposed between the maxillary and mandibular posterior teeth on the affected side.[67,81] In one report, active treatment spanned 6 years of appliance wear, 12–14 hours a day; monthly orthodontic visits for appliance adjustment were made during this treatment period. Therapy was reported to affect mandibular growth, reducing mandibular plane asymmetry. The resultant posterior open bite on the affected side was then treated with fixed orthodontic therapy.

Alloplastic fillers

The use of non-surgical alloplastic filling agents is advantageous for facial contour reconstruction because of the absence of a donor site and their abundant supply. These however, are counterbalanced by their increased susceptibility to local tissue responses, including capsule formation, seroma development, infection, and extrusion as well as their material cost. Examples include silicone gel, hydroxyapatite beads, and hyaluronic acid.

Autogenous filling material, such as fat, is advantageous because fat may be easily harvested from the patient with almost no donor site morbidity. While there is no possibility of rejection, atrophy of some portion of the grafted tissue is a known possibility. As well, in the exceptionally thin patient, subcutaneous fat might be difficult to identify.

Surgical intervention

The surgical treatment options offer larger amounts of tissue for reconstruction and are often used in conjunction with fillers to provide the best possible outcome.[82] These surgical options include dermal fat grafts, local/pedicles flaps, and free tissue transfer.

Dermal fat grafts may be used, and these are larger pieces of free fat grafts attached to the overlying dermis. The skin is first de-epithelialized *in situ*, and the graft is harvested as one unit.

Local pedicled flaps have been described to reconstruct deficits and deformities in the head and neck. However, their lack of significant bulk has limited their role in cases of extensive soft tissue deficit (Fig. 35.9). Soft tissue based on the superficial temporal pedicle may be rotated inferiorly to fill more superficial depressions. Attempts to augment the bulk of a local flap using a free dermal-fat graft, sandwiched between the folded superficial temporal fascia, have been described.[83]

Numerous free tissue transfers, or "free flaps" have been used to correct facial contour deformities in patients with PHA. These include free flaps of omentum, muscle, adipofascial, and often a combination of tissue types, which offer benefits over any single type alone. Smaller deficits may be reconstructed with smaller muscle or fascial flaps, such as the gracilis (Fig. 35.10) and radial forearm adipofascial flap, respectively.[84] Conversely, the deep inferior epigastric perforator (DIEP) flap can provide more soft tissue bulk in patients with significant deformities. In the heavier patient, the omentum, supplied by either the right or left gastroepiploic arteries, provides an adequate source of fat for soft tissue volume.[16,85,86] Of course, harvest requires entering the peritoneal cavity, either by traditional or laparoscopic means, and the lack of internal structure of the free flap often leads to soft tissue descent with time. Other choices include the superficial inferior epigastric artery (SIEA) flap,[87,88] the transverse rectus abdominis muscle (TRAM) flap,[89] and the deltopectoral flap.[90,91] Song *et al.* was the first to report the harvest and application of the anterolateral thigh adipofascial flap in 1984 (Fig. 35.11).[92] Advantages

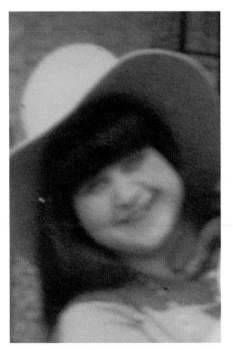
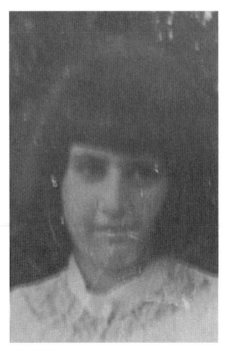
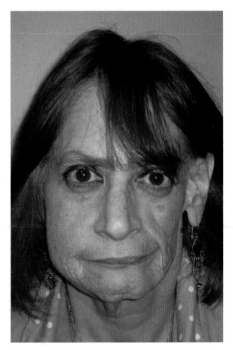

Fig. 35.9 A 59-year-old woman diagnosed with progressive hemifacial atrophy and treated with a tubed pedicle flap from the abdomen to the wrist and eventually to the face, where it was inset via a parotid incision.

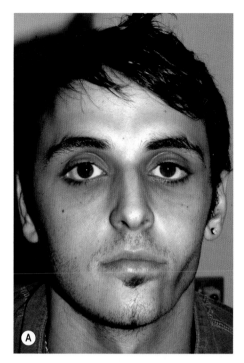
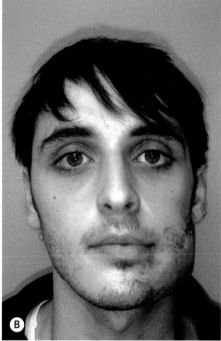
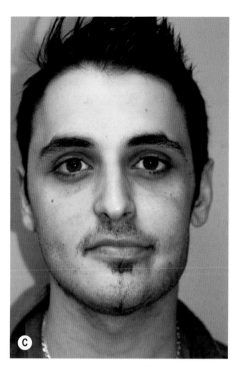

Fig. 35.10 (A) Preoperative photograph of a 20-year-old man with localized progressive hemifacial microsomia affecting primarily the left lower face. **(B)** Postoperative photograph following harvest and inset of a free gracilis flap. **(C)** Postoperative photograph following revision of the free gracilis flap by debulking.

of this flap include the ability to harvest the flap in the supine position away from the area of inset, the large, reliable skin flap that is available, its proximity to larger muscles that may be incorporated into the flap for bulk, and its relatively long vascular pedicle. The donor site defect may be closed directly, in the absence of sufficient tension, or reconstructed with a skin graft. Disadvantages to this flap include the variability of the skin perforators and the potentially tedious dissection of the pedicle if it courses within the muscle for an extended length.[93] If bone augmentation is required, the option of a vascularized costochondral graft taken with a latissimus dorsi musculocutaneous flap has been described.[94]

Scapular and parascapular flap

The scapular and parascapular adipofascial flaps, based on the circumflex scapular pedicle, are among the most useful flaps for restoring facial volume (Fig. 35.12).[95–98] Advantages include its relatively straightforward harvest, posterior torso donor scar, and minimal functional deficit. Disadvantages include the need to position the patient in either a prone or lateral decubitus position in order to harvest the flap. The authors prefer the lateral decubitus position so that the patient does not need to be turned during the case. However, less than adequate exposure of the contralateral face for comparison results.

The technique of soft tissue augmentation of the face begins with marking the patient for reconstruction (Fig. 35.13A). This should be done prior to positioning the patient in the operating room. A transparency of the defect can then be created using transparent X-ray film (Fig. 35.13B). Once anesthetized, the patient is carefully positioned either in a true lateral decubitus position or supine, with the ipsilateral shoulder turned to expose the posterior torso if a scapular or parascapular flap is to be used. The apex of the skin paddle is centered over the triangular space bounded by the teres minor, teres major, and long head of triceps. The vessel within the triangular space is checked with the Doppler. The axillary artery gives off the subscapular artery, which in turn gives rise to the circumflex scapular artery about 1–4 centimeters from its origin. Occasionally, the circumflex scapular artery can arise directly off the axillary artery. The circumflex scapular artery usually travels with paired venae comitantes and the subscapular artery travels with a single vein. The circumflex scapular artery enters the posterior torso via the triangular space and gives off a transverse cutaneous scapular branch and a vertical parascapular branch. The latter supplies the parascapular flap. The transparency made from the defect can then be used to maximize soft tissue harvest (Fig. 35.13C).

The incisions at the donor and recipient sites are injected with lidocaine and epinephrine. Lubrication is placed in the eyes and a temporary tarsorrhaphy can be used to protect the corneas. The face is prepped with dilute Betadine solution. The procedure begins with creation of the subcutaneous pocket at the recipient site deficient in soft tissue volume. The extent of the dissection must extend beyond the borders of the atrophy to allow for adequate contouring. Suitable recipient vessels are identified for the vascular anastomosis. At the conclusion of this portion of the dissection, careful hemostasis is achieved with a bipolar electrocautery and counted sponges are left beneath the dissected skin envelope.

Next, the flap is harvested from the posterior torso. This may be done without having to turn the patient significantly. The trapezius and infraspinatus muscles should be identified early in the dissection since they serve as important landmarks for flap dissection, which should proceed from medial to lateral and inferior to superior. Flap elevation is best performed in the looser areolar tissue just above the muscular fascia. If flap elevation proceeds deep to the fascia, the dissection can become confusing where the pedicle exits the triangular space.

The flap can be completely de-epithelialized and buried or left with a thin cutaneous paddle, incorporated into the closure and available for postoperative flap monitoring (Fig. 35.13D). The flap periphery should be contoured and fixed to the skin with overlying bolsters. Several points of fixation are

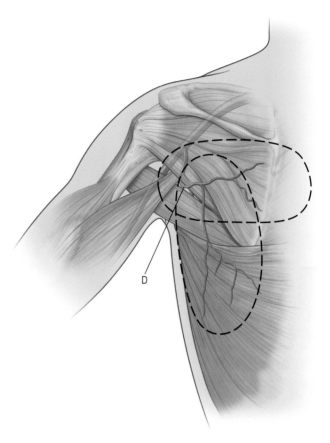

Fig. 35.12 The anatomy of the parascapular flap. D, circumflex scapular artery.

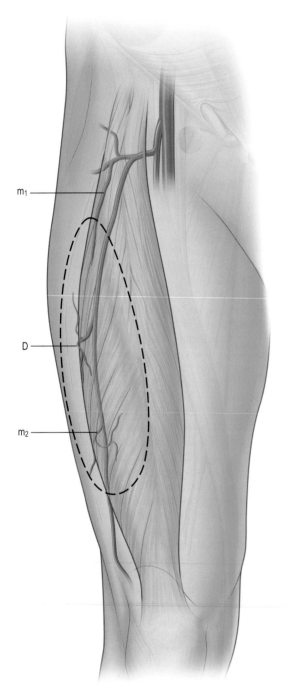

Fig. 35.11 The anatomy of the anterolateral thigh flap. D, septocutaneous perforators of the descending branch of the circumflex femoral artery; m₁, musculocutaneous perforators of the transverse branch of the lateral circumflex femoral artery; m₂, musculocutaneous perforators of the descending branch of the lateral circumflex femoral artery.

required. At each point, a narrow roll of Vaseline gauze is fabricated as a tie-over bolster. Fixation involves passing a smooth nylon or Prolene suture completely through one side of the Vaseline gauze bolsters. It is then passed through the skin and into the pocket for the flap. A mattress suture is used to grab the flap and the suture is passed back into the pocket and out of the skin in proximity to the entrance point. It then passes through the other end of the bolster and is left long while each of the remaining sutures are placed. When all sutures are positioned, each is tied down, making sure the flap is completely passed into each of the pockets that have been dissected out (Fig. 35.13E).

A single small drain is placed in the facial site, and a second larger drain is left in the donor site. The former is removed prior to discharge if the output is sufficiently small. The latter is left in longer because of its tendency to continue to drain serous fluid. The wounds are closed in layers and the face dressed with bacitracin to avoid pressure over the flap.

Even in the absence of a skin paddle, an audible Doppler signal through the skin should be recorded every hour for the first day and then every 2 hours for the second day. Patients are kept NPO for the first night and then gradually advanced to clears and a regular diet.

Orthognathic surgical treatment

It has been observed that the earlier the symptoms appear, the more progressive the bony atrophy becomes.[99] In severe cases, soft tissue augmentation may not be sufficient to camouflage

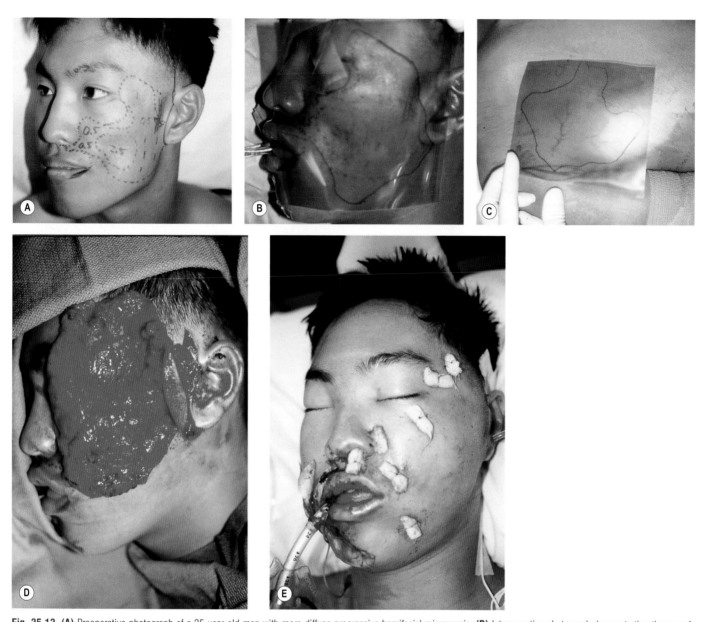

Fig. 35.13 (A) Preoperative photograph of a 25-year-old man with more diffuse progressive hemifacial microsomia. **(B)** Intraoperative photograph demonstrating the use of X-ray film to map the extent of involvement and soft-tissue requirement. **(C)** Intraoperative photograph demonstrating transfer of the template to the posterior torso prior to harvest of a parascapular free flap. **(D)** Intraoperative photograph of the flap positioned over the ipsilateral face prior to inset. Note the thin, vertical skin paddle left over the proximal portion of the flap that is used to monitor the viability of the flap postoperatively. **(E)** Intraoperative photograph following inset of the free parascapular flap. Note the use of Vaseline gauze tie-over bolsters to hold the distal margins of the flap in their respective subcutaneous pockets.

the patient's facial and occlusal asymmetries. The skeletal deformities in PHA that are treated with combined orthodontic and orthognathic surgery include: (1) hypoplasia of the zygomatic complex and maxilla which can cause orbital dystopia and depressive deformities in the zygomaticomaxillary region; the maxilla tilts upward and backward and the volume is reduced; and (2) hypoplasia of the mandible, especially the ramus, which causes obvious deviation of the chin and occlusal plane.[100]

Pre-surgical fixed orthodontic appliances (braces) are typically required to prepare for harmonious postoperative occlusion, and facilitate intraoperative movement and postoperative retention of jaw position. A period of postoperative

orthodontic treatment is required to create an optimal occlusal result. Surgical procedures utilized to address the maxillary and mandibular dysmorphologies of PHA include LeFort I osteotomy, total mandibular subapical osteotomy, MEDPOR implants, bone grafting of osseous defects, rib grafting, mandibular lengthening, genioplasty, and mandibular distraction.[100–102] Typically, reconstructive surgery is deferred until the disease process ceases. The effect of PHA on oral–facial function and appearance can be profound. Orthodontic referral at the time of disease onset is important as treatment during the phase of active facial growth and dental development facilitates the comprehensive goal of optimized functional and cosmetic outcomes.

Outcomes, prognosis, and complications

The outcomes from soft tissue augmentation should be satisfactory, with symmetry as the ultimate goal. At present, free tissue survival is highly successful especially in younger patients with healthy donor and recipient vascularity. Success is predicated more on identifying the tissue types involved, the precise location of the deficit, and subsequently choosing an appropriate intervention strategy. Certainly, incorporating multiple reconstructive strategies is reasonable and often preferable.

Secondary procedures

Following reconstruction with free tissue transfer, secondary revision should be considered part of every treatment protocol. It would be exceedingly unusual for the exact amount of tissue to be harvested and placed at the initial procedure. Edema progresses during surgery and blurs the boundaries between normal and deficient tissue.

The first revision is not planned any sooner than 6 months following the initial flap placement to allow any postoperative edema to resolve and the flap to develop a secondary blood supply from the surrounding tissues. Some patients may benefit from waiting even longer if continued changes in the face are noted. Debulking the flap may be achieved with either direct excision, suction lipectomy, or a combination of the two.

The existing incisions are usually sufficient for access to the flap. At 6 months, it is unlikely that interruption of the pedicle would lead to compromise of the flap. However, the location of the vascular pedicle should be known, so it may be avoided and bleeding minimized. Again, bolsters may be used to fix underlying soft tissue into place. Further refinements of the flap are certainly plausible to address persistent concerns.

Debulking of the flap is usually one component of the revision, along with further addition of soft tissue to areas that remain deficient. In the latter instance, flap tissue from overly bulky areas may be rotated and transferred to areas with a persistent lack of volume. Similarly, additional autogenous fat or alloplastic filler may be used for smaller areas of need.

🌐 Access the complete reference list online at   **http://www.expertconsult.com**

1. Parry C. *Collections From Unpublished Medical Writings of the Late Caleb Hillier Parry*. Vol. I. London: Underwoods; 1825:478.

2. Romberg M. *Trophoneurosen in Romberg's Klinische Ergebrisee*. Berlin: Forstner; 1846:75–81.

3. Eulenberg A. *Lehrbuch der Functionellen Nervenkrakheiten*. Berlin: Hirshwald; 1871.

4. Wartenberg R. Progressive facial hemihypertrophy. *Arch Neurol Psychiatr*. 1945;54:75–96.

5. Pensler JM, Murphy GF, Mulliken JB. Clinical and ultrastructural studies of Romberg's hemifacial atrophy. *Plast Reconstr Surg*. 1990;85:669–676.

6. Rogers BO. *Progressive Facial Hemiatrophy: Romberg's Disease; a Review of 772 Cases*. Third International Congress in Plastic Surgery. Amsterdam: Excerpta Medica; 1964:681.

7. Lewkonia RM, Lowry RB. Progressive hemifacial atrophy (Parry–Romberg syndrome) report with review of genetics and nosology. *Am J Med Genet*. 1983;14:385–390.

8. Blair B, referred to by Padgett E and Stephenson K. *Plastic and Reconstructive Surgery*. Springfield: CC Thomas; 1948:569.

9. Sarnat BG, Greeley PW. Effect of injury upon growth and some comments on surgical treatment. *Plast Reconstr Surg (1946)*. 1953;11:39–48.

10. Neumann CG. The use of large buried pedicled flaps of dermis and fat; clinical and pathological evaluation in the treatment of progressive facial hemiatrophy. *Plast Reconstr Surg (1946)*. 1953;11:315–332.

36

Pierre Robin Sequence

Chad A. Purnell and Arun K. Gosain

Access video and video lecture content for this chapter online at expertconsult.com

SYNOPSIS

- Pierre Robin Sequence (PRS) is a clinical triad consisting of glossoptosis, retrognathia, airway compromise, often with clefting of the secondary palate.
- PRS can be an isolated entity or found in association with many syndromes, most commonly Stickler syndrome.
- The spectrum of symptoms is vast and a multidisciplinary evaluation is necessary.
- This work-up must begin with an airway assessment.
- Respiratory distress can be managed with prone positioning and supplemental oxygen for the majority of children with PRS and isolated base-of-tongue airway obstruction.
- Nasopharyngeal airway is indicated if these measures are inadequate.
- Surgical intervention may be indicated for airway problems refractory to conservative measures, and this primarily consists of tongue-lip adhesion, mandibular distraction, or tracheostomy. There is debate over the preferred surgical management.
- Nutritional support is required for most patients. Specialized bottles, nipples, feeding positions, or feeding tubes may be utilized.
- The PRS patient must be followed throughout childhood by a multidisciplinary team.

Historical perspective

The earliest account of a presentation of PRS dates back to 1822 by St. Hilaire, followed by Fairbain in 1846.[1] Later in the 19th century, attempts were made to subclassify the clinical entity, by Taruffi into those with "hypomicrognathus" and those with "hypoagnathus". These descriptions demonstrate that as early as the 19th century, clinicians understood that a major component of this entity was the mandible. In 1891, Lanneloague and Monard described four cases, two of which had an associated cleft of the palate. In 1902, Shukowsky presented a case of a hypoplastic mandible causing respiratory distress.

Despite earlier descriptions, the condition bears the name of the French stomatologist Dr. Pierre Robin. Dr. Robin lived from 1867 to 1949 and was a professor in the French School of Stomatology as well as the editor of the periodical *Stomatologie*. His main contribution to the body of knowledge regarding PRS was its dissemination. Beginning in 1923, he wrote 17 articles on the problems of "glossoptosis" and is credited with introducing the term. He highlighted the severity of the potential respiratory complications and the difficulty these children have with feeding and weight gain.[2,3] Robin felt that the more severe cases were quite dire and wrote, "I have never seen a child live more than 16–18 months who presented with hypoplasia such as the lower maxilla was pushed more than 1 cm behind the upper." To combat the airway compromise, Robin preferred a "monobloc" dental orthopedic appliance to keep the mandible forward to restore the normal mandibulo-maxillary relationship. Unfortunately, Robin drew many extraneous associations to this cohort and overestimated the incidence of the clinical entity at three out of five live births (Fig. 36.1).

In 1902, Shukowsky performed the first tongue-lip adhesion (TLA) by simply suturing the tongue to the lip, but the description was not published until 1911.[4] This was successful in one patient, but another patient died of asphyxia when the suture pulled through the tongue. The use of TLA was not widely accepted during these initial descriptions. For the next four decades, primary treatment for respiratory distress in this cohort consisted of external traction devices placed on the mandible. One such device consisted of a pediatric back brace with a halo from which traction was applied. This was maintained for 4 weeks and was usually successful in alleviating the airway compromise. This modality, however, led to a significant amount of temporomandibular joint ankylosis. Then, in the 1940s, Douglas published a refined technique of TLA and a resurgence in the technique occurred.[5]

PRS has evolved in name since the early descriptions as the understanding of the etiopathogenesis has advanced. Initially, the clinical constellation was termed "Pierre Robin syndrome". In 1976, Gorlin, Pinborg, and Cohen created the term "Pierre

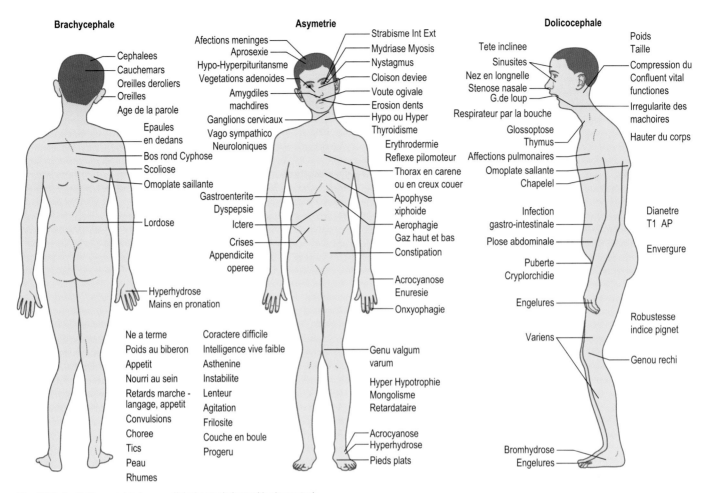

Fig. 36.1 Dr. Robin postulated many clinical associations with glossoptosis.

Robin anomalad", noting that this entity was not a syndrome.[6] The term "anomalad" was used to describe an etiologically nonspecific complex that could occur with various syndromes of known or unknown origin or in isolation. Some authors began to use the phrase "Robin complex" but this was shortly replaced by "Pierre Robin Sequence" (PRS) or "Robin sequence" by Pasyayan and Lewis in 1984.[7] Purists feel that eponyms should not include first names and prefer "Robin sequence".

In the last three decades, significant debate has arisen regarding the diagnosis, natural history, and treatment of PRS. A significant portion of this debate surrounds the rise in popularity of distraction osteogenesis (DO), and the indications for this technique in PRS. At this time, the paradigm of treatment appears to be shifting towards expanding indications for distraction osteogenesis; however, an absence of well-designed studies evaluating long-term outcomes of TLA and DO limit the ability to make definitive decisions regarding these procedures.

Basic science/disease process

PRS is a clinical triad consisting of glossoptosis, retrognathia, and airway obstruction. The term "glossoptosis" refers to a posteriorly displaced tongue that obstructs the airway and does not refer to an enlarged tongue. A cleft palate is not obligatory for the diagnosis. Cleft palate can be U- or V-shaped and is present in approximately 50% of cases (Fig. 36.2). PRS can be an isolated entity or found in the clinical setting of a syndromic child. Some 30–60% of patients with PRS have an associated syndrome.[8–10]

The incidence of PRS is estimated to be from 1:8500 to 1:20000 live births.[10–12] There are no gender differences in incidence, except in extremely rare X-linked syndromic associations.

The etiology of PRS is still unclear and is likely multifactorial. Before any etiological considerations, a clear understanding of the difference between a syndrome and clinical sequence is important. A syndrome refers to a group of signs and symptoms that vary in degree of expression but ultimately result from a single pathologic insult. A sequence describes a spectrum of anomalies that may be instigated by varying disease processes, but ultimately converge in the same phenotypic findings. This differentiation is germane as a portion of patients with PRS will also be syndromic, such as Stickler syndrome. The converse does not hold true, as not all patients with Stickler syndrome have the phenotypic findings of PRS (Fig. 36.3).

The etiology of PRS is not completely clear and is likely multifactorial. Shprintzen[13] classified etiology as "malformational" or "deformational". "Malformational" refers to a mandibular predisposition to be retrognathic, such as in Treacher Collins, Nager, or Stickler syndromes. "Deformational"

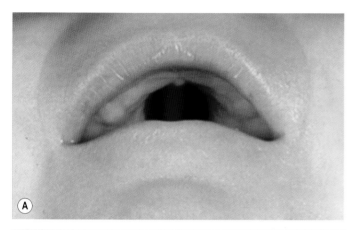

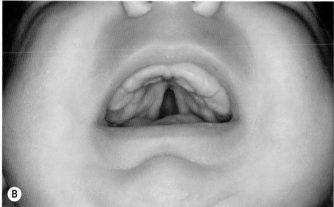

Fig. 36.2 **(A)** This child with Pierre Robin Sequence demonstrates the classic U-shaped cleft palate. **(B)** The cleft palate in Pierre Robin Sequence may also take the form of a V.

formation of PRS. Possible causative teratogens include alcohol, trimethadione, and hydantoin.[17]

Due to the multiple syndromes associated with PRS and its multifactorial etiopathogenesis, analysis of inheritance is complex. Cohen[18] reported up to 18 associated syndromes with PRS in 1978. The current list of recognized associations is quite extensive (Box 36.1).

The most frequently associated syndrome with PRS is Stickler syndrome, which is associated with 11–20% of PRS cases.[8–10,22,23] Multiple subtypes of this connective tissue disorder exist, most commonly with autosomal dominant inheritance. Causative genes include COL2A1 (12q13, accounts for 80–90% of cases), COL9A1, COL11A1 (1p21), or COL11A2 (6p21), which affect type II, IX, or XI collagens.[24] Stickler syndrome is characterized by midline clefting, flattened midface, hypoplastic mandible, flat nasal bridge, long philtrum, epicanthal folds, prominent eyes, retinal detachment, cataracts, joint hypermobility, and sensorineural hearing loss. Molecular genetic testing for causative genes is available; but most often, initial diagnosis is clinical.

The second most commonly associated syndrome with PRS is velocardiofacial syndrome (Shprintzen syndrome), which is associated with 11% of PRS cases.[23] The etiopathogenesis is secondary to a deletion in 22q11.2, hence the updated nomenclature 22q11.2 deletion syndrome. Characteristics include cleft palate, mandibular hypoplasia, long upper lip and philtrum, an elongated face, almond-shaped eyes, a wide nose, small ears, conductive hearing loss, slender digits, hypoparathyroidism, immune dysfunction (thymic aplasia), and learning disabilities. The cardiothoracic anomalies can include pulmonary atresia, ventricular septal defect, and hypoplastic pulmonary arteries. Approximately 21% of patients have micrognathia, and 11% have cleft palate.[25]

Nager syndrome, or acrofacial dysostosis, is a rare syndrome that can demonstrate autosomal-recessive or, more commonly, autosomal-dominant inheritance.[26,27] The majority

refers to an intrauterine growth restriction that places the child's chin in a flexed position into the chest, restricting growth. He hypothesized that restriction could be caused by a multigravid pregnancy, oligohydramnios, or a uterine anomaly.

Chiriac and colleagues[14] postulated three theories regarding the etiology of PRS. In the "mechanical theory", the inciting event is mandibular hypoplasia that occurs in the 7th–11th week of gestational life from various etiologies. The effect is a tongue that rides high in the oral cavity and interferes with the movement of the lateral palatine processes as they progress from a vertical to horizontal orientation (Fig. 36.4). Experimental animal models support this sequence of events.[15,16] Some feel a U-shaped palatal cleft is more common in PRS due to this wide blockage by the tongue; however clinically, both U- and V-shaped clefts have been noted. In the "neurologic maturation theory", a neuromuscular delay occurs in the musculature to the tongue, pharyngeal pillars, and palate. The delay has been noted on electromyogram in PRS. In the "rhombencephalic dysneuralation theory", motor and regulatory organization of the rhombencephalon is related to a major complication in development.

Cohen[17] also described several distinct mechanisms of etiopathogenesis: malformation, deformation, and connective tissue dysplasia. This final mechanism describes a link between diseases of "connective tissue dysplasia" and PRS, such as Stickler syndrome. Many authors also agree upon the potential influence of intrauterine teratogen exposure in the

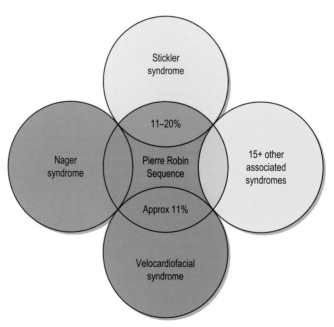

Fig. 36.3 There are many syndromes associated with Pierre Robin Sequence; however, it can also be found in isolation.

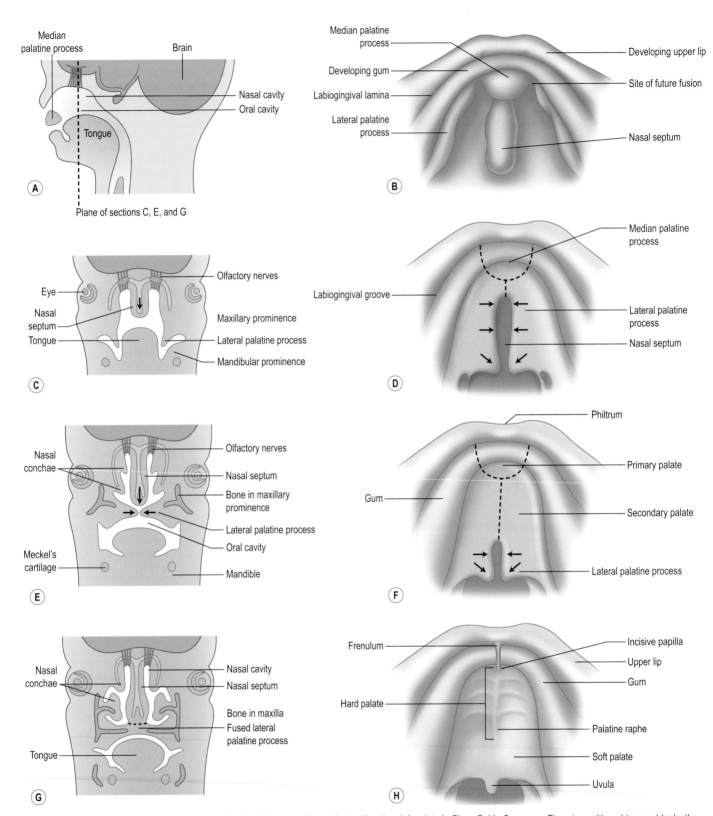

Fig. 36.4 (**A–H**) The embryology of the tongue and palate is important for understanding the cleft palate in Pierre Robin Sequence. The retropositioned tongue blocks the movement of the lateral palatine processes from a vertical to horizontal position.

BOX 36.1 There are many recognized syndromes associated with Pierre Robin Sequence. The postulated or known genetic loci are shown for several syndromes.[8,17,19–21]

- Abruzzo–Erickson syndrome
- Achondrogenesis type II: 12q13.11-q13.2, COL2A1
- ADAM sequence (anionic deformity, adhesions, mutilations)
- Amniotic band disruption
- Andersen–Tawil: 17q23.1-q24.2, KCNJ2 gene
- Beckwith–Wiedemann syndrome: locus 11p15.5, 11p15.5, 11p15.5, 5q35. p57, H19, LIT1
- Bruce–Winship syndrome
- Campomelic syndrome
- Carey–Fineman–Ziter
- Catel–Manzke syndrome
- Cerebrocostomandibular syndrome
- CHARGE association
- Chitayat syndrome
- Collagen XI gene sequence
- Congenital myotonic dystrophy
- Del (4q) syndrome
- Del (6q) syndrome
- Diastrophic dysplasia
- Distal arthrogryposis–Robin sequence
- Donlan syndrome
- Dup (11q) syndrome
- Femoral dysgenesis–unusual facies syndrome
- Fetal alcohol syndrome
- Froster contracture–torticollis syndrome
- Kabuki syndrome
- Larsen syndrome: 3p14.3, mutations in FLNB (Filamin B) gene
- Marshall syndrome: COL11A1
- Martsolf syndrome: 1q41 gene encoding protein RAB3GAP2
- Miller–Dieker syndrome: 17p13.3
- Möbius syndrome: 13q12.2-q13
- Nager syndrome: SF3B4, 9q32
- PARC syndrome (poikiloderma, alopecia, retrognathism, cleft palate)
- Persistent left superior vena cava syndrome
- Popliteal pterygium syndrome
- Postaxial acrofacial dysostosis (Miller syndrome)
- Radiohumeral synostosis
- Richieri–Costa syndrome
- Robin–oligodactyly syndrome
- Sanderson–Fraser syndrome
- Spondyloepiphyseal dysplasia congenital: 12q13.11-q13.2, COL2A1
- Stickler syndrome: 12q13.11-q13.2, COL2A1, COL9A1, COL11A1, COL11A2
- Stoll syndrome
- TARP Syndrome (RBM10, X-linked)
- Toriello–Carey syndrome
- Treacher Collins syndrome: mutation in the "treacle" gene (TCOF1), locus 5q32-q33.1
- Velocardiofacial syndrome: microdeletion at the q11.2 band of chromosome 22
- Weissenbacher–Zweymuller syndrome (otospondylomegaepiphyseal dysplasia) (type II Stickler or "nonocular Stickler Syndrome"): gene COL11A2 locus 6p21.3

---

of cases are caused by haploinsufficiency of gene SF3B4.[28] The craniofacial features are similar to Treacher Collins syndrome, with downward-slanting palpebral fissures and mandibular and malar hypoplasia. Additionally, these patients may have hypoplasia or agenesis of the thumbs, radius, and occasionally lower extremity malformations with short stature. Cleft palate is often present. The mandibular hypoplasia can be severe and patients do not have normal mandibular growth potential.[26,27]

Diagnosis/patient presentation

The spectrum of severity of PRS can be quite varied. Secondary respiratory disturbances are equally varied; these range from mild with subtle findings on polysomnogram to profound, requiring emergent intubation at birth. In severe cases, periodic desaturations may occur, along with retractions, stridor, or hypoxia and hypoxemic neurologic injury. Untreated, these children can progress to develop cor pulmonale. Children with PRS consistently have an obstruction localized to the level of the base of the tongue due to glossoptosis. However, synchronous airway lesions are common in PRS in up to 28% of patients.[29,30] The most common of these is laryngomalacia and 10–15% of infants with PRS have been found to have this loss of support of supraglottic structures.

Cardiac abnormalities are also commonly found associated with PRS. Congenital heart defects are associated with PRS in 14–30% of cases.[31–33] Cardiac findings can be isolated or a result of a syndromic association. The presence of cardiac abnormalities is associated with increased mortality in the population of PRS patients initially admitted to an intensive care unit.[33]

Infants with PRS may also present with feeding difficulties and failure to thrive. Poor feeding, long feeding times, hypoxia during feeding, gagging, vomiting, aspiration, frequent pneumonia, and gastroesophageal reflux disease are possible. The failure to thrive in this cohort has dual causality from both the poor intake and from the increased metabolic demand from increased respiratory effort and prolonged feeding times.[34] Feeding difficulties in PRS are multifactorial. Airway compromise can lead to gastroesophageal reflux through decreased intrathoracic pressure, and reflux can exacerbate respiratory issues.[35] Additionally, children with PRS have abnormal oroesophageal motility, and syndromic PRS patients often have abnormal oral and/or facial muscle innervation.[36–38]

Estimates of mortality have improved as both the understanding of and treatment options for PRS have evolved. As stated above, Robin painted a bleak picture for any child with PRS.[39] In 1946, Douglas reported >50% mortality with conservative treatment.[5] The major cause of mortality was felt to be secondary to aspiration. In 1994, Caouette-Laberge et al.[40]

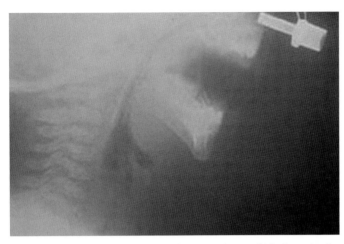

Fig. 36.5 A lateral radiograph demonstrating a nasopharyngeal tube bypassing the base-of-tongue obstruction.

stratified mortality into three groups. For those with adequate respiration in prone positioning and the ability to be bottle-fed, the mortality was found to be 1.8%, increasing to 10% if gavage feeds were required. Mortality increased further to 41% in those with respiratory distress necessitating endotracheal intubation and gavage feeds. More recently, Costa *et al.* describe an 11-year series of 181 patients, with an overall 16.6% mortality rate. Concomitant cardiac and neurologic malformations were the greatest predictors of mortality. There were no deaths in isolated PRS patients.[33]

Patient selection

While prenatal diagnosis of PRS can be successfully accomplished,[41–43] the vast majority of cases are noted on or after the first day of life.[44] The best setting for a child with suspicion of PRS is in a tertiary care institution with a multidisciplinary pediatric team. This team should include a pediatric pulmonologist, geneticist, speech therapist, nutritionist, anesthesiologist, otolaryngologist, and craniofacial surgeon.[45]

As respiratory distress may be lethal, initial management of the airway is of paramount importance. For the child suspected of having PRS, resuscitation according to the American Academy of Pediatrics Neonatal Resuscitation Program begins with prone positioning and supplemental oxygen. If this fails, then a laryngeal mask airway (LMA) or nasopharyngeal airway can be attempted (Fig. 36.5). If this modality fails, then endotracheal intubation may be necessary, and can be aided with a fiberoptic laryngoscope.[46] Intubation is challenging due to retrognathia and glossoptosis, and there have been many descriptions of specialized intubation techniques in this population.[46,47] All the prior steps are contingent on the neonate's cardiopulmonary status, the skill of the physician managing the airway, and the availability of proper equipment. If all else fails in the acute setting, an emergency tracheotomy may be indicated. If a child is prenatally diagnosed with multiple congenital anomalies including micrognathia, an EXIT (*ex utero* intrapartum treatment) airway management procedure may be a viable option.[48] In this scenario, the airway can be secured while the child is still receiving placental circulation. Once the airway is secured, further evaluation may proceed.

The interaction with the PRS child does not necessarily begin in the delivery suite. Patients with more subtle signs may have a more delayed presentation.[49] Once clinical suspicion of PRS is raised, a stepwise work-up should ensue. The work-up should be centered on the significant effects experienced by the PRS patient: the presence of respiratory and feeding difficulties. One must also be mindful of any failed measures previously attempted for the patient. Multiple modalities are required to adequately assess a patient's degree of airway compromise and to guide therapy.

A thorough history should be obtained that includes the mother's history and the patient's prenatal course. Key points to elucidate from the history are maternal alcohol or drug consumption, infections during pregnancy, prenatal care and screening, and a family history of genetic syndromes.

The pathognomonic mandible must be assessed. A metric is needed for initial assessment and growth monitoring of the diminutive mandible in the absence of dentition. This can be simply obtained by using a wooden end of a cotton-tipped applicator or tongue depressor to measure the maxillary-mandibular discrepancy (MMD).[49,50] The stick is pressed against the anterior aspect of the gingiva of the mandibular alveolus and a mark is made at the anterior aspect of the maxillary alveolus (Fig. 36.6). This MMD can be variable if not performed systematically. As the mandible has a tendency to fall posteriorly in the supine position, the MMD should be obtained with the child upright. Some authors have stated that an MMD of 8–10 mm is an indication for surgical treatment. Robin himself stated that no infant lived past 18 months of age when the MMD was >10 mm.[51] However, in practice, this distance should act as a guide and not as an absolute for selecting a treatment modality; surgical indications should arise from the overall clinical picture and additional objective assessments.

Respiratory assessment is essential in selecting the proper treatment for PRS. Respiratory compromise occurs from birth until growth of the mandible allows the base of the tongue to clear the airway and the oropharyngeal musculature gains the control required to keep the airway patent, or occasionally not at all. Some feel that the obstructive events in newborns with PRS increase in frequency in the initial 4 weeks of life; therefore, a false sense of security should not occur after a brief evaluation. In a series by Gosain and colleagues, 18 patients presented in the 1st week of life and three patients presented between 12 and 33 months of age.[49] Initial assessment should include continuous pulse oximetry in different scenarios: while the child is awake, sleeping, and feeding. The monitoring time required during sleep should be a minimum of 12 h for neonates and a regular period of sleep for children. The criteria for desaturations are defined as having any single oxygen saturation value <80% at any time or if oxygen saturation values are <90% for 5% or more of the monitored time.[49] A second portion of the initial airway evaluation is a formal polysomnogram, both with and without a nasopharyngeal airway in place. Polysomnography is useful to identify occult obstructive sleep apnea (OSA), which is present in over 50% of patients with PRS, and is often quite severe.[34,52,53] If OSA resolves with a nasopharyngeal airway in place, this suggests, but does not confirm, that the obstruction is isolated to the tongue base. If the patient has desaturations on continuous pulse oximetry or OSA on polysomnogram, endoscopic evaluation of the airway is performed.

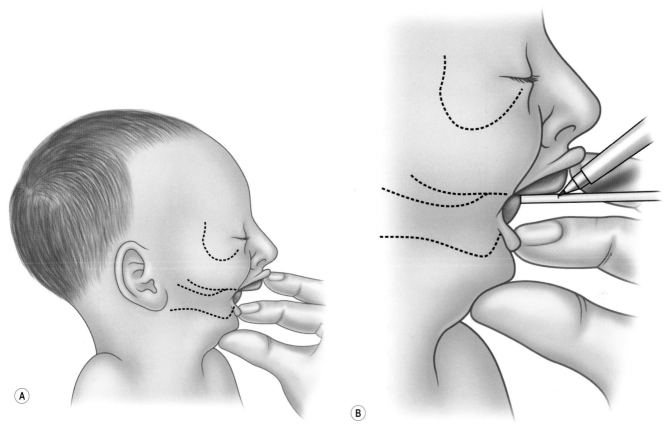

Fig. 36.6 **(A)** The objective measurement of the mandibular-maxillary discrepancy should be standardized with the child in the upright position with the mandible gently supported without translating it out of position. **(B)** The mandibular maxillary discrepancy is then measured by marking the distance from the most anterior aspect of the mandibular alveolus to the most anterior aspect of the maxillary alveolus on a cotton-tipped applicator. This is then measured with a ruler.

Endoscopic evaluation in PRS should include both nasoendoscopy and bronchoscopy. This is paramount to demonstrate the proper level of obstruction. There are three main subdivisions: no visible obstruction, tongue base obstruction, or infraglottic obstruction. Care must be taken not simply to stop after visualizing a tongue base obstruction, because synchronous airway lesions occur in up to 28% of patients. Occasionally, the craniofacial surgeon will be consulted after intubation or tracheostomy. These patients will still require endoscopic evaluation, and if the patient is intubated, nasendoscopy should be done in the setting in which the endotracheal tube can be withdrawn during examination to evaluate the native airway, and replaced immediately following evaluation. If the nasendoscopy in a child suspected of having PRS demonstrates no visible obstruction, one must suspect a central nervous system or pulmonary disorder. It is appropriate to obtain the consultation of a pediatric neurologist and pediatric pulmonologist.

Sher and colleagues[54] described four types of obstruction seen via flexible nasopharyngoscopy in 53 children with neonatal OSA, the majority of whom had micrognathia. Type 1 is described as "true glossoptosis", and consists of a tongue that contacts the posterior pharynx at a level below the soft palate (Fig. 36.7). Type 2 consists of a tongue that is displaced posteriorly as in type 1, but at the level of or above the soft palate, such that the palate becomes sandwiched between the tongue and posterior pharyngeal wall in the upper oropharynx (Fig. 36.8). Type 3 consists of an obstruction caused by a medial collapse of the lateral pharyngeal walls (Fig. 36.9). Type 4 consists of the pharynx collapsing or constricting as a sphincter (Fig. 36.10). In this analysis, 59% of patients were classified as type 1; 21% were type 2; 10% were type 3; and 10% were type 4.

Bronchoscopy is indicated in order to rule out a concomitant subglottic airway obstruction. As stated earlier, synchronous airway lesions are common in PRS, most commonly laryngomalacia.[29] However, not all airway lesions are equal, and laryngomalacia's role in PRS has been debated. As the natural history of this obstruction is that the majority resolves with time, some groups will treat PRS without additional intervention for laryngomalacia unless needed later.[55,56]

All patients with PRS should have a complete feeding assessment, as a majority have some type of feeding difficulty, especially in syndromic associations.[57,58] This begins by plotting the child on a growth chart to determine the starting point and successive trend in weight. Most patients with PRS are below the 50th percentile initially.[45] Additionally, a downward trend in weight can be seen without treatment. The child should also have a formal assessment by a speech therapist, including visual observation of feeding with concurrent pulse oximetry. Children with PRS usually have prolonged feeding times and oroesophageal discoordination.[38] Patients may gag

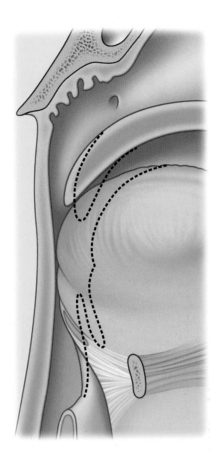

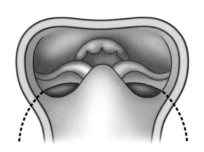

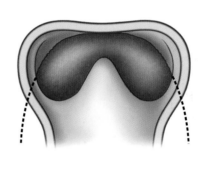

Fig. 36.7 Description of the types of obstruction seen endoscopically in children with Pierre Robin Sequence. Type 1 obstruction is described as "true glossoptosis", and consists of a tongue that contacts the posterior pharynx at a level below the soft palate. *(Reproduced from Sher AE, Sphrintzen RJ, Thorpy MJ. Endoscopic observations of obstructive sleep apnea in children with anomalous upper airways: predictive and therapeutic value. Int J Pediatr Otorhinolaryngol 1986; 11:135.)*

and cough during feeds or even become hypoxic. In addition, it has been suggested that up to 87% of infants with PRS have gastroesophageal reflux.[35,59] The PRS child is already predisposed to aspiration, and the addition of significant reflux only compounds this. A pH probe can be utilized to determine if the child would benefit from medical treatment. However, many PRS patients have reflux that may not be detected on standard pH monitoring, so these results should be interpreted with caution, and manometry should be considered if clinical suspicion is high.[38] Further evaluation with videofluoroscopic swallow studies or upper GI series should be performed at the discretion of speech therapists. A majority of patients with PRS will require temporary supplemental feeding strategies such as a nasogastric tube.[57] Of note, the intrinsic esophageal dysfunction in PRS appears to spontaneously regress by 12 months of age.[38]

Evaluation by a clinical geneticist is indicated and further work-up is guided by physical examination and clinical suspicion. Hearing and ocular evaluation, in particular, should be performed on each child with PRS. The reasons for this are twofold: often PRS is the only initial presentation of Stickler syndrome, and PRS patients in general appear to be at higher risk for hearing loss than other cleft patients.[60,61] In one series, 83% of children with PRS had some degree of hearing loss versus 60% of children with a cleft palate only.[60] The hearing loss was also more profound in children with PRS, and typically conductive in nature. There was also an increased incidence of middle-ear effusions, despite normal middle- and inner-ear anatomy. If cleft palate is present, the anomalous insertion of the tensor veli palatini and levator veli palatini muscles predisposes to eustachian tube

dysfunction. The orifice of the eustachian tube may also be chronically inflamed from continuous reflux secondary to the cleft palate.

Treatment

Treatment of airway obstruction in PRS is a complex decision given the heterogeneity of patient presentation. As in the diagnostic work-up of these patients, one should begin with the least invasive, most appropriate modality first. There are two main categories for airway management: non-surgical and surgical.

To begin a discussion of the treatment of the airway obstruction, the underlying mechanism must be understood. Robin[39] described the mechanism as a tongue that is displaced posteriorly due to the retrognathic mandible. Others have similarly described the tongue base acting as a "ball valve" draping over the glottis (Fig. 36.11). The muscular coordination of the oropharynx also plays a role in the obstruction. Neuromuscular impairment may predispose the airway to collapse. Inadequate functioning of the genioglossus was described by Delorme et al.[62] In this description, the genioglossus is shortened and rotates the tongue posteriorly. Delorme and colleagues went on to postulate that this causes the retropositioned mandible, and not the converse. This theory is not widely accepted, but demonstrates the complexity and lack of consensus of the possible etiology. Secondary airway lesions also exacerbate airway obstruction.

Another point of contention is the role that cleft palate plays in PRS. Some feel that this anatomic finding will

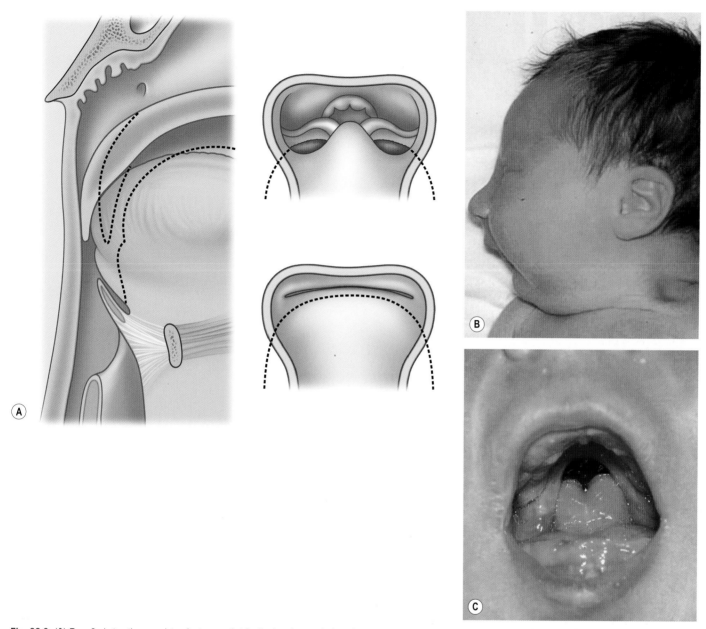

Fig. 36.8 **(A)** Type 2 obstruction consists of a tongue that is displaced posteriorly as in type 1 but at the level of or above the soft palate, such that the palate becomes sandwiched between the tongue and posterior pharyngeal wall in the upper oropharynx. **(B,C)** This child demonstrates a cleft palate with the tongue displaced cranially above the palate.

exacerbate the upper airway obstruction. Hotz and Gnoinski theorized that the tongue may become impacted in the palatal cleft, perpetuating the posterior positioning of the tongue and upper airway obstruction (Fig. 36.12).[63] Others assert that the cleft may be beneficial and act as an oronasal passage for air.

The natural history of the mandible in PRS is a widely debated topic. Pruzansky initially described disproportionately rapid "catch-up" growth of the mandible in patients over time, with a concomitant improvement in the airway.[64] Over time, this finding has been utilized to justify conservative interventions, allowing the mandible in PRS to grow and resolve airway issues. However, later published cephalometric data has added nuance to this idea. While it does appear that in many cases the MMD in PRS improves with time, the maxilla is also smaller than normal, and

therefore a normal dental arch relationship does not necessarily imply normal size of the mandible.[49,65–67] While an increased rate of growth between 3 months and 2 years of age in isolated PRS mandibles was supported in one well-designed study,[68] studies from a smaller cohort have not supported any increased growth rate at all from 2 months to 22 months.[69,70] Different syndromes also appear to have differing mandibular growth potential, with velocardiofacial and Stickler syndrome having more normal growth than Treacher Collins, Nager syndrome, or bilateral craniofacial microsomia.[71] The largest studies to date appear to indicate that faster than normal "catch-up" growth does not occur past 5 years of life; and the mandible, maxilla, and airway remain smaller than normal controls throughout childhood.[67,68,71–74]

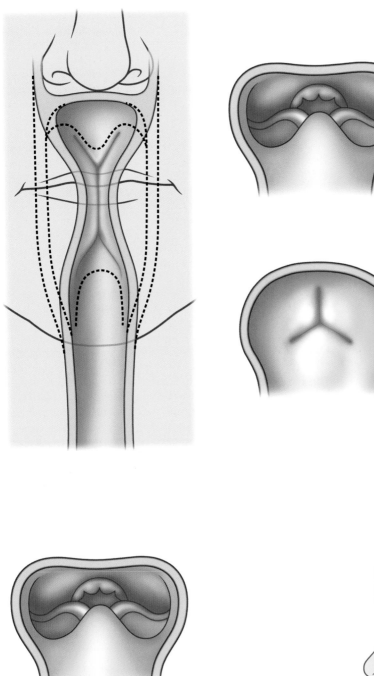

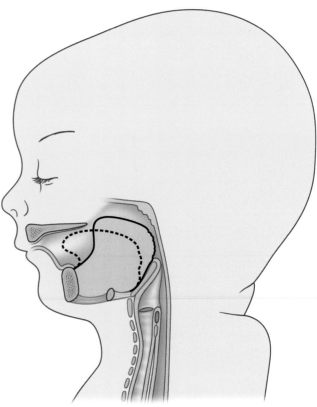

Fig. 36.9 Type 3 obstruction consists of an obstruction caused by a medial collapse of the lateral pharyngeal walls.

Fig. 36.10 Type 4 obstruction consists of the pharynx collapsing or constricting as a sphincter.

Fig. 36.11 The tongue displaces posteriorly and can act as a ball valve. The dashed line demonstrates the normal position of the tongue. The solid line depicts the possible position of the tongue in Pierre Robin Sequence.

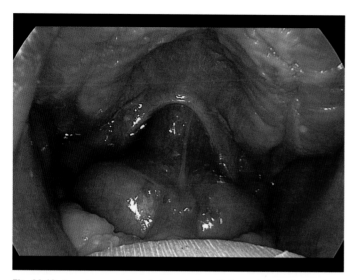

Fig. 36.12 An endoscopic view of glossoptosis, with the posteriorly displaced tongue entrapped in the palatal cleft and completely occluding the oropharynx.

Non-surgical airway management

A majority of patients with PRS (especially isolated PRS) can be managed non-surgically.[9,10,12,57,75] However, the importance of complete evaluation during these maneuvers cannot be stressed enough. Once an intervention is found to improve oxygen saturation acutely, continuous pulse oximetry and polysomnogram should be performed to confirm resolution of obstructive symptoms. The algorithm for the acute management of the airway in this cohort was described earlier. Prone positioning is the initial maneuver attempted in airway management. This acts to displace the chin and tongue base forward. The benefit of this maneuver was described by Robin in 1934[51] and radiographically confirmed by Sjolin in 1950.[76]

Cogswell and Easton[77] showed that the least resistance to airflow for children with PRS is in the prone position. Providing the child with supplemental oxygen can bolster this maneuver. If effective, the prone position must be maintained 24 h a day, even during feeding, baths, and diaper changes (Fig. 36.13). Prone positioning may be the only therapy used in patients with PRS if there is adequate parental understanding and support; however, maintaining this at all times can be challenging.

If prone positioning fails, then a nasopharyngeal airway should be considered.[78] Some authors recommend placement at the epiglottis, or until the resolution of the obstruction occurs. Several centers have had success with long-term management of PRS with nasopharyngeal airway alone.[79–83] Treatment setting for nasopharyngeal airway may be as an inpatient or outpatient.[81,84] In the largest series of nasopharyngeal management of PRS to date, 77 patients had attempted management with nasopharyngeal airway alone. Of these, 63 (81.8%) had successful treatment, with a mean hospital stay of 10 days. Patients were discharged home after parental competence was demonstrated and a post-airway polysomnogram showed significant improvement. The mean time until airway removal was 8 months, as guided by polysomnogram. While nasopharyngeal airway clearly is a viable option for PRS management, it requires significant parental education and involvement, as well as frequent follow-up, or long hospital stays if inpatient management is chosen.[79,81,84]

If nasopharyngeal stenting is not successful, then nasal continuous positive airway pressure can be undertaken, and if successful, has been described for long-term therapy.[85] Further management may include LMA or endotracheal intubation. In the moment of airway compromise, some instruments may not be readily accessible or timely; therefore some steps may be skipped and the child may need immediate endotracheal intubation.

If endoscopic evaluation reveals isolated tongue-base obstruction, a variety of palatal appliances have been described

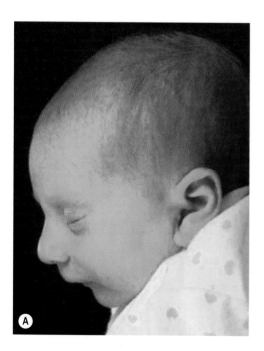

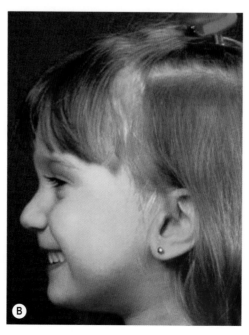

Fig. 36.13 A female with isolated Pierre Robin Sequence treated with prone positioning alone at 1 week old versus 3 years old. Note the improvement in MMD with time.

for treatment.[86–89] These acrylic plates act to push the base of the tongue anteriorly (Fig. 36.14). In the largest report of plate usage, relief of airway obstruction was achieved in 122/134 neonates (91%) diagnosed with PRS. However, the plate was less successful in relieving feeding difficulty, with 26.2% of patients requiring nasogastric or gastrostomy feedings.[88]

Surgical airway management

Surgical management is indicated if conservative measures fail to relieve airway obstruction, if a family is unable to comply with non-surgical home therapy, if a child's syndromic associations predict failure of conservative treatment, if a

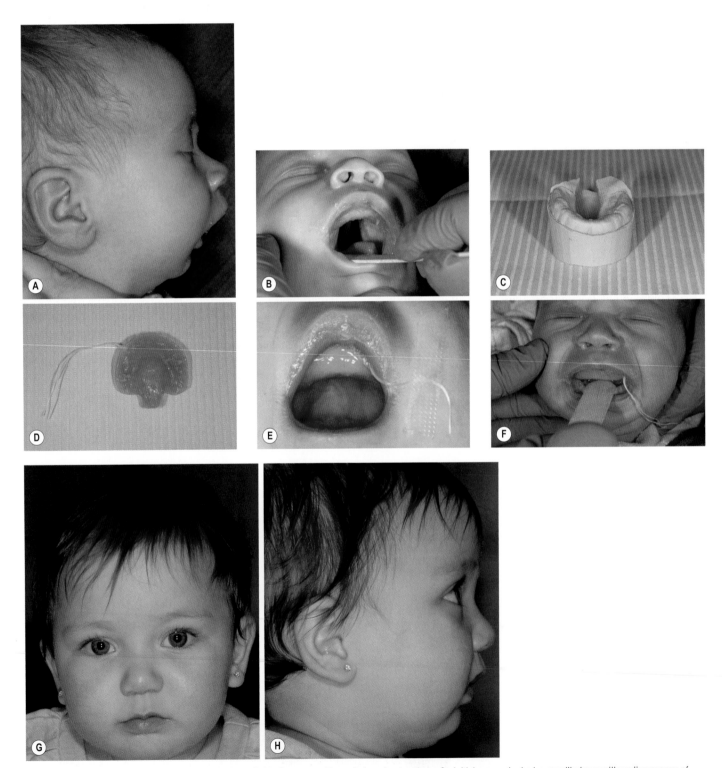

Fig. 36.14 **(A)** A 3-month-old infant with isolated Pierre Robin Sequence with respiratory desaturations. On initial exam, she had a mandibular maxillary discrepancy of 4 mm. **(B)** The patient had a cleft palate. **(C,D)** A mold was made and a dental plate was fashioned. **(E,F)** The plate fits comfortably and is held in place with dental adhesive. **(G,H)** The patient at 6 months of age with a mandibular-maxillary discrepancy of zero. She did not require supplemental oxygen and was feeding well.

child is unable to be extubated, or if the medical team and family agree to pursue a more invasive course of treatment. Airway management can be accomplished with soft-tissue or skeletal techniques, or with tracheostomy. Significant controversy remains as to the optimal management, indications, and contraindications of these procedures.[90,91] Differences also exist between regions of the country and between subspecialty preferences for treatment.[92,93]

Soft-tissue techniques

While many soft-tissue techniques have been developed, all rely on anterior advancement of the tongue to relieve upper airway obstruction. Tongue-lip adhesion (TLA) was originally described by Shukowsky in 1911. In his technique, the tongue was simply sutured to the lower lip.[4] The concept was then popularized by Douglas in 1946.[5] In Douglas' technique, a rectangular area is denuded under the tongue, along the floor of the mouth, on the alveolus, and on to the lower lip. The tongue is then brought forward, and these raw surfaces are sutured together. A mattress tension suture passes from the dorsum of the tongue to the chin. This technique was modified by Routledge in 1960,[94] and more recently modified by Argamaso.[95] TLA remains a common treatment at many centers, with continued modifications. The authors' preferred technique is comprised of elevating a proximally based rectangular mucosal flap from the ventral surface of the tongue and a complementary superiorly based mucosal flap from the labial surface of the lower lip (Figs. 36.15–36.18). These flaps are approximately 1×1.5 cm in size. If a short or tight lingual frenum is present, a frenulotomy or a frenectomy can be beneficial. In the modification described by Argamaso,[95] the genioglossus muscle is detached from the mandible with a small periosteal elevator. The tongue-based flap is sutured to

the inferior side of the opposing defect in the mucosa of the lower lip. The exposed tongue musculature is then sutured to the exposed orbicularis oris and anterior soft tissues through a small incision caudal to the mandibular symphysis. A larger stay or suspension suture is passed in a circummandibular fashion into the muscular substance of the tongue in order to pull the tongue anteriorly. Several authors have described using various methods to accomplish this, including Keith needles or an awl.[95,96] This suture can then be tied over a button or buried in the muscular substance of the adhesion.[97,98] A nasopharyngeal tube may be placed and left indwelling for 2–3 days if there is ongoing airway compromise secondary to swelling. Feeding is often compromised, and can be administered by a nasogastric or orogastric tube. These children should remain in an intensive care setting during the postoperative period as they are extubated in a guarded manner and to ensure that the airway remains patent afterwards.

The timing of the takedown of a TLA is an important aspect of the procedure. Some authors recommended repair of the cleft palate, if present, at the same time as the TLA takedown. This methodology can lead to unnecessary prolongation of the TLA with the potential for oromotor retardation. In addition, a combined cleft palate repair and TLA takedown may produce substantial airway edema and respiratory compromise. Conservative guidelines include evaluation of the child at 1 month of age to assure the TLA was successful. Afterwards, evaluations should be performed every 2 months until the adhesion is taken down. The evaluation focuses on tongue motion, which is infantile and possibly dormant early in life. As the child matures, the tongue will exhibit rhythmic muscular movements. A good clinical indicator of tongue maturity is active motion in response to touch. The decision to take down the TLA should be based on tongue activity in response to stimulus, improvement in the MMD, and the overall

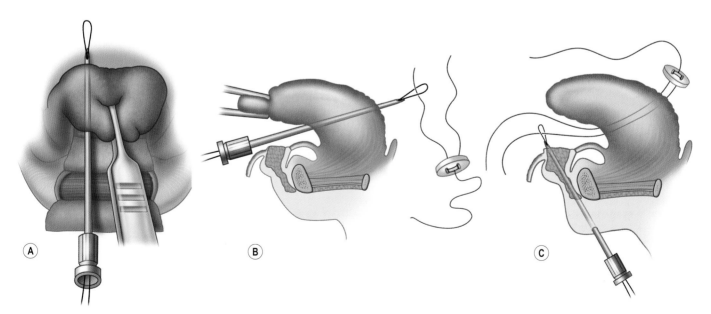

Fig. 36.15 (A–C) In a tongue lip adhesion a posteriorly based flap is elevated from the tongue and a corresponding mucosal flap is elevated from the labial surface of the lower lip. Care is taken not to injure the Wharton's ducts. The tongue-based flap is inset to the caudal margin of the defect created by the elevation of the lip-based flap. A non-resorbable suture is then passed through the tongue and brought through the raw surface created by the flap elevation. The suture is then passed through the raw surface created by the labial flap, taking care to catch orbicularis oris. The suture is then brought out through the submental area by passing anterior to the mandible. The labially based flap is then inset into the tongue defect.

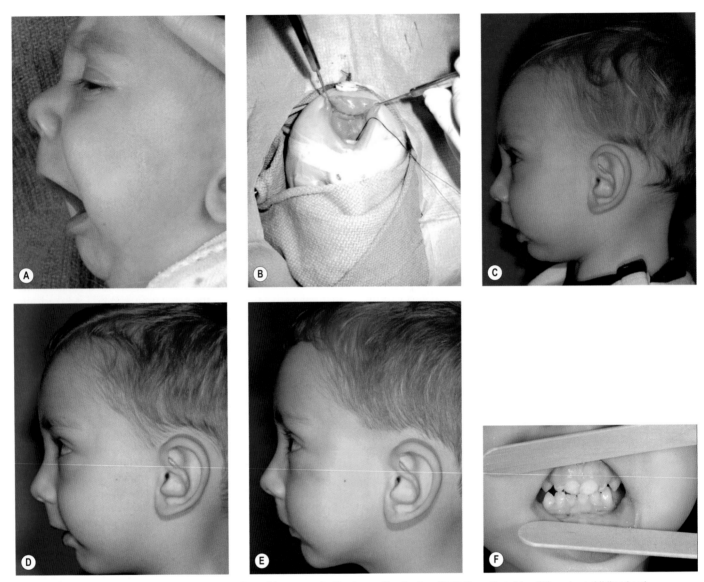

Fig. 36.16 (**A**) A child with Pierre Robin Sequence. (**B**) The child was treated with a tongue-lip adhesion. (**C–F**) The patient did well throughout childhood and demonstrated good mandibular growth over time.

clinical picture. An MMD of 3 mm or less is usually a good prognostic indicator that the TLA can be taken down safely, but larger discrepancies may still be acceptable for takedown of TLA in the face of a very active tongue and a clinically robust child. Using these guidelines, most adhesions are able to be reversed by 6–7 months of age.[49] Elective palate repair

is performed separately at the routine time interval, which is at age 11–12 months at the authors' institution. To takedown the TLA, the two mucosal flaps are incised and the intervening tissue between these flaps is divided by electrocautery. The flaps are then closed such that no raw surfaces remain that could result in scar contracture. Using this protocol, the

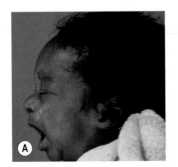

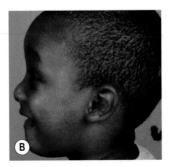

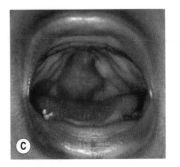

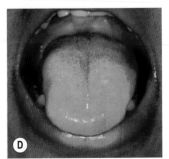

Fig. 36.17 (**A–D**) A child treated successfully for airway compromise and feeding difficulties with tongue-lip adhesion alone.

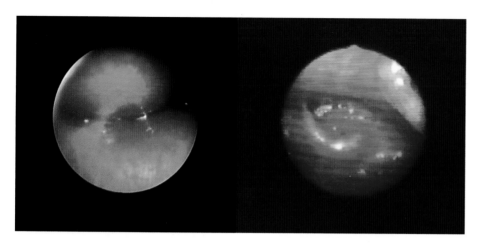

Fig. 36.18 Left: the same patient as in Fig. 36.17 demonstrating glossoptosis on nasoendoscopy. Right: the airway is cleared 3 days after tongue-lip adhesion.

authors have not had any residual tongue dysmorphia or impairment in tongue motility.

Proponents of TLA cite that it is a minimal operation that allows natural mandibular "catch-up" growth to occur without restriction. They also note minimal long-term morbidity and a favorable complication profile if performed by experienced surgeons.

The literature regarding TLA is divided. Studies are retrospective and occur over the course of many years, often with changes in technique, making definitive decisions difficult. One clear point is that TLA is not successful in patients with concomitant lower airway obstruction, highlighting the need for clear bronchoscopic evaluation prior to performing the procedure. Multiple authors have described failure of TLA in patients with synchronous airway lesions such as tracheomalacia.[49,97–100]

The largest series of TLA in the current literature is by Rogers *et al.*, with 53 TLAs with genioglossus release and circummandibular retention suture performed over the course of 11 years.[97] There were six failures and an 89% rate of success. All failures were in patients who were syndromic. The authors conclude that gastroesophageal reflux, preoperative intubation, age >2 weeks, birthweight <2500 g, and syndromic diagnosis are predictors of worse outcomes after TLA, and that the presence of ≥3 of these factors is a predictor of failure of TLA to relieve airway problems. Notably, bronchoscopy was performed preoperatively in all patients, and there was a 4% rate of dehiscence. These findings were supported in a follow-up study.[101]

Critics of TLA state high rates of dehiscence, decreased ability to resolve airway obstruction, speech and swallowing problems later in life, and injury to Wharton's ducts as reasons to avoid the procedure. Dehiscence has been as high as 20–29% in some series.[99,100,102] However, improvements in technique seem to have decreased this rate. Kirschner et al. described a 41% rate of dehiscence with a mucosa-only adhesion, but a 0% rate once a muscular retention suture was added.[98] Other series utilizing a retention suture describe rates from 4–5%.[95–97]

Resolution of airway obstruction is variable in TLA studies, and is difficult to completely characterize given differing indications and preoperative work-up prior to procedure in each manuscript. Success rates as low as 43% and as high as 89% have been reported.[97,103] In Denny and Kalantarian's series of 11 patients with PRS, only two were successfully treated with TLA alone. Five patients required secondary surgical intervention for recurrent airway obstruction within 4 months; however, 7 of the 11 patients were syndromic.[104] Kirschner *et al.* also describe a higher failure rate in syndromic patients.[98] There are only limited data on the effects of TLA on polysomnographic findings in the literature. Sedaghat and colleagues evaluated polysomnograms in eight patients before and after TLA. While seven of the eight patients had improvement in the apnea-hypopnea index after the procedure, only three of the eight patients had reduction to either mild or no OSA postoperatively.[105] Other series describe similar improvements in polysomnography.[106] The only comparative data available is from Flores *et al.*, who also showed improvement in polysomnography and oxygen saturation after TLA in 15 patients, but these improvements were significantly less than those in patients who had mandibular distraction osteogenesis at 1 month and 1 year postoperatively.[107]

LeBlanc and Golding-Kushner examined speech outcomes after TLA and found that patients had minimal long-term effects on speech development.[108] Glossopexy seemed to affect only early speech production by delaying sound production. Once the TLA is taken down, patients have accelerated development and "catch-up" to control patients. Morphologic changes were seen in the TLA cohort, such as thick lower lip mucosa, a blunted lingual apex, and lingual deviation on protrusion, but were temporary. The TLA cohort was equal to patients with cleft palate and syndrome-matched counterparts in the maintenance of articulatory integrity and their development of speech sound production at 18 months.

Other soft-tissue procedures have been described other than TLA, but most are solely of historical interest. Oeconomopoulos[109] described the use of a heavy silk suture through the base of the tongue that is affixed to the cartilaginous portion of the mandible about 1 cm lateral to the midline. Hadley and Johnson[110] also devised a technique where the tongue is pulled anteriorly, then a Kirschner wire is driven through the mandible from angle to angle in order to maintain tongue position (Fig. 36.19). Lewis *et al.*[111] described a tensor fascia latae sling for treatment. In this technique, a long strip of tensor fascia latae is harvested and passed posteriorly through the substance of the tongue through a submental incision. The graft is then tensioned and sutured to the periosteum of the mandibular symphysis. Bergoin and colleagues[112] describe a procedure termed "Hyomandibulopexie". In this technique, the ventral anterior surface of the tongue and mandible is anchored to the hyoid bone with 3-0 braided

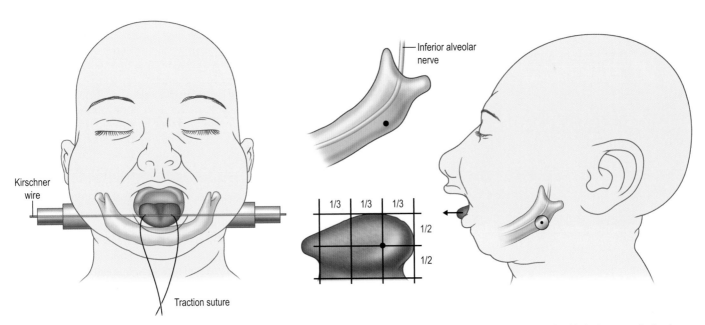

Fig. 36.19 Hadley and Johnson[110] described a technique in which a Kirschner wire is passed from mandibular angle to mandibular angle with the tongue under tension.

nylon sutures. Lapidot and Ben-Hur[113] describe passing 18-gauge steel wire is passed into the most posterior midline portion of the tongue base and tensioned around the hyoid bone (Fig. 36.20). In the Duhamel procedure,[114] heavy nylon suture is passed across the most posterior aspect of the body of the tongue, exits laterally through the cheeks or oral commissures, and is then tied over buttons.

More recently, Delorme and colleagues[62] felt that the musculature of the floor of the mouth is under increased tension in PRS, causing the tongue to rotate cranially and posteriorly. Based on this hypothesis, a full soft-tissue release from the anterior mandible is all that would be required to relieve the airway obstruction through de-rotation of the tongue

(Fig. 36.21). Through a 2 cm submental incision, the periosteum is incised at the lower border of the mandibular symphysis. Then the wide periosteal release of the floor of mouth musculature is done from the mandibular symphysis to bilateral angles. This includes release of the origins of the genioglossus, geniohyoid, and mylohyoid muscles. Caouette-Laberge and colleagues used this technique successfully in 11 of 12 patients, and then reported its success in an additional 26 of 31 patients.[40,106] Breugem and colleagues highlight the need for strict indications for this procedure in their treatment of 14 patients with subperiosteal release. Seven patients failed and required tracheostomy, of which six were syndromic.[115] Dudiewicz et al.[35] felt that success with this technique could

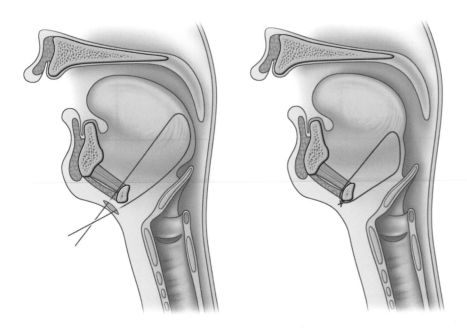

Fig. 36.20 The technique described by Lapidot and Ben-Hur[113] uses an 18-gauge steel wire that is placed into the most posterior midline portion of the tongue base. The steel wire is then directed anterior and caudally to arise below the hyoid bone. The opposite end of the wire is tunneled submucosally to the foramen cecum and then directed inferiorly to emerge at the superior aspect of the hyoid.

applies traction to the mandible. One major drawback of this technique is that the circummandibular wires at the parasymphysis can cut through the thin bone in neonates. One method affixes an acrylic plate to the mandible by circummandibular wires and the tension is distributed evenly, decreasing cut-through (Fig. 36.22). The traction is released for feeds after 1–2 weeks. Over time, the counterweight is decreased. The wires may remain in place for up to 5 weeks. Some centers have had success with this technique on an outpatient basis.[116]

With the advent of distraction osteogenesis, the armamentarium of the craniofacial surgeon was expanded for many purposes. In 1927, Rosenthal[118] performed the first mandibular osteodistraction procedure using an intraoral tooth-borne appliance. The work of Ilizarov with the long bones advanced understanding of distraction osteogenesis exponentially. In 1972, Cosman and Crikelair[119] reported three cases of respiratory difficulty associated with retrognathia that responded to mandibular advancement. In 1989, McCarthy et al.[120] clinically applied the technique of extraoral osteodistraction on four children. In 1997, Guerrero et al.[121] were the first to report the results of intraoral mandibular distraction for widening of transverse deficiencies in 11 patients. In 1994, McCarthy developed a miniaturized bone-borne uniguide mandibular distractor. In 1994, Havlik and Bartlett,[122] and later Haug and

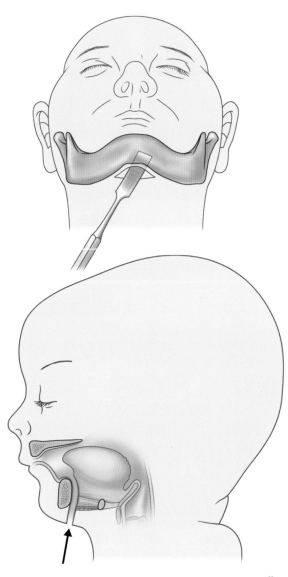

Fig. 36.21 In the procedure described by Delorme and colleagues,[62] a subperiosteal release of the floor of the mouth musculature is done through a 2 cm submental incision. The wide periosteal release is done as far posteriorly as the angles of the mandible. This includes release of the origins of the genioglossus, geniohyoid, and mylohyoid muscles.

be obtained by combining subperiosteal release with closure of the cleft palate. It was felt that a properly repaired cleft palate provides a barrier against the posterior displacement of the tongue.

Overall, all of the soft-tissue techniques strive toward the same goal: to pull the base of the tongue forward relative to the mandible. The authors feel that this is most logically carried out by pulling the tongue longitudinally toward the lip with a TLA.

Skeletal techniques

Skeletal techniques have transitioned from traction procedures to distraction procedures over time. Traction applied to mandible as a treatment for PRS is mainly of historical note, but is still practiced in some institutions.[116,117] Circummandibular wires are placed, and these wires are attached to a pulley that

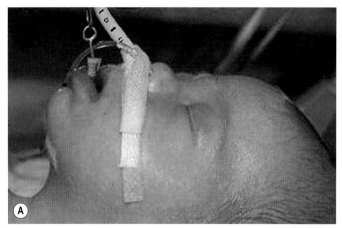
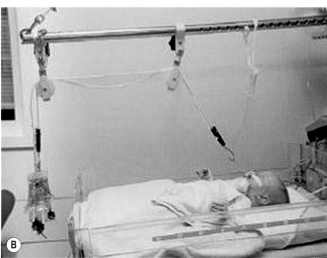

Fig. 36.22 (A,B) A demonstration of using traction on the mandible to relieve airway obstruction. In this technique, an acrylic plate is fixed to circummandibular wires and traction is applied to the plate.

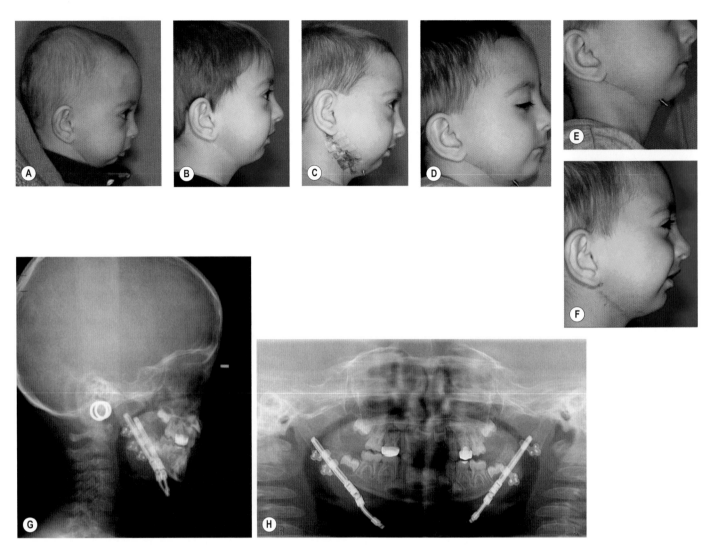

Fig. 36.23 A child with Pierre Robin Sequence treated with mandibular distraction osteogenesis via an intraoral distractor.

colleagues[123] reported on the treatment of severe micrognathia using external distraction devices. Many reports followed on the application of internal appliances (Fig. 36.23).

Mandibular distraction osteogenesis (MDO) results in expansion of the airway through true mandibular lengthening. The tongue base moves anteriorly by its attachments to the distracted mandible, pulling the tongue out of the hypopharynx (Fig. 36.24). The aperture of the airway is increased in anteroposterior and lateral dimensions.[124,125] After approximately 8 mm of distraction, the tongue posture visibly changes. This change in tongue posture to a normal horizontal position on the floor of the mouth is a clinical indicator for the timing of extubation, although definitive evaluation for resolution of tongue-based airway obstruction requires repeat nasendoscopy.

Selection of mandibular distraction to address tongue base position in infants with PRS entails three fundamental decisions: (1) What portion of the mandible is to be lengthened? (2) What vector of distraction is to be used? (3) What type of device is to be used? In answer to the first question, infants with PRS invariably have a short mandibular ramus and body. The mandibular ramus is "safer" to distract due to its lack of tooth buds, but surgical access is significantly more

challenging. The mandibular body is easier to access, but has multiple tooth buds that are difficult to avoid. Not only is one likely to eliminate or injure tooth buds at the site of osteotomy and/or device fixation, but there will inevitably be a gap in the permanent dentition where distraction took place. Therefore, the authors' preference when using internal distraction devices is to make utilize an inverted L-osteotomy on the posterior aspect of the mandibular body and ramus, placing the vertical component posterior to the tooth buds, and the horizontal component above the occlusal plane so as to minimize risk to the inferior alveolar nerve. When using external distraction devices, the authors prefer a transverse osteotomy in the mandibular ramus, placed above the occlusal plane so as to avoid the inferior alveolar nerve. Other types of osteotomy have also been described (Fig. 36.25). Selecting the vector of distraction will depend on patient anatomy. However, neonates with PRS who require distraction to open the airway present during the 1st month of life, and orthodontic assessment cannot be made. Therefore, one must use basic principles rather than orthodontic assessment in selecting the vector of distraction. When utilizing external distraction devices, the authors utilize a vector roughly parallel to the posterior border of the ramus. This usually produces distraction

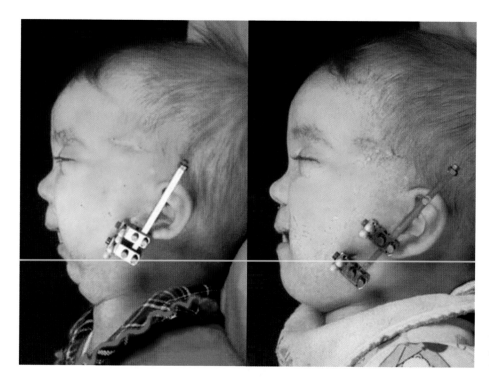

Fig. 36.24 A child with Pierre Robin Sequence treated with mandibular distraction osteogenesis via an external distractor. The mandibular-maxillary discrepancy was dramatically improved.

approximately 60° from the occlusal plane, providing a component of both ramus lengthening and anterior advancement of the pogonion. Autorotation of the mandible secondary to ramus lengthening will also bring the chin point forward. When using internal distraction devices, the authors distract parallel to the body of the mandible for technical ease of distractor placement (Video 36.1 ▶). Regarding which type of device to be used, one may choose between external and internal devices. Advantages of internal distraction over external devices include one-to-one bone lengthening with device activation, whereas external devices may torque at the pin level and not achieve one-to-one distraction. The internal device is also less prone to device dislodgement due to trauma or pin torque in the thin bone of the neonatal mandible, and there are no stretched scars in the skin that are inherent with external distraction pins. Disadvantages of internal devices include the need for wider exposure for device placement, fixed distraction vector at the time of device placement as opposed to multidimensional external units, and the need for a second operation for device removal. As resorbable distraction devices continue to develop, the need for the second

surgery for removal may be obviated.[126,127] If one chooses an external distraction device, the osteotomy may be created through an intraoral or an extraoral incision. If one chooses an intraoral approach, local anesthetic containing epinephrine is injected over the oblique line and the buccal surface of the mandible. A lateral vestibular incision is made on both sides. Subperiosteal dissection is performed to expose the gonial angles and the posterior mandibular body. Selection of pinhole sites is very important as this dictates the vector of distraction. Before placing the percutaneous pins, the skin is bunched and pulled centrally to create laxity during distraction, thereby minimizing pin site stretch and scarring as the device is elongated.

When placing external mandibular distractors, precision in pin placement is critical, as the neonatal mandible is brittle and narrow. The authors prefer accessing the mandible through an intra-oral incision, and placing the distraction pins percutaneously. The pins should be tested and ensured to be in good bone stock. It is prudent to place the pins and temporarily affix the distractor before completing the corticotomies, so as to return the mandible to its original reduction following completion of corticotomies. If distraction is to be performed to elongate the ramus, then a transverse corticotomy is made in the ramus above the occlusal plane to avoid tooth buds and the inferior alveolar nerve. The corticotomy can be made with a mechanical saw at the buccal cortex of the mandible. Following corticotomy, an osteotome is used as a lever to ensure that the proximal and distal segments are independently mobile, therefore ensuring that the osteotomy is complete. Fixation of the distraction device can now be completed to stabilize the mandible. Note that if the distractor was completely fixed prior to this point, one could not ensure completion of the osteotomy, which could predispose to premature consolidation and/or device failure during distraction. When placing the distractor on the contralateral side, it

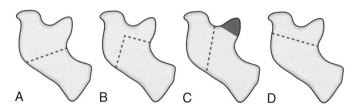

Fig. 36.25 Types of mandibular osteotomy described for treatment of micrognathia in neonates: (**A**) oblique angle osteotomy; (**B**) inverted-L osteotomy (author's preferred internal distraction technique); (**C**) vertical ramus osteotomy with or without coronoidectomy to avoid zygomatic impingement; (**D**) horizontal ramus osteotomy (author's preferred external distraction technique).

is essential to check the placement vector on both sides to place the distractors parallel. Failure to do so will result in midline shift and/or alteration of the mandibular occlusal plane with distraction. The intraoral incisions are then closed with resorbable sutures. The free motion of the distractors is checked while in the operating room and then the device is returned to the starting position. The starting MMD is noted.

Distraction is usually initiated after a latency period of 3 days, and an accelerated rate of distraction of 1.5–2 mm/day is used in children under 1 year of age to prevent premature consolidation. The child recovers in the intensive care unit until the airway is stabilized. The MMD is monitored to ensure effective distraction. The pins are cleaned with peroxide, and antibiotic ointment is applied twice daily. Distraction continues until the desired MMD is obtained and the base-of-tongue obstruction is clinically cleared as confirmed by nasendoscopy. The consolidation timing varies at different centers, but the authors recommend a period of 8 weeks.[128]

When placing internal mandibular distractors, the authors prefer to use bilateral extraoral incisions made in a submandibular skin fold 0.5–1 cm inferior to the mandibular border. An incision length of 2.5 cm is adequate to provide access for device placement; a smaller incision, although feasible, may not permit placement of some devices. The platysma is then divided and care must be taken not to injure the marginal mandibular nerve. One should use a nerve stimulator and avoid the use of local anesthetic so as to maintain motor nerve function. The pterygomasseteric sling is incised and the masseter is stripped, and the buccal cortex of the mandible is exposed. It is important to note that the vector of distraction is fixed once the device is fixed, and therefore positioning of the distractor is critical to the final outcome. Due to limited surface area in the neonatal mandible, fixation of the distal portion of the device will inevitably be in the region of tooth roots, so monocortical screws are recommended. The device is secured prior to completing the osteotomy to ensure correct vector of distraction, and this vector must be parallel to that of the contralateral distractor. Thus, placement must be carefully planned to allow completion of the osteotomy without device removal. The authors complete the transverse component of the reverse-L osteotomy, which is made cephalad to the distractor and above the occlusal plane, after fixation of the device. They do not recommend removing screws once placed, as insertion and removal of the screws can loosen purchase in the hypoplastic bone of the neonatal mandible. If unable to achieve secure screw purchase with the internal device, move to transmandibular pin placement with an external device, as has been described.[129] The authors' preference is to bring the activation unit out through a stab incision inferior and posterior to the lobule of the ear for ease of access during the distraction process, although some surgeons bring the activation out through an intraoral incision and keep the device within the mouth.

Proponents of MDO feel that it is the most efficacious procedure to avoid tracheostomy in PRS. They also believe airway obstruction caused by the tongue base can be relieved, scars are cosmetically acceptable, and the mandible can be redistracted if needed.[104] Other proponents cite improved feeding and polysomnographic outcome compared with TLA.[107] Certainly, MDO has been a successful technique in a majority of cases of PRS. In a recent meta-analysis of MDO for pediatric airway obstruction, there was an 89% success rate, including an 84% rate of tracheostomy decannulation, and a 96% rate of improvement in OSA.[130] These are similar rates of success to those quoted in other meta-analyses of all pediatric MDO for multiple indications, as well as large retrospective series.[128,131–133]

Concerns regarding MDO are related to more gradual improvement in the airway, high rates of complications, and a lack of long-term developmental outcomes data. Depending on the protocol, distraction usually progresses at a rate of 0.5–2 mm/day. The child may still require prolonged intubation or tracheostomy while distraction is being performed. Indeed, a small comparative study of TLA versus MDO found that MDO patients had a longer mean hospital stay, albeit with better feeding and respiratory outcomes than TLA.[134] Recent analyses of the literature have demonstrated an overall complication rate of 20.5–43% for mandibular distraction osteogenesis for varied indications (Figs. 36.26–36.28).[130,131,135] The most common complication after MDO is infection, with a higher rate in external devices. Device failure is also more common in external devices, with a rate of up to 7.9%. Relapse has been reported in up to 65% of cases; however, data until the age of skeletal maturity are lacking. Other significant complications include hypertrophic scarring in 2–15%; nerve injury in 6–11%; and anterior open bite in 3%. Damage/malposition of developing tooth buds is common in MDO, with some abnormality (most minor) in up to 55–76% of cases on long-term follow-up.[136,137] However, this may be technique-dependent, because some authors have reported lower rates of tooth injury.[138]

Finally, long-term data on the natural history of PRS patients undergoing MDO are lacking. The procedure itself requires the periosteum to be stripped and an osteotomy to be made, and in theory, this could restrict growth. Current studies of growth after MDO have included patients with hemifacial microsomia, Nager syndrome, and Treacher Collins, who do not have normal growth potential.[139] Further long-term studies of MDO in isolated PRS patients to full skeletal and dental maturity will greatly enhance our understanding of the complication profile and long-term facial growth potential after this procedure.

There is an ongoing debate over whether to choose initial distraction of the mandible over other methods such as TLA, nasopharyngeal airway, or intraoral appliances. Some authors feel that distraction should be a last resort prior to tracheostomy and less invasive measures be attempted first. These authors express concern over long-term growth of the mandible following osteotomies in the neonate, and the potential for sequelae in mandibular range of motion, dental development, and sensation in the territory of the mental nerve. If the child continues to demonstrate airway difficulties after 6–7 months of age, then the mandibular growth was inadequate to clear the tongue base sufficiently and distraction may be warranted. Some feel that mandibular distraction should be performed earlier in the algorithm for PRS and replace TLA. Dauria and Marsh[140] proposed such an approach. Denny and Kalantarian[104] completed this task successfully in a series of five consecutive neonates with PRS by performing bilateral mandibular distraction osteogenesis using external devices. All neonates avoided tracheostomy, had complete elimination of respiratory symptoms, and were extubated before completion of the active distraction process. All five patients remained extubated without airway support.

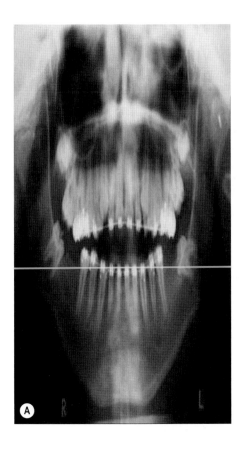

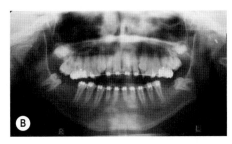

Fig. 36.26 (A,B) Abnormally positioned second molars 8 years after second mandibular distraction osteogenesis.

A recent retrospective series by Flores *et al.* described a single surgeon's 15-year experience performing 15 TLAs and 24 MDOs for PRS.[107] These procedures were not performed in concurrent time periods, so there is likely an experience bias. However, this is currently the largest comparative study of TLA versus MDO. There were no post-procedure tracheostomies in the MDO group and four in the TLA group. The polysomnographic data revealed significantly better apnea-hypopnea indices and oxygen saturation in the MDO group at both 1 month and 1 year postoperatively.

In summary, both soft-tissue and skeletal procedures can successfully clear the airway obstruction in PRS. Current data appear to indicate that more strict indications must be utilized for TLA compared with MDO, and long-term data on both procedures are lacking. In either case, it is important for full airway evaluation, as neither procedure will resolve a subglottic airway obstruction. The role of laryngomalacia in the utilization of either procedure is an evolving concept.[29,55] With appropriate indications and preoperative work-up, good results have been reported with both procedures overall.[29,97,101,107] In a neonate with non-syndromic PRS that has failed non-surgical measures and presents with isolated tongue-based airway obstruction in the absence of laryngomalacia, the authors prefer to attempt a TLA. If the respiratory distress is not alleviated, then mandibular distraction osteogenesis is warranted. If the child has tongue-based airway obstruction with no other synchronous airway lesions besides mild laryngomalacia limited to the supraglottic larynx, or an associated syndrome that conveys poor growth potential, then the authors prefer mandibular distraction osteogenesis over TLA as the initial surgical intervention (Fig. 36.29). Should

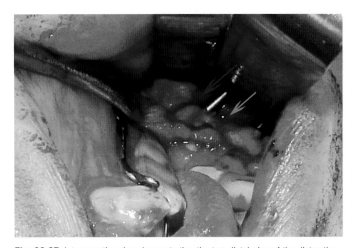

Fig. 36.27 Intraoperative view demonstrating the two distal pins of the distraction device remaining in bone. A fracture has resulted between these pins (small arrow) distal to the site of premature fusion of the initial osteotomy site (large arrow).

this not clear the airway obstruction, tracheostomy is the final alternative.

Tracheostomy

Surgical management of the airway in children with PRS may be required in the acute setting. A tracheostomy may also be unavoidable in certain circumstances, as in the child with PRS with an infraglottic obstruction, multiple comorbidities due to a syndromic diagnosis, central sleep apnea, or failure of mandibular distraction osteogenesis. However,

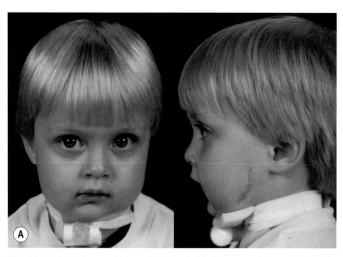
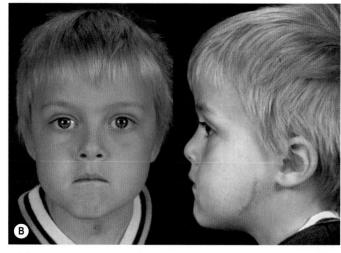

Fig. 36.28 (A) A 3-year-old boy with Pierre Robin Sequence with persistent tracheostomy following one attempt at mandibular distraction. **(B)** Successful decannulation after second mandibular distraction and tracheal reconstruction.

the placement of a tracheostomy involves significant morbidity, as well as a small but well-described rate of mortality.[141] The neonatal tracheostomy tube, because of its small diameter, is prone to mucus plugging and malposition. Some children with PRS may require the tracheostomy for 2–4 years or more prior to decannulation.[142] During this time, significant granulation tissue formation and stenosis can occur. It has been suggested that long-term speech, behavior, and developmental problems are associated with pediatric tracheostomy.[143] Multiple studies have also shown the management of PRS with tracheostomy to be labor-intensive and costly.[142,144,145] For these reasons, it is the authors' preference to avoid tracheostomy whenever possible in children with PRS.

Treatment of the nutritional deficit

One cannot forget to treat the feeding difficulties in PRS, as a malnourished child will have difficulty thriving regardless of any airway intervention. The neonate has minimal skills for coordination of the aerodigestive structures beyond that provided at a reflex level. In PRS, the retrognathia may prevent anteriorization of the tongue and sufficient latching. Additionally, oroesophageal motor dysfunction is common in PRS as previously noted.[36,38] All of these factors predispose PRS patients to feeding difficulty. Involvement of speech and swallowing therapists immediately upon diagnosis of PRS is imperative in order to optimize nutritional intake.

The typical neonate with PRS should be fed 150–165 mL/kg per day of 20 kcal/oz formula or breast milk, which equates to 100–110 cal/kg per day. Optimal weight gain should be 20–30 g/day. If this weight gain is not observed, then the supplementation should be increased, combined with further evaluation. If the child tolerates breast feeding or is bottle-fed breast milk, it should be fortified with powdered term formula or medium-chain triglyceride oil instead of human milk fortifier, as the phosphorus contained may promote neonatal tetany.

There are many described measures that can be attempted to aid in feeding. Manual support of the mandible during feeding can improve the quality of the seal and function of the labial sphincter. This can also help to relieve the base-of-tongue obstruction. Another technique is to move the nipple or bottle in a rhythmic fashion to stimulate better sucking. Benefit has also been seen in placing the nipple on to the substance of the tongue.

Breast feeding is often difficult and requires considerable effort and modification of technique. As a result, many of these neonates are bottle-fed with specialized bottles and nipples. The principle of specialized bottle-feeding is to allow a steady stream of milk, usually by a modified Haberman nipple that prevents negative-pressure build-up, and a soft bottle for the parent to regulate outflow.[57] These nipples are usually softer and longer than traditional nipples. The nipple is long enough to allow contact with the tongue, but not long enough to promote gagging.

If the neonate is unable to take adequate oral feeds with specialized nipples and bottles, then nasogastric or orogastric feeds should be administered. A majority of PRS patients will require these types of feedings for some time.[34,45,57] One must be mindful that the use of a feeding tube may increase the risk for the development of gastroesophageal reflux. The placement of a gastrostomy tube for long-term feeds may be required, but the utilization of these is largely institution-dependent and thus difficult to compare between reports.[146] The placement of a gastrostomy should be decided based on reflux, complete feeding analysis by speech therapy, and the overall syndromic picture of the patient.

Importantly, maintenance of an open airway while trying to feed uses a great deal of calories, contributing to the overall deficit in the Pierre Robin patient. Relieving the airway obstruction will allow the child to overcome feeding difficulties and gain weight. Several studies have shown significant improvement in feeding function after MDO and TLA.[59,98,100,129]

Treatment of otologic conditions

Placement of myringotomy tubes has been shown to be effective in preventing recurrent bouts of otitis media and may restore normal levels of hearing. These children should be followed closely by a pediatric otolaryngologist. The

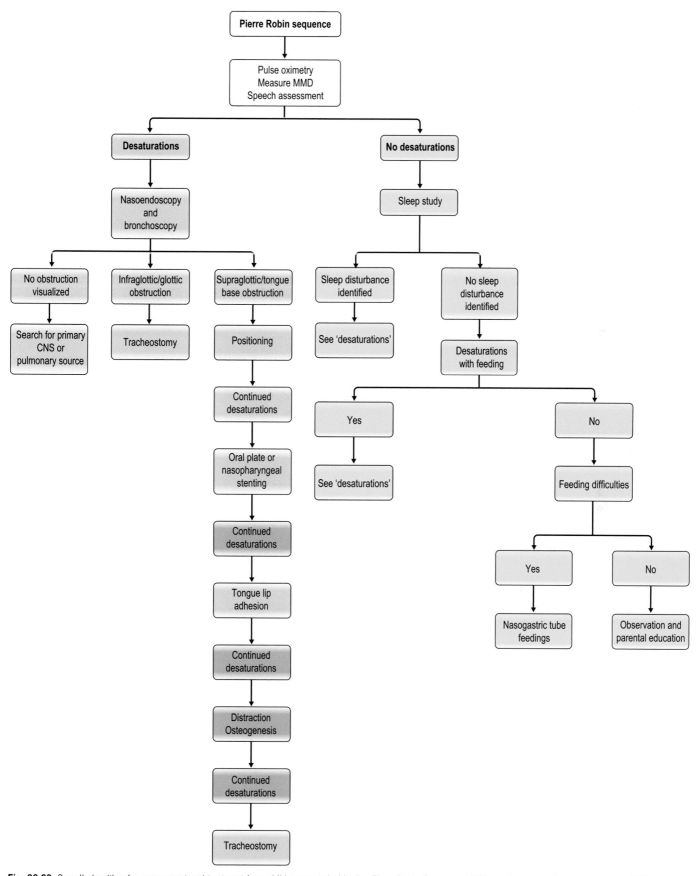

Fig. 36.29 Overall algorithm for assessment and treatment for a child suspected of having Pierre Robin Sequence. MMD, maxillary–mandibular discrepancy; CNS, central nervous system.

treatment plan may be tailored to the associated syndrome if not isolated PRS.

Secondary procedures

As 50% or more of children with PRS will have an associated cleft palate, the timing of palatal repair is an important consideration. Descriptions of palate repair at the time of TLA take-down have been described, and the authors' preference against this has been previously discussed. There are reports of emergent tracheostomy when this combined approach has been performed.[147] At the authors' institution, the cleft palate repair is performed at the routine time interval, which is at 11–12 months of age.

As with other children with cleft palates, the nurturing of speech is important. Later procedures to correct velopharyngeal insufficiency may be required. It has been shown that children with PRS may have a higher risk of requiring surgery for velopharyngeal insufficiency compared with isolated cleft palate patients, although this may be more related to syndromic diagnosis.[45,148]

🌐 Access the complete reference list online at **http://www.expertconsult.com**

1. Sadewitz VL. Robin Sequence: changes in thinking leading to changes in patient care. *Cleft Palate Craniofac J.* 1992;29:246–253.

2. Randall P, Krogman WM, Jahins S. Pierre Robin and the syndrome that bears his name. *Cleft Palate J.* 1965;36:237–246.

8. Izumi K, Konczal LL, Mitchell AL, et al. Underlying genetic diagnosis of Pierre Robin sequence: retrospective chart review at two children's hospitals and a systematic literature review. *J Pediatr.* 2012;160:645–650.e2. *The authors present an analysis of the underlying genetic diagnosis in patients with Pierre Robin Sequence in 125 patients at two different institutions. They also perform a comprehensive literature review of genetic and other causes of PRS.*

9. Evans AK, Rahbar R, Rogers GF, et al. Robin sequence: a retrospective review of 115 patients. *Int J Pediatr Otorhinolaryngol.* 2006;70:973–980. *The authors describe their experience with 115 consecutive patients with PRS over 40 years, including syndromic diagnosis, operative, and nonoperative management.*

45. Filip C, Feragen KB, Lemvik JS, et al. Multidisciplinary Aspects of 104 Patients With Pierre Robin Sequence. *Cleft Palate Craniofac J.* 2015;52:732–742. *In this large retrospective series, the authors report more long-term follow-up for patients with PRS. Interesting observations include a higher rate of both VPI and autism spectrum disorders in this cohort compared to cleft-only controls.*

49. Schaefer RB, Stadler JA, Gosain AK. To distract or not to distract: an algorithm for airway management in isolated Pierre Robin sequence. *Plast Reconstr Surg.* 2004;113:1113–1125. *This paper delineates a comprehensive treatment pathway that provides a safe methodology for treating the child with Pierre Robin Sequence. Many issues are discussed such as airway issues, glossoptosis, and feeding. The paper discusses the difference in treatment options due to differences in severity seen between the isolated and syndromic subsets of PRS.*

Tongue-lip adhesion demonstrated favorable results in the isolated PRS group.

68. Figueroa AA, Glupker TJ, Fitz MG, et al. Mandible, tongue, and airway in Pierre Robin sequence: a longitudinal cephalometric study. *Cleft Palate Craniofac J.* 1991;28:425–434. *In this study, the authors follow cephalometrics in 17 patients with isolated PRS at three time points in the first 2 years of life, compared with isolated cleft palate and normal controls. They demonstrate a dramatic increase in airway size and mandible length compared with controls in PRS over the 1st year of life. Although these measurements did not normalize, this provides some evidence for a possible catch-up growth process.*

97. Rogers GF, Murthy AS, LaBrie RA, et al. The GILLS score: part I. Patient selection for tongue-lip adhesion in Robin sequence. *Plast Reconstr Surg.* 2011;128:243–251. *In the largest series of TLA procedures published to date, the authors identify possible predictors of failure of TLA. They also include a guide for both patient optimization and patient selection for the procedure.*

107. Flores RL, Tholpady SS, Sati S, et al. The surgical correction of Pierre Robin sequence: mandibular distraction osteogenesis versus tongue-lip adhesion. *Plast Reconstr Surg.* 2014;133:1433–1439. *In this comparative study, the authors describe their 15-year experience with both TLA and MDO. With the most comprehensive comparative analysis of both procedures to date, they demonstrate improved avoidance of tracheostomy and polysomnographic outcomes in MDO.*

130. Tahiri Y, Viezel-Mathieu A, Aldekhayel S, et al. The effectiveness of mandibular distraction in improving airway obstruction in the pediatric population. *Plast Reconstr Surg.* 2014;133:352e–359e. *The authors provide a meta-analysis of the existing literature on airway improvement, including tracheostomy decannulation, after pediatric MDO. They highlight complications, distraction techniques utilized, and functional airway outcomes.*

37

Treacher Collins syndrome

Fernando Molina

SYNOPSIS

- Treacher Collins syndrome is a congenital craniofacial malformation that involves the bone and soft tissues of the middle and lower facial thirds. Specifically, the orbits, zygomaticomaxillary complex, and mandible are affected.
- Coloboma of the lower eyelids, inferior obliquity of the palpebral fissures, lateral canthal dystopia, and notching of the upper eyebrows and eyelids are characteristic.
- Surgical reconstruction should include techniques to repair both soft-tissue and skeletal deformities.
- Parietal bone grafts are used to augment the malar eminence. Bilateral distraction osteogenesis corrects hypoplasia of the mandibular ramus and body with simultaneous improvement of respiratory and digestive function.
- Colobomas and macrostomia are repaired prior to bony reconstruction, and microtia is treated between 9 and 10 years of age.

Access the Historical Perspective section online at
http://www.expertconsult.com

Introduction

The abnormal development of the first and second branchial arches results in bilateral Tessier clefts 6, 7, and 8 with the concomitant stigmata of Treacher Collins syndrome. While Treacher Collins syndrome occurs as an autosomal-dominant disorder in 1 per 50000 live births, 60% of cases arise as sporadic mutations. The syndrome is most successfully treated in staged procedures addressing bone and soft tissues.

Airway management is the primary concern when treating infants born with Treacher Collins syndrome. The narrow pharynx and short mandible may cause obstructive sleep apnea and subsequent neonatal death. Early mandibular distraction may avoid the need for tracheostomy in severely affected neonates.

The malar region may be reconstructed with free calvarial bone grafts. Bilateral mandibular distraction, with distraction vectors carefully planned to improve the length of the ascending ramus, will correct micrognathia and an anterior open bite. Orthodontic maneuvers will allow for growth of the posterior vertical dimension of the maxilla.

Colobomas and macrostomia are repaired prior to bony reconstruction. Microtia is usually corrected at approximately 9–10 years of age.

Basic science/disease process

Treacher Collins syndrome, or mandibulofacial dysostosis, is a complex congenital craniofacial malformation that most strikingly involves the middle and lower thirds of the face, affecting both bony structures and soft tissues. It is transmitted by an autosomal-dominant gene of variable penetrance and phenotypic expressivity. The severity of the disease increases in successive generations.[7,8] Half of the cases reported in the literature do not have a documented family history, and thus an influence of exogenous factors on expressivity of the mutation may be inferred. Advanced paternal age is considered a risk factor. These genetic anomalies cause bilateral defects in structures derived from the first and second branchial arches.

Diagnosis/patient presentation

Patients with mandibulofacial dysostosis may present with all or most of the following features (Box 37.1): an inferior obliquity and shortening of the palpebral fissures, coloboma of the lower eyelids, dystopia of the lateral canthi, absence of eyelashes, and notching of the eyebrows and upper eyelids. The craniofacial skeleton is also involved: the malar bone is

The lateral cephalogram demonstrates normal upper anterior face height with a reduced posterior face height, resulting in a vertical occlusal plane and shortening of the choanae. The sphenoethmoid angle is more acute, and the angle between the anterior cranial base and the palatal plane is more obtuse. Mandibular retrognathism is present, with shortening of the ramus and the body of the mandible. The chin is long and retruded.[10]

The absence of the zygomatic bone is responsible for the absence of the lateral orbital rim and for the poor definition of the inferior orbital rim. For the same reason, there is no clear separation between the orbital cavity, the temporal fossa, and the infratemporal fossa. Generally, bony deformity is always symmetrical. The zygomatic arches are hypoplastic or absent, and the aponeurosis of the hypoplastic temporal muscle is in direct continuity with the aponeurosis of the masseter muscle.[11]

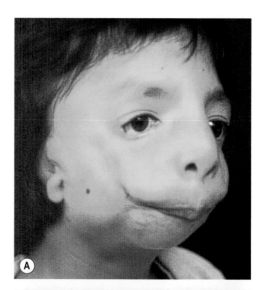

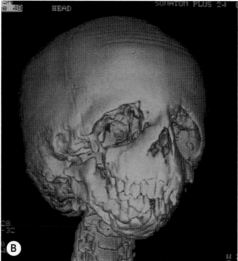

Fig. 37.1 (A) A 7-year-old boy with Treacher Collins syndrome presenting with severe coloboma of the lower eyelids, hypoplastic maxilla, and underprojected and narrow maxilla. There is bilateral microtia and macrostomia. The mandible shows severe hypoplasia, including at the menton. **(B)** 3D computed tomography scan, showing the absence of the zygoma and malar bone and the lack of the inferolateral orbital floor. The mandible has a very short ascending ramus, and the posterior aspect of the maxilla is also very short vertically.

hypoplastic or absent, along with the zygomatic arch. The maxilla is narrow and underprojected, with a high and narrow palate. The mandible is hypoplastic with a severe shortening of the ascending ramus; the condyle is also severely affected. The chin is long and retruded; the mandibular body is short and typically features an exaggerated antegonial notch. Micrognathia of different degrees is also observed, with an anterior open bite. The nose is protruded and broad with a flattened frontonasal angle. Other clinical features include ear deformities or microtia, absence of the external auditory canal, anomalies of the middle ear, and macrostomia (Fig. 37.1).[9]

Radiographically, the Waters and posterior–anterior views, as well as frontal tomograms, show hypoplasia of the malar bones and partial or complete absence of the zygomatic arches. The shape of the orbits is abnormal secondary to the partial or total absence of the lateral wall and floor of the orbits.

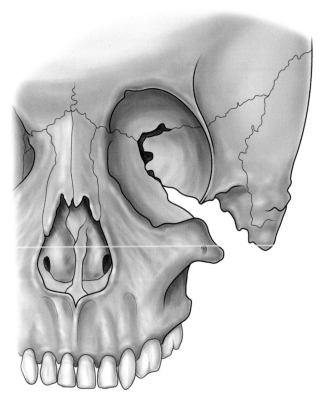

Fig. 37.2 According to Tessier's classification, the confluence of craniofacial clefts 6, 7, and 8 produces the hypoplasia or absence of bony structures, including the zygoma, orbit, maxilla, and ascending ramus of the mandible.

According to Tessier, the zygomatic bone is absent because of the confluence of clefts 6, 7, and 8. The number 6 cleft is situated between the maxilla and the zygomatic bone, opening the infraorbital fissure. The number 7 cleft is a temporozygomatic cleft accounting for the malformations of the ears and the macrostomia. The number 8 cleft involves the frontozygomatic suture (Fig. 37.2).[6] There exists a wide spectrum of phenotypic expressivity, and some clinical features are present in a less evident fashion. Similarly, there are asymmetric cases resulting from different penetrance of the deformity on each side of the face.

Computed tomographic scans with 3D reconstruction show the affected bone structures in detail. Recently, virtual surgical planning (VSP) computer programs are very useful in the sequence of bone reconstruction, especially in more severe patients.

Patient selection

A careful physical exam is required to ensure an adequate functional assessment of the retropharyngeal space. Significant micrognathia can produce respiratory distress, and some patients require a tracheostomy or mandibular distraction at a very early age. It is also important to assess hearing and speech. Dental impressions must be obtained to plan mandibular or maxillomandibular procedures in older patients.

Treatment and surgical technique

Treatment is aimed at correcting the colobomas; reconstructing the malar bones and zygomatic arches; establishing an adequate maxillomandibular relationship with functional occlusion; harmonizing the profile by improving the proportional relationship between the different regions of the face; and correcting the auricular malformations and macrostomia.

Surgical intervention is divided into four stages. The first stage includes the correction of functional emergencies when present. Respiratory distress is addressed with mandibular distraction or tracheostomy very early in life. Corneal exposure is addressed with eyelid reconstruction. The second stage of reconstruction consists of zygomaticomaxillary reconstruction with cranial bone grafts.[12,13] Generally, these procedures are performed between 2 and 4 years of age. The third stage of reconstruction, mandibular distraction, is performed between 3 and 6 years of age. The goal is bilateral elongation of the ascending ramus and closure of the anterior open bite.[14,15] The fourth stage is distraction osteogenesis of the reconstructed zygomaticomaxillary complexes and lateral orbits. This distraction should be performed when zygomaticomaxillary growth is observed to be the limiting factor in global craniofacial growth. This stage is frequently performed between 5 and 8 years of age.

Colobomas

Colobomas usually occur in the lower eyelid and are full-thickness defects. Reconstruction should therefore include all eyelid components. The most popular procedure consists of a myocutaneous flap from the superior eyelid transposed down to cover the defect in the inferior eyelid. Essentially, a Z-plasty is designed along the borders of the coloboma (Fig. 37.3), the defect is defined in the inferior eyelid, and the superior eyelid flap is raised and transposed into the inferior defect. A release of the orbital septum and the lateral canthal ligament is mandatory to correct the position of the lateral canthus. A tarsoconjunctival reconstruction is seldom required.

Zygoma

Zygomaticomaxillary reconstruction has undoubtedly received most of the attention from experts on this topic. Various alloplastic and autologous materials, including silicone, dermis-fat grafts, cartilage grafts, and many others, have been used with varying degrees of success for this reconstruction. Many believe that calvarial bone grafts are the best option for the reconstruction of the zygomatic arch and malar bone. Some characteristic challenges of this procedure include: the large amount of bone required; bone grafts must be adapted to the contour of the defect; the new bone structure must achieve the necessary projection; and secondary bone resorption must be avoided.[12,13,16–18]

The parietal bone is the author's preferred donor site. A paper template is made, including the malar bone, zygomatic arch, and the lateral aspect of the orbit. The template is used to design bilateral bone grafts, each as a single unit, from both parietal regions. The curvature of the donor region will be used to achieve natural contour and projection of the new zygomaticomaxillary structure. The left parietal region is used

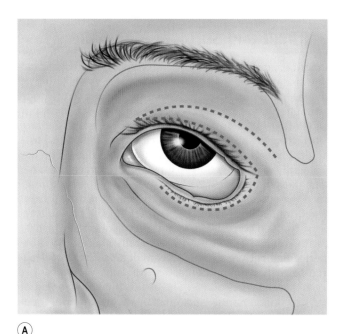

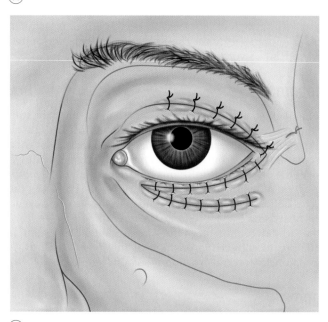

Fig. 37.3 (A) Procedure for coloboma correction. Planning for a simultaneous rotation upper eyelid myocutaneous flap is outlined. **(B)** The result after the flap rotation, including the lateral canthopexy. The ligament has been reattached 4–5 mm superior to its original insertion.

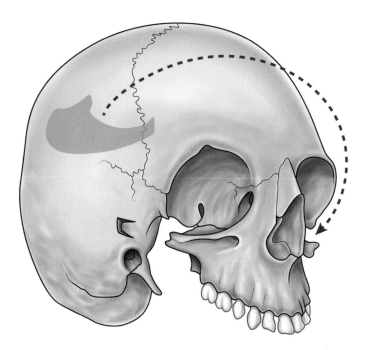

Fig. 37.4 Using a template, a bicortical parietal bone graft is harvested. The right graft will be transferred to the left zygomaticomaxillary region. The natural curvature of the bone will produce an excellent projection of the reconstructed region.

temporalis. If necessary, the lateral canthus is resuspended at this time.

With these techniques, a natural appearance is restored to the zygomaticomaxillary region with good contour and excellent projection. The subperiosteal suspension of overlying soft

to reconstruct the right side of the face and vice versa (Fig. 37.4). The free bone grafts are fixed to the subjacent bone structure at the orbit and the maxilla with 3–4 screws, 16 mm in length. This is usually sufficient for stable immobilization. The new zygomatic arch should reach laterally to the bone ridge at the external auditory canal. In addition to the rigid fixation, the posterior surface of the graft should have good contact with the masseter muscle and the rest of the local soft tissues such that bony resorption is minimized (Fig. 37.5). In addition, a subperiosteal suspension of the cheek soft tissues is performed with 3–4 monofilament sutures attached to the

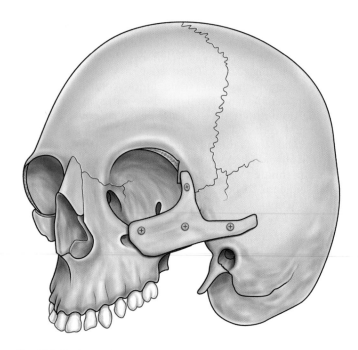

Fig. 37.5 The free parietal bone graft is fixed with 3–4 screws to the deeper bone structures. The bone graft should be adapted to the contour of the receiving bone to reduce bone resorption.

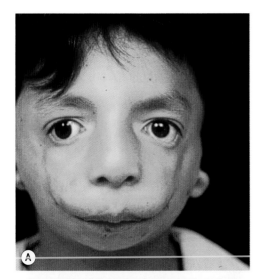

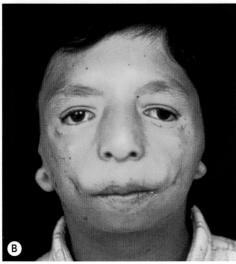

Fig. 37.6 (A) Preoperative frontal view of a 7-year-old boy presenting with all the characteristic features of severe Treacher Collins syndrome. **(B)** Postoperative result after bilateral zygomaticomaxillary reconstruction and coloboma correction. Notice the new structure at the bizygomatic distance. Bilateral bidirectional mandibular distraction has also been performed.

tissues adds volume to the region and redraping of the periorbital skin produces an aesthetic result (Fig. 37.6).

In the past, composite temporoparietal flaps had been widely used; however, the muscle is always hypoplastic and its rotation produced secondary depression at the external temporal fossa.[13,17,18] This procedure also sacrificed precise shaping of the osteomuscular flap to preserve vascularity. Even so, with this technique, only 60% of the muscle's contact with underlying bone can be maintained. This does not represent a considerable blood supply if we consider that 80% of the blood supply of cranial bones comes from the dura mater and only 20% is derived from the periosteum.

Mandible

Micrognathia in Treacher Collins presents a unique problem in which the mandibular anatomy is hypoplastic in all dimensions. Moreover, patients suffer from chronic respiratory and digestive problems. The deformity is usually bilateral, affecting mainly the ramus and the body, both in form and volume. For these patients, a bidirectional, bilateral solution is required.

In these cases, two corticotomies are performed: a vertically oriented one in the mandibular body and a horizontally oriented one in the ascending ramus. Three pins are used: a central one at the mandibular angle, a second in the mandibular body, and a third in the central aspect of the ascending ramus. One bidirectional distraction device is used on each side, each with two distraction rods to allow independent, precise elongation of each segment. The central pin acts as a fixed pivot point for distraction of the ramus and body (Fig. 37.7).

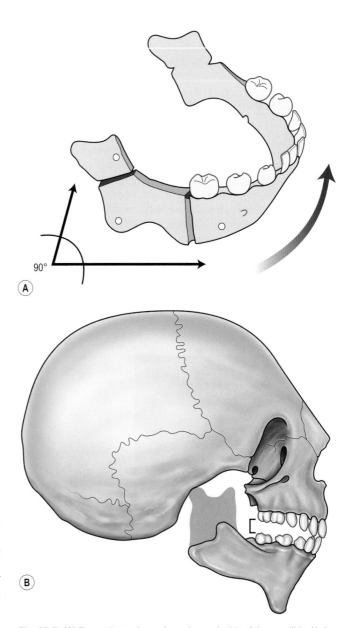

Fig. 37.7 (A) The corticotomies performed at each side of the mandible. Notice the position of pin insertion at the ascending ramus, the angle, and the mandibular body. Also note the relationship that should be obtained between the vertical and horizontal distraction vectors. **(B)** Once elongation of the ascending ramus has been obtained, an important posterior open bite will be produced. The use of bite blocks is gradually diminished to allow for the vertical growth of the posterior maxilla.

Elongation of the ascending ramus produces an important posterior open bite. At the body, the lengthening is minimal: just enough to overcorrect the molar relationship and to close the classic anterior open bite of the deformity. Precisely planned distraction vectors are critical to obtaining the proper degree of mandibular elongation and resultant occlusal changes. The relationship between the vertical (ramus) and the horizontal (body) vectors has to be less than 90°. These vectors will produce an exaggerated counterclockwise mandibular rotation closing the open bite and creating an open bite between the retromolar region and the posterior aspect of the maxilla. Posterior bite blocks are placed and gradually reduced in the vertical dimension to control growth of the posterior maxilla, closing the open bite by increasing the posterior maxillary vertical dimension.

Most of these patients present with a typical facial convexity with deficient soft tissue of the lower third of the face and neck, absence of definition in the submental angle, and shortened suprahyoid muscles. Patients with the most severe phenotype are frequently tracheostomy-dependent, and the ability to open their mouth is minimal or nonexistent. With bone distraction, all tissues from skeleton to skin are simultaneously elongated without the inconvenience of bone grafts or tissue expansion. In contrast, after conventional osteotomies and bone grafts, the contracted muscles and overlying soft-tissue envelope act as a counterforce to the bony advancement, often causing bony relapse and necessitating multiple procedures to achieve optimal aesthetic results. Tissue expansion increases the amount of skin, but other soft tissues such as muscles, vessels, and nerves remain unchanged.

The overall functional and aesthetic results with bidirectional mandibular distraction are satisfying (Fig. 37.8). The neck takes on a more normal shape with a well-defined submental angle, the muscles and soft tissues of the floor of the mouth are elongated, as are the masticatory muscles, and the chin takes on a more prominent position. These anatomic changes reconstruct the inferior third of the face, lending improved proportionality to the entire face. Once a more normal size and shape of the mandible have been achieved, these patients are able to open their mouths to receive orthodontic and dental treatment. Additionally, we have noted improvements in deglutition and respiration. Often, those patients with tracheostomies can be decannulated, and those with feeding tubes are routinely converted to oral feeding.

Distraction of zygomaticomaxillary region

At 7–10 years of age, the grafted zygomaticomaxillary complexes are distracted. The orbitomalar-zygomatic region can be accessed via a coronal approach. An osteotomy is designed to include the zygomatic arch, the posterior aspect of the malar bone, the inferior third of the lateral orbital wall, and the inferior orbital rim medially to the infraorbital foramen. A buried distraction device is fixed to the parietal bone, and its tip is anchored to the posterior aspect of the malar eminence. After 5 days of latency, activation of the device begins at a rate of 1 mm/day. New bone formation is observed and a well-defined malar structure is the result (Fig. 37.9).

Orthognathic procedures

For selected adult patients, classical osteotomies with a combination of midface rotation and mandibular lengthening are still utilized.[19] With a Le Fort III osteotomy, the midface is rotated and placed in proper relationship to the mandible using the frontonasal angle as a fulcrum (Fig. 37.10). As a result, the maxilla has a more pronounced anterior projection. It also approximates a more appropriate horizontal plane,

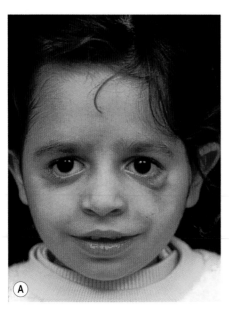 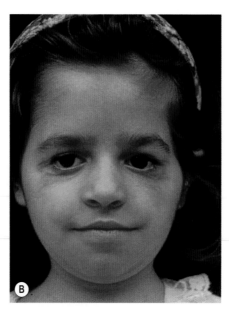 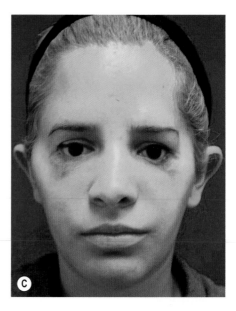

Fig. 37.8 (A) Preoperative view of a 3-year-old girl with Treacher Collins syndrome. Coloboma correction has already been performed. **(B)** Postoperative view at 5 years old. The bilateral bidirectional mandibular distraction has reconstructed the inferior portion of the face. The rotation of the mandible has closed the anterior open bite. **(C)** Postoperative view at 22 years old. The maxilla and the mandible show a nearly normal relationship, demonstrating the kind of craniofacial growth obtained after mandibular distraction and functional orthodontics. The grafted zygomaticomaxillary region, however, demonstrates delayed growth. This situation is likely to be corrected using zygomaticomaxillary distraction and a series of fat injections.

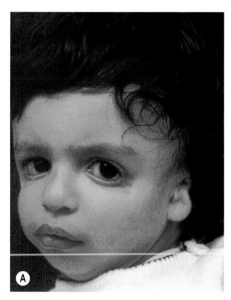
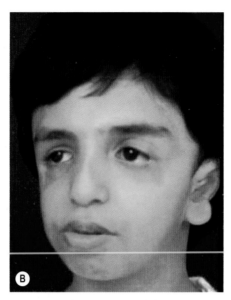
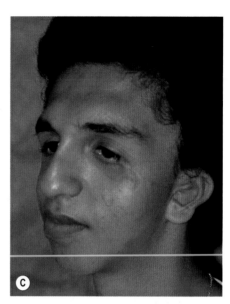

Fig. 37.9 (A) Preoperative view of a 2-year-old boy with classic Treacher Collins syndrome. **(B)** At 7 years old, after coloboma correction, zygomaticomaxillary bone grafting, mandibular distraction, and ear reconstruction. **(C)** At 16 years old, after distraction, new bone formation has produced excellent zygomaticomaxillary volume. Two sessions of fat injection have obtained excellent facial contour and definition.

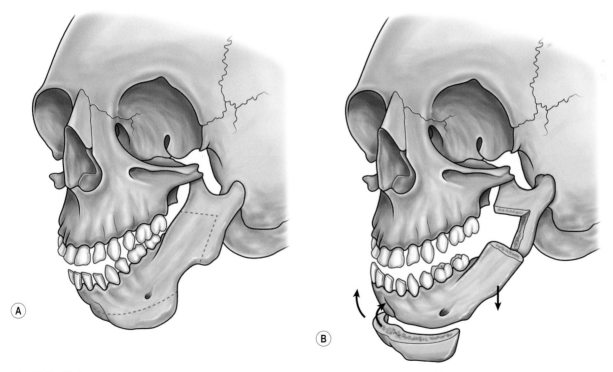

Fig. 37.10 (A) Procedure combining midface rotation and mandible lengthening as proposed by Tessier. **(B)** At the first stage of the surgical procedure, the mandible is elongated and the position of the menton is corrected.

Continued

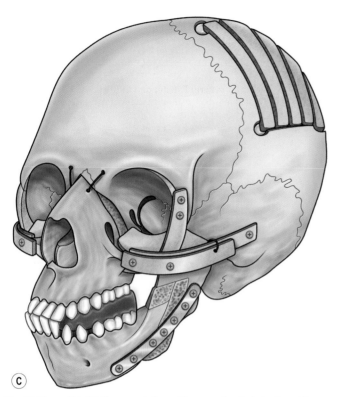

(C)

Fig. 37.10, cont'd (C) The second stage of the procedure includes the midface osteotomy, adapting the occlusion to the new dimension of the mandible. Additional calvarial bone grafts can be added to the orbit and zygoma.

allowing greater lengthening of the mandible, both vertically and sagittally. Unfortunately, the tight soft-tissue envelope sometimes restricts bony repositioning and can be a significant cause of relapse.

Postoperative care

Orthodontic manipulation is absolutely necessary to obtain the final functional occlusion. The use of orthodontic elastics during the consolidation period allows for "callus" manipulation, properly positioning the mandible in relation to the maxilla. Intraoral myofunctional devices, such as the Fränkel III appliance, are used long term to maintain the bone structures and teeth in an excellent relationship.

Secondary procedures

To define the final contour of the cheeks, zygomatic region, and gonial angle, fat grafting is becoming a very important adjunctive technique. In our experience, fat grafting is indicated after 15 years of age to provide the final refinement of soft-tissue contour and volume (Fig. 37.11). With an atraumatic technique, fat is harvested from the abdomen and decanted – preserving growth factors and stem cells. Small parcels of fat are grafted in different planes: the supraperiosteal (30%), muscle (50%), and subcutaneous (20%). In total, 15–20 cc of fat is injected in each side. The procedure is often repeated 2–3 times, at intervals of 4 months between each, to obtain stability of grafted fat.

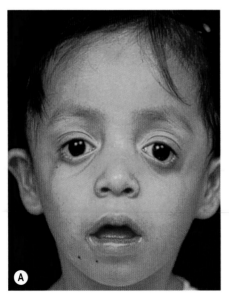
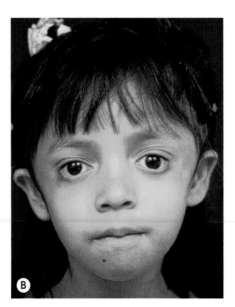
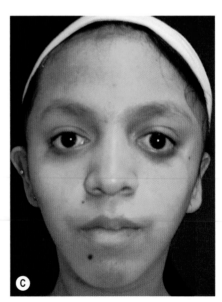

Fig. 37.11 (A) Preoperative fontal view of a 3-year-old girl. Severe colobomas, hypoplastic zygomaticomaxillary region, micrognathia, and anterior open bite are present. **(B)** At 5 years old, after zygomaticomaxillary bone grafting and bilateral codirectional mandibular distraction. Notice the new bone structure at the bizygomatic areas and the inferior third of the face. **(C)** Postoperative view at 20 years old; fat volume has been added, three times to the malar eminences after distraction osteogenesis of the bone grafts. Final permanent refinements of the facial contour have been obtained with fat grafting.

Access the complete reference list online at   **http://www.expertconsult.com**

1. Gorlin RJ, Cohen MM, Levin LS. *Syndromes of the Head and Neck.* 3rd ed. New York: Oxford University Press; 1990.

3. Treacher Collins E. Case with symmetric congenital notches in the outer part of each lid and defective development of the malar bones. *Trans Ophthalmol Soc UK.* 1900;20:109.

4. Franceschetti A, Zwahlen P. Un Syndrome nouveau: La dysostose mandibulo-faciale. *Bull Schweiz Akad Med Wiss.* 1944;1:60–66.

6. Tessier P. Vertical and oblique facial clefts (orbitofacial fissures). In: Mustarde JC, ed. *Plastic Surgery in Infancy and Childhood.* Philadelphia: WB Saunders; 1971:94.

10. Garner L. Cephalometric analysis of Berry–Treacher Collins syndrome. *Oral Surg Oral Med Oral Pathol.* 1967;23:320–327.

11. Marsh JL, Celin SE, Vannier MW, et al. The skeletal anatomy of mandibulofacial dysostosis (Treacher Collins syndrome). *Plast Reconstr Surg.* 1986;78:460–470. *This paper is an observational study of 3D craniofacial CT scans of patients with Treacher Collins syndrome. The authors find that the zygomatic process of the temporal bone is the most frequently aplastic component of these patients' craniofacial skeletons.*

13. McCarthy JG, Zide BM. The spectrum of calvarial bone grafting: introduction of the vascularized calvarial bone flap. *Plast Reconstr Surg.* 1984;74:10–18. *The authors describe traditional methods of bone grafting. A vascularized calvarial flap (based on the temporal vessels) is*

then presented; it is noted that vascularized bone flaps are ideal for devitalized recipient sites, such as may be encountered in midface reconstruction for Treacher Collins syndrome.

14. Molina F, Ortiz Monasterio F. Extended indications for mandibular distraction: unilateral, bilateral and bidirectional. *International Craniofacial Congress.* 1993;5:79.

15. Molina F, Ortiz Monasterio F. Mandibular elongation and remodeling by distraction: A farewell to major osteotomies. *Plast Reconstr Surg.* 1995;96:825–842. *The authors discuss a novel corticotomy-based method for mandibular distraction. Improved facial symmetry was noted in their cohort, with no observed relapse.*

18. Van der Meulen JCH, Hauben DJ, Vaandrager JM, et al. The use of a temporal osteoparietal flap for the reconstruction of malar hypoplasia in Treacher Collins syndrome. *Plast Reconstr Surg.* 1984;74:687–693. *The temporalis muscle provides an axial vascular supply to the temporal periosteal bone flap described in this paper. The osseous component of the flap may seed further bone growth when this flap is used for malar reconstruction in patients with Treacher Collins syndrome.*

19. Tessier P, Tulasne JF. Treacher Collins syndrome. Combined rotation of the midfacial segment and mandibular lengthening. In: Marchac D, ed. *Craniofacial Surgery.* Berlin: Springer-Verlag; 1987:369.

Congenital melanocytic nevi

Sara R. Dickie, Neta Adler, and Bruce S. Bauer

SYNOPSIS

- Congenital melanocytic nevi (CMN) are composed of clusters of nevomelanocytes that are generally present at birth but occasionally arise as late as several years of age. These lesions arise from melanocytic stem cells that migrate from the neural crest to the embryonic dermis and upward into the epidermis. They may also migrate into the leptomeninges.

- Although the bulk of these lesions are small and benign, some cover large portions of the body or can be in conspicuous locations, and may create an aesthetically displeasing appearance, resulting in psychological issues. Furthermore, their potential for malignant degeneration causes anxiety for the parent, primary care physician, and surgeon alike.

- Small pigmented nevi are present in 1 in 100 births; large nevi are present in only 1 in 20 000 births; and the giant lesions are even less common. As a result, most surgeons have little experience with them and little opportunity to develop a rational protocol for their treatment.

Introduction

Congenital melanocytic nevi (CMN) consist of clusters of nevomelanocytes that develop *in utero*. Although many congenital nevi are visible at birth, some are "tardive", probably because they are too small to be detected at birth or do not have sufficient melanin.[1,2] CMN are one of the risk factors for eventual development of cutaneous and extracutaneous melanoma, with larger nevi having greater risk. Based on that, CMN are historically classified according to their estimated largest diameter in adulthood. Small nevi are up to 1.5 cm; medium are 1.5–19.9 cm; and large nevi are those with estimated diameter of more than 20 cm. Giant nevi are 40 cm or larger. Newer classification takes into account size, location, various phonotypical features, and presence of satellite nevi.[3] Congenital nevi present in approximately 1% of births;[4] large CMN occur in approximately 1:20 000 births; and giant lesions (>40 cm) are 1 in 500 000.[5]

While most surgeons are familiar with treating the small and intermediate-sized nevi, it is difficult to gain enough experience when approaching more extensive lesions.

Many strategies have been tried for removal and reconstruction of large and giant nevi. When direct excision and primary closure are not a possibility, then tissue expansion is the "workhorse" treatment modality for many medium to large nevi. Facial nevi that cross multiple aesthetic units as well as involving the periorbital area may require expansion in combination with full-thickness skin graft (expanded or non-expanded). Some unique cases may benefit from a free flap and tissue expansion as an adjunct procedure to close the donor site.

Access the Historical Perspective section online at
http://www.expertconsult.com

Basic science/disease process

The etiology of CMN remains unclear. The development of CMN is determined *in utero* between 5 and 24 weeks' gestation. One of the theories of melanocyte differentiation is that, as the neural tube develops during early embryogenesis, melanoblasts migrate from the neural crest along the leptomeninges to the embryonic dermis.[6] From the embryonic dermis, the progenitor melanocytic cells migrate into the epidermis, where they differentiate into dendritic melanocytes.

Dysregulated migration, proliferation, and differentiation of melanocytes in the skin and leptomeninges are implicated in the pathogenesis of CMN and neurocutaneous melanosis (NCM).[8,9]

Several molecular signaling pathways have been associated with the pathogenesis of CMN. Melanocyte development appears partially under the control of c-met and c-kit proto-oncogenes, which encode met and kit proteins, respectively. Hepatocyte growth factor (HGF), also known as scatter factor (SF), is a multifunctional regulator of epithelial cells expressing the tyrosine kinase receptor encoded by c-met. Overexpression of HGF/SF, which is a ligand for the met protein receptor, is implicated in perturbations of melanocyte proliferation, differentiation, survival, and migration.[10] Transgenic mice overexpressing HGF/SF are born with cutaneous and leptomeningeal melanocytosis.[11] HGF/SF also functions in regulating the migration and differentiation of premyogenic cells during embryogenesis.[11] It has been shown that overexpression of this signaling molecule in mice may lead to rhabdomyosarcoma,[12] a tumor that on rare occasions also arises in patients with large CMN.[13,14] Furthermore, studies with met null mice suggest that met plays a role in NCM, because met knockout mice do not develop NCM.[12] Overexpression of HGF/SF and/or met, and sustained activation of met, could explain the mechanism of cutaneous and leptomeningeal melanoma and rhabdomyosarcoma development in individuals with CMN. C-kit, a proto-oncogene that encodes the kit tyrosine kinase receptor for the ligand known as SCF, also plays a role in melanocyte development. In tissue cell culture, c-kit-expressing neural crest cells give rise to clones containing only melanocytes.[15] Proliferative nodules, consisting of aggregates of epithelioid or spindled immature benign melanocytes in the dermis of CMN, highly express c-kit.[16] Moreover, kit can activate N-RAS, which is an oncogene that is mutated in some cases of nodular melanoma.[17]

Recently, mutations within two oncogenes have been identified within most CMN. Mutations within N-RAS and B-RAF appear to be mutually exclusive to one another and present in up to 85% of lesions.[18] Identical mutations in N-RAS codon Q61 have been found in affected skin lesions and the CNS of patients with NCM, but not in their non-lesional skin.[19] This mosaicism might indicate a somatic versus a germline mutation of these oncogenes. BRAF may be more prevalent in patients with NCM.[18] The identification of these mutations and further research show promise for the development of gene therapies.

The exact risk for development of melanoma in CMN is not clear. While the absolute lifetime risk for the incidence of melanoma in patients with large CMN is reported to be lower than previously thought, around 2–5%,[20–23] the highest risk group in this population is children with giant bathing trunk nevi (12% of CMN >60 cm).[24] Patients with small and medium-sized CMN have a lower risk of melanoma, with a reported absolute risk of <1%.[24,25] Many articles discussing the issue of relative risk of melanoma do not differentiate between cutaneous and extracutaneous melanoma and the presence of NCM may be the greater risk factor in subsequent risk of malignancy.

Neurocutaneous melanosis is characterized by an excess deposition of melanocytes along the leptomeninges (Fig. 38.1). It can occur in both patients with large CMN and those with multiple small or medium-sized CMN. Patients with large CMN located on the posterior axis are thought to have greater risk for NCM but, on a multivariate analysis, the only risk factor for NCM in patients with large congenital nevi is having multiple satellite nevi: >20 satellites had a 5.1-fold increased risk for NCM compared with patients with fewer satellites.[26] The true incidence is not known, but symptomatic NCM may affect 6–11% of patients with large CMN. Symptomatic NCM has a poor prognosis. Symptoms frequently present in early childhood. Neurologic symptoms can manifest themselves as seizures, developmental delay, hydrocephalus, and delayed motor development.

Rarely, other tumors, such as rhabdomyosarcoma and liposarcoma, are associated with CMN.

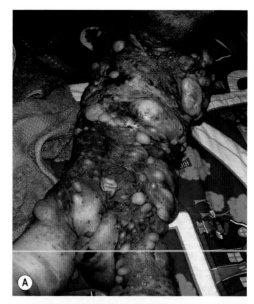

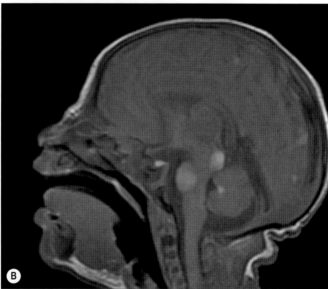

Fig. 38.1 (A) This child with near-total body nevus shows marked variation in nevus thickness, color, and surface architecture. Multiple areas of thick, neural nevus are present. **(B)** A T1-weighted image on magnetic resonance imaging demonstrates several lesions typical of neurocutaneous melanosis.

Diagnosis/patient presentation

Historically, CMN have been categorized by predicted adult diameter as the lone criterion to differentiate one lesion from another. With increasing understanding of the genetic make-up of these lesions and improved, prospective data collection techniques, efforts have been made to standardize the classification system. In 2012, Krengel *et al.*, proposed a schema that has been widely accepted by many experts in the field of CMN (Table 38.1).[3] By using a standardized

Table 38.1 A schema to standardize the description of congenital melanocytic nevi[3]

CMN parameter	Terminology	Definition
CMN projected adult size	Small	<1.5 cm
	Medium	
	M1	1.5–10 cm
	M2	10–20 cm
	Large	
	L1	>20–30 cm
	L2	>30–40 cm
	Giant	
	G1	>40–60 cm
	G2	>60 cm
	Multiple	>3 medium CMN without a single predominant CMN
CMN Localization		
Head	Face, scalp	
Trunk	Neck, shoulder, upper/mid/lower back, breast/chest, abdomen, flank, gluteal region, genital region	
Extremities	Upper arm, forearm, hand, thigh, lower leg, foot	
Number of satellites (refers to the number within the first year of life)	S0	No satellites
	S1	<20 satellites
	S2	20–50 satellites
	S3	>50 satellites
Additional morphologic features	C0, C1, C2	None, moderate, marked color heterogeneity
	R0, R1, R2	None, moderate, marked surface rugosity
	N0, N1, N2	None, scattered, extensive nodules
	H0, H1, H2	None, notable, marked hypertrichosis

Adapted from Table III (Krengel S, Scope A, Dusza SW, et al. New recommendations for the categorization of cutaneous features of congenital melanocytic nevi. *J Am Acad Dermatol.* 2013;68:441–451.)

system to describe these highly variable lesions, clinicians and researchers will be able to correlate morphogenic features with the molecular-genetics underlying this rare disease, eventually leading to improved treatment methods, targeted gene therapy, and better understanding of nevomelanocyte behavior.

Small to medium-sized CMN usually present as round to oval homogeneous pigmented lesions, light to dark brown in color, with sharply demarcated borders, rugous surface, and hypertrichosis. However, larger CMN, in particular, may show asymmetry, irregular borders, multicolored pigment pattern, rugous texture, and a nodular surface. In addition, large CMN are often associated with many smaller satellite nevi. As the child grows, especially at puberty, the CMN may change color, becoming lighter or darker, developing hair, becoming more heterogeneous or more homogeneous. CMN may spontaneously regress, and some patients may develop vitiligo. Nodular proliferation may be present from birth or develop at a later age. CMN are usually asymptomatic;

however, patients with larger lesions may present with pruritus, xerosis, skin fragility, erosions, or ulcerations and decreased ability to sweat from the involved skin (Fig. 38.2).

A review of dermoscopy patterns in congenital nevi found that most nevi demonstrate a reticular, globular, or reticulo-globular pattern. The findings varied with age and the anatomic location of the nevus, with the globular pattern found more often in younger children and the reticular pattern found in patients aged 12 years or older.[27]

Because of the increased risk of melanoma associated with congenital nevi, attempts have been made to distinguish congenital nevi from acquired nevi on the basis of histology. Distinguishing histologic features include: (1) involvement by nevus cells of deep dermal appendages and neurovascular structures (including hair follicles, sebaceous glands, arrector pili muscles, and within walls of blood vessels); (2) extension of nevus cells to deep dermis and subcutaneous fat; (3) infiltration of nevus cells between collagen bundles; and (4) a nevus cell-poor subepidermal zone.[28–30] In contrast to congenital nevi, acquired nevi are usually composed of nevus cells that are limited to the papillary and upper reticular dermis and do not involve the appendages.

In cases associated with a high index of suspicion for the presence of NCM, magnetic resonance imaging of the central nervous system is a useful diagnostic tool (see Fig. 38.1B).

Patient selection

The treatment of large and giant nevi is controversial. Although the risk of malignant transformation in congenital pigmented nevi is well established,[21,31–34] many feel that the risk of developing melanoma is too low to warrant the unsightly scars or grafts that may follow treatment. There is no evidence in the literature that demonstrates decrease in occurrence of melanoma after excision of large congenital melanocytic lesions. Furthermore, these patients have an increased risk of extracutaneous melanoma.[34,35] Others feel that, in the presence of NCM, the greatest risk lies within the central nervous system, so the excision of the cutaneous lesion can only have limited benefits. However, the appearance of these lesions clearly produces a stigma with significant psychological implications. The challenge for the surgeon involved in treating these often-complex lesions is to develop treatment modalities that not only accomplish the excision of all or most of the nevus but also lead to an optimal aesthetic and functional outcome.

Although the lifetime risk of malignant melanoma for small and medium congenital pigmented nevi is reported to be 0–4.9%,[36] the risk of melanoma is nearly nil prior to puberty for small nevi,[37,38] and so one may comfortably wait until the child is old enough to excise the lesion under local anesthesia. If the lesion is located in an area where the excision and reconstruction may not likely be accomplished under local anesthesia, or where there may be the possibility of a better final scar with earlier excision, then early excision under general anesthesia may be warranted. Certainly, many nevi positioned in prominent parts of the face may present as a significant source of peer ridicule starting quite early in the school years, and delaying the excision in an effort to avoid a general anesthetic is not in the child's best interest.

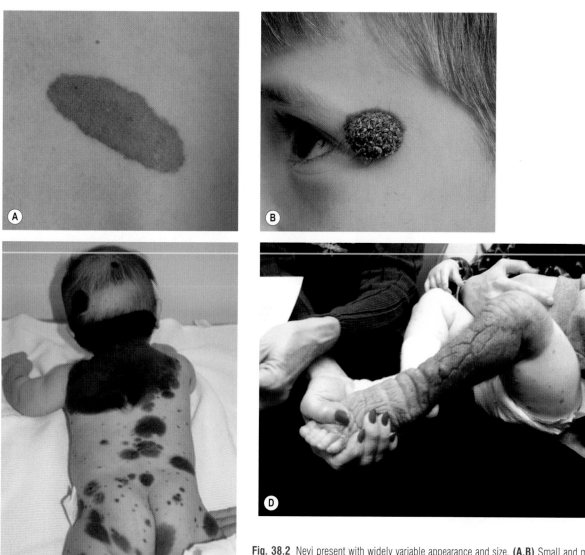

Fig. 38.2 Nevi present with widely variable appearance and size. **(A,B)** Small and medium nevi may be flat with uniform color and border, or thick and verrucous. **(C)** They may present as large nevi with multiple small and medium satellite nevi, or **(D)** on the lower extremity they may become thick, cerebriform-like, and associated with severe pruritus and chronic breakdown.

The authors advocate treatment of large and giant nevi beginning at 6 months of age in most cases. Although many of the tissue expansion procedures used in the treatment of large nevi can be applied to older children and adults, the intolerance for repeated procedures and the decreased elasticity of the skin may make the excision of extensive lesions impractical in older patients. Also, for larger nevi the greatest risk for malignancy is in the first few years.[24,39,40]

Treatment/surgical technique

Many strategies have been tried for the removal and reconstruction of large and giant nevi. Serial excision can often debulk these massive lesions but rarely remove them completely. Excision and split-thickness skin graft have generally poor functional and aesthetic outcomes. Dermabrasion, curettage, chemical peel, and laser treatment all have problems with recurrence, since these modalities only eliminate the superficial portion of the nevus while the cells of congenital pigmented nevi can usually be found as deep as the subcutaneous fat and sometimes even in deeper structures.[32] This group of "partial-thickness" excision, while potentially reducing the overall number of nevus cells and lightening the degree of pigmentation, is commonly associated with later "bleed through" of the deep nevus cells, but may be manifest as both abnormal skin coloration and hypertrichosis (Fig. 38.3). There is also difficulty following the lesions for malignant transformation because of the scarring. The long-term effects of laser treatment on the remaining nevus cells remain to be determined.

Juvenile skin, although elastic, does not have the laxity of an adult skin and local flaps used in adults are often difficult in children. When direct excision and primary closure are not a possibility, then tissue expansion is the "workhorse" treatment modality for many medium to large nevi. Facial nevi that cross multiple aesthetic units, as well as involving the periorbital area, may require expansion in combination with

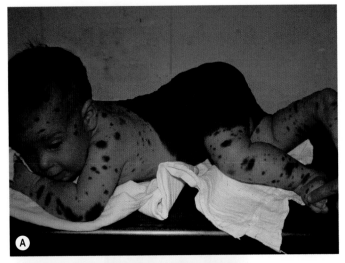

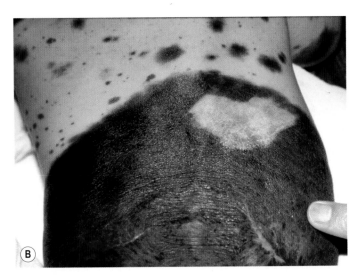

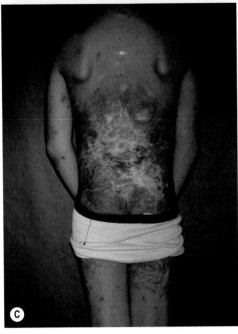

Fig. 38.3 **(A)** This infant has a giant nevus and multiple satellite nevi. **(B)** The light area within the nevus was dermabraded in the neonatal period. **(C)** At 7 years of age, despite partial-thickness excision with a dermatome at 3 months of age, nevus cells are present throughout the back and even in the initially dermabraded area, despite its continued lighter appearance.

full-thickness skin graft (expanded or non-expanded). Finally, some unique cases may benefit from a free flap and tissue expansion as an adjunct procedure to close the donor site.

Partial-thickness excision

Partial-thickness excision of large and giant nevi has taken the form of early dermabrasion, curettage, laser, or more recently, excision, leaving the underlying subcutaneous fat in place, to minimize contour deformities and covering this with a dermal collagen substructure and very thin split-thickness skin graft or even culture skin. These latter approaches have been particularly applied to the extremities where techniques such as expansion are not as readily applied. The potential downside of each of these approaches is that, while the surface nevus population may be reduced, the deeper nevus cells will frequently "bleed through" over time, leaving an even more significant deformity at an age when complete excision may no longer be an option. Circumferential grafting of the

extremities with these approaches can still also result in significant late functional disturbance.

Serial excision

Serial excision is the excision of a lesion in more than one stage. The inherent viscoelastic properties of skin are used, allowing the skin to stretch over time. These techniques enable wound closure to be accomplished with a shorter scar than if the original lesion was elliptically excised in a single stage and to reorient the scar closer to the relaxed skin lines. This technique can be applied to small or medium nevi, depending on the location of the nevus and the laxity of the local skin (Fig. 38.4). However, with each stage of the serial excision there is some recoil, and serial excision alone, near sensitive areas such as the lower eyelid and oral commissure, may create tissue shortage and long-term distortion of structures that would not arise if tissue expansion had been applied rather than serial excision alone.

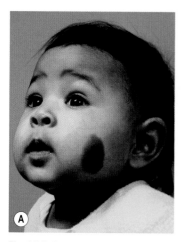
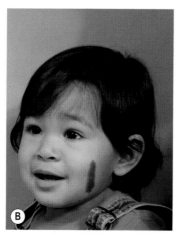
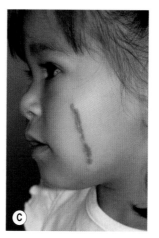
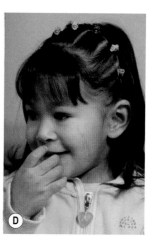

Fig. 38.4 A medium-sized nevus of the cheek is excised in three surgeries with the benefit of reducing the length of the final scar as well as avoiding potential distortion of the surrounding facial structures. **(A)** Preoperatively; **(B)** 6 months after first-stage excision; **(C)** 6 months after second-stage excision; and **(D)** 4 months after the third and final stage.

Excision with skin graft reconstruction

As noted above, the depth of the congenital nevus requires excision to the fascial level if one is to limit the risk of leaving nevus behind, either to "bleed through" later, or to undergo degeneration with potentially late identification. However, skin grafts do have some role in the treatment of congenital nevi.

On the face (periorbital region and ear), expanded and non-expanded full-thickness skin grafts provide good match in both color and thickness for the recipient area. Similarly, expanded full-thickness skin grafts are an excellent choice for coverage on the dorsum of the hand and foot (and distal third of the leg) (Fig. 38.5). However, if the excision is being carried

to the fascial level, the contour deformity produced following excision and skin graft to the extremities and trunk can be significant and result in both aesthetic and functional defects later in life.

Use of split-thickness skin grafting on the trunk, even when done with non-meshed medium-thickness grafts, can still result in considerable late deformity with potential associated functional defects where the graft skin does not keep up with surrounding growth. The one area of the trunk that can be grafted without significant late contour deformity is the back because of the relatively uniform flat surface. Significant contour deformities develop later where the grafting is carried on to the flanks and anterior trunk (particularly in heavier individuals where the border between grafted and non-grafted

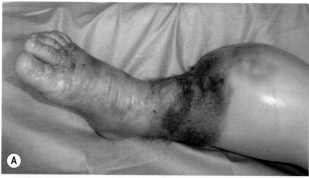
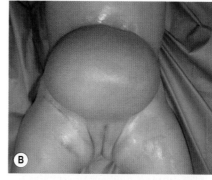
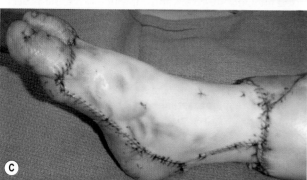
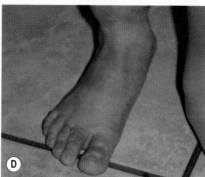

Fig. 38.5 An expanded full-thickness skin graft provides both good functional and aesthetic reconstruction on the dorsum of the foot and lower-quarter to one-third of the leg. **(A,B)** In this patient, expansion was carried out both regionally and at the graft donor site in the lower abdomen and bilateral groin. **(C)** At completion of grafting with the expanded full-thickness skin graft and advancement of the expanded adjacent skin flap to minimize the step-off between flap and graft. **(D)** The result at 1 year post-grafting.

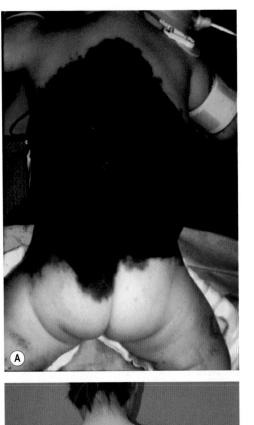

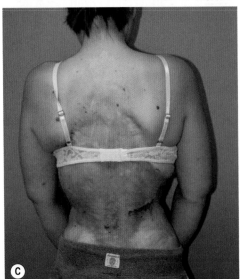

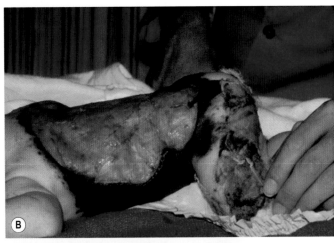

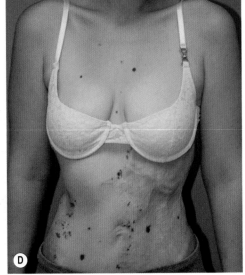

Fig. 38.6 (A) This case, treated early in our giant nevus experience, had the unusual feature of fixation of the nevus to the deep tissues of the back and invasion of the underlying latissimus muscle, requiring a deeper-plane excision. **(B)** At 1 week post-excision, the non-meshed split-thickness skin graft was healing well. **(C,D)** A significant contour deformity is seen 22 years later, after excision of the remaining nevus only to fascial level.

skin can create quite dramatic deformities) (Fig. 38.6). Skin grafting of the back can, however, provide a means of excising a large segment of the nevus, in an area of potentially greater risk of degeneration, and enhance the dermatologist's ability to map and follow the remaining lesion.

Tissue expansion

Several types of tissue expanders exist based on shape, size, and type of filling valve. The shape that the authors most commonly use in treatment of congenital nevi is rectangular. Expander volumes have a wide range and vary according to the anatomic site. Saline is delivered in a controlled fashion via the valve port, which is located at some distance from the

expander, overlying firm tissue. While integrated ports have been used by some surgeons, the authors use remote ports in all cases with none externalized, despite the fact that the parents typically do the expander injections. Since the skin overlying the port can be readily anesthetized with a topical anesthetic, there is no benefit in externalizing the ports.

Consideration for the incisions, expander placement, and flap movement in relation to the defect and postoperative scars requires preoperative planning and discussion with the patient and family. In regard to donor site, one must match color, texture, and contour of the recipient site to maximize the aesthetic and functional outcome. The donor site tissue must be free of infection, or have stable scars, to minimize the risk of expander failure or extrusion. Careful selection of expander size is also imperative in areas with thin donor skin, in order to avoid expander folds or prominence which can create areas of excessive pressure and skin compromise. In the majority of the cases, the expanders are placed through an incision within the border of the lesion. In cases where the expansion has been used repeatedly and scars are present both at the border of the remaining nevus and at junctions of prior flaps, the new expanders should be placed through those scars that are least likely to be stressed by the weight or pull of the new expander (i.e., away from the most dependent points). In other cases, like unstable scar, vascular tumor, and craniofacial deformities, the incisions are planned outside the border of defect or on occasion at a distant site. A pocket is dissected to allow placement of the expander with placement of the port in a separate pocket over a region with firm skeletal support for ease of outpatient filling. Partial fill of the expander (10–20% of the listed volume) ensures the expander is properly positioned without surface folds that can cause pressure against the skin flap to be expanded. Closed suction drains are placed for a few days (3–10 days) to control the potential dead space from wide undermining.

Serial injections are started 7–10 days post-insertion provided the skin flaps are in excellent condition and continue on a weekly basis for about 10–12 weeks. Most pediatric patients go on a home expansion protocol with injections performed by the parents under the direction of our nursing staff and surgeons.

If another set of expanders is needed to excise the lesion fully (serial expansion), the authors usually wait 4–6 months between them.

A broad-spectrum antibiotic is started upon surgery and is continued until the drains are removed. By maintaining a low threshold for placing the expander patient back on antibiotic in the presence of suspected beginning of infection, most infections can be controlled before potential loss of the expander.

The design of an expanded flap is of major importance. While the early dogma of tissue expansion emphasized designing advancement flaps only, experience over more than two decades has demonstrated that expanded transposition and rotation flaps may frequently be preferable. It provides greater versatility in flap design and range.[41,42] The high vascularity of expanded flaps, gained by the process of expansion, makes this design safe. In the expanded transposition flap, the base of the flap is also expanded, which allows advancement of the base of the flap in addition to the transposition of the tissues and thus provides greater coverage than advancement only.

Regional consideration in pediatric tissue expansion

The optimal choice of treatment still varies by body region, and the most pertinent issues and considerations necessary for successful tissue expansion in each body region is now discussed.

Scalp

The expander is placed in a pocket dissected subgaleal but staying above the periosteum. Flaps are designed taking into consideration the orientation of the major scalp vessels (superficial temporal, postauricular, occipital vessels, and contribution from supraorbital vessels). Port placement in the preauricular area is favored when an expander does not encroach on the area because of the ease of palpation, limited risk to the overlying skin, and low risk of migration. The expanders used in scalp reconstruction are usually of 250, 350, or 500 cc volume (although 70 cc expanders may be used for medium-sized nevi). Large and giant nevi might require serial expansion with a larger expander placed after each stage to distribute expansile forces evenly over the hair follicles. As previous studies have shown, tissue expansion itself does not induce proliferation of hair follicles but can more than double the size of the scalp without visible decrease in hair density.[43] Despite former thoughts that expansion may affect cranial vault morphology, it usually self-corrects within 3–4 months.[44,45]

The use of expanded transposition flaps versus simple advancement flap design has greatly reduced the number of serial expansion required and has resulted in improved reconstruction of hair direction and hairline (Fig. 38.7).

Face and neck

Large and giant nevi of the face are the most visible of these lesions and also represent the area where unsightly scarring is most readily visible; consequently, the planning and execution of the reconstructive plan must be very detailed.

To achieve an optimal aesthetic and functional result in the facial and cervical regions, one must adhere to the subunit principle. This dictates incision placement so the final result has the scar hidden in a natural crease (e.g., nasolabial fold). Undue tension on facial structures (brow, eyelid, mouth) can cause disfigurement such as brow asymmetry or ptosis, anterior hairline asymmetry, lower lid and oral drooping, especially when using cervical skin flaps cephalad to the cervicomandibular angle.

Neale and associates report 10% lower eyelid ectropion rate and >10% lower lip deformity in this context.[46] Judicious flap design and the use of expanded transposition and rotation flaps, as well as the use of multiple expanders and overexpansion, are recommended to minimize these complications.

For forehead lesions, in general one should always use the largest expander possible under the uninvolved forehead skin, occasionally even carrying the expander under the lesion. As an initial step to the reconstruction of the forehead, the brow should be set in place using permanent sutures along the supraorbital rim. Thereby the transposition of the forehead does not disrupt the position of the brow as the flap is moved. It is important to avoid elevation of either the ipsilateral or contralateral brow, since it can only be returned to the preoperative position with the interposition of additional non-hair-bearing forehead skin. Expansion of the deficient area alone will not reliably lower the brow once a skin deficiency exists.[47] Over-reaching with the expanded flap both risks flap compromise and increases the risk of brow and hairline distortion. Accepting the need for repeat forehead expansion to complete the forehead reconstruction may also limit the length of the scar above the brow on the uninvolved side.

For eyelid reconstruction, full-thickness skin grafts can also achieve better functional and aesthetic results than split-thickness skin grafts. In the past, the authors used

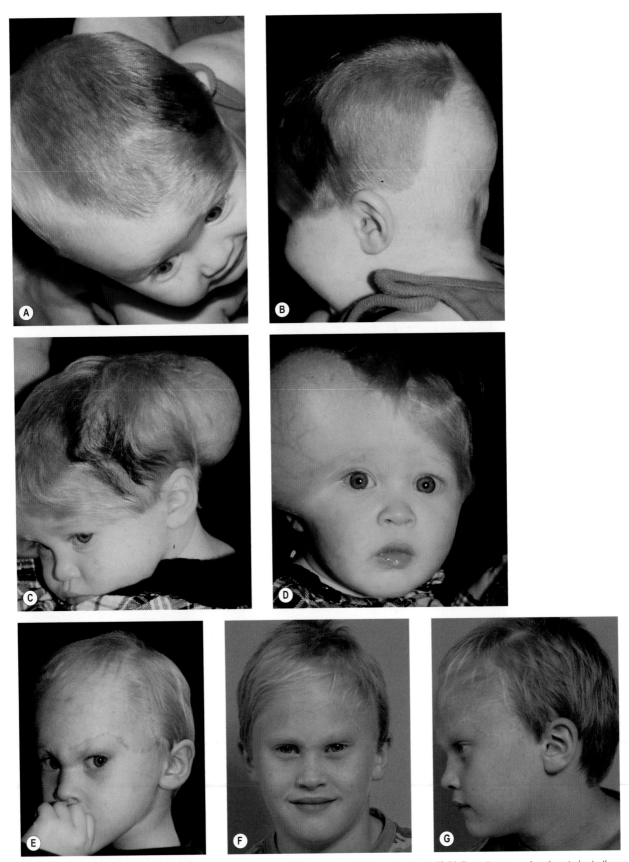

Fig. 38.7 (A,B) This infant was born with a large nevus of nearly half the scalp and left lateral forehead. **(C,D)** Expanders were placed posterior to the nevus and beneath the normal forehead and adjacent scalp at 6 months of age. **(E)** The appearance of the reconstructed scalp and forehead at 2 years of age and 1 year post-excision of the remaining scalp nevus requiring a second expansion. Forehead width, hairline, and hair direction are well-oriented. Some residual excess skin is present in the glabellar area. **(F,G)** At 6 years following completion of the expansion and minor revision of the scars along the brow, the patient has excellent symmetry and a natural hairline and direction of hair growth.

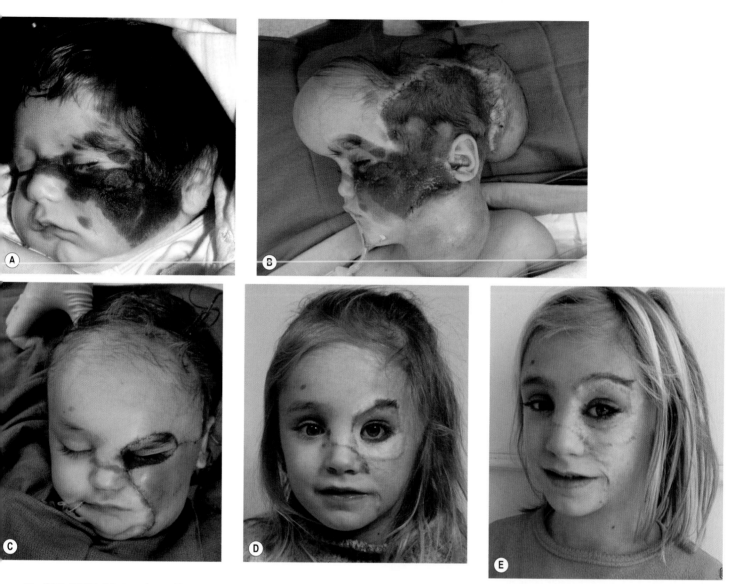

Fig. 38.8 **(A)** This infant was born with a thick mamillated hairy nevus with deeply pigmented areas centrally and light pigmentation along the borders, which gradually darkened. **(B)** Three expanders are shown in place and, with hair trimmed, the full extent of the nevus is visible. **(C)** Nevus of the forehead, cheek, nose, and scalp is excised following well-planned expander placement. The eyelid and brow were not addressed at this point. **(D)** At 3 years post-expansion, prior to further excision of the nevus of the eyelid, revision of graft, and scar of brow and canthal region. The upper and lower eyelids were grafted with a single-piece expanded full-thickness skin graft from the supraclavicular area. **(E)** At 7 years of age, the eye and brow symmetry are good and the patient is ready for minor revision with both surgery and laser.

pre-expansion of a donor site allowing a single, large full-thickness skin graft to be harvested for reconstruction of the eyelids, canthus, and lid between the eyelid fold and brow of the upper lid.[48] In recent years, surgeons have aimed to reconstruct the region between upper eyelid crease and eyebrow with a pedicle flap from the forehead. The tissue likeness is more consistent in young children, whereas a graft in this area can appear too thin and can be aesthetically unpredictable. The supraclavicular and post-auricular areas are the ideal donor sites for grafts to be placed on the face because of excellent color and texture match. For larger grafts requiring expansion, part of the expansion provides for the graft tissue, with the remainder used for primary closure of the donor site. Donor site expansion also allows harvest of free flaps from distant sites to cover complete cheek or forehead aesthetic units when regional tissue is not available. Where previously the surgeons carried the single graft on to the nasal dorsum

when the nevus involved the periorbital area and nose, they now use flaps from the expanded forehead for that coverage (often combined with excision of nevus of the forehead) (Fig. 38.8).

The eyebrow may be reconstructed at the same time as the eyelid, treated after the adjacent forehead or eyelid nevus is excised, or left unresected as an important aesthetic landmark (Fig. 38.8C). When the eyebrow is heavily involved with the nevus, it is the authors' current practice to leave a small portion of the nevus unexcised, to mimic the normal eyebrow. If the nevus is darkly pigmented in a fair-skinned child, the residual lesion may be lightened through laser treatment at a later time. However, the long-term effectiveness of this approach has not yet been established. The residual brow nevus is closely followed, and if changes occur either in surface character or color, leading to concerns about potential degeneration, the involved brow is excised and reconstructed.

A reconstructive option includes an island flap of temporal scalp based on a branch of superficial temporal artery. If the temporal scalp is minimally involved with nevus and there is a plan for simultaneous expansion of the temporal scalp, the island flap can be planned from the area of maximally expanded flap, with the effect that the hair density is lessened in expansion, and the resultant reconstructed brow will not be too dense. However, for patients where the temporal scalp is involved with nevus, reconstruction with micrografts or strip grafts may become necessary. These are decisions that may not be possible to make until the late teens or adult years.

Trunk

The most common location of giant nevi was found to be over the posterior trunk, often extending anteriorly in a dermatome distribution.

Tissue expansion can be very effective on the anterior trunk, provided that the lesion is confined to either the lower abdomen or central abdomen and that there is sufficient uninvolved skin above, or above and below the nevus to expand. Expansion must be avoided in or around the area of the breast bud in females and lesions of the breast should be left until after breast development. Flaps below the chest can be designed as transposition or rotation flaps rather than direct downward advancement to avoid pulling on the nipple areolar complex.

Alternatively, expanded flaps can be advanced transversely across the abdomen, re-insetting the umbilicus in the same manner as in a standard abdominoplasty (Fig. 38.9).

The use of expanded transposition flaps has enabled excision of nevi of the upper back/neck and back/buttock/perineal region, where previously it was thought that only skin grafting was possible. Tissue expanders in the 500–750 cc

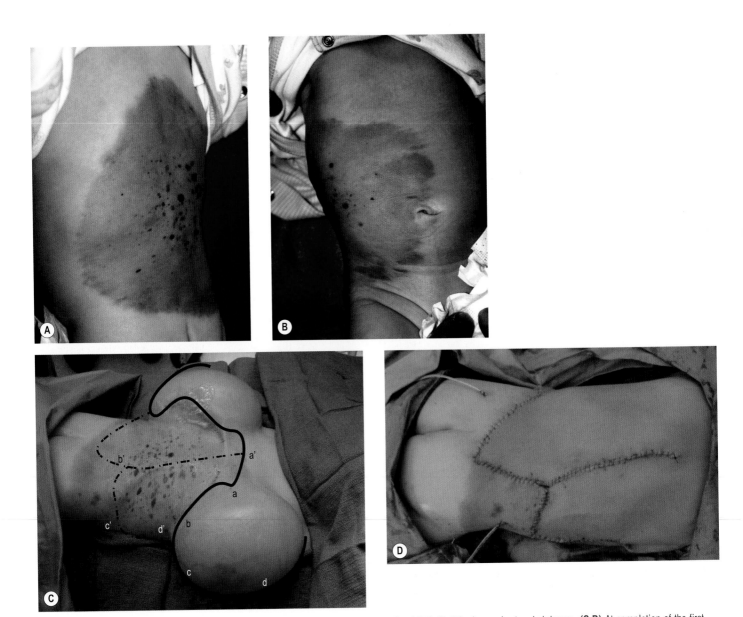

Fig. 38.9 (A,B) This large nevus covers the greater part of the back and wraps around to the right half of the lower chest and abdomen. **(C,D)** At completion of the first expansion of the back, the flaps are transposed to cover most of the back. The flaps are designed with a superomedial base and a back cut across the lateral part of the flap (points c–d). This design allows greater coverage of normal tissue due to the advancement of the base of the flap (points d–d').

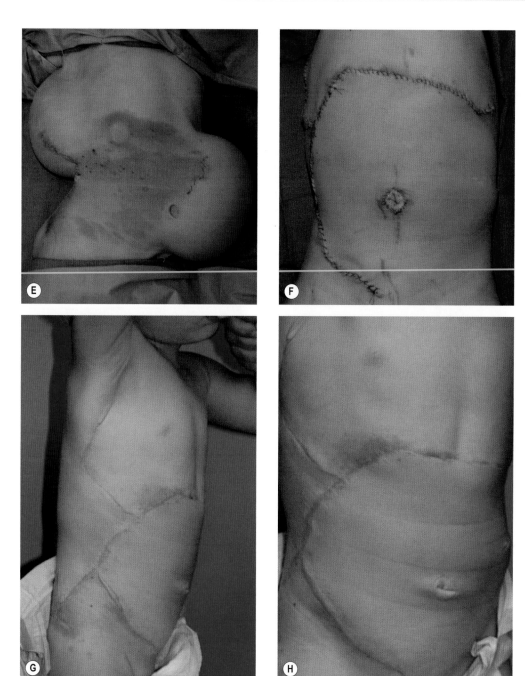

Fig. 38.9, cont'd (E) The second set of expanders is placed beneath one of the previously expanded back flaps and beneath the uninvolved left abdominal skin. **(F)** The expanded flaps, anterior and posterior, join on the right flank as the abdominal flap is advanced transversely across the abdomen and the umbilicus is delivered through the flap. **(G,H)** Anterior and lateral views 2 months postoperatively show only small areas of remaining nevus that can be excised from the upper abdomen without further expansion and without risk of downward pull on the right breast.

range are used most commonly in infants and young children. Serial expansion with careful planning has made possible the excision of progressively larger nevi of the back and buttocks, with excellent outcomes. Subsequent expansions, as a child gets older, are carried out using expanders in the 250–500 cc size for shoulders and upper back and 1000–1200 cc size for the lower back/buttocks (Figs. 38.10 & 38.11).

In patients with giant nevi involving the entire or near-entire back, flanks, and abdomen, and with markedly variegated nevus architecture or color, one may decide to excise the greater part of the nevus of the back alone, and cover this with split-thickness (non-meshed) skin grafts (see Fig. 38.6). Some literature suggests that this is the area at greatest risk of degeneration, and when color, texture, or character of the nevus makes follow-up difficult, excision may be warranted to "simplify" follow-up. It is recognized that split-thickness skin grafts elsewhere on the trunk and extremities may be associated with significant deformity and potential functional disturbance during growth, so the authors recommend against grafting elsewhere. The back is the only area where split-thickness skin grafting may provide a reasonable aesthetic result as long as the graft is not meshed.

Extremities

Tissue expansion of the extremities has been viewed classically as of limited value and is associated with a higher risk of complications.[49,50]

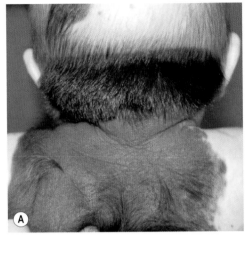

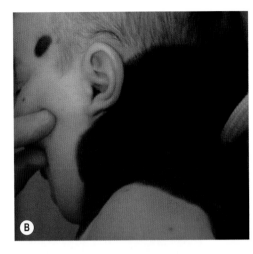

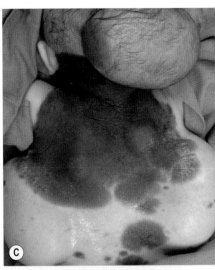

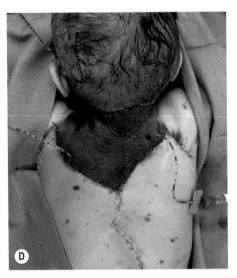

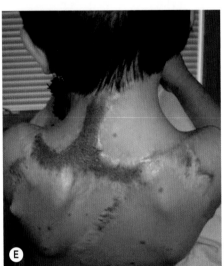

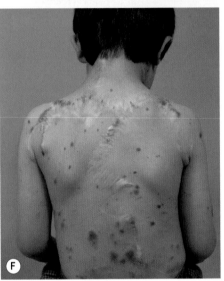

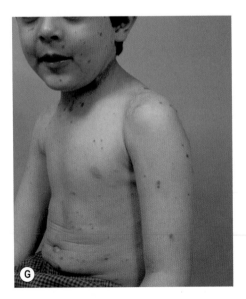

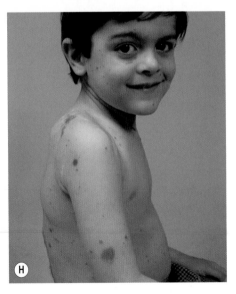

Fig. 38.10 (A,B) This patient, shown fully in Fig. 38.2C, showed thick, deeply pigmented nevus over the occiput, neck, and upper back with multiple satellite nevi on the remaining trunk, extremities, and face. **(C,D)** The first expanders were placed in the occiput above the nevus and bilateral back/flanks below the nevus. This allowed excision of scalp nevus and the lower portion of the back nevus and brought normal back skin to join normal shoulder skin lateral to the remaining neck/shoulder nevus. **(E)** At 3 years of age, the expanded flaps have been advanced further towards the midline of the posterior neck prior to final excision. **(F–H)** As in other patients with some uninvolved skin in the anterior shoulders, he was able to undergo serial expansion of the shoulder flaps to complete the shoulder, neck, and upper back nevus excision. Although some of the satellites remain and scars have widened in the upper back, the shoulder, neck, and upper arm contour are normal and the scars are positioned so as to avoid any inhibition of growth or function.

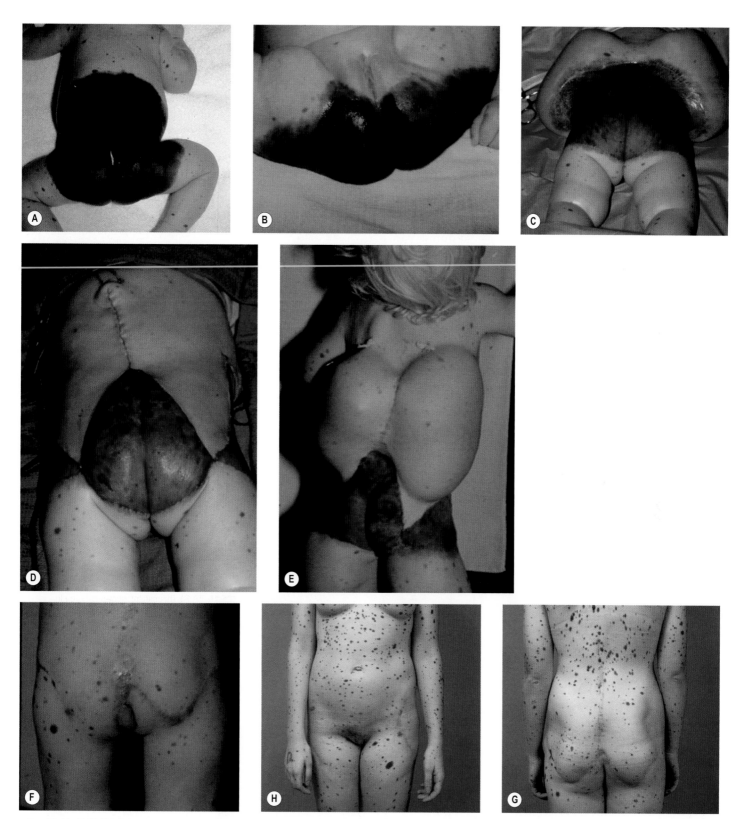

Fig. 38.11 (A,B) This infant was born with a large nevus of the lower half of the back, buttocks, perineum, and upper thigh. **(C,D)** Expanded transposition flaps create the length and flap orientation to allow **(E,F)** repeat expansion and coverage of the remaining buttocks, perineum, and perianal areas. **(G,H)** The patient is seen 13 years later with no additional scar revisions. While she has extensive involvement with small satellite nevi, the scars from the excision and reconstruction were clearly positioned to avoid significant contour deformities and growth disturbance.

The geometry of the extremity, as well as the limited flexibility of the skin (particularly in the lower extremity), makes regional expansion of limited use. Expanded flaps can be moved effectively in a circumferential direction, but move poorly in an axial direction. However, attempts to move a limited amount of skin to reconstruct the defect when the nevus is more than a third of the circumference of the extremity can result in significant constriction of the extremity, particularly in the upper arm (Figs. 38.12–38.14).

In the past decade, the authors have begun to find a way around these limitations.[49] Large expanded transposition flaps from the scapular region are used to cover the upper arm and shoulder. For circumferential nevi from the mid humeral level to the wrist, expansion of the flank creates a large pedicled flap through which the forearm can be placed during vascularization of the flap from the recipient bed. After 3 weeks, the pedicle is divided. Expanded full-thickness skin grafts have been used effectively for the dorsum of the hand, with excellent aesthetic outcome (see Fig. 38.12).

Although pedicled flaps are not readily available for coverage of more extensive lesions of the arm, thigh, or leg, the authors have had success with expanded free flaps from the abdomen and scapular region. Alternatively, when the patient is seen in early infancy, an expanded pedicle flap from the posterior thigh/buttock to the leg from knee to ankle affords the same benefits as an expanded pedicle flap from the abdomen/flank to the upper extremity (see Fig. 38.14). These procedures have been used only in very carefully selected cases, and the optimum timing of these complex reconstructive procedures is still under consideration.

Satellite nevi

Satellite nevi may appear anywhere over the course of the first few years of life, and their number seems to correlate directly with the likelihood of NCM.[26] They may vary in size from small to medium lesions (see Figs. 38.2, 38.3, & 38.11). To date, only one case of melanoma has been reported arising in a satellite nevus.[51] With this in mind, it is generally agreed that the primary reason for excision of satellite nevi is an aesthetic one. A significant benefit may also result from excising multiple satellite nevi on the face before the child enters his or her school years. In addition, some of the larger satellites on the extremities may be excised in infancy and early childhood (simultaneously with other procedures on the major lesion) by relatively simple serial excision techniques; if left to later childhood and adolescence, the reduced subcutaneous fat and added flexibility of the surrounding tissues may no longer allow excision without expansion or grafting.

Postoperative care

Parents are often more comfortable having their child observed for the first night postoperatively. The patients may be monitored for pain or hematoma formation. The dressing is

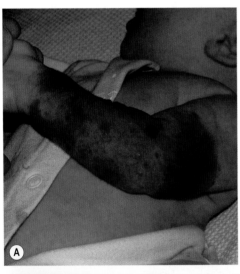
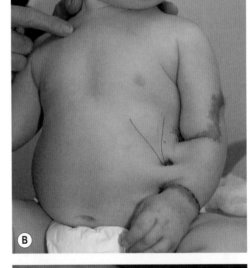
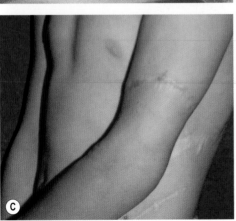
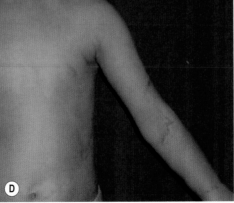

Fig. 38.12 (A,B) This child, with circumferential nevus of the arm, was treated with an expanded pedicle flap from the abdomen and flank. Following 3 months' expansion, the expander is removed, the nevus excised, and the arm passed into a tunnel of expanded skin which is secured around the arm with large bolster sutures. The pedicle is divided at 3 weeks, then additional excision of a narrow strip of remaining nevus both proximal and distal to the flap allows fine-tuning of the scars. **(C,D)** The patient is shown 3 years after division of the flap with excellent contour of the arm, and an aesthetically acceptable donor site.

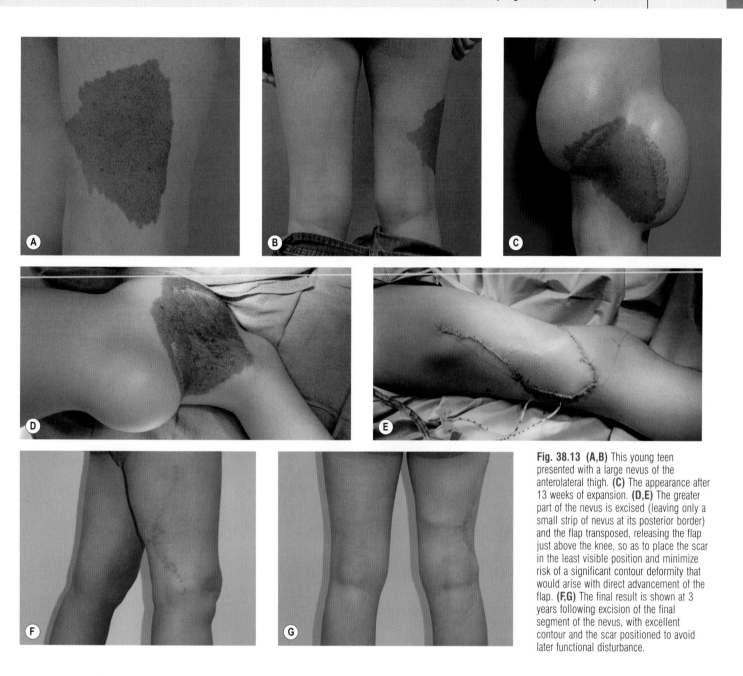

Fig. 38.13 (A,B) This young teen presented with a large nevus of the anterolateral thigh. **(C)** The appearance after 13 weeks of expansion. **(D,E)** The greater part of the nevus is excised (leaving only a small strip of nevus at its posterior border) and the flap transposed, releasing the flap just above the knee, so as to place the scar in the least visible position and minimize risk of a significant contour deformity that would arise with direct advancement of the flap. **(F,G)** The final result is shown at 3 years following excision of the final segment of the nevus, with excellent contour and the scar positioned to avoid later functional disturbance.

changed daily for several days (antibiotic ointment on suture line with Xeroform gauze above and soft padding). The drains are usually removed 3–10 days postoperatively, depending on the amount of discharge. Serial injections are started 7–10 days after insertion, provided the skin flaps are in excellent condition. After one or two postoperative visits and a teaching session, most patients start home expansion directed by the parents or guardians. Parents are provided with a printed card to record the schedule and amount of saline injected throughout the expansion process. They are encouraged to take digital photos and record the process and keep the surgical team well informed.[52] A local anesthetic cream can be put on the skin above the port prior to the injection to minimize pain. The expansion should be performed until the skin is tense but not extremely painful to the patient or of any compromise to the skin.

Outcomes, prognosis, and complications

Beyond site-specific complications of tissue expansion mentioned earlier, major complications may involve infection, expander exposure, and flap ischemia. Traditionally, it has been taught that early postoperative infection should be managed with expander removal and antibiotics; however, early detection of infection and maintaining a low threshold for antibiotic use may avoid expander loss. Small extrusions of the expander when the surrounding wound is stable may allow for some additional expansion and expander salvage. Minor complications include pain during expansion (which is transient), seroma, "dog ears" at donor site, and widening of scars.[53,54]

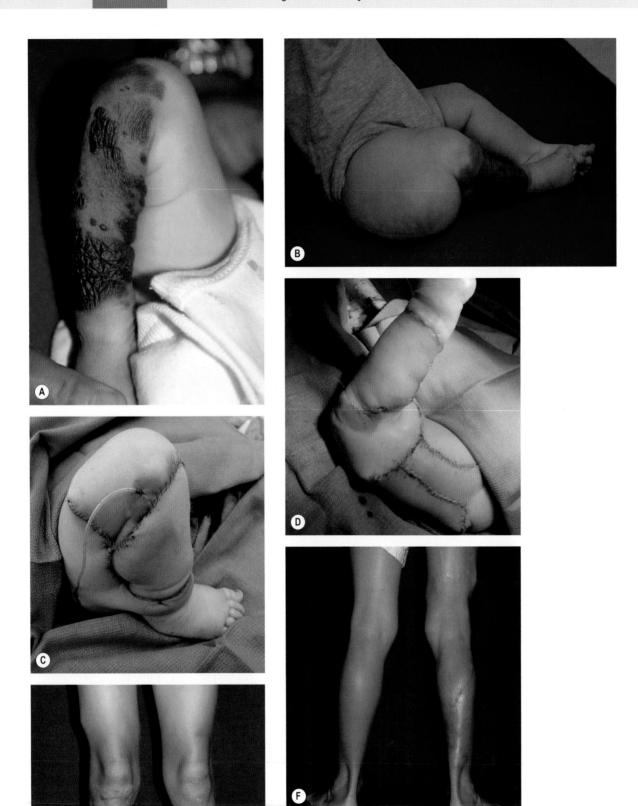

Fig. 38.14 (A) The flexibility of the infant's leg is used to advantage for the excision of this circumferential nevus extending from the knee to just above the ankle. **(B)** The posterior thigh was expanded starting at 4 months of age. **(C)** At 7 months of age, the greater part of the nevus was excised and the defect reconstructed with an expanded pedicled flap from the posterior thigh, held in place by slipping the foot beneath a "bucket handle" of skin, which lay between the initial incision used to place the expander, and the proximal border of the flap. **(D)** The pedicle was divided after 3 weeks and the "bucket handle" bipedicle flap converted to a unipedicle flap and used for partial coverage of the donor defect on the posterior thigh. **(E,F)** The excellent contour of both the leg and proximal thigh is evident on the two views of the patient 6.5 years following the excision and flap reconstruction.

Given the relative scarcity of large and giant nevi, it has been difficult for many surgeons to accumulate large enough numbers of cases to draw conclusions regarding the effectiveness of varied surgical options with respect to risk reduction of degeneration and/or functional and aesthetic outcomes. Since 1988, the authors have closely followed the efficacy of early treatment of large and giant nevi in different body regions with a series of now over 300 patients. Long-term follow-up, and the repetition of patterns of involvement in each affected area, has given us a unique opportunity to compare varied approaches of excision as well as the need for secondary surgical procedures, either to improve the aesthetic outcome or to deal with late functional problems. Modifications are continuing in the treatment protocol to improve outcomes and to minimize the need for secondary surgery.

In regions that do not lend themselves readily to tissue expansion, early in our experience, efforts were directed at excising the nevus and skin-grafting the defect. It became clear after relatively short follow-up that when lesions were excised to a depth assuring complete or near-total removal, split-thickness skin graft reconstruction resulted in poor aesthetic outcomes, and, when carried circumferentially around the trunk or extremities, later growth of the child resulted in a worsening contour defect with potential growth disturbance. In an effort to improve aesthetic outcomes, and provide reconstructions having a greater chance of keeping up with growth, large full-thickness grafts were harvested from expanded donor sites. The relative size constraints of full-thickness grafts were virtually eliminated. However, when following these patients into the teen years, despite relatively normal skin surface appearance and growth, contour deformities were great enough to suggest limiting even full-thickness skin grafting to the dorsum of hand or foot and the periorbital area. In the extremities these late deformities were avoided with the selective use of expanded pedicle flaps, as well as the use of free tissue transfer with subsequent expansion of the transferred tissue to increase its coverage.

Recognizing the increasing difficulty of tissue expansion with age, some of these procedures are only effective if done when the patient is young. While not totally ruling out any procedures (other than the expanded pedicle flap from posterior thigh to lower leg) for reconstruction in older children/adults, one must accept that, at present, many patients with giant nevi extending from waist to knee are best monitored, rather than subjected to unsightly scars and possible functional disturbance. Free tissue transfer, either with or without prior expansion, allows for the harvest of larger flaps with improved ease of donor site closure, and may provide a means of correcting some late deformities secondary to either complications of earlier treatment, or poor choice of the initial treatment option.

🌐 Access the complete reference list online at **http://www.expertconsult.com**

3. Krengel S, Scope A, Dusza S, et al. New recommendations for the categorization of cutaneous features of congenital melanocytic nevi. *J Am Acad Dermatol*. 2013;68:441–451. *An expert consensus-based schema to standardize the description of congenital melanocytic nevi that includes several morphologic features as well as size criterion, the goal of which is to improve intraobserver agreement and aid the development of an international database to collate phenotypic and genetic morphology of CMN.*

9. Kovalyshyn I, Braun R, Marghoob A. Congenital melanocytic naevi. *Australas J Dermatol*. 2009;50:231–240. *A comprehensive review about congenital melanocytic nevi, including pathogenesis, natural history, and complications.*

20. Zaal LH, Mooi WJ, Klip H, et al. Risk of malignant transformation of congenital melanocytic nevi: a retrospective nationwide study from The Netherlands. *Plast Reconstr Surg*. 2005;116:1902–1909. *Retrospective study of a national database of patients with large and giant congenital nevi from the Netherlands. The authors compared melanoma rates between patients with giant nevi and the general population over a 10-year period and revealed an increased rate of melanoma in patients with giant congenital melanocytic nevi when compared with the general population.*

35. Bittencourt FV, Marghoob AA, Kopf AW, et al. Large congenital melanocytic nevi and the risk for development of malignant melanoma and neurocutaneous melanocytosis. *Pediatrics*. 2000;106:736–741.

38. Rhodes AR, Melski JW. Small congenital nevocellular nevi and the risk of cutaneous melanoma. *J Pediatr*. 1982;100:219–224.

41. Bauer BS, Margulis A. The expanded transposition flap: shifting paradigms based on experience gained from two decades of pediatric tissue expansion. *Plast Reconstr Surg*. 2004;114:98–106. *This paper demonstrates the advantages of transposition flaps used in tissue expansion when compared with advancement flaps.*

47. Bauer BS, Few JW, Chavez CD, et al. The role of tissue expansion in the management of large congenital pigmented nevi of the forehead in the pediatric patient. *Plast Reconstr Surg*. 2001;107:668–675. *This paper suggests guidelines for treatment of forehead and scalp congenital nevi with an emphasis on preserving or reconstructing the landmarks of hairline, hair direction, and brow position.*

48. Bauer BS, Vicari FA, Richard ME, et al. Expanded full-thickness skin grafts in children: case selection, planning, and management. *Plast Reconstr Surg*. 1993;92:59–69.

49. Pandya AN, Vadodaria S, Coleman DJ. Tissue expansion in the limbs: a comparative analysis of limb and non-limb sites. *Br J Plast Surg*. 2002;55:302–306.

52. Margulis A, Bauer BS, Fine NA. Large and giant congenital pigmented nevi of the upper extremity: an algorithm to surgical management. *Ann Plast Surg*. 2004;521:158–167.

54. Manders EK, Schenden MJ, Furrey JA, et al. Soft-tissue expansion: concepts and complications. *Plast Reconstr Surg*. 1984;74:493–507. *This paper reviews the early concepts of how and why expansion works and discusses potential complications with avoidance techniques.*

Vascular anomalies

Arin K. Greene and John B. Mulliken

 Access video and video lecture content for this chapter online at expertconsult.com

SYNOPSIS

- Vascular anomalies are divided into tumors or malformations.
- Vascular tumors are comprised of proliferating endothelium; the endothelial lining of malformations is more quiescent.
- Infantile hemangioma is the most common tumor of infancy; it grows rapidly after birth and involutes during childhood.
- Most infantile hemangiomas are observed; problematic lesions are treated pharmacologically or by resection.
- Vascular malformations are present at birth, although not always obvious; they may slowly enlarge during childhood and adolescence.
- Vascular malformations are managed by observation, laser, sclerotherapy, embolization, or resection; pharmacotherapy is not available.

Introduction

Vascular anomalies is a field that incorporates several surgical and medical specialties. Because these disorders usually involve the skin, the initial consultation is often with a plastic surgeon (or a pediatric dermatologist). Development of this field has been impeded by a lack of standardized terminology. For centuries, it was believed that vascular birthmarks were imprinted on the unborn child by a mother's emotions or diet. This was reflected in words for brightly colored foods to describe vascular anomalies. Adjectives such as "cherry", "strawberry", and "portwine" have their roots in these traditional beliefs. Physicians usually preferred the Latin term *naevus maternus* for vascular birthmarks.

In the 19th century, the first attempt was made by Virchow to categorize vascular anomalies histologically. Virchow's *angioma simplex* became synonymous with "capillary" or "strawberry" hemangioma. His term *angioma cavernosum* was used indiscriminately for subcutaneous hemangiomas (that regress) and venous malformations (that never regress). *Angioma racemosum* was modified to racemose (cirsoid) aneurysm or "arteriovenous hemangioma", referring to an

arteriovenous malformation. His student, Wegener, developed a comparable histomorphic subcategorization for "lymphangioma". This nomenclature persisted well into the 20th century. Often the same word was applied to entirely different vascular anomalies. This confusing nosology has been responsible for improper diagnosis, illogical treatment, and misdirected research.

A biologic classification system, introduced in 1982,[1] cleared the terminologic confusion that had long obscured the field. This scheme evolved from studies that correlated physical findings, natural history, and cellular features.[1] The key to this biologic classification is proper use of the Greek nominative suffix *-oma*, which once meant "swelling" or "tumor". In modern times, *-oma* denotes a lesion that arises by upregulated cellular growth. There are two major categories of vascular anomalies, tumors, and malformations (Table 39.1). *Vascular tumors* are endothelial neoplasms characterized by increased endothelial turnover (Fig. 39.1). Infantile hemangioma, a tumor that arises in infants, is the most common. Other vascular tumors are congenital hemangioma, hemangioendotheliomas, tufted angioma, hemangiopericytomas, angiosarcoma, and pyogenic granuloma. *Vascular malformations* are the result of abnormal development of vascular elements during embryogenesis (Fig. 39.2). They are designated according to the predominant channel type as *capillary malformation, lymphatic malformation, venous malformation, arteriovenous malformation,* and complex forms such as capillary-lymphatic-venous malformation. Malformations with an arterial component are rheologically fast-flow; the remainder are slow-flow. This biologic classification was accepted by the International Society for Vascular Anomalies in 1996.[2] It is critical to underscore that vascular malformations, although fundamentally structural disorders, can exhibit endothelial hyperplasia, possibly triggered by clotting, ischemia, embolization, partial resection, or hormonal influences.

History and physical examination should give diagnostic accuracy of more than 90% in distinguishing between vascular tumors and vascular malformations (Fig. 39.3).[3] The most likely error in assigning a clinical diagnosis continues to be

Table 39.1 Classification of vascular anomalies

Tumors	Malformations	
	Slow-flow	Fast-flow
Infantile hemangioma (IH)	Capillary malformation (CM) Cutis marmorata telangiectatica congenita (CMTC) Telangiectasias	Arterial malformation (AM) Aneurysm Atresia Ectasia Stenosis
Congenital hemangioma (CH) Rapidly involuting congenital hemangioma (RICH) Non-involuting congenital hemangioma (NICH) Hemangioendotheliomas Kaposiform hemangio-endothelioma (KHE) Other	Lymphatic malformation (LM) Microcystic Macrocystic Primary lymphedema Venous malformation (VM) Cerebral cavernous malformation (CCM) Cutaneomucosal venous malformation (CMVM) Glomuvenous malformation (GVM) Verrucous venous malformation (VVM)	Arteriovenous malformation (AVM) Capillary malformation-arteriovenous malformation (CM-AVM) Hereditary hemorrhagic telangiectasia (HHT) PTEN-associated vascular anomaly Combined malformations Capillary-arteriovenous malformation (CAVM) Capillary-lymphatic arteriovenous malformation (CLAVM)
Pyogenic granuloma (PG)	Combined malformations Capillary-venous malformation (CVM) Capillary-lymphatic malformation (CLM) Capillary-lymphatic-venous malformation (CLVM) Lymphatic-venous malformation (LVM)	

an inaccurate, imprecise use of terminology (Table 39.2).[4,5] Perhaps the most egregious example is "hemangioma", so often applied generically and indiscriminately to vascular lesions that are entirely different in histology and behavior. There is no such entity as "cavernous hemangioma". The lesion is either a deep infantile hemangioma or a venous malformation.

The terms "congenital" and "acquired" should be used with caution in describing vascular anomalies. The word "congenital" should be restricted to a vascular lesion that is completely expressed at birth. Hemangioma can be nascent or fully-grown in a neonate. Vascular malformations, although present at birth at a cellular level, may not manifest until childhood or in adult life. "Acquired", a term often used for cutaneous lesions that appear after 1 year of life, is inappropriate for a vascular anomaly that is present, but not clinically apparent, at birth.

Vascular tumors

Infantile hemangioma

Pathogenesis

Infantile hemangioma (IH) is a benign endothelial tumor with a biologic behavior that is unique because it grows rapidly, slowly regresses, and never recurs. There are three stages

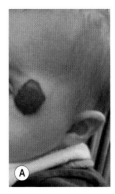 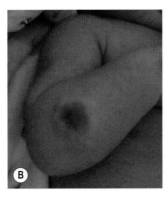 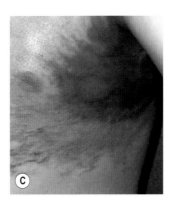 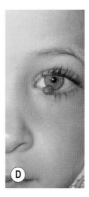

Fig. 39.1 Vascular tumors of infancy and childhood. **(A)** A 3-month-old female with enlarging infantile hemangioma of the cheek first noted at 1 week of age. **(B)** A 6-week-old male with a rapidly involuting congenital hemangioma (RICH). Note purple color and peripheral halo. **(C)** A 1-year-old male with a kaposiform hemangioendothelioma complicated by Kassabach–Merritt phenomenon. **(D)** A 5-year-old with a 2-month history of bleeding pyogenic granuloma of left lower eyelid.

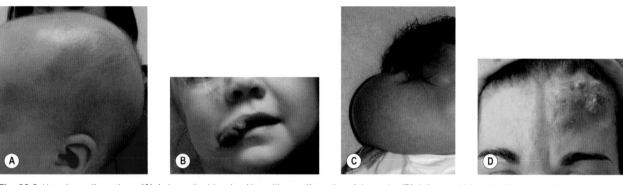

Fig. 39.2 Vascular malformations. **(A)** A 4-month-old male with capillary malformation of the scalp. **(B)** A 3-year-old female with an expanding venous malformation of the lip first noted at birth. **(C)** Infant male with macrocystic lymphatic malformation. **(D)** A 39-year-old female with a bleeding, ulcerated arteriovenous malformation of the forehead.

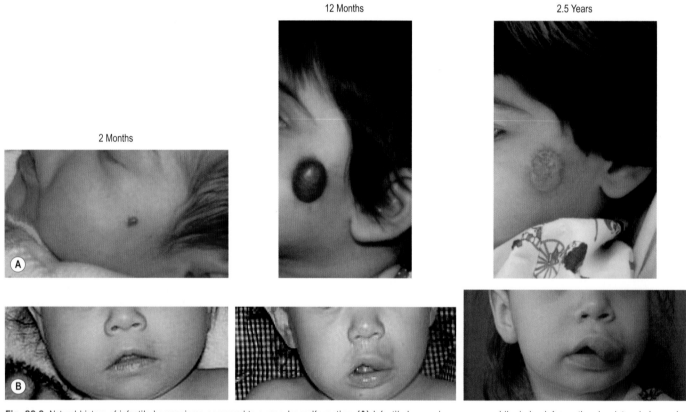

Fig. 39.3 Natural history of infantile hemangioma compared to a vascular malformation. **(A)** Infantile hemangioma grows rapidly during infancy, then involutes during early childhood. **(B)** Venous malformation slowly enlarges over time and does not involute.

Table 39.2 Incorrect terminology commonly used to describe vascular anomalies

Tumors		Malformations	
Biologic name	Incorrect term	Biologic name	Incorrect term
Infantile hemangioma	"Capillary hemangioma" "Cavernous hemangioma" "Strawberry hemangioma"	Capillary malformation	"Portwine stain" "Capillary hemangioma"
Hemangioendothelioma	"Capillary hemangioma"	Lymphatic malformation	"Cystic hygroma" "Lymphangioma"
		Venous malformation	"Cavernous hemangioma"
		Arteriovenous malformation	"Arteriovenous hemangioma"

in its life cycle: the proliferating phase (0–1 year of age); the involuting phase (1–4 years of age); and the involuted phase (after 4 years of age). During the proliferating phase, the histopathologic examination shows clusters of plump endothelial cells with small vascular channels and minimal connective tissue.[6] During involution, mature blood vessels are formed. Vascular channels enlarge and are lined by flattened endothelial cells. Increased extracellular matrix, multilaminated basement membranes, and pericytes are deposited around the vessels. After involution, the majority of the IH is replaced with adipocytes and connective tissue. All that remains are thin-walled vessels with multilaminated basement membranes and larger feeding and draining vessels.[6]

IH appears to arise from vasculogenesis (formation of blood vessels from progenitor cells) rather than angiogenesis (blood vessel formation from pre-existing vasculature).[7] It is likely that IH begins as an intrinsic (genetic) alteration in a stem cell; its life cycle may be influenced extrinsically by up- or downregulated local angiogenic factors. The precursor cell for IH may be a multipotent hemangioma-derived stem cell (HemSC), which has been isolated.[7] They produce human GLUT1-positive microvessels after clonal expansion in immunodeficient mice. They differentiate into endothelium and express CD31.[7]

Several mechanisms may contribute to the rapid enlargement of IH. Hypoxia may stimulate circulating hemangioma-derived endothelial progenitor cell (HemEPC) recruitment to the growing tumor. Increased circulating endothelial progenitor cells have been found in children with IH.[8] Local factors, such as a reduction in anti-angiogenic proteins, also may potentiate tumor growth during the proliferating phase.[9] The mechanism for IH involution is unknown. As endothelial proliferation slows, apoptosis increases, and the IH is replaced by fibrofatty tissue. Apoptosis begins before 1 year of age and peaks at 24 months, causing a reduction in tumor volume.[10] Decreasing circulating maternal estrogens, which are pro-angiogenic, may contribute to involution. Alternatively, increased angiogenesis inhibitors in the epidermis overlying the hemangioma may promote involution.[9] The source of adipocytes during involution are HemSCs, which also may differentiate into pericytes.[7]

Clinical features

Infantile hemangioma occurs in approximately 4–5% of Caucasian infants.[11] IH is more frequent in premature children and in females (4:1).[12] The tumor is typically single (80%) and involves the head and neck (60%), trunk (25%), or extremity (15%).[3] The median age of appearance is 2 weeks; 30–50% are noted at birth as a telangiectatic stain, pale spot, or ecchymotic area.[3] IH grows faster than the child during the first 9 months of age (*proliferating phase*); 80% of its size is achieved by 3.2 (±1.7) months.[13] IH is red when it involves the superficial dermis. A lesion beneath the skin may not be appreciated until 3–4 months of age when it has grown large enough to cause a visible mass; the overlying skin may appear bluish. By age 9–12 months, growth of IH reaches a plateau. After 12 months, the tumor begins to regress (*involuting phase*); the color fades and the lesion flattens. Involution ceases in most children by age 4 years (*involuted phase*).[14] After involution, one-half of children will have residual telangiectasias, scarring, fibrofatty residuum, redundant skin, or destroyed anatomic structures.

Head and neck hemangiomas

The majority of IH are small, harmless lesions that can be monitored under the watchful eye of a pediatrician. However, a minority of proliferating IH can cause significant deformity or complications, usually when located on the head or neck. Ulcerated lesions may destroy the eyelid, ear, nose, or lip. IH of the scalp or eyebrow can result in alopecia. Periorbital hemangioma can block the visual axis or distort the cornea, causing amblyopia. Subglottic hemangioma may obstruct the airway.

Multiple hemangiomas

Approximately 20% of infants have more than one IH.[3] The term *hemangiomatosis* designates five or more small (<5 mm) tumors. These children are more likely to have IH of internal organs, although the risk is low (~16%).[15] The liver is most commonly affected; the brain, gut, or lung are rarely involved. Ultrasonography should be considered to rule out hepatic IH.

Hepatic hemangiomas

The liver is the most common extracutaneous site for IH. There are three subtypes of hepatic hemangioma: *focal, multifocal,* or *diffuse.*[16] Although most hepatic IHs are non-problematic and discovered incidentally, large tumors can cause heart failure, hepatomegaly, anemia, or hypothyroidism. Focal hepatic hemangioma is usually asymptomatic and not associated with cutaneous hemangiomas; the lesion is a rapidly involuting congenital hemangioma (RICH) that regresses immediately after birth.[16] Occasionally, this tumor can cause cardiac overload and thrombocytopenia; however, these symptoms resolve as the tumor involutes. Multifocal hepatic IH are often accompanied by cutaneous lesions. Although usually asymptomatic, intrahepatic multifocal lesions can cause high output cardiac failure, which is managed by oral pharmacotherapy or embolization. Diffuse hepatic IH can cause massive hepatomegaly, respiratory compromise, or abdominal compartment syndrome. Infants are also at risk for hypothyroidism and irreversible brain injury because the large tumor volume expresses enough deiodinase to inactivate thyroid hormone.[17] Patients require thyroid stimulating hormone monitoring and, if abnormal, intravenous thyroid hormone replacement until the IH begins to regress.

Hemangiomas and structural anomalies

There are uncommon presentations of IH with malformations in the head/neck or lumbosacral regions. PHACE association affects 2.3% of patients with IH, and consists of a plaque-like IH in a regional distribution of the face with at least one of the following anomalies: *P*osterior fossa brain malformation; *H*emangioma; *A*rterial cerebrovascular anomalies; *C*oarctation of the aorta and cardiac defects; *E*ye/Endocrine abnormalities.[18] When ventral developmental defects (*S*ternal clefting or *S*upraumbilical raphe) are present, an "S" is added (PHACES).[18] Of infants, 90% are female and cerebrovascular anomalies are the most common associated finding (72%).[18] Because 8% of children with PHACE association have a stroke in infancy, these patients should have an MRI to evaluate the brain and cerebrovasculature.[18] Infants are referred for ophthalmologic, endocrine, and cardiac evaluation to rule out these associated anomalies.

LUMBAR association (Lower body infantile hemangioma, Urogenital anomalies, Myelopathy, Bony deformities, Anorectal malformations, Renal anomalies) is the posterior trunk equivalent of PHACE.[19] The hemangioma is extensive and superficial. The tumor has minimal postnatal growth and a high risk of ulceration. The hemangioma typically affects the sacral area or lumbar region. Patients can have ventral–caudal malformations (omphalocele, recto-vaginal fistula, vaginal/uterine duplication, solitary/duplex kidney, imperforate anus, tethered cord lipomyelomeningocele).[19] Ultrasonography is obtained to rule-out associated anomalies in infants <4 months of age. MRI is indicated in older infants or when ultrasonography (US) is equivocal.[19]

Diagnosis

Most IH are easily diagnosed by history and physical examination. Fast-flow is confirmed using a hand held Doppler device. By formal US, IH appears as a soft-tissue mass with fast-flow, decreased arterial resistance, and increased venous drainage.[20] On MRI, the tumor is isointense on T1, hyperintense on T2, and enhances during the proliferating phase.[20] Involuting IH exhibits increased lobularity and adipose tissue; the number of vessels and flow is reduced. Rarely, biopsy is indicated if malignancy is suspected or if the diagnosis remains unclear following imaging studies. If biopsy is needed, positive erythrocyte-type glucose transporter (GLUT 1) immunostaining differentiates IH from other vascular tumors and malformations.[21]

Nonoperative management

Observation

Most IH are simply observed because they typically are small, localized, and do not involve anatomically important areas. Only 22% of potentially problematic lesions referred to a specialist for management are treated during the proliferating phase.[22] Infants are followed closely, on a monthly basis, during the proliferative phase if a lesion has the potential to cause obstruction, destruction, or ulceration requiring intervention. Once the IH has stabilized in growth, patients are followed annually during the involuting phase if it is possible. Surgical intervention may be necessary in childhood for excess skin, residual fibrofatty tissue, or reconstruction of damaged structures.

Wound care

During the proliferative phase, at least 16% of lesions ulcerate, the median age being 4 months.[23] Superficial IH is prone to ulceration because the skin is damaged by the tumor. In addition, arteriovenous shunting reduces oxygen delivery to the skin, causing ischemia. Consequently, desiccation or minor injury can cause skin breakdown. Tumors located in trauma-prone areas are at greater risk for ulceration; the lips, neck, and anogenital region are the most common locations. To protect against ulceration, IH in these areas should be kept moist with hydrated petroleum during the proliferative phase to minimize desiccation and shearing of the skin. IH in the anogenital area may be further protected by using a petroleum gauze barrier to prevent friction from the diaper.

If ulceration develops, the wound is washed gently with soap and water at least twice daily. Small, superficial areas are managed by the application of topical antibiotic ointment and occasionally with a petroleum gauze barrier. Large, deep ulcers require damp-to-dry dressing changes. To minimize discomfort, a small amount of topical lidocaine may be applied no more than four times daily to avoid toxicity. Bleeding from an ulcerated IH is usually minor, and is treated by applying direct pressure. All ulcerations will heal with local wound care; usually healing takes at least 2 weeks.

Topical corticosteroid

Topical corticosteroid is relatively ineffective; especially if IH involves the deep dermis and subcutis.[24] Ultrapotent agents may be effective for a very superficial IH. Although lightening may occur, if there is deep component, it will not be affected. Adverse effects include hypopigmentation, cutaneous atrophy, and even adrenal suppression.[24]

Topical timolol

This beta-blocker may be effective for superficial lesions, but will not affect hemangiomas with a subcutaneous component. Side effects include alopecia and rash. Because systemic absorption may occur, it should not be used more than twice daily in areas where absorption is greater (e.g., eyelids, mucosa, ulcer).[25]

Intralesional corticosteroid

Small, well-localized IHs (<3 cm in diameter) that obstruct the visual axis or nasal airway, or those at risk for damaging important structures (i.e., eyelid, lip, nose) are best managed by intralesional corticosteroid (Fig. 39.4). Triamcinolone (not to exceed 3 mg/kg) will stop the growth of the lesion; two-thirds will decrease in size.[26] The corticosteroid injection lasts 2–3 weeks, and thus infants may require 2–3 injections during the proliferative phase. Intralesional corticosteroid may cause subcutaneous fat atrophy (2%). Caution injecting upper eyelid lesions should be exercised because blindness has been reported following injection due to embolic occlusion of the retinal artery.[26]

Systemic pharmacotherapy

Problematic IH that is >3–4 cm in diameter (and would require >3 mg/kg of triamcinolone for an injection) is managed by oral prednisolone or propranolol. Oral corticosteroid has been used to treat IH for over 40 years and has proven to be very safe and effective (see Fig. 39.4).[27–30] Patients are given prednisolone 3 mg/kg per day for 1 month; the drug is then tapered by 0.5 cc every 2–4 weeks until it is discontinued between 10–12 months of age when the tumor is no longer proliferating.[30] The drug is given once a day in the morning, and infants have monthly outpatient follow-up. Using this protocol, all tumors will stabilize in growth and 88% will become smaller (accelerated regression).[30] Treatment response usually is evident within 1 week of therapy by signs of involution: decreased growth rate, fading color, and softening of the lesion. Patients do not require prophylaxis against gastric irritation or prophylactic antibiotics. Around 20% of infants will develop a cushingoid appearance that resolves during tapering of therapy.[30] Approximately 12% of infants treated after 3 months of age exhibit decreased gain in height, but

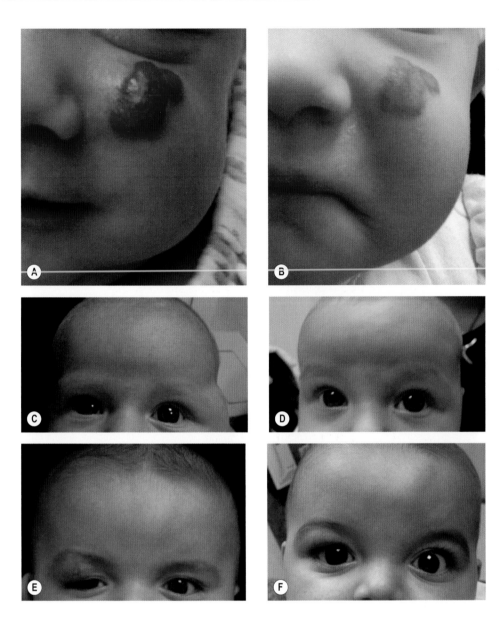

Fig. 39.4 Management of infantile hemangioma with pharmacotherapy. **(A)** Cheek lesion injected with triamcinolone at 3 months of age. **(B)** Accelerated regression at 12 months of age. **(C)** A 3-month-old female with deep infantile hemangioma of left face prior to initiation of oral corticosteroid. **(D)** After 1 month of drug treatment, the tumor has regressed. **(E)** A 4-month-old female with diffuse infantile hemangioma of upper eyelid causing astigmatism and obstruction. **(F)** After 2 months of drug treatment, the lesion has regressed and astigmatism has diminished.

return to their pretreatment growth curve by 24 months of age.[28]

Propranolol is another effective treatment for problematic infantile hemangioma. Typical dosing is 2 mg/kg per day.[31,32] Approximately 90% of tumors will stop growing or regress. Risks (<3%) include bronchospasm, bradycardia, hypotension, hypoglycemia, seizures, and hyperkalemia.[33–36] Preterm infants and those <3 months of age are more likely to have adverse events. Patients usually have cardiology consultation, electrocardiogram, echocardiogram, glucose/electrolyte measurements, and frequent blood pressure, heart rate, and respiratory examinations.[32] Inpatient initiation of treatment is used for premature or infants <3 months of age.[32] Potential contraindications include asthma, glucose abnormalities, heart disease, hypotension, bradycardia, and PHACES association.[32] The drug should be discontinued if the infant is ill because reduced oral intake can increase the risk of hypoglycemia and seizures. Patients treated with propranolol experience much later rebound growth compared with prednisolone, and thus patients may necessitate much longer treatment. Recently,

concern has been raised about potentially negative long-term neurocognitive effects of propranolol when given to infants.[37]

Laser therapy

There is little, if any, role for pulsed-dye laser treatment for proliferating IH. The laser penetrates only 0.75–1.2 mm into the dermis, and thus only affects the superficial portion of the tumor. Although lightening may occur, the mass is not affected.[38,39] These patients have an increased risk of skin atrophy and hypopigmentation.[39] The thermal injury delivered by the laser to the ischemic dermis increases the risk of ulceration, pain, bleeding, and scarring.[40] Nevertheless, pulsed-dye laser is indicated during the involuted phase to fade residual telangiectasias.

Operative management

Proliferative phase

Resection of IH generally is not recommended during the early growth phase. The tumor is highly vascular during this

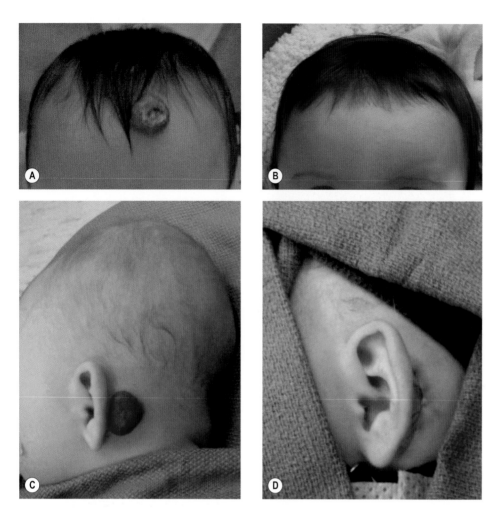

Fig. 39.5 Operative management of proliferating infantile hemangioma. **(A)** A 7-month-old female with a well-localized, ulcerated lesion in an anatomically favorable area. The tumor was removed by transverse lenticular excision and linear closure because of its location near the hairline. **(B)** At 6 weeks postoperatively. **(C)** A 4-month-old female with a rapidly growing, ulcerated retroauricular tumor at risk for causing a prominent ear deformity. **(D)** Following resection and linear closure in retroauricular sulcus.

period and there is a risk for blood loss, iatrogenic injury, and an inferior outcome compared with excising residual tissue after the tumor has regressed. Nevertheless, in experienced surgical hands, there are indications for operative intervention during this phase: (1) failure or contraindication to pharmacotherapy; (2) well-localized tumor in an anatomically favorable area; and (3) if resection will be necessary in the future and the scar would be the same (Fig. 39.5). Circular lesions located in visible areas, particularly the face, are best removed by circular excision and purse-string closure.[41] This technique minimizes the length of the scar as well as distortion of surrounding structures. Lenticular excision of a circular hemangioma results in a scar as long as three times the diameter of the lesion. In comparison, a two-stage circular resection followed by lenticular excision/linear closure 6–12 months later will leave a scar approximately the same length as the diameter of the original lesion.[41] Lenticular excision and linear closure is preferred in certain facial locations, such as the lips and eyelids (Video 39.1 ▶).

Involuted phase

Approximately 50% of IH leave behind fibrofatty tissue or damaged skin after the tumor regresses causing a deformity (Fig. 39.6). Sometimes a child requires reconstruction of damaged structures (i.e., nose, ear, lip). Operative intervention after 3 years of age is much safer than excision during the proliferative phase because the lesion is less-vascular and

smaller. Because the extent of the excision is reduced, the scar is less noticeable. It is preferable to intervene surgically between 3 and 4 years of age. During this period, the infantile hemangioma will no longer improve significantly, and the procedure is performed before the child's long-term memory and self-esteem begin to form, at about 4 years of age.[14] Some parents may elect to wait until the child is older and able to make the decision to proceed with operative intervention, especially if the deformity is minor.

Congenital hemangiomas

Clinical features

There are rare hemangiomas that arise in the fetus, are fully-grown at birth, and do not have postnatal growth.[42–44] Congenital hemangiomas are red-violaceous with coarse telangiectasias, central pallor, and a peripheral pale halo. These lesions are more common in the extremities, have an equal sex distribution, and are solitary with an average diameter of 5 cm.[42–44] There are two forms: *rapidly involuting congenital hemangioma* (RICH) and *non-involuting congenital hemangioma* (NICH). RICH involutes rapidly after birth and 50% of lesions have completed regression by 7 months of age; the remaining tumors are fully involuted by 14 months.[42,44] RICH affects the head or neck (42%), limbs (52%), or trunk (6%). RICH does not leave behind a significant adipose component, unlike

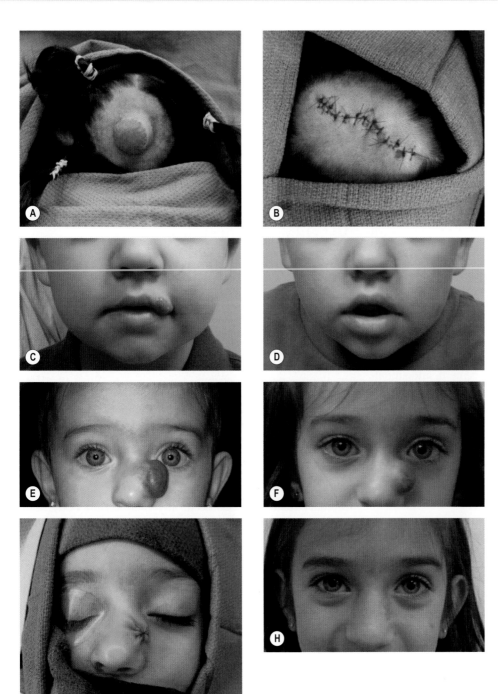

Fig. 39.6 Operative management of involuting phase infantile hemangioma. **(A)** A 2-year-old female with residual fibrofatty residuum and alopecia. A one-stage lenticular excision was chosen because the scalp is an unfavorable location for circular closure, and the linear scar is concealed by hair. **(B)** Note that the length of the scar is approximately three times the diameter of the tumor. **(C)** A 3-year-old male with residual fibrofatty tissue of the upper lip. **(D)** The lesion was removed using a lenticular excision with placement of the scar along the vermilion-cutaneous junction. **(E)** An 8-month-old female with a large nasal hemangioma. **(F)** The same patient at 3 years old. The tumor has involuted facilitating the operative procedure. **(G)** Following circular excision and purse-string closure to limit the length of scar. **(H)** At 3 months following second-stage circular excision and purse-string closure.

common IH. NICH, in contrast, does not regress; it remains unchanged with persistent fast-flow.[44] It involves the head or neck (43%), limbs (38%), or trunk (19%).[43]

Management

RICH usually does not require resection in infancy because it regresses so quickly. Occasionally, RICH is complicated by congestive heart failure, and this is controlled by corticosteroid or embolization as the lesion involutes. After regression, RICH may leave behind atrophic skin and subcutaneous tissue. Reconstruction with autologous grafts (fat, dermis) or

acellular dermis may be indicated. NICH is rarely problematic in infancy; it is observed until the diagnosis is clear. Resection of NICH may be indicated to improve the appearance of the affected area, as long as the surgical scar will be less noticeable than the lesion.

Kaposiform hemangioendothelioma

Clinical features

Kaposiform hemangioendothelioma (KHE) is a rare vascular neoplasm (1/100 000 children) that is locally aggressive, but does not metastasize.[45–47] Although one-half of lesions are present at birth, KHE may develop during infancy (58%), between ages 1–10 years (32%) or after 11 years of age (10%);[48] adult-onset is rare.[49] KHE has an equal sex distribution, is solitary, and affects the head/neck (40%), trunk (30%), or an extremity (30%).[48] The tumor is often >5 cm in diameter and appears as a flat, reddish-purple, edematous lesion.[50] KHE causes a visible deformity as well as pain. Approximately 70% of patients have Kasabach–Merritt phenomenon (KMP) (thrombocytopenia <25 000/mm³, petechiae, bleeding).[51] KHE does not exhibit rapid postnatal growth; however, the tumor can expand with the onset of KMP. KHE partially regresses after 2 years of age, although it usually persists long term, causing chronic pain and stiffness.[51] KHE has overlapping clinical and histopathologic features with another tumor, tufted angioma, suggesting they are on the same neoplastic spectrum. KMP also may complicate tufted angioma, which has a similar anatomic distribution as KHE, but is more erythematous and plaque-like.

KHE is diagnosed by history, physical examination, and imaging. MRI is indicated for diagnostic confirmation and to assess the extent of the tumor. MRI shows poorly-defined margins, small vessels, and invasion of adjacent tissues. T2-hyperintensity, postgadolinium enhancement, and signal-voids may also be present. Histologically, KHE has infiltrating sheets or nodules of endothelial cells lining capillaries.[6] Hemosiderin-filled, slit-like vascular spaces with red blood cell fragments, as well as dilated lymphatics, are present. Tufted angioma is distinguished from KHE by small tufts of capillaries ("cannonballs") in the middle to lower-third of the dermis.[6]

Management

Most lesions are extensive, involving multiple tissues, and well beyond the limits of resection. Patients with KMP require systemic treatment to prevent life-threatening complications. Large, asymptomatic tumors without KMP are also managed with pharmacotherapy to minimize fibrosis and subsequent long-term pain and stiffness. Vincristine is first-line therapy; the response rate is 90%.[52] KHE does not respond as well to second-line drugs, interferon (50%), or corticosteroid (10%).[52] Recently, patients have been treated with sirolimus as first-line therapy with good efficacy.[53] Thrombocytopenia is not significantly improved with platelet transfusion because the platelets are trapped in the tumor. Platelet transfusion also worsens swelling and should be avoided unless there is active bleeding or a surgical procedure is planned. By 2 years of age, the tumor has usually undergone partial involution and the platelet count normalizes.

Pyogenic granuloma

Pyogenic granuloma (PG) is neither "pyogenic" nor "granulomatous". Some pathologists call it *lobular capillary hemangioma*.[54] PG is a solitary, red papule that grows rapidly on a stalk. It is small, with an average diameter of 6.5 mm; the mean age of onset is 6.7 years.[54] The male to female ratio is 2:1. PG is commonly complicated by bleeding (64%) and ulceration (36%).[54] PG primarily involves the skin (88%), but can also involve mucous membranes (11%). It is distributed on the head or neck (62%), trunk (19%), upper extremity (13%), or lower extremity (5%).[54] In the head and neck region,

affected sites include cheek (29%), oral cavity (14%), scalp (11%), forehead (10%), eyelid (9%), or lips (9%).[54]

Once established, PG rarely spontaneously heals. PGs require intervention to control likely ulceration and bleeding. Numerous methods have been described: curettage, shave excision, laser therapy, and excision.[54,55] Because the lesion extends into the reticular dermis, it may be out of the reach of the pulse-dye laser, cautery, or shave excision. Consequently, these modalities have a recurrence rate of approximately 50%.[55,56] Full-thickness excision is a more definitive treatment.[54,55]

Vascular malformations

Capillary malformation

Pathogenesis

Capillary malformation (CM) is the modern term for the antiquated "portwine" stain. The geographic patterns of CMs are often regional or dermatomal (particularly with branches of the trigeminal nerve), suggesting a relationship to the developing nervous system. The cutaneous flush of a CM may, in part, be due to an inability of these vessels to constrict secondary to diminished sympathetic innervation. Recently, the causative mutation for CM has been identified in *GNAQ* in both syndromic (i.e., Sturge–Weber syndrome) and sporadic lesions.[56]

Clinical features

Capillary malformations occur anywhere on the body; they can be localized or extensive. Rarely, they are multiple and generalized, such as in Sturge–Weber syndrome. CM should not be confused with a *nevus flammeus neonatorum*, the most common vascular birthmark, seen in 50% of white neonates. These macular stains are popularly referred to as "angel kiss" on the forehead, eyelids, nose, and upper lip or "stork-bite" in the nuchal area. These predictably fade by 2 years of age, representing a minor transient dilatation of dermal vessels.

The cutaneous discoloration is usually, but not always, evident at birth because the stain may be hidden by the erythema of neonatal skin. CM often causes psychological concerns as the pink color of childhood darkens and the skin thickens, sometimes with raised fibrovascular cobblestoning. Facial CMs often occur in a dermatomal distribution and frequently are noted to overlap sensory dermatomes, crossing the midline or occurring bilaterally. Pyogenic granuloma may develop in CM, causing ulceration and bleeding. CM also can lead to soft-tissue and skeletal overgrowth below the stain. When located on the face, hypertrophy of the lip, cheek, or forehead can occur; the lip is most commonly affected.[57] Enlargement of the maxilla or mandible can result in an occlusal cant (i.e., vertical maxillary overgrowth) with increased dental show and malocclusion.

An extensive CM in an extremity is often associated with increased circumference and limb length discrepancy. CMs in truncal or extremity distributions rarely demonstrate the evolution of textural and color changes seen in facial CMs. CMs often accompany developmental defects of the central neural axis. An occipital CM, often with an associated hair tuft, can overlie an encephalocele or ectopic meninges. A capillary stain on the posterior thorax can signify an underlying arteriovenous malformation of the spinal cord. A CM over the cervical or lumbosacral spine is a red flag for occult spinal dysraphism, lipomeningocele, tethered spinal cord, and diastematomyelia.

Management

In patients with an upper facial CM, as well as V_1–V_2 distribution, the possibility of Sturge–Weber syndrome should be considered. Pulse-dye laser therapy can improve the appearance of CM by lightening the color; the head and neck region responds better than the extremities.[58,59] Outcome also is superior for smaller lesions and those treated at a younger age.[60,61] Of the patients, 15% achieve at least 90% lightening, 65% improve 50–90%, and 20% respond poorly.[62] A higher rate of complications, including pigmentary changes and hypertrophic scarring, is reported in individuals with darker skin. After pulse-dye laser treatment, CM often re-darkens over time.[63]

Facial CM is best treated with pulse-dye laser early in childhood, before memory or self-awareness begins. Intervention in infancy may achieve superior lightening of the lesion, as well as reduce the risk of subsequent darkening and hypertrophy, compared with photocoagulation in later childhood.[61] Infants can be treated with pulse-dye laser while awake (using topical anesthesia), depending on the size and location of the CM. After infancy, it is more difficult to restrain an awake child and general anesthesia is preferred, unless the lesion is small. Adolescents generally tolerate laser treatment while awake, depending on the location and extent of the CM. Multiple treatments, spaced 6 weeks apart, are often required until the CM fails to improve with additional treatments. Some families may elect to wait to treat CM of the trunk or extremities until the child is old enough to make the decision. Similarly, patients may wish to undergo laser therapy only if their lesion darkens and becomes more visible over time.

Because overgrowth often is not present at birth and is progressive, most patients do not require contouring until adolescence or adulthood, more frequently labial (Fig. 39.7). Cutaneous fibrovascular hypertrophy occurs over many years, requiring intervention in adulthood.[64] Malocclusion can be corrected in adolescence with orthodontic manipulation. If orthodontics is insufficient, an orthognathic procedure is considered when the jaws are completely grown. Facial asymmetry caused by overgrowth of the zygoma, maxilla, or mandible can be improved by contour burring.

Trunk or extremity soft tissue overgrowth can be associated with increased subcutaneous adipose tissue.[65] Suction-assisted lipectomy can improve contour while avoiding a large incision. Small fibrovascular nodules or pyogenic granulomas are easily excised. Severe cutaneous thickening and cobblestoning can be resected and reconstructed by linear closure, skin grafts, or local flaps.

Cutis marmorata telangiectasia congenita

Cutis marmorata telangiectasia congenita (CMTC) manifests as congenital cutaneous marbling, even at normal temperatures, and becomes more pronounced with lower temperatures or with crying.[65] The involved skin is depressed in a serpiginous reticulated pattern and has a deep purple color. Differential diagnosis includes cutis marmorata (or livedo reticularis) and reticular hemangioma. Cutis marmorata is merely an accentuated pattern of normal cutaneous vascularity. It is seen as a transient mottling pattern when the child is placed in a low-temperature environment but disappears on warming.

CMTC occurs sporadically in an equal gender distribution. CMTC can cause ulceration and may be localized, segmental, or generalized. It most frequently involves the trunk and extremities; it is typically unilateral (65%) and involves a lower extremity (69%).[65] The affected extremity is often hypoplastic. Almost all infants show improvement during the first year of life that continues into adolescence. Atrophy, pigmentation, and ectasia of the superficial veins often persist into adulthood. CMTC may be associated with hypoplasia of the iliac and femoral veins.

Macrocephaly-capillary malformation (M-CM) is a clinically discrete condition.[66] The vascular lesions are patchy, reticular CM (not CMTC or cutis marmorata). The stains commonly occur on the nose and philtrum, and may be present on the trunk or extremities. Unlike CMTC, the vascular malformation in M-CM does not ulcerate or fade. In addition, the lower limb is often hypertrophied.[66] These children have a high risk for neurologic abnormalities, including developmental delay, megalencephaly, and hydrocephalus.[66]

Lymphatic malformation

Pathogenesis

Investigations support the venous origin of lymphatics, rather than derivation from mesenchymal structures. One etiologic theory for lymphatic malformations (LMs) is that either anlagen of the sacs or their sprouting lymphatic channels become "pinched off" from the main lymphatic system, leading to aberrant collections of lymphatic fluid-filled spaces. Another theory attributes LMs to abnormal budding of the lymphatic system with a loss of connection to the central lymph channels or to development of lymphatic tissue in

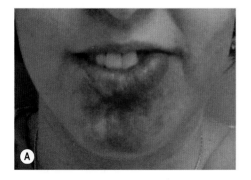

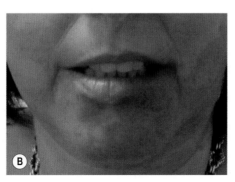

Fig. 39.7 Management of capillary malformation. **(A)** A 48-year-old woman with a capillary malformation of the lower face causing labial overgrowth. **(B)** The appearance after pulsed-dye laser treatment of the chin and contouring of the hypertrophied lower lip using a transverse mucosal excision.

Table 39.3 Vascular anomalies with known genetic mutations

Condition	Mutated gene	Inheritance
Venous malformations		
Sporadic venous malformation (VM)	TIE2 (40–50%)	
Verrucous venous malformation (VVM)	MAP3K3	Somatic
Glomuvenous malformation (GVM)	Glomulin	Dominant
Cutaneomucosal venous malformation (VMCM)	TIE2	Dominant
Cerebral cavernous malformation (CCM)	KRIT1	Dominant
Lymphatic malformations		
Sporadic lymphatic malformation	PIK3CA	Somatic
Familial congenital primary lymphedema	VEGFR3	Dominant
Lymphedema-distichiasis	FOXC2	Dominant
Lymphedema-hypotrichosis-telangiectasia	SOX18	Recessive
Hennekam syndrome	CCBE1	Recessive
Arteriovenous malformations		
Capillary malformation-arteriovenous malformation	RASA1	Dominant
Hereditary hemorrhagic telangiectasia type 1 (HHT1)	ENG	Dominant
Hereditary hemorrhagic telangiectasia type 2 (HHT2)	ACVRLK1	Dominant
PTEN-associated vascular anomaly	PTEN	Dominant

aberrant locations. Recently, sporadic LMs have been found to have a somatic mutation in *PIK3CA*.[67] Lymphedema, a generalized type of lymphatic anomaly in the limbs, can be hereditary, and mutations in *VEGFR3*, *FOXC2*, *SOX18*, *CCBE1* are responsible for some primary forms (Table 39.3).[68]

Clinical features

Lymphatic malformations are characterized by the size of the malformed channels: microcystic, macrocystic, or combined. Macrocystic lesions are defined as cysts large enough to be punctured by a needle and treated by sclerotherapy. LM is most commonly located on the head and neck; other common sites are the axilla, chest, and perineum. Lesions are soft and compressible. The overlying skin may be normal, have a bluish hue, or be studded with pink-red vesicles. LM typically causes deformity and psychosocial issues, especially when it involves the head and neck. The two most common complications associated with LM are bleeding and infection. Intralesional bleeding causes ecchymotic discoloration, pain, or swelling. Infection is common and can progress rapidly

to sepsis. Cutaneous vesicles can bleed and cause malodorous drainage. Oral lesions may lead to macroglossia, poor oral hygiene, and caries. Swelling due to bleeding, localized infection, or systemic illness may obstruct vital structures. Infants with cervicofacial LM may require tracheostomy. Bony overgrowth is another complication; the mandible is most commonly involved resulting in an open bite and prognathism. Thoracic or abdominal LM may lead to pleural, pericardial, or peritoneal chylous effusions. Periorbital LM causes a permanent reduction in vision (40%), and 7% of patients become blind in the affected eye.[69] Generalized lymphatic anomaly and Gorham–Stout disease present with multifocal or osteolytic bony lesions, splenic involvement, as well as pleural and/or pericardial effusions; lymphangiectasia of the bowel with protein-losing enteropathy also may be present.[70]

Lymphatic malformations are diagnosed by history and physical examination. Small, superficial lesions do not require further evaluation. Large or deep LMs are assessed by MRI to (1) confirm the diagnosis; (2) define the extent of the malformation; (3) plan treatment. LM appears as either a macrocystic, microcystic, or combined lesion with septations of variable thickness. It is hyperintense on T2-weighted sequences and does not show diffuse enhancement.[20] Although US is not as accurate as MRI, it may provide diagnostic confirmation or document intralesional bleeding. Ultrasound findings for macrocystic LM include anechoic cysts with internal septations, often with debris or fluid-fluid levels.[20] Microcystic LM appears as ill-defined echogenic masses with diffuse involvement of adjacent tissues.[20] Histologic confirmation of LM is rarely necessary. LM shows abnormally walled vascular spaces with eosinophilic, protein-rich fluid, and collections of lymphocytes. Immunostaining with the lymphatic markers D2–40 and LYVE-1 are positive.[6]

Management

A lymphatic malformation is a benign lesion; intervention is not mandatory. Small or asymptomatic lesions may be observed. An infected LM often cannot be controlled with oral antibiotics and intravenous antimicrobial therapy may be required. Intervention for LMs is reserved for symptomatic lesions that cause pain, significant deformity, or threaten vital structures.

Sclerotherapy

Sclerotherapy is the first-line management for large or problematic macrocystic/combined LMs (Fig. 39.8). Cysts are aspirated followed by the injection of an inflammatory substance, which causes scarring of the cyst walls to each other. Sclerotherapy is preferred and has a lower complication rate than attempted resection.[71] Several sclerosants are used to shrink LMs: doxycycline, sodium tetradecyl sulfate (STS), ethanol, bleomycin, and OK-432. The authors prefer doxycycline because it is effective (83% reduction in size) and safe (<5% risk of skin ulceration).[71] STS is the second-line agent. Ethanol is an effective sclerosant but has the highest complication rate.

The most common complication of sclerotherapy for LM is cutaneous ulceration (<5%). Ethanol is associated with additional systemic toxicity: CNS depression, pulmonary hypertension, hemolysis, thromboembolism, and arrhythmias.[71] Extravasation of the sclerosant into muscle can cause atrophy

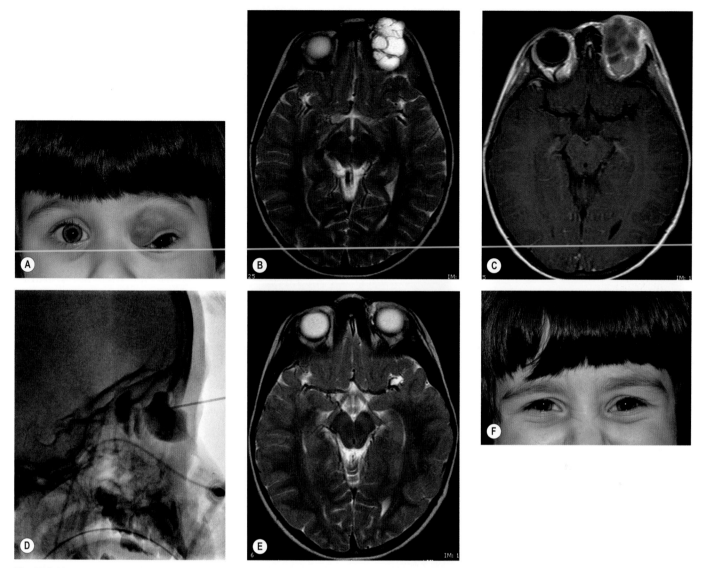

Fig. 39.8 Management of macrocystic lymphatic malformation. **(A)** A 3-year-old female with lymphatic malformation of the left orbit causing exotropia and ptosis. **(B)** Axial T2 MR shows a large hyperintense lesion with multiple, thin internal septations in the superolateral compartment of the orbit. **(C)** Post-contrast T1 MR depicts septal enhancement. There are two different signal intensities due to fluid-fluid levels from intralesional bleeding. **(D)** Fluoroscopic image following needle aspiration and the injection of opacified doxycycline. **(E)** Post-treatment MR demonstrates almost complete resolution of the lymphatic malformation. **(F)** The patient is asymptomatic 4 months following sclerotherapy. *(Reprinted from Greene AK, Perlyn CA, Alomari AI. Management of lymphatic malformations.* Clin Plast Surg. *2011;38:75–82, with permission from Elsevier.)*

and contracture. An LM often re-expands over time and thus patients often need repeated treatment over the course of their lifetime. If a problematic LM recurs and macrocysts are no longer present, resection is the next alternative. Recently, bleomycin sclerotherapy has shown efficacy for microcystic lesions. This modality can be considered for problematic lesions where resection would unfavorable (e.g., face) and where there is a mild/moderate deformity; approximately 10% reduction in the size of the malformation can be expected.[72]

Resection

Attempts at extirpation of LMs can cause significant morbidity: major blood loss, iatrogenic injury, and deformity. Excision is usually subtotal because LM involves multiple tissue planes and important structures; recurrence is common. Resection is reserved for (1) symptomatic microcystic LM causing

bleeding, infection, distortion of vital structures, or significant deformity; (2) symptomatic macrocystic/combined LM that no longer can be managed with sclerotherapy because all macrocysts have been treated; (3) small, well-localized LM (microcystic or macrocystic) that may be completely excised (Fig. 39.9). When considering resection, the postoperative scar/deformity following removal of the LM should be weighed against the preoperative appearance of the lesion.

For diffuse malformations, staged resection of defined anatomic areas is recommended. Subtotal excision of problematic areas, such as bleeding vesicles or a hypertrophied lip, should be carried out rather than an attempting "complete" resection that might result in a worse deformity than the malformation itself. Macroglossia may require reduction to return the tongue to the oral cavity or to correct an open-bite deformity. Bony overgrowth is improved by osseous

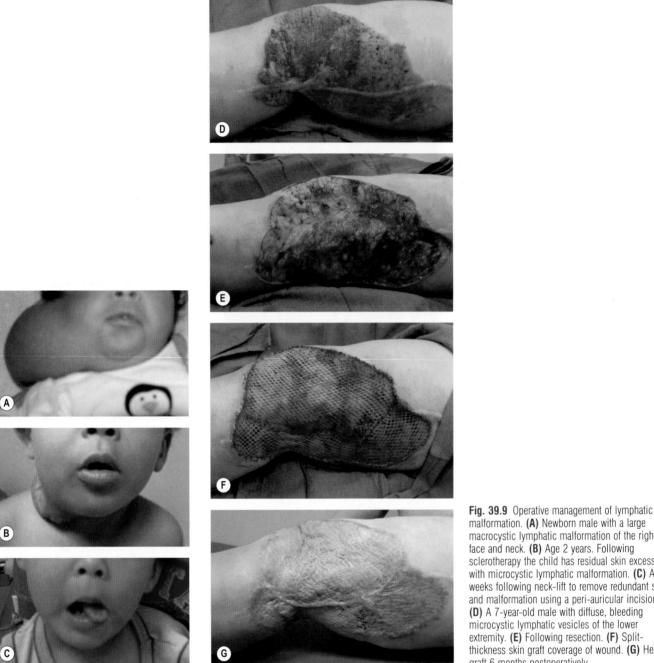

Fig. 39.9 Operative management of lymphatic malformation. **(A)** Newborn male with a large macrocystic lymphatic malformation of the right face and neck. **(B)** Age 2 years. Following sclerotherapy the child has residual skin excess with microcystic lymphatic malformation. **(C)** At 6 weeks following neck-lift to remove redundant skin and malformation using a peri-auricular incision. **(D)** A 7-year-old male with diffuse, bleeding microcystic lymphatic vesicles of the lower extremity. **(E)** Following resection. **(F)** Split-thickness skin graft coverage of wound. **(G)** Healed graft 6 months postoperatively.

contouring and malocclusion may require orthognathic correction.

Bleeding or leaking cutaneous vesicles can be controlled by resection if they are localized and the wound can be closed by direct approximation of tissues. Vesicles often recur through the scar. Large areas of vesicular bleeding or drainage are best managed by sclerotherapy or carbon dioxide laser; alternatively, wide resection and skin graft coverage is required. Microcystic vesicles involving the oral cavity respond well to radiofrequency ablation.[73] Patients and families are counseled that LM can expand following any intervention, and thus additional treatments are often required in the future.

Venous malformation

Pathogenesis

Venous malformation (VM) results from an error in vascular morphogenesis. Lesions are composed of thin-walled, dilated, sponge-like channels of variable size and mural thickness.[6] There is a normal-appearing endothelial lining; it is the smooth muscle architecture that is abnormal. Smooth muscle alpha-actin staining demonstrates decreased smooth muscle cells that are arranged in clumps rather than concentrically.[6] This mural abnormality probably accounts for the tendency of these malformations to gradually expand over time. In addition, intralesional clotting often occurs, ranging from simple fibrin deposition to the later-appearing pathognomonic calcified "phleboliths".

Molecular causes for VMs are known. For example, 50% of patients with a sporadic VM will have a somatic mutation in the endothelial receptor *TIE2*.[74] Approximately 10% of patients with VM have multifocal, familial lesions. *Glomuvenous malformation* (GVM) is the most common type; *cutaneomucosal-venous malformation* (CMVM) is rare.[75] GVM is an autosomal dominant condition with abnormal smooth muscle-like glomus cells along the ectatic veins. It is caused by a loss-of-function mutation in the *glomulin* gene.[75] CMVM is an autosomal dominant condition caused by a gain-of-function mutation in the *TIE2* receptor.[76] *Cerebral cavernous malformation* (CCM) results from mutations in CCM1/(*KRIT1*), CCM2, and CCM3 genes.[68]

Clinical features

Venous malformations are blue, soft, and compressible; calcified phleboliths often can be palpated. VMs range from small, localized cutaneous lesions to diffuse malformations involving multiple tissue planes, vital structures, and internal organs. VM is typically sporadic and solitary in 90% of patients.[75] Sporadic VM is usually >5 cm (56%), single (99%), and located on the head/neck (47%), extremities (40%), or trunk (13%).[75] Almost all lesions involve the skin, mucosa, or subcutaneous tissue; 50% also affect deeper structures (i.e., muscle, bone, joints, viscera).[75]

Glomuvenous malformations are typically multiple (70%), small (two-thirds <5 cm), and located in the skin and subcutaneous tissue; deeper structures are uncommonly affected.[75] GVM involves the extremities (76%), trunk (14%), or head/neck (10%). Lesions are more painful than typical VM.[75] Cutaneomucosal-venous malformations are multifocal mucocutaneous lesions; they are less common than GVM. Lesions are small (76% <5 cm), multiple (73%), and located on the head/neck (typically tongue or buccal mucosa) (50%), extremity (37%), or trunk (13%).[75] CCM is a rare familial disorder with VM involving the brain and spinal cord; patients also may have hyperkeratotic skin lesions.[68] Patients are at risk for development of new intracranial lesions and hemorrhage.

Blue rubber bleb nevus syndrome (BRBNS) is a rare condition characterized by multiple, small (<2 cm) VMs involving the skin, soft tissue, and gastrointestinal tract.[77] Morbidity is associated with gastrointestinal bleeding requiring chronic blood transfusions. *Diffuse phlebectasia of Bockenheimer* is an old eponym to specify an extensive extremity VM involving skin, subcutaneous tissue, muscle, and bone.[78] *Sinus pericranii* refers to a venous anomaly of the scalp or face and transcalvarial communication with the dural sinus. *Verrucous venous malformation (VVM)* (previously called "verrucous hemangioma") is a low-flow vascular malformation that is clinically similar to a hyperkeratotic VM.[79,80] Lesions range from 2–8 cm and are located on an extremity (91%) or trunk (9%).[79] VH involves the skin and subcutis, becomes more hyperkeratotic over time, and frequently causes bleeding. Recently, MAP3K3 mutations have been found in verrucous venous malformations.[80]

Fibroadipose vascular anomaly (FAVA) shares features with intramuscular venous malformation.[81] It affects the calf most frequently followed by the thigh, forearm, gluteal area, and ankle/foot. It is differentiated from intramuscular venous malformation by significant pain, contractures, and a non-spongiform venous cutaneous component (phlebectasia, capillary malformation, or lymphatic vesicles). On MRI FAVA exhibits fat and fibrosis, minimal signal on T2 images, and heterogeneous small channels. Sclerotherapy is not effective because FAVA is solid. Treatment is either corticosteroid injection, cryotherapy, or resection.[81]

Maffucci syndrome denotes the coexistence of cutaneous venous malformations with bony exostoses and enchondromas.[82] Osseous lesions appear first, most often in the hands, feet, long bones of the extremity, ribs, pelvis, and cranium. Recurrent fractures are common.[82] VMs are most commonly located on distal extremities, but may occur anywhere. Malignant transformation, usually chondrosarcoma, occurs in 20–30% of patients at an average age of 40 years (range: 13–69 years).[82] A majority of the chondrosarcomas are low grade and often cured by resection.

Complications of VM include pain, swelling, and psychosocial issues. Head and neck VM may present with mucosal bleeding or progressive distortion leading to airway or orbital compromise. Extremity VM can cause leg-length discrepancy, hypoplasia due to disuse atrophy, pathologic fracture, hemarthrosis, and degenerative arthritis. VM of muscle may result in fibrosis and subsequent pain and disability. A large VM involving the deep venous system is at risk for thrombosis and pulmonary embolism. Gastrointestinal VM can cause bleeding and chronic anemia. Stagnation within a large VM results in a localized intravascular coagulopathy (LIC) and painful phlebothromboses.

At least 90% of VMs are diagnosed by history and physical examination. Dependent positioning of the affected region usually confirms the diagnosis. Small, superficial VM do not require further diagnostic work-up. Large or deeper lesions are evaluated by MRI to (1) confirm the diagnosis; (2) define the extent of the malformation; and (3) plan treatment. VM is hyperintense on T2-weighted sequences.[20] In contrast to LM, VM enhances with contrast, often shows phleboliths as signal-voids, and is more likely to involve muscle.[20] US findings include compressible, anechoic-hypoechoic channels separated by more solid regions of variable echogenicity.[20] Phleboliths are hyperechoic with acoustic shadowing. CT is occasionally indicated to assess osseous VM. Histological diagnosis of VM is rarely necessary, but may be indicated to rule out malignancy or if imaging is equivocal.

Management

Patients with an extensive extremity VM are prescribed custom-fitted compression garments to reduce blood stagnation and minimize expansion, LIC, phlebolith formation, and pain. Patients with recurrent pain secondary to phlebothrombosis are given prophylactic daily aspirin (81 mg) to prevent thrombosis. Large lesions are at risk for coagulation of stagnant blood, stimulation of thrombin, and conversion of fibrinogen-to-fibrin.[83] LIC can become disseminated intravascular coagulopathy (DIC) following trauma or therapeutic intervention. The chronic consumptive coagulopathy can cause either thrombosis (phleboliths) or bleeding (hemarthrosis, hematoma, intraoperative blood loss).[83] Low molecular weight heparin (LMWH) is considered for patients with significant LIC who are at risk for DIC.[83] Patients who develop a serious thrombotic event require long-term anticoagulation or a vena caval filter.

Sclerotherapy

Intervention for VM is reserved for symptomatic lesions that cause pain, deformity, obstruction (i.e., vision, airway), or gastrointestinal bleeding. First-line treatment is sclerotherapy, which is safer and more effective than resection (Fig. 39.10).[71] Good to excellent results are obtained in 75–90% of patients, including reducing the size of the malformation and alleviating symptoms.[71] Diffuse malformations are managed by targeting specific symptomatic areas often the entire lesion is too extensive to treat at one time. Sclerotherapy is repeated until symptoms are alleviated or when injectable vascular spaces are no longer present. Although sclerotherapy effectively reduces the size of the lesion and improves symptoms, the malformation remains. Consequently, patients may have a mass or visible deformity after treatment that may be improved by resection. In addition, VM usually re-expands after sclerotherapy, and thus patients often require additional treatments.

The preferred sclerosants for VM are sodium tetradecyl sulfate (STS) and ethanol; STS is the most commonly used.

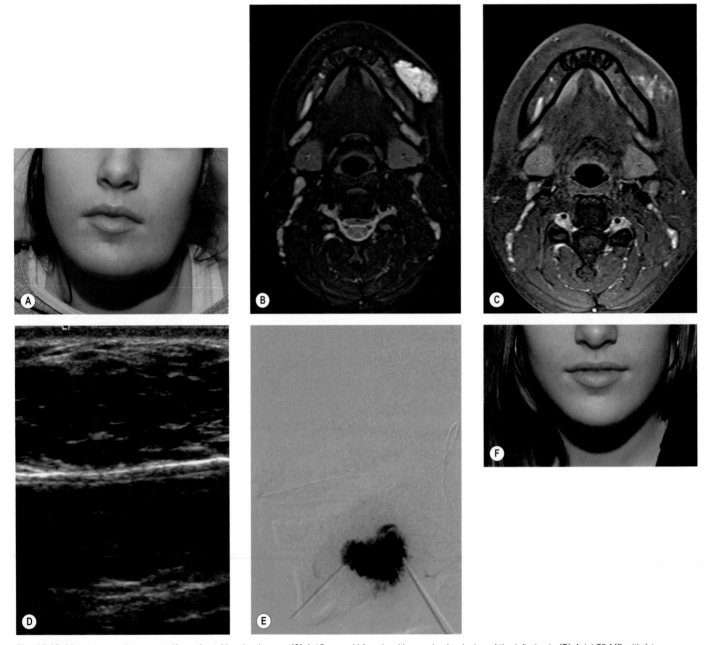

Fig. 39.10 Management of venous malformation with sclerotherapy. **(A)** A 15-year-old female with an enlarging lesion of the left cheek. **(B)** Axial T2 MR with fat suppression illustrates a localized lesion involving the cheek. **(C)** Axial T1 MR exhibits heterogeneous enhancement of the lesion with contrast. **(D)** Ultrasound shows compressible hypoechoic venous spaces with echogenic walls. **(E)** Venogram of the spongiform venous malformation with a minor draining vein. **(F)** Resolution of facial asymmetry 2 months following sclerotherapy with sodium tetradecyl sulfate. *(Reprinted from Greene AK, Alomari AI. Management of venous malformations. Clin Plast Surg. 2011;38(1):83–93, with permission from Elsevier.)*

Although ethanol is more effective than STS, it has a higher complication rate. Most patients, especially children, are managed under general anesthesia using US or fluoroscopic imaging. The most common local complication of sclerotherapy for VM is cutaneous ulceration.[71] Extravasation of the sclerosant into muscle can cause atrophy and contracture. Post-treatment swelling may necessitate close monitoring. Compartment compression is a serious consequence of sclerotherapy for extremity VM. Systemic adverse events following sclerotherapy, including hemolysis, hemoglobinuria, and DIC, are more common with large lesions. Patients with low fibrinogen levels are given LMWH 14 days before and after the procedure.[82] Anticoagulation is held for 24 h perioperatively (12 h before and after the intervention) to prevent bleeding complications.

Resection

In contrast to sclerotherapy, resection is rarely primary treatment because (1) the entire lesion is difficult to remove; (2) the risk of recurrence is high because hidden channels adjacent to the visible lesion are not excised; (3) the risk of blood loss and iatrogenic injury is greater. Resection should be considered for: (1) small, well-localized lesions that can be completely removed, or (2) persistent mass or deformity after completion of sclerotherapy (patent channels are no longer accessible for further injection) (Fig. 39.11). When considering resection, the postoperative scar/deformity following removal of the VM should be weighed against the preoperative appearance of the lesion. Subtotal resection of a problematic area, such as labial hypertrophy, is indicated, rather than attempting "complete" excision of a benign lesion that might result in a worse deformity than the malformation itself. Patients and families are counseled that VM can expand following excision, and additional operative procedures may be required in the future.

Almost all VMs should have sclerotherapy prior to operative intervention. After adequate sclerotherapy, the VM is replaced by scar and thus the risk of blood loss, iatrogenic injury, and recurrence is reduced. In addition, fibrosis facilitates resection and reconstruction. Because GVM is usually small and less amenable to sclerotherapy, first-line therapy for painful lesions may be resection. Gastrointestinal VM with chronic bleeding, anemia, and transfusion requirements is typically managed by resection. Solitary lesions can be treated by endoscopic banding or sclerotherapy. Multifocal lesions of BRBNS require removal of as many lesions as possible through multiple enterotomies, instead of bowel resection, to preserve intestinal length.

Arteriovenous malformation

Pathogenesis

An absent capillary bed causes shunting of blood directly from the arterial-to-venous circulation, through a fistula (direct connection of an artery to a vein) or nidus (abnormal channels bridging the feeding artery to the draining veins). AVM may enlarge because of increased blood flow causing collateralization, dilatation of vessels (especially venous ectasia), and thickening of adjacent arteries and veins.[6] Latent arteriovenous shunts may open, stimulating hypertrophy of surrounding vessels from increased pressure.[6] Alternatively, aneurysms may increase the size of these lesions. *Angiogenesis* (growth of new blood vessels from pre-existing vasculature) and *vasculogenesis* (*de novo* formation of new vasculature) also may be involved in AVM expansion.[83] Although neovascularization may be a primary stimulus for AVM growth, it also could be a secondary event. For example, ischemia, a potent stimulator of angiogenesis, causes enlargement of AVM after proximal arterial ligation or trauma. Alternatively, increased blood flow due to arteriovenous shunting may promote angiogenesis; vascular endothelial growth factor production and endothelial proliferation are stimulated by increased blood flow.[83] Both males and females have a two-fold risk of progression in adolescence; increased circulating hormones during this period may promote AVM expansion.[84]

Clinical features

The most common site of extracranial AVM is the head and neck, followed by the limbs, trunk, and viscera. Although present at birth, AVM may not become evident until childhood. Early lesions present as a pink-red cutaneous stain without a palpable thrill or bruit. Often they are initially mistaken as a capillary malformation or infantile hemangioma. Arteriovenous shunting reduces delivery of capillary oxygen causing ischemia. In time, the patient is at risk for pain, ulceration, and bleeding. AVM also may cause disfigurement, destruction of tissues, and obstruction of vital structures. High-pressure shunting of blood may lead to venous hemorrhage; ruptured arteries can form in weakened areas, such as aneurysms. Arterial bleeding most commonly occurs at skin or mucosal surfaces from erosion into a superficial component of the lesion. AVMs can cause cardiac enlargement and result in high-output cardiac failure by the direct communication

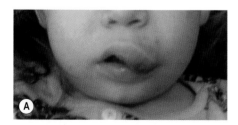 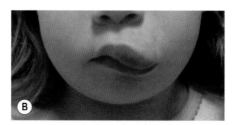 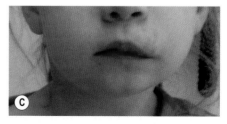

Fig. 39.11 Management of venous malformation with sclerotherapy followed by resection. **(A)** A 2.5-year-old female with an enlarging venous malformation of the upper lip. **(B)** Reduction of the venous malformation after two sessions of sclerotherapy. Further sclerotherapy was not possible because venous spaces had been replaced by fibrosis. **(C)** Improved contour 3 months after resection of residual scarred venous malformation using a transverse mucosal incision.

Table 39.4 Schobinger staging of arteriovenous malformation (AVM)

Stage	Clinical findings
I (Quiescence)	Warm, pink-blue, shunting on Doppler
II (Expansion)	Enlargement, pulsation, thrill, bruit, tortuous veins
III (Destruction)	Dystrophic skin changes, ulceration, bleeding, pain
IV (Decompensation)	Cardiac failure

between the high-resistance, high-pressure arterial system and the low-pressure, low-resistance venous system. While the presence of an AVM may be troublesome, it is the expansion of the lesion that is the primary cause of morbidity. AVM can be classified according to the Schobinger staging system (Table 39.4).[85]

Most AVMs are diagnosed by history and physical examination. Hand held Doppler reveals fast-flow and excludes a slow-flow vascular anomaly. If AVM is suspected, the diagnosis should be confirmed by US with color Doppler examination. MRI also is necessary to (1) confirm the diagnosis; (2) determine the extent of the lesion; (3) plan treatment. To adequately assess the anomaly, MRI with contrast and fat suppression, as well as a T2-weighted sequences, is necessary.[20] MRI shows dilated feeding arteries and draining veins, enhancement, and flow-voids.[20] If the diagnosis remains unclear after US and MRI, angiography is sometimes needed. Usually angiography only is indicated prior to embolization or when resection is planned. Characteristic features are tortuous, dilated arteries with arteriovenous shunting and dilated draining veins.[20] The nidus is angiographically seen as tortuous, small vessels with occasionally ill-defined larger contiguous vascular spaces. CT may be indicated if the AVM involves bone. Histopathologic diagnosis of AVM is rarely necessary, but may be indicated to rule out malignancy or if imaging is equivocal.

Management

Because AVM is often diffuse, involving multiple tissue planes and important structures, *cure* is rare. The goal of treatment usually is to *control* the malformation. Intervention is focused on alleviating symptoms (i.e., bleeding, pain, ulceration), preserving vital functions (i.e., vision, mastication), and improving deformity. Management options include embolization, resection, or a combination. Resection offers the best chance for long-term control, but the re-expansion rate is high and extirpation may cause a worse deformity.[84] Almost all AVMs will re-expand after embolization.[84] Consequently, embolization is used to reduce blood loss during resection or sometimes for palliation of unresectable lesions.

Asymptomatic AVM should be observed unless it can be completely removed with minimal morbidity; embolization or incomplete excision of an asymptomatic lesion may stimulate it to enlarge and become problematic. Intervention is determined by (1) the size and location of the AVM; (2) the age of the patient; (3) Schobinger stage. Although resection of an asymptomatic Stage I AVM offers the best chance for long-term control or "cure", intervention must be individualized based on the deformity that would be caused by resection and reconstruction. For example, a large Stage I AVM in a non-anatomically important location (i.e., trunk, proximal extremity) can be resected without consequence before it progresses to a higher stage where resection is more difficult and the recurrence rate is greater. Similarly, a small, well-localized AVM in a more difficult location (i.e., face, hand) may be excised for possible "cure" before it expands and complete extirpation is no longer possible.

In contrast, a large, asymptomatic AVM located in an anatomically sensitive area is best observed; especially in a young child who is not psychologically ready for major resection and reconstruction. Although the recurrence rate is lower when Stage I AVM is resected, it is still high, and thus, even after major resection and reconstruction the malformation can recur. Some patients (17%) do not have significant long-term morbidity.[84]

Intervention for Stage II AVMs is similar to Stage I lesions. The threshold for treatment is lower if an enlarging lesion is causing a worsening deformity or if functional problems are occurring. Stage III and IV AVMs require intervention to control pain, bleeding, ulceration, or congestive heart failure.

Embolization

Embolization is the delivery of an inert substance, through a catheter into the AVM nidus to occlude blood flow and/or fill a vascular space. Scarring reduces arteriovenous shunting, shrinks the lesion, and diminishes symptoms. Embolization is used either as a preoperative adjunct to resection or as monotherapy for lesions not amenable to extirpation. Because the AVM is not removed, almost all lesions eventually re-expand after treatment. Stage I AVM has a lower recurrence rate than higher-staged lesions. Most recurrences occur within the first year after embolization, and 98% re-expand within 5 years.[84] Despite the high likelihood of re-expansion, embolization can effectively palliate an AVM by reducing its size, slowing expansion, and alleviating pain and bleeding. Preoperative embolization also reduces blood loss during extirpation, but not the extent of resection.

Substances used for embolization are either liquid (n-butyl cyanoacrylate (n-BCA), Onyx) or solid (polyvinyl alcohol particles (PVA), coils). The goal of embolization is occlusion of the nidus and proximal venous outflow. The embolic material is delivered to the nidus, *not* to the proximal arterial feeding vessels. Occlusion of inflow will cause collateralization and expansion of the AVM; access to the nidus also will be blocked preventing future embolization.[86] For preoperative embolization, temporary occlusive substances (Gelfoam powder, PVA, embospheres) that undergo phagocytosis are used. Permanent liquid agents capable of permeating the nidus (n-BCA, Onyx) are employed when embolization is the primary treatment.[86] The most frequent complication of embolization is ulceration.

Resection

Resection of AVM has a lower recurrence rate than embolization alone; it is considered for a well-localized lesion or to correct deformity (i.e., bleeding or ulcerated areas, labial hypertrophy) (Fig. 39.12). Wide extirpation and reconstruction of large, diffuse AVM should be exercised with caution because (1) cure is rare and the recurrence rate is high; (2)

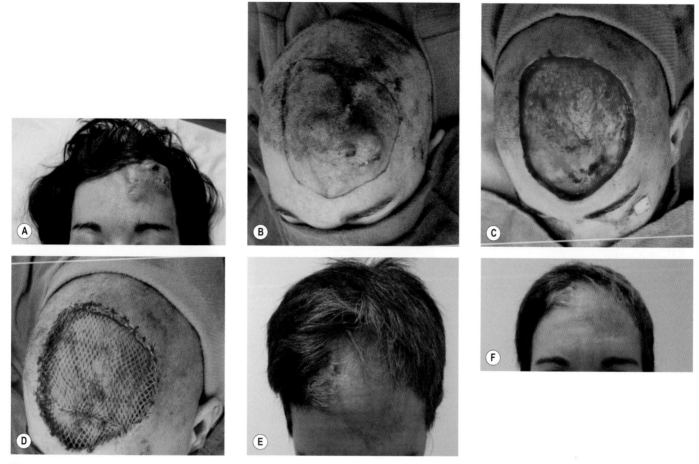

Fig. 39.12 Management of arteriovenous malformation. **(A)** A 39-year-old woman with an enlarging, bleeding, ulcerated stage 3 lesion of the forehead and scalp. **(B)** Intraoperative view following preoperative embolization. **(C)** Wound after extirpation. **(D)** Split-thickness skin graft coverage of periosteum. **(E,F)** Healed graft 4 months postoperatively.

the resulting deformity is often worse than the appearance of the malformation; (3) resection is associated with significant blood loss, iatrogenic injury, and morbidity. When excision is planned, preoperative embolization will facilitate the procedure by reducing the size of the AVM, minimizing blood loss, and creating scar tissue to aid the dissection. Multiple embolizations, spaced 6 weeks apart, may be required prior to resection. Excision should be done 24–72 h after embolization, before recanalization restores blood flow to the lesion.

Resection margins are best determined by assessing the type of bleeding from the wound edges. Some defects can be reconstructed by advancing local skin flaps. Skin grafting ulcerated areas has a high failure rate because the underlying tissue is ischemic; excision with regional flap transfer may be required. Free-flap reconstruction permits wide resection and primary closure of complicated defects, but does not appear to improve long-term AVM control.[84] Despite sub-total and presumed "complete" extirpation, most AVMs treated by resection recur. The majority of recurrences occur within the first year after intervention and 86.6% re-expand within 5 years of resection.[84] Nevertheless, many of these patients remain asymptomatic. Patients and families are counseled

that AVM is likely to re-expand following resection, and thus additional treatment may be required.

Capillary malformation-arteriovenous malformation

Capillary malformation-arteriovenous malformation (CM-AVM) is an autosomal dominant condition caused by a loss-of-function mutation in the *RASA1* gene; the prevalence is 1 in 100 000 Caucasians.[87] Patients have atypical capillary malformations (CMs) that are small, multifocal, round, pinkish-red, and often surrounded by a pale halo (50%) (Fig. 39.13).[84] A total of 30% also have an AVM: Parkes Weber syndrome (PWS) (12%), extracerebral AVM (11%), or intracerebral AVM (7%).[88] A patient presenting with multiple CMs, especially with a family history of similar lesions, should be evaluated for a possible AVM. Because 7% of patients with CM-AVM will have an intracranial fast-flow lesion, brain MRI should be considered.[88] Exploratory imaging of other anatomic areas is not necessary because extracranial AVM have not been found to involve the viscera.[88] Although the CM is rarely problematic, associated AVMs can cause major morbidity.

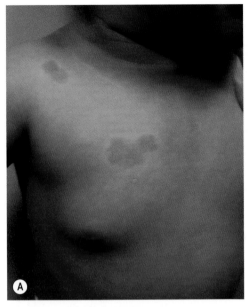
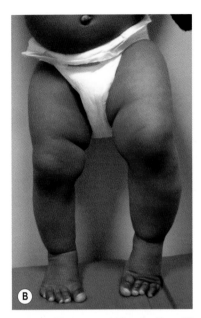
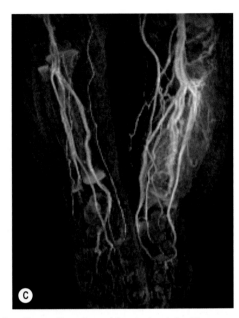

Fig. 39.13 Capillary malformation-arteriovenous malformation (CM-AVM). **(A)** A 1-year-old female with multifocal capillary malformations of the chest and shoulder. **(B,C)** Arteriovenous malformation of left lower extremity with overgrowth.

Eponymous vascular anomalies with overgrowth

Sturge–Weber syndrome

Sturge–Weber syndrome (SWS) is a sporadic neurocutaneous disorder estimated to occur in 1 in 50 000 live births (Fig. 39.14A).[89] The three cardinal features are capillary malformation (CM) in the upper trigeminal neural distribution, ocular abnormalities (glaucoma, choroidal vascular anomalies), and leptomeningeal vascular malformation.[89] Patients also commonly have soft tissue and/or bony overgrowth (60–83%); the frequency is similar to that for glaucoma (65–77%) and for neurologic sequelae (87–93%).[57] In addition to facial capillary staining; extra-craniofacial CMs (29%) and extremity hypertrophy (14%) are frequently present.[57]

In all patients with an upper facial CM, a diagnosis of Sturge–Weber syndrome should be considered on initial presentation. The capillary stain can be in the ophthalmic (V1), extend into the maxillary (V2), or involve all three trigeminal dermatomes. Patients with maxillary or mandibular involvement alone are at low risk for SWS. The leptomeningeal anomalies can be capillary, venous, or arteriovenous malformations. Small foci may be silent, but extensive pial vascular lesions can cause refractory seizures, contralateral hemiplegia, and delayed motor and cognitive development. The anomalous choroidal vascularity can lead to retinal detachment, glaucoma, and blindness. Ophthalmic examination should be performed every 6 months until the age of 2 years and yearly thereafter. MRI best demonstrates pial vascular enhancement in an infant or child thought to have Sturge–Weber syndrome.

Klippel–Trénaunay syndrome

Klippel–Trénaunay syndrome (KTS) denotes a slow-flow, capillary-lymphatic-venous malformation (CLVM) of an extremity in association with soft tissue and/or skeletal

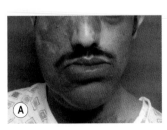
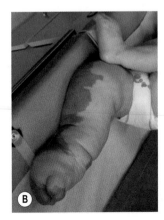
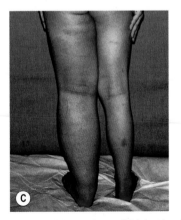
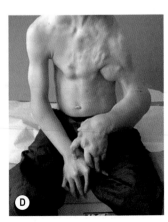

Fig. 39.14 Eponymous vascular anomalies with overgrowth. **(A)** A 36-year-old man with Sturge–Weber syndrome. **(B)** Infant female with Klippel–Trenaunay syndrome. **(C)** A 7-year-old male with Parkes Weber syndrome. **(D)** An 11-year-old male with CLOVES syndrome.

overgrowth (Fig. 39.14B).[90] There is tremendous variability in the presentation of this disorder, from a slightly enlarged extremity with a capillary stain to a grotesquely enlarged limb with malformed digits. KTS affects the lower extremity in 95% of patients, the upper extremity in 5% of patients, and least commonly, the trunk.[90] Sometimes the contralateral foot or hand is enlarged, often with a macrodactylous component and frequently in the absence of a capillary stain. In 10% of patients with KTS, the involved limb is hypoplastic. Pelvic involvement is common with CLVM of the lower extremity. It is usually asymptomatic, although hematuria, bladder outlet obstruction, cystitis, and hematochezia can occur. Upper extremity or truncal CLVM can involve the posterior mediastinum and retropleural space, although this is rarely symptomatic. The capillary malformation is distributed in a geographic pattern over the lateral side of the extremity, buttock, or thorax. Whereas the capillary malformation is typically macular in a neonate, later it becomes studded with hemolymphatic vesicles. The venous component of CLVM manifests as abnormal drainage of the affected area. The lymphatic abnormalities are typically macrocystic in the pelvis and thighs and microcystic in the abdominal wall, buttock, and distal limb.

MRI is obtained to confirm the diagnosis and determine the extent of the anomalies. A large, embryonal vein in the subcutaneous tissue (the marginal vein of Servelle) is often located in the lateral calf and thigh and communicates with the deep venous system. Complications include thrombophlebitis (20–45%) and pulmonary embolism (4–24%).[90] Unlike some other hemihypertrophy syndromes, patients with KTS are not at increased risk for Wilms tumor and screening US is unnecessary.[91,92] By 2 years of age, radiologic surveillance of leg length by plain radiography is indicated. If the discrepancy is >1.5 cm, a shoe-lift for the shorter limb can prevent limping and scoliosis. Epiphysiodesis of the distal femoral growth plate is typically done around 11 years of age. Enlargement of the foot may require a ray, midfoot, or Syme amputation to allow the use of footwear. Management of the VM component is conservative with compressive stockings for insufficiency and aspirin to minimize phlebothrombosis. Symptomatic varicose veins may be removed or sclerosed. Sclerotherapy may be necessary for focal macrocystic lymphatic malformation or to treat cutaneous vesicles. Excision and grafting is occasionally necessary for diffuse bleeding and/or oozing cutaneous vesicles. Circumferential overgrowth may be managed by staged contour resection. Venous insufficiency does not occur following staged subcutaneous excision or removal of the marginal vein of Servelle. A functioning deep venous system is present, although it is often difficult to visualize because of predominant flow in the superficial veins.

Parkes Weber syndrome

Parkes Weber syndrome (PWS) is a diffuse AVM in an overgrown extremity with an overlying CM (Fig. 39.14C).[88] PWS involves the lower extremity approximately twice as often as the upper extremity; patients have microshunting in muscle. The malformation is evident at birth with symmetric enlargement and pink staining of the involved limb. The cutaneous stain tends to be confluent rather than patchy and is typically warmer than a banal capillary malformation. The diagnosis is confirmed by the detection of a bruit or thrill. MRI is obtained to evaluate the extent of the malformation. Overgrowth in an

affected extremity is subcutaneous, muscular, and bony with diffuse microfistulas. The enlarged limb muscles and bones exhibit an abnormal signal and enhancement. Angiography demonstrates discrete arteriovenous shunts.

Treatment is predicated on symptoms. In rare instances, an infant presents with high-output congestive heart failure secondary to shunting through arteriovenous fistulas. This situation mandates emergent embolization with permanent occlusive agents, often followed by repeated procedures. Children are observed annually with careful monitoring for axial overgrowth and development of cutaneous problems. Embolization may be useful for pain or cutaneous ischemic changes. Occasionally, amputation is necessary.

PTEN hamartoma-tumor syndrome (Bannayan–Riley–Ruvalcaba syndrome)

Patients with *PTEN* mutations, a tumor suppressor gene, have PTEN hamartoma-tumor syndrome (PHTS) (Fig. 39.15). This autosomal dominant condition is also referred to as Cowden syndrome or Bannayan–Riley–Ruvalcaba syndrome.[93] Males and females are equally affected, and approximately one-half (54%) of patients have a unique fast-flow vascular anomaly with arteriovenous shunting, referred to as a PTEN-associated vascular anomaly.[93] Patients may have multiple lesions (57%), and 85% are intramuscular.[93]

Suspicion of a PTEN-associated vascular anomaly usually is initiated after reviewing the MRI or angiographic study of a patient suspected of having an AVM. Unlike typical AVM, these lesions may be multifocal, are associated with ectopic adipose tissue, and have disproportionate, segmental dilation of the draining veins.[93] If a patient is suspected of having a PTEN-associated vascular anomaly on imaging, a physical examination is performed. All patients with PHTS have macrocephaly (>97th percentile), and all males have penile freckling.[93] In addition, PHTS is associated with mental retardation/autism (19%), thyroid lesions (31%), or gastrointestinal polyps (30%).[93] Biopsy may aid the diagnosis of a PTEN fast-flow lesion. Histopathology shows skeletal muscle infiltration with adipose tissue, fibrous bands, and lymphoid aggregates. In addition, tortuous arteries with transmural muscular hyperplasia and clusters of abnormal veins with variable smooth muscle are present.[93] Genetic testing is confirmative, although a germline mutation is not found in 9% of families clinically diagnosed with PHTS.[92]

If physical examination is consistent with PHTS, molecular testing is necessary because this mutation is associated with multiple benign and malignant tumors which require surveillance. Patients are followed closely for the presence of tumors, particularly endocrine and gastrointestinal malignancies. In addition, the patient and family are counseled about the risk of transmitting the gene to their offspring. Symptomatic lesions are managed similarly to non-syndromic AVM, with embolization or resection. It is our experience that the recurrence rate after these interventions is even higher than for non-syndromic AVM, possibly because the loss of the tumor suppressor protein favors a more proliferative environment.

CLOVES syndrome

*C*ongenital *L*ipomatosis *O*vergrowth, *V*ascular malformations, *E*pidermal nevi, and *S*coliosis (CLOVES) represents a

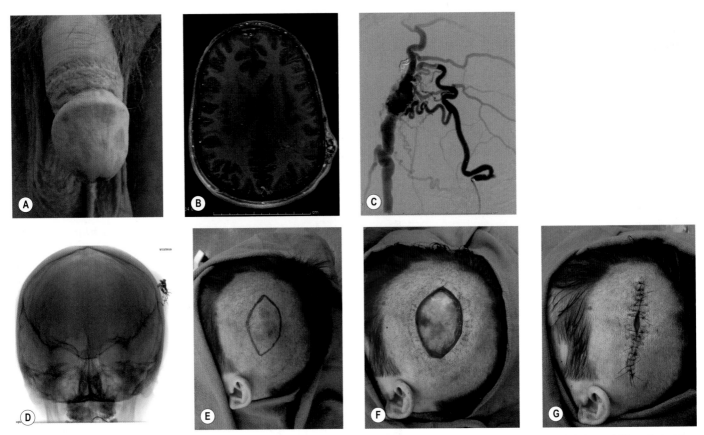

Fig. 39.15 PTEN hamartoma-tumor syndrome (Bannayan–Riley–Ruvalcaba syndrome). **(A)** A 16-year-old male with enlarging, painful scalp lesion and **(A)** penile freckling associated with the syndrome. **(B)** Axial T1 MR image shows enhancing soft tissue lesion consistent with PTEN-associated vascular anomaly. **(C)** Angiogram illustrates arteriovenous shunting without a nidus. **(D)** Onyx cast of lesion following preoperative embolization. **(E)** Intraoperative view. **(F)** A 9×4.5 cm wound following resection. **(G)** Linear closure after wide scalp undermining and subgaleal scoring.

newly described overgrowth syndrome.[94] Many of these patients previously were thought to have "Proteus syndrome". All patients have a truncal lipomatous mass, a slow-flow vascular malformation (most commonly a CM overlying the lipomatous mass), and hand/foot anomalies (increased width, macrodactyly, first web-space sandal gap) (Fig. 39.14D).[94] Patients also may have AVM (28%), neurologic impairment (50%), or scoliosis (33%).[94] Treatment for the lipomatous lesions is resection, but the recurrence rate is high.

Conclusion

Patients with vascular anomalies all too often have been medical "nomads". During infancy and childhood, their parents took them from one physician to another, because no one seemed to understand the condition. The problem usually was that these anomalies lay in the interface between several medical and surgical disciplines. No single specialist had sufficient knowledge to treat the wide variety of disorders.

Terminologic confusion has been replaced with a common language. Interested specialists can now communicate with one another. Vascular anomaly teams, composed of various disciplines on the basis of local interest, enthusiasm, and capabilities, continue to form in many major referral centers. These teams are in a unique position because the collective knowledge of such a group provides a forum for problems that otherwise appear "too complicated" or "insoluble". In addition, they serve as a focus for clinical and basic research in this field.

The future of the field of vascular anomalies is exciting because a significant opportunity exists to improve the lives of these patients. Plastic surgeons are well-positioned to make progress because of their training; management of these lesions requires creativity, surgical problem-solving skills, and a mastery of operative principles. Plastic surgeons, in collaboration with other specialists, will continue to be primary caretakers of patients with vascular anomalies.

Access the complete reference list online at **http://www.expertconsult.com**

1. Mulliken JB, Glowacki J. Hemangiomas and vascular malformations in infants and children: a classification based on endothelial characteristics. *Plast Reconstr Surg.* 1982;69:412–422. *A total of 49 tissue specimens from various vascular lesions were analyzed histologically and by tritiated thymidine uptake. Hemangiomas showed endothelial hyperplasia during the proliferative phase, while malformations had quiescent endothelium. This landmark study clarified the field of vascular anomalies by proposing a binary classification: hemangiomas and malformations.*

4. Hassanein AH, Mulliken JB, Fishman SJ, et al. Evaluation of terminology for vascular anomalies in current literature. *Plast Reconstr Surg.* 2011;127:347–351.

5. Greene AK, Liu AS, Mulliken JB, et al. Vascular anomalies in 5621 patients: guidelines for referral. *J Pediatr Surg.* 2011;46:1784–1789.

13. Chang LC, Haggstrom AN, Drolet BA, et al. Growth characteristics of infantile hemangiomas: implications for management. *Pediatrics.* 2008;122:360–367.

14. Couto RA, Maclellan RA, Zurakowski D, et al. Infantile hemangioma: clinical assessment of the involuting phase and implications for management. *Plast Reconstr Surg.* 2012;130:619–624.

21. North PE, Waner M, Mizeracki A, et al. GLUT1: a newly discovered immunohistochemical marker for juvenile hemangiomas. *Hum Pathol.* 2000;31:11–22. *This is a retrospective immunohistochemical study of 143 hemangiomas, 66 vascular malformations, 20 pyogenic granulomas, and five hemangioendotheliomas. GLUT1 (erythrocyte-type glucose transporter) only was expressed in infantile hemangioma (during proliferation and involution). GLUT1 is a sensitive marker to differentiate infantile hemangioma from congenital hemangiomas, other vascular tumors, and vascular malformations.*

26. Couto JA, Greene AK. Management of problematic infantile hemangioma using intralesional triamcinolone: efficacy and safety in 100 infants. *J Plast Reconstr Aesthet Surg.* 2014;67:1469–1474.

30. Greene AK, Couto RA. Oral prednisolone for infantile hemangioma: efficacy and safety using a standardized treatment protocol. *Plast Reconstr Surg.* 2011;128:743–752.

32. Drolet BA, Frommelt PC, Chamlin SL, et al. Initiation and use of propranolol for infantile hemangioma: report of a consensus conference. *Pediatrics.* 2013;131:128–140.

76. Vikkula M, Boon LM, Carraway KL, et al. Vascular dysmorphogenesis caused by an activating mutation in the receptor tyrosine kinase TIE2. *Cell.* 1996;87:1181–1190. *Two families with inherited multiple venous malformations were found to have an activating mutation in the endothelial receptor tyrosine kinase TIE2, suggesting that the TIE2 signaling pathway is critical for endothelial-smooth muscle cell interaction. This was the first mutation implicated in the pathogenesis of vascular anomalies; the disorder is called cutaneous-mucosal venous malformation.*

40

Pediatric chest and trunk defects

Lawrence J. Gottlieb, Russell R. Reid, and Mark B. Slidell

SYNOPSIS

- Pediatric trunk defects require multidisciplinary comprehensive care in order to maximize patient safety and successful outcome.
- Reconstructive surgery for the pediatric patient requires consideration for the paucity of tissue available in a small body habitus, the necessity for growth, and the tenuous physiology that may accompany children afflicted with congenital defects.
- Closure of ventral body wall defects may pose significant challenges to the neonatal circulation, whereas closure of dorsal body wall defects must address exposed neural elements.

Introduction

Patients with severe congenital trunk defects are frequently diagnosed during prenatal ultrasonography or at birth and require the coordination of multiple disciplines, including reconstructive plastic surgery. Reconstructive surgery for the pediatric patient requires consideration for the paucity of tissue available in a small body habitus, the impact of surgery on future growth of the child, and the tenuous physiology that may accompany children afflicted with congenital defects. Body wall defects have the potential risk of exposing vital structures and subsequent infection. Closure of ventral body wall defects may pose significant challenges to the neonatal circulation, whereas closure of dorsal body wall defects must address exposed neural elements.

Embryology

Development of the body wall begins at 4 weeks' gestation when the mesoderm organizes into the paraxial, intermediate, and lateral plate layers. The paraxial mesoderm, adjacent to the neural tube, differentiates into the skeletal support and surrounding soft tissue that characterize the dorsal body wall and encases the central nervous system. Intermediate meso-derm forms the urogenital structures. Lateral plate mesoderm differentiates into both the soft tissue and skeletal components of the ventral body wall. The lateral plate mesoderm, with ectoderm covering, folds and fuses at the end of the 4th week of gestation.[1,2] Congenital ventral body wall defects result from the lack of lateral plate fusion.

Thoracic wall defects

Pectus excavatum

Pectus excavatum, also known as "sunken chest" or "funnel chest", is the most common congenital anterior thoracic wall deformity. It occurs in 1 in 300–400 live births and makes up ~90% of the thoracic wall defects seen. Pectus excavatum is characterized by a depression of the sternum, as well as costal cartilage displacement. Males outnumber females 3:1 and patients are predominantly Caucasian. Pectus excavatum is often identified within the first years of life although more subtle defects are frequently not noticed until teenage years. Most typically, a mild pectus deformity will become more pronounced in the rapid growth period during puberty.

Pectus deformities often carry a familial component, with 37–47% of patients reporting a family history. Inheritance patterns are not fully understood, but studies of different kindreds have shown autosomal dominant, autosomal recessive, X-linked, and multifactorial inheritance. No definitive genetic mutations have been found, although the frequency of other musculoskeletal deformities such as scoliosis and Marfan syndrome suggest that abnormal connective tissue plays a role. Poland syndrome, scoliosis, clubfoot, and syndactyly are known to be associated with pectus deformities.[3,4]

Clinical presentation and evaluation

Patients with pectus excavatum exhibit a depressed sternum that is frequently greater on the right with sternal retraction on inspiration.[5,6] Both the body of the sternum and the costal

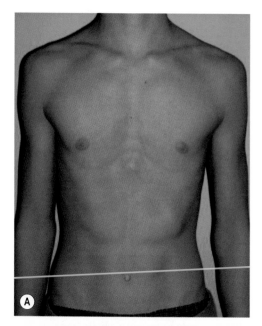

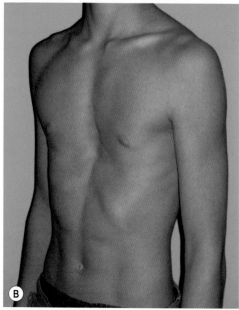

Fig. 40.1 Pectus excavatum is the most common congenital anterior thoracic wall defect and is characterized by a depression deformity in the sternum and costal cartilage displacement. A male predominance exists. **(A)** Anterior view of patient with pectus excavatum. **(B)** Oblique view of patient. Note the decrease in anterior posterior distance between the sternum and the vertebral column.

cartilages at the sternocostal junction have posterior angulation (Fig. 40.1). Rounded sloping shoulders, mild dorsal kyphosis, and a protuberant abdomen are associated findings but may be related to postural changes that patients exhibit secondary to a conscious or subconscious attempt to hide their deformity.

Patients will often complain of subjective dyspnea or chest pain, and may have significant body image concerns. Proper identification of the extent of structural irregularity, physiologic limitations, and psychological responses to the deformity are crucial in treatment decision-making. Basic work-up should include chest CT and/or radiographs, pulmonary

function tests, and echocardiogram or EKG (Fig. 40.2). Haller and others stratified anatomic severity of pectus excavatum by defining a pectus severity index (PSI) using measurements obtained from CT scans.[7,8] The "Haller Index" is calculated by dividing the internal transverse thoracic width by the smallest anterior-posterior distance between the vertebrae and the most depressed portion of the chest wall. Normal values range between 2.5 and 3.25 and an index >3.25 is considered one of the criteria for operative intervention.[9]

Surgical indications

Most patients are asymptomatic and seek elective intervention for the correction of contour deformities, especially when the features become more prominent during the pubertal growth spurt. Although cardiopulmonary compromise is controversial, anatomically severe versions of pectus excavatum are thought to benefit from surgical intervention.[10,11] Kelly suggests that surgery is indicated when two or more of the following occur: a severe, symptomatic deformity; progression of deformity; paradoxic respiratory chest wall motion; CT scan with a PSI >3.25; cardiac or pulmonary compression or pathology; significant body image disturbance; or failed repairs.[12] Historically, many pectus excavatum repairs were performed in younger children, and the optimal timing has been a subject of controversy. The largest single institution series of patients had median age for operative intervention of 14, and most surgeons prefer to operate on children 12–18 years of age, during their pubertal growth spurt.[13]

Treatment

Some patients with very mild deformities can be satisfactorily treated with physical therapy to improve their posture and increase the bulk of their pectoralis muscles. This approach does not correct the deformity, but rather it diminishes its

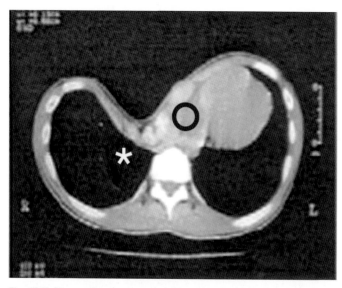

Fig. 40.2 CT scan of pectus excavatum deformities illustrate both the severity of sternal depression as well as the morphology of the depression and its effects on the involved organs. The pectus severity index (PSI) utilized CT scans to stratify deformities by dividing the internal thoracic width by the smallest anterior-posterior distance. Operative intervention is usually performed if PSI >3.25.

prominence by improving posture and emphasizing natural muscle development in other areas.

Surgical correction of pectus excavatum can be categorized into procedures that either camouflage or repair the defect. Camouflage of contour deformities has been successfully accomplished with autologous tissue or custom prosthetics. The disadvantage of autologous tissue is the donor site scar and potential morbidity. Flaps containing muscle should not be relied on for volume correction only unless innervated and able to contract, as the muscle will invariably atrophy if not innervated and contracting. The most common contour camouflage technique is placement of customized silicone implants (Fig. 40.3).[14–17] Satisfactory results are obtained with silicone implants with few short-term complications other than seroma formation. Additional problems with prosthetics are displacement, visualization of edges and potential extrusion, especially in thin patients. Autologous reconstruction has been used as an alternative to prosthetics in selected patients.[17–21] Recently, Sinna *et al.* described a combination of approaches covering a custom implant with bilateral de-epithelialized thoraco-dorsal artery perforator flaps.[22] Injection of autologous fat or prosthetic soft tissue fillers has also been described.[23,24]

Whereas contour camouflage techniques are most appropriate for patients with mild deformities, patients with moderate to severe deformities are better suited for contour repair techniques. Ravitch described an open repair technique of elevating bilateral pectoralis muscle flaps with resection of abnormal costal cartilages followed by transverse osteotomy of the sternum and fixation in a corrected position (Fig. 40.4).[4] The Ravitch procedure has since been modified in many ways: from preserving the perichondrium to minimal cartilage resection and varying technique to support the sternum.[25,26] Haller and colleagues describe supporting the elevated sternum by overlapping the sternal ends of the costal cartilages over the costal ends in a tripod fixation.[27,28] Almost all open techniques utilize a transverse inframammary crease or a short Chevron incision except for older patients or Marfan patients where a vertical midline incision is usually used. Bilateral pectoralis major and upper rectus abdominus muscles are disinserted from the sternum and ribs bilaterally and raised to expose the costal cartilages. With or without sacrifice of the perichondrium, the costal cartilages are resected to a greater or lesser degree. Since Ravitch's initial experience, it has become clear that the most medial and most lateral portions of the costal cartilages should be preserved in young children to minimize secondary growth disturbances. The sternal angulation is corrected with a transverse, wedge osteotomy that is done at the level of the third or fourth intercostal space corresponding to the upper edge of the

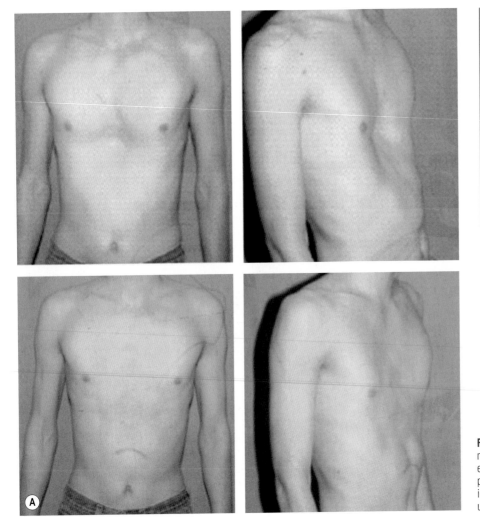

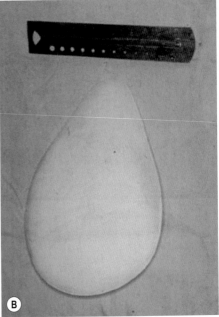

Fig. 40.3 Customized silicone implants are a common method of camouflaging contour deformities in pectus excavatum. **(A)** Preoperative (upper panels) and postoperative (lower panels) photographs following implant insertion. A transverse epigastric incision was used for insertion. **(B)** Custom silicone implant.

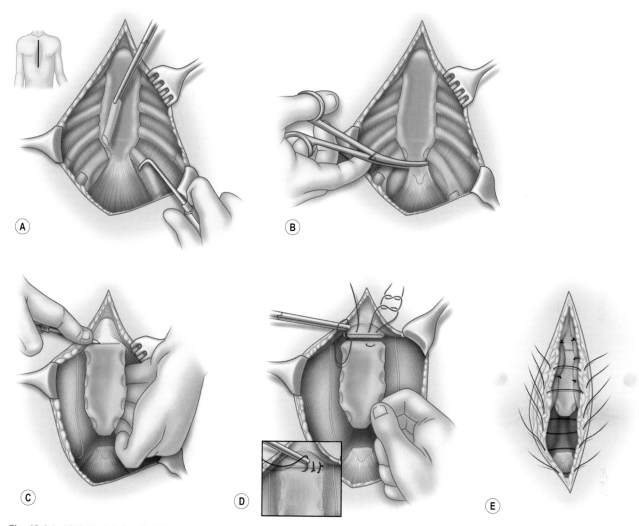

Fig. 40.4 In 1949, Ravitch described his classic approach to pectus excavatum repair. **(A)** Starting with a midline incision, the pectoralis muscles are incised and elevated to expose the sternum and the sternocostal junction. **(B)** The lowest two costal cartilages are resected with perichondrium and the xiphoid is osteotomized to begin mobilization of the sternum. **(C)** Five costal cartilages are divided bilaterally and a single cortex osteotomy is made superiorly. **(D)** The inferior sternum is reapproximated at a corrected position and secured with braided silk mattress sutures. **(E)** The pectoralis muscles are reapproximated midline and the skin incision is closed.

sternal depression. The osteotomy can then be secured with sutures, wire, or rigid fixation plates.[29,30] The xiphoid process is detached from the sternum and allowed to retract down.

Horizontal sternal fixation techniques are not universally used but many surgeons now consider them essential for a durable repair. Most surgeons support the sternum with a metallic strut developed by Adkins and Blades.[31] Fonkalsrud and colleagues report on a modified open technique with minimal cartilage resection and use of the Adkins strut in 450 patients. Most of these patients had retrosternal placement but more recently they have converted to a suprasternal strut to facilitate removal (at 6 months) and minimize the need to enter the pleural cavity.[32] Hayashi and Maruyama describe the use of a vascularized rib strut based on the anterior intercostal branch of the internal mammary artery instead of a metallic strut.[33] Robicsek *et al.* have extensive experience reporting on over 600 patients treated with a retrosternal Marlex mesh "hammock" technique with excellent long-term results.[34]

Recently, bioabsorbable mesh placed for retrosternal support in the Robicsek technique has been reported and found to be associated with decreased inflammatory reaction, decreased postoperative pain, and elimination of the risk of retrosternal metal support device dislodgment.[35]

A radical method to repair contour deformities of the sternum uses a sternal turnover bone graft.[36] This technique has been met with problems of sternal avascular necrosis due to the interruption of blood supply. Vascularized sternal turnover bone flaps with microvascular anastomoses of the internal mammary vessels were later developed to prevent such complications and have been successful in several reports.[37–39] Despite improvements in technique, this approach has never been widely embraced.

With the development and advances in thoracoscopy, minimally invasive repair of pectus excavatum has emerged as a viable option.[40–42] This approach is referred to as the "Nuss procedure" after the surgeon Dr. Donald Nuss, who

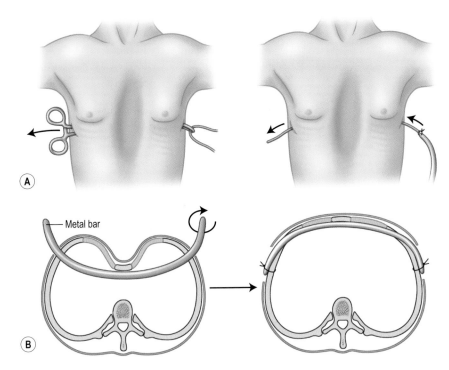

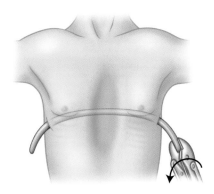

Fig. 40.5 The Nuss repair, also known as the minimally invasive repair of pectus excavatum (MIRPE), is a thoracoscopic method of contour repair using a bent bar. **(A)** A Kelly clamp is advanced across the mediastinum underneath the sternum (left panel). The clamp guides the placement of a bent bar into the substernal space (middle and right panels). **(B)** For the insertion, the bar follows the concave curvature of the deformed thorax (left panel). Once in place, the bar is rotated 180 degrees on its axis such that it forces the sternum anteriorly into a convex formation (right panel).

first developed it. This approach involves thoracoscopic exposure of the sternum and the placement of a custom bent steel or titanium bar (Fig. 40.5). A second procedure to remove the bar is required. Unlike the Ravitch and modified Ravitch procedures, skeletal resection is unnecessary with the Nuss procedure, and this less invasive approach results in less scarring and shorter operative times. However, the operation has less satisfactory results in patients with asymmetric deformities and in these patients, the Ravitch procedure is often a better choice.

Early complications of pectus excavatum repair are infrequent beyond pneumothorax (67%) or suture site infection (1%), and pneumothorax is usually self-limiting, with only 4% requiring chest tube drainage.[13] Longer-term complications of the Nuss procedure, such as bar dislocation (5.7%), overcorrection (3.7%), bar allergy (3%), and bar infection (0.5%) have been reported.[13] Late complications such as recurrent pectus deformity (1%) are very few and have diminished now that most surgeons leave the bar in place for 2–3 years. Secondary thoracic deformity is a serious late complication that has been observed in patients who undergo correction at an early age. Thought to be due to the interruption of growth centers and intrathoracic scar formation, the patients develop narrowed thoraces and severe pulmonary impairment. Haller coined this phenomenon as acquired Jeune syndrome.[43] In the past two decades, most surgeons reserve repair for children who are entering or are already in the pubertal growth phase. Absorbable transsternal bars have been used in the Nuss procedure but they are associated with higher breakage rates and have been mostly abandoned.[44]

There are some novel corrective devices in development, including the Vacuum Bell treatment and implanted magnets with an external magnetic "brace". The Vacuum Bell is a donut-shaped attachment, which the patient wears for several hours daily, and uses negative pressure to raise the sternum. Initial results have been encouraging, but there is limited data so far.[45] Harrison *et al.* have developed the magnetic minimover procedure (3MP), in which implantable magnets are surgically attached to the sternum and the patient wears an external brace which attracts the magnet and pulls the chest wall into a more normal position. The initial FDA sponsored clinical trial enrolled 10 patients and had moderate success. Half of the patients required a second procedure to reposition the magnet on the sternum and 30% of the patients dropped out of the study and opted to undergo the Nuss procedure. In patients who did complete the full treatment with the 3MP device, the costs were nearly half the cost of the Nuss procedure.[46]

Pectus carinatum

Pectus carinatum, also known as "pigeon chest", is less common than pectus excavatum, but is considered to be in the same spectrum of deformities. It is characterized as a protrusion deformity of the anterior thoracic wall (Fig. 40.6). Similar to excavatum deformities, pectus carinatum does not have a defined etiology. The incidence is thought to be about 1 in 10 000, makes up ~5–7% of chest wall deformities, and is six times more common in males.

Clinical presentation and surgical indications

Three types of anterior thoracic protrusion deformities have been described in the pectus carinatum spectrum.[47] The chondrogladiolar type is the most common version and is characterized by anterior displacement of the body of the sternum

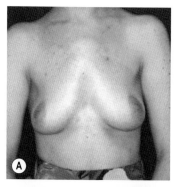

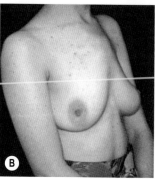

Fig. 40.6 Pectus carinatum is an anterior protrusion thoracic deformity that is the reverse of pectus excavatum but is generally considered to be in the same spectrum of deformities. Shown here are (**A**) anterior and (**B**) oblique photographs of a 28-year-old woman with pectus carinatum.

with costal cartilage concavity. Asymmetric mixed deformities can also occur with displacement of the costal cartilages on one side with normal positioning of the sternum. Prominence of the chondromanubrial junction with a depressed sternum represents the third and least common type. Unlike pectus excavatum, younger patients do not have cardiopulmonary compromise and tend to display subtle findings on clinical exam. Patients tend to be diagnosed at a later age and seek surgical correction for their contour irregularities. Pectus carinatum can also be an acquired defect secondary to pectus excavatum repair.[48] In contrast with pectus excavatum patients, children with carinatum deformities are less likely to have associated symptoms and the most common symptom is chest pain at the costochondral junction. External bracing is usually effective in these patients, and the main indication for surgery is an extreme deformity or the failure to improve cosmetic appearance via bracing.

Treatment

Non-surgical means of correction using orthotics have been described in small case series with improvement of carinatum deformities.[49,50] Successful treatment with external bracing is highly dependent upon the patient remaining compliant with the bracing protocol. Success rates as high as 80% have been achieved using the "Calgary Protocol" for bracing. This requires that the patient be custom-fitted with a lightweight, patient-controlled chest brace that they must initially wear for 23 h per day. Once the convex deformity was corrected, bracing is reduced to 8 h per day and can be accomplished nocturnally. This "maintenance phase" is continued until

axial skeletal maturation ceases. Patients rarely experience discomfort during bracing, and most are very satisfied with their chest wall appearance following bracing and would use the brace again.[51] Significant improvement in self-esteem was also seen after bracing.[52] If bracing fails, operative correction remains an option.

The Ravitch procedure is the operation of choice for pectus carinatum defects. Typically, the approach is through a transverse chevron incision that extends across from one inframammary fold to the other. Classically, the pectoralis and rectus muscles are elevated to expose the costal cartilages and the sternum. For the chondrogladiolar deformity, subperichondrial resection of the costal cartilages is combined with a single or double osteotomy to return the sternum to the correct alignment (Fig. 40.7).[47] For the asymmetric deformities, sternal positioning is corrected after costal cartilage resection with a wedge osteotomy. Recent refinements in this procedure include a method in which costal cartilages are resected through splitting the muscle along its fibers rather than elevating the entire muscle.[49] There are also attempts to develop a minimally thoracoscopic approach to pectus carinatum. In this operation, chondrotomies are made thoracoscopically and a suprasternal bar is placed to compress the carinatum defect and correct the deformity.[53] Only a handful of patients have undergone this procedure, but it proves to be a useful complement to the Ravitch in patients with very symmetric carinatum defects.

Jeune syndrome

Asphyxiating thoracic dystrophy, Jeune syndrome, is the most common thoracic deformity in the diffuse skeletal disorders. The others are spondylothoracic dysplasia (Jarcho–Levin syndrome) and cerebrocostomandibular syndrome, and since there are no surgical interventions developed for these defects, they will not be discussed further in this chapter.

Jeune syndrome is a rare familial autosomal recessive osteochondrodystrophy characterized by a narrow, immobile thorax and a protuberant abdomen (Fig. 40.8).[54] Though the early descriptions were in neonates who succumbed to respiratory insufficiency, subsequent reports have demonstrated that Jeune syndrome has a variable expression and can result in viability.[55] That said, 60–70% will die as infants due to respiratory failure.[56] In patients who have less severe versions of Jeune syndrome, renal and liver disease are common (17% and 22%, respectively) and can lead to organ failure in adulthood.

Clinical presentation and surgical indications

Jeune syndrome can be variably expressed.[57] The neonate with severe Jeune syndrome is generally described to have a narrow, bell-shaped thorax that is narrowed in both the transverse and sagittal dimensions with mild brachydactyly. The ribs are short, wide, and barely reach the anterior axillary line. Histologic examination of the costochondral junction reveals disordered endochondral ossification. These patients have severe restrictive lung disease and frequently require mechanical ventilation and a tracheostomy. In contrast, patients who have a moderate expression of Jeune syndrome tend to have a narrow thorax without respiratory compromise, severe brachydactyly, and renal failure at a later age. These

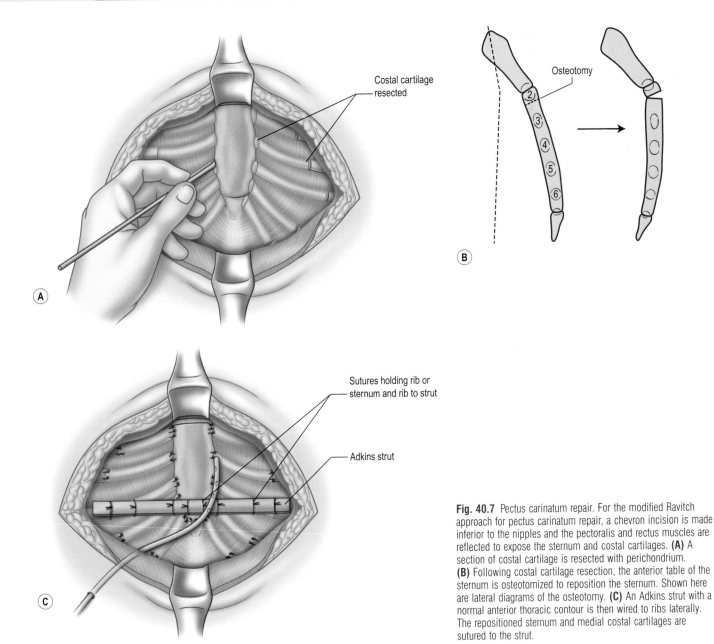

Costal cartilage resected

Osteotomy

Sutures holding rib or sternum and rib to strut

Adkins strut

Fig. 40.7 Pectus carinatum repair. For the modified Ravitch approach for pectus carinatum repair, a chevron incision is made inferior to the nipples and the pectoralis and rectus muscles are reflected to expose the sternum and costal cartilages. **(A)** A section of costal cartilage is resected with perichondrium. **(B)** Following costal cartilage resection, the anterior table of the sternum is osteotomized to reposition the sternum. Shown here are lateral diagrams of the osteotomy. **(C)** An Adkins strut with a normal anterior thoracic contour is then wired to ribs laterally. The repositioned sternum and medial costal cartilages are sutured to the strut.

patients are usually identified upon presentation for renal transplantation or renal replacement therapy. Finally, the mildest form of Jeune syndrome may be manifested with only polydactyly and severe brachydactyly. Surgical enlargement of the thoracic cavity may be attempted in those patients with ongoing respiratory compromise, but it usually is unsuccessful, resulting in prolonged hospitalization and death from respiratory compromise.

Treatment

Operative intervention in Jeune syndrome is focused on expansion of the thoracic cavity. Two methods have emerged as successful options: median sternotomy and lateral thoracic expansion thoracoplasty. The median sternotomy technique

usually requires addition of bone graft, stainless steel struts, or prosthetic spacers.[58–61] Alternatively, Davis and Shah described a lateral thoracic expansion technique (Fig. 40.9). In this procedure, ribs 4–9 are differentially transected, separated from periosteum, and different ribs are secured together in an expanded fashion with titanium plates.[62–64] This is generally performed as a staged procedure with each operation separated by several months. The authors noted good results in patients over 1 year of age and new bone formation with this method. Waldhausen and colleagues report success with a technique in two children using a vertical expandable prosthetic titanium rib (VEPTR) thoracoplasty for the treatment children with thoracic insufficiency syndrome. Long-term follow-up is unavailable for those patients.[65]

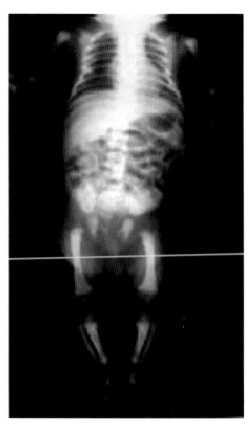

Fig. 40.8 Radiograph of a 3-month-old infant with Jeune syndrome, asphyxiating thoracic dystrophy. Note the horizontal orientation of the ribs, the characteristic "bell-shaped" thorax, shorted lower limbs, and pelvic abnormalities.

Ectopia cordis

Ectopia cordis represents a spectrum of four rare congenital sternal deformities uniformly characterized by a midline sternal defect. The incidence of ectopia cordis is 0.8 per 100 000 live births and can vary from asymptomatic benign clefts to severe conditions with high mortality rates. Many cases can be diagnosed by prenatal ultrasound (Fig. 40.10). The

classification system that is widely accepted today is based upon tissue coverage of the heart and includes: cervical ectopia cordis, thoracic ectopia cordis, thoraco-abdominal ectopia cordis, and cleft or bifid sternum.

Clinical presentation and surgical indications

Cervical ectopia cordis is the most severe variant with superior displacement of the heart and craniofacial deformities. It is distinguished from thoracic ectopia cordis by the extent of superior displacement of the heart. To date, there are no published cases of successful repair of cervical ectopia cordis defects.

Thoracic ectopia cordis describes the classic extrathoracic heart without soft tissue or bony covering. There are also frequently associated congenital heart defects. There are only a handful of survivors among children born with this defect.

Thoraco-abdominal ectopia cordis is a combination of both thoracic wall and abdominal wall defects (Fig. 40.11). These defects are associated with Cantrell's pentalogy, which consists of a midline abdominal wall defect, low sternal defect, anterior diaphragmatic defect, pericardial defect, and intra-cardiac anomalies.[66]

Finally, bifid sternum is a relatively benign finding with a cleft upper sternum that rarely causes significant physiologic disturbance (Fig. 40.12). This is the least severe of the sternal defects, and associated congenital heart defects are rare.

Surgical correction is necessary in thoracic, and thoraco-abdominal defects, with the initial goal of coverage of the heart followed by ultimately returning the heart to the thoracic cavity when patients have developed sufficient reserve. Successful repair is much more likely in thoraco-abdominal ectopia cordis compared with true thoracic ectopia cordis. The absence of concomitant congenital heart disease is another predictor of successful repair. In patients with cleft/bifid sternum, the goal of surgery is to provide a protective bony coverage for the heart and to possibly improve respiratory mechanics. Coordinated multidisciplinary care involving obstetricians, neonatologists, critical care anesthesiologists, cardiothoracic surgeons, and plastic surgeons is critical to reduce mortality in these high-risk neonates.

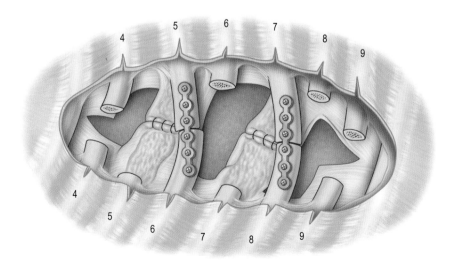

Fig. 40.9 Jeune syndrome repair. The lateral thoracic expansion technique as described by Davis involves transection of ribs 4–9 and rigid fixation of alternate ribs. The thoracic cavity is expanded by increasing the amount of space between ribs.

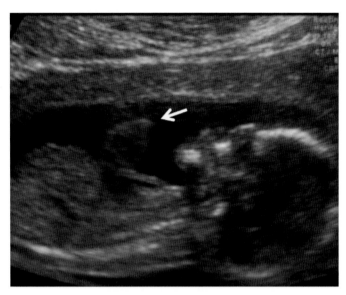

Fig. 40.10 Prenatal ultrasound diagnosis of ectopia cordis. The prenatal ultrasound of a 32-week-old fetus demonstrating an extrathoracic heart (arrow).

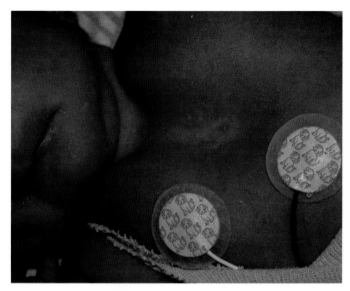

Fig. 40.12 Bifid sternum is a benign condition in the spectrum of ectopia cordis defects. Similar to more severe forms, a failure of sternum fusion is evident. However, the thoracic contents are positioned anatomically and there are no associated physiologic abnormalities.

Treatment

Thoracic and thoraco-abdominal ectopia cordis repair is most successful when performed in a staged manner. The key principles for successful operative management are the construction of tissue coverage surrounding the heart as a partial anterior chest cavity, and also to defer attempts to move the heart to an orthotopic location. The first step is performed within the first several hours of life and involves coverage of the exposed heart with bilateral pectoral skin flaps, split thickness skin grafts (STSG), or synthetic or biologic mesh. There should be no attempt in returning the heart to the thoracic cavity at this point, due to the cardiopulmonary compromise that will occur with compression.[67] At several months to 2

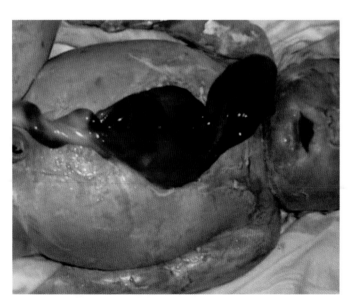

Fig. 40.11 Thoraco-abdominal ectopia cordis. Same patient as in Fig. 40.10 with ectopia cordis, midline supraumbilical defect and low sternal defect.

years of age, the patient receives chest wall reconstruction and repositioning of the heart. Chest wall reconstruction can take the form of musculocutaneous flaps over autologous rib grafts as well as alloplastic custom made struts.[68,69] Hochberg and colleagues[68] described a method of elevating the pectoral and rectus muscles as a unit and transposing bipedicled musculocutaneous flaps medially with relaxing incisions laterally. The resulting donor sites were skin grafted on the lateral aspects of the patient.

Sternal clefts without an exposed heart are significantly less complicated. Surgical repair can often be performed within the first month of life. Bilateral pectoralis major muscle advancement flaps over rib grafts have yielded good cosmetic results.[70] Rigid fixation with titanium plates has also been reported.[71]

Poland syndrome

Poland syndrome is a rare disorder characterized by the unilateral absence of the sternal head of the pectoralis major muscle, breast hypoplasia or aplasia, absence or deformed ribs, axillary alopecia, and ipsilateral upper extremity shortening and brachysyndactyly.[72,73] Poland syndrome has been reported to have an incidence of around 1–30 000 live births, with males outnumbering females.[74] The etiology is unknown. One suggested mechanism for Poland syndrome is subclavian artery insufficiency occurring around the 6th week of gestation, with the right side affected twice as often as the left. Alternatively, unilateral developmental failure of the lateral plate mesoderm has also been proposed.

Clinical presentation and surgical indications

Pediatric patients with Poland syndrome are heterogeneous. The pathognomonic feature is the absence of the sternal head of the pectoralis major muscle with anterior axillary fold deficiency (Fig. 40.13). Varying degrees of chest wall and hand involvement may occur (Fig. 40.14). In rare severe

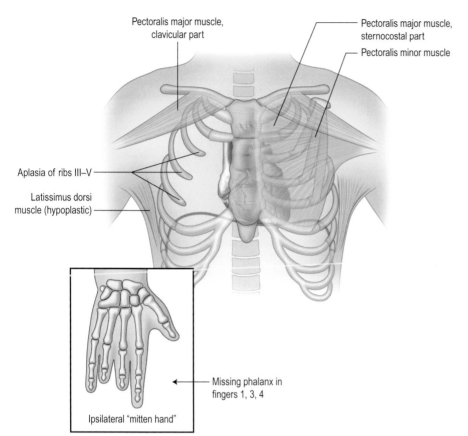

Pectoralis major muscle, clavicular part

Pectoralis major muscle, sternocostal part

Pectoralis minor muscle

Aplasia of ribs III–V

Latissimus dorsi muscle (hypoplastic)

Missing phalanx in fingers 1, 3, 4

Ipsilateral "mitten hand"

Fig. 40.13 Poland syndrome is characterized by a unilateral absence of the sternal head of the pectoralis major muscle, breast hypoplasia or aplasia, absence or deformed ribs, axillary alopecia, and ipsilateral upper extremity shortening and brachysyndactyly.

circumstances, depression deformities can occur with attenuation of ribs 2–5 with absence of anterior cartilage leading to paradoxical motion of the chest wall or lung herniation. Some patients have a pectus carinatum deformity on the contralateral side. Poland syndrome does not preclude correction of the pectus defect. In one-third of patients, the breast is affected and can range from hypoplasia to complete absence.

The latissimus dorsi muscle may be attenuated. Diagnosis of Poland syndrome is possible by prenatal ultrasound but is usually best evaluated with postnatal physical exam.

Basic work-up for Poland syndrome begins with the postnatal physical exam. The trunk and upper extremities need to be examined in its entirety with comparison to the contralateral side. The presence of the pectoralis major, serratus

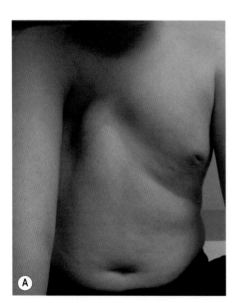
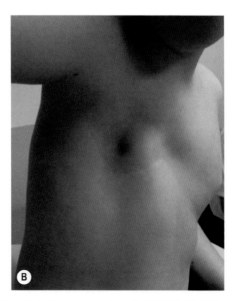
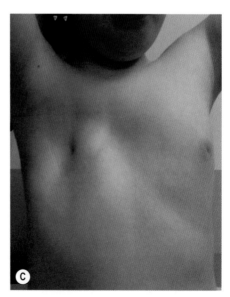

Fig. 40.14 Poland syndrome is a rare disease with a male predominance. A young boy with **(A)** right-sided Poland syndrome. **(B,C)** Note the presence of a hypoplastic nipple and the absence of the sternal head of the pectoralis major.

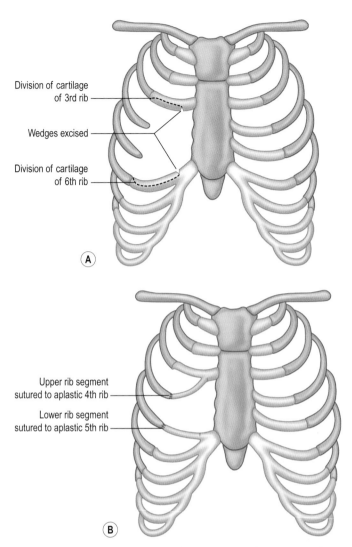

Division of cartilage
of 3rd rib

Wedges excised

Division of cartilage
of 6th rib

(A)

Upper rib segment
sutured to aplastic 4th rib

Lower rib segment
sutured to aplastic 5th rib

(B)

Fig. 40.15 (A,B) Split rib graft repair for Poland syndrome. Skeletal support in Poland syndrome can be achieved by excising the existing superior and inferior costal cartilages, splitting the cartilages, and re-fixation to the abnormal ribs.

anterior, and latissimus dorsi should be confirmed by palpation. A standard chest radiograph is necessary to visualize the ribs. Computerized tomography or MRI with contrast may be helpful for surgical planning. The primary surgical indication for repair at a young age is rib cage aplasia[75] resulting in cardiopulmonary compromise. At later ages, surgery is usually performed for concerns of contour abnormalities in both males and females.

Treatment

A heterogeneous spectrum of reconstructive options exists for correction of Poland syndrome. Mild forms of Poland syndrome generally have a strictly soft-tissue deficiency and may not require any intervention. Similar to adult breast reconstruction, both silicone prostheses as well as autologous tissue reconstruction have been described. Custom prosthetic implants for chest wall deformities have a high incidence of displacement, erosion, discomfort, and edge visibility, especially in thin individuals.[76] Multiple groups have provided

evidence that pedicled latissimus dorsi flaps with or without silicone implants can be accomplished with excellent results improving chest wall contour in a staged fashion. Some groups have modified this method with the use of minimally invasive endoscopy to elevate the latissimus.[77,78] Free tissue transfer such as the transverse rectus abdominis musculocutaneous, deep inferior epigastric perforator, superior gluteal artery perforator (SGAP), and anterolateral thigh perforator flaps have been used for breast reconstruction and soft tissue camouflage/fill of contour defects.[79,80] Contralateral latissimus dorsi microneurovascular transfer has been described for functional replacement of the missing pectoralis muscle, as well as reconstructing a more normal appearance to the anterior axillary fold when the ipsilateral latissimus dorsi muscle is attenuated or otherwise unusable.[81]

In more severe presentations of Poland syndrome, bony support for chest wall reconstruction have traditionally been accomplished with autologous split rib grafts (Fig. 40.15) or Marlex mesh (Fig. 40.16).[82,83] Both techniques have met success; however, Marlex mesh placement tends to result in a flattened appearance and, therefore, tends to be performed in conjunction with latissimus dorsi flaps. Alternatively, mesh prostheses with rib graft, molded silicone prostheses, as well as cryopreserved costal cartilage have been described with varying success.[16,84,85] Symmetry of the carinate deformity on the contralateral side may subsequently be corrected with a sternal osteotomy and rotation.

Abdominal wall defects

Omphalocele and gastroschisis

Congenital defects of the abdominal wall comprise a large spectrum of deformities, ranging from umbilical hernias to giant omphaloceles and the intestinal eventration associated with gastroschisis. These conditions can vary widely in their etiology, associated morbidity, and management.

Omphalocele defects exist along a spectrum ranging from giant omphaloceles to umbilical hernias of the cord. It is important to differentiate between a giant umbilical hernia and an omphalocele. The umbilical hernia is a central abdominal wall defect involving the linea alba, with herniation of intra-abdominal contents into the umbilical stalk. The skin overlying the hernia is intact. In contrast, an omphalocele is characterized by a midline defect of the ventral abdominal wall, resulting in extrusion of intra-abdominal contents, which are covered by a membrane comprised of peritoneum, Wharton's jelly, and amnion. The umbilical cord arises from the membranous sac, and the defect may be located in the central, upper, or lower abdomen. The defect in omphaloceles is due to a failure of the body folds to complete their journey. Purely lateral fold defects will be isolated at the umbilicus, but cephalic fold defects result in associated defects above the omphalocele such as ectopia cordis or the pentalogy of Cantrell. In contrast, caudal fold defects cause defects below the omphalocele such as bladder and cloacal exstrophy. Depending on the size and location of the defect, the hernia may contain bowel, liver, and other organs. Omphaloceles may be termed "minor" or "giant" with the definition of a giant omphalocele typical defined as a 5 cm defect or the presence of the liver within the defect.[86]

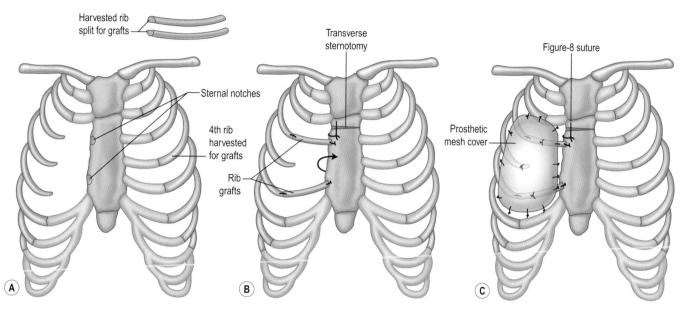

Fig. 40.16 (A–C) Mesh usage in Poland syndrome repair. In addition to autologous split rib grafts, Marlex mesh placed above the rib grafts serve to correct the skeletal contour deformity. However, the appearance of the thorax after either rib grafts alone or Marlex mesh over rib grafts is flattened. The contour deformity also requires addition of soft tissue or prostheses over the bony reconstruction.

Gastroschisis is characterized by a full-thickness defect of the abdominal wall, usually to the right of midline and not involving the umbilicus. This results in evisceration of abdominal contents without any sac or covering. Small intestine is always present, while stomach, colon, and gonads may also be involved. In contrast to omphalocele, it is rare for the liver to herniate outside the abdominal cavity. The exposed organs typically appear normal at birth, but they quickly develop a rind consisting of a fibrinous exudate. The rind is thought to be due to a combination of chronic exposure to amniotic fluid and the air. This inflamed bowel frequently demonstrates dysmotility and malabsorption. The presence of the bowel external to the abdomen precludes normal intestinal fixation *in utero*, and therefore, all children with gastroschisis have an anomaly of intestinal rotation or "malrotation". They do not typically require a Ladd procedure to correct the anomaly of intestinal rotation, but it is important to remember that their intestines are not normally rotated.

Omphalocele and gastroschisis occur at 1–2.5 in 5000 live births and 2–4.9 in 10 000 live births, respectively.[87,88] Omphaloceles have a tendency to be larger in size than gastroschisis and involve the herniation of bowel, liver, and other organs into the umbilical cord with the amniotic sac covering. Males and females are equally affected. The genetic causes of omphalocele and gastroschisis are unknown but the two are thought to be different entities.

Clinical presentation and surgical indications

The abdominal wall defect in omphalocele typically ranges from 4 to 7 cm in diameter, whereas gastroschisis defects tend to be slightly smaller. Infants with omphalocele frequently have concurrent genetic disorders such as chromosomal abnormalities (e.g. Trisomy 18), Beckwith–Wiedemann syndrome (congenital abdominal wall defect, macroglossia, and hypoglycemia with increased abdominal tumors later in life),

ectopia cordis, and OEIS (omphalocele, exstrophy of bladder, imperforate anus, and spinal defect) sequence (Fig. 40.17).[89] Cardiac anomalies are common in patients with omphalocele, occurring in up to 45%. Anomalies range from ventricular septal defects, atrial septal defects, ectopia cordis, tricuspid atresia, coarctation of the aorta, and persistent pulmonary hypertension of the newborn.[90] In patients with giant omphalocele, survival is often predicated on the extant of pulmonary hypoplasia and degree of pulmonary hypertension. In contrast to omphaloceles, patients with gastroschisis are less likely to have other associated defects and approximately 14% of infants with gastroschisis will have associated unrelated genetic defects. The most common associated anomaly is of an intestinal atresia.[91]

Gastroschisis is broadly classified as simple or complex based on the presence of additional bowel anomalies such as intestinal atresias, stenosis, volvulus, or perforation. Intestinal atresias are the most frequent associated anomaly and the full range of intestinal atresias can be found. The size of the defect varies and one occasionally finds a very narrow defect and only a small amount of midgut external to the abdomen. Closer examination often reveals a paucity of bowel, which most likely is due to antenatal volvulus. This is known as a "vanishing gastroschisis" as the defect is so small that it is essentially closed *in utero*.[92]

Treatment

Reconstructive methods for omphalocele and gastroschisis are directly related to the size of the ventral abdominal wall defect and the magnitude of the intra-abdominal "loss of domain" (LOD). Small defects can be closed primarily or with minimal undermining of surrounding soft tissues. Giant omphaloceles usually cannot be closed primarily due to the size of the defect and the severe physiologic consequences of returning the liver and bowel to the abdomen in the setting

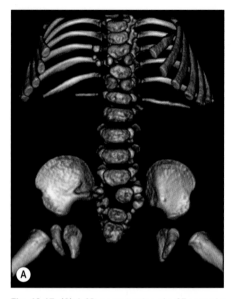
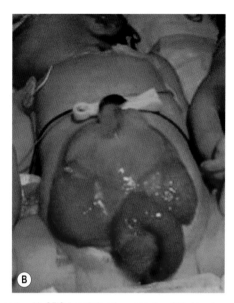
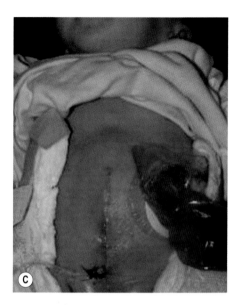

Fig. 40.17 **(A)** A 3D reconstruction of a CT scan of a neonate with OEIS (omphalocele, exstrophy of bladder, imperforate anus, and spinal defect). Note the wide pelvic separation of pubic symphysis and spinal defects. **(B)** Preoperative view of same neonate with OEIS demonstrating extensive abdominal wall defect. **(C)** Postoperative photograph of patient a few weeks after multi-staged omphalocele repair, genitourinary reconstruction, abdominal closure, and orthopedic correction of pelvis.

of decreased abdominal domain. Exacerbation of pulmonary disease and decreased venous return are typical problems encountered.

Small omphaloceles may be closed primarily in the first few days of life. An omphalocele of the cord may benefit from suspension of the defect above the abdomen for 24–48 h to allow gravity to assist with reduction of the omphalocele contents back into the abdomen (Fig. 40.18). Whether early or delayed closure is attempted, it is important to monitor the patient's physiology as the contents of the omphalocele are returned to the abdominal cavity. Methods

of assessing physiologic response to closure are further discussed below.

Giant omphaloceles tend to present unique challenges. A common approach is to apply a sclerosing agent such as 0.25% Mercurochrome or 0.5% silver nitrate to the omphalocele sac until complete epithelialization occurs, and to delay definitive operative management until any problems with pulmonary insufficiency have been stabilized. Silver sulfadiazine (Silvadene) has emerged as an excellent alternative with less potential toxicity (Fig. 40.19).[93] Dressings are performed twice daily until epithelialization is complete, and may potentially be

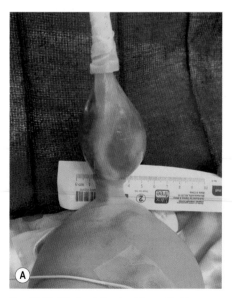
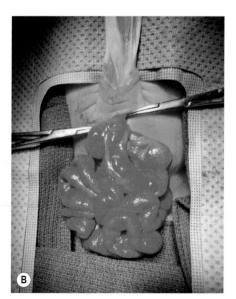
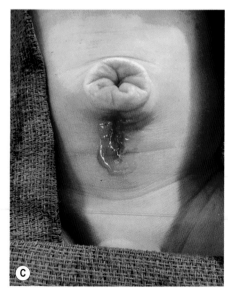

Fig. 40.18 **(A)** Omphalocele of the cord with very narrow defect at the umbilicus. **(B)** Small bowel reduced from omphalocele via an incision below the umbilical ring. This child required a Ladd procedure to remove constricting Ladd bands and broaden the narrow mesentery. **(C)** After closure of the umbilical defect and the incision below the umbilicus.

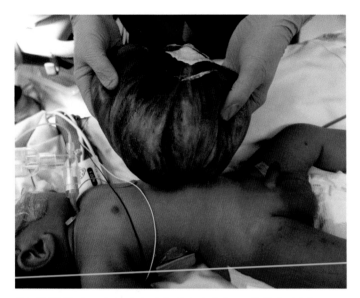

Fig. 40.19 Giant omphalocele treated with topical silver sulfadiazine totally re-epithelialized in approximately 6 months.

completed as an outpatient in selected patients.[94] Alternatively, skin coverage may be expedited through the use of skin grafts directly on the omphalocele sac, avoiding the need for a prolonged period of dressing changes.

Once the new epithelial covering completely envelops the omphalocele, gentle external pressure with an ACE wrap can often gradually compress the abdominal contents back into the abdomen, and definitive closure of the defect can often be achieved in one stage. In complicated cases, there are many creative approaches that have been employed: skin grafting;[95] stretching of the abdominal wall via intentional pneumoperitoneum;[96] tissue expanders to stretch the abdominal wall in preparation for closure;[97–99] partial hepatectomy;[100] lateral relaxing incisions in the fascia;[101] and division of the rectus abdominis muscles.[102]

Surgical closure techniques are frequently staged or delayed. In 1948, the first description of an omphalocele closure with staged skin flaps was reported.[103] Although the closure was successful, the disadvantage of using skin alone was the resultant large ventral hernia. A more definitive closure would necessitate the reapproximation of fascia or the interposition of a synthetic or alloplastic material.

Intraperitoneal tissue expansion is an alternative method of abdominal wall expansion to treat LOD. In two reports, intraperitoneal tissue expansion was performed with an intrapelvic expander over the course of 3–5 weeks.[104,105] Both groups reported successful closure with low complication rates. Finally, the component separation technique has also been described in giant omphalocele closure. In 10 children with giant omphaloceles and a median age of 6.5 months, component separation was performed by incising the external oblique aponeurosis.[106] Unlike the previous techniques, closure was performed after a period of non-operative therapy until complete re-epithelialization of the omphalocele. Complications in three patients included central line sepsis, midline skin necrosis, and hematoma.

Fascial substitution can be accomplished using prosthetic or bioprosthetic materials. The early reports of prosthetic implantation included a Teflon sheet attached to the peritoneum and a Marlex sheet to the anterior rectus sheath as a secondary procedure.[107] Bioprosthetic materials such as pericardial patches[108] and Alloderm have also been described in case reports.[109] The authors' practice has used either Strattice bioprosthetic mesh or a silicone mesh to allow a staged closure. Secondary procedures after abdominal closure are frequently required. In omphalocele patients, umbilicoplasty is performed either in an immediate or delayed fashion.[110,111] Bladder and cloacal exstrophy is often associated with omphalocele. The reconstruction of the urogenital system is addressed in Chapter 43.

In gastroschisis, the lack of amniotic sac covering results in the exposure of a large surface area to the external environment immediately following birth. This can lead to rapid insensible fluid losses and hypothermia, and adequate fluid resuscitation along with early physiologic coverage is crucial to survival of the neonate. Complications from the defect or subsequent closure include pneumonia, bowel obstruction, ileus, sepsis, and necrotizing enterocolitis.

The bowel should be examined for other pathology including atresia, necrosis, or perforation, and the baby examined for other associated anomalies. Tight defects of the abdominal wall may require urgent enlargement, while volvulus may necessitate urgent reduction. In the absence of these findings, the decision must be made whether to attempt immediate reduction and repair, or to perform staged (silo) closure.[112] Primary repair is preferred whenever feasible; however, a number of key variables may potentially prevent this, including: the size of the defect; the degree of abdominovisceral disproportion; the condition of the bowel; extreme prematurity; severe pulmonary disease; and associated conditions or anomalies.

The risk of primary reduction and closure is related to the inevitable increase in intra-abdominal pressure resulting from returning the viscera to the abdomen, which in turn may lead to respiratory compromise, renal insufficiency, and abdominal compartment syndrome.[113] As the degree of abdominovisceral disproportion increases, these risks also rise accordingly. Similarly, in extremely premature infants or infants with severe pulmonary disease, the pulmonary status may be quite tenuous and pulmonary function may be compromised more easily and/or more severely. In these cases, it is often more prudent to undertake staged closure. Several studies have compared the outcomes of primary closure versus silo closure for gastroschisis, looking at overall complication rates, time on the ventilator, time to full feeds, and length of hospital stay. While the results of these studies can be difficult to interpret due to inherent selection bias, it has been shown that with judicious patient selection, the outcomes can be equivalent.[114,115]

Whether closing a giant omphalocele or a large gastroschisis defect, there are risks associated with the acute change in intra-abdominal pressures during closure. There are a few of ways to measure and monitor these changes. A urinary catheter should be placed to periodically measure bladder pressures. Bladder pressure and peak airway pressures are proxies for determining intra-abdominal pressure, and significant elevation of this value following reduction of the viscera may portend the severe complications listed above.

Bladder pressures >10 mmHg are considered elevated in children,[116] and some authors advocate a strict cut-off value of 20 mmHg in deciding whether to proceed with repair. In contrast to bladder pressures indicating intra-abdominal hypertension and acute abdominal compartment syndrome, there are no absolute values for peak airway pressures, which may vary significantly between patients, dependent on age and pre-existing pulmonary comorbidity. As such, relative changes in peak airway pressures are used as a proxy for increased intra-abdominal pressure and the ability to extubate the patient following surgery. Trending the changes in bladder pressure and airway pressures should be continued into the immediate postoperative period.[117]

Near-infrared spectrometry (NIRS) is an additional non-invasive modality that reliably reflects visceral tissue oxygenation and perfusion in neonates <10 kg. Its reliability and usefulness in larger babies, however, is controversial.[118] Our preliminary experience with NIRS in the neonatal ICU setting has been quite promising and we advocate its use in neonates with abdominal fascial defects where bowel vascular supply is at risk.

Posterior defects

Embryology

The neuroectoderm begins as a single sheet of cells. At 4 weeks' gestation, the same time the body wall develops from the lateral plate mesoderm, neural plates emerge and migrate towards each other to form the neural tube.[119] Fusion occurs in an anterior to posterior direction and in a cephalad to caudad manner. Failure of anterior closure results in diastematomyelia and anterior meningocele. Failure of posterior closure results in the spina bifida spectrum.[120]

Spina bifida

Spina bifida is classified into three major groups. Spina bifida aperta is an open myelocele with no covering over the neural elements. Neurologic loss is present at birth. Spina bifida cystica encompasses meningoceles, meningomyeloceles, and syringomyeloceles. Meningoceles account for 14% of neural tube defects and usually occur in the lumbar spine. Meningoceles are defined by the herniation of meninges without cord elements. Meningomyeloceles occur at the conus medullaris and are characterized by a herniation of the meninges with spinal cord through the vertebrae. Meningomyelocele is the most common neural tube defect, accounting for 85% of all neural tube defects with a worldwide prevalence of 0.17–6.39 per 1000 live births.[121] It is frequently associated with motor and sensory deficits. Syringomyeloceles refer to a meningocele with a dilated central canal. Spina bifida occulta is the most benign neural tube defect with minimal clinical significance. Patients frequently present with dermal sinuses, a posterior hair patch, or lipoma but do not usually have neurologic symptoms.

Clinical presentation and evaluation

Patients with spina bifida cystica are frequently diagnosed with prenatal ultrasound and upon birth. Exposed cord in spina bifida cystica have a thin membranous meninges sac and need to be prevented from desiccation with moist dressings to preserve neurologic function.

Evaluation of the neonate should begin with consultation by the neurosurgeon and the reconstructive surgeon for coverage of cord elements. Frequently, neural tube defects are accompanied by other defects such as limb deformities and neuropathic bladder requiring consultations to orthopedics and urology, respectively.

Surgical indications

Prior to the 1960s, meningomyelocele patients bore a mortality rate of approximately 65–75% within the first 6 months of life with rare survival to 6 years of age.[122,123] Since that time, early closure has been recognized to be essential to prevention of infection and is now considered standard of care. Successful closure within 24–48 h of life has resulted in survival to approximately 85% at 3 months, 60–70% at 1 year, and 40–50% at 3 years.[124] Despite advances, patients continue to suffer from significant morbidity due to coexisting conditions such as hydrocephalus and or tethered cord. On the other hand, meningoceles with adequate skin coverage can be deferred until 3 months of age. Bony defects in spina bifida are generally not addressed.

Treatment

As mentioned above, early physiologic closure of exposed spinal elements is essential. The primary goals are to protect cord elements, avoid infection, and seal any cerebrospinal fluid (CSF) leak. Soft tissue closure over the dural repair, whether with muscle, skin grafts, or skin flaps, is important to maintain the integrity of the dural repair.

Historically, primary skin closure of meningomyeloceles accounted for approximately 75% of all repairs.[125] The remaining 25% of large meningomyelocele defects required other means of reconstruction (Table 40.1). Sizable defects up to 20 cm^2 have been accomplished with modest skin undermining. De Brito Henriques, et al. described obtaining primary closure in 15 of 16 patients with defects up to 64 cm^2 using acute intraoperative tissue expansion with an intermittent skin traction technique.[150] The disadvantage in this approach was the increase in operative time necessary to perform the intraoperative slow traction technique.

Variations of random pattern skin flaps and fasciocutaneous flaps have been described by a number of investigators to prevent the skin-edge necrosis common to primary closure. Adjacent tissue rearrangements including rotation, transposition, advancement, Z-plasty, and Limberg flaps have all been described using dermal vascular supply. Cruz and colleagues described a creative double-Z rhomboid skin flap, in which margins of skin were excised in the form of a rhombus with adjacent angles of 60° and 120°. Two sets of 60° equilateral Z-plasty flaps were drawn on opposite sides of defect by extending incisions from the 120° angles and transposed into the defect.[127] Despite the success of this report, local tissue rearrangements relying on random pattern blood supply are generally not reliable for large defects. The amount of skin and subcutaneous tissue required for coverage is usually not well perfused without defined perforator or axial vascular supply thus resulting in frequent wound breakdown.

Although random pattern skin flaps are usually not reliable for large defects, the development of such flaps contributed to the design of geometric pattern fasciocutaneous,

Table 40.1 Meningomyelocele repairs

Type	Method	No. patients (n=74)	Timing	Defect size (avg. or range)	Complications	Ref.
Skin flap, muscle flap, skin graft	Skin flaps, reverse and advancement latissimus, STSG	Skin flap (n=37) Lat flap (n=5) STSG (n=32)	Acute	Primary: 22.7 cm² STSG: 37.3 cm²	Primary: 41% flap necrosis, 13.5% CSF leak, 10.8% sepsis, 2.7% death STSG: 6.3% partial graft loss, 6.3% CSF leak, 3.1% sepsis, no deaths	126
Skin flap	Double-Z rhomboid	10	Acute	4–23 cm²	Partial flap necrosis in one patient, CSF leak in one patient	127
Fasciocutaneous	Modified bipedicled V-Y	11	Acute	7–40 cm²	None	128
Fasciocutaneous	Bilateral rotation advancement	5	Acute	30–80 cm²	None	129
Fasciocutaneous	Bilateral rotation advancement	9	5 acute, 4 delayed	24–48 cm²	Skin necrosis in one patient	130
Fasciocutaneous	Triangular unequal Z-plasty	5	Acute and delayed	54–102 cm²	Hematoma in one patient	131
Fasciocutaneous	Bilobed	20	Acute	38.4 cm²	Partial flap loss with CSF leak in one patient	132
Fasciocutaneous	Bilobed	5	Acute	12.25–36 cm²	None	133
Fasciocutaneous	Z-advancement rotation, bilateral	11	10 acute, 1 delayed	45–114 cm²	None	101
Fasciocutaneous	Rhomboid	1	Acute	42 cm²	None	134
Fasciocutaneous	Modified Limberg flap	4	Acute	16–68 cm²	Wound breakdown in one patient	135
Fasciocutaneous	Bipedicled flap	12	Acute	6–7 cm (width)	None	136
Musculocutaneous	Reverse latissimus island, unilateral	12	7 acute, 5 salvage	Unknown	Two patients with minor wound breakdown at medial aspect of donor site	120
Musculocutaneous	Latissimus transposition, STSG to secondary defect	2	Delayed	Unknown	None	137
Musculocutaneous	Proximally-based latissimus island, bilateral	20	Delayed	6±1.2 cm²	None	138
Musculocutaneous	Unilateral and bilateral latissimus (bipedicled, proximal, and reverse flow)	23	Acute	35–74.16 cm²	Wound dehiscence in two patients, distal flap necrosis in two patients	139
Musculocutaneous	Rhomboid latissimus transposition	30	Acute	Max: 60 cm²	Unknown	140
Muscle and musculocutaneous	Latissimus, gluteus with STSG	8	Acute	97.9 cm²	CSF leak until VP shunting in all cases	141
Musculocutaneous	Latissimus, V-Y advancement	1	Acute	117 cm²	None	142

Continued

Table 40.1 Meningomyelocele repairs—cont'd

Type	Method	No. patients (n=74)	Timing	Defect size (avg. or range)	Complications	Ref.
Muscle	Reverse latissimus, unilateral with STSG over muscle	1	Acute primary repair, salvage	Unknown	None on salvage	143
Musculocutaneous	SGAP	6	Acute	32.64 cm^2	Venous congestion common, epidermolysis in one patient	144
Musculocutaneous	Bilateral latissimus with gluteal fascia, relaxing incisions	19	Most acute, some delayed	20–50 cm^2	None	145
Musculocutaneous	Latissimus and/or trapezius	82	Acute	Unknown	None	146
Musculocutaneous	Bilateral interconnected latissimus and gluteus maximus	9	Acute	42–80 cm^2	None	147
Osteomusculocutaneous	Paraspinous muscle/bifid spine turnover±STSG	Unknown	Acute	Unknown	Unknown	148
Osteomusculocutaneous	Latissimus, trapezius	6	Acute and salvage	Unknown	None	149

SGAP, superior gluteal artery perforator; STSG, split thickness skin graft.

musculocutaneous, and perforator based-flaps providing a more reliable tension-free skin closure techniques (Figs. 40.20 & 40.21).

Doppler confirmation of perforators in the base of these flaps has been helpful in intraoperative planning. Three vascular perforator territories were identified by Iacobucci during the description of bilateral superior and inferior fasciocutaneous transposition flaps.[151] Superolaterally, parascapular and scapular fascial branches of the circumflex scapular artery represent the dominant blood supply to the superior transposition flap. The vascular pattern of the middle-third of the area originates from muscular perforators and lateral cutaneous branches of the costal groove segment of the lower intercostals arteries. The inferior flap receives contributions from the superficial circumflex iliac artery perforators. Permutations of this flap include the fasciocutaneous Z advancement rotation (ZAR) flap and a bilateral rotational transposition flap with curvilinear incisions.[130,134] Both of these flaps are robust flaps based on the preservation of the thoraco-lumbar fascia and the perforating vessels. The curvilinear advancement rotation flap has the added advantage of moving skin incisions such that they do not overlie the dural repair incision line.

One of the most common fasciocutaneous transposition techniques utilizes V-Y advancement from the flanks. Several modifications of this technique have been reported such as placing the apical extensions of the V incisions such that they are supplied by paraspinous perforators, preserving skin bridges at the superior and inferior aspects of the bilateral flaps[129,152,153] and the design of crescentic-shaped flaps in our practice.[154]

Several other fasciocutaneous flap designs reported in smaller numbers of studies include the large bilobed transposition, the rhomboid perforator, and the unequal Z-plasty.[128,132,133,155] Both the bilobed and the rhomboid flaps are elevated in the classical manner with careful attention to the incorporation of perforating vessels. Mutaf's unequal Z-plasty, however, has unique geometric criteria.[131] The advantage of this flap design is that after transposition, the skin incisions are not overlying the dural repair but the excision of skin in the conversion to a triangular defect and the rather complicated design limits its utility.

The unilateral island SGAP flap was described by Duffy for smaller defects averaging 4.8 × 6.8 cm^2.[144] Despite preservation of the perforator pedicle with a cuff of muscle, flaps in this were commonly plagued with venous congestion.

Though bony reconstruction is not thought to be required for meningomyelocele repairs, Mustarde proposed an innovative method of reconstructing a bony spinal canal under turnover paraspinal muscle flaps (Fig. 40.22).[148] Following closure of the dura, the paraspinal muscles are incised and transverse processes are osteotomized. The paraspinal muscles are brought together in the midline and covered with a split thickness skin graft.

Mustarde's paraspinous muscle advancement and turnover flaps have been found to be useful to others in providing a well-vascularized layer above the closed neural placode.[156] Skin closure can then be performed by skin graft, direct closure, or a variety of flaps. The particular advantage of paraspinous muscle flap closure is that it protects the dural repair should there be any overlying skin breakdown.

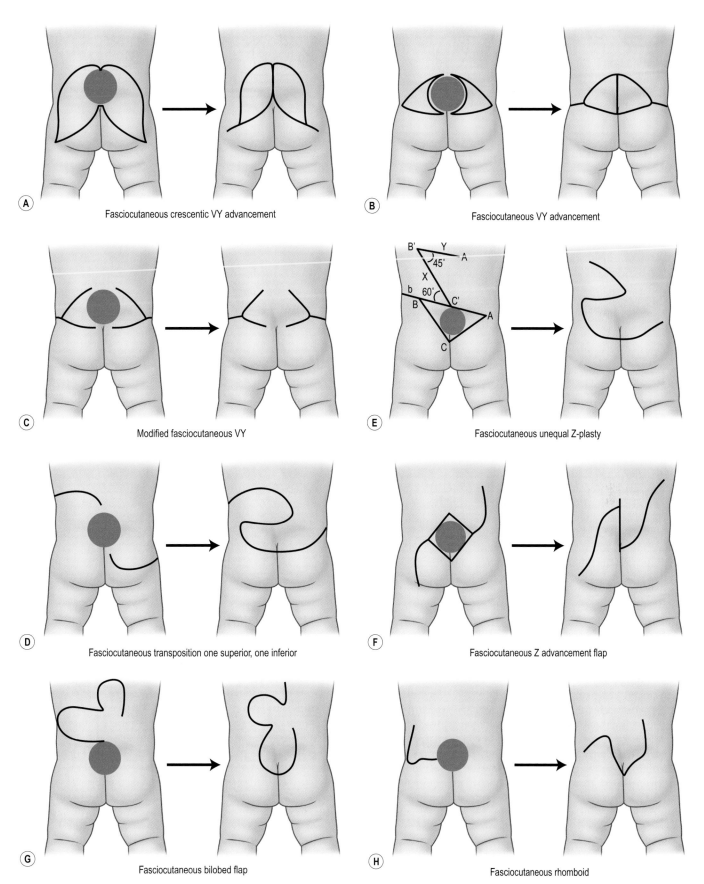

Fig. 40.20 Fasciocutaneous flaps in meningomyelocele repair. **(A)** Bilateral crescentic V-Y advancement. **(B)** Classic bilateral V-Y advancement. **(C)** Modified bipedicle V-Y advancement. **(D)** Superior and inferior rotational transposition. **(E)** Unequal Z-plasty. **(F)** Z advancement. **(G)** Bilobed transposition. **(H)** Rhomboid transposition.

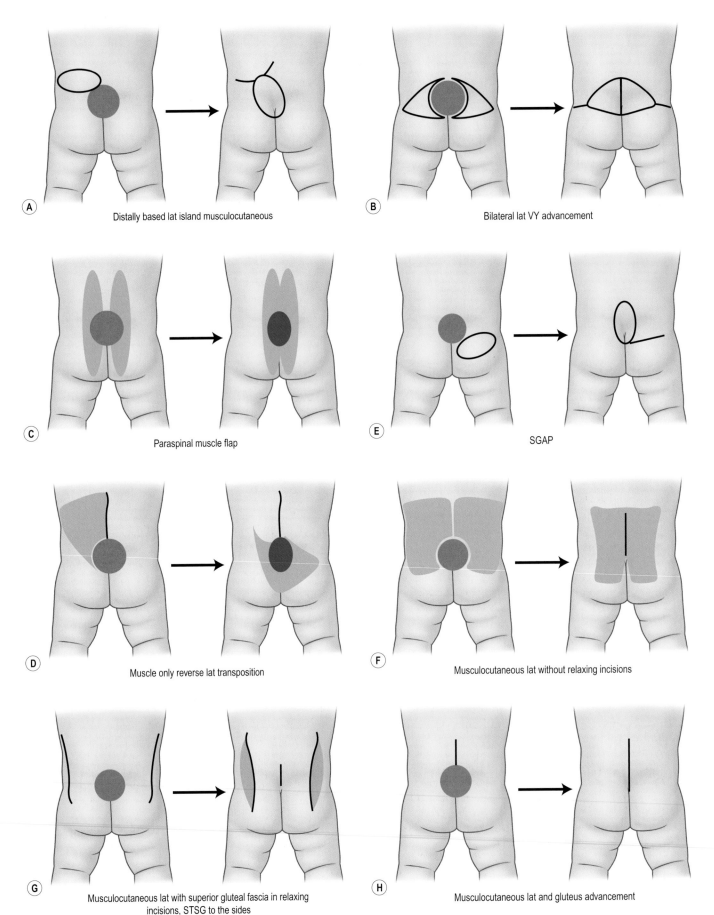

Fig. 40.21 Muscle and musculocutaneous flaps in meningomyelocele repair. **(A)** Distally-based latissimus (lat) musculocutaneous advancement. **(B)** Bilateral latissimus V-Y musculocutaneous advancement. **(C)** Paraspinous muscle advancement or turnover. **(D)** Distally-based latissimus (lat) turnover muscle flap with split thickness skin graft coverage over flap. **(E)** Superior gluteal artery perforator (SGAP) interposition. **(F)** Bilateral latissimus (lat) musculocutaneous advancement. **(G)** Bilateral latissimus (lat) musculocutaneous advancement with lateral relaxing incisions covered with split thickness skin grafts (STSG). **(H)** Bilateral latissimus (lat) and gluteus maximus interconnected musculocutaneous advancement.

The labels within the figure are:

(A) Distally based lat island musculocutaneous

(B) Bilateral lat VY advancement

(C) Paraspinal muscle flap

(D) Muscle only reverse lat transposition

(E) SGAP

(F) Musculocutaneous lat without relaxing incisions

(G) Musculocutaneous lat with superior gluteal fascia in relaxing incisions, STSG to the sides

(H) Musculocutaneous lat and gluteus advancement

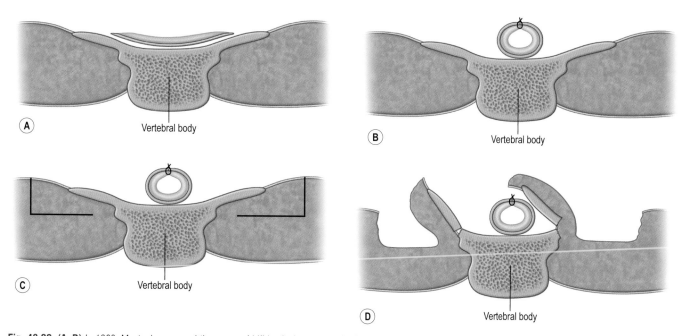

Fig. 40.22 (A–D) In 1968, Mustarde proposed the usage of bifid spinal processes in the reconstruction of the spinal canal. He argued that the skin cover alone was insufficient as a means to protect the spinal cord. Following dural closure, the paraspinal muscles are incised laterally. The spinal processes are osteotomized and the paraspinal muscle flaps with the associated spinal processes are combined into turnover flaps.

Muscle and musculocutaneous flaps frequently involve usage of the latissimus dorsi muscle. Unilateral proximally-based latissimus flaps are most useful for higher lesions, whereas reverse and island flaps can reach low lumbosacral defects.[120,138,143,156] However, many of these defects require bilateral muscle flaps,[157] as recognized first by Desprez and colleagues.[149] The authors documented six children, ranging from neonates to 2 years of age, with large meningomyeloceles that were closed with bilateral bipedicled advancement of the latissimus dorsi and trapezius muscles through lateral skin incisions. The muscles were transected laterally and advanced medially. Bifid spinous processes were osteotomized similar to Mustarde's technique of reconstructing the spinal canal. The lateral incisions were closed with V-Y advancement flaps. Moore and colleagues modified this technique with relaxing incisions along the lateral border of the latissimus in the posterior axillary line.[145] Dissection is carried out under the latissimus muscle with elevation of the thoraco-lumbar fascia in continuity with the superficial gluteal fascia. Intercostal and lumbosacral perforators are divided medially. The paraspinous fascia is incorporated to provide additional strength to the deep layer of the closure. While the authors reported no complications from this series, the maximum defect they closed was 50 cm². The need for skin grafts in the relaxing incisions added scarring to the patient, making this technique less desirable. In contrast, McCraw and colleagues reported 82 patients who received a similar bilateral latissimus dorsi and trapezius musculocutaneous advancement flaps without the need for relaxing incisions.[146,158]

A more extensive version of the bilateral latissimus musculocutaneous advancement was proposed by Ramirez and colleagues.[147] In nine neonates with large thoraco-lumbar meningomyeloceles, the authors elevated the thoraco-lumbar fascia over the paraspinous muscles to the lateral border of the latissimus with perforator obliteration. The gluteus maximus is then de-originated from the iliac crest and sacrum and dissected free from the gluteus medius. The entire unit comprised of latissimus dorsi connected to gluteus maximus is then advanced bilaterally without relaxing incisions and closed in the midline.

Skin grafting over dural closures was popularized by Luce and Walsh.[126] The authors retrospectively reviewed their experience of 74 neonates that included management by primary closure (n=37), latissimus muscle flaps (n=5), and split thickness skin grafts (n=32). The population of patients treated with wide skin flap undermining displayed significant wound healing complications resulting in higher rates of CSF leak, sepsis, and deaths. Despite success with latissimus flaps, the concern for blood loss led these authors to prefer closure with split-thickness skin grafts (either temporary xenograft or immediate autologous skin grafts). They noted that conversion to grafting decreased all immediate complications seen with primary closure and did not cause large volume blood loss. Skin grafting, therefore, offers a simple way to obtain rapid coverage of dural repairs; however, it lacks adequate soft tissue to protect the repair from trauma. In long-term follow-up, lumbosacral skin grafts did not have an increase in skin ulceration, but thoraco-lumbar and thoracic patients covered with split thickness skin grafts not only had an increased incidence of skin ulceration but also had an increased incidence of developing a gibbus deformity when compared with primary skin closure techniques.[159] The etiology of the gibbus deformity and the association with skin graft reconstruction of thoraco-lumbar and thoracic meningomyeloceles are not clear. Considering the results of this long-term follow-up study, skin grafts should only be used in the thoraco-lumbar and thoracic regions as a temporizing measure for immediate neonatal closure. Mustoe et al. reported the use of tissue expansion and delayed primary closure in older children who had poor quality skin coverage over their spinal defects.[160]

Preferred methods

Meningomyeloceles display heterogeneity, therefore necessitating the need for a varied armamentarium of reconstructive options individualized to each patient, with the goal of providing reliable closure using well-vascularized tissue without tension (Fig. 40.23). While many of the studies mentioned above refer to measurements, the size of defects is less important than the relative amount of the uninvolved surrounding back skin (Fig. 40.24).[154]

The primary goals are to protect cord elements, avoid infection, and seal any CSF leak. With that, surgery within the first 24 h of life is routinely performed by a multidisciplinary team of neurosurgeons and plastic surgeons. After closure

of the spinal placode by the neurosurgeon (Fig. 40.25), the plastic surgery team provides a multilayer, tension free, well-vascularized definitive closure. The first layer above the neural closure is paraspinous turnover flaps to help seal and protect the neural repair (Fig. 40.26). Perforator-based crescent-shaped V-Y advancement/rotation flaps are then performed to provide well vascularized tissue. This flap is designed so that the tail of the Y is oriented to where there is most skin laxity laterally. Its goal is to minimize skin tension in the midline. With a paucity of skin lateral to the defect, the crescent design of the V-Y allows for recruitment of tissue from the lateral buttock and thigh area. Flaps used to close lumbar-sacral defects are based on gluteal perforators advancing and rotating the skin from inferior-lateral to midline (Fig. 40.27). Flaps used to close thoraco-lumbar defects are usually based on the paraspinal or latissimus perforators rotating the skin (with or without muscle) from

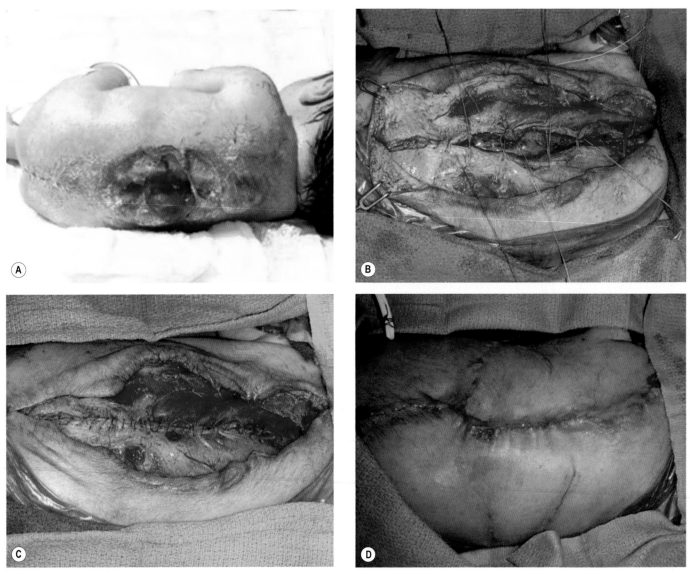

Fig. 40.23 Thoracolumbar meningomyelocele involving most of the back. **(A)** Note the fine membrane covering most of the defect. **(B,C)** After neural tube repair and reinforcement with paraspinous muscles, gluteus, latissimus, and trapezius muscles advanced to midline with minimal undermining. **(D)** V-Y relaxing incision through skin and subcutaneous tissue to allow for tension-free midline closure.

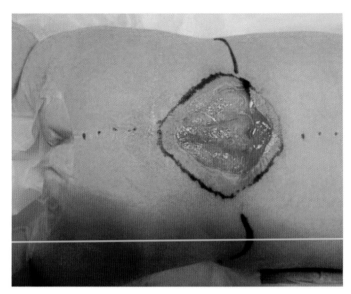

Fig. 40.24 Lumbosacral meningomyelocele. Not enough skin lateral to the defect to allow for primary closure without tension. The location of the iliac crests are marked, as is the midline (dotted line) and edge of the compromised skin.

superior-lateral to midline, similar to the case report described by Sarifakioglu *et al.*[157]

Sacrococcygeal teratoma

Sacrococcygeal teratomas are the most common congenital tumors in the posterior trunk with an incidence of 1 in 40000 live births with a female predominance.[161] Teratomas are thought to originate from embryonic cell material derived from totipotent cells, thus organ parts are frequently found with elements or various different tissue types. Most sacrococcygeal teratomas are benign and consist of well differentiated mature tissues. They uniformly can undergo malignant transformation with increasing age and therefore usually removed shortly after birth. When the tumors are excised during the

neonatal period, the patients tend to recover well with rare incidence of malignancy and recurrence. Malignant tumors require adjuvant chemotherapy.

Clinical presentation and surgical indications

Patients are usually identified at birth with a midline round, cystic, or solid mass attached at the sacrum or coccyx. Teratomas grow in the posterior and inferior direction with stretching of the muscles surrounding the tumor. Large tumors may cause difficulty in delivery. There is occasional intra-abdominal extension. Dr. Altman and colleagues developed a classification system based upon anatomic location of the teratoma. Type I (46.7%) is predominantly external with minimal extension in the presacral region; Type II (34.7%) is also predominantly external, but has a significant intrapelvic component; Type III (8.8%) is primarily a pelvic and abdominal mass, but also has a smaller external component; finally, Type IV (9.8%) consists of a presacral mass without any external portions visible.[162] Teratomas can usually be detected by elevated maternal AFP levels and routine prenatal ultrasound. Types I–III are readily classified on prenatal ultrasound. It is common to also find polyhydramnios on the prenatal ultrasound.

Treatment

Resection is usually performed shortly after birth when the neonate is deemed medically stable to undergo surgery. The

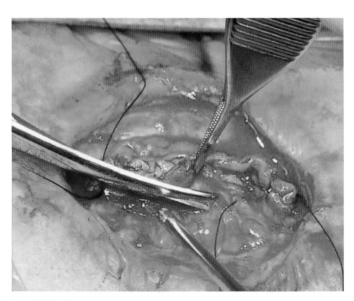

Fig. 40.25 Meningomyelocele. Neurosurgeons preparing to close the neural elements prior to any soft-tissue closure.

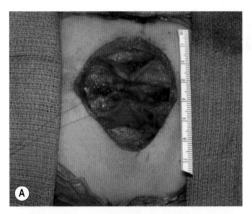

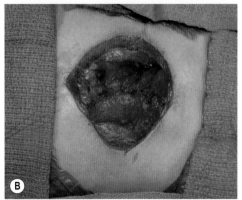

Fig. 40.26 Paraspinal muscle flaps. **(A)** Lateral edge of paraspinous muscles are incised and advanced to ward midline. **(B)** Paraspinous muscle flap closure completed providing a well vascularized layer to protect the spinal closure beneath it.

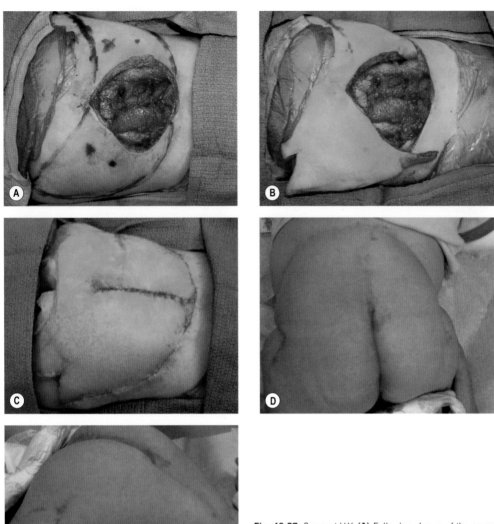

Fig. 40.27 Crescent V-Y. **(A)** Following closure of the paraspinal muscle flaps, the skin defect is addressed. With a paucity of skin lateral to the defect, the crescent design of the V-Y allows for recruitment of tissue from the lateral buttock and thigh area. An intraoperative hand held Doppler helps identify perforating vessels and facilitate flap planning and elevation. **(B)** The superior limbs of the fasciocutaneous crescent V-Y advancement flaps with V-Y back-cuts are incised and the flap is isolated on its main perforators. The inferior limbs are only completed (to islandize a true V-Y flap) if needed to release tension. **(C)** Skin closure accomplished without tension in the midline. V-Y back-cut converted to a Z to facilitate insetting of the lateral tip of the flap. **(D,E)** Incisions at 3 months postoperatively.

resulting defect usually can be closed primarily via a chevron incision with local tissue rearrangement. One case report of a giant sacrococcygeal teratoma resection with a resulting skin defect has required advancement of gluteal musculocutaneous flaps for closure.[163]

Other posterior malformations

Dermal sinus and postanal pits are congenital back lesions that rarely require extensive reconstruction.[164] Dermal sinuses are found in the midline back between the occiput and the sacrum and are sometimes associated with an angioma. Infection of the sinus tract can result in recurrent meningitis.

Postanal pits occur over the coccyx and appear to tract similar to pilonidal cysts. Asymptomatic pits pose no danger and can be observed. When infected, postanal pit resection usually only requires primary closure.

Neonates with tethered cord frequently present with a tuft of hair or an angiomatous lesion at the site of tethering. Neurosurgical repair is important for prevention of future neurologic dysfunction. Skin is virtually always primarily closed.

Diastematomyelia presents similarly to tethered cord.[165] The spinal cord is divided with a median septum and patients tend to have focal neurologic deficits. Prognosis is excellent for such patients and primary closure is routine.

Access the complete reference list online at **http://www.expertconsult.com**

1. Netscher DT, Peterson R. Normal and abnormal development of the extremities and trunk. *Clin Plast Surg*. 1990;17:13–21.

2. Sadler TW, Feldkamp ML. The embryology of body wall closure: relevance to gastroschisis and other ventral body wall defects. *Am J Med Genet C Semin Med Genet*. 2008;148C:180–185.

3. Kelly RE Jr, Shamberger RC, Mellins R, et al. Prospective multicenter study of surgical correction of pectus excavatum: Design, perioperative complications, pain, and baseline pulmonary function facilitated by internet-based data collection. *J Am Coll Surg*. 2007;205:205–216.

4. Creswick HA, Stacey MW, Kelly RE Jr, et al. Family study of the inheritance of pectus excavatum. *J Pediatr Surg*. 2006;41:1699–1703.

5. Ravitch MM. The operative treatment of pectus excavatum. *Ann Surg*. 1949;129:429–444.

6. Ravitch MM. New trends in pediatric surgery; pectus excavatum, esophageal atresia, intussusception, Hirschsprung's disease. *Surg Clin North Am*. 1949;29:1535–1550.

7. Garcia VF, Seyfer AE, Graeber GM. Reconstruction of congenital chest-wall deformities. *Surg Clin North Am*. 1989;69:1103–1118.

8. Haller JA Jr, Kramer SS, Lietman SA. Use of CT scans in selection of patients for pectus excavatum surgery: a preliminary report. *J Pediatr Surg*. 1987;22:904–906.

9. Fonkalsrud EW, DeUgarte D, Choi E. Repair of pectus excavatum and carinatum deformities in 116 adults. *Ann Surg*. 2002;236:304–314.

10. Beiser GD, Epstein SE, Stampfer M, et al. Impairment of cardiac function in patients with pectus excavatum, with improvement after operative correction. *N Engl J Med*. 1972;287:267–272.

41

Pediatric tumors

Sahil Kapur and Michael Bentz

SYNOPSIS

Neurofibromatosis
- Neurofibromatoses are a group of inherited disorders with established diagnostic criteria based on symptoms of presentation.
- Craniofacial presentation of this disease is classified based on the surgical treatment options available.

Juvenile aggressive fibromatosis
- Fibroblastic or myofibroblastic neoplasms are locally aggressive lesions.
- Different presentations include:
  - Fibromatosis colli
  - Congenital solitary or generalized fibromatosis
  - Infantile digital fibroma
  - Gingival fibromatosis
  - Juvenile nasopharyngeal angiofibroma.

Dermoids
- They are present from birth and consist of both ectoderm and endoderm.
- They commonly arise in the head and neck. They can grow large to compress adjacent structures.
- Different types include: nasal dermoids, intradural dermoids, extra-angular dermoids and dermoid cysts of the neck.

Branchial cleft anomalies
- Each branchial arch, pouch, and groove complex forms a particular area of the head and neck.
- The 1st and 2nd branchial cleft anomalies comprise 98% of all such anomalies. The 3rd and 4th brachial cleft anomalies form the other 2%. Definitive treatment involves surgical excision.

Thyroglossal duct cysts
- A persistent embryological remnant of the descending thyroglossal duct gives rise to a cyst.
- This clinically presents in the first two decades of life.
- Treatment involves excision using the Sistrunk technique.

Pilomatrixoma
- These are ectodermal in origin and arise from the outer root sheath cells of the hair follicle.
- These tumors usually occur in the head and neck region of children.
- Treatment is surgical excision, with radiation therapy for malignant lesions.

Rhabdomyosarcoma
- This is a malignant tumor of mesenchymal origin.
- In the head and neck, the most common presentations are in the orbit, nasopharynx, paranasal sinuses, and middle ear.
- Four histologic types include embryonal, spindle-cell alveolar, and pleomorphic rhabdomyosarcoma.

Synovial soft-tissue sarcoma
- These sarcomas arise from synovioblastic differentiation of pluripotent mesenchymal stem cells.

Alveolar soft part sarcoma
- A rare tumor that occurs primarily in skeletal muscles or musculofascial planes of extremities.

Lymphadenopathy
- Acute bacterial lymphadenitis presents with mild fever, tender, indurated, and erythematous lymph nodes, or systemic toxicity.
- Chronic regional lymphadenopathy is observed in diseases such as cat scratch disease.
- Cervical tuberculous adenitis (Scrofula) begins with a pulmonary infection that spreads to the lymph nodes.

Neurofibromatosis

Introduction

Neurofibromatoses are a set of inherited disorders comprising neurofibromatosis-1 (NF-1), neurofibromatosis-2 (NF-2), and

Schwannomatosis. All of these lead to the formation of benign nerve sheath tumors.[1]

Basic science/disease process

Neurofibromatosis-1 is an autosomal dominant disorder with complete penetrance and variable expression. Chromosome 17 is involved. The incidence is 1/3000, and the average age of children at the time of presentation is 7 years.[1–3]

Café-au-lait spots

Diagnosis/patient presentation

Café-au-lait spots are characterized as cutaneous, hyperpigmented lesions, typically 20–30 mm in diameter. They contain keratinocytes with increased macromelanosomes. Greater than six lesions are found in 90–99% of cases.[4,5]

Treatment/surgical technique

Surgery is rarely recommended. Laser treatment can be considered for cosmetic improvement.[6,7]

Lisch nodules

Diagnosis/patient presentation

Lisch nodules are dome-shaped, melanocytic hamartomas found on the surface of the iris.[4,5] They appear around age 10 years and are present in nearly all people with NF-1 by age 20.

Treatment/surgical technique

No treatment is required.

Optic nerve gliomas

Diagnosis/patient presentation

Optic nerve gliomas are the most common central nervous system tumors in NF-1 patients. They occur in 15% of cases and are histologically identified as low-grade pilocytic astrocytomas.[4,5,8] They are relatively indolent and sometimes asymptomatic. If symptomatic, they can cause proptosis, squint, abnormal color vision, visual field loss, pupillary abnormalities, and hypothalamic dysfunction.[7]

Treatment/surgical technique

Treatment involves vincristine and cisplatinum.[9] Surgery is necessary if proptosis is present and if there is a need to debulk extensive chiasmal gliomas.

Glomus tumors

Diagnosis/patient presentation

Glomus tumors are usually solitary lesions, but occur in multiples in individuals with NF-1. They present under fingernails with symptoms of cold sensitivity and increased localized tenderness.[10]

Treatment/surgical technique

Treatment is local excision.

Craniofacial manifestation

Diagnosis/patient presentation

In the craniofacial region, the orbitotemporal area is most commonly involved. Orbitotemporal neurofibromatosis associated skeletal malformations and deformities include:[11–17]

- Sphenoid wing hypoplasia, which leads to expansion of the middle cranial fossa into the posterior orbit and causes proptosis
- Remodelling and/or decalcification of the posterior orbit
- Supraorbital tumors, which cause defects of the orbital roof and lead to a downward and outward displacement of the globe
- Thinning of the lateral and inferior orbital rims
- Depression of the orbital floor and elevation of the orbital roof and supraorbital rim, which increases orbital volume
- Dysplasia and downward dislocation of the zygoma
- Progressive plexiform neurofibromatosis of the temporal area, which leads to continued enlargement of the eyelids, excessive mechanical ptosis, pulsating proptosis, eye pain, and epiphora.

Treatment/surgical technique

Treatment is based on Jackson's Classification:[11,14]

Class 1: Significant soft tissue involvement with minimal bone involvement and normal vision. Treatment involves debulking of the soft-tissue component of the tumor through an anterior, lateral, or anterolateral orbitotomy. If blepharoptosis is present, levator resection is performed.[16] In cases where only a partial resection is carried out, a technique of netting the remaining tissue using Teflon mesh has been proposed (Fig. 41.1).[18]

Class 2: Soft tissue and bone involvement with normal vision. Treatment involves an intracranial approach for tumor debulking and posterior orbital wall reconstruction.[16] After the tumor is debulked, the herniated temporal lobe is reduced and bone grafts, obtained from splitting the contralateral frontal bone, are used to reconstruct the posterior and superior orbital walls. Orbital volume is increased with osteotomies and the globe is elevated by raising the canthal ligaments and building the floor. A two-stage approach has been suggested in which the intracranial portion of tumor debulking and orbital reconstruction is completed in stage one. A second-stage procedure is performed in which subcutaneous debulking, eyelid, face, and orbital reconstruction is completed (Fig. 41.2).[19]

Class 3: Soft-tissue and bone involvement with blindness or an absent globe. Treatment involves debulking the tumor with exenteration. An orbital approach is used to reduce the herniated temporal lobe into the middle cranial fossa. The bony defect is covered with a split-rib/bone graft. The orbital volume is reduced and its position is adjusted with

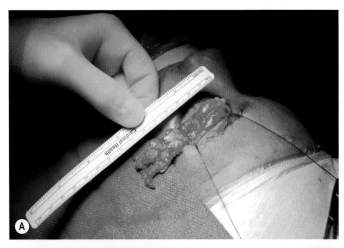

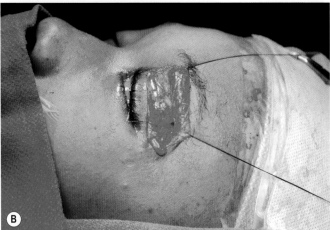

Fig. 41.1 (A,B) Anterior orbitotomy with debulking of left orbitotemporal neurofibromatosis. *(Courtesy of Dr. Delora L. Mount.)*

osteotomies and bone grafts. Finally, an orbital prosthesis is fitted.

Neurofibromas

Diagnosis/patient presentation

Nerve sheath tumors arise between the dorsal root ganglion and terminal nerve branches.[4,5,20] They are composed of schwann cells, fibroblasts, mast cells, and perineural cells.[7,20,21] Localized cutaneous neurofibromas are the most common nerve sheath tumors. They present as multiple slow growing, pedunculated lesions that progressively increase in prominence.[7] These lesions can be surgically excised for symptomatic benefit. This, however, may lead to hypertrophic scarring. The benefits of carbon dioxide laser treatment have not been clearly established. Diffuse cutaneous neurofibromas present as a plaque-like thickening of the dermis and subcutaneous tissue and are most frequently found in the head and neck region. These are non-destructive, soft, compressible lesions that grow along the fibrous septae in children and young adults. Removal of these subcutaneous lesions may lead to neurologic deficits in the region of the concerned nerve. Localized intraneural fibromas are the second most frequent

type of neurofibroma and represent fusiform enlargement of peripheral nerves. These are the most common neurofibromas of the upper extremity and account for 85% of cases.[22] Spinal and cranial nerves may also be involved. Massive soft-tissue neurofibromas (elephantiasis neurofibromatosa) lead to distortion of the face and require complete excision.[23] Plexiform neurofibromas are composed of nerve sheath cells proliferating along the length of the nerve and are associated with hypertrophy of the overlying soft tissue, hyperpigmentation, and hypertrichosis of the overlying skin. Plexiform neurofibromas occur in 16–40% of patients with NF. These lesions involve the trunk (43–44%), extremities (15–38%), and head and neck (18–42%).[20] They are congenital in origin and become evident by 2 years of age. Plexiform neurofibromas are locally destructive lesions that grow during periods of hormonal change, and may involve multiple nerve branches and plexi.[24]

Treatment/surgical technique

Preoperative contrast-enhanced CT, MRI, angiography, and embolization have been recommended.[20–22,25] The highly vascular nature of these lesions makes surgical removal complicated.[24] Multiple non-surgical management options such as farnesyl transferase inhibitors, antiangiogenesis drugs, and fibroblast inhibitors are being explored.[26] Since the mechanistic target of rapamycin (mTOR) pathways are a major mediator of tumor growth in NF-1, drugs such as sirolimus are demonstrating beneficial effects such as the halting of tumor progression and reduction of pain.[27] Recent studies have demonstrated the benefits of farnesyl transferase inhibitors such as Tipifarnib in reducing rate of tumor progression.[28] Tumors resected in children below the age of 10 years re-occur in 60% of the cases, while those resected above the age of 10 years re-occur in 30% of the cases.[29]

Malignant degeneration of peripheral nerve sheath tumors

Diagnosis/patient presentation

There is an 8–13% lifetime risk for these tumors to undergo malignant degeneration. This occurs predominantly between ages 20 and 35.[4,7] Medium and large nerves of the thigh, buttock, brachial plexus, and paraspinous areas are involved. Signs of malignant degeneration include increased pain, new neurologic deficits, sphincter disturbance, rapid increase in the size of the neurofibroma, or change in texture.[30] Fluorodeoxyglucose positron emission tomography helps with the quantification of glucose metabolism in the cells and can help distinguish between benign and malignant lesions.[31,32]

Treatment/surgical technique

Prompt surgical intervention is necessary, which consists of debulking and nerve grafting. Complete removal with tumor-free margins is necessary. Adjuvant radiotherapy for tumors >5 cm, high-grade lesions, or incompletely excised tumors is recommended.[7,30] Chemotherapeutic regimens consisting of tamoxifen and trifluoperazine are proving to be efficacious in halting progression of the tumor in rodent models.[33]

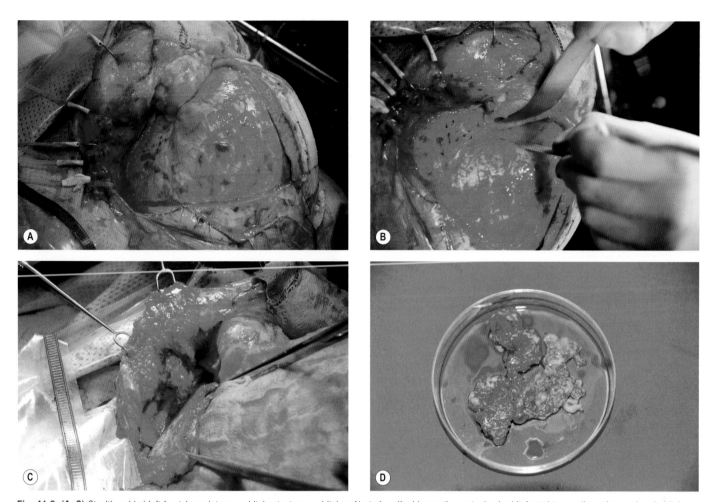

Fig. 41.2 (A–C) Stealth-guided left frontal craniotomy, orbital osteotomy, orbital roof/anterior clinoid resection, extradural orbitofrontal tumor dissection, and periorbital cranial reconstruction for craniofacial neurofibromatosis. **(D)** Specimen: neurofibroma lesion. *(Courtesy of Dr. Delora L. Mount.)*

Malignant schwannomas (neurofibrosarcomas)

Diagnosis/patient presentation

Neurofibrosarcomas can involve either the cervical vagus nerve or the sympathetic chain and present as parapharyngeal masses, with paresthesias, pain, and muscle weakness.[34] They may also be of parotid origin. Children with NF-1 are at increased risk for developing these lesions.[35]

Treatment/surgical technique

Surgery is the primary treatment modality. Adjuvant chemotherapy and radiation may be indicated. Local recurrence and lung metastases are common.[36,37]

Juvenile aggressive fibromatosis

Basic science/disease process

Fibroblastic or myofibroblastic neoplasms are locally aggressive lesions. The average age of onset is the third decade of life. These tumors, however, may also occur during the 1st month of life. About 5% of cases are found in the hand.[38]

Fibromatosis colli

Diagnosis/patient presentation

Fibromatosis colli are solitary tumors of the sternocleidomastoid muscles (SCM) and present as a cervical mass during infancy. They are the most common cause of neonatal torticollis. The tumors are first seen between 3 and 4 weeks of age. They develop in the lower portion of the SCM and may involve both sternal and clavicular heads of the muscle. The diagnosis is made through fine-needle aspiration that yields fibroblasts, degenerative atrophic skeletal muscle cells, and numerous giant muscle cells. Ultrasound can also be used as a non-invasive modality to facilitate diagnosis. Natural regression of the tumor is seen during the first 6 months of life. Torticollis is associated with fibromatosis colli in 23–33% of patients and may continue after treatment in 17% of patients because of progressive fibrous replacement of the muscle tissue.[39]

Treatment/surgical technique

Surgery involves releasing both heads of the SCM through a limited transverse incision. The clavicular head is readvanced and attached to the sternal head to lengthen the muscle and preserve the anatomic landmarks of the sternal column.

Surgery is performed on patients in whom torticollis persists for 1 year.[40]

Congenital fibromatosis

Diagnosis/patient presentation

Congenital fibromatosis can present in a solitary or generalized form. Solitary lesions can be seen as well-demarcated, firm, palpable masses (<3 mm) in skin, subcutaneous tissue, muscle, or as hyperlucent masses in bone. These lesions are usually present at birth, but additional lesions may develop later.

Treatment/surgical technique

Treatment is surgical resection. The rate of recurrence is about 32%.[41]

Infantile digital fibroma

Diagnosis/patient presentation

These generally appear as single or multiple gelatinous or firm nodules on fingers or toes. They are rare and are seen in both males and females. They are generally harmless but are removed because of the discomfort they cause by rubbing on footwear. The diagnosis can be confirmed with a skin biopsy that shows spindle-shaped cells and collagen fibers in the dermis. A radiograph is usually taken to determine the extent of the lesion (Fig. 41.3).

Treatment/surgical technique

Surgical procedure is relatively simple and calls for shaving off the lump. Recurrence rate after surgery is high.

Outcomes, prognosis, and complications

A conservative approach can also be undertaken because many fibromas can resorb and disappear by themselves over 2–3 years.

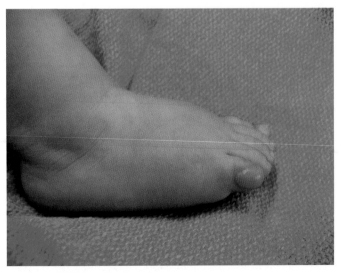

Fig. 41.3 Infantile digital fibroma. *(Courtesy of Dr. Michael L. Bentz.)*

Gingival fibroma

Diagnosis/patient presentation

Gingival fibromas are common lesions of the oral cavity caused by chronic irritation that leads to connective tissue hyperplasia. They occur on any oral mucosal surface, including the tongue, palate, cheek, and lip. The lesions are pale, smooth and firm, with sessile or pedunculated bases, and are usually <1 cm in diameter.

Treatment/surgical technique

Treatment is surgical excision. Recurrence is rare if the source of irritation is removed.

Juvenile nasopharyngeal angiofibroma

Diagnosis/patient presentation

Juvenile nasopharyngeal angiofibromas are benign, locally aggressive, vascular lesions, typically found in adolescent males between the ages of 10 and 17. They originate in the posterolateral nasopharynx, near the sphenopalatine foramen, and present with nasal obstruction and epistaxis. About 66% of patients present with local disease and 20% have intracranial invasion. CT scans show widening of the pterygopalatine fossa and the pterygomaxillary fissure. MRI is used to delineate the soft tissue invasion, while angiography helps determine the vascular supply. Given the highly vascular nature of these tumors, biopsy should not be attempted.

Treatment/surgical technique

Treatment involves embolization followed by surgery. A transpalatal, transfacial, midface degloving or LeFort I osteotomy approach can be used. An anterior subcranial approach is used for transcranial lesions.[42–44]

Endoscopic approaches are becoming more popular due to progresses made in instrumentation, skull base anatomy, and surgical strategy. A recently published systematic review comparing open and endoscopic treatment approaches found that endoscopic approaches are associated with lower blood loss and recurrence rates.[45,46]

Outcomes, prognosis, and complications

The recurrence rate is 73%, but can be as high as 90% with positive margins. Recurrence usually occurs within 3 months of excision.[38]

Dermoids

Introduction

Dermoids are present from birth, and form due to embryonic inclusion of germ cells between fusing tissue layers. They commonly arise in the head and neck.

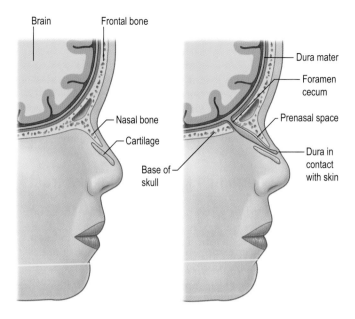

Brain   Frontal bone

Nasal bone
Cartilage
Base of
skull

Dura mater
Foramen
cecum
Prenasal space
Dura in
contact
with skin

Fig. 41.4 Dermoid embryology.

open rhinoplasty approach. This approach has been reported to have improved exposure of the osteotomies, the upper lateral cartilages, and the septum (Fig. 41.5).[50]

A closed rhinoplasty technique has been proposed for the excision of superficial distal nasal tip dermoids. Since the majority of nasal dermoid cysts are confined to the superficial nasal area, this technique can prove to be beneficial.[51] For lesions with suspected/confirmed intracranial extension, failure to completely excise the tract can lead to abscess formation, meningitis, or osteomyelitis.[52,53] Multiple approaches have been proposed.[54–67] The traditional approach calls for combining an intracranial procedure such as a bifrontal craniotomy, with an extracranial procedure, such as a transverse, vertical, inverted U, lateral rhinotomy, or rhinoplasty to address the entire sinus tract.[54,55]

A second approach, described as the "keystone" technique, involves a bifrontal craniotomy superior to the supraorbital rims, two paramedian sagittal osteotomies extending down the length of the nasal bones, followed by out-fracturing of the keystone component. This technique allows complete exposure of the sinus tract and enhanced exposure of the

Nasal dermoids

Basic science/disease process

Between the 3rd and 8th week of embryogenesis, when the neural groove deepens to form the neural tube, incomplete sequestration of the neuroectoderm from the somatic ectoderm leads to a persistent connection of the foramen cecum with the fonticulus nasofrontalis, and the foramen cecum with the prenasal space. These connections cause the formation of nasal dermoids, dermal sinuses, gliomas, and encephaloceles.[47] Nasal dermoids can be present at any point between the glabella and the base of the columella. Intracranial extension can exist via the tract through the nasal septum and foramen cecum, or through the widened frontonasal suture (fonticulus nasofrontalis) and foramen cecum. In these cases, the presence of the dermoid between the leaves of falx and a bifid crista galli are noted (Fig. 41.4).

Diagnosis/patient presentation

Dermoids present as firm, cystic lesions, or infected persistent abscesses. They expand slowly and cause destruction of the nasal bones and widening of the nasal ridge. MRI can help differentiate between normal anatomic variants of the anterior cranial base versus the intracranial extension of dermal sinus tracts. CT scans can help delineate the bony anatomy of the nose and the cranial base, and help in operative planning with the use of 3D reconstruction.[48,49]

Treatment/surgical technique

Dermoid cysts or sinuses that are present at the columella usually extend to the nasal spine. Resection involves a circumscribed removal of the sinus tract. If a cyst is associated with it, it is dissected through the labial sulcus. Sinuses and cysts that are present from the radix to the nasal tip, but are without intracranial extension, are excised in combination with an

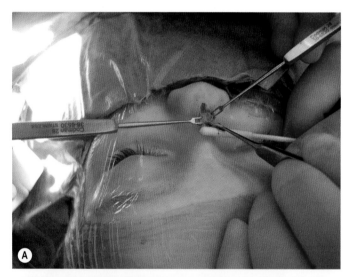
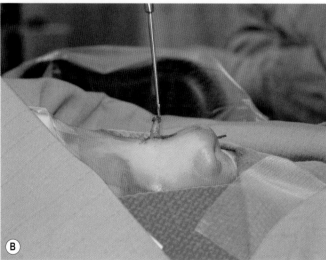

Fig. 41.5 (A,B) Excision of nasal dermoid without intracranial extension. *(Courtesy of Dr. Diane G. Heatley.)*

anterior cranial base.[59] A similar subcranial-transglabellar approach involves horizontal osteotomies above the supraorbital rims and at the level of the nasal bones, and vertical osteotomies at the supraorbital rims to expose the intracranial portion of the dermoid. This technique allows one to approach the lesion from one direction, thereby maintaining a single field. It is also attributed to require decreased frontal lobe retraction and therefore has a lower risk of contusions, cerebral edema, and long-term neurologic defects.[61] The osteotomy size is smaller than the traditional frontal craniotomy approach, which reduces the risk of dural tears or CSF leaks (Fig. 41.6).[64]

Outcomes, prognosis, and complications

The recurrence rate of nasal dermoids after surgical excision is 12%.[67] A meta-analysis showed that the rate of complications with the traditional craniofacial approach was 30%, while the subcranial approach reduced the complication rate to 16%.[63] Complications included tension pneumocephalus, CSF leakage, subdural hematoma, longer operative times, and longer ICU stays.[64,65]

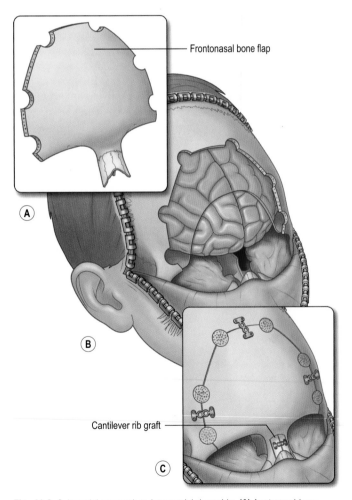

(A)

(B)

Frontonasal bone flap

Cantilever rib graft

(C)

Fig. 41.6 Subcranial approach to intracranial dermoids: **(A)** frontonasal bone fragment; **(B)** subcranial approach with simultaneous access to the frontal lobe, the anterior skull base, and the nasal cavity; **(C)** reconstruction with replacement of the frontonasal bone fragment, cantilever rib grafts to the nasal dorsum, and orbital floor reconstruction with split calvarial bone graft.

Secondary procedures

Immediate reconstruction is preferred and may involve the use of conchal or costal cartilage grafts, as well as bone grafts for reconstruction of the cartilaginous skeleton of the nose. Reconstruction of "keystone" skull base defects can be carried out with bone grafts taken from the parietal bone of the skull. The origin of the frontal sinus may be disturbed, and the resulting defect, if not in continuity with the sinus, can occasionally be corrected, some reporting the use of hydroxyapatite.

Intradural dermoids and dermal sinus tracts

Basic science/disease process

The incomplete sequestration of neuroectoderm and somatic ectoderm during embryogenesis, can lead to persistent dermal sinus tracts from the occiput to the sacrum.[68,69] About 1% of these tracts are found in the cervical spine, 10% in the thoracic spine, 41% in the lumbar spine, and 35% in the lumbosacral spine.[70] These sinus tracts are cephalically oriented, lined with stratified epithelium, and may lead to the vertebral column, ending as intradural dermoid cysts.[68]

Diagnosis/patient presentation

Dermal sinus tracts can present as hypertrichosis, skin tags, abnormal pigmentation, subcutaneous lipomas or angiomata.[71,72] The presence of these tracts can also lead to recurrent bacterial meningitis. Additionally, traction on the spinal cord can occur and can lead to symptoms of motor weakness, autonomic irritation, or sphincter dysfunction. MRI is the imaging tool of choice, and helps with the evaluation of other associated pathologies such as inclusion tumors, dermoids, epidermoids, teratomas,[73–80] split cord malformations, and tethered cords (Fig. 41.7).[81–83]

Treatment/surgical technique

Surgical excision involves tracing the tract through the subcutaneous tissue, lumbosacral fascia, and bony defect. If the dura is involved, laminectomy is necessary to open the dura and explore the intradural space. Laminectomy may be required to inspect the intradural extension within the subarachnoid space. Intramedullary dermoids located at the conus are usually associated with cephalic extension. Occasionally, there is an associated thickened tethered cord, which requires sectioning of the filum.[83] The presence of adhesions at the site of previous resection and associated progressive neurologic deficits, require re-exploration and lysis of adhesions.[84,85]

External angular dermoids

Basic science/disease process

External angular dermoids are usually fixed to the orbital rim periosteum and the frontozygomatic suture, with very rare intraosseous extension. Intraosseous extension presents as intraosseous cysts that can very rarely erode intracranially.[86] External angular dermoids usually lie along the trajectory of the Tessier No.10 cleft. They may also be present more medially at the brow and supraorbital region. If they approach the

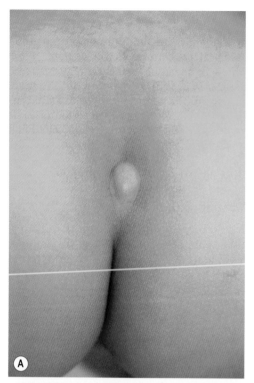
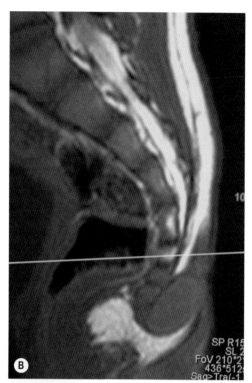
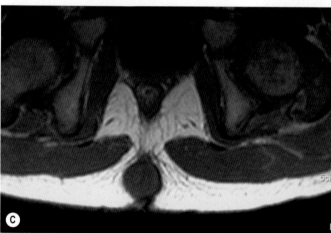

Fig. 41.7 **(A)** External manifestation of intradural dermoid. **(B,C)** MRIs showing intradural dermoid. *(Courtesy of Dr. Dennis P. Lund.)*

frontonasal junction, they need to be evaluated as frontonasal dermoids.

Diagnosis/patient presentation

External angular dermoids are slow growing and rarely exceed 4 cm in size. Size varies based on sweat gland activity.[86]

Treatment/surgical technique

Most lesions are excised through an incision in the lateral portion of the upper lid. Dermoids are generally found underneath the orbicularis muscle. If the dermoid is large with extension temporally, a hairline incision can be made

to gain access. Endoscopic assisted excision is discouraged laterally because it has been associated with injury to the facial nerve.

Dermoid cysts of the neck

Basic science/disease process

In contrast to dermoids of the head, which are found in different fusion planes, these present as subcutaneous masses. About 28% of them are dermal in origin. They are located in the midline of the neck and are composed of ectodermal tissue, sebaceous glands, and hair.[87–89] The epidermoid cyst is the most common dermoid cyst.[89]

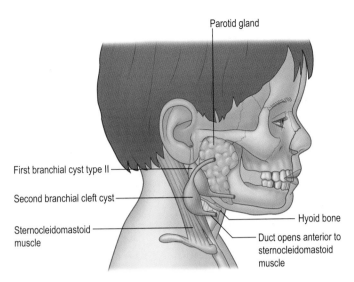

Parotid gland

First branchial cyst type II

Second branchial cleft cyst

Sternocleidomastoid muscle

Hyoid bone

Duct opens anterior to sternocleidomastoid muscle

Fig. 41.8 Branchial cleft.

Diagnosis/patient presentation

In newborns, these can present as masses in the floor of the mouth, with extension to the midline of the neck.[90]

Branchial cleft anomalies

Introduction

Fusion of branchial arches takes place 3–6 weeks' gestation. Failure of fusion of these arches leads to branchial cleft anomalies, which present as cysts, internal sinuses, external sinuses, fistulas or combinations of the previous. A branchial anomaly is present inferior to all the embryonic derivatives of its associated arch, and superior to all the embryonic derivatives of the next arch.[91] Cysts are the most common and are lined by squamous or columnar epithelium. Cysts and the masses associated with them are usually found in the anterior cervical triangle near lymph tissue.[92] Internal sinuses present with infection and halitosis. External sinuses present as openings in the middle to lower neck in the anterior cervical triangle or by the external ear.

The 2nd branchial cleft anomaly (90%)

Basic science/disease process

A complete 2nd branchial cleft begins near the sternal origin of the SCM, passes along the anterior border of the SCM lateral to the hypoglossal and glossopharyngeal nerves, and ends at the tonsillar fossa, superior to the hypoglossal and glossopharyngeal nerves (Fig. 41.8).

Diagnosis/patient presentation

Cystic masses are more common. Sinuses and fistulas may be present along the superior two-thirds of the tract.[93] The tract may be a blind sinus, or may extend all the way up to the tonsillar fossa, leading to chronic salivary drainage problems. These lesions also present as recurrent deep neck infections, and CT scans are helpful in recognizing them (Fig. 41.9).[94]

Treatment/surgical technique

Fistulous tracts can be identified by injecting methylene blue or radio-opaque material into the tract followed by a CT scan.[95] This step can be avoided since the tract may easily be followed during the excision. While dissecting out the tract, care is taken to preserve the hypoglossal and glossopharyngeal nerves, and the internal and external carotid arteries. If the tract extends into the base of the tonsillar fossa, the tonsil may need to be resected (Fig. 41.10).

The 1st branchial cleft anomaly (8%)

Basic science/disease process

Normal fusion of the 1st branchial arch, presents as the external auditory meatus. A complete non-fusion of the 1st arch leaves a cleft extending from the external auditory canal traveling along and under the border of the mandible up to the midline.

Diagnosis/patient presentation

About 66% of the associated lesions are cysts. These usually present as masses in the parotid region along with pits or depressions near the external auditory meatus.[96] Sinuses and fistulas are less common. These tracts may pass through the parotid gland and their excision may jeopardize facial nerve branches. Fistulas can be traced from the junction of the ear and cartilaginous canal, to the overlying skin (Fig. 41.11).

Fistulas present as two types:

The *type 1* anomaly is a duplication of the membranous external meatal canal and is composed of ectodermal elements. The tract begins medial, antero-inferior or posterior to the pinna and conchal cartilages. It then runs parallel to the external canal and has a blind end in the middle tympanic region.

The *type 2* anomaly is a duplication of the membranous ear canal and the auricle and therefore contains both ectodermal and mesodermal structures. The tract begins with an opening in the anterior neck, superior to the hyoid

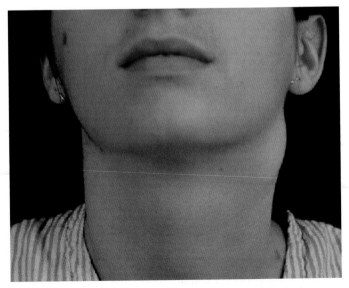

Fig. 41.9 Second branchial cleft cyst. *(Courtesy of Dr. Diane G. Heatley.)*

deep to the carotid artery, toward or through the thyrohyoid membrane. It originates at the base/cranial end of the pyriform sinus and then passes above the superior laryngeal nerve.[100]

The 4th branchial cleft anomaly

The 4th branchial cleft anomaly begins at the apex of the pyriform sinus and passes through the cricothyroid membrane beneath the superior laryngeal nerves. It then travels inferiorly in the tracheoesophageal groove, posterior to the thyroid gland and into the thorax. The tract then loops around the arch of the aorta on the left and the subclavian artery on the right and courses superiorly, posterior to the common carotid artery. It finally makes another loop around the hypoglossal nerve and terminates at the medial border of the SCM. The descending portion of the tract has the highest likelihood of being infected. Patients present with respiratory distress, mediastinal abscesses, and suppurative thyroiditis.[101,102]

Outcomes, prognosis, and complications

Recurrence rates are increased when there is a history of multiple preoperative infections associated with the anomaly, and when there is no epithelial tissue found in the specimen.[91]

Thyroglossal duct cysts

Introduction

Thyroglossal duct cysts are the most common tumors of the anterior cervical region, which are usually located in the midline at or below the level of the hyoid. They are persistent embryologic remnants of the descending thyroglossal duct.

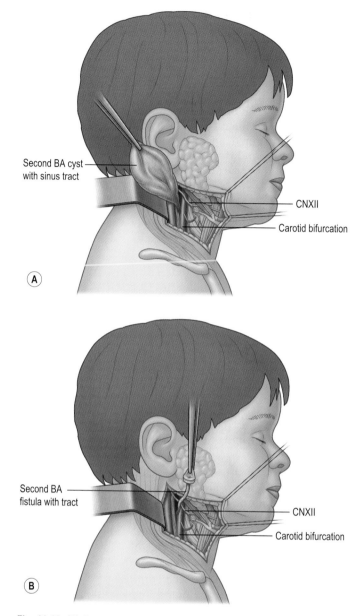

Fig. 41.10 (A) Excision of second branchial cleft cyst. **(B)** Excision of second branchial cleft fistula. BA, branchial arch.

bone and anterior to the SCM. It extends superiorly through subcutaneous tissue, pierces the substance of the parotid gland, and then passes superficial, deep, or in between two branches of the facial nerve.[97,98]

Treatment/surgical technique

Incision and drainage of infected cysts may be necessary before definitive surgery. The sinus/fistulous tracts extend into the parotid gland and their excision may jeopardize the facial nerve.[93,98,99] Complete excision consists of a superficial parotidectomy with facial nerve dissection.

The 3rd branchial cleft anomaly

The 3rd branchial cleft anomaly presents with a tract that has an opening along the anterior border of the SCM and extends

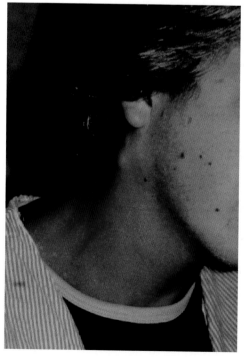

Fig. 41.11 First branchial cleft cyst. *(Courtesy of Dr. Diane G. Heatley.)*

Basic science/disease process

During the 3rd week of gestation, thyroid gland development begins at the foramen cecum, at the junction of the tongue and pharynx. As the thyroid anlage begins to descend, the fusion of the 2nd branchial arch causes the gland to move more anteriorly. The thyroglossal duct passes superficially, through or just deep to the hyoid bone. The duct tissue differentiates into the thyroid gland and the mid-portion of the duct disintegrates. If this middle area persists, then it can differentiate to give rise to columnar, ciliated, or squamous epithelium, thereby forming a cyst. These cysts are found anterior and inferior to the hyoid bone and present during the first or second decades of life.

Diagnosis/patient presentation/patient selection

Thyroglossal duct cysts are tethered to the hyoid bone and therefore move with swallowing and tongue protrusion (Fig. 41.12). They are usually painless masses unless they get infected. If the cysts get infected or rupture, thyroglossal duct sinus tracts can form. These sinus tracts then drain clear or cloudy mucus.[93,103,104]

Treatment/surgical technique

Treatment involves surgical excision using the Sistrunk technique. A curvilinear incision is made over the cyst followed

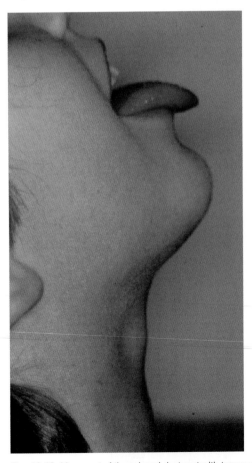

Fig. 41.12 Movement of thyroglossal duct cyst with tongue protrusion. *(Courtesy of Dr. Diane G. Heatley.)*

by excision of the full duct up to the foramen cecum along with the central 1 cm of the hyoid bone.[105] Thyroid scans should be done to ensure that the tissue is not a functioning ectopic thyroid gland. Hormonal evaluation, CT, or ultrasound scans may also be performed.[103,106]

Outcomes, prognosis, and complications

Recurrence is possible if lingual thyroid tissue is left behind. In this case, treatment may involve a transoral excision of tongue tissue around the foramen cecum. The Sistrunk technique reduced the recurrence rate from 20–49% to <5%.[107]

Pilomatrixoma

Introduction and history

In 1880, this lesion was first described by Malherbe and Chenantais who thought this arose from sebaceous glands and called them "calcifying epitheliomas of Malherbe". In 1961, Forbis and Helwig proposed this to be a benign lesion and gave it the name "pilomatrixoma".[108–112]

Basic science/disease process

Pilomatrixomas originate from the outer root sheath cells of the hair follicle in the lower dermis and form a connective tissue capsule. Histologically, these tumors are seen as non-invasive islands of basaloid cells with hyperchromatic nuclei and no nucleoli. The other major component of the tumor consists of cells that show a central unstained area, representing the shadow of a lost nucleus, called ghost cells. These tumors are well-demarcated and are completely or partially surrounded by fibrosis or an inflammatory reaction.[109] Malignant transformation has not been reported in children but it has in adults. In adults, pilomatrical carcinoma behaves similar to basal cell carcinoma and has similar metastatic potential.[110] Pilomatrical carcinomas show invasive nests of tumor cells with irregular borders, large vesicular nuclei, prominent nucleoli, multiple mitotic figures, and focal necrosis.

Diagnosis/patient presentation

The average age of presentation is 7 years, with a peak between ages 8 and 13 years.[111,112] These tumors commonly occur in regions of fine vellus hair growth in children, such as the cheeks and periorbital area (Fig. 41.13).[111] Female preponderance of the tumor and a history of regional trauma in 9% of patients have been reported.[109,112] The frequency of having multiple tumors is about 2–3%, although rates of as high as 10% have also been reported.[110] Multiple tumors are noted in patients with Gardner syndrome, Steinert disease, myotonic dystrophy, and sarcoidosis.[112–115] When the skin is tented and the tumor is palpated below it, one can feel multiple nodules.[116] The freely mobile characteristic of the mass rules out dermoid cysts, and its nodular nature helps rule out epidermal cysts. Fine-needle aspiration determines cytology and the presence of ghost cells, basaloid cells, and/or calcium deposits and helps solidify the diagnosis.[117] Ultrasound is cheap, effective, and helps determine the relationship of the tumor with the parotid gland.[118]

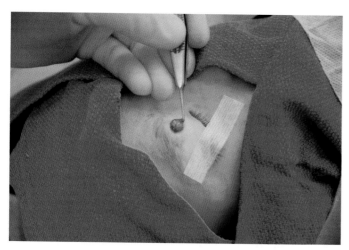

Fig. 41.13 Excision of pilomatrixoma. *(Courtesy of Dr. Delora L. Mount.)*

Treatment/surgical technique

Treatment for the malignant lesion is wide local excision. Reconstruction is deferred for 1 year while observing for recurrence. Radiation may help for locoregional control.[110]

Benign lesions are completely excised. When the tumor adheres to the skin, overlying skin is resected. Surgery is generally curative and recurrence is rare.[119] Treatment with incision and curettement have been reported for large tumors in cosmetically significant areas.

Postoperative care

Malignant lesions have a high likelihood of recurrence; thus patients need to be observed for recurrence.

Outcomes, prognosis, and complications

The rate of recurrence of benign lesions is very low and patients have an excellent prognosis. Metastatic spread occurs in 6% of patients with malignant lesions.[120] Metastatic lesions are usually found in the lungs, but have also been reported in the lymph nodes, liver, pleura, kidney, and heart.[121]

Soft-tissue sarcomas

Rhabdomyosarcoma

Introduction

Soft-tissue sarcomas account for 10% of all pediatric malignancies, 50% of which are rhabdomyosarcomas.[122] These tumors are the third most common solid, extracranial, pediatric tumor (after Wilm's tumor and neuroblastoma) and are diagnosed in about 250 patients annually.

Basic science/disease process

Rhabdomyosarcomas generally originate from mesenchymal cells committed to becoming skeletal muscle cells. They have, however, also been found to arise from viscera such as the prostate, gallbladder, and urinary bladder. The tumors resemble different stages of prenatal muscle formation. There are four histologic types: embryonal, spindle-cell, alveolar, and pleomorphic. Rhabdomyosarcomas have also found to be present in multiple syndromes such as Li-Fraumeni, Beckwith Wiedemann, and a subset in Gorlin syndrome.[123]

Diagnosis/patient presentation

Patients most commonly present with lesions in the head and neck, genitourinary tract, and extremities.[124] In the head and neck, the most common presentations involve the orbit (20–40%), nasopharynx, paranasal sinuses, and the middle ear.[125] Embryonal tumors are found in 60% of cases, alveolar tumors in 20%, and pleomorphic and spindle-cell tumors in 10% of cases. Embryonal rhabdomyosarcomas occur between birth and age 15 years and have a relatively favorable prognosis. They are usually found in the head and neck and genitourinary system. Spindle-cell rhabdomyosarcomas have a bimodal distribution and are found in both children and adults. They usually occur in the head and neck or paratesticular region. Their prognosis is more favorable in children. Alveolar rhabdomyosarcomas are relatively aggressive and are found in adolescents and young adults. These tumors occur in the extremities, head, and neck and genito-anal areas. Pleomorphic rhabdomyosarcomas usually affect adults in the sixth and seventh decades of life.[123] In general, the median age of presentation for rhabdomyosarcomas is 5 years.[126] These tumors tend to present as fungating masses in the conjunctiva and vagina or as obstructive masses in the genitourinary tract and biliary system. They cause proptosis and diplopia when they involve the orbit and neurologic manifestations when they involve nerve roots in the paraspinal region. Rhabdomyosarcomas of the temporal bone present with hearing loss, otalgia, and otorrhea (Fig. 41.14). CT scans of the head and skull base, and lumbar puncture are used to evaluate for extension of the disease into the skull, meninges, and brain.

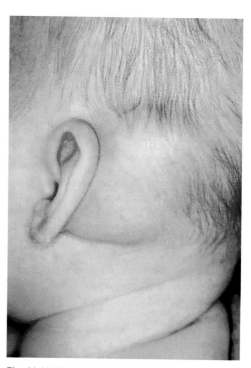

Fig. 41.14 Rhabdomyosarcoma. *(Courtesy of Dr. Diane G. Heatley.)*

Treatment/surgical technique/postoperative care

Risk stratification is determined by pretreatment staging, post-surgical clinical grouping, and tumor histology. All non-metastatic embryonal rhabdomyosarcoma (ERMS) at favorable sites and completely resected tumors at non-favorable sites are considered low risk. Non-metastatic alveolar rhabdomyosarcoma (ARMS) and incompletely resected ERMS at non-favorable sites are intermediate risk, and distant metastases are considered high risk. Primary treatment modalities are multidrug chemotherapy and external beam radiation therapy and protocols are adjusted based on risk stratification. If complete remission is not obtained, adjuvant radiation therapy and surgery are carried out. Surgical involvement (staging and treatment) is mutilating and leads to functional loss as a result. Primary excision should be attempted only if complete excision can be accomplished without functional or cosmetic consequences.[127]

Outcomes, prognosis, and complications

Patients undergoing the primary treatment modality have a 74% 5-year survival rate, while 33% have recurrent metastatic disease that is fatal. Metastases occurs through blood or lymphatic channels to lymph nodes, lungs, bones, or brain.[126]

Secondary procedures

Secondary excision may be considered after chemotherapy, based on the judgment of the surgeon. If the tumor still remains unresectable, then radiotherapy is employed.

Synovial soft-tissue sarcoma

Introduction

Synovial soft-tissue sarcomas are the most common soft-tissue sarcoma of the hands and feet, and represent 8–10% of all malignant somatic soft tissue neoplasms.

Basic science/disease process

These sarcomas arise from synovioblastic differentiation of pluripotent mesenchymal stem cells. Histologic studies show a biphasic pattern of pseudoepithelial cells and spindle cells with a fibrosarcomatous appearance.[128]

Diagnosis/patient presentation

Synovial soft-tissue sarcomas present as solitary, well-circumscribed lesions in the upper or lower extremities (80%). They are para-articular, never arise within the joint, and are not associated with normal synovial tissue. Non-extremity sites include the trunk (8%), retroperitoneum/abdomen (7%), and head and neck (5%).[129] Common locations in the neck include: parapharyngeal/retropharyngeal spaces, larynx, pharynx, tongue, and tonsils.[130] The most common symptom is a painless mass that has existed for several weeks to years. These lesions may also present as chronic contractures, acute arthritis, bursitis, or as tumors following trauma. Up to 30% of synovial soft-tissue sarcomas have calcifications on radiographs. MR is the imaging modality of choice and it shows the tumors to be sharply marginated and largely cystic.

Treatment/surgical technique

The treatment of choice is surgical excision, with pre- or postoperative radiation therapy. Adjuvant chemotherapy may improve local control if the tumor size is >5 cm. The goal of surgery is to obtain tumor-free margins of 1–3 cm.[131–134]

Outcomes, prognosis, and complications

The overall survival rates with surgery and radiation therapy are shown to be 76% at 5 years and 57% at 10 years. Disease-free survival rates have been shown to be 59% at 5 years and 52% at 10 years. The rate of local failure is below 20% but the rate of metastatic spread at 10 years has been shown to be 44%. Tumors >5 cm in size have worse survival rates.[134] Complications at 5 years are 7%, and at 10 years are 9%. These include fractures, fibrosis, soft-tissue necrosis, neuropathy, and edema. Most common sites of metastases are lung (74–81%), lymph nodes (12–23%), and bone (10–20%).[135]

Alveolar soft-part sarcoma

Introduction

Alveolar soft-part sarcoma is a rare neoplasm of unknown etiology or histogenesis but has a poor prognosis.

Basic science/disease process

Alveolar soft-part sarcomas account for 1% of all soft tissue sarcomas. They occur primarily in skeletal muscles or musculofascial planes of extremities, and in the head and neck region in children.

Diagnosis/patient presentation

Children, adolescents, and young adults between the ages of 15 and 35 years are more likely to carry this diagnosis. The tumor has a predilection for females and usually presents as a soft, painless, slow-growing mass. The majority of patients have metastases at the time of diagnosis.

Treatment/surgical technique

Wide local excision is the mainstay of treatment. Metastatic spread occurs to lungs, bone, central nervous system, and liver.

Outcomes, prognosis, and complications

Survival has been reported as 82% at 2 years, 59% at 5 years, and 47% at 10 years.[136–138] Alveolar soft-part sarcomas can recur more than 10 years after primary resection.

Lymphadenopathy

Introduction

About 30% of lymph nodes are found in the head and neck region.[139] Posterior auricular and occipital lymph nodes drain the posterior scalp and the superficial portion of the postero-superior neck.[140] Preauricular and infraorbital nodes drain the temporal scalp, lateral eyelids, conjunctiva, and cheek. These nodes are connected to the parotid lymph nodes in the lateral parotid gland. Submandibular and submental nodes drain the teeth, gum, tongue, and buccal mucosa. The deep cervical lymph node chain runs along the internal jugular vein, deep to the sternocleidomastoid muscles. Its superior portion drains the tongue and the posterior pharynx. Its inferior portion drains the larynx, trachea, thyroid, and esophagus. Superficial cervical nodes lie superficial to the SCM. The anterior chain of nodes runs along the internal jugular vein, while the posterior chain is present in the posterior triangle. These nodes receive drainage from the superficial tissues of the neck, mastoid process, posterior auricular nodes, and the nasopharynx. The tonsillar nodes drain the palatine tonsils.

Bacterial lymphadenitis

Basic science/disease process

Bacterial lymphadenitis usually occurs in children under 4 years of age and is preceded by an upper respiratory tract infection or pharyngitis. It can present with mild fever, tender, indurated, and erythematous lymph nodes, or systemic toxicity. Submandibular nodes are affected in half of the patients. Upper cervical nodes are affected in 25% of patients. The most common causative organisms in children under the age of 3 years include *Staphylococcus aureus* and *Streptococcus agalactiae* (Group G *Streptococcus*). Sepsis is most likely in this age group. In children over the age of 3 years, *Staphylococcus aureus* and *Streptococcus pyogenes* (Group A *Streptococcus*) are the most common organisms. Bacterial lymphadenitis can also be caused by *Escherichia coli* and anaerobes in the setting of periodontal disease.

Diagnosis/patient presentation

Staphylococcus aureus adenitis is most likely to cause an abscess. About 30% of acutely infected lymph nodes suppurate in 2 weeks.[141,142] Group A *Streptococcus adenitis* causes bilateral jugulodigastric node enlargement, fever, severe sore throat, frontal headache, abdominal pain, toxic appearance, and exudative tonsillitis. It may also present with minimal systemic symptoms and non-tender adenopathy.

Treatment/surgical technique

Treatment of acute lymphadenitis abscess involves incision and drainage. This prevents migration of the disease into the chest and abdomen via fascial planes.

Chronic regional lymphadenopathy

Basic science/disease process

Cat scratch disease is the most common cause of chronic regional lymphadenopathy affecting the head and neck region in children and young adults.[143–146] Up to 50% of the cases involve head and neck nodes. The bacterial organisms involved are *Bartonella henselae* and *Afipia felis*, which are transmitted via a cat scratch or bite.[147]

Diagnosis/patient presentation

The clinical course of this disease begins with the formation of a red papule at 3–12 days at the site of inoculation.

The papule progresses to a vesicle, then to a pustule, which develops an eschar and then resolves. This is followed by lymphadenopathy 1 week later. About 85% of patients develop a deep enlarged lymph node at the site of inoculation. Proximal lymph nodes may be skipped, with distal level nodes developing lymphadenopathy.[148,149] The disease is self-limiting, but may lead to complications in 5–13% of cases.

Treatment/surgical technique

Antibiotic therapy is used for highly symptomatic patients. Surgical excision of enlarged lymph nodes is advocated if the nodes become fluctuant.[146]

Outcomes, prognosis, and complications

Complications include encephalopathy, erythema nodosum, thrombocytopenic purpura, Parinaud oculoglandular syndrome, and hepatitis.[146,150] If the patient is immunocompromised, then lymphadenopathy may progress to bacillary angiomatosis, which is characterized by disseminated disease and cutaneous nodular lesions.

Cervical tuberculous adenitis (scrofula)

Basic science/disease process

Cervical tuberculous adenitis is caused by inhaled mycobacteria, which lead to a pulmonary infection. The infection eventually spreads to regional lymph nodes via lymph vessels or distal lymph nodes via blood vessels.[151]

Diagnosis/patient presentation

Scrofula typically presents in children under the age of 6 as painless enlarging masses. Lower anterior and posterior cervical lymph nodes are involved bilaterally. Tonsillar and submandibular lymph nodes may also be involved. Symptoms include fever, weight loss, night sweats, and decreased appetite. Lymph nodes will occasionally develop suppurative changes and produce draining sinuses. Generalized lymphadenopathy can develop from miliary spread of the disease. The diagnosis is made using ESR, tuberculin skin tests, chest radiographs, and fine-needle aspiration.[152]

Treatment/surgical technique

Surgical excision is recommended to prevent the formation of chronic draining fistulas, especially if open wounds are present. If the tuberculin skin test is positive, cultures are sent and four-drug therapy consisting of rifampin, isoniazid, pyrazinamide, and ethambutol is started. The course of treatment is 6 months. Treatment may be tapered to two-drug therapy, based on culture results.

Atypical non-tuberculous mycobacteria

Basic science/disease process

Mycobacterium scrofulaceum and *Mycobacterium avium-intercellulare* are the most common atypical non-tuberculous mycobacteria responsible for this lymphadenopathy. Both organisms are commonly found in the southeastern US. The site of entry is the mouth, followed by spread to the regional lymph nodes.

Diagnosis/patient presentation

Patients present with unilateral lymphadenopathy mainly involving submandibular nodes. Nodes are initially painless and mobile but eventually become inflamed, fixed, and suppurative (Fig. 41.15). Infection spreads locally to subcutaneous surrounding tissues leading to chronically draining sinus tracts. The age of presentation is between 1 and 5 years, and patients usually do not have systemic symptoms. They have a normal ESR, chest radiograph, and white cell count. Definitive diagnosis is made through culture.[153]

Treatment/surgical technique

Definitive treatment involves surgical excision with or without medical therapy. These organisms are more resistant to anti-tuberculosis drugs. If there exists a suspicion for an atypical mycobacterial infection, the treatment consists of a combination of clarithromycin, ethambutol, rifampin, and ciprofloxacin while awaiting results.[154]

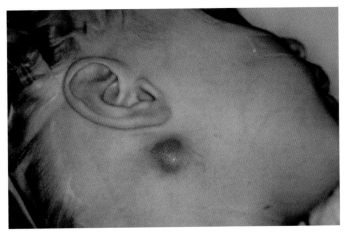

Fig. 41.15 Atypical mycobacterial abscess. *(Courtesy of Dr. Dennis P. Lund.)*

Access the complete reference list online at **http://www.expertconsult.com**

11. Jackson IT, Carbonnel A, Portparic Z, et al. Orbitotemporal neurofibromatosis: classification and treatment. *Plast Reconstr Surg.* 1993;92:1–11. *This article divides the clinical presentation of orbitotemporal neurofibromatosis into three groups based on orbital and soft tissue involvement and the state of the eye. The treatment methods differ based on the severity of presentation and therefore this classification helps guide the treatments used. The article presents 24 patients who are followed for a maximum of 12 years.*

31. Ferner RE, Gutmann DH. International consensus statement on malignant peripheral nerve sheath tumours in neurofibromatosis 1. *Cancer Res.* 2002;62:1573–1577.

47. Sessions RB. Nasal dermal sinuses: new concepts and explanations. *Laryngoscope.* 1982;92:1–28. *This is a classic paper that describes, evaluates, and unifies the various existing theories describing the etiology of dermoids. The paper shows how dermoids and encephaloceles are a continuum in the manifestation of congenital anterior cranial base defects. The diagrams in the paper clearly illustrate the surgical anatomy of these defects.*

56. Hanikeri M, Waterhouse N, Kirkpatrick N, et al. The management of midline transcranial nasal dermoid sinus cysts. *Br J Plast Surg.* 2005;58:1043–1050.

63. Kellman RM, Marentette L. The transglabellar/subcranial approach to the anterior skull base: a review of 72 cases. *Arch Otolaryngol Head Neck Surg.* 2001;127:687–690. *This paper describes the transglabellar/subcranial approach to the anterior skull base in patients who have dermoids with intracranial extension. Through a retrospective analysis of 72 cases in two academic medical centers it*

analyses parameters such as average operating room time, complication rates, and length of ICU stay, and compares them with results published for traditional craniofacial approaches.

91. Schroeder JW, Mohyuddin N, Maddalozzo J. Branchial anomalies in the pediatric population. *Otolaryngol Head Neck Surg.* 2007;137(2):289–295. *This paper reviews the presentation, evaluation, and treatment of branchial anomalies. It accomplishes this task through a retrospective study involving 97 pediatric patients with branchial anomalies who were treated over a 10-year period. The associated complications and the rates of recurrence after treatment are also discussed.*

105. Sistrunk WE. The surgical treatment of cysts of the thyroglossal tract. *Ann Surg.* 1920;71:121–122.

114. McCulloch TA, Singh S, Cotton DWK. Pilomatrix carcinoma and multiple pilomatrixomas. *Br J Dermatol.* 1996;134:368–371.

119. Prousmanesh A, Reinisch JF, Gonzalez-Gomez I, et al. Pilomatrixoma: a review of 346 cases. *Plast Reconstr Surg.* 2003;112:1784–1789. *This article examines the cause, clinical, and histologic presentation, management, and treatment outcomes of pilomatrixoma. A retrospective review of patient records spanning a period of 11 years is conducted, during which 346 pilomatrixomas were excised from 336 patients at Children's Hospital in Los Angeles. The study concludes that the treatment of choice is surgical excision and that the rate of recurrence is low.*

121. Aslan G, Erdogan B, Aköz T, et al. Multiple occurrence of pilomatrixoma. *Plast Reconstr Surg.* 1996;98:510–533.

42

Conjoined twins

Oksana Jackson and David W. Low

SYNOPSIS

- Conjoined twins are one of the most uncommon congenital anomalies, with an incidence between 1 in 50 000 and 1 in 100 000 births.
- Conjoined twins are classified by dorsal or ventral site of fusion and anatomic region of fusion.
- Separation of conjoined twins requires a multidisciplinary team approach.
- Understanding the shared anatomy through preoperative imaging studies and investigations is critical to successful separation.
- Careful planning and insertion of tissue expanders is almost always necessary to accomplish wound closure.
- Intensive care monitoring and support, nutritional supplementation, and pressure-reducing strategies are essential for successful separation.

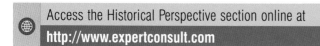

Access the Historical Perspective section online at

http://www.expertconsult.com

Figs. 42.1–42.3 ⊕ appear online only.

Basic science/disease process

Incidence

Conjoined twins are one of the most uncommon congenital anomalies. The typical form of monozygotic twinning occurs in 4 per 1000 live births, and dizygotic fraternal twinning in approximately 10–15 per 1000. Twin births therefore occur in about 1 in 90 live births.[12] The incidence of conjoined twins has been estimated at between 1 in 50 000 and 1 in 100 000 pregnancies. Spencer has reported that 1% are stillborn and 40–60% die shortly after birth, so the true incidence is closer to 1 : 200 000 live births.[5,13] Recent reports of prenatally diagnosed conjoined twins indicate that more than one-quarter of cases die *in utero* and one-half die immediately after birth, leaving only 20% potential survivors who are candidates for separation.[14] In all reports, females predominate over males by approximately 3 : 1. However, in reports of stillborn conjoined twin pairs, males predominate over females.[5,10,15–17]

Classification

A number of classification systems exist and each categorizes conjoined twins by their most prominent site of union together with the suffix *pagus*, a Greek word meaning "that which is fixed". The most commonly used system, both clinically and historically in the literature, was adapted from that proposed by Potter and Craig, and simplified to include the five most common forms of conjoined twinning, listed here in order of decreasing frequency: thoracopagus, omphalopagus, pygopagus, ischiopagus, and craniopagus.[18] These five types are summarized below and illustrated in Fig. 42.4. Additionally, the number of shared anatomic structures can be described with the prefixes "di-", "tri-", and "tetra-", combined with the involved parts, "prospus" (face), "brachius" (upper extremity), and "pus" (lower extremity). For example, ischiopagus twins may have three (*tripus*) or four (*tetrapus*) legs.

The *thoracopagus* type is the most common, occurring in 74% of cases. Infants with this form of twinning face each other, have major junctions between the chest and abdomen, and may have conjoined livers, hearts, and upper gastro-intestinal structures (Fig. 42.5; Case 6, below). Separation may be limited by the degree of cardiac involvement. Conjoined six-chamber hearts are common in thoracopagus twins and have never been separated successfully; only a single successful case of separation of twins with conjoined atria has been reported.[19] Advances in prenatal diagnosis and the development of fetal surgery have improved perinatal survival in cases where separation is deemed appropriate. For example, the EXIT procedure (*ex utero intrapartum treatment*) has been recently used at the Children's Hospital of Philadelphia in the separation of thoracopagus twins. In this case, one twin had a normal heart that perfused a co-twin with a rudimentary heart, and EXIT allowed prompt control of the airway and

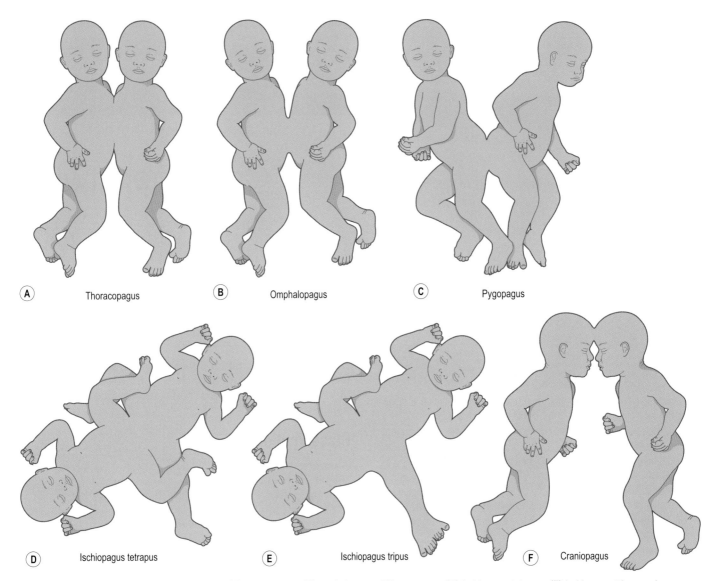

Fig. 42.4 Clinical classification of conjoined twins: **(A)** thoracopagus, **(B)** omphalopagus, **(C)** pygopagus, **(D)** ischiopagus tetrapus, **(E)** ischiopagus tripus, and **(F)** craniopagus.

circulation prior to clamping the umbilical cord, leading to survival of the normal co-twin.[14]

In omphalopagus twins, there is fusion in the abdominal area with variable connections of the liver, biliary tree, and gastrointestinal tracts. In isolated omphalopagus forms, there is no cardiac connection (Case 8, below).

Pygopagus twins are joined at the level of the sacrum and commonly face away from each other. There is usually a shared spinal cord, and the perineal structures and rectum also may be fused. Pygopagus twins represent about 17% of conjoined twins.[12]

In the *ischiopagus* type, the junction is at the pelvic level with sharing of the genitourinary structures, rectum, and liver (see Fig. 42.5; Cases 5 and 7, below). These twins may each have a single normal leg and a common fused leg, referred to as a tripus, or four legs may be present. The tripus, when present, usually has dual neural and vascular supply and preoperative determination of perfusion is important in planning separation. Often, the tripus is sacrificed and the soft tissue used for closure of each twin, leaving each with a single

leg. In a unique case, Zuker *et al.* reported successful transplantation of an entire extremity from a dying twin to her sister, thus leaving the surviving one with two functional legs.[20]

The least common and perhaps the most difficult to separate is the *craniopagus* type because the cranial union often involves a variety of neural and vascular connections.[12,21,22] Craniopagus twins represent 2–6% of conjoined twins and occur with an incidence of one in 2.5 million births.[9] They can share scalp, calvarium, dural sinuses, and surfaces of the brain, but the face, foramen magnum, and spine remain separate. Even when the cerebral cortices are contiguous, craniopagus twins do not share neuronal pathways, as demonstrated by completely independent behavior and by electroencephalogram studies. Facial and skull asymmetry can occur, as well as other intracranial and extracranial abnormalities. The site of fusion can vary significantly, and rotation about this site of union can produce a variety of anatomic orientations.[3,8,21,23] A number of authors have classified craniopagus twins by the site, degree of fusion, or alignment of the twins.[24,25] The more

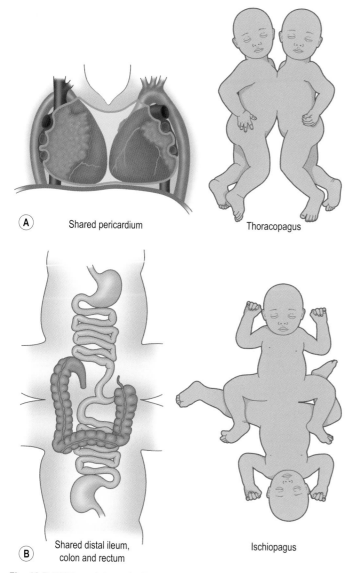

(A) Shared pericardium

Thoracopagus

(B) Shared distal ileum, colon and rectum

Ischiopagus

Fig. 42.5 Within each type of union, the anatomy of conjoined twins can be quite variable. The anatomic features on the left of the illustration describe the anatomy of the twins depicted on the right. These are examples of two common types, amenable to surgical separation. **(A)** Thoracopagus twins with separate hearts but a shared pericardium. **(B)** Tetrapus ischiopagus twins with shared intestine from distal ileum and single colon, rectum, and anus.

common phenotypic variations described in case reports in the literature are illustrated in Fig. 42.6.

An alternative classification system was proposed by Spencer, based on the analysis of embryologic data and the teratology of over 1200 cases. She divided conjoined twins into *dorsal* and *ventral* forms of union, joined in one of eight anatomic sites (Fig. 42.7). This classification system specifically defines and restricts the anatomy of fusion between the different types of conjoined twinning, thus attempting to standardize the nomenclature for purposes of predicting separability, surgical planning, and outcomes after surgery, as well as for consistent documentation for research purposes.[26] In Spencer's embryologic classification system, ventral unions are oriented ventrally or ventrolaterally, and the union always includes the umbilicus, whereas dorsal unions are united dorsally or dorsolaterally and do not include the thoracic or

abdominal viscera or the umbilicus. Ventral unions are further subdivided into rostral, caudal, or lateral. These eight types with their definitions and restrictions are listed below.[26]

Ventral

Rostral

1. *Cephalopagus*: fused from the top of the head to the umbilicus.
2. *Thoracopagus*: united from the upper thorax to the umbilicus and always involving the heart.
3. *Omphalopagus*: joined primarily in the area of the umbilicus and never including the heart.

Caudal

4. *Ischiopagus*: united from the umbilicus through the pelvis and sharing external genitalia and anus.

Lateral

5. *Parapagus*: sharing a conjoined pelvis with one symphysis pubis and one or two sacrums (see Fig. 42.7E).

Dorsal

6. *Craniopagus*: united on any portion on the skull except the face or foramen magnum, and the trunks are never united.

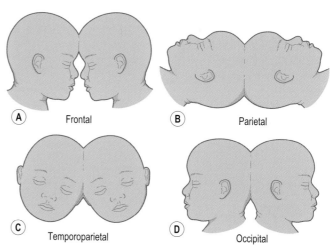

(A) Frontal   (B) Parietal

(C) Temporoparietal   (D) Occipital

O'Connell's classification of vertical craniopagus

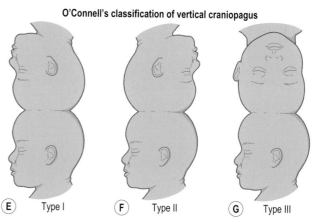

(E) Type I   (F) Type II   (G) Type III

Fig. 42.6 The more common phenotypic variation of craniopagus conjoined twins.

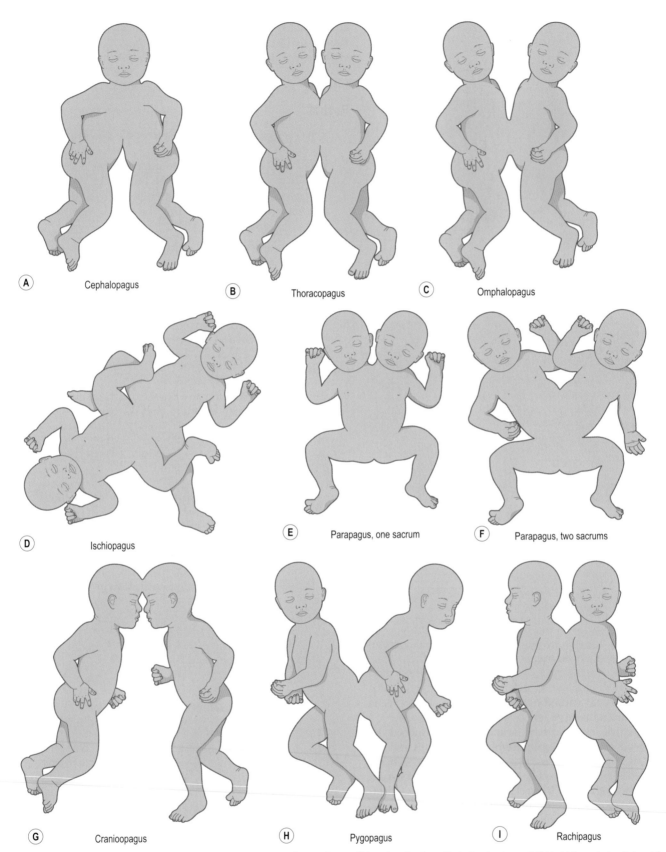

Fig. 42.7 (A–I) The eight types of conjoined twins, as classified by Rowena Spencer[26] based on the theoretical site of union and divided into ventral and dorsal forms of junction.

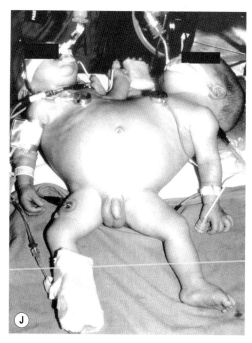

Fig. 42.7, cont'd (J) Parapagus conjoined twins with a single pelvis.

7. *Pygopagus*: sharing sacrococcygeal and perineal regions, and sometimes the spinal cord.
8. *Rachiopagus*: fused dorsally above the sacrum, and exceedingly rare.

Asymmetrical forms of conjoined twinning often occur, resulting in a smaller and larger twin; these are termed "parasitic" followed by their closest classification. When one twin is significantly smaller and less well developed, it is often malnourished and has other physiologic problems which can complicate potential separation. On some occasions, the smaller twin may die and much of the deceased twin may be absorbed. Conjoined twins whose union and anatomy are intermediate between different types are termed "atypical conjoined twins".[26]

Etiology

Two theories have been proposed to explain the embryology resulting in conjoined twins. The classic theory of incomplete fission, described by Zimmerman,[27] proposes that there is incomplete separation of the embryonic discs of twins arising from a uniovular gestation between 13 and 16 days after fertilization. More recently, Spencer[28] proposed an alternative theory of secondary fusion of two originally separate monovular embryonic discs. This theory postulates that, during the 3rd or 4th week of development, previously separate embryonic discs reunite either dorsally or ventrally at specific sites where the surface ectoderm is either absent or normally programmed to fuse or break down. These sites include the anlage of the heart, the diaphragm, the oropharyngeal and cloacal membranes, the neural tube, and the periphery of the embryonic discs, each site corresponding to specific types of conjoined twinning. The unions are always homologous, meaning the fusion occurs head to head, tail to tail, front to front, back to back, or side by side – but never head to tail or front to back. Spencer's "spherical theory" proposes that

conjoined twins united dorsally "float" in a shared amniotic cavity, and those united ventrally "float" on the sphere of a shared yolk sac. In both cases, they can be oriented from rostral to caudal, depending on the relative temporal–spatial relationship of the embryonic discs during fusion (Fig. 42.8).[28]

Diagnosis/patient presentation

Prenatal evaluation

The diagnosis of conjoined twins can be made as early as the 12th week of gestation on prenatal ultrasound. First-trimester or early second-trimester ultrasound findings suggestive of conjoined twins include a fixed position of the twin bodies on serial examinations; lack of a separating membrane between the twins; and inability to separate the fetal bodies and skin contours.[29,30] Once the diagnosis is suspected, evaluation should continue with serial ultrasound, magnetic resonance imaging (MRI), and echocardiography to define better the extent of the union and the anatomy of the shared organs, to determine the presence of any associated abnormalities, and to monitor the pregnancy for complications (Fig. 42.9).[14]

Careful cardiac evaluation is essential, given the high incidence of thoracopagus types. Both ultrafast fetal MRI with 3D reconstruction and echocardiography are useful in determining the cardiac structure and function. Prenatal echocardiography may be superior to postnatal scans because the amniotic fluid provides a good buffer for scanning, and positioning of the transducer may be difficult postnatally against the small pericardial window. Delineation of the conjoined cardiac anatomy has been achieved as early as the 20th week of gestation, although third-trimester studies are most reliable; even those may underestimate the severity of disease when compared with autopsy studies.[12,14,29] Echocardiography can also be utilized while on placental support during the EXIT procedure, as was reported by Mackenzie *et al.* at the Children's Hospital of Philadelphia and proved critical in delineating the relationship of the great vessels in preparation for immediate separation.[14]

The presence of other anomalies, even in organ systems not related to the conjoining, may affect survival, and need also to be ascertained prenatally. Observed anomalies include congenital diaphragmatic hernia, abdominal wall defects, neural tube defects, club foot, imperforate anus, esophageal atresia, and cystic hygroma.[14] Serial scans are also necessary to monitor the pregnancy for the unique complications that are known to occur in multifetal gestations such as twin–twin transfusion syndrome, co-twin demise, and oligohydramnios-polyhydramnios sequence, as well as for the effects of cross-circulation on the pregnancy such as polyhydramnios and hydrops. Polyhydramnios is noted in 50% of cases of conjoined twin gestations and may require treatment during pregnancy to prevent complications such as preterm labor.[12,31]

Ethical, religious, and moral issues surrounding conjoined twin pregnancies and separation are complex. Accurate prenatal diagnosis and early determination of the extent and severity of the twin union enable determination of the feasibility of separation and prediction of postnatal outcomes. This is critical in early counseling of families, so that the options of termination versus near-term cesarean delivery can be discussed. Elective termination is recommended in cases

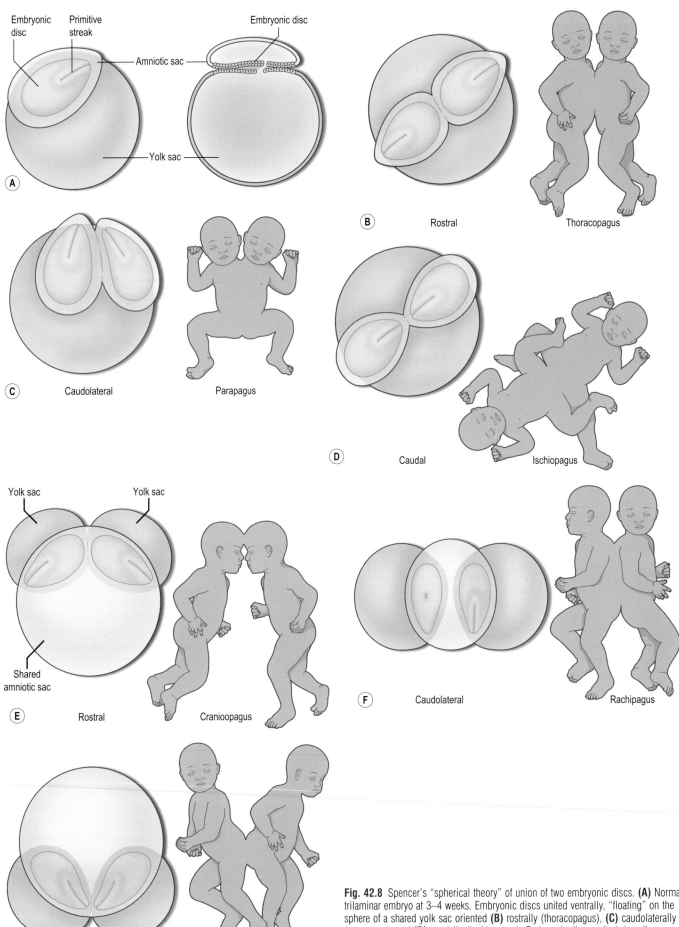

Fig. 42.8 Spencer's "spherical theory" of union of two embryonic discs. **(A)** Normal trilaminar embryo at 3–4 weeks. Embryonic discs united ventrally, "floating" on the sphere of a shared yolk sac oriented **(B)** rostrally (thoracopagus), **(C)** caudolaterally (parapagus), and **(D)** caudally (ischiopagus). Embryonic discs united dorsally, "floating" in a shared amniotic cavity oriented **(E)** rostrally (craniopagus), **(F)** mid-dorsally (rachipagus), and **(G)** caudally (pygopagus).

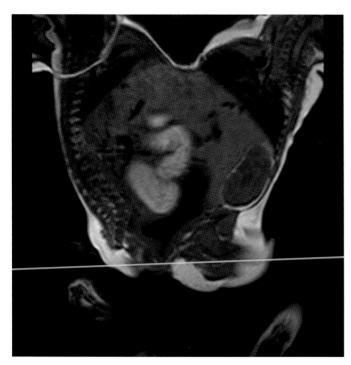

Fig. 42.9 Prenatal magnetic resonance imaging of ischiopagus twins with conjoined livers and colon and a cloacal malformation (Case 7).

where there is cerebral or cardiac fusion, and parents may also elect termination when the anticipated severity of deformity and quality of life following separation is unacceptable.[12] Early assessment also provides time for parental adjustment and predelivery planning; the involvement of psychologists, social workers, and ethicists may be beneficial in this decision-making and counseling process.

Treatment/surgical technique

Obstetric management

Near-term cesarean delivery at 36–38 weeks' gestation after confirming lung maturity and delivery at or near a pediatric surgical center is the recommended obstetric management. Although a number of vaginal deliveries have been reported in the literature, cesarean section is preferred for the safest management of the fetuses and the mother. Cesarean section also provides the opportunity for utilizing the EXIT procedure for the management of twins expected to have rapid cardiac deterioration.

Twins who survive delivery fall into three groups, determined predominantly by their cardiac anatomy: those who die shortly after birth, those who survive to planned separation, and those who require emergent separation after birth. Those who do not require emergent separation have a survival rate of 80–90% in most series. Emergent separation is required when one twin is dead or dying and threatening the survival of the other twin, or when a life-threatening and correctable congenital anomaly is present in one or both twins such as intestinal atresia, malrotation, ruptured omphalocele, or anorectal agenesis. Survival in this situation falls to 30–50%.

The obvious advantages of delayed separation include diminished risks of anesthesia, ability to confirm the anatomy and evaluate for other congenital anatomies, and the ability to ensure adequate wound coverage with preseparation tissue expansion.[12,14,15,32]

Preoperative planning

Elective separation may take place as early as 2–4 months after delivery. Maintenance in an intensive care setting during this time allows for close monitoring and stabilization of the infants, and nutritional supplementation as necessary to optimize growth and development preoperatively. Detailed postnatal investigations continue to confirm the conjoined anatomy and other possible congenital anomalies. Computed tomography scanning in addition to MRI may provide useful information about shared organs as well as skeletal anatomy, while MRI is preferred for delineating vascular anatomy; gastrointestinal contrast studies and angiography also may be utilized but have been less helpful.[3,10]

Assembly of a multidisciplinary team of various surgical subspecialists, neonatologists, anesthesiologists, and nurses, as well as the development of a comprehensive surgical and perioperative management plan, is critical to the success of twin separation. Two distinct anesthesia and surgery teams should be assembled, and the anesthetic management plan and operative steps in separation should be predetermined and reviewed. Both schematic diagrams as well as 3D models may be useful in planning separation.[3,33] Logistic details, including patient positioning, placement of lines and monitors, and operative room set-up and instrumentation, should not be overlooked.

Essential preoperative planning also includes proposed management of the soft tissues at the time of separation. If the shared anatomy allows for separation and survival of both twins, then wound closure becomes a critical issue. Assessment of the anticipated soft-tissue deficiency will determine the need for preseparation tissue expansion to accomplish stable wound closure. Without adequate skin coverage, the child is at risk for exposure of important viscera, frank evisceration, and sepsis. If the closure is too tight, embarrassment of cardiac and pulmonary function can occur, which can be fatal. Additional support materials may be necessary when large defects of the body walls, particularly the chest, abdomen, and pelvic floor, are created after separation. The plastic surgeon, therefore, is an essential member of the surgical team attempting twin separation.

Delineation of the vascular skin territories is important in planning the line of separation between co-twins, especially in cases of ischiopagus tripus where the common leg is to be sacrificed and the soft tissue divided for reconstruction and closure of both twins. Although magnetic resonance angiography and angiographic studies can illustrate large-vessel anatomy and extremity perfusion, they are inadequate at assessing the precise vascular territories of the skin at the level of the pelvis and along the extremity. Fluorescein previously has been used to evaluate perfusion and viability of skin flaps, ischemic extremities, injured bowel, and burn wounds.[34–38] The traditional fluorescein test uses qualitative visual assessment of tissue fluorescein delivery by inspection under ultraviolet light. A quantitative technique of intravenous fluorescein mapping employing a fiberoptic perfusion fluorometer

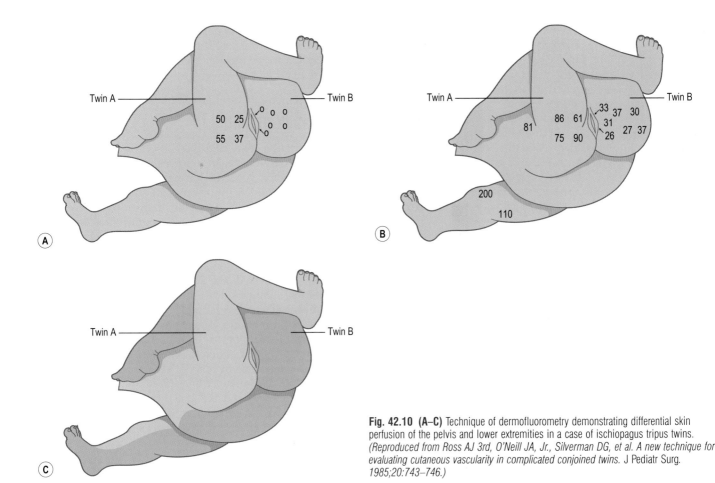

Fig. 42.10 (A–C) Technique of dermofluorometry demonstrating differential skin perfusion of the pelvis and lower extremities in a case of ischiopagus tripus twins. *(Reproduced from Ross AJ 3rd, O'Neill JA, Jr., Silverman DG, et al. A new technique for evaluating cutaneous vascularity in complicated conjoined twins. J Pediatr Surg. 1985;20:743–746.)*

was reported by Ross *et al*.[39] as helpful in defining the vascular territories and the line of separation between a pair of complicated ischiopagus twins at the Children's Hospital of Philadelphia in 1984 (Fig. 42.10).[39,40]

Role of the plastic surgeon

The separation of conjoined twins challenges the plastic surgeon to provide sufficient soft tissue to cover a significant area of intrinsic deficiency. Twin separation is analogous to separation of a simple or complex syndactyly, a congenital anomaly well known to plastic surgeons. As in the separation of syndactyly, insufficient tissue is present for resurfacing the conjoined interface so that skin grafts are generally needed, except in the simplest types. Similarly, the soft-tissue deficit in conjoined twins is twice the surface area of the canal joining the twins.[41] A variety of methods for providing soft-tissue coverage have been reported in the literature and include the use of skin grafts and skin substitute products, local skin flaps, pneumoperitoneum, and tissue expansion.

Skin grafting represents the least useful primary method of coverage in these patients. Skin grafting can be used only in the smallest of defects and requires an intact body wall for a bed. Only under the most extreme circumstances would a skin graft primarily be applied to abdominal viscera, although skin grafting is often used secondarily to treat wound-healing complications, not uncommon after twin separation. Today, various skin substitute products are available and can be used

to cover deficient areas of skin and also to reconstruct fascial defects.[42–44] As in traditional abdominal wall and chest wall reconstruction, both synthetic and biologic materials can be utilized, although biologics are much preferred in the pediatric population and where soft-tissue coverage may be precarious. Dermal replacement materials and other biologic meshes are favorable because they are quickly revascularized and promote ingrowth of new tissue; thus they are compatible with growth and are easily managed if exposure occurs.[45–47] Random-pattern or arterialized flaps of skin or skin and muscle can be used for coverage of small defects. Few case reports from the literature describe their use for coverage other than utilization of the third leg with fillet and sacrifice of the tripus. Indeed, many of the successful ischiopagus tripus separations have used the third leg for soft-tissue coverage.

Pneumoperitoneum has been reported by several surgical groups in the past. Mestel *et al*. utilized pneumoperitoneum in an ischiopagus tripus twin pair. They injected 500–1500 cc of air every 3 days and were able to increase the abdominal circumference by 12 cm. At separation, there was insufficient skin and the tripus was sacrificed to achieve a successful closure.[48] Yokomori *et al*. used pneumoperitoneum in conjunction with tissue expanders in an ischiopagus tripus twin pair, but again the tripus was sacrificed for successful coverage at the time of separation.[49] Wen-Sung Hung and co-workers also utilized pneumoperitoneum in an ischiopagus tripus with twice-weekly injection of 500–1500 cc of air. The circumference was increased by 19 cm, but again, the third leg was sacrificed for closure.[50] Although infection was felt to be a potential risk of pneumoperitoneum, it was not encountered by any of the investigators. In all three cases, however, an insufficient amount of soft tissue was generated to achieve successful closure without sacrifice of the third shared leg.

Tissue expansion represents a great advance in the ability to provide adequate soft-tissue coverage for the separation of conjoined twins. Although Neumann first introduced the concept in 1957, it was not until 1976 that tissue expansion became popular, with the introduction of the Radovan expander.[51,52] Since then, tissue expansion has been used widely by plastic surgeons for a variety of conditions where additional skin is needed. The first report of the successful use of tissue expansion for the separation of conjoined twins was by Zuker and his co-workers in 1986 for the successful separation of an ischiopagus conjoined twin pair. Five subcutaneous and two intraperitoneal expanders were used. One twin was closed successfully, but in the second, Marlex mesh reinforcement of the abdominal wall and split-thickness skin grafting were needed to complete the closure.[53] Numerous reports have followed, utilizing tissue expansion in both the intraperitoneal and subcutaneous positions.[41,53–55]

We advocate subcutaneous tissue expansion with placement of the maximum number of tissue expanders possible in all areas surrounding the canal separating the infants. They should be placed on the extremities in tripus cases as well, to facilitate harvest of adequate skin and subcutaneous tissue flaps without sacrifice of the lower extremities. Smooth-walled over-textured tissue expanders should be used for two reasons. In infants, the subcutaneous tissue layer is thin. Tissue expanders with a hard backing produce sharp edges, which can gradually erode through the skin at the margin of the expander. In addition, capsule formation is reduced with a textured implant surface, and thus prevent further thinning of the skin. Distant ports rather than integral ports are also preferred for the same reason. The thin skin overlying the tissue expander is subject to breakdown from repeated injections during the expansion process, thus increasing the risk of expander exposure with integral ports.

Clinical experience

The following 10 cases review the authors' experience with the separation of conjoined twins at the Children's Hospital of Philadelphia between 1980 and 2012. These examples highlight the lessons learned and present principles in surgical technique and patient management that may be helpful to future teams attempting conjoined twin separation.

Case 1 Thoracopagus and ischiopagus twins (1980)

Separation of this male thoracopagus and ischiopagus twin pair (Fig. 42.11) was performed at 2.3 years of age and represented the first use (1980) of tissue expanders in this series. One large circular 1000 cc Radovan expander was inserted beneath their shared abdominal skin through an incision in the xiphoid region and the umbilicus was released from its attachment to the abdominal wall. Despite the extra skin generated, it was inadequate and resulted in a tight closure on the smaller twin, resulting in

cardiopulmonary insufficiency and death. His skin was harvested and was frozen for eventual use for coverage of open wounds on the surviving twin. The skin grafts were frozen in liquid nitrogen after sequential passage through increasing concentrations of glycerol in saline, as described by Lehr and co-workers.[56] Closure of the surviving twin was achieved using the capsule along with the expanded skin. Granulation tissue developed on the capsular surface over the ensuing days and was successfully grafted with skin that had been harvested from the deceased twin.

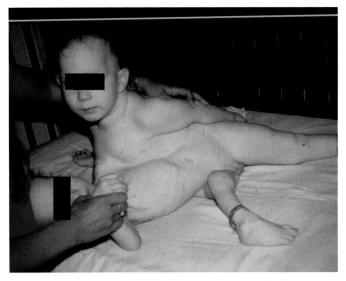

Fig. 42.11 Thoracopagus and ischiopagus twins prior to separation. Tissue expanders were used for the first time at the Children's Hospital of Philadelphia in 1980 to generate additional skin prior to separation.

Case 2 Ischiopagus twins (1984)

This ischiopagus tripus conjoined twin pair were joined from the sternum to the pelvis with a shared liver, terminal ileum, and colon. Each twin had a separate normal lower extremity and a shared extremity. Fluorescein studies were used in this case and proved quite helpful in assessing the territories of skin perfusion and determining the lines of separation. Preoperative studies demonstrated a clear line of separation along the pelvis and extremity with the blood supply to the extremity predominantly coming from twin A. The twins were separated along this line and the extremity was given to twin A. A pedicled flap from the shared thigh based on the lower abdomen of twin B was used to complete the cutaneous closure of twin B. Injection of fluorescein was performed again intraoperatively to assess the viability of this pedicled flap prior to closure and any non-viable tissue was trimmed. Because the knee joint of the shared extremity was not stable, the knee was disarticulated and the distal flap of skin and muscle used to complete the closure of twin A (see Fig. 42.10).

Case 3 Omphalopagus and ischiopagus twins (1988)

This omphalopagus and ischiopagus twin pair had a less complex connection between the infants from xiphoid to pelvis. They were treated with a single 1000 cc Radovan expander beneath the shared abdominal skin. The expander was introduced through a single incision in the xiphoid region with release of the umbilicus. Expansion was initiated in the hospital but was completed on an outpatient basis. A successful surgical separation with complete skin coverage was achieved without difficulty at 14.5 months of age, without the need for skin grafts.

Case 4 Ischiopagus twins (1992)

In this ischiopagus twin pair, additional expanders were used because of the soft-tissue inadequacy experienced in the first twin pair separation. At 3 months of age, a 700 cc round Radovan expander was used to expand the conjoined abdominal region and two smaller 250 cc rectangular expanders were used on the back, all with remote ports. At 4 days postoperatively, some skin necrosis was evident in the upper abdomen and the twins were taken back to the operating room. The area of necrosis was excised and the single abdominal tissue expander was replaced with two smaller 250 cc expanders. The patients were initially treated on a regular bed mattress with frequent, regular rotation from the abdomen to the back. Despite this, chronic pressure on their backs caused a threatened exposure of the posterior expanders. Transfer to a Clinitron bed improved the situation to some degree but the skin continued to thin over the posterior expanders. This prompted earlier surgical separation, which was performed at 5 months of age. The expanded abdominal skin was converted into bipedicled flaps to achieve closure and the remaining defects were grafted with autogenous split-thickness skin grafts. Once again, despite the use of additional expanders, there was insufficient soft tissue for complete wound coverage with the expanded skin. Further expansion would have been desirable.

Case 5 Ischiopagus tripus twins (1993)

This ischiopagus tripus twin pair were treated at 3.5 years of age using multiple rectangular tissue expanders. Two expanders were placed on the shared lower extremity, one on the anterior aspect and the other on the posterior aspect of the upper thigh; another was inserted on the back; and two more were placed in the abdominal region (Fig. 42.12). They were expanded over a period of 3 months with a total of 6 L of saline. During the expansion process, there was threatened erosion of the skin from the firm backing on the rectangular abdominal expander, and it was replaced with a smooth-walled expander. The twins were treated in a Clinitron bed for the entire expansion period, thus eliminating the problems with skin breakdown on the back. However, continuous movement of the legs caused chronic abrasion of the expanded skin overlying the tissue expander in the tripus against the expanded abdominal skin, and therefore, the legs were immobilized in a cast. Separation was successful with sufficient soft tissue to cover both twins without sacrifice of the tripus.

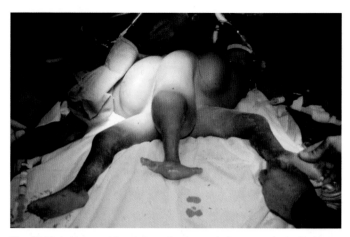

Fig. 42.12 Ischiopagus tripus twins – the abnormal tripus extremity is clearly demonstrated.

Case 6 Thoracopagus and omphalopagus twins (1999)

This thoracopagus and omphalopagus twin pair were separated at 6 months of age. They were joined from the level of the manubrium to the umbilicus with a shared liver, diaphragm, and chest cavity, although their hearts were not joined (Fig. 42.13). At 3 months of age, three rectangular-shaped 500 cc remote port tissue expanders were placed, one superior to the area of union in the thoracic area, and the other two at the inferior lateral aspect of the junction in the lower abdomen. These were filled over the next 3 months and produced ample expanded skin. At the time of separation, Gore-Tex patches were used by the general surgeons to close the chest cavities in both twins; there was sufficient soft tissue for uneventful and stable closure over these prostheses.

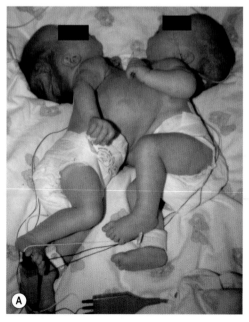

Fig. 42.13 (A) Thoracopagus and omphalopagus twins.

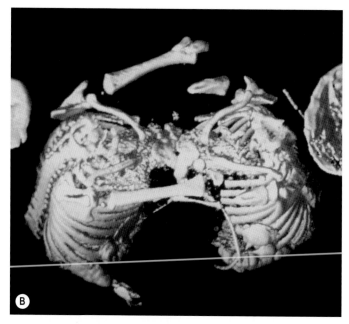

Fig. 42.13, cont'd (B) A 3D computed tomography scan was helpful in demonstrating shared skeletal structures.

Case 7   Ischiopagus twins (2001)

This ischiopagus twin pair were separated at 7 months of age. They had joined livers, a shared colon, and both had a cloacal malformation requiring a shared colostomy shortly after birth. Four expanders originally were placed in the thoracic and abdominal regions at 3 months of age (Fig. 42.14A). The patients were taken back to the operating room twice during the expansion process because of expander complications. The thoracic expander was removed due to some overlying skin necrosis and one of the lateral abdominal expanders was removed due to threatened exposure and a seroma. One month later, two additional expanders were placed in the thoracic and abdominal regions since a greater soft-tissue requirement was anticipated. Expansion was resumed uneventfully, and separation was performed 3 months later. Vicryl mesh was used in closure of the abdominal wall due to contamination from the colostomy during the procedure with a plan for more definitive abdominal wall reconstruction in the future. Local advancement and rotation flaps of the expanded thoracic and abdominal skin were used and complete coverage of the abdominal defect was obtained in one twin. In the second twin, a small lateral defect remained after rotation of the abdominal skin flap; vacuum-assisted closure therapy hastened wound healing, and the defect was eventually covered with an autologous skin graft (Fig. 42.14B).

Case 8   Omphalopagus twins (2007)

This pair shared a portion of liver and duodenum. Four expanders were placed in subcutaneous pockets, but one developed a leak during the expansion process. Acellular dermal matrix was used to compensate for insufficient skin coverage over the central abdomen (Fig. 42.15).

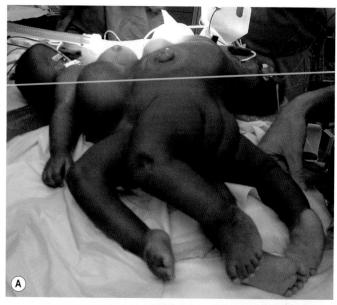

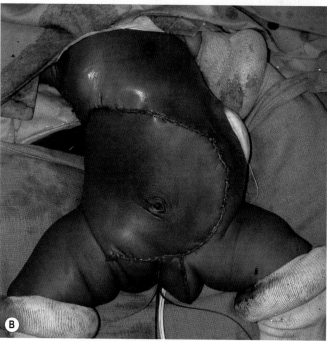

Fig. 42.14 (A) Ischiopagus twins with shared liver and colon, with tissue expanders in place. The shared colostomy is visible. **(B)** Twin A with complete skin closure of abdominal wall.

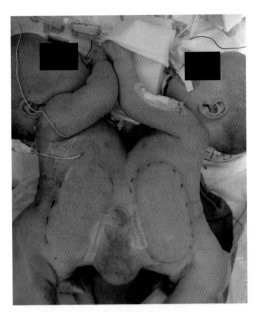

Fig. 42.15 Omphalopagus twins with newly placed expanders. The injection ports are dorsally located. Two additional expanders were placed on the contralateral side.

Case 9   Thoracopagus and omphalopagus twins (2011)

This complex pair were fused from chest to abdomen including conjoined pericardium, diaphragm, communicating cardiac structure, long segment jejunum, and biliary tree. One of the twins required cardiac surgical intervention through a right thoracotomy at 2 months of age due to a hypoplastic right ventricle and pulmonary stenosis. Four expanders were placed at 3.5 months and separation occurred at 8 months of age. Thoracoplasty was performed in one twin to reposition the ribs and partial manubrium, then Gore-Tex patches were used in both twins to complete chest closure. After complex hepatobiliary and intestinal reconstruction, the large abdominal defects in both twins were closed with absorbable Vicryl mesh followed by Strattice porcine dermal matrix. Despite aggressive mobilization of the skin flap, defects remained which were treated with vacuum-assisted sponge devices. In one twin, the area was granulated and re-epithelialized without the need for skin grafting. The second twin with the hypoplastic right heart suffered a complicated postoperative cardiac and respiratory course, with eventual demise 8 months post-separation.

Case 10   Thoracopagus and omphalopagus twins (2012)

This pair shared pericardium, diaphragm, and liver. At 3 months of age, four tissue expanders were placed on the lateral chest and abdominal walls adjacent to the central conjoined area, with care taken to avoid trauma to the breast bud, and 5 months later, the twins were separated successfully. Large chest and abdominal wall defects with exposed heart and areas of the liver, diaphragm, and intestines in both twins were reconstructed with Vicryl

---

absorbable mesh covered by Strattice porcine dermal matrix and expanded skin. One twin developed a partial wound dehiscence with exposed Strattice. After slow secondary healing, this site developed a ventral hernia, which was successfully repaired at age 2 years with permanent mesh.

Postoperative care

Supportive care in an intensive care unit setting with meticulous monitoring is essential for postoperative stabilization of the separated infants. Elective paralysis and ventilation for 24–48 h are preferable during the immediate postoperative period for fluid and electrolyte replacement and cardiac stabilization. Perioperative antibiotics and strict infectious precautions are also recommended to avoid sepsis.

Perioperative pressure reduction strategies are critical for successful management of the soft tissues. A Clinitron bed is recommended during tissue expansion to optimize soft-tissue viability and prevent pressure-related ulcerations in dependent areas or over the expanders. This should be continued during the early postoperative period of immobilization to augment postoperative wound healing, especially when flaps and grafts have been utilized in closure. Adjunctive techniques such as frequent turning, supportive gel padding, and immobilization of the extremities when necessary to prevent traumatic ulcerations, should also be employed.

Continued nutritional support is equally critical. More often than not, one of the infants is smaller and less well nourished. The stress of prolonged treatment and repeated operations compounds this problem, placing the infants at greater risk for wound-healing and infectious complications. In this situation, the use of supplemental parenteral or enteral feedings is beneficial, and should be considered in most cases.

Outcomes, prognosis, and complications

Wound-healing complications are common postoperatively. Postoperative vacuum-assisted closure therapy can be useful in managing wound dehiscence or flap losses, and secondary skin grafting and surgical revision are frequently necessary to manage soft-tissue wounds and unacceptable scarring.

The overall success of conjoined twin separation depends on the experience and preparedness of the treating team and the resources available at the pediatric specialty center. Recent advances in imaging techniques for prenatal diagnosis, pre- and postoperative critical care management, and anesthetic care have improved outcomes and survival rates in general. Comprehensive long-term care by a multispecialty team is critical in the management of these patients from prenatal diagnosis to postoperative follow-up to address their complex issues. Follow-up at the same institution is recommended due to the anatomic complexity of these patients, and it also allows for determination of long-term outcomes.

Access the complete reference list online at **http://www.expertconsult.com**

1. Bates AW. Conjoined twins in the 16th century. *Twin Res.* 2002;5: 521–528.

3. Redett R, Zucker RM. Conjoined twins. In: Bentz M, Bauer BS, Zucker RM, eds. *Principles and Practice of Pediatric Plastic Surgery.* St. Louis: Quality Medical Publishing; 2008:185–212. *A well-rounded account of perioperative and operative considerations relating to the separation of conjoined twins is presented.*

5. Spitz L. Surgery for conjoined twins. *Ann R Coll Surg Engl.* 2003;85:230–235.

6. Spitz L, Kiely EM. Conjoined twins. *JAMA.* 2003;289:1307–1310. *The authors begin with an account of conjoined twin reports in history. A review of classification, diagnosis, and management follows.*

10. Spitz L. Conjoined twins. *Br J Surg.* 1996;83:1028–1030. *This brief reports offers the author's perspective from an experience of 10 sets of conjoined twins over a decade. Special mention is made of the potential for heavy intraoperative blood loss and the fragility of these patients after separation.*

12. O'Neill JA Jr. Conjoined twins. In: Grosfeld JL, O'Neill JA Jr, Fonkalsrud EW, et al., eds. *Pediatric Surgery.* Philadelphia: Mosby; 2006 *This chapter is a review of topics ranging from prenatal diagnosis to ethical considerations related to conjoined twins. Particularly useful is the authors' systems-based approach to surgical technique.*

14. Mackenzie TC, Crombleholme TM, Johnson MP, et al. The natural history of prenatally diagnosed conjoined twins. *J Pediatr Surg.* 2002;37:303–309.

21. Walker M, Browd SR. Craniopagus twins: embryology, classification, surgical anatomy, and separation. *Childs Nerv Syst.* 2004;20:554–566.

28. Spencer R. Theoretical and analytical embryology of conjoined twins: part I: embryogenesis. *Clin Anat.* 2000;13:36–53. *This review spans over 1200 cases of conjoined twins. Observations drawn from these cases form the basis for a discussion of the embryology leading to this pathology.*

41. Zubowicz VN, Ricketts R. Use of skin expansion in separation of conjoined twins. *Ann Plast Surg.* 1988;20:272–276.

43

Reconstruction of urogenital defects: Congenital

Mohan S. Gundeti, Michael C. Large, and William R. Boysen

 Access video content for this chapter online at expertconsult.com

SYNOPSIS

- Hypospadias is common, perhaps increasing in incidence, and may be managed through multiple surgical approaches. Penoscrotal transposition and chordee commonly accompany hypospadias and may be treated concomitantly.
- Reconstruction of cloacal or urogenital sinus abnormalities is complex, often requiring multiple surgical disciplines and stages to obtain optimal functional outcomes. Timing of reconstruction for ambiguous genitalia remains controversial, but advancement in knowledge of the neuroanatomic innervation has allowed for reconstruction with good preservation of function.
- Technique for repair of bladder and cloacal exstrophy continues to evolve, with debate over single versus staged repair.

Introduction

The reconstructive techniques for congenital urogenital defects are broad ranging, and the indications for intervention vary from emergent to elective. Herein the authors will discuss the normal development of the urogenital tract, followed by a discussion of some common female and male disorders and their surgical repairs. The spectrum of hypospadias disorders will be addressed first, followed by cloacal and urogenital sinus disorders, and a brief discussion of variant presentations that may include clitoromegaly, exstrophy, and/or epispadias. For each condition, attention will be given to diagnosis and evaluation, representative surgical techniques, potential complications, and expected short-term and long-term outcomes. In general, reconstructive techniques for urologic disorders have satisfactory outcomes, but the importance of proper surgical timing and patient selection may not be understated.

Normal development

The cloaca appears during the 2nd gestational week, with the urorectal septum forming during week 4 (Fig. 43.1). The urorectal septum fuses with the cloacal membrane by week 7. Defects of the cloacal membrane may result in bladder or cloacal exstrophy and epispadias. The Mullerian ducts fuse to become the uterovaginal canal. Distally, the urogenital sinus forms the vestibule and the intervening sinovaginal bulbs canalize to form the distal vaginal canal. Paramesonephric abnormalities are frequently associated with ipsilateral renal anomalies, partly based upon their proximity during development. Anomalies of agenesis and fusion may occur. When the urogenital sinus fails to develop into the distal vagina, atresia results; agenesis occurs when the proximal third of the vagina fails to develop in a 46XX phenotypic female. Transverse septa arise from failure of fusion or canalization of the urogenital sinus and Mullerian ducts. Mayer–Rokitansky–Kuster–Hauser syndrome consists of Mullerian aplasia, often accompanied by renal and cervicothoracic dysplasias.

Differentiation of the external genitalia begins around 7–8 weeks' gestation. The male gonads differentiate secondary to the transcription of the *SRY* gene, thereby producing testosterone. The distance between anus and genitalia increases, the phallus elongates, the genital folds fuse, the preputial folds form and fuse dorsally, and during the 11th gestational week, the urethral folds fuse ventrally. If the genital folds fail to fuse, as in hypospadias, the preputial folds also fail to fuse ventrally, resulting in excessive dorsal preputial tissue. By week 16, the glandular urethra forms. The glandular portion of the urethra is lined by squamous epithelium, which likely also arises from urogenital sinus origin, but then undergoes differentiation.[1] Histologically, the hypospadiac urethral plate contains sinusoids of urethral spongiosum and no scar tissue. The innervation of the hypospadiac penis is like that of the normal penis: the pudendal nerve gives off the dorsal nerve, which travels as two bundles on either side of 12 o'clock.

In females, the folds of the urogenital sinus remain open and become the labia majora, the labioscrotal folds form the labia minora, the genital tubercle becomes the clitoris, and the urogenital sinus becomes the lower vagina and urethra. An excess or absence of intrauterine androgens at 9–14 weeks can alter this process, leading to ambiguous external genitalia.

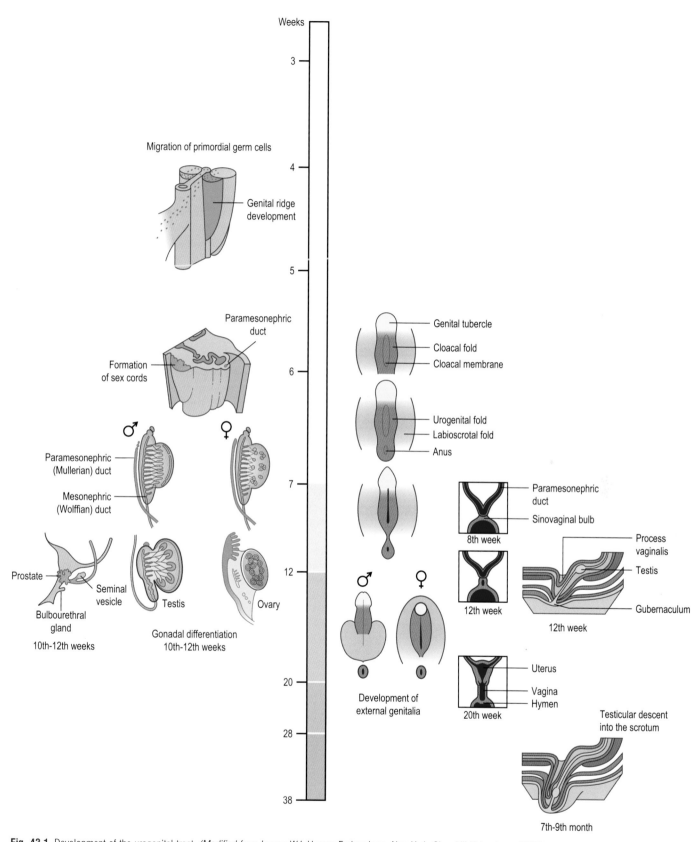

Fig. 43.1 Development of the urogenital tract. *(Modified from Larsen WJ.* Human Embryology. *New York: Churchill Livingstone; 1997.)*

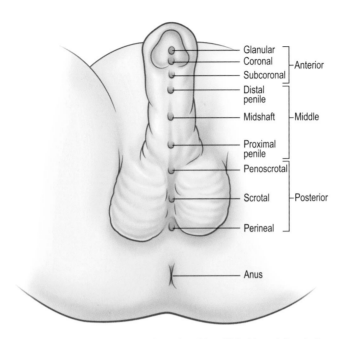

Fig. 43.2 Spectrum of hypospadias. *(Reproduced from Wein AJ, et al.* Campbell-Walsh Urology, *9th edn. Philadelphia: Saunders; 2007.)*

The clitoral innervation travels along the dorsal surface of the clitoris before entering the corporal tissue, and care must be taken not to dissect or mobilize this area during reconstruction to preserve innervation and future sexual function.

Hypospadias

Background, diagnosis, and patient selection

Hypospadias occurs when the development of the urethral spongiosum and prepuce halts, resulting in a meatal location proximal to that of the distal glans. A hypospadiac meatus is often accompanied by penile chordee as the normal embryologic correction of curvature is arrested. The severity of hypospadias is dictated by associated chordee, urethral plate width, glans volume, phallus size, and meatal location, which can range from perineal to glanular (Figs. 43.2 &

43.3). The more severe the hypospadias, the more likely it is accompanied by chordee and penoscrotal transposition (Figs. 43.4 & 43.5).

The incidence of hypospadias is roughly 1:300 male births, an increase from 2:1000 male births in 1970. There is nearly a nine-fold increase in hypospadias in monozygotic twins. A polygenic, multifactorial etiology is most likely. Some cases may be caused by testosterone, dihydrotestosterone, or androgen receptor deficiencies, but these are found in only 5% of cases. There are also hypotheses that maternal environmental exposures such as phthalate in some plastics and estrogens in food, cosmetics, and pesticides can increase the risk of hypospadias, though there is not definitive evidence to support this. Theories of chordee include incomplete development of the urethral plate, abnormal urethral meatal mesenchyme, and disproportional corporal growth.

Hypospadias is frequently diagnosed at birth on physical examination, although later diagnoses are not uncommon. Patients with bilateral impalpable gonads and hypospadias have a disorder of sexual differentiation until proven otherwise, and karyotype is indicated.

Patient selection is most pertinent to hypospadias repair. The meatal location, glans volume, penile length, presence of penoscrotal transposition and/or chordee, and width and depth of the urethral plate all weigh in the surgeon's selection of technique. In general, distal hypospadias with favorable features may be treated by tubularized incised plate (TIP) procedure with meatoplasty and glanuloplasty (MAGPI) techniques, while proximal hypospadias are frequently treated by two-staged graft or onlay island flap repairs.

The optimal timing for hypospadias repair is 6 months of age in a full-term male, allowing the glans and phallus to grow during the testosterone surge that occurs naturally between 4 and 6 months of age. Some 92% of pediatric urologists perform a TIP procedure for distal hypospadias.[2] Proximal hypospadias without curvature is repaired by TIP or onlay island flap by equal proportions of urologists, while proximal hypospadias with severe chordee is most often repaired by a staged repair.[3] Intramuscular testosterone injections of 25 mg/dose or 2 mg/kg per dose may be administered up to three times prior to repair, in an attempt to improve penile vascularity and tissue robustness, thereby facilitating subsequent surgery. However, studies assessing the effect of

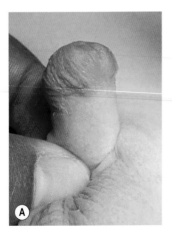
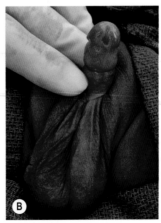
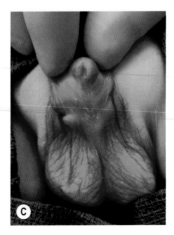
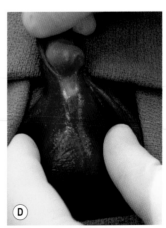

Fig. 43.3 (A) Glanular, **(B)** coronal, **(C)** penoscrotal, and **(D)** perineal hypospadias.

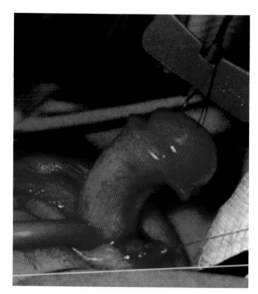

Fig. 43.4 Intraoperative depiction of chordee.

preoperative testosterone on postoperative complication rate have yielded mixed results, leaving the role of preoperative hormone stimulation unclear.[4] In the authors' experience, there is a role for preoperative testosterone in patients with unfavorable preoperative factors such as small glans size and narrow urethral plate. Outcomes for these patients will likely be impacted by many factors in addition to preoperative testosterone, including surgical technique.

Treatment/surgical technique

The goal of hypospadias repair is to allow for standing urination and normal ejaculatory function, while providing a slit-like terminal meatus. The technique should be simplistic with readily reproducible results. The prepuce may or may not be reconstructed depending upon cultural and patient expectations. Scrotoplasty may be performed for significant penoscrotal transposition (Fig. 43.6). Baskin and Ebbers delineate five steps apparent in all hypospadias repairs: orthoplasty (straightening of the penis), urethroplasty, meato- and glanuloplasty, scrotoplasty, and epithelial coverage.[5] Herein the authors will highlight some of the more common repair techniques.

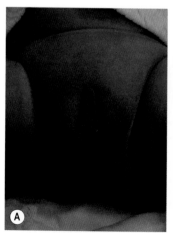

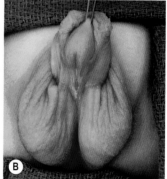

Fig. 43.5 (A,B) Penoscrotal transposition.

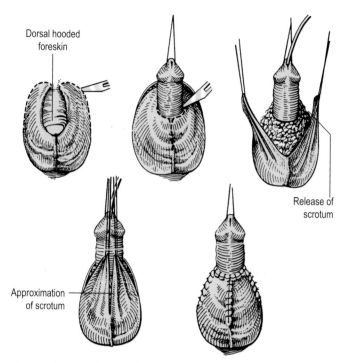

Fig. 43.6 Penoscrotal transposition correction. *(Reproduced from Wein AJ, et al. Campbell-Walsh Urology, 9th edn. Philadelphia: Saunders. 2007.)*

Meatoplasty and glanuloplasty

The MAGPI repair is best suited for the individual with a distal or anterior hypospadias. Often, these patients are able to void with a straight stream, but the repair is requested for social, cultural, or parental concerns. The initial incision is circumferential, 5 mm proximal to the glans, and degloving is performed, allowing for orthoplasty (Fig. 43.7). Any bridge within the urethral plate is incised and then repaired in Heineke–Mikulicz fashion so that the distal glanular groove and the more proximal hypospadiac meatus are in continuity. A stay stitch allows for distal advancement of the meatus, and the glans edges are subsequently trimmed and approximated in two-layer fashion.

Tubularized incised plate repair

For all distal variants of hypospadias, it is recommended that surgeons choose a single technique that allows for reproducible outcomes with 95% success rates. Easily reproducible, the TIP repair is the authors' initial choice for patients with distal hypospadias. The urethral plate is measured in width, and diluted epinephrine may be injected prior to incision (though this is not the authors' practice). A vertical incision is made alongside each edge of the urethral plate, and a crossing incision connects the two at the proximal extent of the meatus. The depth of the lateral incisions is based upon the glans volume and plate size; the crossing incision should be exceptionally thin, serving simply to disconnect the ventral penile skin from the underlying urethra, while avoiding entrance into the urethral lumen (Fig. 43.8). Similar to the MAGPI repair, a circumferential incision extends each side from the crossing incision, approximately 5 mm from the coronal margin. The penis is degloved, chordee is assessed, and orthoplasty is performed if indicated. The midline of the plate is then incised utilizing an ultrafine-tipped

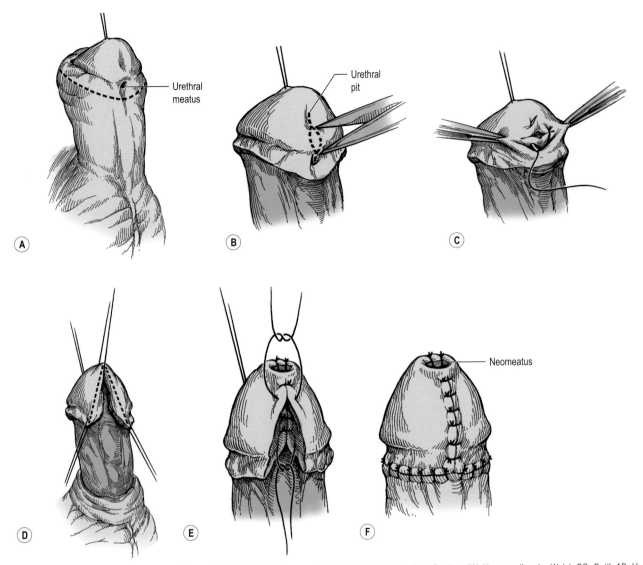

Fig. 43.7 (A–F) Meatoplasty and glanuloplasty (MAGPI) for distal hypospadias defects. *(Reprinted from Duckett JW. Hypospadias. In: Walsh PC, Retik AB, Vaughan ED Jr, Wein AJ (eds). Campbell's Urology, 7th edn. Philadelphia, WB Saunders; 1998.)*

ophthalmologic knife, and the plate is tubularized around a 5 or 8 French feeding tube, which serves as a urethral stent. Glans flaps are created laterally, making sure the tissue is thick enough to provide food coverage and a tension free closure. A second layer of dartos tissue or spongiosal tissue is rotated to cover the urethral suture line. The glans is reapproximated in two layers, and the shaft is closed at midline to complete the repair. In the case of a very shallow urethral groove or small glans, a free graft may be interposed between the posterior TIP defect, thereby allowing for larger ultimate circumference.[6]

Onlay island flap repair

Onlay island flap repair is commonly employed for midshaft hypospadias defects, although distal applications also exist.[7] Two stay stitches are placed at corners of the prepuce (Fig. 43.9). Similar to a TIP repair, U-shaped and circumferential subcoronal incisions are performed. Degloving and orthoplasty follow, after which the distance from meatus to distal glans tip is measured. A rectangular preputial onlay graft is

Hints and tips

- A glans traction suture helps with intraoperative manipulation of the penis
- Placement of a penile tourniquet aids in visualization and can be safely used for 45 min without compromising outcomes (in the authors' experience)
- Minimization of tissue handling and creation of tension-free anastomoses optimize tissue health
- Bipolar electrocautery forceps are preferable to monopolar forceps for hemostasis
- A 2.5× or greater loupes or the surgical microscope may improve tissue manipulation

harvested and rotated to the ventrum along its pedicle. A second layer of vascularized inner preputial tissue may be utilized for coverage before glans approximation and closure. The authors have rarely used this technique, as they prefer either the TIP or two-stage repair when TIP is not feasible.

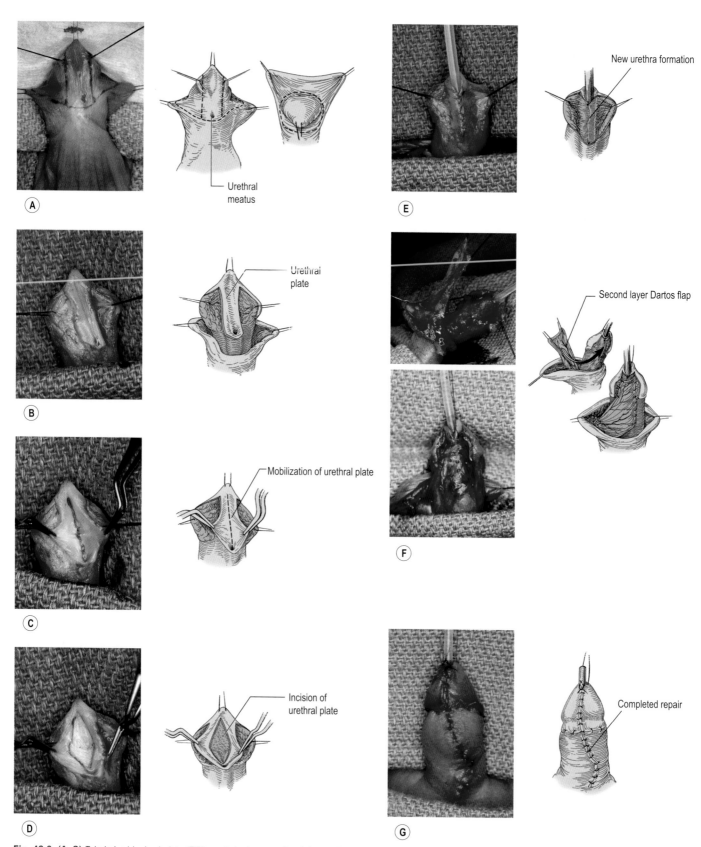

Fig. 43.8 (A–G) Tubularized incised plate (TIP) repair for hypospadias defects. *(Reprinted from Retik AB, Borer JG. Primary and reoperative hypospadias repair with the Snodgrass technique.* World J Urol. *1998;16:186.)*

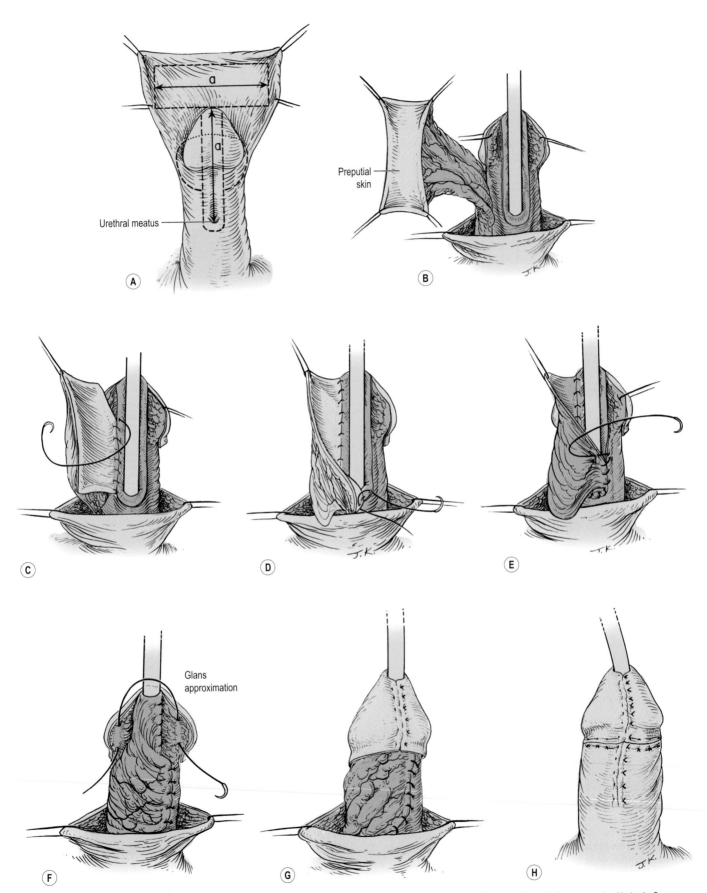

Fig. 43.9 (A–H) Onlay island flap repair for hypospadias defects. *(Reprinted from Atala A, Retik AB. Hypospadias. In: Libertino JA (ed.). Reconstructive Urologic Surgery, 3rd edn. St. Louis: Mosby–Year Book; 1998.)*

Two-stage repair

For proximal hypospadias, a two-stage repair often affords the greatest chance for long-term success, albeit with the limitation of multiple surgeries separated by 6 months or more. A subcoronal circumferential incision is made, as well as a longitudinal incision from glans tip to hypospadiac meatus (Figs. 43.10–43.12). Once the healthy urethral plate is identified, the remaining distal plate is excised. The glans is split longitudinally, and the resulting urethral defect measured. If of sufficient size, the prepuce may be utilized as either a pedicled flap or free graft (Video 43.1 ▶). If insufficient, a free graft of buccal mucosa is performed with a 1:1 ratio of graft to site sizing. The buccal tissue has an extensively vascularized lamina propria, so long-term shrinkage is minimal. Second-stage repair is performed by tubularization of the graft with second-layer coverage before final epithelial approximation (see Fig. 43.11 and Video 43.2 ▶).

Orthoplasty

While discussion of chordee repair is contained elsewhere (Vol. 4, Chapter 13), a brief description of the authors' chosen approach to orthoplasty will follow. After complete degloving of the penis, <10% of patients with hypospadias require penile straightening.[8] A Gittes test is performed, during which a penile tourniquet is tightened, and a small-gauge butterfly needle is placed through the glans directly into one of the corpora cavernosa. Sterile saline is slowly injected into the corpus until an erection is achieved, and any chordee is elucidated. As anatomic studies have shown, a paucity or absence of neural structures at the 12 o'clock position of the penile shaft, the authors repair all instances of chordee by simple midline dorsal plication (Fig. 43.13) and no longer perform historical, more elaborate techniques.[5] The authors prefer to avoid Nesbit corporal plication or corporal grafts due to concerns for neuronal damage, erectile dysfunction, and venous leak. However, long-term data on outcomes for these techniques are lacking.

Postoperative care

Hypospadias repair is primarily an outpatient procedure. Pain control is ameliorated by a preoperative caudal nerve block. A soft 5 or 8 French feeding tube is utilized to stent the urethra. A dressing consisting of three supportive DuoDerm strips followed by a Tegaderm wrap serves to keep the penis elevated, thereby minimizing swelling.

Hints and tips

- Glans-to-glans approximation is critical in preventing meatal regression after meatoplasty and glanuloplasty (MAGPI) repair
- After degloving and orthoplasty of the penis, an initially distal hypospadias may now appear proximal and require a more extensive repair. Similarly, in a patient with poor distal urethral tissue, proximal dissection to healthy spongiosum may convert a distal hypospadiac meatus to a proximal defect
- Urinary diversion with catheter for 5–7 days is crucial for optimizing outcomes

---

Complications and outcomes

The mantra of "the first chance being the best chance" is certainly true for hypospadias repair. While successful outcomes are the norm, those who have poor surgical outcomes are at risk for scarring and abnormal-appearing genitalia, difficulty in urinating, and long-term sexual and relationship difficulties. Bleeding and catheter dislodgement are the most common issues encountered immediately postoperatively. A second layer of coverage is the single best measure for preventing urethrocutaneous fistula formation. Less common complications include meatal stenosis, infection, urethral diverticula and stricture, and balanitis xerotica obliterans (BXO). Diverticula, strictures, and BXO are more common with two-stage repairs or those with replacement urethroplasty with buccal mucosal graft.

With regard to the MAGPI repair, Duckett and Snyder have described 1000 patients with fistulae in 0.5%, meatal retraction in 0.06%, and chordee in 0.1% at mean follow-up of 2 months.[9] These results have failed to be reproduced, with other groups noting that at 2 years nearly 15% had complete meatal regression.[10] Data for the TIP repair are evolving. A multicenter review of over 2000 patients suggested a complication rate of 9%.[11] Fistulae occur in 5%, meatal stenosis in 2%, and glans dehiscence in 5%.[12]

A large series of onlay island flap repairs shows a 6% urethrocutaneous fistula and 9% reoperation rate.[13] In a review of 600 patients with two-stage repair, the majority preputial, a first-stage revision was required in 4%, and second-stage fistulae occurred in 6%, although the use of a dartos flap for second-layer closure may serve to limit this rate further.[14]

Secondary procedures for hypospadias are sometimes required in the event of primary failure. Distal or midshaft hypospadias repairs should be single-staged and definitive. When complications such as urethrocutaneous fistulae do occur, primary repair, while attempted by some, is cautioned. Our experience has echoed that of Bracka, where two-stage buccal mucosa repair has yielded good results for those with previous failed hypospadias repair.[14]

Data regarding long-term cosmesis, urinary function, and sexual function remain quite limited, though this is an area of ongoing study. Numerous validated outcome assessment scales have been developed including the Penile Perception Score[15] and the Hypospadias Objective Penile Evaluation (HOPE) score,[16] which will hopefully facilitate future studies assessing these outcomes among men who have undergone hypospadias repair. Regardless of the assessment scale used, the data on long-term outcomes are limited and mixed, with some series reporting higher rates of sexual dysfunction among men who have undergone hypospadias repair and others showing no difference compared with matched controls.[17] As expected, severity of hypospadias prior to surgery correlates with the degree of sexual dysfunction and dissatisfaction with cosmetic result.[18]

Ambiguous genitalia, persistent cloaca, and urogenital sinus disorders

Background, diagnosis, and work-up

Urogenital sinus abnormalities may be isolated or associated with congenital adrenal hyperplasia (CAH), most often due

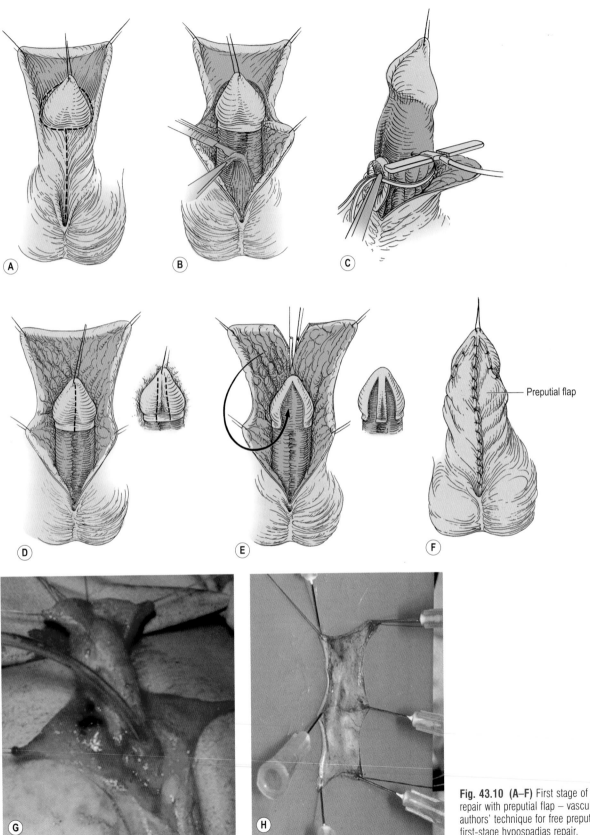

Preputial flap

Fig. 43.10 (A–F) First stage of two-stage hypospadias repair with preputial flap – vascularized. **(G,H)** The authors' technique for free preputial/buccal graft for first-stage hypospadias repair.

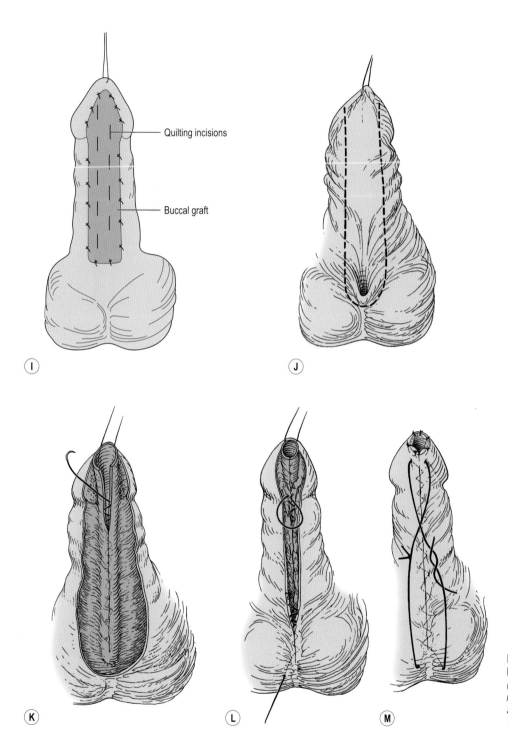

Quilting incisions

Buccal graft

Ⓘ Ⓙ

Ⓚ Ⓛ Ⓜ

Fig. 43.10, cont'd (I–M) Second-stage
hypospadias repair of two-stage repair.
*(Reprinted from Retik AB, Borer JG. Primary and
reoperative hypospadias repair with the
Snodgrass technique.* World J Urol.
1998;16:186.)

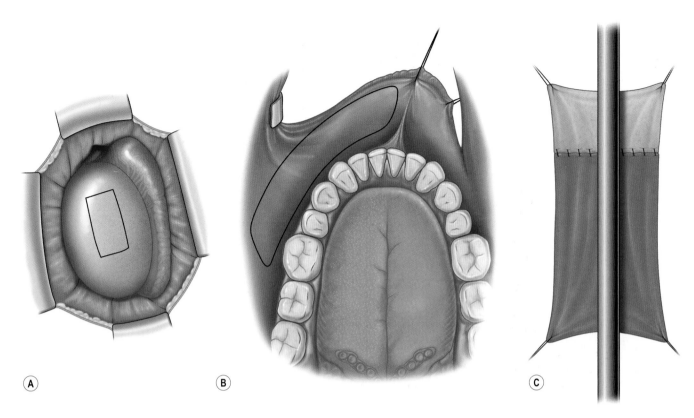

Fig. 43.11 **(A,B)** Harvesting the buccal mucosal graft. **(C)** Buccal mucosal onlay graft with catheter overlying.

to 21-hydroxylase deficiency. These conditions are rare, with incidence of CAH approximately 1:5000–15000, UG sinus abnormality 0.6:10000, and persistent cloaca 1:20000.

The work-up of a newborn with ambiguous genitalia should involve multidisciplinary teams and critical associations such as CAH should be ruled out. Fluid and electrolyte balance and blood pressure control should be maintained. Examination should note any suprapubic mass or ascites, sacral dimples, genitalia curvature and size, palpability of gonads, location of anus and perineal orifices, and pigmentation. Karyotype and adrenal biochemical studies should be undertaken, with prompt replacement of cortisol and fludrocortisone in cases of congenital adrenal hyperplasia. *In utero* exposure to androgenic substances should be investigated, as should a family history of infantile death. Radiographic and endoscopic evaluations of the genitalia and urinary tract are indicated, including abdominal X-ray and ultrasound, genitography, echocardiography, lumbar magnetic resonance imaging (for patients with isolated cloacal malformation due to association with VACTERL malformations), and cystoscopy with vaginoscopy for planning approach to surgical repair.

The Prader classification system has classically been used to describe urogenital sinus abnormalities, which can range widely in severity and degree of feminine or masculine appearance.[19] An updated classification system has been described to further delineate the spectrum of disorders that exist, with attention paid to the phallic length/width and true vaginal location in addition to the external appearance described by Prader.[20] The clinical utility of this updated classification system remains unclear.

Treatment/surgical technique

The optimal timing of surgical repair remains controversial, and consideration must be made to the child's long-term psychosexual development and gender satisfaction.[21] Consultation with an experienced multidisciplinary team is recommended prior to surgery. In particular, a pediatric surgeon with experience in gastrointestinal surgery is needed for the anorectoplasty component of cloacal repair.

Abnormalities of the urogenital sinus may be divided into low or high confluence defects. A confluence of the urogenital sinus distal to the urinary sphincter is considered low; those proximal are high. Common channel length of 3 cm is also used to differentiate low and high confluence defects. Goals of feminizing genitoplasty should include creation of normal appearing external female genitalia, creation of an unobstructed urinary tract free of incontinence and recurrent infection, and allowance of normal adult reproductive and sexual function.[22] Repair may involve nerve sparing reduction clitoroplasty, development of labial folds, and construction of a capacious vagina. The perineal approach is commonly preferred except in high variant cases, where prone positioning is preferred initially.

Lower confluences may be repaired by cut-back vaginoplasty for simple labial adhesions, flap vaginoplasty, or vaginal pull-through. In a flap vaginoplasty, a posterior perineal flap is fashioned anterior to the rectum (Fig. 43.14). The posterior urogenital sinus wall is incised and subsequently sutured to either side of the interposing posterior skin flap. The anterior vaginal wall remains intact.

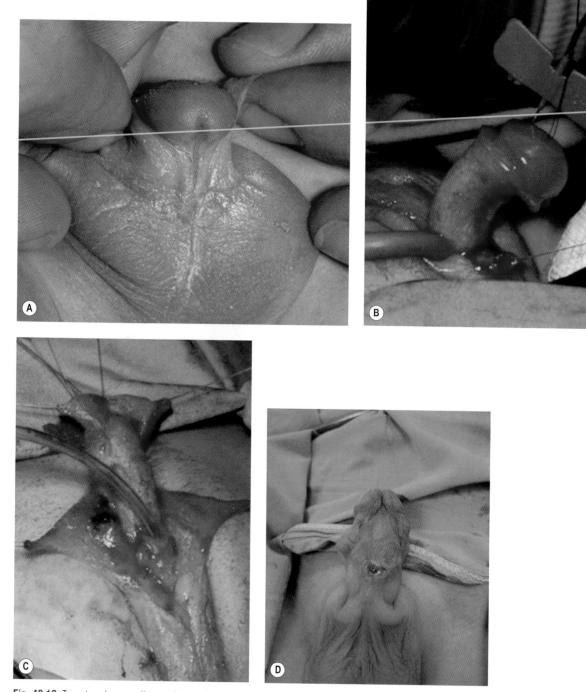

Fig. 43.12 Two-stage hypospadias repair with chordee correction. **(A)** Perineal hypospadias; **(B)** chordee; **(C)** corrected chordee; **(D)** completed first-stage repair 6 months postoperatively;

Continued

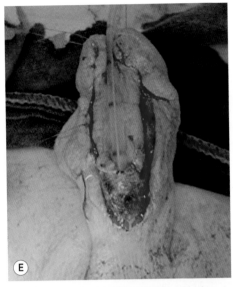

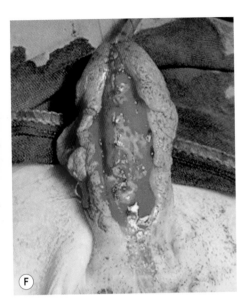

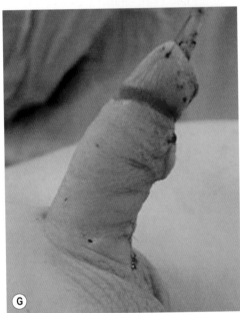

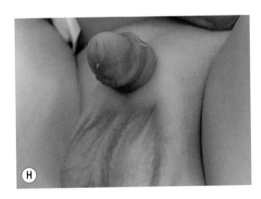

Fig. 43.12, cont'd (E–G) second-stage hypospadias repair depicting free preputial and delayed tubularization. (H) The final appearance 1 year after the second-stage repair.

For some low and all high confluence sinuses, total urogenital mobilization may be indicated with subsequent pull-through vaginoplasty. Partial urogenital mobilization has also been described and can be considered in cases where adequate mobilization is achieved without dissection under the pubic bone and up to the bladder neck. To perform urogenital mobilization, the authors prefer the technique described by Rink and Cain.[23] With the child in the lithotomy position, cystoscopy and vaginoscopy is performed to assess the common channel. A Fogarty catheter is placed in the vagina and a Foley catheter in the bladder to facilitate manipulation as needed. The child is then returned to the supine position and a traction suture is placed through the clitoris. Clitoroplasty, described below, can be performed at this time if desired. To begin total urogenital mobilization, the sinus is dissected circumferentially. The dissection is carried to the pubourethral ligament anteriorly behind the pubic bone and posterior to the vagina, to allow mobilization of the entire urogenital complex down to the perineum. In partial urogenital mobilization, the dissection is stopped at the pubourethral ligament. The urogenital sinus is then dissected from the corporal bodies. Traction sutures can be placed around the sinus meatus to aid in exposure. An omega flap is then raised posteriorly to expose the posterior aspect of the UG sinus. The posterior dissection can be challenging, and care must be taken to avoid injury to the rectum or entry into the UG sinus. Next, the posterior wall of the vagina is opened over the Fogarty catheter between stay sutures. If a tension-free anastomosis to the perineum cannot be achieved without further mobilization, then total urogenital mobilization must be performed with additional dissection anteriorly behind the pubic bone followed by pull-through vaginoplasty. Interrupted absorbable sutures are used to approximate the vagina to the perineal skin flap or to the distal redundant sinus membrane rotated to bridge any gap between vaginal ostium and skin.

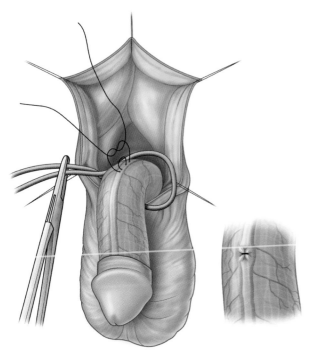

Fig. 43.13 Approach to chordee correction, showing suture placement at 12 o'clock to avoid neurovascular structures. *(Reproduced from Baskin LS. Hypospadias: anatomy, embryology, and reconstructive techniques. Braz J Urol. 2000;26:621.)*

With regard to clitoroplasty, the glans clitoris, the tunics, and the neurovascular bundles are preserved, while excess erectile tissue may be left intact or debulked laterally.[24] Salle *et al.* advocate for corporal body preservation, while Poppas *et al.* have demonstrated that debulking can be performed without damaging the dorsal nerves or impacting clitoral sensation.[25,26] To begin, a U-flap is created anterior from the perineum to each lateral ventral aspect of the phallus (Fig. 43.15). A single incision connects the two flaps along the perineal raphe. The phallus is then degloved, leaving the ventral strip intact. Buck's fascia is incised, and the cavernosa are separated from the tunics and suture-ligated. The glans is then approximated to the ends of the foreshortened cavernosa.

Hints and tips

- Endoscopic elucidation of the confluence is critical in planning urogenital sinus repair (Fig. 43.16)
- Identification and preservation of the neurovascular bundles are critical for successful clitoroplasty
- Total or partial urogenital mobilization without separation of vagina from urethra allows for optimal outcomes

---

Complications and outcomes

As previously mentioned, the goals of surgery for persistent urogenital sinus and persistent cloaca include creation of normal appearing external female genitalia, creation of an unobstructed urinary tract free of incontinence and recurrent infection, and allowance of normal adult reproductive and sexual function/sensation. One series reviewed outcomes of 22 girls undergoing total urogenital mobilization for cloaca repair, with complications including urethral stenosis (9%), urethrovaginal fistula (4.5%), residual common channel requiring urethral revision (4.5%), and a need to re-do posterior sagittal anorectoplasty for complete vaginal and anal closure (4.5%).[27] Another small series of seven patients undergoing total urogenital mobilization demonstrated a postoperative continence rate of 86%, with half of those patients voiding spontaneously and the other half requiring clean intermittent catheterization. In this same small study of seven patients, urodynamic studies showed detrusor underactivity or acontractility, with normal compliance in 86% of patients and poor compliance in the remaining 14%.[28] With respect to urinary continence, another series has demonstrated that there is no significant difference in rates of continence between children undergoing total urogenital mobilization versus partial urogenital mobilization. They report an overall continence rate of 95.5% by 3 years of age, regardless of surgical approach. Continence rates are slightly lower in children undergoing urogenital mobilization for persistent cloaca (87.5% at 3 years of age) compared with those with persistent urogenital sinus (96.4% continent at age 3 years).[29]

Genetic, social, hormonal, and psychological factors all impact sexual outcomes. Long-term data on sexual outcomes are limited but preliminary studies do suggest that, despite efforts to preserve the neurovascular bundles during surgery, sensation is markedly impaired in woman having undergone feminizing genitoplasty relative to controls. One series identified 37 women with ambiguous genitalia, of which 24 had undergone feminizing genitoplasty and 13 had not undergone surgery. Rates of anorgasmia were higher among women who had undergone surgery (26% vs 0%), but sexual function scores based on a standardized questionnaire were not different between the groups. Sexual function scores were significantly lower among all women with ambiguous genitalia regardless of surgical history relative to the overall population, suggesting that the disease process itself may play a role in the diminished sexual function and not surgery alone.[30] Numerous other studies have examined this issue, but are limited by small numbers and lack of standardized assessment tools. Despite these limitations, it is clear that children born with ambiguous genitalia tend to have diminished sexual satisfaction and desire, though dyspareunia is rare.[31]

Exstrophy–epispadias complex

Background and diagnosis

Bladder exstrophy tends to occur in nulliparous, young females' offspring, with a recurrence risk of 1:275 and a risk of 1:70 in progeny. Incidence is approximately 1:30000 with a male-to-female ratio of 3:1. Patients have a low-set umbilicus and wide pubic diastasis. The pubic bone is shortened by 30%, with external rotation of the posterior pelvis. The clitoris or penis is short and bifid due to separation of the pubis, and the urinary sphincter mechanism is underdeveloped. Nearly all patients have radiographic evidence of vesicoureteral reflux, and the incidence of inguinal hernias is increased. In

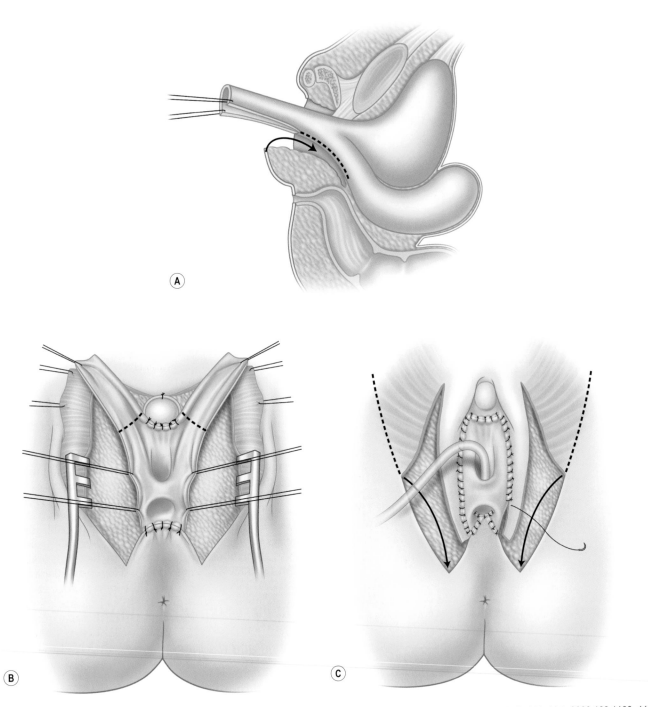

Fig. 43.14 (A–C) Urogenital sinus repair. *(Reproduced from Rink RC, Cain MP. Urogenital mobilization for urogenital sinus repair. Br J Urol Int. 2008;102:1182–1197.)*

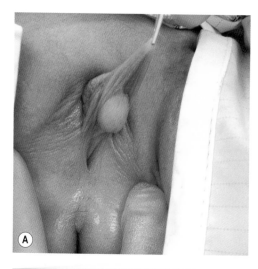

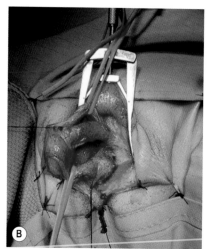

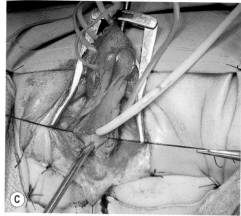

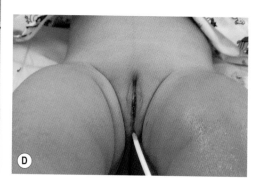

Fig. 43.15 (A–D) Corresponding intraoperative sequence of urogenital sinus repair with feminizing genitoplasty.

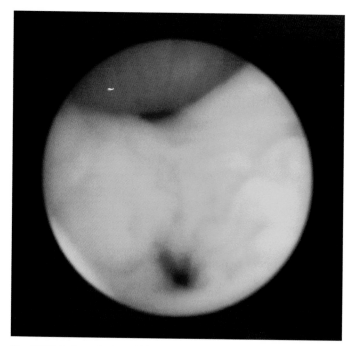

Fig. 43.16 Endoscopic view within common channel of urogenital sinus demonstrating urethral (ventral) and vaginal (dorsal) orifices.

females, epispadias ranges in severity from simply a patulous meatus to a complete dorsal separation of urethra and urinary sphincter (Fig. 43.17). The clitoris may be bifid, the mons shallow, and the labia minora underdeveloped. Repair often involves tapering of the urethra with excision of dorsal redundancy and subsequent genitoplasty (Fig. 43.18). The urethra is reconstructed over a catheter, and the mons tissue is utilized as a second layer for closure. In the Ransley–Gundeti modification, the dorsal redundant tissue is excised, the posterior urethral plate tubularized, and the anterior urogenital diaphragm reconstructed; however, additional sutures are placed to anchor the distal urethra to the reconstructed urogenital diaphragm (see Fig. 43.18). This modification is thought to recreate more readily the physiologic anterior angulation of the distal female urethra.

Treatment/surgical technique

Patients presenting with the exstrophy–epispadias complex are managed with a staged procedure.[32] Plastic cling film or Tegaderm is utilized to keep the bladder mucosa moist between birth and repair. In the neonatal period, bladder and abdominal closure is performed similar to that for second-stage cloacal exstrophy repair and is combined with bilateral osteotomies (Fig. 43.19). Epispadias repair occurs 6–12

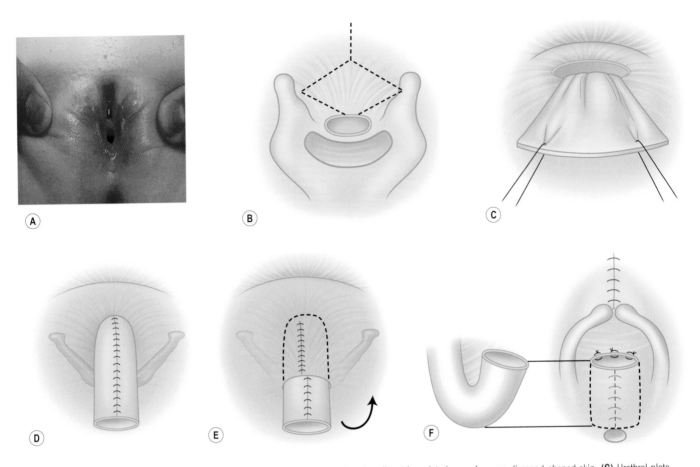

Fig. 43.17 (A) Ransley–Gundeti technique of female epispadias repair. **(B)** Female epispadias: triangulated area of excess diamond-shaped skin. **(C)** Urethral plate mobilization. **(D)** Neourethra formation. **(E)** Pelvic floor tissue approximation over the neourethra. **(F)** Completed female epispadias urethral reconstruction, showing the urethral angulation technique.

months later, and bladder neck reconstruction with ureteral reimplantation and possible bladder augmentation in another 4–5 years if indicated. Complete primary repair of bladder exstrophy has been described in recent years, but the authors favor the staged approach. (For a more complete description, please see Vol. 4, Chapter 13.)

Complications and outcomes

Important goals in managing exstrophy are urinary continence, sexual function, and aesthetic appearance, which often require multiple procedures to achieve. Compared with the staged repair, the one-stage repair has a high incidence of loss of the glans or corpora, though the exact incidence of this complication is unknown. One series of 48 patients undergoing staged repair for bladder exstrophy demonstrated a continence rate of 90%, though 70% of patients did require bladder augmentation to achieve continence. Only a third of patients achieved continence with bladder neck reconstruction alone.[33] Data on long-term outcomes are lacking, but small series suggest men who undergo repair of bladder exstrophy assess their own genital appearance as good or fair in 71% of cases, have a normal sperm count in 63% of cases, are able to achieve orgasm in 75% of cases, and tend to have

normal social integration.[34,35] These children require close follow-up and may need additional surgery in the future including bladder augmentation or revision of repair.

Vaginal agenesis

Background and diagnosis

Vaginal agenesis occurs in 1 : 5000 female births and is associated with Mayer–Rokitansky–Kuster–Hauser syndrome, wherein the proximal two-thirds of the vagina is absent. A mesonephric duct abnormality has been proposed as the etiology, with diagnosis often occurring in the work-up of primary amenorrhea.

For the patient with vaginal agenesis, the techniques and timing of surgery remain controversial. It is apparent that the majority of patients undergoing vaginoplasty as infants require additional vaginal surgery. When vaginal defects are associated with clitoromegaly, as in congenital adrenal hyperplasia, the surgeon has two fundamental options: perform an uncomplicated clitoroplasty with deferred vaginoplasty or a complex clitorovaginoplasty with deferred minor introitus repair in postpuberty.

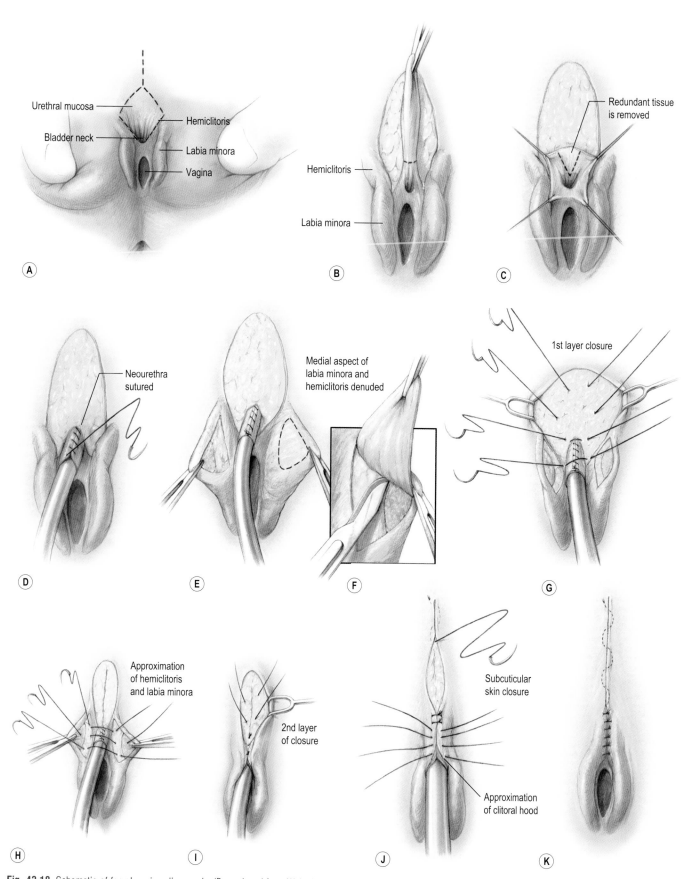

Fig. 43.18 Schematic of female epispadias repair. *(Reproduced from Wein AJ, et al. Campbell-Walsh Urology, 9th edn. Philadelphia: Saunders; 2007.)*

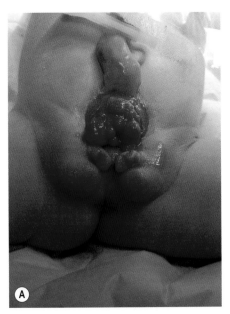
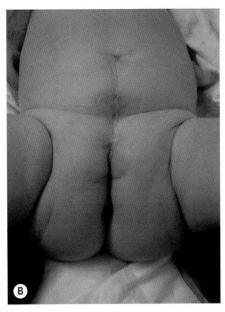
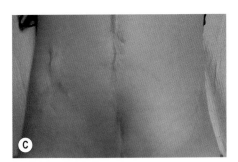

Fig. 43.19 (A,B) Female bladder exstrophy repair. **(C)** Final late appearance.

Treatment/surgical technique

Reconstruction may involve grafts of the skin, intestine, or buccal mucosa. Buccal mucosal vaginoplasty has been reported with good success and durability.[36,37] The buccal mucosa grafts may be quilted, and after development of the neovaginal space, single or multiple grafts are utilized to line the cavity. A stent or mold is placed following suturing of the graft to the vaginal bed. Others advocate usage of minced $0.5 \, mm^2$ micromucosal grafts derived mechanically from bilateral buccal grafts.[38] These micromucosal grafts are spread onto five gelatin strips, each $2.5 \times 6 \, cm^2$, to line the anterior, posterior, apical, and lateral walls with a 5 mm interpatch distance. Similarly, a silicone vaginal stent with drainage holes and luminal packing is placed to maintain counterpressure. Regardless of technique, the surgeon must place tantamount importance on patient compliance as disuse or failure to dilate may result in atrophy. It is the authors' practice that vaginoplasty is best performed once the patient is considering sexual activity or of appropriate age for performing periodic manual dilations.

The use of bowel results in mucus production, which may require daily douching and result in odor or ulcerations.[39] While bowel preparation has historically been advised, the authors have found it to be unnecessary.[40,41] A Pfannenstiel incision is appropriate, although a midline incision may also be employed. A 10 cm segment of mobile sigmoid or ileum may be taken out of continuity and anastomosed directly to the skin dimple (Fig. 43.20). While some surgeons detubularize and subsequently fold the bowel to form the neovagina, the authors find this unnecessary and perform a simple proximal-limb closure with 2-0 absorbable suture. The distal aspect of the bowel limb is anastomosed in recessed fashion to skin flaps or the rudimentary vagina is cases of proximal atresia. The bowel anastomosis may be hand-sewn or stapled. With recent adoption of minimally invasive surgery among pediatric patients, this can be undertaken with robotic assisted laparoscopic approach.

Within bowel constructs, stenosis occurs more often with the ileum than with the colon.[42] The type of bowel utilized depends upon surgeon preference and patient anatomy (e.g., cloacal exstrophy will require ileal vaginoplasty). Some advocate the usage of sigmoid colon as the proximity of its mesentery allows for free passage into the low pelvis.[43] Vaginal reconstruction is cautioned in patients with cervical agenesis, as severe ascending bacterial infections can result.

The neovaginal walls can also be formed by partial-thickness skin grafts harvested from the hip and buttock, though this is not as commonly performed in current practice. Vulvobulbocavernosus, gracilis, or rectus myocutaneous flaps are frequently utilized for vaginal reconstruction in the adult population following radical pelvic surgery.

Non-operative management with serial dilation can also be considered. Ideal candidates are highly motivated and compliant, with a shallow vaginal dimple. Most patients treated with dilation have good functional outcomes, as defined by ability to satisfactorily achieve intercourse or accommodate largest dilator without pain. Reported disadvantages include insufficient vaginal lubrication, decreased frequency of orgasm, and rarely dyspareunia.[44]

Hints and tips

- The proximal extent of the bowel vaginoplasty limb may be sutured to the sacrum or paraspinous ligaments to minimize potential prolapse[43]
- For buccal mucosal repairs, each cheek may yield a graft of approximately 3×7 cm. The graft should be harvested from inside the vermillion border extending posterior, inferior to Stensen's duct

Complications and outcomes

Potential problems after vaginoplasty may include graft foreshortening, injury to adjacent urinary structures, and

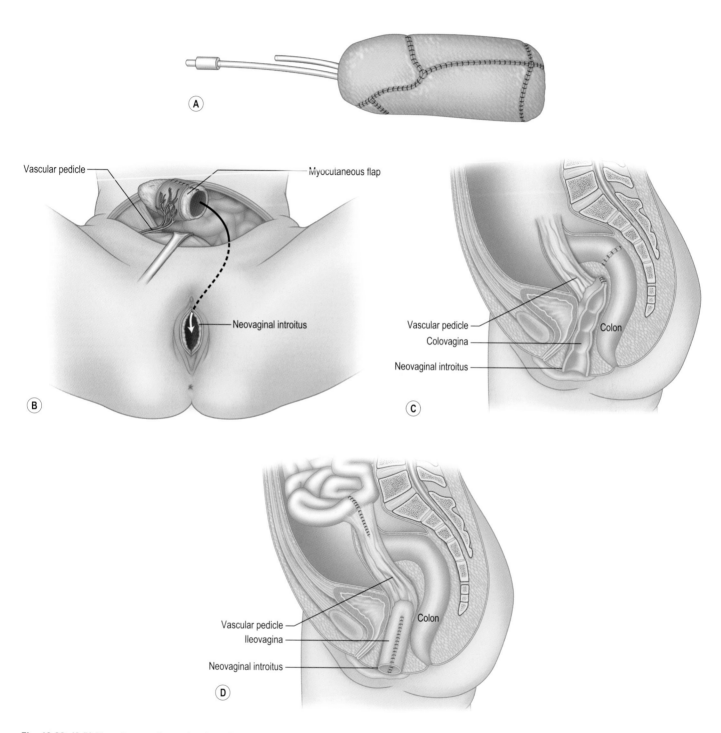

Fig. 43.20 (A,B) Myocutaneous flap vaginoplasty. Schematic depiction of bowel vaginoplasty: **(C)** colovaginoplasty and **(D)** ileovaginoplasty.

problems secondary to prolonged postoperative immobilization. Long-term studies on outcomes and complications are limited by the rarity of conditions requiring vaginoplasty. Stenosis or stricture of the intestinal segment can occur, and is typically managed by dilation. Delaying vaginoplasty until after puberty is associated with a lower overall complication rate (56.8% pre-pubertal vs 14.8% post-pubertal), though pre-pubertal vaginoplasty may be performed in children undergoing other genital surgery or children experiencing symptoms such as recurrent urinary tract infections or post-void dribbling.[45] A review of 57 patients who underwent bowel replacement vaginoplasty demonstrated reasonable sexual function, with 78% reporting sexual desire, 33% reporting sexual arousal, 33% reporting sexual confidence, and 78% reporting sexual satisfaction. Only 5% reported dyspareunia.[46]

Conclusion

Congenital anomalies of the urogenital tract vary widely in severity and incidence but generally result from failure of key steps in normal embryogenesis. When any reconstructive procedure is being considered, careful thought should be given to the timing of surgery and the potential need for a multidisciplinary approach. Outcomes tend to be quite good overall, although long-term data are lacking due to the rarity of these conditions.

⊕ Access the complete reference list online at   http://www.expertconsult.com

4. Snodgrass W, Bush N. Recent advances in understanding/management of hypospadias. *F1000Prime Rep.* 2014;6:101.

5. Baskin LS, Ebbers MB. Hypospadias: anatomy, etiology, and technique. *J Pediatr Surg.* 2006;41:463–472. *A comprehensive review of hypospadias, highlighting recent advancements in surgical technique.*

9. Duckett J, Snyder H. Meatal advancement and glanuloplasty hypospadias repair after 1000 cases: avoidance of meatal stenosis and regression. *J Urol.* 1992;147:665–669.

12. Snodgrass W, Koyle M, Manzoni G, et al. Tubularized incised plate hypospadias repair: results of a multicenter experience. *J Urol.* 1996;156:839–841. *Results of 148 patients undergoing TIP repair at six centers are reported.*

14. Bracka A. Hypospadias repair: the two stage alternative. *Br J Urol.* 1995;76:31–41. *A single surgeon's experience of 600+ two-stage hypospadias repairs.*

23. Rink RC, Cain MP. Urogenital mobilization for urogenital sinus repair. *BJU Int.* 2008;102:1182–1197. *This article provides an excellent overview of the technical aspects of urogenital mobilization for management of urogenital sinus.*

27. Leclair MD, Gundeti M, Kiely EM, et al. The surgical outcome of total urogenital mobilization for cloacal repair. *J Urol.* 2007;177:1492–1495.

29. Palmer BW, Trojan B, Griffin K, et al. Total and partial urogenital mobilization: focus on urinary continence. *J Urol.* 2012;187:1422–1426.

30. Creighton SM. Long-term outcomes of feminizing surgery: the London experience. *BJU Int.* 2004;93:44–46.

41. Rajimwale A, Furness PD 3rd, Brant WO, et al. Vaginal construction using sigmoid colon in children and young adults. *Br J Urol Int.* 2004;94:115–119. *A large retrospective review of the surgeons' experience with sigmoid vaginoplasty, comparing pre- and postpubertal patient outcomes.*

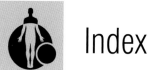

Index

Page numbers followed by "f" indicate figures, "t" indicate tables, "b" indicate boxes, and "e" indicate online content.